The Infusion Nurses Society

INFUSION THERAPY

IN CLINICAL PRACTICE

The Infusion Nurses Society

INFUSION THERAPY

IN CLINICAL PRACTICE

SECOND EDITION

Judy Hankins, BSN, CRNI
Coordinator, IV Admixture
Moses H. Cone Memorial Hospital
Greensboro, NC

Rose Anne Waldman Lonsway, BSN, MA, CRNI
Director
Around the Clock Home Care, Inc.
Lake County General Health District Home Care
Painesville, OH

Carolyn Hedrick, BSN, CRNI
Director, IV Therapy-System
Moses Cone Health System
Greensboro, NC

Maxine B. Perdue, BSN, MHA, MBA, CRNI, CNAA
Director of Clinical Support Services
High Point Regional Health System
High Point, NC

W.B. SAUNDERS COMPANY
A Harcourt Health Sciences Company
St. Louis   London   Philadelphia   New York   Sydney   Toronto

Vice President and Publishing Director, Nursing: *Sally Schrefer*
Executive Editor, Nursing: *Darlene Como*
Developmental Editor: *Tamara Myers*
Project Manager: *John Rogers*
Designer: *Kathi Gosche*

W.B. Saunders Company
A Harcourt Health Sciences Company
The Curtis Center
Independence Square West
Philadelphia, Pennsylvania 19106

Printed in the United States of America

Library of Congress Cataloging in Publication Data

Infusion therapy in clinical practice / Judy Hankins . . . [et al.].—2nd ed.
　　　p. cm.
　　Includes bibliographical references.
　　ISBN 0-7216-8716-4
　　　　1. Intravenous therapy.　2. Nursing.　I. Hankins, Judy.

RM170 .I525　2001
615′.6—dc21　　　　　　　　　　　　　　　　　　　　　　　00-068798

01　02　03　04　05　GW/MVY　9　8　7　6　5　4　3　2　1

Contributors

MARY C. ALEXANDER, BS, CRNI
Legal Aspects of Intravenous Nursing
Product Selection and Evaluation

MARY A. BANKS, BS, BSN, CRNI
Patient Education

REBECCA KOCHHEISER BERRY, RN, MS
Patient Education

CYNTHIA H. BLACKBURN, RN, CCM
Case Management

KATHLEEN M. BROTHERTON, RN, MS, CCM
Case Management

KATHRYN CARLSON, BS, CRNI
Infection Control

KIMBERLY A. CHRISTOPHER, PhD, RN, OCN
Research

BARBARA A. CIANO, RN, MSN
Hemodynamic Monitoring

ANN M. CORRIGAN, BSN, MS, CRNI
History of Intravenous Therapy

NANCY M. DELISIO, RN, CRNI
Intravenous Nursing as a Specialty

JEAN B. DOUGLAS, BS, PharmD, FASHP
Pharmacology

BRENDA DUGGER, RN, MS, CRNI, CNA
Documentation

ANNE MARIE FREY, BSN, CRNI
Intravenous Therapy in Children

LYNN C. HADAWAY, MEd, RNC, CRNI
Anatomy and Physiology Related to Intravenous Therapy
Entrepreneurial Roles in IV Therapy

JUDY HANKINS, BSN, CRNI
Fluids and Electrolytes
Infection Control
Parenteral Fluids

CAROLYN HEDRICK, BSN, CRNI
Parenteral Fluids
Pharmacology

MARY R. HEISEY, CRNI
Management of Hazardous Materials in IV Therapy

NANCY L. JORDAN, RN, BS
Parenteral Nutrition

ROSE ANNE WALDMAN LONSWAY, BSN, MA, CRNI
Fluids and Electrolytes
Patient Assessment
Intravenous Therapy in the Home

GLORIA PELLETIER, CRNI
Intravenous Therapy Calculations

MAXINE B. PERDUE, BSN, MHA, MBA, CRNI, CNAA
Infection Control
Intravenous Complications
Management of Hazardous Materials in IV Therapy

ROXANNE PERUCCA, MSN, CRNI
Infusion Therapy Equipment: Types of Infusion Therapy
    Equipment
Obtaining Vascular Access
Infusion Monitoring and Catheter Care
Changing and Discontinuing Infusion Therapy

CRYSTAL MILLER, RN, BSN, MA, CRNI
IV Therapy in the Acute Care Setting

NANCY MORTLOCK, CRNI, OCN
Intravenous Therapy in the Alternative Care Setting

LORYS ODDI, EdD, RN
Ethics

BARBARA ST. MARIE, MA, CNP
Pain Management

GAIL EGAN SANSIVERO, MS, ANP, AOCN
Vascular Access in Interventional Radiology

KRISHA S. SCHARNWEBER, BSN, CRNI
Intravenous Therapy Equipment: Preparation, Maintenance,
    and Problem Solving

GRACE P. SIERCHIO, MSN, CRNI
Quality Management

KATHERINE V. VANDEGRIFT, CRNI, OCN
Oncologic Therapy

KATHLEEN WALTHER, RN, BSN, CRNI
Intravenous Therapy in the Older Adult

HUGH K. WEBSTER, ESQ.
Legal Aspects of Intravenous Nursing

SHARON M. WEINSTEIN, MS, RN, CRNI
Future of Intravenous Therapy

JANE A. WEIR, BA, BSN, CRNI
Blood Component Therapy

JEANNE M. WILSON, RN, BSN, CRNI
Parenteral Nutrition

LORY YOUMANS, RN, MS
Conscious Sedation

Reviewers

JOHN G. AKER, CRNA, MS
Department of Anesthesia
University of Iowa Hospitals and Clinics
Iowa City, IA

JOANNE VENTURELLA, RN, BA
Emergency Department
St. Agnes Hospital
Baltimore, MD

MARY L. MCCARTHY, RN, BSN
Mercy Health System
Janesville, WI

MARLYS KAY HUNT, RN, BS, MSN
Director of Infection Control and Employee Health
Navapache Regional Medical Center
Show Low, AZ

D. DANIEL HASSELL III, MD
Section Head, Vascular and Interventional Radiology
Greensboro Radiology, P.A.
Greensboro, NC

STEVEN B. OGLEVIE, MD
Associate Professor of Radiology
University of California, San Diego
Chief, Radiology Service
VA San Diego Healthcare System
San Diego, CA

MARY C. ALEXANDER, BS, CRNI
Chief Executive Officer
Infusion Nurses Society
Cambridge, MA

Preface

The practice of infusion therapy is a multifaceted, vitalizing process. It is a specialty that plays an extensive role in the care of patients. In addition to its traditional domain—intravenous delivery of therapy—the specialty has expanded to encompass other therapies, including arterial, intraosseous, epidural, intrathecal, and other treatment modalities. Infusion therapy incorporates the clinical needs of the patient and the physician's treatment plan with valuable input from many other health care providers.

As the practice of infusion therapy expands, there is an increasing need for additional information, from the basic to the more sophisticated. This is evidenced by the questions that are continuously posed about the many facets of infusion therapy. *Infusion Therapy in Clinical Practice* was developed with this need for information in mind.

Beginning with the history of intravenous therapy, this book travels forward to a discussion of current infusion therapy practice and professionals providing this care. The foundation on which the infusion specialty is built includes knowledge of anatomy, physiology, and infection control.

With this foundation securely established, various treatments can be used to achieve the desired patient outcomes. Infusion-related treatment involves a host of different modalities, such as parenteral fluids, blood and blood components, pharmacologic agents, nutritional solutions, antineoplastic agents, and pain medications, all of which are covered here. Legal and ethical aspects of infusion practice are reviewed, along with maintenance of quality.

The technology and procedures used to deliver infusion therapy provide a framework for the clinical practice of the specialty. Technology involves the selection and preparation of infusion-related equipment. The discussion of procedures begins with patient assessment and follows through to posttherapy monitoring with documentation at every level. Important considerations for patient assessment, treatment, monitoring, complications, and patient education are addressed.

Because certain patient populations require different infusion approaches, information on providing care for children and older adults is included. Also, with infusion-related treatment no longer being administered solely in the hospital setting, the provision of care in other surroundings continues to expand.

The specialty's evolution has resulted in an expanded role for nurses providing infusion therapy. This edition addresses the recent changes to infusion practice. Information is provided on hazardous materials, including proper handling and disposal, as well as regulatory agencies involved. Other new chapters are related to the role of the infusion nurse in case management, radiology, and conscious sedation. Because of the rise in entrepreneurial activity in the areas of product design and development, education, and patient care services, this edition addresses the development of the infusion nurse's entrepreneurial role.

Our intent has been to provide answers to the many questions and concerns related to the practice of infusion therapy. This text can help ensure that quality care is delivered and can help infusion nurse professionals prepare for the many profound changes that are occurring and will continue to occur. The valuable assistance and expertise of all those who contributed to this text are greatly appreciated.

Judy Hankins
Rose Anne Waldman Lonsway
Carolyn Hedrick
Maxine B. Perdue

Foreword

This authoritative text is a comprehensive, research-based reference for *all* health care professionals involved in the delivery of infusion therapy. It addresses fundamental to advanced concepts that reflect the increased responsibility and accountability placed on health care professionals. A vast body of knowledge is necessary to provide safe care, and readers are encouraged to use this information to build on their knowledge and enhance their practice. Incorporation of current research findings into the clinical arena leads to "best practice," delivery of the highest-quality care, and increased patient and provider satisfaction.

The new title of the second edition of this textbook, *Infusion Therapy in Clinical Practice,* is intended to reflect the ongoing changes in infusion therapy practice. Infusion care has become a key component of a diverse array of therapies and supporting practices, including oncology, infection control, emergency care, risk management, quality assurance, legal and ethical issues, and research. Delivery of infusion therapy takes place across the continuum of health care settings, in hospitals, ambulatory infusion centers, skilled nursing facilities, and the home. Infusion therapy providers are now caring for a wider spectrum of patients—from neonatal to geriatric—with higher degrees of acuity. These health care professionals represent varied levels of education, skill, and competence in infusion practices; in addition to infusion nurse specialists, there are physicians, pharmacists, nurse generalists, and nurses in other specialties such as oncology or intensive care who contribute to infusion therapy delivery. Moreover, the role of the infusion nurse specialist is no longer bound by the clinical area: they make an impact as educators, entrepreneurs, and legal consultants, to name a few. Rapid technologic advances and increasingly sophisticated equipment constantly reinforce the need for nurses' education and professional development.

A new approach to the specialty is needed, one that is compatible with the recent changes in health care. The following chapters do not just address intravenous access and management but describe the broader scope of infusion practice, including nonvascular routes of therapy delivery, alternative care settings, and the expanded role of the infusion nurse. In this way, we hope to reflect the infusion specialty's impact on the entire continuum of health care.

To meet the challenges of the future, all infusion professionals must be prepared to become more deeply involved in the advancement of the specialty. This means not only using research to change and improve practice, but becoming active participants in research efforts and expanding the specialty's knowledge of new technology and techniques. We need to stimulate global discussion to develop appropriate initiatives for each country's health care environment. We must determine and validate continued competence in infusion practice in a rapidly changing health care environment. In the current context of health care reform, cost control, rising patient acuity, and new technology, the infusion specialty needs resources that promote and guide the delivery of safe, effective patient care and increase the confidence of the practitioner. This book is intended to be such a resource, with the ultimate goal of excellent infusion care for every patient.

Mary C. Alexander, BS, CRNI
Chief Executive Officer
Infusion Nurses Society

Acknowledgments

The specialty of infusion therapy encompasses a variety of areas, including physiologic aspects, medications, equipment, nursing care, special considerations, expanded roles, and professional issues. Incorporating this vast array of information into a textbook is an enormous undertaking that has been accomplished only through the efforts of many dedicated individuals.

First, I would like to acknowledge the associate editors, Rose Anne Waldman Lonsway, Carolyn Hedrick, and Maxine Perdue, for their dedication to the practice of infusion therapy and for their role in planning and completing this endeavor.

Without the contributing authors who were willing to share their knowledge and time, there would be no textbook. Their contributions are greatly appreciated.

I would like to thank the Infusion Nurses Society's Board of Directors for giving the editors the opportunity to be involved with this project. The help of the INS staff was invaluable throughout the process. The support of Tamara Myers, Developmental Editor from Harcourt Health Sciences, and Suzanne Kastner, Production Editor from World Graphic Publishing Services, was appreciated as we entered and completed the final phase.

Finally, sincere appreciation is expressed by the editors to their departmental administrations, staffs, and families for their patience and support in bringing this project to fruition.

Judy Hankins, BSN, CRNI

Dedication

The second edition of *Infusion Therapy in Clinical Practice* is dedicated to Leslie Baranowski. Leslie's theme as the 1995-1996 Intravenous Nurses Society President was "Take Ownership." This theme was not only a dream but was also her way of life.

The specialty of infusion nursing was certainly influenced by her knowledge, expertise, and day-to-day practice. The enthusiasm for infusion nursing was shared far and wide through her profession and many other INS activities on both local and national levels.

Leslie was instrumental in the development of the first edition as she assumed many roles, including an associate editor and author. Except for an untimely death, she would have been a valuable part of this edition. Hopefully, she is proud of the work and dedication of her colleagues and this second edition of *Infusion Therapy in Clinical Practice.*

Contents

Chapter

1

History of Intravenous Therapy

Ann M. Corrigan, BSN, MS, CRNI

EARLY EXPERIMENTS
19TH CENTURY
20TH CENTURY
    Advances in agents
    Advances in equipment
    Nurse's role in intravenous therapy

Intravenous (IV) therapy as we know it today is a technical, highly specialized form of treatment. It has evolved from an extreme measure used only on the most critically ill to a therapy used for almost 90% of all hospitalized patients. No longer confined to the hospital, IV therapies are now delivered in alternative care settings such as the home, skilled nursing facilities, and physician offices. IV therapy refers to the parenteral administration of fluids and medications, nutritional support, and transfusion therapy. Although the major advancements in IV therapy occurred in the past 150 years, the practice of using veins to inject substances essentially began in the 17th century.

EARLY EXPERIMENTS

The first documented use of blood as a treatment was in 1492, when blood from three young boys was administered to Pope Innocent VIII.[1] It was not until 1615, however, that the concept of infusing blood from one person to another was considered again, by Libavious,[1-3] but at that time, it was still impossible in practice. This concept constituted the beginning of IV therapy. It was several centuries before person-to-person transfusion became possible, and even longer before it became a safe practice.

In 1628, William Harvey's experimental work with blood expanded on the findings of earlier physicians.[1-3] As a result, the theory of circulation was developed, which led to an understanding of blood flow and of the presence and importance of valves. This new information about the circulatory system led others to experiment with injecting substances into the vascular system to observe the effect on the recipient. One of the earliest to document this type of experiment was Sir Christopher Wren,

of England. In 1656, he experimented with injecting opium and wine into the veins of dogs using a quill and an animal bladder.[2-4] The first successful injection into humans was accomplished in 1662, by J. D. Major.[4]

About this time, Richard Lower presented a paper before the Royal Society in England on IV feeding and blood transfusion in dogs. He was able to demonstrate his transfusion theory with a successful animal-to-animal transfusion,[1,3] and in 1666, Lower attempted the first known animal-to-human transfusion.[1]

The first documented transfusion is credited to Jean Baptiste Denis. In 1667, Denis, a physician to the French royalty, successfully transfused 9 ounces of lamb's blood into a 15-year-old boy suffering from madness.[1,2,4] Subsequent transfusions to the boy were not successful and resulted in the first transfusion reaction. The initial success of Denis, however, led to the promiscuous use of transfusions, with fatal results. As a result of the many fatalities, the church and the French parliament banned the transfusion of blood from animals to humans in 1687.[1,4]

During these early trials with transfusion therapy, scientists and physicians used feather quills (sometimes with metal tips), animal veins, and animal bladders. This equipment has been described in a 1670 Amsterdam publication *Clysmatic Nova*.

Following the 1687 edict banning blood transfusions, little growth in the field of IV therapy was noted for the next 150 years. The one significant event in the 18th century occurred in 1795, when Philip Syng Physick, from the University of Edinburgh, noted that the use of blood transfusions in obstetric hemorrhage had some success in decreasing mortality from this complication.[1,2] It must be remembered, however, that the success or failure of these transfusions was totally without scientific understanding and can only be considered luck.

19TH CENTURY

IV therapy, as practiced today, had its beginnings in the 19th century, which was a time of rapid advancement in medicine. A first major accomplishment occurred in 1818, when James Blundell performed the first man-to-man transfusion in London.[1-4] In 1834, Blundell again used human blood to transfuse women during childbirth who were threatened by hemorrhage.[4] Blundell is further credited with the correlation between blood loss and hypoxemia during hemorrhage.

One complication of early transfusions was blood clotting during the transfusion. In 1821, Jean Louis Prevost, a French physician, experimented with preventing this coagulation. Prevost and Jean B. Dumas were the first to use defibrinated blood in animal transfusion.[1,4] By 1875, Landois had discovered lysing between the serums of different animals, which later resulted in an understanding of antigen-antibody reactions.[4]

The cholera epidemic of 1831 in Leith, Scotland, was an important event in the advancement of IV therapy. Dr. William O'Shaughnessy, an Edinburgh physician, identified the significance of water and salt loss from the blood of cholera victims.[2,3,5] In 1832, Thomas Latta used this information and experimented with administering a saline solution to a patient. He described the patient as one who "apparently had reached the last moments of her earthly existence and now nothing could injure her. Indeed, so entirely was she reduced that I feared that I shall be unable to get my apparatus ready, ere she expire."[2,3,6] Latta successfully treated the patient, who eventually recovered and survived. The success of the saline injection led to extensive use of this therapy during the epidemic, but these efforts met with only limited success.

Further work continued, and in 1843, Claude Bernard, a French physiologist, experimented with injecting sugar solutions into dogs. For the next two decades, he continued to experiment and infused not only sugar solutions but also egg whites and milk into animals, with some success.[2] During this time, Bernard also discovered that cane sugar, injected intravenously, soon appeared in the urine, whereas ingested sugar, which was acted on by gastric juices, disappeared.

In 1852, the importance of protein in relation to nitrogen balance, weight gain, and general well-being was first observed by Bidder and Schmidt and confirmed by Voit in 1866. This correlation between protein and health led to the concept of nutritional support, although the effect of this relationship would not be fully known for another 75 to 100 years.

During the 1860s, major advances were made that would have an impact on IV nursing and on all of medicine. In 1860, Louis Pasteur developed the germ theory of disease and demonstrated that fermentation and putrefaction result from the growth of germs.[2] Building on this theory, Joseph Lister, Professor of Surgery at the University of Glasgow, hypothesized that microbes might be responsible for wound suppuration. He further postulated that infection could be prevented by destroying organisms and preventing contaminated air from coming into contact with the wound.[2,6] In 1867, Lister published the results of his studies using carbolic acid spray as an antiseptic.[2] He initially used the spray as a dressing material and eventually advanced to using carbolic acid as a soak for the hands and ligatures and for cleaning the site before surgery. Lister's work led to the use of cleaner instruments in surgery and provided the framework for the theory of antisepsis and asepsis.

Many physicians, including Lawson Tait of London, observed strict rules of cleanliness without understanding the implications. In France, surgeons continued to focus on the use of antisepsis during procedures instead of asepsis.[6] Not until the early 1900s were the principles of asepsis fully understood. By then, it was common practice for everything coming into patient contact to be sterile.

The use of gloves for procedures was introduced in 1889, when William Halsted of Johns Hopkins Hospital had the Goodyear Rubber Company make a pair of rubber gloves for his operating room nurse.[2,6,7] This nurse, who Halsted later married, was allergic to the hand rinse being used before procedures (a corrosive sublimate), and Halsted's only intention was to protect her hands.[7] The use of gloves became popular, and by 1899, rubber gloves were being used on all clean cases. Today, gloves are used not only to protect the patient but also to protect the practitioner. The gloves used in health care today are no longer made of rubber but are composed of various synthetic materials.

The last half of the 19th century also saw advances in the field of nutritional support. In 1869, Menzel and Perco of Vienna wrote a paper on the use of fat, milk, and camphor injected subcutaneously.[2] By 1878, the use of oil and a protein extract to treat a patient suffering from anorexia nervosa was reported by Krug, and cow's milk was being injected for volume expansion and nutritional support.[2] Hodder, of Canada, used cow's milk to correct fluid and nutritional losses caused by cholera.[2] Although the results were generally considered good, Hodder was subsequently barred from the practice of medicine by his colleagues. The successful administration of a glucose solution is credited to Biedl and Krause, in 1896.[3]

20TH CENTURY

For almost 250 years, experiments with injecting different substances into the body had yielded limited results. As with most of medicine, the major advances that would bring IV therapy to its current level of sophistication occurred in the 20th century. By this time, the use of saline and glucose solutions was a more widely accepted practice, although they were still used only on the critically ill patient. Equipment was cleaned and sterilized between uses as a routine measure with the advent of heat sterilization in 1910, and with the medical profession's acceptance that everything coming into contact with the patient needed to be sterile. The discovery of pyrogens in 1923 led to measures that helped eliminate them from fluids and drugs. Dr. Florence Seibert of the Phipps Institute in Philadelphia solved the serious problem of pyrogenic reactions to IV infusions in 1925, thus paving the way for safer practice.[1,2,6]

Advances in agents

Early in the 20th century, Landsteiner discovered naturally occurring antibodies in the blood that led to a reaction when mixed with blood from another subject. This discovery eventually led to the identification of the ABO blood groups in 1901.[1,2] By 1907, Reuben Ottenberg began using blood type differences as a basis for donor selection. By 1908, Epstein had set forth the hypothesis that ABO blood groups are inherited.[1,2] Even with this information, transfusion therapy was still potentially fatal. Matching donor and recipient blood types helped reduce the incidence of transfusion reactions, but coagulation during the procedure continued to be a problem. During World War I, Oswald Robertson introduced the use of preserved anticoagulant blood, and by 1915, sodium citrate was being successfully as an anticoagulant in blood transfusions.[1]

Levine and Stetson discovered the anti-Rh antigen in 1939, and in 1941, Levine and Burnham recognized that the anti-Rh antigen is responsible for alloimmunization during pregnancy and causes hemolytic disease of the newborn.[6] These developments were important steps in the safe transfusion of blood. An understanding of the effects of the anti-Rh antigen led to the decreased risk of hemolytic disease for children.

World War II is important in the history of transfusion therapy because the practice was used more widely during this time than ever before. Out of necessity, blood was being administered to the wounded troops in an effort to save more lives. Plasma was the first component to be used, and new techniques for the separation of plasma were developed in 1941.[1] It was soon recognized, however, that plasma transfusions could not meet all the needs of the wounded. By 1943, red blood cells were being salvaged and transfused. In 1962, the first filter to reduce white cell contamination and help screen out fibrin clots was designed.[1] This helped solve an undesirable effect of transfusion therapy that had been recognized for more than four decades.

Today, transfusion therapy is a common medical practice. Blood can be separated into many different components, and each component is administered to correct a specific deficiency. Improved techniques make it possible to obtain, test, store, and administer these components. The risk of transfusion therapy has diminished as a result of the discovery and understanding of antigen-antibody reactions and of the development of improved methods for detecting blood-borne diseases. Administration sets, filters, infusion and warming devices, and other types of equipment are constantly being modified and improved. Pharmaceutical agents, such as erythropoietin, are being developed to stimulate the body's own production of blood, thereby reducing the need for transfusions and further reducing risks.

During the 20th century, advances were also being made in the area of nutritional support. Between 1904 and 1906, research on maintaining nitrogen balance for general well-being was conducted, and the rectal administration of protein for nutrition was documented. By 1918, Murlin and Riche were experimenting with the administration of fats to animals as a source of nutrition.[6] The 1930s was a time of intense experimentation in nutritional support. In 1935, Emmett Holt of Baltimore administered an infusion of cottonseed oil and has since been credited with the first infusion of a fat emulsion.[6] The administration of a hydrolyzed casein solution was first attempted by Henriques and Anderson in 1913.[6] In 1936, Dr. Robert Elman attempted further administrations of this solution. By 1939, Elman, along with Weiner, infused a solution of 2% casein hydrolysate and 8% dextrose without adverse effects.[6] Following this success, various protein hydrolysates were studied, and in 1940 Schohl and Blackfan infused synthetic crystalline amino acids into infants.[4] By 1944, Helfich and Abelson provided nutritional support to a 5-day-old infant with a solution of 50% glucose and 10% casein hydrolysate, alternated with a 10% olive oil-lecithin emulsion.

Stanley Dudrick's name is synonymous with parenteral nutrition. With the assistance of Dr. Harry Vars at the Harrison Department of Surgical Research at the University of Pennsylvania, Dudrick conducted a series of experiments on beagle puppies in an attempt to support them totally by the parenteral route.[2,3] By the early 1970s, Dudrick had proven the effectiveness of protein and dextrose solutions for nutritional support. Today, primarily because of Dudrick's work, patients can receive total nutrition through the IV route and survive diseases and conditions that had formerly resulted in death.

The use of fat emulsions as a caloric source was also investigated, but the severe adverse reactions encountered with the IV administration of these substances led the U.S. Food and Drug Administration (FDA) to ban their use in the United States in 1964. However, fats were still being administered in Europe, and an emulsion derived from soybean oil was developed. This refined product, which produced no significant side effects, led the FDA to reverse its ban on the IV administration of fat emulsions in 1980, and soybean and safflower oil emulsions were approved for IV administration.

Advances in equipment

The advances in fluids and medications used for IV administration continue today. Medical science has provided the information necessary for us to replace and maintain the body's fluid and electrolyte balance, to maintain or improve nutritional status, and to treat many disease states intravenously. The technology for administering IV fluids and medications has also advanced since Sir Christopher Wren used the quill, vein, and bladder of an animal for his treatments.[2-4]

The crude apparatus of Wren was later replaced by metal needles, rubber tubing, and glass containers. Originally, the equipment was designed to be reused and required cleaning and eventually sterilization between uses. The first fluid containers consisted of an open glass flask that was covered with a piece of gauze. By the 1930s, the container had evolved into a closed, vacuum glass bottle. The technology for refining plastics has also done much for the improvement of IV therapy equipment. Use of rubber gave way to the use of the plastic, polyvinyl chloride, with this knowledge being applied to administration sets first. Today, plastic containers and administration sets are state of the art for infusion therapy.

Devices for accessing the vein have also progressed rapidly in the last 50 years. Metal cannulas, crude metal needles that required cleaning and resharpening between uses, were first used in the 19th century. Problems with infiltration, however, led to the development of the plastic cannula in 1945.[3,4] These first catheters were made of flexible plastic tubing that required either a cutdown or needle for introduction into the vessel. In 1950, the Rochester needle was introduced by Gautier and Maasa, and revolutionized the IV catheter.[3,4] Today, this over-the-needle type of catheter is used to deliver almost all peripheral infusions.

The metal needle is still available, but it is now a disposable device modified for short-term use. It has plastic attachments at the hub to assist in handling, and a short piece of plastic tubing is attached. Another piece of equipment available for infusion therapy is the through-the-needle device, which allows the plastic catheter to be threaded into the vein through the needle after venipuncture has been completed. This device was first introduced in 1958, and its successors are used today, especially for peripherally inserted central lines.[3,4]

Today, IV cannulas, both metal and plastic, are available in varying sizes (gauges) to deliver different therapies. Gauges range from a large lumen (12 gauge) to a neonatal size (27 gauge). Cannulas are also available in varying lengths, from 0.75 to 30 inches or longer. The length is generally determined by the route of administration, peripheral or central, and the size and age of the patient. The Intravenous Nurses Society recommends that the shortest length, smallest-gauge cannula be used to accommodate the therapy prescribed.[8]

Before 1949, IV therapy could be administered only through a peripheral vein. At that time, Meng and colleagues documented the use of a catheter placed in the central venous system of a dog for administering a hypertonic dextrose and protein solution.[9] The subclavian puncture for accessing the central veins was more frequently used after its description by Aubaniac from Vietnam in 1952.[9] In 1967, Dudrick adapted the subclavian approach for the administration of high concentrations of dextrose and proteins, which produced minimal side effects caused by the tonicity of the solution.[2]

Further expansion on this concept led to the development of a catheter that is placed in the subclavian vein and then tunneled under the subcutaneous tissue to exit on the chest wall. Originally designed for use with children, this catheter became known as the *Broviac catheter*. A size appropriate for adults, the Hickman catheter, was developed soon after. The evolution of the Hickman-Broviac catheter has allowed for the administration of therapies over long periods, with minimal technical complications. It has also revolutionized IV therapy by allowing safer administration of solutions in the home setting.

The 1980s saw further evolution of the use of central venous access with the introduction of the totally implanted system. This system consists of the central catheter, which is still placed by percutaneous puncture into the subclavian vein and then tunneled under the subcutaneous tissue, but the catheter end is attached to a device referred to as a *port,* which is placed under the subcutaneous tissue on the chest wall. Access to this port is by puncture through the skin with a specially designed needle for the portal septum.

Peripheral catheters primarily consist of a single lumen, although experiments have been carried out with dual-lumen peripheral catheters. Central catheters—percutaneous, tunneled, and ports—are available in both single-lumen and multilumen design. The multilumen design makes it possible for multiple therapies to be delivered through one device, thus sparing the patient from numerous venipunctures.

To make the delivery of IV therapy safer, various infusion devices have been developed. Filters were first used in 1943 to screen out fibrin clots during blood transfusions.[1] Filters are now of two types, screen and depth, and are available in a number of micron sizes. Filters remove particulate matter from the infusion and, depending on the micron size, can also eliminate air and remove endotoxins.

In addition to filters, infusion devices that allow for the closer regulation of flow rate have been developed. Before the use of this technology, infusions were administered by gravity pressure and the flow rate was regulated primarily by a screw or roller clamp on the administration set. The development of electronic infusion devices has improved the accuracy of administration. Factors that affect flow rate, such as head height and internal pressure, can be overcome by the use of these devices.

The first infusion device developed was the syringe pump, and the quantity of solution it delivered depended on the syringe size used. It was used primarily to administer fluids at a slow rate, especially to infants and children. This type of device is still available and is often used to control medication administration. The concept of the syringe pump was modified further to allow large volumes of fluid to be administered. The controller, first developed by IVAC in 1972, allowed for gravity infusion but controlled it through a drop-counting system that set off an alarm when the number of drops deviated from the preset number. Subsequently, infusion pumps were designed to deliver a solution at a prescribed rate under positive pressure. Infusion device technology now allows the user to adjust the pressure setting to administer the therapy under varying conditions. Infusion devices can also deliver simultaneous or multiple infusions at prescribed intervals.

Ambulatory infusion devices currently available allow for continuous or intermittent infusions outside the hospital setting. These devices allow patients to receive necessary therapy while maintaining as normal a lifestyle as possible. The quality of life for many patients has been dramatically improved by the use of these ambulatory devices.

Another technologic advance that has improved the quality of patient care is the patient-controlled analgesia (PCA) pump. This device enables patients to control their pain by allowing them to administer their pain medication as they need it. This method of control has proven especially effective in postoperative pain management.

During the 1970s, the administration of pain medication was expanded by alternative routes. As early as 1976, Yaks and Rudy had demonstrated the successful administration of morphine directly into the subarachnoid space of animals.[2] In 1977, Wang proved that an intrathecal injection of morphine provides profound relief in humans. Today, the intrathecal and epidural routes have proven effective for the administration of specific therapies, especially the control of postoperative and cancer pain. The intrathecal route has also been used for administering some antineoplastic agents.

A method of fluid administration that regained some popularity in the 1980s, especially for emergency fluid resuscitation in pediatrics, is intraosseous administration. The bone marrow as a route for transfusion was first advocated by Drinker in 1922.[2] In the 1940s, Tocantins established the basis for the widespread use of this technique for fluid administration,[2] but it was used only briefly. By the late 1950s, intraosseous infusion had fallen into obscurity. The resurgence of this method of administration occurred as a result of advances in pediatric resuscitation, and its use is generally limited to young children in the emergency setting. The successful use of this type of administration has proven it to be an important advancement in IV therapy.

Nurse's role in intravenous therapy

By the 1980s, administering IV fluids and medications had become a specialized practice involving the introduction of fluids and medications not only into the circulatory system but also into the bone marrow and epidural and intrathecal spaces. Nursing involvement in the practice of IV therapy is relatively new; it is only since the 1940s that nurses have been allowed to perform IV procedures. Before this, nursing's only role in IV therapy was in assisting physicians with venipuncture and the administration of fluids.[2,4] Massachusetts General Hospital of Boston was the first to allow a nurse, Ada Plumer, to be responsible for the administration of IV therapies.[2,4] Plumer became the first IV nurse, and she eventually developed the first IV team.

IV nursing is now a technical, highly specialized field that requires advanced clinical knowledge and technical expertise. Nurses involved in the practice of IV therapy need to be knowledgeable in the areas of technical and clinical applications, fluid and electrolytes, pharmacology, infection control, pediatrics, antineoplastic therapy, transfusion therapy, parenteral nutrition, and quality assurance to perform their duties competently. The professional practice of IV nursing was formally recognized in 1980, when the United States House of Representatives declared January 25 as IV Nurse Day.

Several professional organizations for IV therapy have been established over the last 25 years. The Intravenous Nurses Society, founded in 1973, promotes the specialty practice of IV nursing. It seeks to educate the practitioner and protect the public through the development of the *Infusion Nursing Standards of Practice*.[8] The Intravenous Nurses Certification Corporation also seeks to protect the public by developing and administering a certification-recertification program that meets judicial, regulatory, and professional testing standards.

The administration of fluids and medications has improved considerably since 1492. Advances continue to be made in this practice—in the equipment used, in the fluids and medications administered, and in the techniques used to deliver them. Those involved in the delivery of IV therapies must remain current in the field to provide their clients with high-quality care.

References

1. Greenwalt TJ: A short history of transfusion medicine, *Transfusion* 37:550, 1997.
2. Philips LD: *Manual of I.V. therapeutics,* ed 2, Philadelphia, 1997, FA Davis.
3. Millam D: The history of intravenous therapy, *J Intravenous Nurs* 19:5, 1996.
4. Weinstein SM: *Plumer's principles and practice of intravenous therapy,* ed 6, Philadelphia, 1997, Lippincott-Raven.
5. Holliday M: The evolution of therapy for dehydration: should deficit therapy still be taught? *Pediatrics* 98:171, 1996.
6. Lyons AS, Petrucelli RJ: *Medicine: an illustrated history,* New York, 1987, Harry N Abrams.
7. Bennett JV, Brachman PS: *Hospital infections,* ed 4, Boston, 1997, Little, Brown.
8. Intravenous Nurses Society: Infusion nursing standards of practice, *JIN* (suppl) 23(65), 2000.
9. Andris DA, Krzywda EA: Central venous access: clinical practice issues, *Nurs Clin North Am* 32(4):719, 1997.

Intravenous Nursing as a Specialty

Nancy M. Delisio, RN, CRNI*

PROFESSIONAL ORGANIZATIONS
SCOPE OF PRACTICE
COMPETENCY
    Educational requirements
    Role and qualifications
    Curriculum
    Clinical evaluation
CERTIFICATION
    The examination
    Recertification
IV NURSE SPECIALISTS
ROLE DELINEATION: BENEFITS OF THE IV NURSE SPECIALIST

It has been nearly 500 years since Sir William Harvey, an English physician generally considered the father of modern medicine, completely and accurately described the circulatory system.[1] His widespread lecturing in Europe caught the attention of his fellow physicians and other professionals. Through his discoveries and the work of others such as Sir Christopher Wren, an architect who together with a chemist produced the first hypodermic needle,[2] experimentation with intravenous (IV) injection began.

Success with IV injection was slow. In 1687, a fatal attempt at animal-to-human blood transfusion led to an edict from the church and parliament prohibiting further such experimentation.[3] Nearly 150 years passed before James Blundell, an English obstetrician, resurrected the idea of transfusion therapy. In 1834, recognizing that hemorrhage often claimed the lives of young women during childbirth, he successfully treated women by transfusing human rather than animal blood.[3] IV treatment was refined over the next 100 years until in 1940, Drs. Karl Landsteiner and Alexander Wiener discovered the Rhesus blood group system. Today blood and blood products are routinely administered in various practice settings, with few reported complications.

While the details of safe transfusion evolved, advances were occurring in other areas. Robert Koch, along with predecessors and contemporaries such as Ignaz Semmelweiss, Louis Pasteur, and Lord Joseph Lister, advanced the science of bacteriology, developing the process of pasteurization and the drying and staining method of examining bacteria, and establishing the

principles of asepsis. In 1895, Wilhelm Röntgen discovered x-rays and established the foundations of radiology.[1] Saline was identified as a reasonable treatment for dehydration, and the caloric value of dextrose was recognized. It was not until 1923, however, when the discovery and elimination of solution pyrogens made IV fluid administration safer, that use of IV treatment became more common. Until 1940, the administration of IV solutions remained the domain of physicians and, because it was considered a major procedure, was used to treat only critically ill patients.[3] From the mid- to late 20th century, however, progress exploded.

The health care needs of soldiers during World War II stimulated medical innovation and rapid advances in technology. This war and those subsequently fought in Korea and Vietnam necessitated large-scale fluid resuscitation, multiple medication infusions, improved methods of venous access, and innovative disposable medical supplies to treat those who survived injuries that previously led to almost certain death. The steel needle gave way to the flexible catheter, reducing infiltration. Glass bottles were replaced by nonvented plastic containers, reducing the risk of air embolism and airborne contamination. By 1952, the percutaneous approach to subclavian vein catheterization was developed in France,[3] permitting both central venous access for infusion and the monitoring of central venous pressure.

Advances were also being made in our understanding of fluid and electrolyte balance and human nutritional needs. In the mid-1870s, Hodder and Thomas discovered that the IV infusion of cow's milk into humans could expand intravascular volume and provide nutritional support. Because the freshness of the milk was believed to be a critical factor, cows were often brought to the steps of the hospital to be milked,[4] an interesting forerunner to today's practice of delivering total parenteral nutrition and lipid solutions to the patient's refrigerator.

Throughout the 20th century, experimentation with amino acids, sugar, and fat continued. In 1968, in the Department of Surgical Research at the University of Pennsylvania, Dr. Stanley Dudrick used nothing more than IV dextrose and amino acid solutions as a nutritional source to successfully achieve normal growth and development in children and maintenance in adults.[4] This classic work marked the beginning of the clinical application of IV nutritional support.

Where was nursing in these continuing attempts to use the bloodstream as a route to calm and cure? It is fitting that Boston,

---

*The author and editors wish to acknowledge the contributions made by Christine A. Pierce, author of this chapter in the first edition of *Intravenous Nursing: Clinical Principles and Practice*.

home of "America's first trained nurse" in 1863,[1] should also attain notoriety for the development of infusion nursing as a specialty. In 1940, the Massachusetts General Hospital developed a new nursing position, which included the following general responsibilities:

- Administering IV solutions and transfusions
- Cleaning and sharpening needles
- Cleaning infusion sets
- Maintaining patent needles and unobstructed infusion flow[1]

Although the emphasis was on technical performance and the ability to perform a successful venipuncture, this new nursing role established initial autonomy from the physician and conferred the specialty title of "Intravenous Therapist."

Over the next 50 years, the role of the nurse in infusion therapy has evolved to the modern IV practitioner, no longer a technician but a multifaceted specialist capable of integrating holistic principles of medicine, nursing, management, marketing, education, and quality improvement into the patient's plan of care. Since the early 1980s, there has been a particularly rapid growth of the IV nursing specialty, as evidenced by the following:

- Publication of the National Intravenous Therapy Association's (NITA's) recommendations of practice (1980)
- Recognition of IV Nurse Day by the United States House of Representatives (October 1, 1980) to honor IV nurses on January 25 of each year
- Offering of the first national certification examination for intravenous nurses (March 1985)
- Development by the Centers for Disease Control and Prevention of "universal precautions" to reduce the risk of transmitting the human immunodeficiency virus and hepatitis B virus to health care workers (1987)
- Evolution of the multibillion dollar home infusion business, made possible by the specialty practice of infusion nursing

Today more than 85% of hospitalized patients receive some form of IV therapy during their stay, and many continue therapy after discharge. Pharmacologic and technologic advances provide the patient with improved quality of care but concurrently demand a more specialized and detailed nursing knowledge to offset risks and maximize value. Factors such as the growing elderly population, the economic need to service patients outside the hospital, and changes brought by health care reform provide expanding possibilities for the prepared and flexible infusion nurse. By pursuing continuing education, specialty certification, and membership in professional organizations, today's successful IV nurse specialist can create opportunities for career advancement and personal reward.

PROFESSIONAL ORGANIZATIONS

One November day in 1972, two IV nurses, Ada Plumer from the Massachusetts General Hospital in Boston and Marguerite Knight from the Johns Hopkins Hospital in Baltimore, wrote an organizational letter asking interested individuals to join in forming the American Association of IV Nurses. By the time 16 charter members assembled in Baltimore on January 25, 1973,

there was already some concern that the use of "nurse" in the organization's name would restrict membership to nurses exclusively, whereas the proposed bylaws were more expansive.[5] Because of this concern, the charter members decided to name the organization the National Intravenous Therapy Association (NITA). NITA's purpose was to standardize the specialty practice of IV nursing and to ensure the provision of quality, cost-efficient patient care.

Over the next 6 years, NITA expanded rapidly. The addition of new members facilitated the formation of local chapters and affiliations with other national organizations. In 1979, the demands of rapidly increasing membership heralded the need for a professional full-time staff to work with elected and appointed officials. A national office was established in Cambridge, Massachusetts.

By 1987, many milestones had been achieved by NITA. The "Standards of Practice," unifying the specialty approach to infusion nursing, was developed in 1980. In response to rapid changes in health care and emerging technology, the standards served to increase the recognition of the IV specialty nationwide. In October 1980, the United States House of Representatives acknowledged the practice of IV therapy as an independent specialty and declared January 25 each year to be National IV Nurse Day. The first specialty certification examination was offered in 1985, and successful candidates were awarded the designation of Certified Registered Nurse Intravenous (CRNI).

Although nurses made up 99% of NITA's membership in the mid-1980s, there remained some confusion among fellow professionals, consumers, and legislators about what group this organization represented. In 1987, a letter from one of NITA's own CRNIs described her experience at the "Nurse in Washington Internship Program" and stated that NITA would be recognized by other professional nursing organizations only if the word *nurse* was reflected in its name.[5] In 1987, by a majority vote of the members, NITA officially became the Intravenous Nurses Society (INS). This name was chosen to more accurately reflect the organization's nature and focus.

Within the INS, there are local chapters with a membership composed primarily of registered nurses, as well as other professionals, including physicians, pharmacists, and licensed practical/vocational nurses. The growing interest in global initiatives is evidenced by international members and international IV nursing professional organizations. INS continues to work on an international level to help facilitate excellence and quality worldwide.

Because INS is committed to reviewing and revising its standards as required by modern practice and technologic advances, *Infusion Nursing Standards of Practice* has undergone five revisions since the original document was written in 1980. INS publishes a peer-reviewed journal bimonthly, highlighting clinical, management, ethical, and technologic issues. In 1999, to ready its members for the opportunities and challenges of the 21st century, INS revised its Mission Statement (Box 2-1) and the underlying values (Box 2-2). "The revised mission statement emphasizes advocacy, professional development, resource networking and opportunities to enhance the knowledge of intravenous nurse professionals. Underlying values of the revised mission statement are integrity, excellence, and commitment."[6]

A blueprint to assist the organization in meeting the challenges of the changing health care environment was also developed.[6] This plan allows the organization to respond to the changing environment of health care reform and helps INS offer its members a wide range of professional services that support infusion nursing practice.[6]

More than 25 years of INS success have contributed significantly to the growth and recognition of the specialty of IV nursing and its ongoing goal of quality health care.[5] Having stepped firmly into the 21st century, INS is prepared not only to continue developing the IV specialty but also to fashion it into a collaborative practice with other nursing specialties for the holistic welfare of its consumers worldwide.

SCOPE OF PRACTICE

Basic nursing education is designed to prepare the *nursing generalist,* a nurse with a global approach to nursing practice. Although there are three primary education entries to registered nursing practice—associate degree, diploma, and baccalaureate degree—all are designed to provide entry-level nurses with a foundation on which to build more specialized practices in their areas of competence and interest. Nursing practice advances by means of specialization, which requires detailed knowledge and skills within a circumscribed area. Although specialization can be achieved by formal education at the graduate level and beyond, it is also a product of concentrated study, continuing education, and skill development in a specific area of clinical interest. The practice of IV nursing is a specialization.

The IV nurse may be an RN or a licensed practical/vocational nurse (LPN/LVN) who has acquired knowledge and skill in IV nursing and is committed to providing safe, quality IV nursing care to the patient. The IV nurse's practice is based on the six major foundations listed in Box 2-3.

The nursing process is pervasive in the practice of IV nursing. The cycle of assessment, problem identification, intervention, and evaluation enhances the ongoing expansion of knowledge and practice in this and all other specialties. By constantly monitoring patient and process outcomes, the nurse is able to refine the process of data collection and problem identification, thereby improving the quality of care. Continuous improvement causes a paradigm shift, moving the nurse from the role of technician to the expanded role of colleague and collaborator. This shift enables the IV nurse to interact with other members of the health care team, particularly those who regulate or influence nursing practice.

Education and research should have a place in the practice of every IV nurse. Research is the foundation for nursing's body of knowledge and a general prerequisite to the recognition of nursing as a profession. This distinct knowledge sets nursing apart from medicine and the social and biologic sciences, and it is the nurse's responsibility to continually contribute to this base. Sharing information through presentation and publication ensures the dissemination of practice-based specialty learning, and encourages an influx of new practitioners into that specialty. Only then can collaborative nursing truly exist.

COMPETENCY

The practice settings for IV therapy delivery are as disparate as the patient populations served by this specialty. From the hospitalized neonatal patient to the geriatric patient in an extended care facility, IV nurses serve patients with wide-ranging clinical diagnoses at a variety of locations. In a critical care setting, one might find the nurse transfusing blood products and interpreting hemodynamic data gained from transvenous monitoring. Another nurse may be training a mother to administer total parenteral nutrition to her toddler in a suburban home. A colleague is fighting downtown traffic to reach a working executive in time to change a cassette on an ambulatory antibiotic pump, while yet another is recommending vascular access devices to the new oncology patient in the physician's office. At first glance, the scenes appear to be unique. What are consistent, however, are the basic competencies of the nurse; the combination of knowledge, skills, and abilities necessary to administer IV infusion therapy.

Basic competencies are intended to serve as guidelines for the practicing nurse and to help design orientation and continuing education programs. They provide a valid foundation for professional IV nursing practice.

Clinical. The nurse should be proficient in the clinical aspects of infusion nursing with validated competency in clinical judgment and practice.

IV nursing is defined as the use of the nursing process as it relates to technology and clinical application, fluids and electrolytes, pharmacology, infection control, pediatrics, transfusion therapy, oncology, parenteral nutrition, and quality assurance. An organization must define in policy and procedure that clinical competencies are the responsibility of the RN. It must also define tasks that may be delegated to and performed by the LPN/LVN. Clinical competencies must be in accordance with state Nurse Practice Acts and *Infusion Nursing Standards of Practice*.[7] To demonstrate the full range of clinical competencies, the nurse should be able to do the following:

- Validate the physician's order for infusion therapy
- Initiate, monitor, and terminate infusion therapy
- Prepare IV solutions with the addition of medications in the absence of an admixture service
- Recognize medication and solution incompatibilities and factors affecting stability
- Administer and monitor antineoplastic agents
- Administer and monitor investigational drugs
- Administer and monitor parenteral nutrition
- Administer and monitor blood and its components
- Administer and monitor pain management
- Perform venous and arterial punctures
- Perform phlebotomies
- Maintain infusion site, administration set, and dressing
- Maintain established aseptic practices and infection control
- Initiate IV therapy in emergency situations
- Demonstrate knowledge and proficient technical ability in the use of infusion-related equipment
- Evaluate and maintain infusion-related equipment
- Observe and assess all adverse reactions and complications related to parenteral therapy and initiate appropriate nursing interventions
- Document infusion therapy as appropriate
- Perform initial and ongoing assessment and care planning
- Coordinate care
- Educate patient or caregiver regarding infusion therapy
- Understand the psychosocial implications of infusion therapy
- Collect and analyze data
- Communicate with other members of the health care team

- Monitor and evaluate outcomes
- Demonstrate knowledge of quality improvement and risk management

Communication. The IV nurse should have the verbal and written communication skills necessary to translate ideas and facts to individuals within and beyond the scope of the specialty.

Patient education. In keeping with the holistic approach to patient care, it is the IV nurse's responsibility to educate the patient and significant others about the prescribed therapy. This education and an assessment of the patient's comprehension are documented, communicated to the appropriate people, and stored in a system that allows retrieval. Also, the nurse's teaching effectiveness should be evaluated and continually observed.

Technology. Technology continually advances. Consequently, the IV nurse must evaluate products for clinical application. The nurse must be cognizant of new technologic advances and should help evaluate, select, and implement new products in the clinical setting.

Continuing education. Continuing education is essential to sustain and advance nursing and is required of all nurses. Active participation in continuing IV education programs is vital for the growth of the IV specialty and nursing profession. The IV nurse should share the knowledge obtained from these programs with colleagues in collaborative disciplines to improve care.

Legal. Nursing standards for the delivery of infusion therapy include the following:

- Establishing a framework for monitoring the care given and products used
- Providing a frame of reference that distinguishes among malpractice, product failure, and unfortunate medical result
- Helping resolve ethical conflicts between the IV nurse's duty to the patient and employer

Adherence to nursing standards for the delivery of infusion therapy achieves the following:

- Reduces the patient's risk of unnecessary trauma or complications
- Reduces the risk of malpractice claims against the physician, nurse, or health care organization
- Reduces the risk of product liability claims against manufacturers

Quality improvement. Patients requiring infusion therapy receive quality care through the nurse's compliance with outcome criteria. Nurses are responsible for quality improvement as it relates to this specialty and should document pertinent statistics relative to infusion therapy. Nurses must also evaluate any deviation from optimal care in IV nursing practice and take corrective action. All infusion policies and procedures should be reviewed and/or revised annually and approved by the appropriate organizational committee.

Research. Research is an inherent component of IV nursing that allows the continual investigation, validation, and development of this specialty. Through the dissemination of research results, the IV nursing specialty will be advanced.

Consultation. The IV nurse is an essential consultant to health care professionals, the patient's family, the community, and related industries. The nurse's principal concerns in each of these relationships are patient advocacy and delivery of safe, optimal IV nursing care.

Clinical management. Clinical management encompasses all aspects of the nursing process. The goal of clinical management is to meet the needs of the patient and achieve the established therapeutic outcome.

Budgetary process. To manage costs while rendering quality IV care, the nurse should be actively involved in and accountable for establishing and maintaining the budgetary process that encompasses staffing, education, and products used in IV nursing.

Educational requirements

Besides demonstrating characteristics such as accountability, reliability, initiative, sound judgment, and effective communication and technical skills, the IV nurse must complete certain educational requirements before practicing infusion therapy. The educational curriculum, including theory and clinical components, is fundamental to preparing for practice in IV nursing. The nurse's role within the specialty is based on education, experience, and technical and clinical expertise.

Role and qualifications

The RN may function as a nurse specializing in infusion therapy within the scope of a state's Nurse Practice Act. The LPN/LVN who is educated in IV therapy is the minimum level practitioner able to assist in tasks delegated by the RN for the delivery of IV therapy. A state's Nurse Practice Act and a health care organization's policies and procedures define the scope of the LPN/LVN's involvement. The RN, even when assisted by an LPN/LVN, is responsible for all aspects of patient care specific to infusion therapy. The RN remains accountable and responsible for delegated tasks and must have clear knowledge of the nursing scope of practice relative to assessment, planning, implementation, and evaluation within IV nursing. The RN must also be cognizant of the legal ramifications of delegating nursing care activities.[7]

RN specializing in infusion therapy. Currently, the Intravenous Nurses Certification Corporation (INCC) does not require the Bachelor of Science in Nursing (BSN) degree for the RN to sit for the CRNI Certification Examination. The INCC, the sole governing organization for this test and the CRNI program, has never required a BSN as a prerequisite and has no future plans to incorporate it into the requirements.[8] To enter the specialty and become an IV specialist, the RN should meet the following requirements.[7]

Entry level
- A current RN license in the United States or Canada
- Two years of medical/surgical nursing experience

Specialist level
- A current RN license in the United States or Canada
- A minimum of 1600 hours of experience in IV therapy as an RN within the 2 consecutive years before the date of applica-

tion. *Note: RNs functioning as educators, administrators, or researchers in IV nursing meet the experience criterion if they have spent the equivalent of 1600 hours in their position within 2 years before the date of application for certification.*

LPN/LVN practicing in intravenous nursing. To enter the specialty and become an IV nurse, the LPN/LVN should meet the following requirements.

Entry level
- A current LPN/LVN license in the United States
- Two years of medical/surgical nursing experience

Curriculum

The revised *Infusion Nursing Standards of Practice* describes the detailed curriculum and implementation of that curriculum that is thought to best prepare the IV nurse specialist.[7] The following discussion highlights those recommendations.

Establishing objectives. The nurse wishing to practice in this specialty should undertake a course of study that is based on outcome criteria established by behavioral objectives from the cognitive, affective, and psychomotor domains.

The educational program should consist of the following curriculum:
- *Program goal or purpose:* statement of intent to describe how this activity will be beneficial
- *Learning objectives:* written statements describing the learner-oriented outcomes expected to result from the activity
- *Cognitive behaviors:* behaviors that place primary emphasis on the mental or intellectual processes of the RN and the LPN/LVN
- *Affective behaviors:* behaviors that primarily emphasize attitudes, emotions, and values of the RN and the LPN/LVN
- *Psychomotor behaviors:* behaviors that place primary emphasis on the various degrees of physical skills and dexterity as they relate to the thought process

The following categories of learning objectives should be represented:
- Acquisition of knowledge
- Enhancement of critical thinking skills: purposeful, goal-directed thinking oriented toward judgment based on evidence, not conjecture
- Development of psychomotor skills
- Changes in attitude, values, or feelings

Program planning. The following are objectives of an educational program:
- Identifying needs of the targeted audience
- Selecting and sequencing content related to the objectives
- Selecting instructional techniques, strategies, and methods appropriate for the learning objectives, instructor's skill, and learner's characteristics
- Creating or assembling instructional materials such as audiovisual aids, workbooks, and equipment for demonstration and practice sessions
- Arranging for clinical experience under direct and indirect supervision
- Validating initial competency in both theory and prac-

tice through the organization's competency assessment program

- Participating in the ongoing competency assessment program as determined by each organization

Curriculum description

Theoretical. The theoretical aspect of IV nursing includes the IV nurse's knowledge and understanding of general organizational policies. The nurse should be cognizant of responsibilities to the patient, employer, nursing profession, and health care community.

Theoretical aspects should provide a formalized instruction program to enhance communication, both written and verbal, and expand knowledge. The formalized instruction program for the LPN/LVN should be modified to ensure compliance with state Nurse Practice Acts.

Curriculum content. A comprehensive theoretical curriculum in IV therapy nursing should include technology and clinical application, fluids and electrolytes, pharmacology, infection control, pediatrics, transfusion therapy, oncology, parenteral nutrition, and quality assurance. These same topics are the basis for the certification examination offered through the INCC as an assessment of specialty knowledge. Before discussing certification, however, it is necessary to take a more detailed look at each content area and to understand the specific objectives needed to determine competency within that subject. The following descriptions are taken from the revised *Infusion Nursing Standards of Practice.*[7]

Technology and clinical application. This curriculum should prepare the IV nurse in the skills, techniques, and clinical aspects of delivering parenteral therapies. The instruction in skills and techniques should be interactive; educational aids, actual equipment, and hands-on practice sessions should be used.

This instruction should present the proper function, use, care, and maintenance of supplies and equipment used in the delivery of parenteral therapies. Knowledge and understanding of potential hazards and possible complications related to the use of supplies and equipment should be included.

This instruction should provide in-depth focus on the vascular system and its relationship with other body systems. A thorough knowledge and understanding of the neurologic system should be included, with emphasis on the layers and compartments of the spinal cord and brain and diffusion of medication through this system. In addition, knowledge of the skeletal system should be included to help the nurse recognize those bones appropriate for intraosseous use. The nurse must know and understand all applications of parenteral therapies and be able to recognize complications and initiate interventions to achieve desired patient outcomes.

Fluid and electrolyte balance. This curriculum should include an understanding of the nature, pathophysiology, clinical manifestations, and principles of maintenance, replacement, and corrective therapy. This instruction should include the distinct body systems and their related diseases with relationship to the major objectives of therapy.

Pharmacology. This curriculum should address classifications of IV medications, including investigational drugs. The knowledge and understanding of IV drugs should include indications for use, pharmacologic properties, contraindications, dosing, clinical mathematics, anticipated side effects, potential complications/antidotal therapy, compatibilities, stabilities, and any other special considerations.

Infection control. This curriculum should include a general overview of microbiology, with instruction on microorganisms pertaining to infusion therapy, transmission of disease-causing organisms, surveillance, preventive measures, precautions, and aseptic technique.

Pediatrics. This curriculum should include the safe administration of infusion therapy to the pediatric patient. It should include growth and development; fluids and electrolytes related to the pediatric population; appropriate IV solutions; special considerations in delivery systems; treatment modalities, such as dosing; site selection; and psychologic implications.

Transfusion therapy. This curriculum should include immunohematology, blood grouping, blood and its components, equipment, and reactions. This curriculum should also include the selection of blood donors, confidentiality of blood donors, fractionation of blood into its components, and laboratory testing required to determine compatibility. Emphasis should be placed on the administration of blood, its cellular components, and plasma derivatives and recognition and management of any adverse reactions.

Oncology. This curriculum should include knowledge and understanding of the cell cycle; types of cancer; purpose of therapy, such as curative or palliative; assessment of laboratory values; antineoplastic agents and their indications for use in both single and combined therapy; and all related aspects of antineoplastic agent use, such as dosing, anticipated side effects, potential complications, administration and safe handling of these agents, patient education, nursing interventions, psychosocial implications, and the disease continuum.

Parenteral nutrition. This curriculum should include indications for use, types and composition of solutions available, patient assessment, and administration and termination techniques. This instruction should emphasize patient education, metabolic processes, potential complications, psychosocial implications, and measures to ensure the desired outcome.

Quality assurance, performance improvement, and risk management. This curriculum should include structural components; legal aspects; criteria to measure outcome based on policy and procedure; participation in the process, such as planning, implementation, evaluation, and monitoring for desired outcomes; standards of practice; and principles of continuous quality improvement.

Clinical evaluation

All clinical aspects of IV nursing should be supervised until proficiency is determined to be acceptable and competency has been validated through a competency assessment program.

CERTIFICATION

The history of certification actually spans the greatest portion of the 20th century, although most are familiar with it as a buzz word during the early 1990s. Believed to have first been used as a credentialing measure for public health nurses as early as 1912,[9] certification was created out of concern for the inadequacy of hospital-based training for diversified roles. The nurse was required to complete a particular program of postgraduate education to earn a certificate. By the late 1950s, the American Nurses Association (ANA) began to examine a certification mechanism to acknowledge achievement in various areas of clinical practice.[9] The ANA identified certification as a method for regulating and protecting specialized practice, but also claimed that it effectively ensured expert quality to the public. It was not until 1974 that the ANA began certifying RNs officially, and then only for three practice areas.[10] By 1987, that number had grown to 17, and today the ANA offers certification in 27 specialties.

Soon other organizations began considering certification for their areas of specialty practice. One of the earliest to establish a certification program was the American Association of Critical Care Nurses. Established in 1976, this program awards the Critical Care Registered Nurse (CCRN) credential and now has more certified nurses than any other specialty.[10] In 1984, there were only 85,000 certified nurses nationwide.[10] Between 1985 and 1990, however, 20 new certifications were developed (for a total of 60 certifications) and the total number of certified nurses rose to nearly 250,000.[11] Just what does certification mean today, and why is there an increasing number of nurses following their "RN" with a credential?

The primary goal of certification has always been consumer protection. Licensure declares someone qualified to perform, whereas certification identifies those who practice on a higher, more sophisticated level than that determined by license.[12] Licensure is mandatory, but certification is voluntary.

By design, licensure ensures only a minimal degree of competency. It is the oldest mechanism by which occupations are regulated in the United States and was defined by the Department of Health, Education, and Welfare as "the process by which an agency of government grants permission to an individual to engage in a given occupation, upon finding that the applicant has obtained the minimal degree of competency necessary to ensure that public health, safety and welfare will be reasonably protected."[12] Nurses are licensed to practice under the Nurse Practice Act within each state.

Certification is the process by which a nongovernmental agency or association grants recognition to an individual who has met its qualification requirements for specialty practice. Such qualifications may include the following: (1) graduation from an accredited or approved program, (2) acceptable performance on a qualifying examination or series of examinations, and/or (3) completion of a work requirement.[1] Whereas licensure addresses competence for the general practice of nursing, certification signifies competence in specialized professional practice based on the acquisition of additional knowledge and skills.

Although each specialty group has its own objectives, certification programs generally seek to accomplish the following:

- Assessment of advanced knowledge and skill
- Demonstration of excellence in practice
- Insurance of the public's welfare
- Standardization of the qualifications necessary for specialty practice

- Advancement of the knowledge and standards of the specialty[13]

It is clear that certification programs instill a system of accountability that directly affects the quality of care consumers can expect to receive. Certification protects not only the public but the nurse as well by providing control over a specific sphere of practice and limiting the inward migration of those who are unqualified. Certification provides control to the professional association granting the credential by forcing it to establish a clear identity, define the area of practice, and set performance standards.[12]

The early 1990s witnessed a virtual explosion in the number of certification programs and nurses participating in the credentialing process. There were a number of reasons for this trend. It has been shown that over time voluntary processes have the tendency to become institutionalized and legalized and that voluntary agencies with no legal power may gain access to power through rules and regulations that are subsequently developed.[12] An example of power without law is the requirement to pass the survey from the Joint Commission on Accreditation of Healthcare Organizations, a voluntary accreditation process, to qualify for Medicare reimbursement—a necessary fiscal survival mechanism.[10] In the psychiatric/mental health specialty, certification makes the nurse eligible for third-party reimbursement,[14] and the advanced roles of nurse anesthetist, nurse midwife, and nurse practitioner require certification to practice. As trends continue toward increased professionalism and accountability to provide quality care for health care consumers, certification is certain to gain even more popularity. There is a growing effort by nursing organizations and associations to direct reimbursement by third-party payers to care delivered by certified nurses, and health care organizations are beginning to recognize the importance of supporting nurses seeking certification, if only for long-term institutional survival.[13]

Beyond the predicted employment and financial implications of certification and the obvious consumer benefits, there are many additional motivations for a nurse to seek it. The literature is filled with reports of increased job satisfaction, improved self-esteem, increased employment opportunities, clinical advancement, and the pride of peer recognition and respect, all attributable to certification.[12-14] Although informal surveys and spot checks suggest that most hospitals do not directly increase nursing salaries as a result of certification, some provide a one-time bonus or use the credential as a component of advancement on the clinical ladder, ultimately leading to higher compensation.[10] Others encourage and reward their nurses by providing on-site review courses and paid workshop days during test preparation, refunding test fees for successful passing, and recognizing achievement with certificates, recognition in the organization's newsletter, and new name pins with the certification designation clearly printed.[13]

The INS, then known as the *NITA*, offered the first national certification examination for IV nurses on March 23, 1985. At 17 sites around the country, 540 RNs sat for this examination. Successful completion led to the CRNI designation. This examination has been offered annually ever since, extending the CRNI credential to thousands of IV nurses in a variety of practice settings.

The Intravenous Nurses Certification Corporation (INCC), established in 1983 as a separate corporation from the INS, is responsible for preparing and administering the certification examination. Although working collaboratively within the IV specialty, these organizations have different missions. As previously mentioned, the INS focuses on its membership, whereas the INCC is concerned with protecting the public (Box 2-4).

The RN Examination Council for the INCC consists of RNs who have passed the written CRNI Certification Examination, received the CRNI designation, and are widely recognized as experts in the content areas of the examination. This examination council works in conjunction with a national testing agency to develop, administer, and evaluate tests. The council also consults with a psychometrician, a professional with a doctoral degree with an emphasis in statistics, research, and theory of testing.[8] To become certified, an RN involved in the specialty practice of infusion therapy must pass the written CRNI Certification Examination. The following eligibility criteria must be fulfilled before applying for the examination:

- A current RN license in the United States or Canada
- A minimum of 1600 hours of experience in IV nursing as an RN within the 2 consecutive years before the date of application

RNs functioning as educators, administrators, or researchers in IV nursing meet the experience criterion if they have spent the equivalent of 1600 hours in their position within the 2 consecutive years before the date of application.[8]

The examination

Preparation for the examination is best undertaken with a well-defined plan implemented months in advance of the actual testing date. Because of the differences among the various practice settings and clinical situations encountered, the nurse should not rely exclusively on work experience to prepare for this broad examination. It is helpful to assemble reference material that includes a comprehensive, basic nursing text and publications specific to the IV specialty practice and test content areas. A number of helpful publications and a recommended bibliography are available through the INS and the INCC.

Once the study materials have been gathered, the nurse should plan to devote a specific amount of time each day for reading and review. Some nurses find it helpful to form a study group with colleagues who are also preparing for the test. This can be particularly helpful if the group members represent different areas of expertise and can share information. Certification review courses are offered in conjunction with national INS educational programs and may occasionally be presented by a local INS chapter. Some nurses find this classroom instruction structure to be most familiar and comfortable. Other certified nurses should be sought out in the workplace and asked to act as mentors. A successful CRNI can offer much advice and guidance for test preparation and enjoys the opportunity to serve as a recognized expert in the IV specialty.

There are nine major content areas covered on the certification examination. The content tested is identical to that recommended for the basic curriculum of IV nursing[7] and should serve as the foundation for any IV nursing practice. Candidates who successfully pass this examination are awarded the CRNI designation.

Recertification

The CRNI credential is valid for a 3-year period and always expires on December 31 of the third year. To become recertified, one must be an active CRNI, possess a current RN license, and be able to document 1000 hours of clinical practice in the IV nursing specialty within 3 years of the recertification date. The nurse must either document 40 recertification units earned during the 3 years preceding the recertification date (recertification by continuing education) or successfully pass the CRNI certification examination during the year preceding the recertification date (recertification by examination).[8]

Under the recertification program, CRNIs are required to meet the 40-unit specification to renew their credentials for an additional 3-year period. Of the 40 units, 30 must be obtained by attending INS educational meetings, 1-day programs, or INCC's Item Writers Workshops. The remaining 10 units may be obtained by several options approved by the INCC Board of Directors. General nursing education credits do not currently apply toward recertification credit. Retaking the CRNI certification examination is always a recertification option for CRNIs.[8]

IV NURSE SPECIALISTS

INS's ultimate goal is to ensure that patients receive high-quality, cost-effective nursing care. In any practice setting where infusion therapy is delivered, it is necessary to have highly trained and knowledgeable IV nurse specialists place, monitor, and assess IV products. IV nurse specialists provide consistent high-quality IV care to their patients, thereby ensuring that guidelines of competent practice are observed. INS recommends that nurses practicing in the IV specialty achieve and maintain IV certification.

The IV nurse specialist practices IV therapy with autonomy and accountability and is instrumental in establishing IV therapy policy and procedure. The IV nurse specialist's responsibilities may include inserting IV cannulas; administering prescribed IV solutions, medications, and blood products; monitoring and maintaining IV sites and systems; evaluating response to prescribed therapy; educating patients and families and evaluating comprehension; documenting pertinent information on the patient's record; collaborating with other members of the health

---

Box 2-4   Intravenous Nurses Certification Corporation Mission Statement

The Intravenous Nurses Certification Corporation (INCC) exists to benefit and protect the public through assessment, validation, and documentation of the clinical eligibility and continued clinical competency of nurses practicing infusion therapy in all practice settings worldwide. INCC supports education and research and validates the reliability of credentialing mechanisms and their relationship to clinical practice. INCC promotes recognition of its credentialed nurses and programs to the public, to other healthcare organizations, and to the nursing profession.

care team; and compiling statistics to quantify, qualify, and justify the specialist's performance and IV services rendered. The IV nurse specialist possesses the experience and theoretical knowledge to determine conditions, patient population, and proper use of IV therapy devices.

INS recognizes the IV-educated LPN/LVN as having the minimum level of education and training to perform IV therapy. If used under the supervision of a qualified RN, competent LPNs/LVNs educated in IV nursing can provide efficient, high-quality, and cost-effective IV therapy. When the LPN/LVN practices IV therapy, all job functions must, as defined in their licensure, be under the supervision of the RN, and these job function limitations must be recognized.

LPNs/LVNs have a limited role in IV therapy and may not perform advanced technical procedures, such as inserting peripherally inserted central catheters. After completing education and training requirements, the LPN/LVN may be permitted to perform venipuncture, monitor IV administration and sites, change dressings, and administer certain solutions according to state Nurse Practice Acts. LPNs/LVNs practicing IV therapy should demonstrate clinical competency and meet educational requirements. The RN specializing in IV therapy, assisted by the LPN/LVN educated in IV nursing, is the best qualified health care provider to manage and administer high-quality IV nursing care.[7,15-19]

ROLE DELINEATION: BENEFITS OF THE IV NURSE SPECIALIST

The CRNI credential identifies the IV nurse as a highly knowledgeable and skilled practitioner in the delivery of infusion therapies, indicates that the practitioner is prepared to be accountable for his or her professional development, and serves as objective and measurable evidence of clinical expertise in a specialty practice.[20] From the public point of view, the designation of certified infusion specialist ensures that the nurse has been educated to provide IV services and should be selectively sought, much as board-certified physicians are sought in medical subspecialties.[20] Physician colleagues evaluate the CRNI from a perspective of minimal risk and high patient satisfaction, convinced that certain complex infusion therapies should be handled only by the infusion specialist,[21] and are selectively requesting these nurses in hospital and alternate site settings. The CRNI has shown positive outcomes in facility and agency quality management and has decreased liability and risk in areas of high-volume, high-technology procedures. IV specialty nurses have extended that benefit to manufacturers by using products as intended, in a safe and appropriate manner.[20]

Not surprisingly, use of the certified IV nurse specialist has also proved cost-effective. A CRNI requires less orientation and in-service time and can also have a positive impact on equipment and supply costs by proper and effective utilization. With the increasing attention given to total quality management and continuous quality improvement, the process of specialty credentialing becomes more important daily. Within that environment, the certified IV nurse specialist is prepared to serve as a benchmark against which all those in IV nursing practice can be evaluated.

REFERENCES

1. Kelly LY: *Dimensions of professional nursing,* ed 4, New York, 1981, Macmillan.
2. Phillips LD: *Manual of IV therapeutics,* ed 2, Philadelphia, 1997, FA Davis.
3. Weinstein SM: *Plumer's principles and practice of infusion therapy,* ed 6, Philadelphia, 1997, Lippincott-Raven.
4. Grant JP: *Handbook of total parenteral nutrition,* ed 2, Philadelphia, 1992, WB Saunders.
5. Larkin M: From the editor, *NITA* 10(5):319, 1987.
6. Intravenous Nurses Society: INS develops strategic plan initiatives, *INS Newsline* 22(2), 2000.
7. Intravenous Nurses Society: Infusion nursing standards of practice, *JIN* (suppl) 23(65), 2000.
8. Intravenous Nurses Certification Corporation: CRNI program summary, *INCC Chronicle* 3(1):6, 1999.
9. Beecroft PC, Papenhausen JL: Certification for specialty practice? *Clin Nurse Specialist* 3:161, 1984.
10. Collins ML: Certification: is the payoff worth the price? *RN* 50(7):36, 1987.
11. Fickeissen J: 56 ways to get certified, *Am J Nurs* 90(3):50, 1990.
12. Crudi C: Credentialing for I.V. nurses, *NITA* 7(3):234, 1984.
13. Simpson KR: A specialty certification incentive program: cost versus benefits, *J Nurs Staff Dev* 6(4):180, 1990.
14. Winter EJS et al: Is certification for you? *Nursing '92* 22(1):88, 1992.
15. Intravenous Nurses Society: Position paper: the intravenous nurse specialist's role in the evolving healthcare environment, *JIN* 20(3):119, 1997.
16. Intravenous Nurses Society: Position paper: the registered nurse's role in product purchase, *JIN* 20(2):69, 1997.
17. Intravenous Nurses Society: Position paper: the registered nurse's role in vascular access device selection, *JIN* 20(2):71, 1997.
18. Intravenous Nurses Society: Position paper: the role of the licensed practical nurse and the licensed vocational nurse in the clinical practice of intravenous therapy, *JIN* 20(2):75, 1997.
19. Intravenous Nurses Society: Position paper: the use of unlicensed assistive personnel in the delivery of intravenous therapy, *JIN* 20(2):73, 1997.
20. Interview: A conversation with Paul Creager, *JIN* 15:34, 1992.
21. Interview: The value physicians place on nursing certification: the Journal speaks with George Ritter, MD, *JIN* 15:237, 1992.

Case Management

Kathleen M. Brotherton, RN, MS, CCM, Cynthia H. Blackburn, RN, CCM

Case management is a functional area of practice within the nursing profession, which has an interdisciplinary relationship with all members of the multidisciplinary health care treatment team. The term *case management* has many meanings and models depending on the health care practice setting, but it supports a universal goal of improving quality of care and containing cost.[1]

Case management in intravenous (IV) nursing practice is designed to benefit patients, families, and caregivers through education and advocacy for those in need of short- and long-term infusion therapy services. The infusion case manager's goal is for the patient to reach his or her maximum functional level and maintain an acceptable quality of life.

MANAGED CARE
Defining managed care

To fully understand the process of case management, one must first have a basic understanding of the concept of managed care. Managed care is an evolving health care process that integrates the delivery of health care services between purchaser, provider, and payer. There are several elements involved in this integration:

- Established medical management and quality assurance programs based on established criteria and guidelines
- Arrangement with predetermined health care providers to deliver comprehensive health care services for the members
- Contracted reimbursement fees for health care services
- Established incentives for members to encourage participation in the health care plan

In today's managed health care environment, every nurse—even the infusion nurse—providing care to a patient covered by a managed care plan must, in essence, become a managed care nurse. The managed care nurse works directly with the patient as a liaison between the physician, payer (managed care organization), and providers (Fig. 3-1). Functions of the managed care nurse include those listed in Box 3-1.

History of managed care

Managed care is a change in the traditional fee-for-service health care system, and as such, it involves changes in corporate structures, U.S. health care policy, and demographics; all have contributed to the evolution of managed care. In the last century, society has transformed from rural to urban, from an industrial to an institutional-based orientation, and from an agricultural to an industrial and service economy. During the same period, physicians have moved from general practitioners to specialists, from solo to group practice, and from direct patient payment to group health insurance programs, most of them employer sponsored.

Managed care is not a new idea in the delivery of health care in the United States. It has roots back to the 1920s, when precursors of health maintenance organizations (HMOs) started in farm communities as part of cooperatives. In 1929, Elk City, Oklahoma, started a prepaid health plan. In 1934, Dr. Donald Ross and H.C. Loos agreed to provide comprehensive prepaid health care to a group of water company employees in Los Angeles. The Kaiser Foundation Health Plan was started in 1937 by Dr. Sidney Garfield at the request of the Kaiser construction company, which sought to finance medical care for workers constructing the Grand Coulee Dam in Washington State. Kaiser expanded services in 1942 to shipbuilding plants in the San Francisco Bay area. Following World War II, Kaiser further expanded the health plan by allowing nonemployees to participate.[3]

Prepaid health plans gained slow but steady acceptance in the 1940s. By the mid-1950s, fee-for-service physicians were competing with these prepaid health plans for patients. During this period, the *independent practice association* (IPA) model evolved. Physicians continued their fee-for-service practices but also began to offer a prepaid product. Prepaid group and individual practice associations were the prototypes for a new kind of

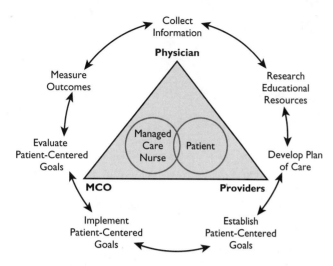

FIG. 3-1 *Managed care nursing model.* (Reprinted from the American Association of Managed Care Nurses: *Managed care nursing practice standards,* Glen Allen, Va, 1998, AAMCN.)

Box 3-1   Common Functions of the Managed Care Nurse

- Collect information.
- Research educational resources.
- Develop a plan of care.
- Establish patient-centered goals.
- Implement patient-centered goals.
- Evaluate patient-centered goals.
- Measure outcomes.[2]

---

health care delivery system. Under these new models, physicians shared the risk of financing care for enrollees. The physician could choose to bill and collect a fee-for-service payment from the patient or be paid by the HMO out of capitated service dollars. This fundamentally changed the way health care was financed and structured.[3]

Health care costs increased dramatically in the 1960s. As a result, business and government officials began to express great interest in prepaid health plans. Medicare was developed as a social program that provides health insurance to the elderly, those who have permanent kidney failure, and people with certain disabilities. Medicaid is a social program developed to provide health insurance coverage for the uninsured and underinsured population. These programs were signed into law in 1965.

The Health Maintenance Organization Act of 1973 recognized the promise of HMOs and encouraged their growth nationwide by removing legal impediments to their development. During this time, the Health Care Financing Administration of the Department of Health, Education, and Welfare approved the first Medicaid managed care program in Arizona. This program provided Medicaid services to beneficiaries on a prepaid, capitated payment basis.

In the 1970s and 1980s, prepaid, capitated managed care systems experienced steady growth and acceptance as a new

vision of health care to supplement the traditional acute care medical model. HMOs embraced new information technology in the belief that effective and efficient service was impossible in an environment where decisions were often made on supposition rather than credible objective information. Information translated into efficiency, which in turn translated into power in the competitive HMO marketplace.

The 103rd Congress addressed issues related to the current state of health care in the United States under a proposed health care reform initiative. The reform failed, however, and the pressure for health care reform shifted from the political arena to the payers of health care—the federal government (Medicare and Medicaid), state governments, and private businesses. The harsh reality is that we had exceeded our ability to pay for the fee-for-service model of health care. A better solution had to be found. Payers of health care are demanding a cost-effective, prepaid, and accountable system that provides high-quality and cost-effective care.[4]

Types of managed care

Health maintenance organization.
HMOs are organized health care systems that are responsible for both the financing and the delivery of a broad range of comprehensive health services to an enrolled population. The original definition of an HMO also included the aspect of financing health care for a prepaid fixed fee, hence the term *health plan*.

In many ways, an HMO can be viewed as a combination of a health insurer and a health care delivery system. Whereas traditional health care insurance companies reimburse covered individuals for the cost of their health care, HMOs provide health care services to their covered members through affiliated providers, who are reimbursed in a variety of ways.

HMOs must ensure that their members have access to covered health care services. This access is most commonly administered through a *gatekeeper* approach: except for emergencies, all care from providers other than the primary care physician (PCP) must be authorized by the PCP in advance. In addition, HMOs generally are responsible for ensuring the quality and appropriateness of the health care services they provide to their members.

The five common models of HMOs are (1) staff, (2) group practice, (3) network, (4) IPA, and (5) direct contract. The primary differences among these models are based on how the HMO relates to its participating physicians.[5]

Preferred provider organization.
A preferred provider organization (PPO) is a loosely managed fee-for-service managed health care model. In a PPO plan, contracts are established directly with medical care providers. Providers under contract are called *preferred providers*. Usually, the benefit contract provides significantly better benefits (lower copayments) for services received from preferred providers, thus encouraging their use. PPO plans generally provide benefits for services provided by nonparticipating providers, usually on an indemnity basis with higher copayments. A PPO plan can be insured or self-funded.

Providers may be, but are not necessarily, paid on a discounted fee-for-service basis. In this model, physicians are defined as participating "in network" or as nonparticipating providers. Discounts are applied to traditional fee-for-service charges as long as services are within the provider network. If services are obtained outside the network, reimbursement covers only a maximum allowable charge under fee-for-service arrangements.

Physicians and advanced practice registered nurses practice in solo or group settings in PPO arrangements. The incentives for providers to stay within the network are its large practice and high volume of patients. The consumer, who often subscribes to this model of managed care because the employer selected it, receives lower deductibles and copayments for in-network services, as well as some preventive care coverage. The quality of providers' practices is monitored. Information gathered is paired with cost and patient satisfaction data to determine best-practice patterns within a group of providers.

Exclusive provider organization. Exclusive provider organizations (EPOs) are similar to PPOs in their organization and purpose. Unlike PPOs, however, EPOs restrict their subscribers to participating providers. Beneficiaries covered by an EPO are required to receive all their covered health care services from providers who participate with the EPO. The EPO generally does not cover services received from other providers, although there may be exceptions.

Some EPOs resemble HMOs, not only by requiring exclusive use of the EPO provider network but also by using a gatekeeper to authorize nonprimary care services. In these cases, the primary difference between an HMO and an EPO is that the former is regulated under HMO laws and regulations, whereas the latter is regulated under insurance laws and regulations or the Employee Retirement Income Security Act of 1974 (ERISA). ERISA governs self-insured health plans.

EPOs are usually implemented by employers whose primary motivation is cost savings. These employers are less concerned about the reaction of their employees to severe restrictions on the choice of a health care provider and offer the EPO as a replacement for traditional indemnity health insurance coverage. Because of the severe restriction on choice, few employers have been willing to convert to an EPO format.[5]

Point of service. A point of service plan (POS) eases the member's entry into a strict managed health care model by allowing the member to opt out of the plan if needed. The member can choose among in-network providers with a reduced copayment or can opt for an out-of-network provider with higher copayment fees. This option was originally used as a marketing strategy by mature, established HMOs to increase membership.

The POS plan allows members to choose from participating and nonparticipating providers, with different benefit levels associated with IPA, staff-model, or group-model HMOs. Physician credentialing is similar to that for the PPO model. Consumers gain more rights, including clearly defined and well-established complaint and grievance procedures.[4]

Provider-sponsored network. Provider-sponsored networks (PSNs) were developed by physicians and hospitals, who form a legal entity and contract with purchasers to provide members of specific populations with a range of medical services. In this type of network, the providers own the network.

A physician-sponsored organization (PSO) is a type of PSN comprising physicians who contract separately with hospitals and ancillary service providers. Physician-only networks may include PCPs and specialists.

Capitation is the most common form of contracting within a PSN. This form of contracting provides a set monthly prepaid fee per member; thus the PSN bears responsibility for the use of services.[6]

Defining Case Management

The origin of case management can be traced back to the early 1900s, when people became interested in coordinating community services. This trend was soon followed by legislation affecting the public sector and was later propelled by the insurance industry into the private sector.

Case management was initially developed to deal with the many issues and challenges that arose within our complex health care delivery system. These issues include risk-based reimbursement models, a multitude of new and expensive technologies, numerous benefit plan designs, service fragmentation, variable quality and outcomes, and medical malpractice. Many different case management models have evolved over the past decade to address the needs of specific organizations and populations.[7] Case managers function in a multitude of settings as coordinators, facilitators, impartial advocates, and educators.

The role of the IV nurse case manager varies with the organizational setting and the job title. IV nurse case managers may work in outpatient clinics, physician offices, home care settings, or hospices, or they may work for insurance companies. In some cases, the IV nurse case manager assumes both clinical and administrative responsibilities for all aspects of the patient's care.

Case management process

The Commission for Case Manager Certification defines case management as follows:

> A collaborative process which assesses, plans, implements, coordinates, monitors and evaluates the options and services to meet an individual's health needs, using communication and available resources to promote quality, cost-effective outcomes.[8]

The case management process has become more involved as our health care system has grown more complex. Nursing case management is evolving into its own specialty apart from the traditional modes of care because it requires specialized knowledge. Negotiating the modern health care system to procure services for patients is beyond the scope of a nurse generalist.[9] Nurse case managers must have excellent interpersonal skills, a working knowledge of related community-based programs, effective problem-solving abilities, and relevant experience with different cultural groups. The active participation of the patient and many health care professionals, including but not limited to physicians, other medical providers, treatment facilities, case managers, and insurance or third-party payers, is required to achieve positive case outcomes. A helpful way to envision the roles of the many participants in the case management process

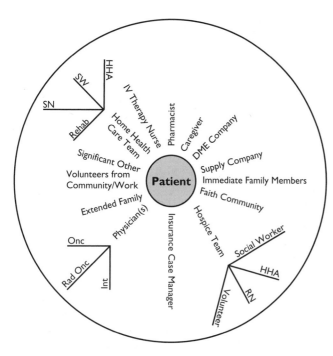

FIG. 3-2 *Infusion case management model.*

Box 3-2   **Components of the Initial Assessment Process**

- Demographic information about the patient and family
- Patient's past and current health issues and problems
- Current medications
- Patient's functional status
- Physical and nutritional care needs
- Patient's mental health status, memory, and behavior
- Patient's psychosocial function and perception of the illness or injury
- Financial data
- Caregiver capabilities
- Home environment
- Resources and providers

Table 3-1   **Sources of Assessment Data**

- Patient interview
- Family/primary caregiver interview
- Discussion with attending physician and/or consulting physician
- Home visit
- Medical records review
- Discussion with allied health professionals providing care to the patient (e.g., dietitian, respiratory therapist, rehabilitation therapists)

is to use the analogy of a wheel with the patient at the center (Fig. 3-2).

Components of the case management process

Assessment. Assessment is the first and perhaps most important component of the case management process. The accuracy of the entire case management plan depends on the information gathered during the assessment phase. Assessment is the ongoing process of analyzing and integrating data obtained from the patient and family, relevant treatment providers, caregivers, and funding sources to identify the plan of care, current and anticipated needs, and problems or obstacles that may be resolved through case management intervention.[8] The initial assessment process should include at least the components listed in Box 3-2.

Most case management organizations have established standards that require case managers to complete the initial clinical assessment within a specified time. The time frame should be realistic enough to allow the case manager to capture as much relevant data as possible because the primary purpose of the assessment is to determine needs and the corresponding resources to meet these needs.

The family assessment is best accomplished in the home (Table 3-1). Case managers who are able to provide on-site assessments have an advantage; they are often able to obtain first-hand knowledge of the home environment and the family members' interaction with each other. Home interviews allow the case manager an opportunity to observe such things as the following:

- Environmental risks and barriers

- The setting in which activities of daily living occur (bathroom, bedroom, kitchen)
- Interactions between all parties

Regardless of where the interview is conducted, family assessments should include the following details:

- Names, addresses, and phone numbers of spouse and identified caregivers (including work phone numbers)
- Family health problems and limitations
- Perceptions of the patient's illness or injury
- Emotional status of family
- Transportation mode and availability
- Potential barriers within the home, if the home is to be the discharge destination
- Identification of the person who will be the primary caregiver
- Identification of patient, family, and caregiver teaching needs in relation to the plan of treatment
- Caregiver's physical, emotional, and mental capabilities and availability
- Cultural, ethnic, and religious beliefs[10]

Planning. Once the assessment is complete, the next step is developing and writing the case management plan. A written case management plan (which may also be called a *map, care map, critical pathway,* or *clinical pathway*) must be developed for every patient. This plan should be updated and changed as the patient's condition shows evidence of progression, regression, or failure to change, or as goals are reached. The frequency of change depends on the changing needs of the patient.[11]

To be effective, the case management plan must be centered on the patient and family and should be developed using an interdisciplinary health care team approach. Patients' rights laws mandate that the patient and family be actively involved throughout the plan of care; this also helps reduce anxieties and alleviate crises. In addition, patient and family involvement encourages positive participation in the plan and contributes to a positive outcome. A case management plan cannot be successfully created without input from all members of the health care team involved in the patient's care. This involvement is fundamental to case management as outlined by the Commission for Case Management Certification.

When developing a plan, the case manager must always be aware that the patient's problems may have been present before the case manager began working with the family and, as such, may never be resolved. The key to the success of the case management plan is to list all pertinent problems, list recommendations for solutions to each problem, and then establish realistic, achievable, specific, and measurable short- and long-term goals. Ideally, the case management plan should be shared among all members of the multidisciplinary treatment team, especially the patient.

Additional factors that must be considered in the final plan include the following:

- Benefits available through the patient's health insurance coverage
- Exclusions or limitations to the patient's health insurance coverage
- Patient and family financial resources and ability to pay out-of-pocket expenses
- Patient and family level of motivation to participate in the plan[10]

In today's managed health care system, costs are important, but costs should not be the most important driving factor for the final plan; quality of care must be.

Documentation. Documentation is required to support the individualized patient care plan. Documentation must be clear, concise, pertinent, and accurate; all actions and resultant reactions should be briefly summarized (Box 3-3). Most case managers develop a format that can be used to summarize the details of the plan.

Obtaining approval. The case management plan needs to meet the approval of all participants to be effective. The patient, physician, health care providers, and payer must be working together toward common patient-centered goals to ensure a positive outcome. Open communication and dialog is vital to developing and implementing an effective individualized case management plan. Before sharing patient information, the case manager needs to secure the patient's approval in the form of a signed consent for treatment. Lack of approval from the patient, physician, provider, or payer necessitates the revision of the case management plan. The case manager cannot serve the provider, payer, and/or employer first and the patient last; the interests of the patient must always come first.[8]

Implementation. The case management plan is implemented by coordinating and achieving timely transfer of the patient to the most appropriate, cost-effective provider or level of care in lieu of more costly care. The Commission for Case Management Certification defines *coordination* as "the process of organizing, securing, integrating, and modifying the re-

---

Box 3-3   Essential Data Elements of the Patient Care Plan

- Patient's name and identification number
- Diagnosis and date of onset of illness or injury
- Date case was opened to case management
- Health care payer or other coverage or alternative funding programs
- Brief overview of patient's medical history and care
- Identified problems, recommendations, and time frames for resolution
- Types of providers and community resources to be used
- Teaching required, identification of the teacher, and completion date
- List of equipment required and sources
- Clear and specific short- and long-term goals that can be objectively measured toward a desired outcome[10]

---

sources necessary to accomplish the goals set forth in the case management plan."[10] *Implementation* is further defined as "the process of executing specific case management activities or interventions that will lead to accomplishing the goals set forth in the case management plan."[10] Case management plans vary from patient to patient, even though the medical treatment plan may be the same; what works for one patient does not always work for another. There is no "recipe" for dealing with any one problem because all individual and family situations differ.

Follow-up. Attention must be paid to each detail of the case management plan. A case manager responsible for recommending services owes it to himself or herself, the patient, and the referral source to ensure that the plan works and that it provides high-quality, cost-effective, and necessary services. Although obtaining approval for monitoring from a client company can be difficult, managing a case without appropriate follow-up can lead to liability exposure.

The follow-up process varies from case to case. It may include on-site visits for patients requiring multiple services or complex coordination, or it can be as simple as periodic phone call monitoring for patients with single-service needs.

Continued follow-up and reports are especially important because they help maintain the case manager's link to the patient and support the case manager's role throughout the process. During this stage, barriers to achieving the goals outlined in the plan of care can be identified.[8]

Evaluation. In addition to monitoring the medical treatment plan and its effectiveness, the case manager must evaluate and reevaluate the case management plan throughout the course of the intervention. The questions in Box 3-4 can serve as a guide for evaluating a plan.

Because modern research provides an abundance of breaking technologic advances, therapies, and medications, the case manager may be dealing with cases that fall outside the limits of his or her expertise. When this occurs, the case manager has the responsibility to become knowledgeable about the unfamiliar disease entity and treatment options.

When things start to look questionable or when results are uncertain, it is important to seek the advice of the treating physician or to acknowledge a need for more information. It is

---

Box 3-4   Questions Used to Evaluate a Patient Care Plan

- Is the treatment plan sound?
- Is the treatment plan promoting the desired outcome?
- Does it appear that the treatment plan will lead to eventual recovery or resolution of the problem, or have there already been too many complications?
- Does the plan need to be modified or changed to achieve the desired outcome?
- Are the patient and family compliant with the care plan?
- Is the treatment plan appropriate and reasonable for the patient?
- Does the treatment plan impose any undue hardship or discomfort on the patient?
- Is the desired outcome realistic for this patient?

---

also the case manager's responsibility to comment on treatments (provide feedback) that, based on his or her experience, may seem unusual or strange. In doing so, tone is vital; constructive feedback and offering alternative suggestions works best.

The patient's interests should always come first. If the case manager notes that a patient is in a poor system of care (e.g., the physician is not communicating, the patient is having multiple complications, or the therapist is unapproachable), part of the case manager's role is to serve as patient advocate. If the patient's needs are not being met, the case manager has a moral and ethical responsibility to help create a better system of care. Patients often do not have the information they need to see their position or options clearly to make informed decisions. They are often not even aware of what constitutes appropriate care. They might not know that they are entitled to a second opinion or that they do not have to stay in a hospital where their care may be less than adequate. The case manager must be careful when presenting treatment options not to recommend a single provider.

Case managers must always remember their role in the managed health care system: they are there to empower patients, to promote patient involvement in their own treatment and destiny, and to help the very young and very old achieve the highest level of independence they can. Often, the more catastrophic and irreversible the situation, the more strategic the case management plan must be. Sometimes, the best thing a case manager can do is directly ask the patient and family what it is they want, what they hope to achieve as a result of this care, and if they could change the patient's care in any way, how they would do it. By examining the patient's and family's thoughts and feelings, the case manager can often help them cope with a difficult or catastrophic situation.[8]

Role and interfacing with other members of the health care team

Advocacy. The case manager is an advocate for the patient and family at both the service-delivery level and the policy-making level. As such, the case manager has an ethical responsibility to the patient to ensure high-quality care. The nurse case manager must serve as a patient advocate, helping the patient move along the continuum of care through the organizational red tape that is so often part of a large organization. The nurse case manager can facilitate this process by doing the following:

- Establishing a working relationship with the patient, family, physician, provider, and payer
- Fostering independence in decision making along with growth and development within the patient and family
- Educating and supporting the patient and family toward self-care
- Educating and facilitating patient and family access to necessary health and human services
- Advocating for patients with long-term care needs at local, state, and federal levels:
  - Participation in professional organizations
  - Self-education on new laws and policies that effect patient care and case management practice
  - Active participation in changing policies or laws that adversely affect health care delivery and reimbursement[12]

Communication. The most critical management skill for the case manager is the ability to communicate. Communicating clearly, directly, honestly, and positively with all participants in the case management plan cannot be emphasized enough. The frequency of communication with various members of the health care team, patient, and family depends on case variables (Fig. 3-3). The patient and family should be kept informed every step of the way.

To achieve an atmosphere of receptivity and cooperation between team members, information and ideas must be communicated and shared. Letters, memos, and reports have their place, but the ideal method of communication is speech, either in person or via telephone. By talking with each other, information and ideas can be exchanged as needed to clarify details and develop an appropriate plan.

Timing is everything when planning to communicate with the patient or family about even basic information. Matching the timing with the emotional readiness of a patient or family is important to their understanding of the information. Patients and families vary in their resistance and ability to grasp reality.

Some patients and families are unable to communicate their wants, needs, or feelings. When this is the case, it is essential that the case manager build trust and take on the role of patient advocate until the patient and/or family is able to do so. It is vitally important in this situation that the case manager have continual communication with the patient and family and encourage their questions, input, and presence in the process. When the case manager assumes the role of advocate, he or she must not lose sight of the fact that the patient (or sometimes the family) is the final decision maker and that nothing can be implemented until approval has been granted.[8,10]

Problem solving. Problem solving is another important skill required to be an effective case manager. The case manager needs a variety of skills to cope with unexpected situations. To effectively deal with problems that arise during the course of treatment, the case manager must have access to current information on which to base decisions. In addition, the case manager must have a strong educational and clinical experience background. The case manager often serves as the eyes and ears for other members of the health care team. Maintaining open

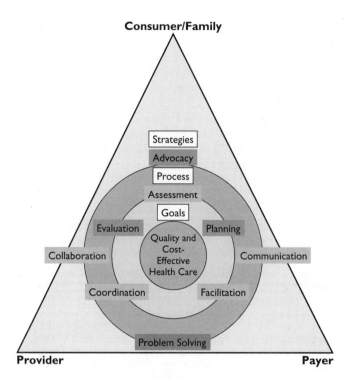

FIG. 3-3 *Health care participants.* (From McCollum PL, Sager D: Case management. In Hoeman SP, editor: *Rehabilitation nursing: process and application*, ed 2, St Louis, 1996, Mosby.)

Table 3-2	**Benefits of Case Management**

- Increased patient/family satisfaction
- Increased physician satisfaction
- Decreased length of treatment as plan of treatment remains on track
- Improved collegial relationships among interdisciplinary care team members
- Improved communication/collaboration among health care providers
- Improved continuity of care throughout duration of treatment
- Increased focus on quality
- Fosters appropriate use of health care resources
- Increased practitioner accountability
- Improved patient outcomes
- Increased cost-effectiveness
- Improved coordination of care
- Empowers patient/family to take charge of their health care destiny

communication with all members of the treatment team can often avert problems that may develop during care.

Collaboration. The case manager's role requires collaborative, proactive, and patient-focused relationships that facilitate and maximize patient health care outcomes. Collaborative practice enhances communication, which supports improvement and continuity of care and increases problem solving abilities as issues arise throughout the case management process.

Case management skills that support a collaborative effort include the following:

- Cooperating with interdisciplinary team members before and throughout the plan of treatment
- Placing the patient and family outcomes as primary
- Demonstrating communication and leadership with health care team members to facilitate maximal patient outcomes
- Demonstrating creativity, care, balance, and commitment to the people served
- Being knowledgeable and educated regarding the roles and capabilities of various professionals and conducting research to determine the type and quality of those resources[12]

Using a collaborative approach to patient care increases the health care team's responsiveness to the patient. The benefits of this approach include improved patient satisfaction and improved quality of care (Table 3-2).

Empowerment. A primary focus of case management is to empower patients, giving them and their families access to a greater knowledge of their disability or disease, a larger voice in the delivery of their care, and more personalized attention to their particular needs. Empowerment is derived in part from awareness. Hence, the case manager, as patient advocate, must respect patients' rights to understand their situation, disability, disease, or injury. Obtaining data on the particulars of each patient's case, case managers enable patients and their families to make informed decisions. Through their role as advocate, case managers can help the patient navigate the complexities of the health care system.[8]

TYPES OF CASE MANAGEMENT
Clinical case management

Clinical case managers are employed in hospitals, rehabilitation facilities, home health care agencies, and infusion companies, to name but a few. Most clinical case managers have been trained as nurses or social workers. They may oversee treatment while a patient is in a particular facility or receiving a certain type of service, such as clinic-based infusion therapy, but generally they are not involved with the patient's care once the patient moves to the home setting. Depending on the employer, a case manager may never make a home visit or manage care outside a facility. This type of case management is most often event based or episodic in nature because the clinical case manager usually does not follow a patient throughout the continuum of care.[8]

Insurance case management

Payers employ insurance case managers, who work for employer groups through third-party administrators, self-administered programs, HMOs, or major insurance carriers. In these settings, case managers identify and track all hospital admissions and other events for which there is a likelihood of costly or high-risk conditions. Although employers' emphasis may seem to be on reducing overall costs, these case managers are also dedicated to helping employees and their dependents use available and beneficial services. Sophisticated computer tracking systems provide the insurance case manager with a more complete historical perspective regarding potential interventions that might result in better outcomes.[8] In some managed care companies, there is a designated IV nurse case manager who follows patients with diagnoses requiring long-term or complex infusion therapy (e.g., those with Crohn's disease, hyperemesis gravidarum, osteomyelitis, or cancer).

Independent case management

Although all forms of case management are valuable, clinical and insurance case management are significantly different from independent case management. Independent case managers are not affiliated with insurance companies or providers of service. They fall outside the medical care provider and claims payer systems. They have the opportunity to make totally objective assessments while coordinating a program of care. Because they do not have a vested interest in a particular company or provider group, independent case managers can remain impartial advocates for their patients.

Independent case management has emerged in response to the needs and growth of the older population. Concern over health service costs, increase in the types of services commercially available, the entrepreneurial spirit of health care professionals, and a realization that health care professionals cannot meet all the care coordination needs of older people—all of these factors have encouraged the growth of independent case management.

Independent nurse case managers help patients with needs that are not served by public programs. The benefits of having this type of case manager include a long-term relationship with the patient and family and the ready availability of care 24 hours per day, 7 days a week.[9]

Clinical expertise in infusion services is a valuable skill that allows the infusion nurse to help the patient deal with the complexities of today's managed health care environment. Hence, we can anticipate the number of independent case managers to increase in the future as infusion therapies become increasingly complex and costly.

Demand management

Demand management programs are designed to reduce the requirement for health care services by ensuring that necessary services are provided at the appropriate level of care. Demand management services typically include around-the-clock telephone access to registered nurses, who provide immediate feedback using computer-based algorithms when responding to inquiries. Patients also have access to on-line medical information and a list of health care providers and facilities within a managed health care organization. This service is designed to provide information and education to patients and answer their health care questions.[2]

The goal of a demand management program is to reduce the need for and use of costly or clinically unnecessary medical services and arbitrary managed care interventions, while enhancing the overall health status of an entire population. Changes to effect the demand side of the health care equation require that wellness, health, and prevention information be shared with managed health care members so that they can learn how to reduce particular risk factors, adopt more healthful lifestyles, and make appropriate decisions regarding their health care needs.

There are four basic services by which a demand management program shares information.
1. Decision support by telephone
2. Self-care resources
3. Group and individualized educational programs
4. Traditional health promotion programs (e.g., programs focused on nutrition or dieting, and parenting classes)[1]

Demand management and case management programs are offered in different situations to different patients; blending the two together increases the effectiveness of case management. Making case management services available to outpatients with complex needs and significant risk factors can potentially avert the need for hospitalization. It is important to recognize that patients may increase their use of some outpatient or home care services. However, the overall cost, quality, and satisfaction outcomes should improve over time in response to this educational approach.[13]

Disease management

Disease management programs were developed in the 1990s as a proactive approach to managing disease. A disease management program provides guidelines and interventions that include both patient and provider education. This approach can best be defined as the integration of services across the continuum of care to treat a given disease with the goal of improved outcome and reduced cost. Utilization data used to determine patient outcome include risk profiling (scoring on risk assessment tools) and encounter data (including hospitalization, PCP and provider contacts, and claims review). Diseases conducive to this type of approach include asthma, congestive heart failure, and diabetes.[2]

A disease management program requires extensive research to define and measure good outcomes and the treatment protocols that will most likely lead to them. Measurements that must be tracked include the following:
- Utilization outcomes for all members enrolled in the disease management program
- Patient satisfaction and perceptions of general health and well-being
- Specific clinical outcomes for each program

Research, analysis of data, and planning are integral to the development of a disease management program. The following six steps should be considered:
1. Identify key processes for patient care according to severity.
2. Examine the current system of care from the patient's perspective and modify it to be more user friendly.
3. Use research to define appropriate systems of care.
4. Compare the current process to that which is identified by research as more appropriate.
5. Modify or create new systems of care as needed.
6. Establish an oversight committee to monitor success and facilitate continuous improvements.

The role of the IV nurse case manager in a disease management program is similar to that in traditional case management.

Box 3-5   Three Classifications under Population Case Management

Well: patients with no chronic illness

At risk: patients with primary or independent risk factors for chronic illness

Unstable: patients with chronic illness that has progressed to the point of significant interference with functional abilities

---

The involvement begins with screening patients to assess their ability to benefit from this type of program, coordinating care, monitoring care across the continuum of the health care delivery system, and assisting with critical pathway compliance.[14]

Population management

The focus of population case management (PCM) is to affect the movement of individuals along the continuum from the *well* condition to the *medically unstable* condition. The traditional focus of IV nursing has been on treating an illness or disease to promote a return to the well condition. In the PCM model, the focus shifts to keeping the patient as healthy as possible for as long as possible and to prevent exacerbation of disease.

The movement from well to unstable is inevitable in all persons, but with proper attention to current medical trends, the time spent on the wellness side of the health care continuum can be prolonged. The biggest drawback with this type of approach is cost, in both money and resources.

The three classifications of people who exist under the PCM umbrella are listed in Box 3-5.

The components of a PCM model include population identification, a health profile, condition-specific modules, medical logic, and an intervention plan.

Population identification. Population identification requires a system for tracking patient movement in and out of a given health care system. Methods commonly used are claims analysis, member contact, health screening tools, enrollment calls, and physician or self-referral.

Health profile. A health profile is a record of common health-related data relevant to all persons in a given population. Examples of data collected include medications, allergies, surgeries, family history, preventive care activities, and functional scales.

Condition-specific modules. Condition-specific modules ask questions that measure and track condition-specific information such as symptoms, condition control, and health practices. This information supplements a patient's health profile and allows condition-specific tracking of utilization and outcome data.

Medical logic. *Medical logic* refers to a collection of medical algorithms that process health profile and condition-specific information in a manner consistent with established medical practice.

Intervention plan. An intervention plan flows from the outcome of a medical logic calculation. The intervention plan is the "to do" list for the population case manager. Common interventions include medical reevaluation, education, preven-

---

Box 3-6   Tasks to Be Accomplished by a Worker's Compensation Case Manager

- Obtain a history of past education, employment, hobbies, and job skills and identify vocational interests and future goals.
- Oversee psychosocial testing, work evaluations, schooling, transportation, on-the-job situations, and anything else needed to help the patient become or remain gainfully employed.
- Help the patient use the recuperative period constructively to study, upgrade skills, prepare for job interviews, and so on.
- Visit the patient's place of employment and speak with the personnel director or immediate supervisor about the employer's expectations and the patient's needs.
- Complete a job analysis and discuss the possibility of the patient's return to work in the same job, perhaps after job modifications or lightening of duties.
- Share this information with the physician at the appropriate time.[8]

---

tive care reminders, specialty consults, and referral to specialized case management programs.[15]

These five components of a PCM model are designed to be tracked by an automated system, are physician and nurse driven, and can be conducted within a scalable infrastructure.

Workers' compensation/vocational case management

Workers' compensation is a state-mandated insurance program that provides benefits for health care costs and lost wages to qualified employees and their dependents if an employee suffers a work-related injury or disease; in turn, the employee cannot normally sue the employer unless true negligence exists. Workers' compensation has undergone dramatic increases in cost as group health has shifted into managed care, resulting in workers compensation carriers adopting managed care approaches. Workers' compensation is often heavily regulated under state laws that are significantly different from those used for group health insurance and can be subject to intense negotiation between management and organized labor.[6]

The case manager's focus in workers' compensation case management is on the patient's vocational rehabilitation, with return to employment as the primary goal. To achieve this goal, the case manager must accomplish the tasks listed in Box 3-6.

MEASURING THE EFFECTIVENESS AND BENEFITS OF CASE MANAGEMENT

Outcome assessment

Outcome assessment permits the case manager to assess the performance of a plan of care over time and to identify variations within the plan of care. An outcome assessment can provide a quantitative comparison among treatment programs, map the typical course of a chronic disease across a continuum, or identify variations in the outcome of care as potential markers of process variation. The following are representative of outcome assessment:

- Outcome measurements are "point-in-time" observations.
- Outcome monitoring includes the process of repeated measurements over time, which permits causal inferences to be drawn about the observed outcome.
- Outcome management is the application of the information and knowledge gained through outcome assessment to achieve optimal outcomes through improved decision making and care delivery.[16]

Case managers are challenged with providing quality outcomes for their referral sources. The IV nurse case manager receives referrals from many sources—acute care hospitals, outpatient infusion centers, skilled nursing facilities, home care and hospice agencies, physician offices, and insurance companies.

Effecting quality outcomes has a very direct impact on health care costs, an impact that often cannot be seen by calculating cost savings on individual cases. Outcomes have an impact on the costs of the *aggregate* of cases. The following outcome statistics are important for a case manager when making a provider referral.

- Length of stay
- Ability to live independently
- Number of rehospitalizations
- Morbidity
- Ability to return to work

Several data collection tools have been developed for collecting objective clinical data. Uniform Data System for Medical Rehabilitation's Functional Independence Measure (FIM) emerged from the rehabilitation field, Outcome Assessment Systems Information Set (OASIS) emerged from the home health care field, and Minimum Data Set (MDS) was developed to facilitate outcome measurement in the skilled nursing facility level of care.[17]

The case manager must exercise caution when evaluating a provider's outcome data. Providers that specialize in patients with chronic or comorbid disease processes often have less positive outcome data. It is important to compare like programs using similar data collection tools and similar reporting methods.[14]

Goals are met when optimal treatment or service is rendered by the most appropriate providers within a predetermined period at a reasonable cost (Table 3-3).

Table 3-3 The Case Management Report Card	
QUESTIONS ASKED FOR EVERY PATIENT	**CHECK IF YES**
Was the right care delivered?	
By the right clinician and mix of staff?	
At the right time?	
In the right setting?	
With the right resources?	
With the right intensity of service?	
With the right outcome, both clinically and financially?	

FUTURE DIRECTIONS FOR CASE MANAGEMENT

Case management continues to evolve as a beneficial model of health care delivery. As health care reform continues to bring about change, the fundamental characteristics of case management will remain the same.

There are two major trends in health care driving the redesign of case management. The first is a trend toward disease prevention and wellness; the second trend is increased use of advanced practice nurses in health care delivery settings.

The trend toward wellness and disease management is very strong. The World Health Organization has promoted a move toward a wellness-based system for many years. Managed care was conceived in the wellness delivery model. Recognizing the financial impact of time lost from work, employers are spending more money and expending more effort to keep employees and their families healthy. Wellness programs such as weight reduction, smoking cessation, regular exercise, nutrition, and stress management classes are a few examples of the types of programs employers are implementing. This growing trend toward wellness will soon reshape case management models. Protocols will be developed to manage the care of populations throughout the life span, with a focus on maintaining wellness and healthy lifestyles. Nurse case managers must be prepared to take the lead in facilitating this transition.

Utilization of advanced practice nurses is expected to escalate over the next few years. Studies have shown that advanced practice nurses provide high-quality and cost-effective care. Thus, as health care reform continues to unfold, we will witness advanced practice nurses taking on major roles in our health care system. They will become more intensely involved in case management methodologies, and many will assume advanced case management roles.[8]

The White House Paper prepared by the National Coalition of Associations for the Advancement of Case Management and presented to the Clinton Administration's National Health Care Task Force perhaps best attests to the unlimited potential of case management in the years to come:

> Clearly, these federal health objectives require coordination of all health services, knowledge of the full continuum of services available to assist people in moving efficiently through the health system, and the ability to facilitate full community integration regardless of health status. Case management is a logical process for addressing these needs.
>
> Health care reform and the changing population of health system users will create new challenges. Proactive use of case management can anticipate needs, design solutions and facilitate changes that will benefit the efficacy and cost-effectiveness of the health system. The need for case management services will increase in the future.[18]

REFERENCES

1. Coleman JR: Integrated case management: the 21st century challenge for HMO case managers: Part 1, *Case Manager* 10(5):28, 1999.
2. American Association of Managed Care Nurses: *Managed care nursing practice standards*, Glen Allen, Va, 1998, AAMCN.
3. Fox PD: An overview of managed care. In Kongstvedt PR, editor: *Essentials of managed health care*, ed 2, Gaithersburg, Md, 1997, Aspen.

4. May CA, Shraeder C, Britt T: *Managed care and case management: roles for professional nursing,* Washington, DC, 1996, American Nurses Publishing.

5. Wagner ER: Types of managed care organizations. In Kongstvedt PR, editor: *Essentials of managed health care,* ed 2, Gaithersburg, Md, 1997, Aspen.

6. Academy for Healthcare Management: *Managed healthcare: an introduction,* Washington, DC, 1997, AHM.

7. Kuklieris A, Mayer G, Day T: Case management: a new market focus for tertiary medical centers, *Case Manager* 10(6):45, 1999.

8. Mullahy CM: *The case managers handbook,* ed 2, Gaithersburg, Md, 1998, Aspen.

9. Gerber LS: Case management models: geriatric nursing prototypes for growth, *J Gerontol Nurs* 20(7):18, 1994.

10. Rossi P: *Case management in health care: a practical guide,* Philadelphia, 1999, WB Saunders.

11. Spooner SH, Yockey PS: Assessing clinical path effectiveness: a model for evaluation, *Nurs Case Manage* 1(4):188, 1996.

12. Case Management Society of America: *Standards of practice for case management,* Little Rock, Ark, 1995, CMSA.

13. Geary CR, Smeltzer CH: Case management: past, present, future—the drivers for change. In Fantle LA, editor: *Case managers desk reference,* 1999 ed, Gaithersburg, Md, 1999, Aspen.

14. Siefker JM et al: *Fundamentals of case management: guidelines for practicing case managers,* St Louis, 1998, Mosby.

15. Howe RS: Population case management emerging as significant approach to case management: a brave new world for case managers. In Fantle LA, editor: *Case managers desk reference,* 1999 ed, Gaithersburg, Md, 1999, Aspen.

16. Siren PB, Laffel GL: Quality management in managed care. In Kongstvedt PR, editor: *The essentials of managed health care,* ed 2, Gaithersburg, Md, 1997, Aspen.

17. Mateo MH, Newton C: Managing variances in case management, *Nursing Case Management* 1(1):45, 1996.

18. McCollum PL, Sager D: Case management. In Hoeman SP, editor: *Rehabilitation nursing: process and application,* ed 2, St Louis, 1996, Mosby.

Quality Management

Grace P. Sierchio, MSN, CRNI*

Quality management is the commitment to achieving excellence in health care. It is not a singular activity, but a ceaseless effort that seeks to improve outcomes by improving the processes involved in the delivery of patient care.[1] By means of ongoing monitoring, opportunities for improvement are identified, strategies for change are formulated, planned actions are implemented, and the results of those actions are assessed. The approaches to quality management may vary, but the underlying goal is always the provision of effective and efficient patient care services that results in positive outcomes.[2]

Quality management in intravenous (IV) nursing seeks to ensure that the desired outcomes of IV therapy are achieved. Realistic objectives for IV therapy include preventing complications, reducing morbidity from IV-related complications, promoting patient comfort, and providing effective patient education. To achieve these goals, the IV nurse must understand and apply the basic principles of quality management. This chapter emphasizes quality management as it relates to IV nursing.

Throughout this chapter, there are numerous references to the Joint Commission on Accreditation of Healthcare Organiza-

*The author and editors wish to acknowledge the contributions made by Donna R. Baldwin, as author of this chapter in the first edition of *Intravenous Nursing: Clinical Principles and Practice.*

tions (JCAHO). JCAHO was established as a voluntary, nongovernmental accrediting body for hospitals, but it has since expanded accreditation to all health care organizations. Quality management requirements have always been part of JCAHO's accreditation process, but introduction of the *Agenda for Change* in 1986 shifted the focus from problem-solving endeavors to continuous improvement of quality.[3] Because this shift is consistent with proven quality management techniques, JCAHO standards are a benchmark for quality in health care. The Joint Commission's most recent publication of standards in the latter part of 1998 introduced the term *performance improvement.* Performance improvement (PI) shifts the focus away from measuring quality (which can be at times vague and indiscrete), to measuring an organization's elements of performance (which can be easier to define, dissect, and measure).

DEFINING QUALITY

There is an ever-greater emphasis on quality health care, but the concept is difficult to define. *Quality* has been broadly described as the comprehensive positive outcome to a product.[4] In health care, however, the product is multifaceted, which contributes to different perceptions of quality. A precise definition of quality health care acknowledges these differences and includes the care *and* services delivered and their perceived value to the consumer (Fig. 4-1).

Quality of care

Quality of care has been defined as "the appropriate technical application of medical science to diagnose, treat, and cure disease."[5] This is the simplest description of quality because it concentrates on the technical aspects of patient care. Care is a product or process that can be observed, measured, tested, and controlled through statistical methodologies. For this reason, it is understandable that the National Association of Quality Assurance Professionals originally described *quality* as the levels of excellence produced and documented in the process of delivering patient care.[6]

The quality of IV nursing care relates to the technical aspects of care. IV nursing requires the performance of procedures based on established standards. Compliance with procedure is relatively easy to observe, measure, and evaluate. An example is venipuncture, which requires appropriate selection of an insertion site and cannula, suitable preparation of the intended insertion site, correct insertion of the cannula, proper securing of the device, and accurate documentation of the procedure. If any steps of the procedure are omitted or inappropriate, quality IV nursing care has not been delivered.

One problem with an emphasis on the quality of care is the tendency to overlook outcomes. If, in the previous example, performance of the procedure was absolutely correct but the venipuncture was unsuccessful, the outcome was not achieved and quality care was not delivered. Therefore quality of care requires that the technical interventions be appropriate *and* that the intended results be achieved.

Quality of service

Quality care is the major product delivered in health care, but *service* is the subjective aspect that influences the consumer's perception of quality.[5] The nursing procedure may be technically correct, but the patient judges the care according to how the service was delivered. In the case of IV nursing, explaining the venipuncture procedure before it is performed, considering the patient's preferences in selecting the IV site, and timely restarting the infusion after infiltration all influence the patient's perceptions of the quality of care.

JCAHO refers to this as *patient perception of care.* Measuring patients' perceptions of the care they receive is an important component in the performance improvement program of any health care organization.

From the patient's perspective, patient education is a major factor in providing quality service. Although patients often cannot give a definition of quality, most can instinctively perceive whether they have received quality services. Sources often describe the relationship between the quantity and quality of patient education and the perception of care received. The more quality education provided, the higher the patient rates the overall quality of care. For example, consider a patient with an IV infusion that becomes infiltrated. If the nurse has not instructed the patient about the signs and symptoms of infiltration, the patient may presume that there is something wrong with the way the cannula was inserted and that the infiltration is the result of poor-quality service. In contrast, if the possibility of infiltration had been discussed with the patient when the cannula was inserted, the patient could promptly alert the nurse if signs of infiltration are noted. A timely restarting of the infusion then contributes to the patient's perception that quality service has been provided.

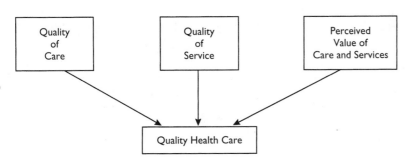

FIG. 4-1 *Scope of quality in health care.*

Perceived value

Quality is also influenced by the *perceived value* of the care to the consumer. Consumers are now more conscious of the value of the care they receive, and they expect the highest caliber care in relation to the cost. This is the basis of managed care, which attempts to create the perception of acceptable value in return for the cost of health care.[7]

Perceived value is sometimes a challenge in IV nursing. A nurse may routinely rotate the IV site on a pediatric patient (quality service) following the established procedure (quality care), but the child's parents may not perceive the value of this practice. In their eyes, the child is being subjected to an unnecessary painful experience. As with quality of service, the nurse must educate the parents about the value of routine site rotation and problems that may occur if this practice is eliminated.

Quality health care

The quest for a universal definition of quality health care continues, but the most accepted description has been offered by the JCAHO. According to JCAHO, *quality of care* is "the degree to which patient care services increase the probability of desired outcomes and are consistent with current professional knowledge."[8] This definition represents the emphasis on outcomes that was introduced with JCAHO's *Agenda for Change,* and it encompasses all aspects of quality.

LEADERS IN QUALITY MANAGEMENT

Three names often mentioned in discussions of quality are Juran, Crosby, and Deming. These leaders defined, refined, and popularized the concept of quality in the business world, but their teachings serve as the groundwork for the quality initiative in health care.

J. M. Juran

Dr. Juran was among the first to recognize that product quality requires careful planning, control, and improvement. He conceptualized these basic managerial processes as the *Juran trilogy.* Although his teachings were initially applied to Japanese business, Juran's principles of quality planning, quality control, and quality improvement have since been used in American industry.[9]

Quality planning. Quality does not occur by accident; it is the result of meticulous preparation. The major aspects of planning are determining customer needs and developing products that meet those needs. The primary emphasis is on external customers, who are the end users of the product, but consideration must also be given to the internal customers, who assist in product development.

Quality control. The process of quality control requires that product performance be evaluated and compared with product goals and that differences between performance and goals be resolved. To achieve quality control, all employees must be accountable and make use of the feedback loop.

Quality improvement. Quality improvement requires organized change to attain unprecedented levels of performance. It represents a transition from little *q* (narrow scope of quality limited to clients and products) to big *Q* (broad concept of quality that defines *customer*s as those who are affected and *products* as all goods and services). In addition, it exchanges the reactionary practices of "putting out fires" and "ready, fire, aim" for a proactive, systematic process that concentrates on improving all aspects of business. One of the best known methods for achieving quality improvement is by means of quality councils, also known as *quality circles.*

Philip B. Crosby

Crosby is a management consultant who worked his way up through the ranks of business. He introduced the philosophy of "do it right the first time," which conveys his belief that quality is free; it is the nonquality products that cost money because they require rework. To explain the concept, Crosby used the phrase *zero defects.* This expression emphasizes that compliance with defined standards and specifications is necessary to achieve quality; poor quality is the result of lack of compliance and nonconformance. However, it was also Crosby's contention that conformance requirements must be based on input from the workers who produce the product.[10]

Most quality experts in health care agree that the concept of zero defect is not applicable to most aspects of the health care industry. Providing health care services is, by its nature, very different from manufacturing a product. Although the latter can be controlled by specifications and procedures to the degree that a 100% perfection rate can be attained, the unpredictability of human physiology, psychology, and circumstances make this an impossible challenge in health care, including IV nursing.

W. Edwards Deming

Dr. Deming, the "guru" of quality, is best known for helping the Japanese achieve world-class quality in product manufacturing, but many American industries have since adopted his teachings. Like Crosby, Deming's philosophy of quality is based on the premise that problems with quality reside predominantly in an organization's systems and processes, not in its employees.[11] Deming's strategy stresses continuous quality improvement and is based on the 14-point system for managing quality (Box 4-1).[12]

APPROACHES TO QUALITY MANAGEMENT

With the increasing emphasis on quality in health care, organizations have initiated programs to control, ensure, assess, improve, and manage quality. The focus of each program is quality, but the inherent strategies to promote quality care services are considerably different. As a result, the terms *quality control, quality assurance, quality assessment, continuous quality improvement,* and *total quality management* are not synonymous and represent a paradigm shift in the approach to quality management.

It was once assumed that health care was of high quality, so the primary objective was to ensure that the level of care was maintained. When it was determined that the assumption of quality was inaccurate, health care began to adopt components of the industrial models of quality management. During the transition, quality programs in health care progressed from quality control to continuous quality improvement, and we are now embarking on an era of total quality management.[13]

Quality control

Quality control (QC) is the evaluation of the production of quality goods, the provision of services, or the outcome of services by means of statistical methodologies. It was originally used for the inspection of manufacturing equipment and has been referred to as *statistical quality control*. The approach consists of retrospective inspection that compares a random sample of products with a predetermined, acceptable level of defects. Primary components of QC include data collection and statistical analysis of data.[14]

The major disadvantages of QC are its emphasis on statistical methods and the retrospective nature of the process. Data analysis should serve as the basis for decision making, but in quality control, there is a tendency for the statistical tools to become an end in themselves. Results are monitored and reported after goods or services have been produced, without emphasis on improving outcomes. Hence, this tool-oriented approach is being replaced by problem-oriented and results-oriented techniques.[9]

An example of QC in IV nursing is the monitoring of phlebitis rates. Some organizations place great emphasis on collecting and analyzing data regarding the occurrence of phlebitis. However, once it is determined that the incidence of phlebitis is within the accepted range of 5% or less, no action is taken to further reduce the phlebitis rate.

Quality assurance

Quality assurance (QA) may be defined as the determination of the degree of excellence through monitoring and evaluation to detect and resolve problems.[13] It is the most widely known of the approaches to quality because QA requirements have been included in the JCAHO standards since the 1950s. JCAHO accreditation is a voluntary process, but most states have now enacted mandatory QA requirements for licensure of health care facilities. In fact, in many states, the department responsible for licensure of health care facilities is titled the Quality Assurance Division.

In addition, most third-party payers require service providers to have an active and effective QA program. This requirement, partly to minimize risk and to meet standards of the National Committee on Quality Assurance, have greatly increased the participation of health care providers in QA activities.

Over the years, the QA activities required by JCAHO have evolved from performance of chart audits to problem-focused studies to ongoing monitoring and evaluation of patient care services. In 1986, JCAHO developed the *Agenda for Change,* which initiated the transition from QA to continuous quality improvement. The goal was to create outcome monitoring and evaluation processes to help organizations improve the quality

---

Box 4-1   Deming's 14-Point System for Managing Quality

1. *Create consistency of purpose for product improvement.* The vision of the organization must be directed at continual refinement of the product. For an organization to become and remain competitive, there must be a strategy for achieving continuous improvement.
2. *Adopt the new philosophy.* Mistakes and negativism cannot be tolerated. Instead, the philosophy of the organization must be dedicated to improving quality.
3. *Cease dependence on inspection.* Quality is the result of improved production processes, not the identification of defective products. Prevention reduces the need for inspection to produce a quality product.
4. *Avoid awarding business on price alone.* If the concentration is on quarterly dividends alone, quality and productivity suffer.
5. *Constantly improve.* Quality improvement is a continual process, not a one-time activity. Improvement is the result of a never-ending pursuit to reduce waste and improve systems.
6. *Institute training.* Workers must be properly trained to perform effectively and efficiently. The organization must invest in training; failure to do so may be detrimental to survival of the organization.
7. *Institute leadership.* Management and leadership are different. Managers tell the worker what to do; leaders create a vision and guide the workers in achieving progressively improved outcomes.
8. *Drive out fear.* Fear inhibits innovation. If workers are fearful of expressing their ideas or asking questions, the job may continue to be done ineffectively or incorrectly.
9. *Break down barriers between staff areas.* Competition and rivalry between departments stem from conflicting goals. A unity in mission and promotion of teamwork within and among departments help identify opportunities for improvement.
10. *Eliminate slogans, extortions, and targets for workforce.* Quality is not a management-defined slogan and is not achieved by coercing workers to achieve optimal results. Workers must be involved in identifying methods to improve quality and determining how these expectations are communicated to others.
11. *Eliminate numerical quotas.* Quotas are counterproductive because they concentrate on numbers instead of processes that can be improved.
12. *Remove barriers to pride of workmanship.* Workers need to be empowered to have pride in the quality of their work. To accomplish this, the organization must eliminate barriers, such as defective materials, that hinder the quality of the product.
13. *Institute vigorous program of education.* Quality improvement activities require that both managers and workers be educated about statistical techniques and team-building exercises.
14. *Take action to achieve transformation.* All workers must be involved in the change from quality control to quality improvement. The change must be led by a dedicated team of those in top management who have established a precise plan of action to improve quality.

"14-Point System," from *Deming Management at Work* by Mary Walton, © 1990 by Mary Walton. Used by permission G.P Putnam's Sons, a division of Penguin Putnam, Inc.

Table 4-1   Quality Assurance versus Quality Improvement

QUALITY ASSURANCE	QUALITY IMPROVEMENT
Problem-oriented	Results-oriented
Focuses on inspection	Focuses on prevention
Uses data to evaluate performance	Information trended to identify opportunities for improvement
Focuses on negative aspects of care	Focuses on positive aspects of care
Monitors nursing tasks	Monitors patient outcomes
Retrospective	Concurrent
Evaluates documentation	Evaluates care and services
Random monitoring	Planned, systematic monitoring
May be unrelated to standards	Based on standards
Fixed process	Dynamic process
Concentrates on compliance	Customer-driven
Reactionary	Proactive
Responsibility of QA coordinator/designee	Organizationwide commitment

of care provided.[15] Consistent with this change, JCAHO renamed their quality assurance standards *Quality Assessment and Improvement.*[16,17]

JCAHO explained that the underlying rationale for the shift to assessing and improving quality was to overcome several weaknesses inherent in QA practices. First, QA is often focused solely on the clinical aspects of care rather than on the interrelated managerial, governance, support, and clinical processes that affect patient care outcomes. Second, QA is typically discipline specific or service specific instead of concentrating on the interdisciplinary or cross-service nature of patient care. Third, QA is often individual- or problem-oriented instead of examining the processes and systems involved in the delivery of patient care. Each of these tendencies inhibits the organization's ability to improve processes and thus improve patient care outcomes.[16,17] Table 4-1 highlights the differences between QA and quality improvement.

The term *quality assurance* may still be used, but it does not appropriately convey the intent of the current quality management programs. Quality cannot be ensured; it can only be assessed, managed, or improved. Even the president of JCAHO, Dennis O'Leary, has admitted that, in retrospect, QA was an "unfortunate semantic selection" because it does not accurately reflect JCAHO's vision of quality.[18]

The clinical record reviews performed by some home health agencies are examples of QA. Such reviews consist of a retrospective chart audit that evaluates a random sample of documentation. The data collection tool is typically a checklist on which the presence or absence of the required elements of documentation is noted. The form is appropriate if the objective is to monitor documentation. However, it is of little value in the evaluation of care.

Additional disadvantages of this example of QA are the fact that it concentrates on the negative, it may be punitive, and it does not have an impact on patient care outcomes.[19] The clinical record review focuses on the absence of documentation and the

identification of those responsible for the omissions. The collected data may then be used to address the deficiencies with the responsible individuals and evaluate their performance. Such practices promote the punitive nature of QA. If, on the other hand, the documentation is excellent, there is a perception that the individuals "passed the QA audit." In reality, the documentation, not the care, has been evaluated, and the data are insufficient to induce improvements in patient care.

Quality assessment

Quality assessment consists of monitoring, data collection, and data analysis to determine the quality of the care and services provided. Because assessment is not directed at changing or improving outcomes, this activity is typically coupled with quality improvement. Quality improvement is the component necessary to initiate corrective actions or seize opportunities to improve the effectiveness and efficacy of services.[13]

Using the initials *QA* for both quality assurance and quality assessment may be confusing. Quality assessment is an element of quality assurance; it is the measurement component. More often, quality assessment is combined with quality improvement to denote activities that both assess and improve the quality of patient care. To reduce the confusion with acronyms, it is the consensus that *QA* stands for quality assurance, whereas quality assessment is typically linked with quality improvement and designated *QA/QI.* Some organizations have further eliminated the confusion by substituting the term *continuous quality improvement* for QA/QI.

As nurses, we understand assessment; it is a basic component of the nursing process. Assessment requires observation and measurement of a problem or condition, and in quality assessment, we observe and measure the quality of nursing care. An example of quality assessment in IV nursing is the monitoring of phlebitis rates. Quality assessment is similar to quality control, but the merging of QA/QI ensures that assessment is not the only activity performed. QA/QI is a comprehensive process that identifies opportunities for improvement, initiates corrective actions, and evaluates the effectiveness of the corrective actions.[14] For example, if during the QA/QI process it was determined that the incidence of phlebitis was 3%, methods to further reduce the phlebitis rate would be identified and implemented and a follow-up evaluation would determine whether a reduction was achieved.

Continuous quality improvement

Continuous quality improvement (CQI) is an approach to quality management that builds on traditional QA methods. An effective QA program provides a sound foundation for ongoing quality review in the transition to CQI. However, CQI broadens the focus from only the clinical aspects of care to all the facets of the organization that affect patient outcomes.[14] Inherent in this transition is a change in management philosophy and organizational culture, because there must be a visible commitment to CQI for the process to be effective. Current JCAHO standards emphasize that managers and leaders in the organization contribute to the CQI process by establishing expectations, providing necessary resources, and fostering communication and coordination of activities.[16,17]

The scope of CQI is more extensive than the activities of quality assessment and improvement. CQI considers processes by determining how well they are performed, coordinated, and integrated and by developing strategies for further improvement; it recognizes both internal customers (all employees) and external customers (patients, physicians, third-party payers) and values their perceptions of the care and services delivered; and it promotes the pursuit of objective data to evaluate and improve patient outcomes.[20] An essential characteristic of CQI is that it is a continuous process. Quality is not achieved and then discarded; quality is the result of long-term commitment to the ongoing evaluation and improvement of patient outcomes. CQI is based on the assumption that outcomes are never optimized but may be constantly improved.[21] This concept is best expressed by Dennis O'Leary's philosophy, "Even if it ain't broke, it can still be improved."[22]

Assuming that care can be continually improved, CQI may be applied to IV nursing. As with all aspects of clinical care, numerous procedures are performed simply because "we always do it that way." CQI encourages creativity in practice; however, nurses must be cognizant of the inherent risks in altering practice unless the innovations are based on valid research. Research is the foundation of IV nursing practice and has precipitated significant changes to improve patient outcomes. An example is the routine rotation of peripheral IV catheters based on research findings demonstrating an increased incidence of phlebitis when peripheral catheters made of Teflon are left in place more than 48 to 72 hours. There is now controversy regarding the time frame for rotating peripheral catheters made of other polymers. In the quest to improve quality, valid research is needed to address this issue.

A distinctive feature of CQI is that it emphasizes improvement in the interdisciplinary processes involved in patient care delivery, not just individual activities. Applying this concept to IV nursing requires that all factors contributing to the quality of care be examined. An example is the administration of IV medication. Steps involved in this process in the hospital setting include prescription of the medication by the physician, transcription of the order on the nursing unit, preparation and delivery of the medication by the pharmacy, and administration of the scheduled dose(s) by the nurse. Coordination of these various steps affects the quality of the desired outcome, which is efficient and effective administration of IV medication. Therefore, with CQI, monitoring IV medication administration entails all functions contributing to the actual nursing procedure.

Performance improvement

JCAHO continues to influence how organizations design and implement quality management programs. As a result, terminology and theoretical models recommended by JCAHO have significant impact, much like the proverbial ripples on a pond's surface.

With the publication of their hospital and home care standards for 1999 and 2000, JCAHO introduced the term *performance improvement*. Its standards on quality referred to the "assessment and improvement of organizational *performance*" rather than on the assessment and improvement of *quality*.

Changing the focus to specific elements of an organization's performance may make it easier for quality management teams. Rather than trying to define and measure *quality*, which can be subjective at times, the team can define and measure specific aspects of its performance. Examples of performance measures used in IV therapy (hospital or home care) include incidence of peripherally inserted central catheter (PICC) phlebitis per 1000 catheter days, proportion of patients satisfied with their venipuncture experience, or the incidence of adverse drug reaction per 1000 drug doses administered.

Other than shifting the conceptual framework toward evaluating *performance* versus *quality*, the elements of monitoring, assessment, and improvement remained relatively unchanged from CQI. In addition, like CQI, performance improvement is leadership driven; crosses all key functional areas of an organization, including clinical, managerial, and support; and recognizes both internal and external customers.

Total quality management

With the shift from QA to CQI and now PI, health care organizations have recognized that quality is not a fixed commodity defined by health care professionals but is a strategic mission that must be shared by the entire organization. As a result, several health care organizations have adopted a management system that fosters continuous improvement at all levels and for all functions by focusing on maximizing customer satisfaction. This system is aptly named *total quality management* (TQM).

Because TQM and CQI are based on the teachings of the quality gurus Deming, Crosby, and Juran, the two approaches to quality management share several characteristics. First, both programs are customer focused. The goal is to meet the expectations of internal and external customers. Second, continuous process improvement is stressed. A culture conducive to ongoing quality improvement is the critical link between customer requirements and outcomes. Last, and most important, there must be total organizational involvement. Those in top management must be committed to the program and provide a clear vision for the organization; employees must be empowered to participate actively in the quality improvement process.[23]

Unlike CQI, TQM is not unique to health care. It has been successfully implemented as a strategic resource management system in various sectors of the service industry. Application of the system to health care has been prompted by the current regulated, cost-competitive environment of the health care industry. No longer can health care providers deliver merely *acceptable* care and services. Health care affects patients' lives, so any outcome that is less than optimal may have serious ramifications. Box 4-2 illustrates the effects of reducing quality by just $\frac{1}{10}$ of 1%.

There are several distinctive characteristics of TQM. First, TQM contributes to a positive work environment by emphasizing horizontal cross-functional coordination and vertical integration. The clinical, managerial, and support staffs within the organization function as an interconnected network linked

---

Box 4-2   Examples of Less Than 100% Quality

If you settle for 99.9% quality, you get:
- 1 hour per month of unsafe drinking water
- 16,000 pieces of mail lost per hour
- 20,000 wrong prescriptions per year
- 500 incorrect surgical operations per week
- 50 newborns dropped by physicians per day
- 22,000 checks deducted from the wrong account per hour
- Two unsafe landings per day at O'Hare International Airport
- 3200 missed heartbeats per person per year

---

laterally, over time, in a collaborative culture. This is in contrast to the typical functional hierarchy in which the organization is a loose collection of separate individuals or departments. Second, TQM fosters collaboration by recognizing the underlying psychosocial principles affecting individuals and groups within the organization. There is a natural tendency for individuals to make judgments based on biases, but through careful and continual training, TQM overcomes these biases and creates an environment of trust. Third, TQM promotes teamwork as a means to break down barriers to communication and enhance interdepartmental collaboration. Active involvement and cooperation within the organization creates a common bond among team members by encouraging them to reach consensus on goals and collaborate on solutions.[24]

To realize total quality as a strategic management vision, the costs of quality versus the cost of not supporting quality must be acknowledged. The cost of not supporting quality has been depicted as an iceberg. Above the surface are the visible costs (e.g., patient complaints, repeat work, loss of revenue because of customer dissatisfaction); the less obvious but larger costs (e.g., excessive employee turnover, lack of teamwork) are hidden below the surface. Applying the principles of TQM helps uncover and eliminate these hidden costs. The visible costs of quality (e.g., quality management team expenses) may then be deemed as either necessary or avoidable so that unnecessary expenditures are reduced.[25]

TQM is also effective because it strengthens the customer-supplier chain. All employees are customers *and* suppliers, linked in a chain that runs through the organization to the ultimate, external customer. Alignment and execution determine the strength of the chain. *Alignment* is defined as "doing the right thing," whereas *execution* is "doing the thing right." When both alignment and execution are achieved throughout the chain, "right things are done right."[26]

As an integrated internal management system, TQM focuses on organizational improvement. The system is broader than the clinical aspects of IV nursing, but an organizational culture fostered by TQM facilitates improvements necessary to deliver quality IV nursing care.

Other quality acronyms

The programs implemented in the management of quality have been described as an alphabet soup—there are QC, QA, QA/QI, CQI, PI, and TQM. Still other acronyms describe lesser-known

quality management programs. These include QRM (quality resource management), QAA (quality assessment and assurance), TQC (total quality care), QAI (quality assessment and improvement), and IQM (integrated quality management). The terminology differs, but the goal of all these programs is continuous improvement of processes, products, and services. Perhaps confusion could be avoided if health care organizations followed Crosby's suggestion to use the term *quality management.*[27]

MEASURES OF QUALITY

Effective quality management is based on well-defined measures of quality. The measures are the criteria by which the levels of excellence are established and are a basis for quality improvement. However, establishing measures of quality in health care is a complex process. The delivery of patient care services does not result in a tangible product; the service is consumed as it is delivered. Traditional technical quality-of-conformance measures are therefore ineffective unless they are combined with behavioral norms that describe how the service is to be provided and criteria that outline the intended results of care.[23]

Measures of quality that integrate the technical features, behavioral aspects, and desired outcomes of health care are known as *standards.* Standards represent the agreed-on levels of excellence. They do not necessarily depict the optimal level of achievement but refer to the levels of achievement that are acceptable based on the realistic availability of resources and the current state of knowledge. Discrepancies between optimal and acceptable levels of performance are catalysts for continual improvement. As a result, standards are dynamic and reflect progressively higher levels of acceptable achievement in the continual refinement of quality patient care.[13]

Standards have several distinguishing characteristics. First, they are predetermined. Levels of acceptable achievement are established before the delivery of care, not after the care is rendered. Second, standards are written. Accountability to standards requires written communication of the defined rules, actions, and conditions. Third, standards must be approved by an authority. Unless there is proper sanctioning by an entity empowered to enforce the standard and to which the individual is accountable, the standard may be ignored. Fourth, standards must be accepted by those individuals affected by the standards. Standards serve no purpose unless they represent an acceptable level of achievement. Fifth, for standards to be used as assessment tools they must be measurable and achievable. Because of these characteristics, a *standard* is defined as an accepted written statement of predetermined rules, actions, and conditions that are measurable and achievable and that have been sanctioned by an authority.[19] (Additional information regarding standards is available in Chapter 5.)

Types of standards

Standards determine whether the delivery of health care services is properly established, implemented, and evaluated. *Properly established* means that the structure of the organization is sufficient to support the acceptable levels of achievement; *properly implemented* signifies that the process by which the services are delivered reflects the established norm; and *properly evaluated* indicates that emphasis is placed on the outcomes of service.[28] Hence, standards may be divided according to the structures, processes, or outcomes that affect patient care.[29]

Structure standards. *Structure standards* refer to the conditions and mechanisms that provide support for the actual provision of care. They are the framework that facilitates patient care by defining the rules of the organization and its governance. Examples of structure standards are the mission, philosophy, and goals of the organization, which serve as a foundation for the commitment to quality.

Policies are a critical component of structure. They are the established rules that guide the organization in the delivery of patient care. A unique characteristic of policies is that they are not negotiable. This means that under no circumstances may a policy be modified.[19] If an organization's policy specifies that only registered nurses are permitted to administer IV medications, a licensed practical nurse may not perform the procedure.

Process standards. *Process standards* have been described as "working" standards because they describe the functions performed by health care providers in the delivery of patient care. Structure standards specify what may be done, but process standards describe how it is done. As such, process standards focus on the practitioner and include job descriptions, performance standards, procedures, practice guidelines, and protocols.

A *job description* is a written record of the job qualifications, scope of responsibilities, and principal duties. It is a generic instrument that describes the basic functions of the position.[30]

Performance standards evolve from the job description and define the level of performance required for the job.[28] For example, the job description for an IV nurse may state that a basic function is the performance of venipuncture, but the performance criteria specify that the IV nurse must adhere to aseptic technique, follow established policies and procedures, and demonstrate proficiency in the insertion of peripheral IV catheters.

Procedures involve psychomotor skills performed by health care providers in the delivery of patient care. Written procedures contain a series of precise steps that outline the recommended manner in which the skills should be performed.[30] Some organizations also have practice guidelines, which are based on the nursing process and further delineate care delivery.

Protocols complement procedures and practice guidelines because they provide a basis for clinical decision making in specific patient care issues.[30] For example, the IV nurse follows the written procedure and practice guidelines for the performance of venipuncture but complies with an established protocol for the use of a local anesthetic at the intended venipuncture site.

Although structure standards are not negotiable, process standards may be modified based on the decision of the practitioner and as the situation demands.[19] For example, the written procedure specifies that the intended insertion site is to be prepared with povidone-iodine solution before venipuncture, but the patient is allergic to iodine. In such a situation, alcohol may be substituted to prepare the intended venipuncture site.

Outcome standards. *Outcome standards* concentrate on the end results of patient care. They are patient focused and reflect the desired goals of the care provided.[13] However, outcome standards are usually expressed in negative terms such as *mortality rates, infection rates, phlebitis rates,* and *medication errors.* To describe the desired outcomes accurately, positive criteria are preferable. Statements such as *patient satisfaction, resolution of infection, control of pain,* and *maintenance of desired nutritional status* better communicate the ultimate goal of patient care.

Because the outcome of care is typically a consequence of how the care was delivered, outcome standards are linked to process standards. For every process standard, there is an associated outcome; the process influences or determines the results to be achieved. For example, preparation of the insertion site, stabilization of the catheter, and rotation of peripheral catheters all influence the outcome of IV nursing care.

Standards and organizational key functions

The delivery of patient care services encompasses three domains: clinical, professional, and administrative. There is a patient who receives the service (clinical domain), the nurse who delivers the service (professional domain), and organizational leaders who manage the service (administrative domain). These three domains parallel the types of standards (outcome, process, and structure). However, terminology that more appropriately describes the measures of quality in health care are *standards of care, standards of practice,* and *standards of governance.*[19]

Standards of care. The recipient of care, the patient, is the focus of the standards of care. The patient expects a predetermined level of care from the health care provider, and standards of care describe these expectations and imply the expected outcomes. To measure quality based on expectations, JCAHO has indicated that standards of care must be developed within the organization. The standards either may be generic, addressing patient care throughout the organization, or may be specific to the care delivered in or by a specialty area.[31] For example, a generic standard of care might state, "patients can expect to acquire no infections resulting from nursing care"; a specific standard of care, relative to IV nursing, further stipulates that "patients can expect to receive IV therapy without complications of infection."

Standards of practice. Standards of practice focus on the provider of care and represent acceptable levels of practice in patient care delivery. Like the standards of care, practice standards address the clinical aspects of patient care services and imply patient outcomes. However, standards of nursing practice define nursing accountability and provide a framework for evaluating professional competency in the delivery of patient care services. They are consistent with valid research findings, national norms, and legal guidelines, and they complement expectations of regulatory agencies. In Table 4-2, fundamental aspects of IV therapy are written as both standards of care and standards of practice.

Based on the premise that nurses, individually and collectively, are responsible and accountable for their practice, professional nursing associations have researched, developed, and

Table 4-2   **Examples of Standards of Care and Standards of Practice Regarding Fundamental Aspects of IV Therapy**

Aspect of Care	Standard of Care	Standard of Practice
Plan of care	Patient has health care needs identified.	Nursing care plan is established within 24 hours of completion of initial patient assessment.
Initiation of infusion	Patient has infusion initiated for therapeutic or diagnostic purpose.	Therapy is initiated on physician's order using the nursing process.
Cannula site preparation	Patient is free of infection related to IV therapy.	Peripheral insertion site is aseptically cleansed with antimicrobial solution before cannula insertion.
Monitoring infusion	Patient receives infusions at prescribed flow rate.	Patient assessments are performed at routine intervals and as required during the infusion.
Disposal of sharps	Patient is safe from preventable hazards in the environment.	Needles and stylets are disposed of in nonpermeable tamper-proof containers.
Patient education	Patients have the right to receive information on all aspects of their care.	Patients are informed of each treatment in clear, concise terminology.

published standards of nursing practice. These standardized methods reflect commitment to quality patient care and include generic *and* specialty standards of practice.[32] Generic standards, such as the *Standards of Nursing Practice* from the American Nurses Association, are universal for all types of nursing; specialty standards are applicable to a specific area of practice, such as the *Infusion Nursing Standards of Practice* by the Intravenous Nurses Society.[33]

Because published standards of nursing practice define criteria relative to nursing accountability and professional competency, they may be adopted by health care organizations. This differs from standards of care, which must be developed and individualized by the organization in which the care is delivered.[13] For example, *Infusion Nursing Standards of Practice* defines the autonomy, accountability, and requirements of the specialty practice of IV nursing and are applicable to all practice settings where IV therapy is delivered.[33] Box 4-3 is an example of the standard of practice for handwashing as presented in the 2000 revision of *Infusion Nursing Standards of Practice.*[33]

Box 4-3   Standard Practice of Handwashing

STANDARD
Handwashing shall be performed before and immediately after all clinical procedures and before applying and after removal of gloves.
PRACTICE CRITERIA
- Handwashing should be a routine practice established in organizational policy and procedures.
- Bar soap should not be used because it is a potential source of bacteria; however, liquid soap and water are adequate for handwashing.
- Dispensers of liquid soap/antiseptic solutions are recommended with the caveat that the containers are routinely inspected for bacterial contamination; these containers should be discarded and replaced according to organizational policy and procedures.
- Single-use soap scrub packets or waterless antibacterial products should be used when running water is compromised or unavailable.

Modified from Intravenous Nurses Society: Infusion nursing standards of practice, *JIN* (suppl) 23(6S), 2000.

Standards of governance. JCAHO is placing greater emphasis on the role of the health care organization's leaders in providing the necessary support and resources to improve patient care. Such expectations and responsibilities of managerial and other key leaders can be established by means of standards of governance. Standards of governance define the administrative domain and establish parameters to measure the levels of excellence in leadership.[19] An example of a standard of governance is the statement, "Organizational leaders will provide an environment that fosters the highest quality of patient care and employee satisfaction."

METHODS OF MEASURING PERFORMANCE

In the past, literature written about the QA model described the use of *indicators* as statements of performance that are measured and monitored to see whether the organization met predetermined goals. The term *indicator* is used less often today, and instead performance improvement teams refer to *performance measures.* Measures are numerical (statistical) representations of one aspect of care or an outcome of care that has been evaluated.[34]

No performance improvement can occur without the ability to measure current performance. How can a hospital's managers know improvement is necessary if they can't measure performance? In addition, most areas of performance should be monitored over time, looking at the trends and patterns inherent in the performance.

Today's accreditation standards demand the use of more complex statistical methods than in the past. Leaders and performance improvement teams in hospitals and home care need to become familiar with the terminology and methods of performance measurement and statistical process control that have been used for decades in other industries. Staff and IV team nurses should help monitor performance trends and patterns as part of their unit or team's PI activities.[35] To this end, the remaining chapter sections provide an overview of some of the important principles of using performance measures and the statistical methods used to display and analyze those measures.

Types of performance measures

There are two different ways of looking at how measures are categorized. One is by placing measures into categories based on what aspect (domain) of patient service is being evaluated, and the other is to look at what *statistical* type of measure it is.

Performance measures by domains of care.
There are at least three types of "aspect of care" or "domain" categories: structure measures, process measures, and outcome measures. The previous section in this chapter provided detailed definitions of the terms *structure, process,* and *outcome,* which will not be repeated here.

A *structure measure* is a quantitative tool to measure an aspect of the organization's infrastructure that can impact patient care. An example is the percentage of infusion pumps audited that met rate reliability criteria when tested by technicians between patient use. Assuming that you consider equipment as part of the organization's structures, this would be a structure measurement.

A *process measure* is a quantitative tool to measure an aspect of actual patient services that can impact patient outcome. An example is the percentage of PICCs inserted within 12 hours of the physician's request for the insertion.

An *outcome measure* is a quantitative tool to measure the outcome of the patient's treatment. An example is the incidence of extravasation in patients receiving chemotherapy per 1000 chemotherapy treatment days.

Of the three measures, JCAHO recommends the use of outcome measures as the most accurate measurement of the organization's overall performance. One important difference to note is that outcome measures tend to cross departmental lines. In other words, patients who have positive outcomes generally do so because all departments worked effectively and in unison for the welfare of the patient. Patients with poor outcomes may have had complications as a result of the actions of one or of several departments. Because of this universal nature of outcome measures, they lend themselves to the principles of TQM, which requires performance improvement to be viewed as an organizationwide process, and not as a process isolated to an individual department or unit.[34]

There are two other measures that are sometimes used to evaluate an organization's performance but are not strictly clinical in nature. These are patient perception measures and utilization or financial measures.

The appropriateness of using patient perception measures has been debated by health care experts for some time. Should an organization use the opinions and customer satisfaction ratings provided by patients as a measurement of its quality? An organization could provide patient care according to all best practice standards and the patient might still not be satisfied. Conversely, a patient may have received substandard care and, not knowing this, provide high marks on his or her questionnaire. In addition, the sampling of the responses may be affected by the opinions of the patient. It may be human nature to complete a survey questionnaire more completely if you have had a negative experience and wish to report it, versus having had an acceptable or positive experience.

Nursing has endorsed the use of a satisfaction measure if it is composed of four different functional perspectives. These include health status, knowledge function, skill function, and psychosocial function. When a satisfaction survey includes each of these elements, it offers a comprehensive evaluation of how the care was delivered (processes) and the patient's perceptions of the results (outcomes).[36] JCAHO recommends that the organization use either clinical performance measures or patient perception measures to meet accreditation requirements.

Organizations may also choose to measure and monitor utilization and financial performance. Every well-run organization should be able to report its financial performance and act on negative or positive trends to increase financial efficiency and profitability. However, measures of this kind are not related to the quality of care provided to patients and are therefore not customarily accepted by licensing agencies, accrediting bodies, or payers as part of a clinical QA program. An example of a financial measure is billing days outstanding, also called *DSO,* which is the number of days between the billing of services and the receipt of payment from a third-party payer.

Performance measures by statistical type.
Another way to categorize performance measures is by how they are expressed numerically.

Continuous variable measures.
A continuous variable measure (sometimes called a *measure of central tendency*) is a measure that is expressed as a number along a continuous scale. The value is a single discrete number that rises and falls at each measurement.[37,38]

A hospital-based example of a measure of central tendency or continuous variable would be the average wait time between the ordering of a PICC placement by a physician and the time of PICC placement. This month an evaluation of all patients who had PICCs ordered and placed may indicate an average wait time of 6.3 hours. This value might rise and fall each month as staffing, volume, or other variables affect the system. An example for home care might be the time elapsed between an initial referral and the delivery of home medical equipment.

Rate-based proportion measures.
Rate-based measures are measures that compare the total number of times something occurred to the total number of times that it could have occurred. This type of measure has a numerator and denominator and is often expressed as a percentage. Note that the numerator is a subset of the denominator.

A home care–based example of a rate-based proportion measure is the percentage of patients who received home pain management infusion therapy who expressed satisfaction with their pain relief. In this outcome/patient-perception measurement, the PI team assesses the total number of high satisfaction ratings for pain management returned on surveys, compared with the total number of patients who received pain management. Assuming that all questionnaires are returned, this would give an accurate measurement of the success of the pain management program.

Rate-based ratio measures. A rate-based ratio measure compares the number of times something occurred with an unrelated phenomenon. This type of measure also has a numerator and a denominator, but the numerator is not a subset of the denominator as in the previous type. (Therefore this measure is never expressed as a percentage.) Rather, the denominator is usually a common denominator used for comparison purposes and benchmarking.[37,38]

An example of a rate-based ratio measure often used by hospitals and home care organizations is the number of cases of catheter infections (numerator) per 1000 catheter care days (denominator). Another common example is the number of adverse drug reactions per 1000 drug therapy days, or the number of adverse drug reactions per 1000 drug doses administered.

Selecting appropriate measures

One of the most difficult decisions for an organization is which measures to use as indications of quality and performance. Writers have described a health care "dashboard," or the development of a concise set of performance measures that can be reviewed regularly to give the "driver" (or leadership) of the organization a clear view of its performance. This area of quality management in health care is still evolving. Much needs to be learned about the development and use of measures that not only can assess an organization's performance, but also can be used by similar organizations to compare themselves with each other. These are sometimes referred to as *core* measures.

The best recommendations available from experts are to use measures that do the following:

- Reflect areas of service that are high risk, problem prone, high cost, or high volume
- Directly reflect the outcome or potential outcome of the patient's care
- Address (cross over to) all key functions of an organization: managerial, clinical, and support services
- Cross departmental lines so that the use of the measure becomes an interdisciplinary and interdepartmental process
- By consensus, are meaningful and useful for the improvement of the organization
- Can be used to benchmark (compare) your performance against another organization's[8,34]

Characteristics of good measures

Because the criteria for acceptable measures can be demanding, performance improvement teams often elicit the help of statisticians or research designers when developing measures.

For a measure to be statistically appropriate and useful, it must possess the following characteristics[34,38]:

- *Reliability* denotes the ability to measure the variable regardless of who is gathering the data, when the data are collected, or from which source the data are obtained.

- *Validity* means that the indicator measures what it is intended to measure. A valid indicator identifies situations in which quality is lacking or confirms circumstances in which quality is present.
- *Measurability* is the ability to translate the important aspects of care into measurable, quantifiable terms to detect the level of quality.
- *Specificity* implies that indicators characterize a specific event. Each indicator must be precise and unique to the event to be measured.
- *Relevancy* requires that the indicator relates to and only to the critical aspect of care being measured.

Sentinel events

Another type of performance measure that should always be monitored is the sentinel event measure. A *sentinel event* is "an unexpected occurrence involving death or serious physical or psychologic injury, or the risk thereof." Serious injury specifically includes loss of life or function. The phrase *risk thereof* includes any process variation for which a recurrence would carry a significant chance of a serious adverse outcome.[39]

Examples of sentinel events used by hospitals are the death of a patient because of a hemolytic blood transfusion reaction, the removal of an incorrect limb or body organ, or a patient suicide.

Sentinel events used by home care agencies and home care pharmacies include the death of a patient related to administration or dispensing of an incorrect drug or incorrect dosage, violence perpetrated on a patient by a home care worker, or permanent organ dysfunction as a result of insufficient or incorrect drug monitoring.

Because of the very serious nature of a sentinel event, any occurrence must instigate a performance improvement project by the QI/PI team. After a sentinel event, the organization's leaders generally assemble a task force comprised of QI/PI, leadership, and risk management staff to investigate and act on the issue. A root cause analysis must be performed and corrective measures taken.[39]

The threshold, or acceptable level, for sentinel events in any organization should always be 0%.

Reporting of a sentinel event is a controversial issue. Experts in risk management have voiced concern over any policy or standard that mandates the reporting of a sentinel event to an outside organization, whether it be a governmental or consulting agency. JCAHO has encouraged the voluntary reporting of these occurrences as part of the accredited organization's performance improvement efforts. However, the reporting is voluntary and not mandated. Each organization must develop its own internal policies on this issue.

Establishing thresholds

Once performance measures are selected and approved, the next difficult decision is what the acceptable level should be for each measure. In some cases the answer is self-evident. As described earlier, the acceptable threshold for sentinel events should always be 0%. In this way, even a single occurrence would raise a quality improvement "flag" and initiate investigation and action.

However, most events are not sentinel in nature. They are "rate-based" events that can and will occur from time to time. The PI team must determine the extent to which rate-based events can occur and still be deemed acceptable.

Establishing this threshold depends on the seriousness of the event, the effect of the event on quality patient care, customer expectations, published research, and baseline data.[13] Each of these factors is considered when determining the realistic level at which all manageable variables may be controlled. For example, if the nationally accepted phlebitis rate is 5% and historical information reveals that the incidence of phlebitis within the organization is between 4.45% and 5.35%, the threshold for evaluation could realistically be set at 5%.

Thresholds for evaluation are not static, but rather change as the quality of care continuously improves.[13] For example, if the threshold (of compliance) over the past year was between 94% and 95%, the threshold may be increased to 95%. This is a positive approach to establishing thresholds for evaluation because it represents a realistic determination of levels of compliance and demonstrates the ability to improve outcomes over time.

In addition to comparing a performance measurement with a predetermined threshold, there are other recommended statistical methods to detect positive or negative changes in the organization's processes. These are discussed further in the section on display and analysis of data.

Determining sample size

Standard research methodologies should be used when designing performance measures for performance improvement. One of the most important considerations is the sampling technique, sampling frequency, and sample size to be used. The technique selected should ensure the accuracy and reliability of the data. The sample size should be sufficient so that conclusions can be drawn from the data.

Possible sampling techniques include probability and non-probability methods. Probability methods are the most scientific because they involve random selection of the sample. By using numerical tables, each case has an equal chance of selection for the review process. Nonprobability sampling reflects qualitative judgment and does not ensure selection based on chance. Convenience and quota sampling are examples of nonprobability methods.[40]

Sample size is a controversial issue. Because the sample size must be representative of the total population under examination, application of the research process is the most accurate means to determine an appropriate sample size. However, some authors have offered general guidelines for sampling. They have suggested a sample size of 5%, or 20 cases (whichever is greater), for routine review; 10%, or 40 cases (whichever is greater) if the threshold for monitoring has been triggered; and 15%, or 60 cases (whichever is greater), for intensive review.[19] Because of the seriousness of sentinel events, a 100% review is always required.

Collecting data

Data collection may involve either retrospective or concurrent review. Retrospective review entails collecting data after the care has been provided. In the past, such data collections were known as *chart audits* because they focused on the documentation of care after the patient was discharged. Retrospective reviews are the easiest to perform but are the least effective in changing practice. In contrast, concurrent reviews are done while patients are still hospitalized or on service. Interviews and observations are examples of concurrent review, and the timeliness of such activities is instrumental in improving the quality of the care delivered.

METHODS OF DISPLAYING AND ANALYZING DATA

To get the most benefit from the data collected, the QI/PI team should monitor data over time. Monitoring data over time allows the team to detect trends and patterns that can lead to problem identification and resolution.

The methods of displaying and analyzing data reviewed in this section have been used extensively in other industries for decades. The health care industry is now evolving to a level of sophistication where statistical techniques are used to detect variations in the system, prioritize problems and possible solutions, and evaluate the effects of changes. The IV nurse, whether direct caregiver or manager, is now expected to be familiar with basic statistical models so that he or she can participate in performance improvement cycles. Nurses and other quality team members should no longer rely on "gut feelings" or informal observations of problems to design improvement projects. Projects and improvements should be based on sound statistical design, collection, and analysis. JCAHO has several standards specifically related to the appropriateness of the data aggregation, display, and analysis used by an organization.

Run chart

A run chart displays a numerical value over a period of time. The number on the chart might represent anything from the incidence of PICC infections, the wait time for special meal orders from the hospital food service, or the adverse drug reaction rate on a pediatric unit.

Most persons are familiar with run charts in either their workplace or an outside setting because they offer an easy, at-a-glance view of a trend. Many people use run charts to monitor stock prices, average daily temperatures, and so on. Fig. 4-2 depicts a run chart of medication variances.

Run charts are useful in that the viewer can easily see if the trend is upward, downward, or static. Unfortunately, run charts have limited value outside of this. Some experts believe that run charts can be analyzed for statistically significant patterns. However, most PI practitioners use them only to demonstrate the most basic and obvious of trends.

Most experts in statistical process control agree that to best detect variations in a system (and to determine whether the

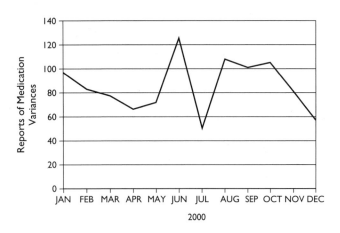

FIG. 4-2 *Run chart of medication variances for 1992.*

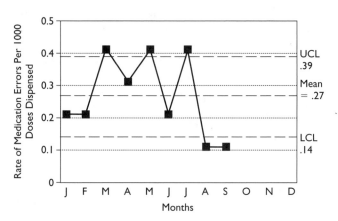

FIG. 4-3 *Control chart of rate of medication dispensing errors per 1000 doses dispensed.* (From Joint Commission, Oakbrook Terrace, Ill: Joint Commission on Accreditation of Healthcare Organizations.)

variation is statistically significant), the run chart's more complex relative, the control chart, should be used.

Control chart

The control chart is one of the most valuable, versatile, and informative tools that health care providers can use to detect variations in the system. These variations might be positive or negative (improvements or problem areas).[35,37] Fig. 4-3 shows an example of a control chart.

At first glance, a control chart appears similar to a run chart. A numerical value is plotted on the chart over time, and the movement of this value can be easily observed for upward or downward movement. Upon closer inspection, however, the user will note two *thresholds,* usually indicated as colored lines or dotted lines. One of these thresholds, referred to as the *upper control limit* (UCL), is found somewhere above the average (mean) numerical value on the chart. The other, the lower control limit (LCL), is found below the mean numerical value on the chart.

Researchers and performance improvement experts use the UCL, LCL, and mean to tell them when the organization's process has gone "out of control," referring here to statistical control. The UCL and LCL values are *not* arbitrarily set by the QI/PI team. Unlike thresholds of performance measures discussed earlier, these values are not determined by literature review or benchmarking. They are set statistically by the values on the chart. The values of the UCL and LCL are determined by using the mathematical formula for standard deviation (sometimes referred to as *sigma*). Most PI teams set the UCL and LCL for a total of two or three standard deviations (or two or three sigma) from the mean or average.

An important point that control charts teach as they are used is that there is always movement upward and downward in a system. Upward movement is not always positive, and down-

ward movement is not always negative. This constant fluctuation is a result of the normal variations in a system, such as hospital staffing, changes in equipment, and so forth. It is referred to as *common cause variation* and should not concern the PI team. However, control charts can show us when significant fluctuations are out of the ordinary. These changes, referred to as *special cause variations,* may be cause for concern if they negatively affect patient welfare.

There are many ways that a control chart can tell you if the process is statistically out of control (if special cause variation exists). The most obvious is if one of the observed values falls above the UCL or below the LCL. (There are many other trends and patterns that PI teams look for on control charts that are beyond the scope of this text. Readers interested in learning how to use control charts for performance improvement are encouraged to read references on statistical process control.)

Pareto chart

The Pareto chart is considered by many experts in performance improvement to be the most useful type of bar graph.[35,37] It is named for its creator, Vilfred Pareto, who is also credited with development of the Pareto Principle, commonly known as the *80/20 rule.* Supporters of the Pareto Principle believe that, in most cases, 80% of the root cause of a problem are attributed to 20% of the factors.

When data are displayed on a Pareto chart, they are always ranked in sequence from the most common result or cause to the least common. Therefore the bar on the extreme left will always be the largest, and each bar will gradually decrease in size. Therefore users of Pareto charts will focus their attention on the one or two bars immediately to the left of the y axis. Fig. 4-4 is an example of a Pareto chart.

The Pareto chart is used to help the PI team prioritize. The chart helps distinguish between the one or few possible causes of

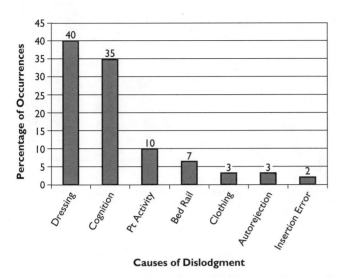

FIG. 4-4 *Pareto chart of causes of midline dislodgment.*

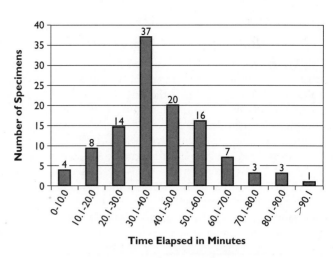

FIG. 4-5 *Histogram of time elapsed for stat laboratory results.*

a problem that have the most impact and cost, from the many other possible causes that have little significance.

For example, the PI committee of an area hospital needed to begin an improvement cycle. A control chart created from an outcome measure on catheter dislodgment showed that for the last 2 months the rate of catheter dislodgment of midline catheters had been above the upper control limit, signaling that the process was "out of control" and required correction. To determine the most common causes of dislodgment, the team brainstormed, listed eight possible causes, and collected data through survey to determine the distribution of the causes. The Pareto chart in Fig. 4-4 shows the results. The team determined that 75% of the dislodgment occurred for one of two reasons: the dressing technique used did not hold the catheter in place securely, or cognitive impairment of patients caused them to remove the catheter. By using the Pareto Principle, the team was able to concentrate its efforts to these two causes, rather than spending valuable time and resources correcting other causes that had little bearing on the overall picture.

Histogram

The histogram is also a bar graph. Instead of showing prioritization of causes, the histogram shows the distribution of data, or patterns in variation.[35,37]

The histogram in Fig. 4-5 shows the distribution of the following data: time elapsed between delivery of specimen to the laboratory and return phone report of results for stat chemistry values.

On viewing the histogram, we see that the majority of laboratory results were returned between 30 and 40 minutes from the time of specimen delivery, with a normal distribution both above and below this time frame.

If the laboratory director wished to improve this elapsed time and implement corrective (improvement) actions, he or she could repeat the same survey 2 months later and look at the distribution of the results. Has the distribution changed by moving toward the lower values of the time interval?

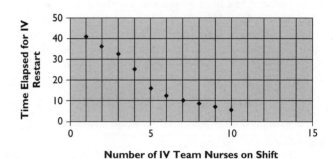

FIG. 4-6 *Scatter diagram of staffing effect on IV team response time.*

Scatter diagram

The scatter diagram is a useful tool that illustrates the relationship (or lack thereof) of two variables.[35,37] On a scatter diagram, each of the two variables is assigned an axis. The point where the two intersect is marked with a dot or other symbol.

By looking at the clustering of these symbols, one can hypothesize whether there is a relationship between the variables. Points clustered in an area going from lower left to upper right indicate a positive correlation. Points clustered in an area going from upper left to lower right indicate a negative correlation. If the points do not cluster at all but are randomly located throughout the grid, it is presumed that there is no correlation at all.

For example, the scatter diagram in Fig. 4-6 shows the possible relationship between the number of IV nurses staffing the hospital at any given time and the time elapsed between a request for an IV start and the actual insertion. We can observe that as the number of nurses increased, the wait time decreased. There is a negative correlation between these two variables, showing the organization leadership that staffing most probably does affect the efficiency of services.

Note that a relationship cannot be absolutely proven by the use of a scatter diagram. However, the probable relationship or lack thereof between two variables can be supported.

METHODS (CYCLES) FOR IMPROVING PERFORMANCE AND QUALITY

The Shewhart cycle (PDSA or PDCA)

The PDSA cycle (also called the *Plan-Do-Study-Act cycle*) is attributed to Walter Shewhart, a quality improvement specialist with Bell Laboratories in the 1920s and 1930s. This cycle model was introduced to Mr. Shewhart's student, W. Edwards Deming, who then described the PDSA cycle in many of his writings and teachings. This cycle, which has also been referred to as the *PDCA cycle* (Plan-Do-Check-Act), is depicted in Fig. 4-7.[34,35,39,41]

The PDSA cycle has been adopted by many organizations in health care and other industries because of its flexibility, logic, and simplicity. It is adaptable to many different situations, making it a powerful and convenient tool. The following description provides an overview of the process.

Plan. The plan phase of the PDSA cycle calls for the development of a plan for implementing and testing the changes that will be made. It is recommended that the number of improvements agreed to during this phase be limited to less than four. In addition to deciding what changes should be made, the QI/PI team must decide how to test the changes. In other words, how will the team know that the change they made in fact led to an improvement? What type of data or observations will need to be collected and recorded to show the team the effect of the changes?

Other questions answered during the planning phase of the cycle include the following:

- What is the team trying to accomplish?
- What staff members will be involved in these changes?
- What resources are available to make the changes?
- What obstacles may prevent the changes?
- What time frames will be in effect for making the changes and collecting the data?

Do. During the do phase of the cycle, the changes are actually made, and the team collects data or makes observations to determine whether the changes created an improvement. Many references refer to this phase as the *pilot test* phase because many teams will make changes on a limited scale and observe the results before making a change on a large scale. For example, a hospital may institute a change in patient admission assessment procedures on a medical unit and test the results. If successful, the changes would then be phased into all medical units. Likewise, a home infusion company might make changes to the type of equipment dispensed by one branch, evaluate the results, and then expand the change to all branches of the company.

Check or study. During the study or check phase of the cycle, the team must objectively review data collected during the previous phase and ask itself, "Did the changes we made improve our process or our outcomes?" The team must assess whether it met its objectives.

A question often asked is, "How do we know how much of a change to expect?" The degree of success must be assessed by comparing the baseline data to the data collected after the changes were made. Did the degree of change meet the team's target? The target must be mutually agreed upon and described

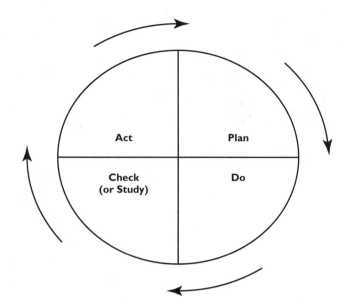

FIG. 4-7   *The PDCA (plan, do, check [or study], act) cycle.*

in the plan phase of the cycle. It may be based on group consensus or national benchmarking data.

Act. During the act phase of the cycle, the team must decide whether to move forward with the changes that were made, incorporating them fully into the organization's structure, policies, procedures, and educational processes. Changes that brought about improvements should be phased into all applicable areas of the organization as part of its standard operating procedures. Those that did not should be either abandoned or redesigned and tested again.

FOCUS-PDSA

The FOCUS-PDSA model is an extension of the PDSA model. The FOCUS subcycle was developed by the Hospital Corporation of America and is used as a prelude to the PDSA cycle to identify elements of performance that would most benefit from improvement.[35] The following explanations provide an overview of the FOCUS process.

Find a process to improve.
Organize a team that knows the process.
Clarify current knowledge of the process.
Understand causes of process variation.
Select the process improvement.

Once the team completes the steps in the FOCUS process, the improvements and staff members identified are used as the basis of the plan phase of the PDSA cycle.

The Joint Commission cycle for improving performance

Recent publications by JCAHO introduced a new cycle methodology for improving performance. Replacing the traditional Ten Step Model was a cyclical model that integrates several theories of performance improvement.[8,35,41] This new model, depicted in Fig. 4-8, differs from its predecessor in that the model is

Improving Organization Performance Function

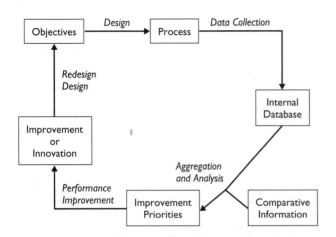

FIG. 4-8 *The Joint Commission cycle for performance improvement.* (From Joint Commission: *1999-2000 comprehensive accreditation manual for home care,* Oakbrook Terrace, Ill, 2000, Joint Commission on Accreditation of Healthcare Organizations.)

cyclical in nature, can be entered at any point in the cycle, and is flexible enough to meet the needs of many types of organizations, from large projects to small.

The four basic components of the Joint Commission's cycle are as follows:

- Design
- Measure
- Assess
- Improve

For the sake of consistency with JCAHO publications, the discussion of this improvement cycle begins with the design phase. Remember, however, that the improvement process can begin at any point in this cycle.

Design. The design phase of the cycle refers to the design of a new process within the organization to meet the needs of the consumer. Infusion-related examples are the creation of an assessment procedure and documentation form for epidural analgesia patients, the creation of a 24-hour help line for postdischarge surgical patients with central catheters, and development of patient education materials for patients going home with parenteral nutrition.

There are many issues that the leadership and staff of an organization should take into account when designing a process, including the following:

- The organization's mission, vision, and goals
- Expectations and needs of the consumers
- Preexisting knowledge about the same type of process at other organizations (which can be obtained from the literature or through peer networking)
- The necessary data, resources, and time to make the process successful
- The cost versus the benefit of creating the process
- The benefit to the consumer resulting from function, process, product, or service

Measure. To determine whether a process is meeting its intended goal of benefiting the consumer, data must be collected

and analyzed. Without data it is impossible to objectively determine whether a process, product, or service is "good enough" as it exists or whether it requires redesign for improvement. In addition, data should be collected after changes are made to assess the degree to which improvement occurred as a result of the changes.

JCAHO recommends that an organization continually collect performance measurement data related to services that have significant impact on the patient or consumer. The guideline of measuring processes that are high risk, high volume, and problem prone applies to this segment of the cycle. Variations or unacceptable levels of performance would then initiate an improvement process.

The results of this phase of the improvement cycle are statistical data. There are many methods of collecting and displaying data for performance improvement. These were discussed earlier in the section on displaying and analyzing data.

Assess. The assessment phase of this cycle involves using the collected data to make judgments to determine whether an opportunity for improvement exists. The data is translated into usable information. The analysis of data can answer the following questions:

- Where can the organization improve? What are its strengths versus weaknesses?
- How can the organization prioritize improvement activities? Certain statistical graphs, such as a Pareto chart, can point out areas that require more immediate attention.
- How can the organization improve? If an opportunity for improvement is found, planning methods (discussed later) such as root cause analysis and brainstorming will find reasons for the organization's weaknesses and strategies for improvement.
- Did the organization improve? Once changes are made, assessment can determine whether the change resulted in improvement.

The result of this phase of the cycle is a list of improvement priorities.

Improve. This is the action phase of the improvement cycle, during which the team actually institutes the changes proposed during the assessment phase. During this phase, the team determines what must be done, who should do it, how it should be done, and how to decide whether the action was successful. JCAHO recommends instituting changes on a limited test basis and measuring their effect before instituting them throughout the entire organization. The result of this phase of the cycle is actual change to the process being improved upon.

TOOLS FOR PLANNING IMPROVEMENTS

Regardless of the conceptual model used to guide the improvement process, the organization can use any one of several tools available for planning improvements. In other words, whether the organization uses the JCAHO cycle for improvement, the PDSA cycle, or FOCUS-PDSA, there will be a certain phase of the cycle where the team must decide what improvements need to be made and how they should be made. When that time comes, the QI/PI team can select from many available tools to

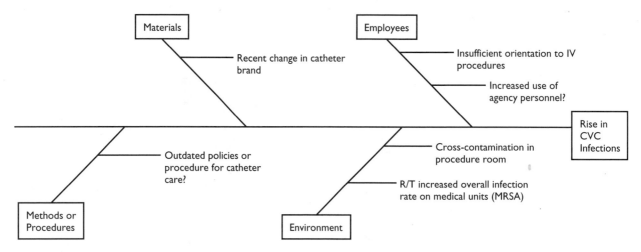

FIG. 4-9   *Cause-and-effect diagram (Ishikawa diagram) of central venous catheter infections. CVC, Central venous catheter; MRSA, methicillin-resistant Staphylococcus aureus; R/T, related to.*

guide the planning process. Some of the most well known and commonly used tools are described next.

The Ishikawa diagram (cause-and-effect diagram)

The Ishikawa diagram, named for its originator Kaoru Ishikawa, is often referred to as the *cause-and-effect diagram,* or the fishbone diagram.[35,42] The cause-and-effect diagram is an excellent tool for documenting why things happen. For example, if a hospital notes an increase in its central venous catheter infection rate, the QI/PI team might draw a cause-and-effect diagram to document the possible reasons why the infection rate has risen. Being able to view the list of reasons on a cause-and-effect diagram can help the QI/PI team decide which reasons merit the most attention and require corrective action.

The Ishikawa diagram is used extensively in what is termed *root cause analysis,* meaning the development of hypotheses of why an event occurred.[35,39,41] The importance of root cause analysis has increased since JCAHO has required every organization to have a method for root cause analysis for any sentinel event.[35,39,41]

An example of a cause-and-effect diagram is found in Fig. 4-9. In the original popularized by W. Edwards Deming, the segments of the "fishbone" were materials, methods, manpower, management, and machines. Users of the diagram assigned and listed potential root causes into one of these five sections. As this diagram became adapted to health care situations, the segments were listed in JCAHO literature as materials, people, equipment, and methods. Some versions of the diagram included a fifth segment titled *environment.* Users can create or delete segments to the fishbone as warranted by the specific setting and information.

When all the potential causes have been listed on the diagram, the team should study the diagram to determine any obvious root causes and causes that can be readily solved. A plan for correcting each cause is then developed.

Brainstorming

Brainstorming is a group process used to develop a list of ideas for improvement in a minimal amount of time. It is often a starting point for teams faced with a problem that needs resolution. Many teams brainstorm regularly but do not recognize it as an accepted tool for improvement and therefore do not document the activity in performance improvement records. However, brainstorming is an effective tool, especially at the beginning of the planning phase of the improvement cycle.[35,43]

Brainstorming should be directed, not haphazard. Usually, the QI/PI team leader directs the group. The leader should define the subject and keep the brainstorming session on track by steering members back to the subject as needed. Team members should be given time to think about the subject at hand, but the time should be limited. The goal of this creative process is to have members contribute ideas without overanalyzing them. Too much analysis of an idea can hamper the creative flow.

The leader should set a short time limit (10 to 20 minutes is adequate) during which the team members contribute ideas to the list. An unstructured approach has members voicing ideas as they come to mind, in no apparent order. The leader must carefully guide this group to encourage participation from everyone while staying on track. In a structured approach, members voice ideas by going around a circle or in some order until all ideas are exhausted.

Many groups write the ideas down as they are contributed onto a wipe board, easel and pad, or overhead projector, or they use computer technology to project the typed ideas onto a screen. No matter which method is used, members can benefit from seeing the submitted ideas (Fig. 4-10). No effort should be made to discuss the ideas, rank them, or analyze them in any way.

Affinity diagrams

Many teams use affinity diagrams after a brainstorming session. Affinity diagrams are used to organize large volumes of ideas or

The performance improvement team and the home care agency's IV team was asked to brainstorm for possible improvements to be made to increase patient satisfaction ratings with the education provided. The following list was generated:

- Spend more time on initial visit.
- Have an in-service for staff on teaching skills.
- Provide a fourth teaching visit instead of the usual three.
- Develop new patient education literature for IV teaching.
- Use videos.
- Use practice models (to practice procedures).
- Call the patient before his or her first independent dosing to review steps.
- Hire an education specialist for teaching only.
- Ask the patient to have a caregiver or family member attend teaching visits.
- Make the pamphlets easier to understand.
- Find out what the patients don't like if they give a bad rating (what are the causes of dissatisfaction).
- Prepare patient before hospital discharge for the fact that they will need to learn skills (minimize fear, frustration).

FIG. 4-10   *Brainstorming session: how to improve patient satisfaction with IV teaching.*

How can we improve our patient satisfaction rating for teaching IV therapy skills to patients?

Staff Development and Resources	*Teaching Aids*	*Teaching Procedures Revised*
Hire education specialist	Revise written teaching materials	Spend more time on initial visit
Staff in-service on teaching skills	Purchase teaching models	Schedule a routine fourth teaching visit
	Use manufacturer videos	Call patient before first independent procedure to review steps
		Ask patient to have a caregiver/family member present at all teaching visits to reinforce teaching and help
		Explain learning expectations before hospital discharge

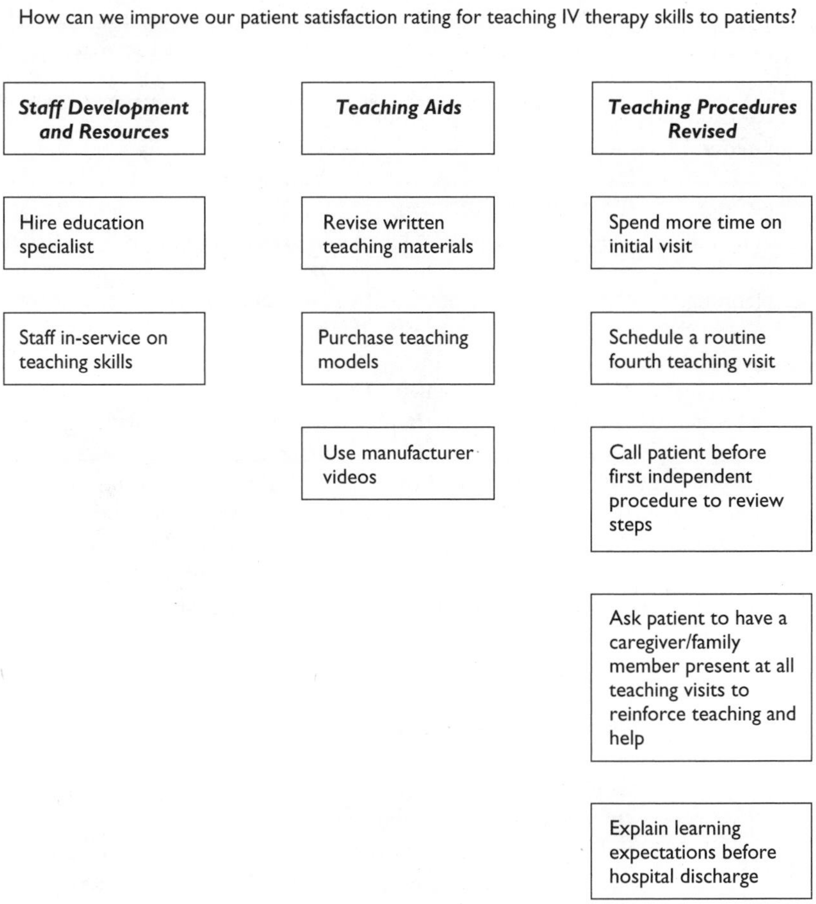

FIG. 4-11   *Affinity diagram: how to improve patient satisfaction with IV teaching.*

issues into logical groups.[35,43] Once a brainstorming session generates a list of ideas, an affinity diagram can help the team organize those ideas into manageable projects or subgroups, as shown in Fig. 4-11.

Most often, affinity diagrams are created by listing each brainstorm idea onto an index card or sticky note.[42] The ideas are displayed on an easel or on a table top. Team members then sort the ideas into groups silently. The ideas should not be discussed. Team members can move a card into another grouping. Once all the cards are sorted and a consensus is reached, the sorting ends. The team then creates headers for each group and draws the diagram using the groups created.

Multivoting

Multivoting is a strategy used to narrow down a large list of ideas to a list that is more manageable, uses resources more wisely, and will lead to better improvement.[35] By using this technique, the team can rank ideas in an order that will guide the improvement planning process toward ideas with greatest impact.

The principle of multivoting is that each member of the team is given a certain number of points to distribute to the ideas on the list. A general guideline is to take the total number of ideas on the list and divide by four. For example, if there are 20 ideas on the list, each member is given five points to distribute.

The team members independently assign number values to items on the list, up to five (in this example) in any way they choose. They can give one item all five points or distribute points as they wish to any or all of the items. The points for each idea are tallied, and the ideas are ranked in order of total points assigned, as shown in Fig. 4-12.

Flowcharting

Another tool used extensively for root cause analysis is the flowchart. A flowchart is a graphic representation of a process. It is "a simple form of process mapping that uses symbols to represent points of decisions and events that collectively form a 'picture' of an organizational process."[44] Flowcharts help team members understand steps in a process, identify costly redundancies and omissions, and plan for changes.[44]

Flowcharts are often drawn or reviewed during the planning phase of the improvement cycle to detect weak links in the process that may cause problems and therefore warrant improvement. Flowcharts can also be used during the planning phase when designing new processes or solutions.[43]

An interesting observation has been that many important and valuable issues are raised for discussion during the creation of a flowchart because team members may have different concepts of how a process is intended to run. Flowcharting and brainstorming often occur simultaneously. Flowcharting can take some time, especially when there is a problem in the process and resulting confusion about how it should be charted. However, because this is a very effective PI tool, the time is well spent.

To create a good flowchart, the team must determine the start and end points of the process, list all of the steps or events and decision points in the process, arrange them in sequence, and then use universal flowchart symbols to create a flowchart that can be analyzed. A sample flowchart is depicted in Fig. 4-13.

Other tools for planning improvements

Some of the more common tools used by performance improvement teams to plan what must be improved and how improvements can be prioritized and implemented have been described. This is only a partial listing, however, and library sources on quality management can provide detailed descriptions of additional tools and methodologies. Two other tools are briefly discussed here.

The IV team and PI team were given the list created during the brainstorming session. They were asked to consider which ideas were feasible and would improve the satisfaction ratings most significantly. Each member (total of 10 members) was allowed three points to allot to one or more items on the list. The result of the multivoting was as follows:

Points	Item
5	Spend more time on the initial visit.
0	Provide a fourth teaching visit instead of the usual three.
10	Develop new patient education literature for IV teaching.
0	Use videos.
6	Use practice models.
2	Call the patient before first independent dose to review the steps of the procedure(s).
1	Hire an education specialist for teaching only.
2	Ask the patient to have a caregiver or family member attend teaching visits.
0	Make the pamphlets easier to understand.
0	Find out what the patients don't like if they give a bad rating (determine the causes of dissatisfaction).
4	Have a staff in-service on teaching skills.
0	Review teaching plan in the hospital before discharge.

FIG. 4-12 *Multivoting: how to improve patient satisfaction with IV teaching.*

Hoshin planning. Hoshin planning is an organization-wide process of creating a vision and taking action.[35] The term *hoshin* is derived from the Japanese *hoshin kanri,* meaning "policy deployment." A tree diagram is used to document a strategic plan, transform the plan into action steps, and audit the plan.

The development of a vision and associated breakthrough areas and projects is driven by organization leadership and should include all members of the organization. The focus on the development of these strategies is always on the customer. JCAHO's reference publication *Using Performance Improvement Tools in Home Care and Hospice Organizations*[35] has a more comprehensive discussion of the steps of hoshin planning. Although this method is not used extensively, it has great value in organizational strategy and planning.

Critical paths. Critical paths are comprehensive process frameworks that guide a specific patient care process, procedure, or service. The path details the actions required or expected of each member of the health care team (e.g., nurses, physicians, social services, pharmacists). The actions are placed on a day-by-day sequencing for quick reference.[35]

A *variance* refers to the deviation of the patient's progress from the critical pathway. It can also refer to the deviation of the health care team's actions from the critical pathway. Variances are documented, categorized, and analyzed (for cause) by the use of variance reporting mechanisms. If you consider that variance reports contain data about how patients fare on a specific path, you can also say that the use of critical paths is both an improvement planning tool and a data measurement (outcome measurement) tool.

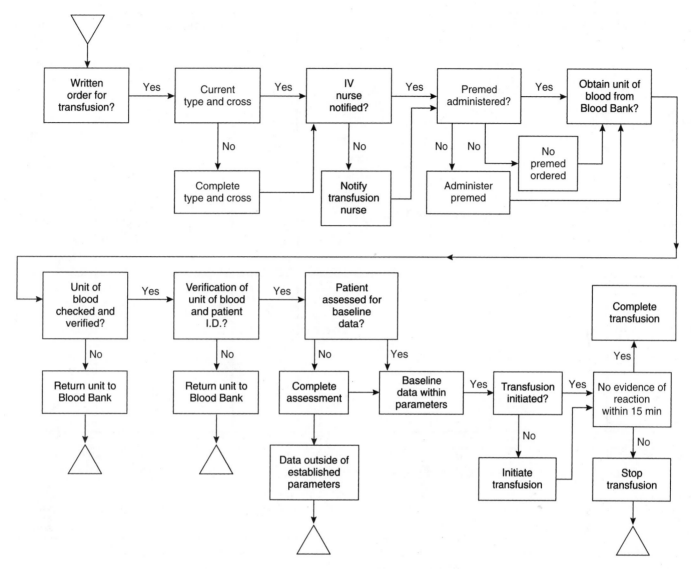

FIG. 4-13   *Flowchart of administration of transfusion.*

TOOLS FOR DOCUMENTING IMPROVEMENT ACTIONS

All improvement cycles, whether PDSA or the JCAHO cycle, include a phase for implementing the planned improvements or changes. This occurs after the team delegates responsibility for tasks to specific team or staff members.

To expedite the activities and document that they are completed according to the team's desired time frame, many teams use a documentation tool. The two most common tools are task lists and action plans.

Task lists

A task list is simply a list of things to be done or obtained. They are used to keep track of what needs to be completed. In some situations, a task list can be expanded into an action plan.

Action plans

Action plans contain more detail than simple task lists. Most action plans include a detailed description of the task, the person to whom the task has been delegated, and the target completion date. Some action plans also have a column for the initials of the person who has completed the task and the date of completion A suggested format for an action plan is shown in Fig. 4-14.

Action plans and task lists are important quality improvement documents that should be kept with the organization's performance improvement records.

Story boards

A story board is a posterlike display of the steps of an improvement project. It is intended for public display. Some story

ISSUE	DESIRED OUTCOME	TARGET DATE	ACTIONS	COMPLETION DATE		RESPONSIBLE PERSON	ACTUAL OUTCOME
				PROJECTED	ACTUAL		

FIG. 4-14 *Action plan format.*

boards are laid out using the specific improvement cycle method used, such as PDSA or FOCUS-PDSA. Other boards simply use a timeline sequence to tell the viewer the story of how an improvement was planned, implemented, and evaluated.[35]

Story boards provide an easy, visual way of explaining the PI team's accomplishments to other members of the organization and keep the PI team members focused on the project.

EXAMPLES OF IMPROVEMENT PROJECTS
A hospital-based performance improvement project using the PDSA cycle

Patient surveys on the oncology unit for the first quarter of 1999 indicated a problem with response time when nurses were asked to administer pain medication. Of the surveys returned, 20% included a comment concerning the wait time for pain medication. The QI/PI team assembled an interdisciplinary team of nurses, clinical pain specialists, pharmacists, and administrative staff to discuss the potential for improvement.

Plan. Using brainstorming and a root cause analysis, the team developed a list of three possible causes for the sudden increase in wait time. After evaluating work processes and staffing, the following three were listed:

1. Fewer physicians were ordering patient-controlled analgesia (PCA) pumps for patients, resulting in the need for medications to be administered as needed by the nursing staff.
2. Patients were waiting until the pain was moderate to severe before asking for a medication dose, possibly resulting in the perception of an increased wait time.
3. The hospital had adopted a "satellite pharmacy" system, where a small pharmacy substation located between three nursing units dispensed individual analgesia doses upon request. This method of increasing control over the dispensing of controlled substances sometimes resulted in increased wait times for the nurse requesting the dose.

The following changes were selected from a brainstorming list of 30:

- The pain management team, together with sales representatives from drug companies, would provide lunchtime continuing medical education (CME) programs on pain management, highlighting the increased effectiveness of PCA modalities.
- A new patient education pamphlet and poster would be developed reminding patients not to wait until pain was severe before asking for their next dose of medication. The pain management team would target one visit per pain management patient during the initial 48 hours of hospitalization to review the principles of preventive dosing.
- A meeting was scheduled between the Director of Pharmacy, Director of Nursing, and a representative of the QI/PI team to discuss alternative ways of dispensing unit

doses of analgesics from the satellite pharmacies. After the meeting, a plan was developed to prepare one day's number of doses in the morning, based on the previous day's consumption. A nurse would be able to sign out a dose from a locked patient drawer at the substation without placing a request with the pharmacist.

A timetable for the changes was established, and it was decided that the effectiveness of the changes would be assessed by surveying 100% of patients discharged from the oncology unit for 6 months. An acceptable threshold of surveys with negative comments about wait time would be 2%.

Do. During the do phase, the interdisciplinary team divided responsibilities and carried them out. Checklists were completed as tasks were finished and were forwarded to the QI/PI team leader for this project. The tasks were completed within 60 days. The QI/PI team began to collect patient surveys about wait time for analgesia once the changes were implemented. The data from the following quarter showed improvement, but 5% of surveys still indicated a problem with wait time. The results from the subsequent data indicated further improvement. Only 1% of surveys indicated a problem.

Check. During the check phase, the QI/PI team evaluated the surveys and found the level of improvement to be within acceptable range. The patient satisfaction rate with analgesia wait time increased from 80% to 99%, indicating a tremendous improvement to the process.

Act. The QI/PI committee recommended to the hospital leadership that the tested strategies be implemented on all oncology units and units where a high volume of patients use pain medication, such as postsurgical units.

A home care–based improvement project using the JCAHO cycle

A national home infusion pharmacy company recently noted an increase in the number of nonreimbursable nursing visits being provided to patients receiving total parenteral nutrition (TPN). This was noted on analysis of utilization data provided by the company's billing center. Interviews with managers at branches with the highest utilization disclosed that on-call nurses were reporting a higher number of after-hour visits since the company switched to a new ambulatory infusion pump for TPN. The nurses reported an increased number of phone calls from patients, caregivers, and home care nurses with complaints that they were unable to properly prime the disposable infusion tubing used with this new pump. As a result, customer satisfaction with equipment had fallen, and nursing costs had increased. Additional nursing visits were required to troubleshoot the problem and deliver additional infusion sets.

Although this situation called for an improvement study, the company's QI/PI team entered the cycle at a different place than you might expect. The function or process in question, the use of a new infusion pump for TPN, was already in place. The beginning phase for this team's project was therefore the *measure* phase.

Measure. By comparing current information in the internal database to previous quarters, the company had detected a significant variation, namely a sudden 18% increase in nonreimbursable after-hours nursing visits. The comparative information came from previous month's data, rather than from an external source. Interviews with the branch Directors of Nursing uncovered a second variation, a decrease in customer satisfaction with equipment, as noted by patient grievances and discharge patient surveys. Previous satisfaction ratings with equipment had ranged from 4.1 to 4.9 on a scale of 1 to 5, with a mean of 4.6. Over the last 2 months, however, patients had rated their satisfaction from 2.0 to 4.9 with a mean of 3.5.

Assess. The company's QI/PI committee scheduled a conference call with six local branch Directors of Nursing, the Purchasing Director, and the QI/PI department. During this conference, the group brainstormed and performed a root cause analysis of the problem. The following assessment was made:

- The nursing personnel agreed that the new pump, although less expensive, used an inferior disposable product as its dedicated set. The new infusion tubing sometimes had insecure Luer-Loc fittings near the filter assembly that prevented proper priming of air.
- The Purchasing Director emphasized the need to reduce costs to stay competitively priced and agreed to discuss the situation with the manufacturer.
- The group agreed that special labels could be printed to attach to the outside of the tubing wrapper, reminding all personnel and patients to secure all connections before attempting to prime the tubing.
- The group agreed that the improvement would be tested in 2 months, after the labels were attached by these six branches. The target improvement would be a satisfaction rating of at least 4.1 (mean) on discharge surveys, as reported by patients or their caregivers.

Improve. The QI/PI committee worked with the manufacturer to create bright warning labels, which were shipped to the six branches agreed upon. The pump manufacturer agreed to address the problem internally to see if a change in the assembly of the set or the use of a new set manufacturer was in order.

On the local level, delivery technicians and nurses placed the stickers on each tubing wrapper before delivery. They also reinforced the instructions with each patient, caregiver, and home care agency by memorandum or by a personal phone call.

One month after the initiation of label use, the local branches began to measure customer satisfaction with equipment and the number of after-hours nursing visits. Two months after the change was made, the mean value of customer satisfaction with equipment had risen back to 4.4, and the number of after-hour visits had decreased to within 3% of the baseline.

Design. When the QI/PI team noted the success of the changes, they began to redesign the process for all branches of the company. All branches were instructed to provide warning labels until a change in the manufacturing process occurred and to provide additional verbal instructions regarding the tubing. Nine months later, the manufacturer informed the infusion company that a different factory was being used to manufacture the tubings and that the ill-fitting connection issue had been addressed with the engineers.

INTEGRATED QUALITY MANAGEMENT

As quality management continues to evolve, the trend is to integrate monitoring and evaluation activities within the health care organization.[14] JCAHO standards specify that infection control, utilization review, and risk management be included in the organizationwide performance assessment and improvement activities.[17] Although each activity has a distinct purpose, they all indicate trends that are useful in identifying opportunities for improvement. Infection control is directed at the surveillance and control of the transmission of disease; utilization review relates to the appropriate use of the patient care services; and risk management focuses on identifying and preventing potential risks to the patient, health care worker, and organization. Merging these various functions under the umbrella of quality management services offers a comprehensive approach to quality improvement.

Integration of quality management activities is not new to IV nursing. Monitoring and evaluation of IV nursing care has always included trending of IV-related infections, determination of appropriateness of IV therapy, and prevention of IV-associated risks and complications. In fact, Cheryl Gardner, one of the pioneers of IV quality management, endorsed comprehensive monitoring as early as 1981. The current trend of integrating infection control, utilization review, risk management, and other quality management activities within health care organizations reduces the complexity of data collection and ensures that all aspects of quality IV nursing are evaluated.

Quality management integration also poses a challenge for IV nursing. As stated earlier, JCAHO advocates that performance measurement and improvement activities be interdisciplinary and cross-service rather than compartmentalized within departments or services. In the hospital setting, this means that the IV quality management program can no longer be limited to care provided by the IV team. Patients receive IV nursing care on units and in departments other than those serviced by the IV team, such as the critical care unit and emergency, surgery, and radiology departments.

In the home care setting and other alternative sites, this means that the IV quality management program must integrate the organization's pharmacy staff, nursing staff, associated professionals (e.g., physical therapists, occupational therapists, dietitians), nonprofessional staff (e.g., nurse aides), and administrative personnel. Each member of the team provides important and valuable services to the patients and should contribute to the IV team's PI process.

Integrating quality assessment and improvement activities requires that the IV team work with others to identify opportunities for improvements in IV nursing care throughout the organization.

REFERENCES

1. Freeland B: Moving toward continuous quality improvement, *JIN* 15:278, 1992.
2. Ives JR: Quality initiates in health care, *Boston Nurse News* 2:5, 1993.
3. Roberts JS, Coale JG, Redman RR: A history of the Joint Commission on Accreditation of Hospitals, *JAMA* 238:936, 1989.
4. Graham NO: *Quality assurance in hospitals: strategies for assessment and implementation,* Rockville, Md, 1990, Aspen.
5. Bradford L: Total quality management: doing it wrong the first time, *Med Interface* 4:61, 1992.
6. Kibbi P: *The National Association of Quality Assurance Professionals, utilization review and risk management: a study guide and primer,* Chicago, 1986, National Association of Quality Assurance Professionals.
7. Gillen TR: Deming's 14 points and hospital quality: responding to the consumers' demand for the best value health care, *J Nurs Qual Assur* 2:70, 1988.
8. Joint Commission on Accreditation of Healthcare Organizations (JCAHO): *1999-2000 comprehensive accreditation manual for home care,* Chicago, 1998, JCAHO.
9. Juran JM: *Juran on leadership for quality,* New York, 1989, Free Press.
10. Crosby PB: *Quality is free: the art of making quality certain,* New York, 1979, New American Library.
11. Deming WE: *Out of crisis,* Cambridge, Mass, 1989, MIT Center for Advanced Engineering Study.
12. Walton M: *Deming management at work,* New York, 1990, Putnam.
13. Meisenheimer CG: *Improving quality: a guide to effective programs,* Gaithersburg, Md, 1992, Aspen.
14. Koch MW, Fairly TM: *Integrated quality management,* St Louis, 1993, Mosby.
15. Joint Commission on Accreditation of Healthcare Organizations: *Agenda for change,* Chicago, 1990, JCAHO.
16. Joint Commission on Accreditation of Healthcare Organizations: *Accreditation manual for home care, 1993,* Chicago, 1992, JCAHO.
17. Joint Commission on Accreditation of Healthcare Organizations: *Accreditation manual for hospitals, 1992,* Chicago, 1991, JCAHO.
18. O'Leary DS: CQI: a step beyond QA, *Qual Rev Bull* 17:4, 1991.
19. Katz J, Green E: *Managing quality: a guide to monitoring and evaluating nursing services,* St Louis, 1992, Mosby.
20. Joint Commission on Accreditation of Healthcare Organizations: *Transitions: from QA to CQI,* Chicago, 1992, JCAHO.
21. Berwick DM: *Continuous improvement as an ideal in health care,* N Engl J Med 320:53, 1989.
22. O'Leary D, Ripple H: Responding to harsh criticism of the JCAHO, *Nurs Econ* 7:126, 1989.
23. Milakovich ME: Creating a total quality health care environment, *Health Care Manage Rev* 16:9, 1991.
24. Milakovich ME: Total quality management for public service productivity improvement, *Public Productivity Manage Rev* 14:19, 1990.
25. Labovich GH: *Managing quality and productivity in healthcare,* Burlington, Mass, 1988, Organizational Dynamics.
26. Labovich GH: Keeping your internal customers satisfied, *The Wall Street Journal* July 6, 1987.
27. Crosby PB: *Let's talk quality,* New York, 1990, McGraw-Hill.
28. Marker CG: The Marker model for nursing standards: implications for nursing administration, *Nurs Admin Q* 12:4, 1988.
29. Donabedian A: Structure, process, and outcome standards, *Am J Public Health* 59:1833, 1969.
30. Gillies DA: *Nursing management: a systems approach,* ed 2, Philadelphia, 1989, WB Saunders.
31. Joint Commission on Accreditation of Healthcare Organizations: *Implementation of the revised standards to nursing care, 1990, workshop materials,* Chicago, 1990, JCAHO.
32. Thompson MW, Hylka SC, Shaw CF: Systematic monitoring of generic standards of patient care, *J Nurs Qual Assur* 2:9, 1988.
33. Intravenous Nurses Society: Infusion nursing standards of practice, *JIN* (suppl) 23(6S), 2000.
34. Joint Commission on Accreditation of Healthcare Organizations (JCAHO): *Using performance measurement to improve outcomes in home care and hospice settings,* Chicago, 1999, JCAHO.
35. Joint Commission on Accreditation of Healthcare Organizations (JCAHO): *Using performance tools in home care and hospice organizations,* Chicago, 1996, JCAHO.

36. Wilson AA, Hartnett M, Ferrari R: Outcome measurement from the functional status perspective, *Home Health Care Nurse* 10:32, 1992.

37. Murray S, Murray OB, editors: *Total quality tools for health care,* Miamisburg, Ohio, 1997, Productivity-Quality Systems Inc.

38. Joint Commission on Accreditation of Healthcare Organizations: *ORYX outcomes: technical implementation guide for performance measurement systems,* Oakbrook Terrace, Ill, 1997, JCAHO.

39. Joint Commission on Accreditation of Healthcare Organizations: *Sentinel events: evaluating cause and planning improvement,* Oakbrook Terrace, Ill, 1997, JCAHO.

40. Polit DF, Hungler BP: *Nursing research: principles and methods,* ed 4, New York, 1991, JB Lippincott.

41. Joint Commission on Accreditation of Healthcare Organizations: *A guide to performance improvement for pharmacies,* Oakbrook Terrace, Ill, 1997, JCAHO.

42. Walton M: *The Deming management method,* New York, 1986, Putnam.

43. Straker D: *Rapid problem solving with Post-It Notes,* Tuscon, Ariz, 1997, Fisher.

44. Greer T, editor: The art of flowcharting, *Synapse* vol 1, no. 3, Knoxville, 1998, The Quality Management Group.

Chapter

5

Legal Aspects of Intravenous Nursing

Mary C. Alexander, BS, CRNI, Hugh K. Webster, Esq.*

Nowhere in professional nursing has the role of the nurse grown as fast, as effectively, and as favorably as in intravenous (IV) nursing. The development of IV nursing reflects a general trend in the nursing profession. Nurses today monitor complex physiologic data, operate sophisticated lifesaving equipment, and coordinate the delivery of health care services. More importantly, nurses now have responsibility for exercising discriminatory judgment. No longer do nurses blindly follow physicians' orders; they collaborate with physicians to ensure that their patients receive the highest quality of care.

The expanding responsibility of IV nurses has advantages and disadvantages. The nurse's emerging role offers rewards such as intellectual stimulation and professional satisfaction. However, the heightened status also means increased legal risks for the nurse and the added potential for liability. It is therefore the intent of this chapter to broaden awareness of the legal aspects of IV nursing. Four major topics are discussed: the legal standard of care, legal terminology, legal principles, and risk management.

LEGAL STANDARD OF CARE

Nurses have a duty to provide reasonable, prudent patient care as required by the situation. The care delivered by the nurse must comply with what is expected, given the circumstances in which the care is provided. This is known as the *legal standard of care.*

The legal standard of care is used to evaluate the quality of nursing conduct and has several important characteristics.[1] First, the standard of care is a reasonable expectation of the nursing care. This means that it represents the typical performance of a professional nurse who has special knowledge and skill beyond that of an ordinary person. For example, an IV nurse is expected to calculate the flow rate for an IV infusion. Second, the standard of care is measurable. The care can be evaluated based on what a similarly prepared nurse would do in the same situation. For example, all nurses who have earned the credentials CRNI are evaluated by the same standard as a result of the successful completion of the IV nursing certification examination. Third, the standard of care is valid based on where the care was delivered. There is variability based on the state where the care is delivered, thus influencing the established standard by which the care may be evaluated. An illustration of such variability is the insertion of a peripherally inserted central catheter (PICC). Until recently, some states did not consider this procedure within the realm of nursing practice, whereas other states allowed it to be performed by professional nurses. Fourth, the standard of care must be applicable based on the current state of knowledge. Standards evolve with increasing knowledge and experience, so the care must be evaluated within the historical context of when the care was delivered. For example, the 2000 revision of the *Infusion Nursing Standards of Practice* is applicable only to IV nursing care delivered since this document was published.

Standards can be voluntary, such as those promulgated by professional groups, or they may be mandated legislatively. Nursing, like most other professions, is regulated by these dual controls, both of which are aimed at providing quality patient care. Professional standards are the forerunners of legal standards. What has become the customary, usual nursing practice, as defined by the profession, later translates into the legal duty the nurse owes to the patient.

The nurse must demonstrate a familiarity with standards to deliver safe, competent nursing care. However, in IV nursing,

*The authors and editors wish to acknowledge the contributions made by Donna R. Baldwin and Donna Lee Mantel, as coauthors of this chapter in the first edition of *Intravenous Nursing: Clinical Principals and Practice.*

myriad standards are applicable, depending on the facts and issues involved in the situation. The location where the care is provided, the qualifications of the nurse, the procedure performed, and the type of product involved influence the applicability of the standard. As a guideline, the legal standards of care for IV nursing are derived from four sources: federal statutes and regulations, state statutes, professional standards, and institutional standards. A summary of some sources of the legal standards of care is presented in Table 5-1.

Federal statutes and regulations

Federal statutes are laws that have been enacted by Congress and are published in the *United States Code*. Regulations interpreting

Table 5-1	**Legal Standards of Care Relative to IV Nursing**	
SOURCE	**AGENCY**	**EXAMPLE**
Federal statutes and regulations	OSHA	Hazard Communication Standard
		Guidelines for Antineoplastic Cytotoxic Drugs
		Occupational Safe Exposure to Bloodborne Pathogens: Final Rule
	FDA	Safe Medical Device Act of 1990
	DEA	Controlled Substance Act
State statutes	Department of Health	Licensure of health care facilities
	Board of Nursing	Nurse Practice Act
Professional standards	JCAHO	*Comprehensive Accreditation Manual for Hospitals*
		Comprehensive Accreditation Manual for Home Care
		Comprehensive Accreditation Manual for Ambulatory Care
		Comprehensive Accreditation Manual for Long Term Care
	ANA	*Standards of Nursing Practice*
	INS	*Infusion Nursing Standards of Practice*
	AABB	*Technical Manual*
	ECRI	*Health Devices* (journal)
Institutional standards	Department of Nursing	Nursing policies Nursing procedures

OSHA, Occupational Safety and Health Administration; *FDA,* Food and Drug Administration; *DEA,* Drug Enforcement Agency; *JCAHO,* Joint Commission on Accreditation of Healthcare Organizations; *ANA,* American Nurses Association; *INS,* Intravenous Nurses Society; *AABB,* American Association of Blood Banks.

and implementing these laws are promulgated by numerous federal agencies, including the Occupational Safety and Health Administration (OSHA), Food and Drug Administration (FDA), and the Department of Health and Human Services. Agency regulations are published in the *Code of Federal Regulations*. The most applicable federal statutes and regulations relative to IV nursing concern occupational safety and health, infection control, environmental hazards, medical device safety, control of drug abuse, federally funded insurance programs, and patient self-determination.

Occupational Safety and Health Administration.
By law, OSHA has the authority to both establish and enforce regulations to promote job safety and protect the health of workers. One of OSHA's regulations is the Hazard Communication Standard, or "right-to-know" law, which requires that employees be informed of the hazardous potential of chemicals encountered in the workplace.[2] Hence, IV nurses must be trained as to warning labels on hazardous chemical containers used within the health care organization and in the use of material safety data sheets (MSDSs).

OSHA has addressed the hazardous potential of cytotoxic drugs with *Guidelines for Antineoplastic Cytotoxic Drugs*.[3] Cytotoxic drugs, including many of the antineoplastic agents, have genotoxic, mutagenic, or teratogenic potential. Because such drugs may be harmful to the health care worker, protective equipment is required to prevent skin exposure and aerosolization of the drug. OSHA recommendations include the use of a biologic safety cabinet to prepare cytotoxic drugs; the use of latex gloves and a lint-free, long-sleeved, cuffed, nonpermeable gown for drug administration; and special procedures in the event of a drug spill.[3]

To protect health care workers from human immunodeficiency virus (HIV) infection, OSHA, in 1987, expanded the interpretation of its "general duty clause." OSHA originally used precautions issued by the Centers for Disease Control and Prevention (CDC) as the basis for compliance interpretation. As a result, IV nurses were required to comply with standard precautions to prevent exposure to HIV. In 1991, OSHA established the standard *Occupational Safe Exposure to Bloodborne Pathogens*, which expands on standard precautions and addresses the risk of occupational exposure to blood-borne pathogens, including HIV and hepatitis B virus. The standard specifies that all body secretions can be potentially infectious and that personnel having contact with patients must adhere to strict guidelines.[4] These precautions are a combination of engineering and work-practice controls, and compliance with the guidelines are subject to comprehensive enforcement procedures.[4] Box 5-1 summarizes the rules the IV nurse must follow to minimize or eliminate the risk of exposure to blood-borne pathogens.

Infection control.
The CDC was established in 1946, under the Public Health Service, to prevent disease by means of surveillance, research, and demonstration projects. The CDC comprises 11 centers, institutes, and offices, including a National Center for HIV, STD, and TB Prevention. Although this agency does not regulate health, the CDC is responsible for providing guidance in the form of recommendations, which are considered voluntary standards. An example is the *Guideline for Prevention of Intravascular Device-Related Infections*.[5] Some-

Box 5-1   Regulations Regarding Occupational Exposure to Blood-Borne Pathogens[4]

STANDARD PRECAUTIONS

Standard precautions are based on the premise that blood and certain body fluids (e.g., mucus, saliva, urine, feces, drainage) are considered potentially infectious. Training must be conducted in a manner appropriate to the employees' educational backgrounds so that they understand this concept.

HEPATITIS B VACCINATIONS

If an employee is exposed to blood on the average of at least once per month, the employer must offer hepatitis B vaccine to the employee free of charge.

SHARPS DISPOSAL

Contaminated needles and sharps must be disposed of in puncture-resistant, leak-proof containers that are easily accessible and appropriately labeled.

GLOVES

Vinyl or latex gloves must be worn if exposure to blood or body fluids is anticipated. The gloves must be of appropriate quality for the procedure to be performed and of appropriate size for the health care worker. If the employee is allergic to standard gloves, hypoallergenic gloves must be provided by the employer.

PROTECTIVE EQUIPMENT

Equipment such as gowns, masks, and eye protectors must be available and used if exposure to skin, eyes, mouth, or clothing is anticipated.

HAZARD COMMUNICATION

Infectious waste must be labeled "Biohazard" to prevent accidental injury or exposure.

Table 5-2   Product Problem Reporting Program

WHEN TO REPORT

Problems with medical devices should be reported if the event observed involves, or has the potential to cause, a death, serious injury, or life-threatening malfunction. This includes problems such as the following:

- User error is the cause (the design of the device or unclear/incomplete labeling may have contributed to the problem).
- A decision is made to no longer use the device because of a malfunction that has occurred.
- Repeated repairs fail to solve the problem.
- Design or repair changes by the manufacturer have adversely affected the performance, safety, or efficacy of the device.
- The problem was the result of incompatibility between devices of different manufacturers and labeling failed to warn the user of this potential for problems.
- The malfunction results in prolonged hospitalization, readmission, or repeated surgical procedures.

WHAT TO REPORT

A complete description of the problem and information regarding the device needs to be submitted, including the following:

- Product name
- Manufacturer's name and address
- Identification numbers of the device (lot number, model number, serial number, expiration date)
- Problem noted (including any actual or potential adverse effects)
- Name, title, and practice specialty of the user of the device

HOW TO REPORT

Problems are reported to MedWatch, the Food and Drug Administration (FDA) medical products reporting program. Reports can be made by telephone, 800-FDA-1088; by facsimile, 800-FDA-0178; or by mail: MedWatch, Food and Drug Administration, 5600 Fishers Lane, Rockville, Maryland, 20852-9787. A MedWatch reporting form is available at www.fda.gov/medwatch/index.html, and reports can be made online at the same Web address.

---

times, the voluntary guidelines issued by the CDC may be adopted by a federal agency and, in effect, become regulations. Such was the case when OSHA adopted the standard precautions developed by the CDC for compliance interpretation.

Environmental Protection Agency. The Environmental Protection Agency (EPA) is a federal regulatory agency responsible for overseeing the enforcement of laws enacted to protect the environment. It was created in 1969 pursuant to the National Environmental Policy Act.[6] There are five federal laws administered by the EPA that have particular importance in health care: (1) Toxic Substance Control Act,[7] which grants EPA control over chemical hazards; (2) Resource Conservation and Recovery Act,[8] whereby the EPA tracks the movement of hazardous waste from creation to disposal, or "cradle to grave"; (3) Medical Waste Tracking Act,[9] which grants the EPA authority to establish practices for the handling and disposal of infectious waste; (4) Comprehensive Environmental Response, Compensation and Liability Act,[10] whereby the EPA has the authority to implement and finance the cleanup of hazardous waste; and (5) Emergency Planning and Community Right-to-Know Act,[11] which focuses on the community's "right to know" about hazardous materials.

Medical device safety. Since 1938, the FDA has been responsible for regulating products such as food, cosmetics, prescription and over-the-counter medications, and biologic agents to ensure that they are safe and effective for their intended purposes. In 1976, this authority was extended to medical devices.[12] With enactment of the Safe Medical Device

Act of 1990, hospitals, ambulatory surgical facilities, nursing homes, and outpatient treatment facilities are legally required to report to the FDA incidents in which a medical device may have contributed to the serious injury, serious illness, or death of a patient. The term *device* is broadly defined and may include IV-related equipment such as vascular access devices, solution containers, and electronic infusion devices.[13] It is the IV nurse's professional responsibility, regardless of the practice setting, to inspect product integrity before use and to report any suggested or potential medical device problems. Medical device regulation within the FDA is administered by the Center for Devices and Radiological Health. Guidelines for reporting product problems to the FDA are listed in Table 5-2.

Control of drug abuse. The Comprehensive Drug Abuse Prevention and Control Act, also known as the Controlled Substances Act, was passed in 1970.[14] The act provides for the control of drug abuse and the enforcement of its provisions by the FDA and the Drug Enforcement Agency (DEA) of the Department of Justice. By law, controlled substances are classified according to five schedules based on the potential for abuse, accepted medical uses, and potential for physical or psychologic dependence.[15] The DEA, however, has the authority to reschedule drugs, schedule a previously unlisted drug, or remove a drug from the schedule.[15,16] IV nurses must be aware of the schedules and subsequent revisions because of the stringent requirements regarding handling, storing, and documenting controlled drugs.[17]

Federally funded insurance programs. The Health Care Financing Administration (HCFA) is a federal agency created in 1977 to administer the Medicare program and the federal portion of the Medicaid program. Because the HCFA is responsible for ensuring the quality of health care for beneficiaries participating in these federally funded health insurance programs, the agency sets standards for health care providers receiving Medicare-Medicaid reimbursement. Nurses employed by such providers must comply with the applicable standards, which are commonly referred to as *HCFA regulations.*

Patient self-determination. The Patient Self-Determination Act of 1990[18] requires that all health care providers accepting Medicare and Medicaid payments provide written information regarding advance directives. An advance directive is a document by which an adult patient may legally decide about future medical treatment. The information is provided at the time of admission to the facility, and it recognizes the patient's rights as a competent adult to decide about the use of do-not-resuscitate orders and the withdrawal of life-sustaining equipment.[19] Although this requirement is federally mandated, each state is responsible for overseeing this program, thus there may be implementation variations from state to state.

State statutes

A *jurisdiction* is a legally established geographic area, such as a state. Variations exist among state statutes because each state government may enact laws specific for that geographic area. A state cannot enact a law that conflicts with federal laws, but it may pass additional regulations.[20] The primary types of state statutes that affect the delivery of IV nursing care are the Nurse Practice Acts, requirements for nurse licensure, joint policy statements, and licensing of health care facilities.

Nurse practice acts. The Nurse Practice Act defines the practice of professional and licensed practical nursing within the state. Although each state has a Nurse Practice Act that describes the nurse's role and function, the definition of nursing is typically generalized. This allows the employer to delineate additional functions and activities that the nurse may perform during employment.

Relative to IV nursing, a state Nurse Practice Act may be general or specific in its guidance. Those states that publish only general standards in the Nurse Practice Act announce specific criteria for nursing behavior in bulletins or newsletters.

Requirements for nurse licensure. Each Nurse Practice Act specifies that the nurse must be licensed to practice nursing within the state. The minimum requirements for licensure are established by the State Board of Nursing. The State Board of Nursing is also empowered to suspend or revoke the license of any nurse for violation of the specified norms of conduct for that state. For example, the nurse must meet the minimum requirements to be licensed as a registered nurse in the state of New York, but the license may be revoked if the nurse fails to comply with New York's established rules of conduct.

Joint policy statements. When questions regarding the professional responsibility of nurses to perform specific therapeutic procedures cannot be answered by existing state statutes, a joint policy statement may be issued. Sponsors of joint policy statements include the state's nursing association, medical society, and hospital association.[21]

Licensing of health care facilities. Each state has a Department of Health that sets standards for the licensing of health care facilities. Although these standards are generally directed toward the physical facilities, qualifications of employees, and maintenance of records, they are interrelated with the nursing process. For example, the state health department may mandate how and where medications are to be stored, and the nurse's conduct must not violate these standards.

Professional standards

Professional standards are not merely the minimum criteria enacted by the legislature but represent an attempt by a peer group to establish a level of competency that is expected by the profession[22] and has been recognized as such by courts.[23] (Additional information on professional standards is provided in Chapter 4.)

In health care, professional standards may apply to the entire industry or may pertain only to a specific profession or specialty. The accreditation standards published by the Joint Commission on Accreditation of Healthcare Organizations (JCAHO) exemplify national health care industry standards. In contrast, specific standards that affect IV nursing have been developed by the American Nurses Association (ANA), the Intravenous Nurses Society (INS), the American Association of Blood Banks (AABB), and the American Society of Health-System Pharmacists (ASHP). Criteria developed by the Association for the Advancement of Medical Instrumentation (AAMI) and the Emergency Care Research Institute (ECRI) also influence professional standards for intravenous nursing.

Joint Commission on Accreditation of Healthcare Organizations. JCAHO is a nongovernmental accrediting body that defines optimal, achievable standards for health care organizations such as hospitals, home care services, nursing homes, and ambulatory care centers. The intent of the standards is to improve the quality of health care provided to the public by stimulating health care organizations to meet or exceed the standards through accreditation.[24]

American Nurses Association. The ANA has published generic standards for nursing practice that focus on the delivery of nursing care related to the six steps of the nursing process: assessment, diagnosis, outcome identification, planning, implementation, and evaluation.[25] As such, they may be considered the foundation for nursing practice.

Intravenous Nurses Society. INS introduced the first standards for IV nursing in 1980. The standards are reviewed annually, and subsequent revision reflects changes in practice and technologic advances. The *Infusion Nursing Standards of*

Practice are specific to the specialty practice of IV nursing but are applicable to all practice settings in which IV therapy is delivered.[26]

American Association of Blood Banks. The AABB publishes standards regarding the professional practice of blood donation, blood processing, and transfusion therapy.[27] These standards address the safe and effective replacement of blood and blood components. Criteria from the AABB standards that relate to IV nursing are included in *Infusion Nursing Standards of Practice.*

American Society of Health-System Pharmacists. The ASHP is the national professional association that represents pharmacists in organized health care settings. Based on published research, ASHP has offered guidelines that affect IV nursing. An example is the set of guidelines concerning the handling of cytotoxic drugs published in 1990.[28] As with the AABB standards, the ASHP standards relative to IV nursing are reflected in *Infusion Nursing Standards of Practice.*

Association for the Advancement of Medical Instrumentation. The AAMI is a professional organization that promotes interdisciplinary interaction regarding the use of medical devices. By generating information, services, and forums, AAMI helps determine criteria for selecting and using medical instruments such as electronic infusion devices.

ECRI. ECRI, an independent nonprofit agency is dedicated to improving the safety, efficacy, and cost-effectiveness of health care technology. ECRI publishes a monthly journal, *Health Device System,* which provides comparative evaluations of medical devices, including infusion devices.[29]

Institutional standards

In addition to governmental and professional standards, each institution or agency also specifies its own standards in a policy and procedure manual. *Policies* are guidelines or general statements as to when a particular procedure, method, or action is to be used. In contrast, *procedures* are step-by-step outlines of how actions or methods are to be performed.[30] Box 5-2 contains an example of a policy and the corresponding procedure.

LEGAL TERMINOLOGY

In an age that greatly emphasizes the legal rights of people, nurses have a responsibility to understand the basic precepts of law. Our society is founded on a system of legal principles and processes by which people can resolve problems and disputes without resorting to physical force. To comprehend this legal system and apply the principles to the practice of IV nursing, the nurse must be cognizant of the terminology commonly used to discuss legal matters.

Origins of law

The term *law* has been broadly defined as those standards of human conduct that are established and enforced by the authority of an organized society through its government. In the United States, there are four sources of law: constitutions, legislation, regulations, and judicial opinions.[31] The federal

---

Box 5-2 **Example of a Policy and Corresponding Procedure: Changing of IV Administration Set**

POLICY
IV administration sets will be changed every 24 to 48 hours (including in-line filters, extension tubing, volume-control sets, and secondary piggyback administration sets) and as required. Every effort will be made to perform the set change at the time a new IV solution container is hung.
PROCEDURE
1. Prepare new solution container.
2. Close flow control clamp on new administration set.
3. Remove protective cover from spike and insert spike of new administration set into new solution container.
4. Fill drip chamber half full and prime tubing.
5. Close flow control clamp on old administration set.
6. Remove tape securing old administration set.
7. Disconnect old administration set from cannula and insert new set.
8. Secure new administration set with tape.
9. Adjust flow rate as prescribed.
10. Discard contaminated equipment.

Note that, for clarity, nursing actions generic to all procedures (i.e., identify patient, assemble equipment, wash hands, glove, and document) have been omitted from this example.

---

constitution is the highest form of law and is considered "organic law" because it defines the organization of our government. The constitution provides the framework of government by establishing the Legislative, Executive, and Judicial branches that are responsible for the other three sources of law.

In addition to the federal government, every state has a constitution and the three branches of government. The powers of state governments are subject to limitations defined in the federal constitution, the stipulations of state constitutions, and restrictions necessary for the operation of the federal systems. Local governments are created by the state and may exercise only those powers conferred on them by the state government.

Categories of law

There are numerous types of laws and various methods by which they are categorized (Fig. 5-1). Often, laws are categorized in relation to the four sources from which they originate and may be identified as follows: (1) *constitutional law,* originating from the federal and state constitutions; (2) *statutory law,* enacted by the legislative branch of government; (3) *administrative law,* issued by administrative agencies that have been established by the legislature or appointed by the executive branch; and (4) *common law,* which results from interpretation of the laws by the judicial system.[32] Some texts also classify laws as public and private law. Constitutional, statutory, and administrative laws are considered *public law* because they deal with public welfare. In contrast, *private law* is concerned with the rights, duties, and legal relations involving private individuals. Contractual law and laws regarding negligence and malpractice are components of private law.[33]

Laws may also be categorized as to their intent. Such a classification emphasizes how the law affects nurses and which laws are applicable to practice. Therefore the categories of law

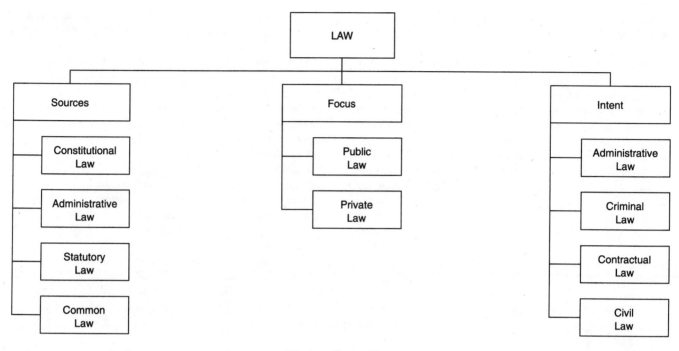

FIG. 5-1   *Types of laws.*

relative to IV nursing include administrative, criminal, contractual, and civil law.

Administrative law. Statutes are laws that are enacted by the legislature and are known as *statutory law*. When the legislature enacts statutes to regulate business or confer benefits on its citizens, it may be difficult to foresee variations necessary for proper execution of the law. To provide for this eventuality, the legislature may establish an administrative agency empowered to make rules and regulations that have the force of laws. OSHA, the FDA, and HCFA are examples of federal administrative agencies. Regulations from these agencies affect the practice of IV nursing. Rules issued by OSHA focus on protection of the health care worker, FDA regulations emphasize product safety, and HCFA guidelines affect providers participating in the Medicare program.

States may also have administrative agencies that are created by the legislature. The primary example is the State Board of Nursing, also referred to as the Board of Nurse Examiners, Nurse Licensing Board, or Nursing Board. These boards set requirements for and grant approval to nursing schools, conduct licensing examinations, and issue and renew licenses for nurses. In addition, they are empowered to revoke or annul a nurse's license if there is evidence of incompetence, fraud, or deceit in securing the license; unprofessional conduct; practicing while impaired; criminal acts; or gross negligence.

Criminal law. Laws relating to an offense against the general public that results in a harmful effect against society as a whole are classified as *criminal law*. The primary emphasis of criminal law is defining behaviors that are prohibited or controlled by society. Criminal offenses are prosecuted by a governmental authority and punishment may result in fines and/or imprisonment. Performing IV nursing procedures in a manner that violates the Nurse Practice Act or the Medical Practice Act is an example of a criminal offense.

There are two types of criminal actions: misdemeanors and felonies. A *felony* is a criminal act of a particularly serious nature. Under many state laws, any crime punishable by imprisonment for more than 1 year generally is considered a felony. There are also different classes of felonies. A *misdemeanor* is simply any criminal act that does not rise to the level of a felony.

Contractual law. A *contract* is an agreement between two or more persons that creates, changes, or eliminates a legal right or obligation. Most nurses do not have employment contracts, but rather enter into general, flexible arrangements with their employers. However, even if the employing agency has no written contract, there is still a binding legal commitment based on a mutual understanding. The nurse has a duty to perform the nursing assignment in accordance with the standards of professional nursing practice; the employer's duty is to provide a safe workplace and properly trained and qualified coworkers.

As more IV nurses become entrepreneurs, there is an increasing need for nurses to understand how to negotiate written contracts for their services. Consideration must also be given as to how the contract may be terminated. If the nurse fails to perform the obligations required by the contract, a breach of contract may be committed and the nurse may be required to pay damages. The term *damages* usually refers to a sum of money awarded to a person or organization whose rights have been violated by another.

Civil law. The legal rights and obligations of private citizens are the focus of civil law. This category is commonly referred to as *case law* because it is decided by a judge and/or jury. By law, individuals and groups are protected from harm and, if injured by the actions of another, may file a civil action seeking damages. If the civil offense is a private wrong against another's person or property, it is referred to as a *tort*. Torts are the result of a private act or omission and may be further classified as intentional, unintentional, or quasi-intentional.

Intentional torts.   An intentional tort involves the purposeful invasion of a person's legal rights. The two best known intentional torts are assault and battery. Although the two terms are often linked, they have separate and distinct meanings. *Assault* is the unjustifiable attempt to touch another person or the threat to do so, communicated in such a way as to cause the person to believe it will be done. For example, if a competent adult patient refuses to have a venipuncture performed but the nurse proceeds to assemble the venipuncture equipment and to prepare to perform the procedure, the patient has been assaulted. *Battery* is defined as the unlawful carrying out of threatened physical harm. If, in the previous example, the nurse proceeds to apply the tourniquet and actually perform the venipuncture, the action would be considered battery.

The term *coercion* is often used to explain assault and battery. Coercion is the forcing of another person to act in a certain manner by means of threat or intimidation. Hence, coercing a rational adult patient to accept a venipuncture constitutes assault and battery.

Another example of intentional tort is *false imprisonment*, which involves placing individuals in a confined area against their will. In the practice of IV nursing, it is sometimes necessary to restrain a patient's extremity to stabilize and secure the IV cannula. In such situations, the nurse must follow policies and procedures governing the use of restraints and resort to restraints only when the patient's safety is in jeopardy. Failure to follow these guidelines may result in allegations of false imprisonment.

Unintentional torts.   An inadvertent act, or failure to act, that results in injury or harm to a person is an *unintentional tort*. An unintentional tort may involve an action that is unreasonable and inappropriate or the lack of an action that is reasonable and appropriate. Two types of unintentional torts are negligence and professional malpractice.

Negligence is not doing something that a reasonable layperson would do given the situation. For example, if a store owner knows that the store parking lot is icy, yet takes no corrective action and a customer slips and falls, the owner may be deemed to have been negligent. However, the opposite also constitutes negligence, because a person who does something that a reasonable person would not do in similar circumstances is also negligent.

When negligent conduct occurs on the part of a member of a profession, it is considered *malpractice*. Medical malpractice has been further defined as deviation from the professional standard of practice that a qualified health care provider of the same specialty would follow given similar circumstances. In this context, malpractice may be considered synonymous with *professional negligence* because the failure to act in a reasonable and prudent manner, as defined by the profession, may result in harm to the patient.[20] For example, the death of a patient as a result of the administration of 1000 ml of 3% sodium chloride infusion, instead of the prescribed 1000 ml of 5% dextrose in 0.33% sodium chloride, may be ruled as malpractice.

Although malpractice implies the failure to act in a reasonable and prudent manner, it also denotes stepping beyond one's authority. Each state has a Nurse Practice Act that defines the scope of nursing practice. If the nurse performs a procedure outside the boundaries of nursing practice, it may be ruled an illegal "practice of medicine" in violation of the Medical Practice Act for that state. For example, removing a tunneled or implanted vascular access device is a medical act; if a nurse performs this procedure, it could be malpractice.

Quasi-intentional torts.   The categories of civil wrongs that involve a person's reputation or peace of mind are considered quasi-intentional torts. *Defamation* damages a person's reputation through false and malicious statements. If the statements are written, they are known as *libel*, and if spoken as *slander*. A person's peace of mind may be violated through *invasion of privacy* or by a *breach of confidentiality*. Patients are vulnerable to unauthorized release of private and confidential information concerning their diagnosis, prognosis, treatment, and plan of care. Hence, nurses have a legal duty and professional responsibility to ensure that these civil rights of patients are not violated.

Legal processes

In our legal system, there are three forums in which legal disputes are settled, and each has unique rules of procedure and rules of evidence. Disciplinary disputes and violations of regulations set by an administrative agency are settled within the administrative law forum. For example, State Board of Nursing decisions are governed by the state administrative laws. Criminal charges are heard in a criminal law forum. An example is the use of criminal laws to try a nurse charged with a criminal offense. Tort disputes, such as negligence or malpractice, are referred to a civil law forum, which is typically a court. In a civil action, the person who has been wronged seeks compensation for the harm or injury suffered. This differs from criminal or administrative law, which seeks to punish the wrongdoer.

Two basic legal rights are paramount in the legal process. First, as Americans, we have a right to use courts to settle disputes. There are two sides to the dispute—the plaintiff and the defendant—and both have the right to use the legal system to settle the conflict. In a case questioning the nurse's care, the *plaintiff* may be the injured patient who initiated a civil suit, or the state agency or prosecutor if the offense involves an administrative or criminal action. The *defendant* is the person accused of violating the standard of care (civil law), acting unprofessionally (administrative law), or committing a criminal offense (criminal law).

The second basic legal right is the right to due process. This means that certain principles must be followed within a fair and just forum, including proper notice, arrangement of an opportunity to be heard, presentation of evidence, and cross-examination of witnesses.

LEGAL PRINCIPLES

As a result of the growth and increasing complexity of IV nursing, the greatest legal risk for nurses practicing this specialty is negligence, also known as *negligent conduct* or *malpractice*.[34]

The plaintiff may believe the nurse was negligent, but legal action cannot be initiated unless several rules are followed.

Elements of negligence

If a patient (plaintiff) believes that an act performed by a nurse or the nurse's failure to act has resulted in injury or harm, the legal process begins once he or she selects a lawyer to represent his or her interests. The counsel for the plaintiff (the allegedly injured patient or heirs) must then determine whether there is a basis for the lawsuit. This involves reviewing the medical record, collecting data, interviewing witnesses, and arranging for the case to be reviewed by an expert. Because the plaintiff has the burden of proof, counsel must determine whether there is evidence of the elements of negligence.

In a lawsuit, the plaintiff (patient) must present evidence that the defendant (nurse) failed to use the degree of skill and judgment commensurate with the nurse's education, experience, and position. In other words, there must be evidence of failure to conform to what a reasonably prudent nurse would have done, or would not have done, if placed in the same situation. As stated by one court, "A nurse who undertakes to render professional services is under a duty to exercise reasonable care and diligence in the application of her knowledge and skill to the patient's case and to use her best judgment in the treatment and care of patients."[35] The four elements necessary to prove negligence are duty of care, breach of duty, causation, and legally compensable injury.

Duty of care. The first element that must be proven by the plaintiff is that the defendant owed a duty of care. This means that the nurse was in some way responsible for the patient. For example, if the nurse performs a venipuncture on a patient to initiate an infusion, there is a duty of care to the patient. However, if the mother of the patient becomes faint during the venipuncture procedure and falls, injuring her wrist, the duty of care to the patient's mother is questionable. The nurse owed a duty of care to the patient but not to the patient's mother, unless there was a prior realistic agreement to do so. Hence, the mother (as a plaintiff) will probably not be successful in proving duty of care.

Breach of duty. The second critical element that must be proven is that the defendant violated, or breached, the duty of care owed to the patient. The breach of duty may be the result of an act (commission) or of a failure to act (omission). For example, necrosis and tissue sloughing resulting from infiltration of a peripheral infusion of 10% dextrose in water may be the result of failure to monitor a peripheral IV site, an act of omission. On the other hand, injury caused by initiating an infusion without a physician's order is an act of commission. Both may be considered breaches of duty. Other examples of breach of duty relative to IV nursing are as follows:

1. *Delay in drug administration:* A lidocaine infusion has been prescribed for a patient experiencing ventricular tachycardia. Although the infusion is to be initiated immediately, the order is not communicated to the IV nurse and there is a 3-hour delay until the infusion is initiated.
2. *Failure to administer infusion at the prescribed rate:* A dehydrated patient is to receive an IV infusion at 150 ml/hr, but the drop rate is incorrectly calculated and the solution infuses at 50 ml/hr.
3. *Inappropriate administration of a drug:* Phenytoin is administered at a rate of 100 mg/min and the patient experiences a severe adverse reaction.
4. *Failure to provide patient education:* A patient is discharged home with a long-term central venous catheter. No arrangements are made for home health care and the patient is not instructed regarding care of the catheter.

Breach of duty may also result from barriers to the delivery of patient care. In home infusion therapy, for example, a patient who refuses to follow the treatment regimen may affect the agency's ability to manage the patient's care. However, termination of care without reasonable notice and adequate time for the patient to secure additional care may be interpreted as patient abandonment. When an agency contracts to provide services, a duty is owed to the patient. Regardless of the reasons, termination of care without adequate notice or provision for continued care represents a breach of duty.

In the case of a private citizen, such as a landlord, the jury can generally comprehend what a reasonably prudent landlord would have done based on the circumstances, and the law allows jurors to use their common sense in reaching a verdict. A nursing negligence case, however, is far more complex because the allegation is that the nurse breached the standard of reasonable nursing care. Because the law recognizes that the average juror does not understand medical terminology, the nursing process, or the legal standard of nursing care, it is often mandated that qualified witnesses educate the jury as to the circumstances of the case.[36] This is the role of the expert witness. An *expert witness* in a medical or nursing malpractice case is a health care provider who is called on to educate the judge and jury regarding the appropriate standard of care and to identify any deviation from the established standard. Typically, the expert witness is of the same profession, has similar experience as the defendant, and has demonstrated expertise in the specialty practice.[37] For example, a CRNI with extensive experience in home infusion therapy would be qualified to offer expert testimony in a case involving the actions of a home care IV nurse.

In offering expert testimony, the witness may rely on personal knowledge and experience, professional articles, published standards of practice, and nursing documentation contained in the patient's medical record to educate the jury. Once the jury understands the applicable standard of care, the expert may offer an opinion as to whether the defendant deviated from that standard. Because nursing negligence is a complex issue, expert witnesses may be used to testify both for and against the defendant. The plaintiff's expert witness will attempt to convince the jury that the defendant (nurse) deviated from the accepted nursing standards; the expert witness for the defense will testify that the defendant's actions represented reasonable nursing care. The jury, however, is not governed by the opinions of the experts and can reject either or both testimonies.

Causation. The third element that must be proven is causation or proximate cause.[38] By law, the injury to the plaintiff must be the result of negligent conduct on the part of the defendant. Patients may be injured because of the conduct of the nurse, but if the nurse was performing in a reasonable, safe manner, the nurse is not responsible for the harm. For example, if a nurse administers penicillin intravenously to a patient and an allergic reaction ensues, the nurse is responsible only if he or she failed to check for possible allergies before administration of the drug. However, if the patient had no known allergies, there is no liability on the part of the nurse.

An important criterion in establishing proximate cause is *foreseeability*. It is often easier to determine what *should* have been done in a given situation after the fact. Foreseeability requires that the defendant's actions be judged based on the facts known at the time of the occurrence.

Legally compensable injury. The final element of negligence is that the patient suffered injury and that the injury is a type for which the law allows compensation. Because the plaintiff must prove that negligent conduct was actually responsible for harm or injury, it is possible to have severe negligence but no lawsuit. For example, the nurse performs a venipuncture to initiate an infusion of 5% dextrose in 0.225% sodium chloride, but 5% dextrose in 0.45% sodium chloride was prescribed. If the nurse discovers the error before initiating the infusion and no harm has come to the patient, then there can be no lawsuit. Often, potential clients contact malpractice attorneys and relate how they were "almost" injured by a nurse or physician. However, the common reply is that by law, "almost" doesn't count. If there is no injury, there can be no lawsuit.

Common areas of nursing negligence

To avoid the risks of negligence, the nurse needs to be aware of those areas most commonly associated with negligent conduct and act in such a way as to prevent liability. Areas of negligence specific to IV nursing include medication administration, equipment use, failure to act, lack of communication, and negligent conduct of another.

Medication administration. The actions of nurses relating to the administration of medications have been the subject of more lawsuits than any other area of nursing. Examples include giving the wrong medication,[39] not being familiar with the possible harmful effects of a medication,[40] failure to administer medication at proper intervals,[41] administering medication in an improper manner,[42,43] and failure to obey a physician's instructions.[44] However, there also can be a duty to correct the erroneous orders of a physician.[45] If the nurse fails to meet the professional expectations relative to medication administration and the failure results in injury to the patient, the nurse is liable. Many cases involving medication errors are settled before reaching a jury because the health care organization's records furnish ample proof of the error.

Equipment use. Protecting the patient from equipment hazards is a responsibility the nurse assumes when using items such as vascular access devices, solution containers, administration sets, and electronic infusion devices. The nurse has the duty to reasonably inspect, maintain, use, and supervise equipment to prevent obvious harm to the patient. Nurses have been held responsible for improper use and disposal of equipment, for not supervising the use of equipment, and for leaving equipment in an inappropriate area. If the patient cannot prove when, where, or by whom he or she was injured, courts have found nurses

responsible by applying a doctrine called *res ipsa loquitur.*[46,47] This doctrine means that the injury is so obvious that it "speaks for itself." For example, when an unconscious patient sustains injury from a hematoma caused by an unsuccessful venipuncture attempt, he or she certainly is unable to testify as to how or by whom the injury occurred. In this situation, the law allows the patient to prove, by virtue of the obviousness of the situation, that it was the negligence of the nurse performing the venipuncture that caused the injury.

If, however, the nurse can prove that ordinary precautions were taken to protect the patient from danger, the nurse is not liable, even though the patient was subsequently injured. Such may be the case when a peripheral IV catheter breaks off and harms the patient during an IV infusion. If the nurse inspected the catheter before insertion and detected no visible defect, the nurse is not responsible for the manufacturer's defective product.

Failure to act. Affirmative actions are the subject of most lawsuits against nurses, but the nurse's failure to act may also injure the patient. An example of negligent failure to act is a nurse who receives an order to administer a potassium infusion to a patient experiencing cardiac arrhythmia but who fails to respond to the order. If the arrhythmia becomes life-threatening because of the failure to act and subsequently results in death, the nurse is liable for the patient's demise.

Lack of communication. Although failure to communicate is closely related to the failure to act, it may be the sole specific cause of injury. Examples of nursing negligence resulting from lack of communication are the failure to inform the physician of abnormal findings noted during the nursing assessment[48] or the failure to notify the physician of a patient's deteriorating condition.[49] Clearly, nurses have an obligation to exercise sound clinical judgment as to what is significant regarding the patient's status and to communicate that information.[50]

Negligent conduct of another. Along with the person who is primarily responsible, a nurse may be liable for allowing or aiding the negligence of that other person. For example, if a physician fails to specify the route of administration for a drug and the nurse administers the drug without checking the route with the prescribing physician, the nurse and physician are jointly responsible if an injury occurs. Merely attempting to contact the physician is not enough to release the nurse from liability. If there is a lack of action by the physician, the nurse is required to advise authorities within the organization to ensure intervention on behalf of the patient.

Time constraints

The statute of limitations is often referred to as a *rule of repose* because cases not filed within the legally required time are automatically rejected by the courts. Although all citizens are allowed their day in court, plaintiffs cannot abuse this right and hold the defendant in suspense long after an incident occurs. The reason for the time constraint is fairness to all parties. If a plaintiff waits beyond the legal time limit to file a lawsuit, the defendant may be unable to locate coworkers or witnesses who can testify on his or her behalf. Critical records may have been destroyed, memories of the incident may have faded, and justice cannot be served.

Time limits differ according to the type of lawsuit and the state in which the suit is filed. For example, in some states, lawsuits regarding nursing negligence must be filed in court within 2 years of the injury, but clients have 6 years to file attorney malpractice cases. Because a patient may not be aware of the negligence until a delayed injury manifests itself, an exception to rigid time frames is mandated by the *discovery statute*. This means just what it implies; the statutory time begins only once the injury is discovered.

Tools of discovery

Once the complaint is filed in court and served on the defendant, the discovery phase of litigation begins. Two tools of discovery often used are interrogatories and depositions. The first step in discovery is for both sides of a lawsuit to develop lists of questions called *interrogatories*. Interrogatories can be presented to the plaintiff, defendants, and witnesses for either side, and the questions must be answered in writing. Although the questions can encompass more than the issues of the specific case, the goal of interrogatories is to uncover relevant facts regarding the dispute. The following is a list of sample questions that might be found in an interrogatory:

1. State fully (1) your name, (2) date of birth, (3) residence, (4) professional address, (5) area of specialization if any, and (6) board-certified specialty if any.
2. State your professional nursing training, qualifications, and experience in detail, including (1) each university or college attended by you; (2) each degree awarded to you and the date(s) of same; (3) each hospital with which you have been affiliated at any time up to the present, including the nature of such affiliation and inclusive dates; (4) each nursing society or association of which you have ever been a member and the inclusive dates of membership; and (5) bibliography of all your publications, including titles, dates, and publishers.
3. State the date and place where you first saw the patient, Ms. O, and indicate (1) a detailed account of the nursing, physical, or other history you received about the plaintiff; (2) a description of the nature and scope of any and all examinations or procedures performed by you on this occasion of the plaintiff's first treatment; (3) your observations regarding the plaintiff's condition; (4) a description of all treatments and/or therapy, medication, or instructions rendered by you on June 25, 1999; and (5) nursing diagnoses rendered as to the nature of Ms. O's condition.
4. State in chronologic order each and every date that you thereafter saw the patient and indicate (1) a description of all examinations or procedures performed by you on each such visit; (2) a description of all treatments and/or therapy, medication, or instructions rendered by you on each visit; and (3) a nursing diagnosis rendered as to the nature and/or cause of any disease, bodily impairment, disabilities, conditions, or symptoms.
5. State the names and addresses of any and all persons who have knowledge of any facts related to the issues in this case, and for each person so named, state to the best of your knowledge the substance of all information or knowledge known about this case.
6. State in full and complete detail what you contend are the cause or causes of the injuries as mentioned in Ms. O's complaint, identifying each person responsible for any cause.

In contrast, a *deposition* is a statement taken from the witness under oath but outside the courtroom. This is a formal procedure in which the opposing party's attorney asks questions of the witness and the entire exchange is recorded by a court reporter.

The following are excerpts taken from the deposition of a nurse who was the defendant in an IV-related lawsuit. The plaintiff was the father of an infant whose right foot had been severely damaged by infiltration of an IV infusion. The nurse was charged with negligence because of her failure to appropriately monitor the infusion. During the deposition, the questions were asked by the plaintiff's attorney; the answers were supplied by the defendant (nurse).

Q. Do you have any memory of what IV solution the patient was receiving on April 10, 1999?
A. Dextrose in water 10%.

Q. 10% dextrose in water, is that the same concentration as in the blood?
A. No, that's a hypertonic solution.

Q. By hypertonic, do you mean that the solution going into the patient's vein was stronger chemically than what he already had in his body?
A. Yes.

Q. Is it fair to say that this is a reason why it could be very irritating to the patient's veins and tissues?
A. Yes.

Q. So then, it's fair to say that the tonicity would be one reason why you wouldn't want that concentrated solution to get out into his body tissues?
A. Right.

Q. On April 10, 1999, who was responsible for observing the IV on the patient?
A. If you mean on the 7-3 shift, I was assigned to the patient.

Q. That means, as the nurse assigned to the patient, you were responsible for observing that the IV was infusing correctly.
A. Yes.

A key component of the discovery phase is the use of written standards of care. Interrogatories and depositions of the defendant concentrate on the extent of the nurse's familiarity with professional standards of practice. A lack of familiarity with applicable standards seriously detracts from the defendant's credibility as a witness. Conversely, a well-prepared defendant can take advantage of the opposing attorney's questions. By effectively communicating familiarity with the standards cited, the nurse may retaliate against any inference of negligence, and point out how the nursing actions met or exceeded the written guidelines.

Responsibility for the nurse's actions

Liability denotes that a person has a legal responsibility to fulfill an obligation. Because nurses are responsible for delivering reasonable, prudent nursing care, they are liable for deviations from the established standard and any resultant harm. This is known as the *rule of personal liability.* For example, the nurse administers a prescribed medication, but rapid injection of the drug results in harm to the patient. In this situation, the physician who prescribed the medication is not responsible for the nurse's negligence in administering the drug; the harm was the result of the nurse's actions, not the physician's.

Although the nurse is responsible for nursing actions, in select circumstances, the physician may be held jointly accountable for the negligence of a nurse. This primarily concerns the operating room, where the nurse is considered the "borrowed servant" of the physician. This legal principle is derived from agency law, and it places responsibility on the person who is clearly in charge of the situation and who has the greatest control over all present. It is often referred to as the *captain-of-the-ship* doctrine because it analogizes the surgeon to a captain who is the master of the operating room "crew." Outside the operating room, physicians have rarely been found to be responsible for nurses' negligent acts.

Another concept that must be considered in determining responsibility is the doctrine of *respondeat superior,* or "let the master answer." According to this legal principle, an employer is liable for damages caused by a servant's wrongful act performed within the scope of his or her employment. As a result, even when the nurse is held liable for negligence, the employer may also be held responsible for the nurse's actions. The doctrine does not absolve the nurse from responsibility, but it allows both the nurse and employer to be named in the lawsuit. Application of this legal principle is most common in cases in which a nurse does not have liability insurance and the plaintiff must rely on the employer's insurance to cover the injury.

Locality rule in nursing litigation

The courts have, at times, imposed a uniform definition of reasonable conduct on medical malpractice cases. This is known as the *locality rule.* The rule is a uniquely American legal doctrine and is specific to the medical profession. Based on the rule, the conduct of members of the medical profession may be measured only against the conduct of other medical professionals in that locality.[51] The underlying rationale is that although physicians practicing in smaller towns and rural areas may possess adequate theoretic knowledge, they are not able to observe and practice many of the sophisticated techniques that are common in urban hospitals. This rule has come under serious attack because the wide circulation of medical information, such as professional journals and postgraduate courses, has effectively established national standards for medical care. Some courts have abandoned the rule altogether.[52]

Reasons for being named defendant when no negligence exists

The fact that a nurse is named as a defendant in a negligence case does not necessarily mean that the nurse was negligent. Indeed, the nurse may be an innocent victim who is sued even though not directly involved in the care of the patient who filed the lawsuit. There are legal complexities that play a hidden role in the lawyer's decision to name a nurse as a defendant, and they involve more than the nurse doing something wrong. The lawyer's responsibility to the client is similar to that of the nurse to the patient; he or she has a responsibility to do everything possible to obtain the best results for the client according to accepted standards of professional practice. To accomplish this, three legal technicalities may be used.

Statute of limitations. As previously stated, there is a time frame within which a plaintiff may file a lawsuit or lose the chance to have a day in court. If the plaintiff does not contact an attorney until shortly before the statute of limitations expires, there may not be enough time to investigate the facts of the case fully. To protect the client's interests, the attorney may name every person who could possibly be responsible for the injury. For example, if a patient dies as a result of an overdose of heparin and four different nurses administered the medication to the patient during the last 2 days of the patient's life, the attorney may name all four nurses as defendants. Those nurses determined to be fault free are then removed from the lawsuit before the trial.

Fear of the "empty chair" defense. In the so-called empty chair defense, the defendant claims that someone not named in the lawsuit was responsible for the injury. To prevent this type of defense strategy, the attorney for the plaintiff may name other nurses involved in the patient's care. There are overlapping responsibilities in health care, and often no one person is solely responsible for what happens to the patient.

Charitable immunity statute. A third reason a nurse may be named as defendant is an immunity statute that has been enacted by many states to protect charitable institutions. This statute protects such institutions from excessive liability by setting limits on the amount of compensation for which they are responsible in a negligence lawsuit. For example, an immunity statute may place the limit on awards against charitable institutions at $250,000. Unfortunately, no such limit typically applies to the nurse defendant. Because the institution may be liable for damages if a nurse employee harms the patient through negligent conduct (*respondeat superior*), the plaintiff's attorney can name the nurse as a defendant to override the limits set on the institution's liability.

RISK MANAGEMENT

Risk management is a system used by health care organizations to identify, analyze, and implement strategies for eliminating, minimizing, and coping with liabilities. Although the discipline of health care risk management did not emerge until the mid-1970s, several states now mandate such programs for health care facilities, and JCAHO standards require risk management activities for hospital accreditation.

Concepts

The initial phase of risk management is the identification of the organization's exposures to loss. The four areas that expose an organization to loss are liability, property, personnel, and net income. In health care, liability is the greatest concern because of the risk of medical malpractice and negligence. However, the organization must also consider property exposures caused by physical damage to the facility and the equipment contained within it, personnel exposures related to employee injuries and occupational diseases, and net income exposures resulting from theft or embezzlement.

The second step in risk management is evaluation of the potential loss based on the exposures. By means of a series of complex calculations, the likelihood and potential severity of loss from liability, property, personnel, and net income exposures can be determined. The most appropriate strategy is then selected to manage each potential risk.

The primary emphasis of risk management is managing the exposures. This is the third step in the process of reducing or preventing unplanned loss and may require either risk financing or risk control. *Risk financing* is based on transferring the risk of financial loss from the organization to others through agreements, contracts, or insurance. Purchasing commercial insurance and establishing a self-insurance fund are examples of risk financing. In contrast, *risk control* focuses on activities within the organization that can reduce or eliminate the risk. Risk control activities include exposure avoidance, risk shifting, loss prevention, and loss reduction.

Because an exposure that has been completely avoided cannot produce a loss, *exposure avoidance* is an effective risk control technique. However, in health care, it may not be an effective option. For example, if a hospital determined that IV medication administration posed the greatest threat of nursing negligence, eliminating this practice would exemplify risk avoidance, but such an action would be neither possible nor realistic.

A more feasible method of controlling risk is by *risk transfer,* which shifts the responsibility and liability by means of a contractual agreement. Instead of the organization providing services that subject it to risk, the services may be contracted from another organization that accepts responsibility for the potential exposure to loss. For example, a nursing home may contract professional nurses from an outside agency to administer IV medications within the facility. As part of the agreement, the agency would assume responsibility for the nurses' actions.

Although the first two methods of controlling risks are directed at eliminating risk exposure, the third technique focuses on preventing the exposure. *Loss prevention* is therefore any measure that reduces the probability or frequency of a particular type of loss. For example, identifying trends (e.g., the incidence of phlebitis) and interventions (e.g., measures to reduce the current rate of phlebitis) are two preventive programs that may avert a loss-producing event.

The final method, *loss reduction,* comprises measures to reduce the severity of losses. Loss prevention reduces the frequency of loss but does not completely eliminate it. Therefore loss reduction measures are designed to lessen the size or extent of a loss. If a patient develops an IV-related complication, loss reduction measures include appropriate care following the injury, safeguarding the patient from further injury, and courteous treatment of the patient.

Strategies

In practice, risk management strategies combine the elements of loss reduction *and* loss prevention. Through a series of reactive and proactive activities, the potential for risk exposure is managed. The following are examples of risk management strategies that may decrease the risk of potential liability.

Patient rights. A critical responsibility of nurses is the duty not to violate patient rights. State and federal regulations governing health care mandate that every patient receiving health care be afforded certain rights. Hence, nursing care should be delivered in a manner that honors the rights of the patient. The five major topics pertaining to these rights are informed consent, refusal of treatment, discharge planning, freedom from restraints, and confidentiality. These issues, which are based on a professional obligation to the patient, carry legal consequences.

Informed consent is one of the most effective proactive risk management strategies. Patients must be provided with sufficient information to enable them to rationally decide whether to undergo treatment. For the consent to be valid, the patient must be capable of granting consent, receive sufficient information to make an informed decision, and freely grant consent without coercion.

An example of informed consent involves the insertion of a PICC. The nurse must provide accurate and complete information, including a description of the procedure, potential benefits of such a catheter, possible risks associated with the procedure, and available alternatives. This information must be provided in a language understood by the patient, and there must be an opportunity for dialog between the patient and nurse regarding the information. Only after the patient has considered all options can consent be obtained, and it must reflect the patient's voluntary agreement to the procedure.

Although consent may be obtained verbally, a written agreement may also be required. Such may be the case with specialized procedures such as a PICC insertion. Documentation of the consent generally consists of evidence that the patient has received the necessary information and that the patient has agreed to the proposed procedure. Because such documentation may protect both the patient and the nurse, consent forms are used as a risk management tool. However, the patient's signature on the form does not necessarily imply understanding of the informed consent.

Refusal of treatment refers to the right of every competent adult patient to decline therapy. Because the patient's wishes are paramount to any decision regarding health care, health care professionals are legally required to honor the patient's decisions and any advance directives. For example, a patient has the right to refuse a transfusion. The patient must be informed of the consequences of such a decision and should be required to sign forms documenting receipt of the information and confirming the decision.

Refusing care may also take the form of leaving the health care facility against medical advice. Unless patients pose a danger—to themselves or others—that necessitates emergency detention for observation or psychiatric care, patients cannot be held against their will. Patients must be informed of the consequences of leaving, provided with adequate discharge instructions, and requested to sign forms confirming that they are leaving the facility against medical advice.

Discharge planning concentrates on preparing the patient for eventual discharge from the health care facility. Because patients are discharged when care is no longer medically necessary, governmental regulations mandate that patients be informed of and prepared for their date of discharge.

Preparing the patient for discharge begins at the time of admission to the facility and continues throughout the patient's stay. For example, if a patient is admitted for insertion of an implanted port, instructions regarding care of the port should be initiated at the time of admission and continued until discharge. By doing so, the patient may be adequately prepared to care for the port, and discharge does not need to be postponed until patient teaching has been completed.

Freedom from restraints is a basic right of every patient. The only exceptions are in behavioral management situations or if the patient's safety is in jeopardy. All restraints must be ordered by a physician, with face-to-face evaluation of the patient within 1 hour if the purpose is behavioral management. The patient must be continually monitored, and the reason for and the need to continue the use of restraints must be documented. For example, a restraint may be required to stabilize and secure an IV cannula, but the restraint must be prescribed by the physician for this specific purpose and for a set time. In addition, because of the potential risks associated with the use of restraints, the patient's extremity must be closely monitored.

Confidentiality means that information about the patient must be kept private and should not be released without the patient's permission. This includes information contained in the patient's medical record and details regarding the patient's diagnosis, treatment, and expected length of stay.

Because of the risk of exposure to blood-borne pathogens, IV nurses may be concerned if a patient is HIV positive. If the results of HIV screening are available on the patient's medical record, the nurse must ensure that this information is kept confidential. Unauthorized disclosure carries fines, and if the disclosure results in economic, bodily, or psychologic harm, the person who disclosed the information may be liable for damages.

Unusual occurrence reports.
Documenting an unusual occurrence is a reactive risk management strategy that provides the facts concerning an event that may result in risk exposure. It is an internal reporting mechanism that notifies the organization that an event has occurred and provides an opportunity to investigate the situation while the circumstances are still clear. Such documents were once referred to as *incident reports,* but because of the negative connotation, the terminology has been replaced with *reports of an unusual occurrence* or *variance reports.*

Reporting unusual occurrences can be crucial to the organization's risk management program if several key principles are

followed. First, the report must be an objective account of the event. The purpose of the report is to record the facts; personal opinions should never be included in the document. To ensure that the reports are factual and nonjudgmental, some organizations have converted to a checklist format to record the information, as shown in Fig. 5-2. Second, the type of occurrence must be noted. This assists in a trending analysis to monitor patterns of occurrences. Third, the report must include an assessment of the patient's condition before *and* after the occurrence. This helps evaluate the extent of the injury or severity of the risk exposure. Fourth, no reference to the report should appear in the patient's medical record. Unusual occurrence reports are confidential internal reporting mechanisms. If the patient's medical record contains evidence of a report and the patient later files a lawsuit, the report must be presented in court.

Documentation.
Accurate documentation in the medical record objectively describes the care rendered and the patient's response. Because a lawsuit may be filed years after the event occurred, the documentation in the medical record is often the only factual information available to determine whether there was a deviation from the standard of care. However, the reliability of the medical record may be discredited if there are inconsistencies, contradictory entries, unexplained time gaps, alterations, obliterations, omissions, or illegible entries.

Nurses know that documentation in the medical record must be objective, legible, timely, complete, and accurate. The problem with documentation is often the result of a lack of compliance, not a lack of education. As nurses deliver patient care, they often become frustrated with the amount of paperwork required by their jobs. However, documentation is the only evidence to demonstrate that nursing actions met the legal standard of care. (For additional information, refer to Chapter 26.)

Professional liability insurance.
Insurance is a risk management strategy whereby the nurse may transfer financial risk to an insurer. Because of the doctrine of *respondeat superior,* health care facilities and agencies usually carry insurance for negligent acts of their employees performed within the scope of their job responsibilities. However, many nurses also carry their own individual professional liability insurance.

The decision to purchase liability insurance is a personal one, and many factors must be considered. First, without insurance, the nurse may be required to use personal assets to compensate for a patient's injuries. However, if the actions were within the scope of employment, the damages may be covered by the employer's insurance policy. Second, potential risks must be evaluated. If there is high risk of personal liability because of the practice setting and nursing interventions employed, purchasing individual insurance may be warranted. Third, purchasing insurance requires that the nurse enter a contract with the insurer. As part of the contract, the nurse agrees to pay premiums and the insurer agrees to compensate the patient if the nurse is found guilty of malpractice. The nurse must evaluate the price of the premiums and understand that compensation is limited to the terms set in the insurance policy. Because insurance can be complex, the nurse must consider all benefits and risks before purchasing professional liability insurance.

A. STAFF MOST CLOSELY INVOLVED (circle one)	B. IV VARIANCE (circle one)
1. Attending physician 2. RN 3. LPN 4. Pharmacist 5. Pharmacy technician 6. IV nurse 7. Delivery technician	1. Incorrect compounding 2. IV not checked properly 3. Incorrect rate 4. Infiltration 5. Phlebitis +1 6. Phlebitis +2 7. Phlebitis +3 8. Phlebitis +4
C. DELIVERY VARIANCE (circle one)	D. MEDICATION VARIANCE (circle one)
1. Nondelivery 2. Delivery off schedule 3. Incomplete delivery 4. Wrong product delivery 5. Product damaged	1. Adverse effect 2. Omission 3. Duplication 4. Incorrect time 5. Incorrect route 6. Incorrect medication 7. Incorrect patient 8. Incorrect dose 9. Documentation incorrect

FIG. 5-2 *Example of categorizing IV-related variances on an unusual occurrence report form.*

Patient relations. It has been said that it is easier to sue an enemy than a friend. A patient who perceives the nurse as an impersonal, aloof person who is unconcerned with the patient's welfare is more apt to initiate legal action if an injury occurs. However, if the lines of communication are open between the nurse and patient and expressions of anger, fear, and complaints by the patient are promptly investigated and resolved, claims of negligence may be avoided.

Quality management. Quality management is the continuous effort to improve patient care. It serves as a risk management strategy because it is a proactive approach to identify opportunities for improvement. Not only are problems identified and resolved, but outcomes are improved by enhancing the processes involved in patient care. (For additional information, see Chapter 4.)

In today's increasingly cost-conscious and litigious health care environment, IV nurses must provide quality IV nursing care. Excellent nursing care is the best method of preventing liability. If care is rendered appropriately, the patient adequately monitored, actions accurately documented, and the physician informed of changes in the patient's condition, patient injury and litigation may be avoided.

References

1. Beare PG, Myers JL: *Principles and practice of adult health nursing*, ed 3, St Louis, 1997, Mosby.
2. 29 C.F.R. §1910.1200, et. seq.
3. OSHA PUB. 8-1.1., OSHA Office of Occupational Medicine (Jan. 1986).
4. 29 C.F.R. §1910.1200, et. seq. *See also*, "Occupational Exposure to Bloodborne Pathogens," OSHA PUB. 3127 (1996).
5. 24 Am J Infect Control 262-93, 1996. *See also*, Bennett J, Brachman P: *Hospital infections*, ed 4, Philadelphia, 1998, JB Lippincott.
6. 42 USC §§ 4321-4347.
7. 5 USC § 2601, et. seq.
8. 42 USC § 321, et. seq.
9. 42 USC § 6992, et. seq.
10. 42 USC § 9601, et. seq.
11. 42 USC § 11011, et. seq.
12. Medical Device Amendments.
13. 21 USC § 301 et. seq. *See also*, 21 CFR parts 803 and 807. The Safe Medical Device Act was further amended by the FDA Modernization Act of 1997.
14. 21 USC § 801, et. seq.
15. 21 USC § 811, 812.
16. Shafler M, Marieb EN: *The nurse, pharmacology, and drug therapy*, Redwood City, La, 1999, Addison-Wesley.
17. 21 CFR §§ 1301-1312.
18. 42 USC § 1395 cc. *See, generally*, Parkman C: The Patient Self-Determination Act: measuring its outcomes, *Nursing Mgt* Oct 1997.
19. Fletcher JC: The Patient Self-Determination Act, *Hastings Center Rep* 20:33, 1990.
20. Rhodes AM, Miller RD: *Nursing and the law*, ed 5, Rockville, Md, 1997, Aspen.
21. Weinstein S, Plumer A: *Plumer's principles and practices of intravenous nursing*, ed 6, Boston, 1997, Little, Brown.
22. Katz J, Green E: *Managing quality: a guide to monitoring and evaluating nursing services*, St Louis, 1992, Mosby.
23. *Koeniguer v. Eckrich*, 422 NW2d 600 (S.D. 1988) ("standards published by the ANA and various general practices treatises" relevant in nurse malpractice cases).
24. Joint Commission on Accreditation of Healthcare Organizations: First Annual Invitational Forum for Liaison Network Organizations, Workshop Materials, Chicago, JCAHO, 1993.

25. American Nurses Association: *Standards of nursing practice,* ed 2, Washington, DC, 1998, American Nurses Association.

26. Intravenous Nurses Society: Infusion nursing standards of practice, *JIN* (suppl) 23(6S), 2000.

27. American Association of Blood Banks: *AABB technical manual,* ed 13, Philadelphia, 1999, JB Lippincott.

28. American Society of Health-System Pharmacists: ASHS technical assistance bulletin on handling cytotoxic hazardous drugs, *Am J Hosp Pharm* 47:1033, 1990.

29. Ritter HT: Evaluating and selecting general-purpose infusion pumps, *JIN* 13:156, 1990.

30. Gillies DA: *Nursing management: a systems approach,* ed 3, Philadelphia, 1994, WB Saunders.

31. Creighton H: *Law every nurse should know,* ed 5, Philadelphia, 1986, WB Saunders.

32. Fiesta J: *The law and liability: a guide for nurses,* ed 2, New York, 1988, John Wiley & Sons.

33. Holmes HN, managing editor: *Nurse's legal handbook,* ed 4, Springhouse, Pa, 2000, Springhouse Corp.

34. *Vassey v. Burch,* 262 SE2d 865 (NC Ct. App. 1980). *See also,* Sweeney P: Proving nursing negligence, *Trial* 27:34, 1991.

35. *See, generally,* Miller-Slades D: Liability theories in nursing negligence cases, 33 *Trial Liability* 43 Clev. St. L. Rev. 57 (1995).

36. *Gibson v. Bossier City General Hospital,* 594 So. 2d 1332 (La. Ct. App. 1991) ("[T]he events and circumstances [of the case] were beyond the knowledge of the average person" and therefore an expert witness was needed regarding alleged improper injection of medication).

37. Popp P: Experts in malpractice litigation: what about nurses, *Legal Med* 165, 1992.

38. Fiesta J: Nursing malpractice: cause for consideration, *Nurs Manage* 30(2):12, 1999.

39. *Habuda v. Trustees of Rex Hospital, Inc.,* 164 SE2d 17 (N.C. Ct. App. 1968) (nurse administered pHisoHex antibacterial scrub, instead of Milk of Magnesia, which was similar in appearance and location).

40. *Polonsky v. Union Hospital,* 418 NE2d 620 (Mass. Ct. App. 1981) (nurse found negligent for not knowing of dangers of giving sleeping drug Dalmane to elderly patient recovering from a heart attack.)

41. *Harrington v. Rush Presbyterian-St. Lukes Hospital,* 569 NE2d 15 (Ill. App. 1990).

42. *Hill v. Ohio University,* 610 NE2d 634 (Ohio Ct. Cl. 1988) (alleged failure to give "deep intramuscular injection" of Kenalog, as required).

43. *Belmon v. St. Francis Cabrini Hosp.,* 427 So.2d 541 (La. App. 1983) (failure to notice hemorrhage at needle puncture sites, a "major known complication" and "well-known" risk of certain anticoagulant).

44. *Georgetti v. United Hospital Medical Ctr.,* 611 NYS2d 579 (1992) ("It is clear that when an attending physician gives direct and explicit orders to hospital staff, nurses are not authorized to unilaterally depart from them.")

45. *Jensen v. Archbishop Bergen Mercy Hosp.,* 459 NW2d 178 (Neb. 1991).

46. *Dixon v. Taylor,* 431 S.E. 2d 778 (N.C. Ct. App. 1993) (failure to keep code cart restocked). *Guilbeaux v. Lafayette General Hospital,* 589 So. 2d 629 (La. Ct. 1991) (nurse committed malpractice by improperly removing Jackson-Pratt drain, leaving a strip of tube in the patient's back).

47. *Maciag v. Strato Medical Corp.,* 644 A.2d 647 (N.J. Super. Ct. 1994) (*res ipsa* applied when subclavian venous catheter fractured inside unconscious patient).

48. *Roach v. Springfield Clinic,* 585 NE2d 1070 (Ill. App. 1991) (failure to notify physician of abnormal fetal heart tones detected by monitoring system).

49. *Vogler v. Dominguez,* 624 NE2d 56 (Ind. Ct. App. 1993) (failure to report "abnormalities" or changes in a patient's condition can be negligent).

50. *Berdyck v. Shinde,* 613 N.E. 2d 1014 (Ohio 1993) (nurse who did not report nausea, headaches, and stomach pain of patient was negligent).

51. *Alef v. Alta Bates Hospital,* 6 Cal. Rptr. 2d 900 (Cal. App. 1992) ("It is well-established that a nurse's conduct [should] be measured by the standard of care of other nurses in the same or similar locality and under similar circumstances.").

52. *Berdyck v. Shinde,* 613 N.E. 2d 1014 (Ohio 1993) (court expressed "serious doubts as to whether any locality rule is applicable to registered nurses").

Chapter

6

Anatomy and Physiology Related to Intravenous Therapy

Lynn C. Hadaway, MEd, RNC, CRNI

Knowledge of the anatomy and physiology of the skin, peripheral vasculature, and cardiopulmonary and neurologic systems is crucial for the safe administration of any parenteral therapy. Many factors related to these body functions can encumber or increase the success of infusions. Conversely, parenteral therapy administration can have a detrimental effect on the anatomy and

physiologic function of all body systems. Our goal is to consider all pertinent factors in an effort to manage the risk of parenteral therapy and ensure a positive outcome for the patient.

When an IV device is inserted, the skin is the first organ affected. Skin serves several functions: it is a mechanical barrier against microorganisms and radiation, provides sensory and temperature regulation, and helps maintain fluid and electrolyte balance. Breaking this natural barrier increases the risk of infection. The use of antiseptic solutions, ointment, and dressing materials can affect the skin's natural composition of bacteria, oils, and sweat. Factors such as age, chronic disease, and the environment can produce changes in the skin, making entry through the skin a difficult process.

Vascular anatomy is of primary importance when locating and cannulating veins or arteries. Both the insertion site and location of the cannula tip are important considerations. Extreme variations in pH, osmolality, volume, and rate can alter the risk of complications if consideration is not given to the size of the vessel lumen and the amount and type of blood flow. Fluid volume status and general cardiopulmonary condition can limit the volume and rate of infusion and lead to a negative patient outcome when not monitored closely.

The neurologic system affects all other systems and can influence the success or failure of any parenteral therapy. The sensory receptors in the skin, the innervation of the walls of veins and arteries, the systemic responses evoked by emotion and pain, and the use of the epidural space for infusions necessitate knowledge of the central nervous system.

Finally, variation in personal technique used for insertion, infusion, injection, and withdrawal is another vital component affecting anatomy and physiology. The impact of differences in cannula types and components and solution composition can be evaluated and monitored more easily than the nuances of individual technique. A thorough working knowledge of the anatomy and physiology of multiple body systems, combined with a carefully crafted expertise, are necessary to ensure a positive patient outcome.

INTEGUMENT AND CONNECTIVE TISSUE

The integument, or skin, is a highly specialized organ that protects the body from its environment. It ranges in thickness from 1.5 to 4.0 mm, with the thickest skin appearing on the palms of the hands and plantar aspect of the feet.[1] Skin is divided into two layers: the epidermis and the dermis. Lying immediately under the dermis is the hypodermis, which is composed of adipose tissue. This layer cushions and protects the underlying structures and acts as insulation for the body (Fig. 6-1).

Loose connective tissue lies under the skin and is composed of several types of fibers and cells. Its primary functions include providing structure and defense. Superficial veins for venipuncture lie in this layer of loose tissue.

Structure

Epidermis. The epidermis is composed of five layers, or strata, of squamous cells. These layers represent different stages of the maturation process. Individual cells are constantly maturing, moving upward to the surface and being replaced by new cells from the base. These cells, or keratinocytes, contain keratin, a protective protein found in epithelial tissue that is subject to drying and other mechanical stresses. As keratinocytes mature, they change in shape and content, becoming a dense layer of mechanically strong parallel fibers.[1] Stressful agents such as prolonged exposure to sunlight, habitual pressure, and abrasion may cause thickening of the keratin layer. This may explain difficult venipunctures in some patients, especially those who are manual laborers or others whose lifestyle involves excessive exposure to sunlight.

Three other types of cells can be found in the epidermis:

Langerhans' cells, melanocytes, and lymphocytes, each functioning in symbiotic fashion with keratinocytes. Symbiotic interactions are important in growth, development, inflammation, immunology, and wound healing.[1] Langerhans' cells function in cellular defense by detecting antigens and bringing them in contact with T lymphocytes. This process may be clinically responsible for skin reactions such as allergic contact dermatitis or graft rejection. Patients with some types of skin diseases and those exposed to ultraviolet radiation may have a reduced number of Langerhans' cells, or the cells may be functionally impaired.[2] Melanocytes contain the pigment that imparts color to the skin. Variation in color depends on the number and composition of melanocytes and on genetic, hormonal, and environmental factors.

Between the epidermis and dermis is a basement membrane, or lamina. This membrane has a mechanical function, providing additional support and flexibility to the skin. It contains adhesive materials that help anchor the epidermis to the dermis. Other cellular activities, such as antigen-antibody complex development and the filtration of other large molecules, occur in this membrane.

Dermis. The dermis, the thickest layer of the skin, is soft connective tissue with varying amounts of elastin fibers, collagen fibers, blood, and lymphatic vessels. Collagen is arranged in bundles and is the largest component of the dermis. Sebaceous glands, sweat glands and ducts, hair follicles, and arrector pili muscles surrounding the follicles are also located in the dermis (see Fig. 6-1).

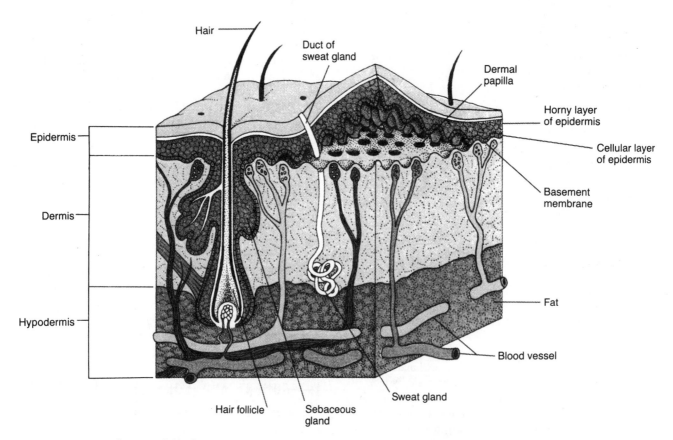

FIG. 6-1 *Anatomy of the skin.* (From Ignatavicius DD, Bayne MV: *Medical-surgical nursing: a nursing process approach,* Philadelphia, 1991, WB Saunders, p. 1134.)

The dermis is divided into the papillary and reticular layers. The papillary layer is immediately under the epidermis and serves to anchor the epidermis mechanically and support it metabolically. Fingerlike projections extend into the base of the epidermis to enhance the bond between the two layers. The reticular layer is the deepest and is characterized by dense, irregular, connective tissue. This type of connective tissue is formed by strong collagen fiber bundles arranged in a multilayered network, providing the ability to stretch. Elastin fibers are usually thinner and have almost perfect recoil.

The hair bulb, responsible for generating the growth of hair, is located in the dermis and is surrounded by the hair follicle. Arrector pili muscles extend at an angle from the follicle into the dermis. When these muscles are stimulated by cold or emotion, the hair shaft is pulled upward and the skin appears dimpled.

Sebaceous glands are located in the angle between the muscle and follicle and the muscular action expresses sebum, the secretion from the sebaceous glands. Sebum passes through a duct, into the hair follicle, and onto the skin surface. The complete function of sebum, composed of glycerides, cholesterol, and wax esters, is not known, but it is believed that it lubricates and protects the hair and skin and contributes to body odor.

Sweat glands and ducts arise from the dermis and communicate with the skin surface. These glands secrete a clear, odorless fluid containing urea, lactate, amino acids, and ions such as sodium, chloride, calcium, and bicarbonate. Secretion is stimulated by temperature elevation and emotional stimulation.

Subcutaneous tissue. Continuing downward to the next layer, the superficial fascia is a layer of loose connective tissue (Fig. 6-2). This layer contains the same collagen and

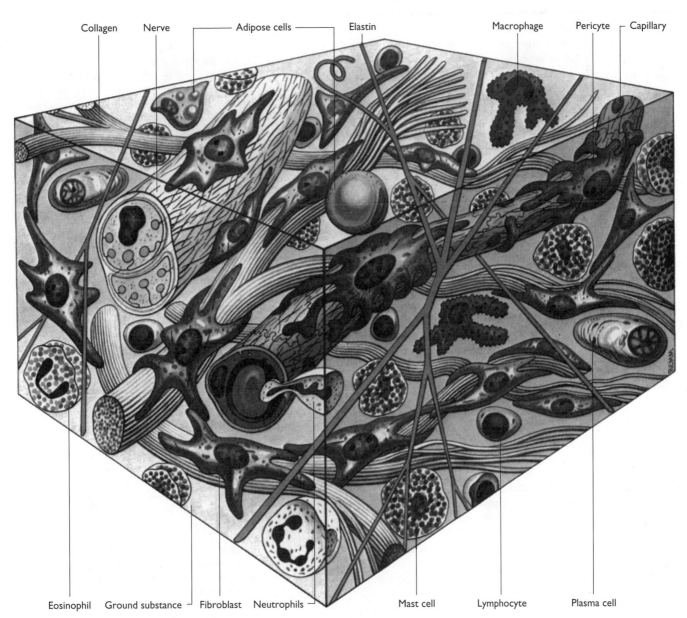

FIG. 6-2 *Schematic reconstruction of loose connective tissue showing the characteristic cell types, fiber, and intercellular spaces.* (From Williams PL et al, editors: *Gray's anatomy*, ed 37, New York, 1989, Churchill Livingstone, p. 59.)

elastin fibers as the dermis. Adipose tissue or fat cells are located in this layer, where they serve as energy stores and thermal insulation. A large variety of defensive cells similar to those found in the blood are found in this tissue. Among all these important components lie the superficial veins used for peripheral venipuncture.

Defense cells include fibroblasts, macrophages, lymphocytes, and mast cells. Fibroblasts, the most abundant, are involved with the synthesis of proteins and help create a fibrous matrix that forms granulation tissue during wound healing. Macrophages play an important role in the defense mechanisms of the immune system by attacking and engulfing foreign substances. These cells can be mobile or attached to other fibers and are similar in action to circulating monocytes and Langerhans' cells in the epidermis. Macrophages are responsible for bringing antigens in contact with lymphocytes.

Lymphocytes are present in loose connective tissue, but their number can increase greatly during pathologic states. They synthesize and secrete antibodies after stimulation from an antigen. There are two types of lymphocytes: B and T. B lymphocytes originate in the bone marrow and travel to various locations through the lymph. They mainly produce antibodies or immunoglobulins when stimulated by an antigen. T lymphocytes are formed in the bone marrow and migrate to the thymus gland before moving into the lymphatic system. Their function is not completely known, but they do destroy viruses, fungi, and tumor cells.

Mast cells are specialized cells found in all connective tissue. They originate in the bone marrow and are similar to basophils in the blood. Their protective actions include defense against parasites, promote phagocytosis, and stimulate connective tissue repair. They are also the principal mediators of allergic reactions. The mean number of mast cells in the skin ranges from 7000 to 20,000/mm^3.[2] They can be found in large numbers around blood vessels and nerves.

Blood is supplied to the skin through small arteries that penetrate from the superficial fascia to the reticular layer of the dermis and then branch into a sheetlike plexus. Arterioles supply sweat and sebaceous glands and hair follicles with another plexus that is formed as arterioles pass through the reticular and papillary layers of the dermis. Capillaries loop upward to the base of the epidermis and venules pass back through the dermis to join small veins in the superficial fascia.[1] The skin is also served by a large number of small lymphatic vessels with numerous anastomoses at all levels.

Cutaneous circulation serves as a thermoregulator. Blood flow to the skin is 10 times greater than its nutritional requirements. In response to the need for heat loss or conservation, cutaneous blood flow can be increased or decreased by 20 times the normal capacity. Cold conditions can quickly cause vasoconstriction, making venipuncture difficult, yet heat application rapidly causes vasodilation.[1]

The extensive nerve supply in the skin acts as a sensory organ and regulator of response to thermal stimuli. Sensory receptors in the form of free nerve endings provide needed information about the external environment. Encapsulated mechanoreceptors are found in the deep dermal layer and respond to weight, pressure, and vibration.

Normal resident flora on human skin includes four bacterial groups and a fungal group. Coryneforms and staphylococci are the major bacterial groups, with *Micrococcus* and *Acinetobacter* as the minor bacterial group. *Acinetobacter* species can easily be found in the antecubital fossa. *Malassezia* is the primary fungus found on skin. Microorganisms are found in pilosebaceous ducts and on the skin surface in microcolonies. These colonies are larger in men than in women and are found at different quantities depending on the type of skin. For instance, the dry skin of the forearm may have only 100 organisms per colony, whereas the shoulder area may have colonies containing 10^5 organisms.[2] Factors affecting the growth of skin microorganisms include the amount and type of nutrients such as lipids, adherence properties of the flora, and humidity at the skin surface. Presence of water at the skin surface leads to rapid microbial growth in short periods.

Effects of aging

The normal aging process, a physiologic process, can have a distinct affect on the appearance and performance of the skin. An environmental source of skin changes is habitual sun exposure, called *photoaging,* and is considered to be preventable damage.[2]

Changes in the appearance of skin attributed to age include wrinkling, dryness, and looseness. These effects can be found in all layers and cells of the skin (Table 6-1). Such changes indicate that the skin has a continually decreasing capability to respond to forces and strain, becoming more rigid and inflexible. The common clinical picture of these problems as related to parenteral therapy includes bleeding from venipuncture sites, shearing of skin layers when tape or dressing materials are removed, and excessive skin dryness with the use of alcohol and other antiseptic agents.

Table 6-1	**Anatomic and Physiologic Changes Related to Aging**
LOCATION	**CHANGE(S)**
Epidermis	Flattening of projections between the two layers; widening space between keratinocytes; slower maturation of keratinocytes; decreased thickness of layer
Dermis	Decreased thickness of layer; thicker and calcified elastin fibers, sometimes with complete fragmentation; decrease in total amount of collagen; reduction in vascular network around hair follicles and glands; decreased number of blood vessels and shorter capillary loops; decreased amount of mucopolysaccharides, resulting in changes in turgor; decreased number of nerve endings; decreased number of sweat glands and sweat production
Cells	Decreased number of melanocytes, resulting in decreased protection from ultraviolet light; decreased number of mast cells and reduction in histamine release

Photoaging from exposure to the sun differs with the length of exposure, gender, and individual differences in the skin. However, the same problems are seen as those that occur with the normal aging process.

Role in infection control

The three most important factors in infection control are immunocompetence, nutritional status, and the maintenance of an intact integument. Therefore careful attention must be given to the condition of the skin under dressings, the patient's response to various antiseptic solutions and dressing materials, and the number of venous, arterial, or epidural cannulations with the necessary break in the skin.

The skin's primary function in the control of infection is as a mechanical barrier to the invasion of pathogenic organisms. Chemical barriers include sebaceous secretions that have antibacterial and antifungal fatty acids, the role of circulating im-munoglobulins, cellular immunity and delayed hypersensitivity, and the acidic pH of the skin (usually between 3 and 5).[2] The inflammatory process and subsequent infections are influenced by these factors.

Wound healing

Because initiating any parenteral therapy requires breaking the skin, it is appropriate to consider the process for the healing of that wound. The anatomy of skin has been presented from the outer surface inward. However, to understand the process of restoring the dermis and epidermis after injury, it is necessary to discuss the repair of the dermis and the regeneration of the epidermis.

Immediately after any wound is sustained, the initial phase is one of inflammation in response to stimulation of platelets and mast cells (Fig. 6-3). Bleeding is controlled by activation of the complex clotting cascade and the activation of platelets. The

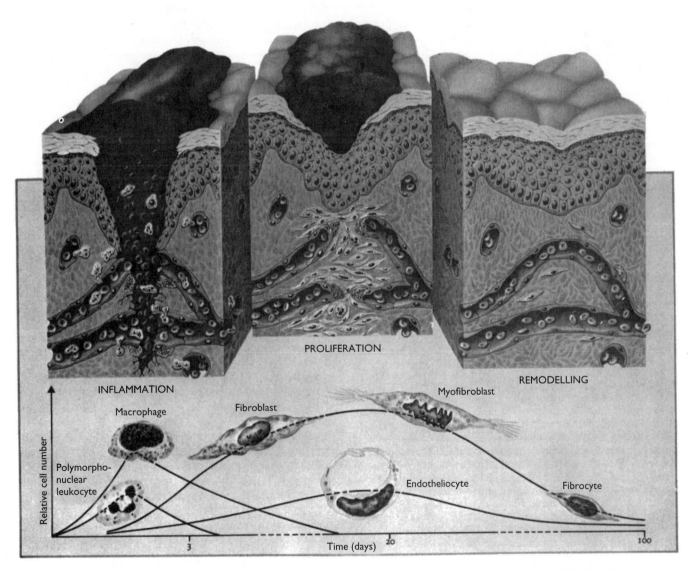

FIG. 6-3 *Normal response of skin to incision.* (From Williams PL et al, editors: *Gray's anatomy,* ed 37, New York, 1989, Churchill Livingstone, p. 85.)

permeability of local blood vessels increases and causes plasma proteins to leak into the wound, forming an extravascular clot. Neutrophils, which control bacteria, and monocytes enter the wound. Monocytes become macrophages and have a phagocytic action; in addition, they release chemicals necessary for granulation.

The second phase, proliferation or granulation, is characterized by the formation of a large number of capillaries. These are embedded in a thick matrix of fibronectin, a glycoprotein that acts like glue. Macrophages are present in this stage and act to debride the wound. Collagen is synthesized, which adds more strength to the tissue.

Within a few hours after injury, the epidermis begins to regenerate new epithelial cells. Keratinocytes use a "leapfrog" action, moving over each other to reach the bed of the wound. They then stop moving and begin to divide, forming new epidermal cells. This process seals and protects the healing wound and severs the connection between the underlying clot and wound surface.

Two factors may inhibit the healing process at this point. The presence of antiinflammatory steroids prevents macrophages from entering the wound, thus slowing the formation of granulation tissue. A lack of ascorbic acid (vitamin C) can interfere with the production of collagen.

The final stage of dermal repair is remodeling. Granulation tissue, containing a large number of cells and blood vessels, is gradually replaced with scar tissue, which contains fewer cells and vessels. Fibronectin is removed and replaced with randomly cross-linked collagen fibers. Over time these fibers become more organized, and the tensile strength of the new tissue improves, although it will regain only about 80% of its original tensile strength.[3] This entire process usually occurs over several months.

Healing of wounds is delayed when there is excessive or prolonged bleeding during the initial injury. Red blood cells and fibrin must be cleared away before the repair begins. Lack of oxygen in the tissue causes vasoconstriction and decreases the deposit of cells necessary for the inflammatory process. Improper nutrition and underlying diseases such as diabetes also slow wound healing.

NEUROLOGIC SYSTEM

The human nervous system acts as an information loop. When changes in the environment are picked up by the sensory organs of the body, information is fed back to the controlling organ, or brain, which coordinates this with numerous other pieces of information, decides what response to make, and then communicates that response back to the body.

The system can be studied in many ways. Distinct functional divisions of the nervous system include the following: (1) the sensory ability to transmit information from tactile, visual, and auditory receptors; (2) the motor functions, controlling all skeletal and smooth muscles; and (3) the autonomic system, which controls glands and smooth muscles. Anatomic divisions are the central system, composed of the brain and spinal cord, and the peripheral system, composed of 12 cranial and 31 spinal nerves.

Functional divisions

Sensory receptors. There are five types of sensory receptors (mechanoreceptors, thermoreceptors, nociceptors, electromagnetic receptors, and chemoreceptors), with corresponding stimuli for each (Table 6-2). Except for electromagnetic receptors, all have an affect on parenteral therapy. Many types of stimulation, such as heat, light, cold, pressure, and sound, must be processed appropriately. All these variations in modalities of sensation are transmitted along different afferent fibers, ending at a specific point in the central nervous system. This is called the *labeled line principle,*[4] which means that pain receptors transmit a painful response whether it is caused by puncture, crushing, or electricity. The sensation of touch is transmitted along a single path, no matter how the stimulation occurs.

The sensation of pain can have a profound impact on parenteral therapy. Pain can be felt quickly or slowly. Fast pain is felt within 0.1 second after stimuli, but slow pain takes seconds to be felt and may increase over minutes.[4] Pain receptors in skin, subcutaneous tissue, and vessel walls are free nerve endings. Fast pain is associated with skin punctures, cuts, or electrical shock. Slow pain is more intense, occurring over a prolonged period, and is usually associated with tissue destruction. Mechanical, thermal, and chemical stimuli can activate pain receptors. Fast pain is evoked primarily by mechanical and thermal means, whereas slow pain is associated with all three. Histamine, bradykinin, potassium ions, serotonin, and various acids can stimulate pain receptors, and all are found in damaged tissue.

Motor function. Information controlling muscular and secretory functions is sent from the central nervous system along efferent nerve fibers. These motor functions are controlled by specific areas of the cerebral cortex and brain stem. The pyramidal tract (or corticospinal tract) is the principal pathway for the transmission of impulses from the motor cortex through the brainstem and down the spinal cord. Other pathways for impulses include the mesencephalon (midbrain) and the cerebellum. The term *extrapyramidal motor system* has been used clinically to describe those motor functions outside the pyramidal system. Because there are many functions and pathways included in this term, it is difficult to use it for physiologic purposes. However, the term *extrapyramidal side effects* is used to describe uncoordinated motor movements of the neck, jaw, and extremities that are associated with the administration of some types of medications.

Autonomic nervous system. The autonomic system regulates the body's internal organs and controls such functions as glandular secretions, arterial blood pressure, sweating, and body temperature. Perhaps the most astonishing factor about this system is the speed with which changes occur. The heart rate can double within 3 to 5 seconds, the blood pressure can drop enough to cause fainting within 4 to 5 seconds, and sweating can occur within seconds.[4] The two major divisions of this system are the sympathetic and parasympathetic (Fig. 6-4). The vagus nerve contains about 75% of all parasympathetic nerve fibers.

It is difficult to generalize about the effects of each of these systems on an individual organ. Sympathetic stimulation may cause excitation in some organs but have an inhibitory effect on others. The same can be said for the parasympathetic system.

Table 6-2   Sensory Receptors and Related Parenteral Therapy Procedures

TYPE OF RECEPTOR	SENSATION	EFFECT OF PARENTERAL THERAPY
Mechanoreceptor	Skin tactile sensibilities	Palpation for veins and arteries; application of antiseptic solutions and dressings; removal of tape and dressings
	Deep tissue sensibilities	Puncture of vein or artery; tight or constricting dressing
	Arterial pressure control through the baroceptor or pressure receptor system in all large arteries	Excessive infusion of intravenous fluid, increasing circulating blood volume, and activating pressure receptors
	Hearing	
	Equilibrium	
Thermoreceptor	Cold, warmth	Application of heat or cold to treat phlebitis and/or infiltration
Nociceptor	Pain	Puncture of vein or artery for insertion of any cannula; puncture of lumbar area for epidural catheter insertion; removal of dressings; infusion of irritating medications subcutaneously; application of extreme heat or cold
Electromagnetic receptor	Vision	None
Chemoreceptor	Decreased arterial pressure stimulates receptors in aorta and carotid arteries to respond to low oxygen levels and increased carbon dioxide levels	Inadequate amount of solution infused, resulting in decreased circulating blood volume
	Osmotic changes in blood	Infusion of extremely hypertonic or hypotonic solutions
	Taste	
	Smell	

Also, the two systems may work in a reciprocal arrangement, with one causing excitation and the other producing inhibition. For example, sympathetic stimulation increases the rate and force of heart contraction, and parasympathetic stimulation has the opposite effect. Systemic blood vessels, especially in the skin of extremities, are constricted by sympathetic stimulation and thus increase the difficulty of peripheral venipuncture. Parasympathetic stimulation has no effect on blood vessels except for those in the face that react in the form of a blush.[4]

Anatomic divisions

Central nervous system. The spinal cord extends from the medulla oblongata and occupies about two thirds of the length of the vertebral column. In most adults, the cord terminates between the first and second lumbar vertebrae. The cord is enclosed within three protective layers. The pia mater is the most proximal to the cord, the arachnoid mater is next, and the dura mater is the most distal. Between the pia and arachnoid mater is the subarachnoid space, which contains cerebrospinal fluid. The subdural space lies between the arachnoid and dura mater and does not contain fluid. The subdural space, below the level of the cord, can be used for the epidural infusion of medication, such as for pain management.

Peripheral nervous system. Twelve pairs of cranial nerves and 31 pairs of spinal nerves compose this system. Cranial nerves originate at the base of the brain and have four functions: motor, somatic sensory, special senses, and parasympathetic.

Of primary importance for parenteral therapy is the vagus nerve, which has the longest course of any cranial nerve. Numerous branches extend to the pharynx, larynx, heart, lungs, esophagus, stomach, liver, pancreas, spleen, small intestines, and kidneys. The heart is innervated by six branches of the vagus nerve. Stimulation leads to a depressant effect on the cardiac muscle, with clinical symptoms of bradycardia and hypotension. This syndrome is known as *vasovagal syncope,* and it may be preceded by weakness, nausea, vomiting, and pallor. The nervous and cardiovascular systems react together, but the exact physiologic mechanisms are unknown. This reaction could be triggered by pain, fear of pain, emotional stress, or the Valsalva maneuver.

The brachial plexus arises from cervical and thoracic spinal nerves, passing posteriorly to the clavicle in close proximity to the subclavian artery and veins. There are two large branches of this plexus: the supraclavicular and infraclavicular (Fig. 6-5). These branches bifurcate into smaller nerves that serve the muscles and cutaneous areas of the shoulder, chest, and upper and lower arm. The close proximity of this group of nerves to the puncture sites of the subclavian vein make damage to the nerves and ultimately the areas served by that nerve a real possibility.

The median, ulnar, and radial nerves are all branches of the brachial plexus. The median nerve passes laterally to the brachial artery and then crosses the artery, descending medially into the antecubital fossa and then into the forearm and palm of the hand. Branches of the median nerve can be superficial in the volar aspect or palm side of the wrist (Fig. 6-6). Veins in this

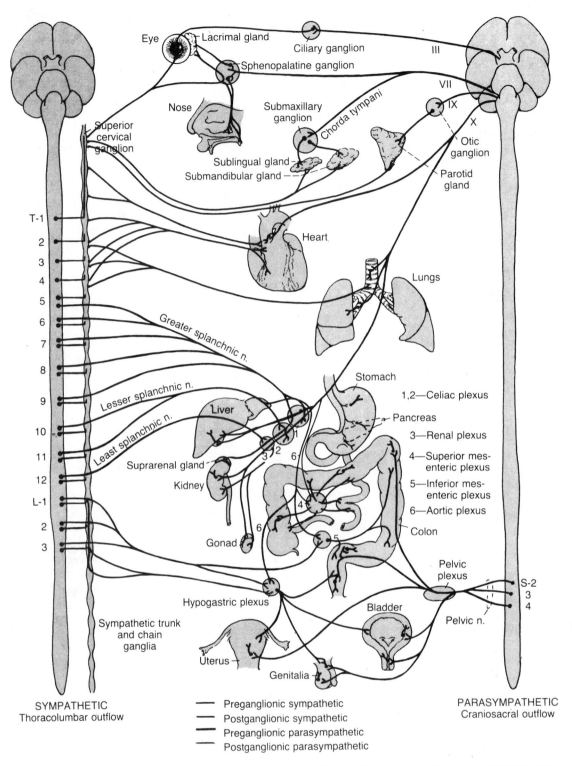

FIG. 6-4 *Autonomic nervous system.* (From Jacob SW, Francone CA: *Elements of anatomy and physiology,* ed 2, Philadelphia, 1989, WB Saunders, p. 129.)

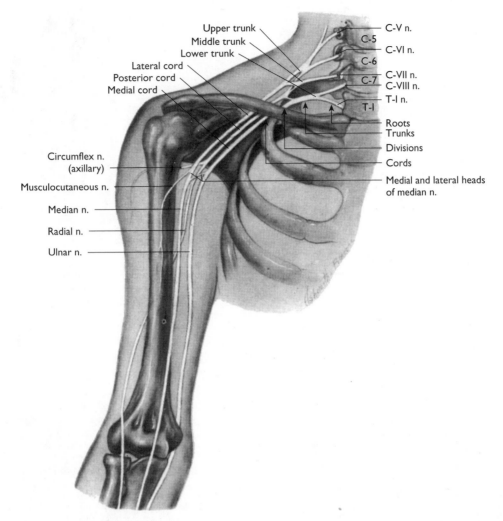

Upper trunk
Middle trunk
Lower trunk
Lateral cord
Posterior cord
Medial cord

C-V n.
C-5
C-VI n.
C-6
C-VII n.
C-7
C-VIII n.
T-I
T-I n.
Roots
Trunks
Divisions
Cords
Medial and lateral heads
of median n.

Circumflex n.
(axillary)
Musculocutaneous n.
Median n.
Radial n.
Ulnar n.

FIG. 6-5 *Brachial plexus and its skeletal relations.* (From Jacob SW, Francone CA: *Elements of anatomy and physiology,* ed 2, Philadelphia, 1989, WB Saunders, p. 126.)

area appear to be good for cannulation, but venipuncture is usually painful in this area because of the close proximity of the nerve.

In the lower extremity, the sacral plexus arises from the sacral vertebrae and descends the leg in much the same manner as the brachial plexus in the arm. Of particular importance is the medial plantar nerve, which passes on the medial aspect of the foot near the ankle. The saphenous nerve passes close to the saphenous vein on the anterior aspect of the foot. When the foot of an infant is used for venipuncture, with subsequent immobilization of the joint, the nerves can be damaged if adequate padding and range of motion exercises are not used.

THE THORACIC CAVITY

The borders and boundaries of the thorax help determine the optimal locations for cannula insertion and cannula tip placement. The presence of any cannula and the solutions infused can affect the physiology of the heart and lungs, in addition to the anatomy of the vessels.

Bony thorax

The first rib curves from the first thoracic vertebra to the upper border of the sternum. This junction is difficult to palpate because the clavicle joins the sternum immediately in front of and superior to it (Fig. 6-7). The costoclavicular ligament connects the first rib with the lower border of the clavicle close to the sternum. Motion of the sternoclavicular joint is involved with all shoulder movement. The first rib moves with respiration.

Subclavian vein cannulation in the medial aspect or close to the junction of the clavicle and first rib can have a negative outcome. Known as the *pinch-off syndrome,* the scissorlike action of these bones can sever the cannula, causing a catheter emboli.[5,6] Positioning the patient in the Trendelenburg position with a rolled towel or sheet between the scapulas helps open the

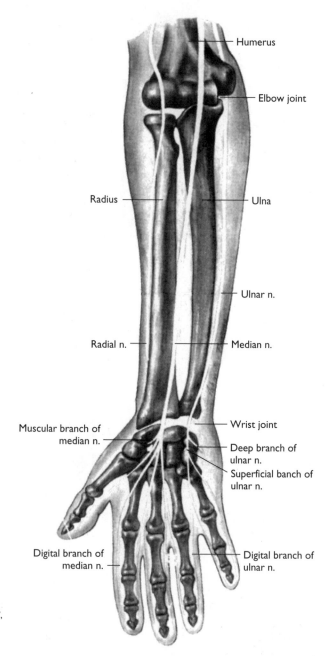

FIG. 6-6 *Nerves of the right forearm and hand (palmar view).* (From Jacob SW, Francone CA: *Elements of anatomy and physiology,* ed 2, Philadelphia, 1989, WB Saunders, p. 127.)

angle of these bones. When the patient is moved from this position, the angle is closed. The minimal clinical problem is compression of the cannula, causing difficult infusion. Irritation to the tunica intima of the vein could compound the problem, with the possibility of a thrombosis developing. This can be eliminated by making the venipuncture in a more lateral location, at the axillary vein, and then advancing into the central system.

The nerves and vascular structures in the thoracic outlet can be compressed by changes in normal anatomy brought about by posture, chronic illness, and occupation. Pain, muscle weakness and atrophy, and sensory changes result from these thoracic outlet syndromes. Arterial compression causes pallor of the fingers while venous compression leads to edema and cyanosis.[7]

Venous cannulation can increase the risk of thrombosis in these patients.

The kidney-shaped opening formed by the first rib, sternum, and vertebra is the *thoracic inlet.* It measures about 5 cm from front to back and about 10 cm from side to side and is angled downward toward the anterior side.[1] This small opening must accommodate many important structures, including the subclavian arteries and veins, carotid arteries, internal jugular vein, thymus gland and its muscles and nerves, trachea and esophagus, part of the brachial nerve plexus and vagus nerve, and the upper part of the pleura and apex of the lungs. Venous cannulas inserted, terminating, or passing through the veins in this area could lead to complications affecting all these structures.

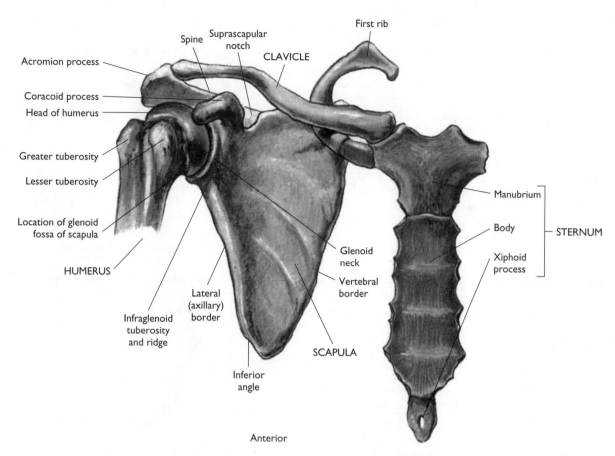

FIG. 6-7 *Anterior view of the scapula, sternum, and shoulder girdle.* (From Solomon EP, Phillips GA: *Understanding human anatomy and physiology*, Philadelphia, 1989, WB Saunders, p. 87.)

Respiratory system

Anatomically, the primary components of the respiratory system with regard to parenteral therapy include the trachea, bronchi, and lungs. Functionally, the purpose here is to examine the exchange of air between the environment and the lungs, the diffusion of oxygen and carbon dioxide between the lungs and the blood, and the movement of gases into and out of the various cells of the body.

Pulmonary anatomy. The top of the lung, or apex, arches upward into the thoracic inlet and extends about 3 to 4 cm above the first costal cartilage and 2.5 cm above the medial aspect of the clavicle.[1] This is extremely close to the subclavian vein, thus creating the risk of pneumothorax with puncture of the subclavian vein. The base of the lungs is immediately above the diaphragm, which separates the thoracic cavity from the abdominal cavity.

The blood flows into the lungs through the pulmonary arteries, which carry deoxygenated blood. Pulmonary arteries and arterioles are short segments of vessels with large diameters. They have thin walls and are capable of distension, thus allowing for a large blood volume capacity. They follow the path of the bronchi, branching into smaller arterioles with the network of capillaries surrounding each alveolus. The venous side of this same pathway, carrying oxygenated blood, follows the path of bronchioles, and becomes larger as it returns to the pulmonary

veins. These veins are short and their ability to distend is about the same as the veins in the systemic circulation.

IV solutions contain many types of particulate matter. Undissolved drug particles, precipitate from incompatible drugs, rubber cores of vials or solution containers, glass particles from ampules, and plastic particles from administration sets make up this particulate matter. The most likely place for these particles to stop during intravenous infusion is the microcirculation of the lungs. The average diameter of pulmonary capillaries is about 5 μm,[1] which act as a trap for infused particles and requires the red blood cells to change shape in order to pass through.

One study has provided information about the examination of autopsied lung tissue from 11 patients who had lengthy stays in an intensive care unit.[7] Samples of lung tissue were taken from 12 locations in each patient, mainly from the apex, base, and close to the pulmonary hila. The study used a scanning electron microscope and was the first to demonstrate particles as small as 0.8 μ. Embolism of the microcirculation, damage to the capillary endothelium, and the formation of thrombi and granulomas around these particles were noted. More acutely ill patients, immunocompromised patients, and those with a prolonged need for IV infusion can benefit by final filtration of solutions. Avoiding respiratory complications can lead to a more positive patient outcome.

Physiology of respiration. Because the lungs expand and contract like balloons, pressures inside the chest are of great importance. The negative pressure in the pleural space becomes more negative during inspiration. Alveolar pressure, or the pressure inside the alveoli, is equal to atmospheric pressure when no air is moving in or out and the glottis is open. When the alveolar pressure falls, inspiration occurs. With about 500 ml of air inside, the pressure rises above atmospheric pressure and expiration occurs. The Valsalva maneuver increases the chest pressure by holding air in the lungs against a closed glottis.

To prevent an air embolus, positive pressure in the chest is necessary when manipulating the line of a cannula whose tip lies within the thorax. Cannula insertion, changing administration tubing, inadvertent disconnection of the tubing, and cannula removal can place the patient at risk for an air embolus.

Gases, such as oxygen, carbon dioxide, and nitrogen, dissolved in water or body fluids exert the same pressure and movement as in the gaseous state. Gas molecules in the alveoli are still in the gaseous state, whereas gas molecules in the blood are dissolved. Transfer of the molecules occurs because of the partial pressure exerted by each gas. The partial pressure of oxygen in its gaseous state inside the alveoli is greater than the partial pressure of oxygen in the blood, so this pressure forces oxygen to move into the pulmonary membrane and into the capillary. The same is true for carbon dioxide—its partial pressure is greater in the blood so the transfer is in the opposite direction, from the blood across the membrane and into the alveolar sac.

Although the respiratory membrane is extremely thin, it is composed of several layers (Fig. 6-8). The capillary is so small that a red blood cell must squeeze through the wall, with the gases diffusing directly into and out of each red cell without passing through plasma. Although this individual unit is extremely small, there are about 300 million alveoli in both lungs. The surface area of the respiratory membrane covers about 70 m^2 in a normal adult.[4] With gaseous exchange over such a large area, the speed of diffusion is understandable.

The heart

Heart wall. The heart is enclosed in a protective sac, called the *pericardium,* which extends between the second and sixth costal cartilages. The great vessels leading away from and into the heart are also enclosed in the pericardium (Fig. 6-9).

The pericardium has two layers: an outer fibrous layer and an inner serous layer. The fibrous layer is composed of strong collagen fibers and covers the aorta, superior vena cava, right and left pulmonary arteries, and the four pulmonary veins. The serous layer is further divided into the parietal and visceral layers, with the latter also being known as the *epicardium.* Between these two layers is a thin film of fluid that allows the heart to move. Vascular access devices within the great vessels and heart inside the pericardium have the potential to erode through the wall. Two clinical conditions can occur: (1) pericardial effusion, with fluid leaking between the layers of the pericardium, or (2) cardiac tamponade, with the blood and fluid exerting pressure on the heart.

The endocardium is the innermost layer of the heart and is composed of a single layer of endothelial cells. This is a continu-

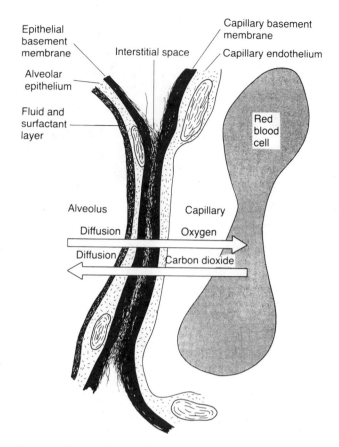

FIG. 6-8 *Cross section of the ultrastructure of the respiratory membrane.* (From Guyton AC: *Textbook of medical physiology,* ed 8, Philadelphia, 1991, WB Saunders, p. 429.)

ation of the same endothelial layer as that found on the internal surface of all arteries and veins.

Right side of the heart. The superior and inferior vena cava joins the atrium of the right side of the heart on the posterior aspect. The superior vena cava returns blood from the upper part of the body and has no valve. The inferior vena cava returns blood from the lower part of the body, is larger than the superior vena cava, and has a semilunar valve near the opening into the atrium. The atrium acts as a reservoir and has only enough pumping ability to move blood through the tricuspid valve into the right ventricle.

Cardiac function. Cardiac output, the quantity of blood pumped into the aorta each minute, is regulated by changes in the volume of blood flowing into the heart and control of the heart by the autonomic nervous system. *Venous return* is the amount of blood flowing into the right atrium each minute. The heart has a unique ability to pump out all that is returned, avoiding any pooling of blood in the veins. This is known as the *Frank-Starling mechanism.* For this reason, the heart can adapt easily to normal changes such as increased exercise. The force of the contractions increases as the heart chambers stretch to accommodate larger volumes. Stretching the right atrium also stretches the sinoatrial node, which signals an increase in the heart rate. It also initiates a nervous reflex that passes to the brain and back to the heart through the sympathetic nerves and the vagi to increase the rate.

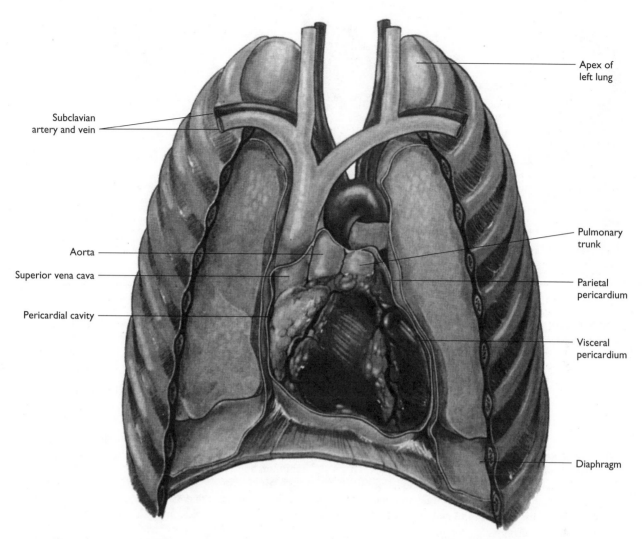

Subclavian
artery and vein

Aorta

Superior vena cava

Pericardial cavity

Apex of
left lung

Pulmonary
trunk

Parietal
pericardium

Visceral
pericardium

Diaphragm

FIG. 6-9 *The heart lies in the mediastinum between the lungs. The heart and the roots of the great vessels are loosely enclosed by the pericardium.* (From Solomon EP, Phillips GA: *Understanding human anatomy and physiology*, Philadelphia, 1987, WB Saunders, p. 210.)

PERIPHERAL VASCULAR SYSTEM

For oxygen and carbon dioxide to be transferred at the cellular level, blood must reach all tissues of the body through an immense network of interconnecting tubes. Anatomic names for these tubes, based on size and structure, include arteries, arterioles, capillaries, venules, and veins. They may also be described in functional terms as vessels of distribution (arteries), resistance (arterioles), exchange (capillaries), and capacitance, or reservoir (veins). Small venules act as exchange vessels and larger venules act as reservoirs.

Blood vessel structure

The walls of all arteries and veins are arranged in three layers: the tunica intima (innermost layer), tunica media (middle layer), and tunica adventitia (outer layer) (Fig. 6-10). These layers have structural differences determined by the location and function of each vessel (Table 6-3).

The tunica intima is made up of a single layer of smooth flat endothelial cells that lie along the length of each vessel, subendothelial connective tissue, and a basal lamina or basement membrane. The tunica media contains smooth muscle and other fibrous tissue and is arranged around the circumference of the vessel. The tunica adventitia is connective tissue whose fibers are arranged along the length of the vessel. There is much variation in these tunicas, depending on the type of vessel.

All blood vessels, lymphatic vessels, and the heart are lined with endothelium, which is a single layer of flat, smooth cells with a thickness usually less than 10 μm,[2] arranged along the length of the vessel. This layer of cells rests on a basement membrane to provide additional support. Each cell is linked together to form occluding or tight junctions, which prevent the leakage of fluids and cells from the vessel. Capillary walls are characterized by a thin endothelial structure, the presence of more junctions between cells, and fenestrations or openings in the cells, which allow for the rapid transfer of fluid and other substances (Fig. 6-11). Biochemical mediators such as histamine, serotonin, leukotrienes, prostaglandins, and brady-

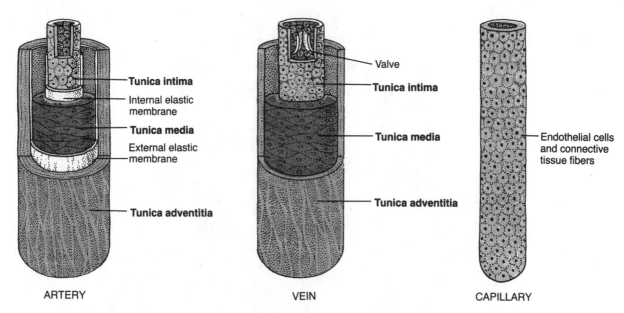

FIG. 6-10 *Microscopic anatomy of an artery, vein, and capillary.* (From Ignatavicius DD, Bayne MV: *Medical-surgical nursing: a nursing process approach,* Philadelphia, 1991, WB Saunders, p. 2083.)

kinin alter vascular permeability by creating a separation of these cells.

Endothelial cells have three important functions. First, they maintain homeostasis of the blood by preventing clot formation inside the vessel and are ready to stimulate appropriate cellular responses, such as during infection or physical injury. Their second function is to isolate the circulating blood from other tissue while permitting limited passage of fluid and macromolecules to nourish the tissue. The third function is to regulate local blood flow by producing potent vasodilating and vasoconstricting factors.[2]

Prostacyclin, a prostaglandin formed in the endothelium from arachidonic acid, promotes relaxation of vascular smooth muscle, although the mechanism that causes its release is unknown. Nitric oxide or endothelial-derived relaxing factor is released when the endothelium is stimulated. Studies assessing the effect of nitric oxide have primarily been conducted by measuring arterial flow and vasomotor tone following infusion of neurotransmitors such as acetylcholine, substance P, and serotonin. Endothelial dysfunction can be found in patients with hypercholesterolemia, systemic and pulmonary hypertension, diabetes, arteriosclerosis, sepsis, chronic heart failure, posttransplantation, and chronic cigarette smoking.[8]

Endothelin is a strong vasoconstrictor that has been isolated from endothelial cells in cardiovascular and noncardiovascular tissue. During periods of hypoxia, ischemia, or shear stress, endothelin-1 is secreted within minutes. It binds with the smooth muscle in the tunica media to produce vasoconstriction.[9] Other endothelial-derived contracting factors exist, although little is known about their function at present.[3]

Because of its smoothness, the endothelial surface is designed to prevent clotting inside the vessel. There is also a layer of glycocalyx, a mucopolysaccharide, on the endothelial surface that repels clotting factors. Thrombomodulin, a protein bound

to the endothelial cells, slows the clotting process by removing thrombin and activating protein C, a plasma protein with anticoagulant properties.[4] Numerous other factors that promote or prohibit coagulation can be found in the endothelium, including tissue plasminogen activator, plasminogen activator inhibitor, and von Willebrand factor.[10] Damage to these cells is the beginning of the inflammation process of phlebitis and of the clotting process that can cause thrombosis. The endothelial cells of veins and arteries can be damaged by the following:

- Rapid cannula advancement
- Cannula advancement without anchoring skin and vein by holding traction on skin
- Insertion of cannula too large for lumen of vein
- Insertion of cannula close to area of joint flexion without adequate support from hand boards
- Inadequate taping, allowing for motion of cannula
- Inadequate skin preparation, allowing for invasion of microorganisms
- Nonocclusive, dirty, or wet dressing, allowing for invasion of microorganisms
- Location of cannula tip that causes impingement of tip on vein wall
- Infusion of particulate matter
- Infusion of hypertonic or hypotonic fluids
- Infusion of solution with an extremely high or low pH
- Rapid infusion of quantities too large for vessel lumen to accommodate

Smooth muscle in the tunica media is composed of long, tapered spindles of muscle fibers. These spindles are arranged in bundles or layers around the circumference of the vessel and contract together as a single unit. Each bundle is closely arranged so that their cell membranes adhere in numerous places. The action potential for each bundle stimulates the remaining ones by communicating gap junctions through which ions flow

Table 6-3   Structural Differences in Blood Vessels in Arterial and Venous Walls

	BLOOD VESSELS				
LAYER	**ARTERIES**	**ARTERIOLES (LUMEN DIAMETER, <0.5 MM)**	**CAPILLARIES**	**VENULES**	**VEINS**
Tunica intima	Elastic arteries—elongated endothelial cells, multiple layer subendothelial tissue, and fenestrated elastic membrane; thicken with age and fatty deposits; contain baroreceptors and chemoreceptors Muscular arteries—thinner, allowing diffusion of metabolites; contain other afferent nerve fibers	Thin layer of endothelial cells with basal lamina	Single cell layer of endothelium and thin basal lamina	Endothelial layer and basal lamina	Endothelial layer of shorter, broader cells and basal lamina
Tunica media	Elastic arteries—thicker with more elastic and fibrous tissue arranged in circular bands; responds to pumping action of heart Muscular arteries—smooth muscle fibers controlling constriction and relaxation	Decreasing amounts of elastin; muscle cells form communicating (gap) junctions, allowing diffusion of ions and electrical stimulation	No middle layer	Small venules—no middle layer Larger venules—thin layer of smooth muscle	Thick layer of connective tissue with elastin fibers and smooth muscle fibers, although thinner than same layer in arteries
Tunica adventitia	Elastic arteries—thin layer of collagen fibers Muscular arteries—contain collagen and elastin; contain vasa vasorum, lymphatic channels, and both efferent and afferent nerve fibers	Fine collagen fibers; contain vasa vasorum, lymphatic channels, and efferent nerve fibers	Thin reticular tissue with occasional fibroblasts and mast cells	Thin fibrous tissue	Loose connective tissue, with elastin fibers; contain vasa vasorum, afferent and sympathetic nerves

freely. Smooth muscles of blood vessels are capable of maintaining contraction or a state of tension for lengthy periods. Several other differences exist between the function of smooth muscles and skeletal muscles. The force of contraction is greater in smooth muscles and less energy is required to maintain contraction. Also, smooth muscles can shorten by two-thirds during contraction, thus allowing the vessel lumen to change from very large to extremely small. This strong venous contraction makes it difficult to remove some midline and peripherally inserted central catheters.[11]

The stress-relaxation phenomenon of smooth muscles is another important aspect of blood vessel physiology. When a tourniquet is placed on the extremity to distend peripheral veins, the muscle fibers elongate to accommodate the increased volume collecting in the veins. The pressure increases quickly and then, within a few seconds, falls back toward the normal level, even with the increased volume. When the tourniquet is removed, the volume and pressure suddenly fall, and within several minutes, the normal pressure is reestablished. Knowledge of this process is crucial when timing the removal of a tourniquet and advancing long cannulas into the vein. Obstruction may be encountered if not enough time has elapsed to allow equilibrium to return.

Another characteristic of smooth muscles is excitation by stretch. When smooth muscles have been excessively stretched, the muscles contract to automatically resist that stretch. This

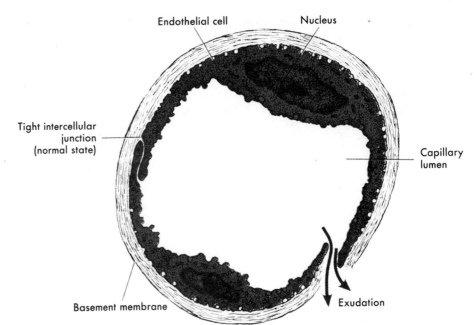

FIG. 6-11 *Cross section of a capillary.*
(From McCance KL, Huether SE: *Pathophysiology: the basis for disease in adults and children,* St Louis, 1990, Mosby, p. 219.)

explains what happens when a tourniquet has been left in place for an extended period and the veins can no longer be palpated.

Stimulation of the tunica media by trauma or changes in temperature and pressure can lead to vascular spasm. If an artery is affected, the result is an interruption in the flow of blood to the area served by that artery, with possible necrosis of that tissue. When this occurs in a vein, the outcome is not as negative, but the patient experiences pain at the site from a change in the blood flow.

Studies with balloon catheters used during angioplasty have demonstrated the effect of removing the endothelial layer that exposes the basal lamina and smooth muscle. Platelets are immediately deposited and vasoconstriction occurs. Smooth muscle cells begin to grow toward the intima, causing the wall to thicken. Function of the endothelium may not return to normal and is dependent on the severity of the injury to the endothelium and the degree to which the vessel wall has thickened.[9]

The aorta, its major branches, and the pulmonary arteries are elastic arteries; the flow of blood is rapid and under high pressure, so these vessels need to be composed of a large amount of elastic tissue. This allows for a high degree of distensibility, especially during ventricular systole when blood is forced out into these arteries. Medium and small arteries are muscular arteries, containing more muscular tissue, and are capable of controlling blood flow by constriction and dilation. Distension and recoil keep blood flowing during diastole in a smooth yet pulsatile manner.

As arteries branch and become smaller in diameter, they are known as *arterioles*. They further subdivide into terminal arterioles and metarterioles. All are considered resistance vessels. On the capillary end of each metarteriole is a precapillary sphincter, which controls the flow of blood through the capillary bed (Fig. 6-12).

The venous side of the circulation is known for its compliance or the ability to increase in volume with a given increase in pressure. The amount of elastic tissue found in the wall of the vessel is the primary reason for the difference in compliance or capacitance. About three times more of the circulating volume of blood is located on the venous side than the arterial side. Because of the ability of the venous walls to distend about 6 to 10 times more than the arterial walls, a small increase in pressure results in a much larger quantity of blood in any vein. The same pressure increase in a corresponding artery would not result in a volume increase.

Blood is supplied to the vessel walls by the vasa vasorum, a dense capillary network within the tunica adventitia of each vessel. This capillary network may be a branch of the artery it serves or may be from a distant artery. In veins, this network may penetrate to the tunica media.

Sympathetic nerves are located in the adventitia of large arteries and veins. A steady flow of impulses is sent from the vasomotor center in the medulla and pons of the brain to maintain the vasomotor tone, which is a partial state of contraction of all vessels. Norepinephrine, the neurotransmitter at the synapse of these sympathetic nerves, acts on the α-adrenergic receptors of the smooth muscles in the vessels to cause contraction. This state of contraction supports the arterial pressure and keeps blood moving back to the heart. There are no nerve endings in vessels that directly cause vasodilation. Instead, a decrease in the impulses causing vasomotor tone leads to vasodilation. Also located in the intima and adventitia of systemic arteries are afferent peripheral nerves. Some of these may carry pain impulses, whereas others are baroreceptors and chemoreceptors (see Table 6-2).

Valves are found in veins but not in arteries. Valves are semilunar folds, extending from the tunica intima into the lumen of the vein (see Fig. 6-10). They are composed of collagen and elastin fibers covered with endothelial cells. Usually, valves are arranged in pairs, but there can be three folds or leaflets together as well as a single leaflet at other locations. Valves can

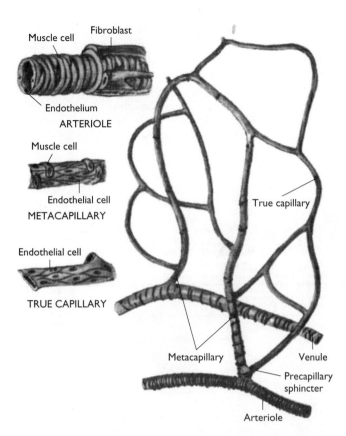

FIG. 6-12 *Diagrammatic representation of a portion of a capillary bed typical of many tissues. Precapillary sphincters regulate the flow of blood from the metacapillary into true capillaries.* (From Jacob SW, Francone CA: *Elements of anatomy and physiology,* ed 2, Philadelphia, 1989, WB Saunders, p. 184.)

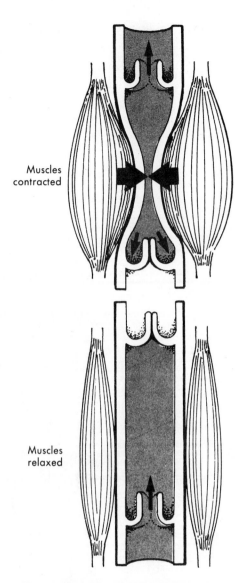

FIG. 6-13 *The muscle pump.* (From McCance KL, Huether SE: *Pathophysiology: the basis for disease in adults and children,* St Louis, 1990, Mosby, p. 889.)

be found in most veins, except for extremely small or large ones. They can be found at bifurcations or where two veins unite. However, there is little or no documentation about any specific locations for valves within the superficial veins used for venipuncture, probably because of the great variations among individuals. On the proximal side of each valve the vein wall expands, creating a sinus above each valve. When veins are distended, such as with the application of a tourniquet, blood flow is temporarily stopped. This creates a pooling of blood in these sinuses and yields a "knotted" appearance externally.

The purpose of valves is to keep blood moving toward the heart by way of the muscle pump, sometimes called the *venous pump* (Fig. 6-13). With the contraction of each muscle during movement, pressure is applied to the vein, forcing blood back toward the heart. This pumping action opens the proximal valve and closes the distal valve, preventing a backward flow. Venous blood flow in all extremities is against gravity, resulting in a great rise in venous pressure if this pumping system fails. When valves become damaged or incompetent, pressure rises in the distal end of the extremity. The pooling of blood in capillaries causes fluid to leak outside the circulatory system, resulting in edema and a decreased blood volume.[3] This muscle pump may have an impact on cannulas made of soft, flexible material, causing them to migrate out of the vein. This may occur more

often with patients in the home care setting who are engaged in normal activities of daily living.

The normal pattern of blood flow is through the aorta, which branches into smaller arteries, but there are some deviations from this pattern. Rather than ending in an arteriole, two arteries may anastomose and bypass the capillary bed. This occurs in some arteries in the brain, intestines, and joints. An arteriovenous anastomosis is a small artery and vein connected together. These may be found in mucous membranes and deep in the dermis of the hands and feet. The venous side is affected by the higher pressure from the arterial side, and may result in unsuccessful venipuncture attempts in this area.[1]

Location of important arteries

The axillary artery extends from the first rib to the lateral edge of the chest in the axilla. The axillary sheath is a neurovascular bundle containing the axillary artery, axillary vein, and parts of the brachial nerve plexus controlling the arm. The continuation of the axillary artery is the brachial artery, which moves down the arm to immediately below the elbow. There it divides into the ulnar artery, on the medial side of the arm, and the radial artery, on the lateral side of the arm (Fig. 6-14).

Although the radial artery is smaller than the ulnar artery, it is preferred for arterial puncture for blood withdrawal and cannula insertion because it is more superficial and can be stabilized for easier entry. It is imperative that the Allen test be performed to assess the collateral circulation. This is done by locating and compressing both arteries and noting the blanching that occurs. When only the ulnar artery is released, color should return to the entire hand, indicating the ability of this artery to supply blood to the whole hand. If this positive assessment cannot be made, another site should be chosen.

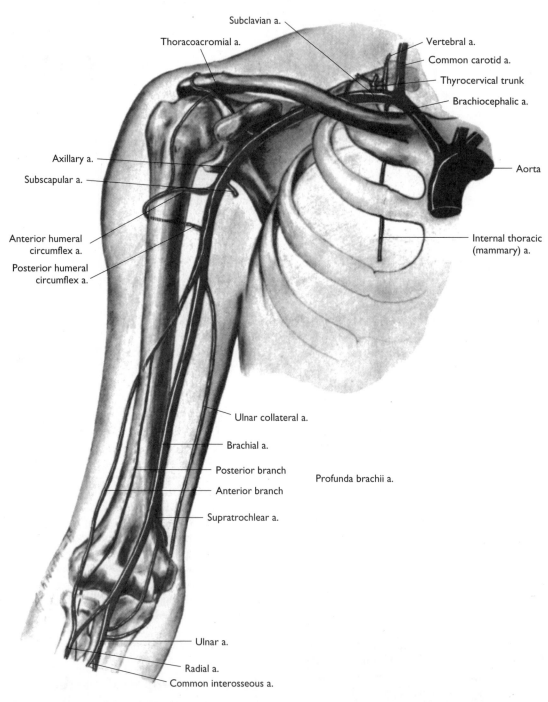

FIG. 6-14 *Arteries of the right shoulder and upper arm.* (From Jacob SW, Francone CA: *Elements of anatomy and physiology,* ed 2, Philadelphia, 1989, WB Saunders, p. 191.)

Location of important veins

Systemic veins can be divided into two types: superficial and deep. Deep veins accompany arteries, usually of the same name, and both are enclosed in a protective sheath of connective tissue, known as *venae comitantes*. Superficial veins, best suited for venipuncture, lie in loose connective tissue under the skin. This location allows for easy movement of these veins. Therefore, during any attempt to cannulate a vein, some method must be used to anchor the vein. Without securing the vein, puncture and advancement of the cannula result in unnecessary damage to the endothelium of the vein and could lead to phlebitis. Using one hand to hold traction on the skin over the vein during complete cannula advancement secures the vein (Fig. 6-15).

The primary veins used to initiate IV therapy are the superficial veins in the hand and forearm. Both upper extremities should be assessed carefully (Table 6-4). Small digital veins line the borders of the fingers and unite on the back of the hand to form the dorsal venous network (Fig. 6-16). On the lateral aspect of the wrist, proximal to the thumb, the cephalic vein rises from the dorsal veins. Close to this area are perforating

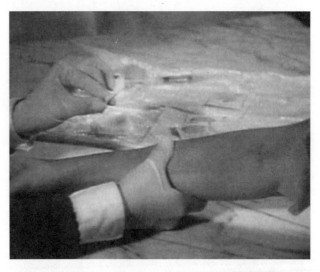

FIG. 6-15 *Holding traction on the skin over a vein during complete cannula advancement will secure the vein and prevent damage to the endothelium of the vein.*

Table 6-4   Short Peripheral Cannula Insertion Sites for Children and Adults

SITE	ADVANTAGES	DISADVANTAGES
Dorsal venous network of hand	Most distal site, allowing successive sites in a proximal location; can be visualized and palpated easily; easily accessible	Should be stabilized on hand board; smaller than veins in forearm; diminished skin turgor and loss of subcutaneous tissue in geriatric patients; excessive subcutaneous fat in infants; limited ability to use hand may present problems for patients at home
Cephalic vein	Large vein; easy to stabilize; easily accessible for caregiver and patient; may be palpated above antecubital fossa	May be obscured by tendons controlling thumb; puncture sites directly in wrist and antecubital fossa can increase complications because of joint motion
Accessory cephalic	Medium to large vein(s); easy to stabilize; can be palpated easily	Valves at junction of cephalic may prohibit cannula advancement; length of vein may be too short for cannula; may not be located on children
Median	Medium vein; easy to stabilize; easily accessible for caregiver and patient	Puncture in wrist may be excessively painful because of close proximity of nerve; may be slightly more difficult to palpate and visualize
Basilic	Large vein; can be palpated easily; may be available after other sites have been exhausted	More difficult to access because of location; may be difficult for patient to access and observe site; puncture site directly in antecubital fossa may result in increased complications because of joint motion; cannot be palpated above antecubital fossa
External jugular	Large vein; easily accessible for emergency situations	Increased complications because of motion of neck; occlusive dressing difficult to maintain
Dorsal venous network on foot	Easily accessible	May not be easily palpated because of age or disease-related changes; higher incidence of complications related to impaired circulation; difficult to stabilize joint; greatly limits ability to walk
Medial and lateral marginal veins of foot	May be large; usually easy to palpate and visualize	Higher incidence of complications related to impaired circulation; difficult to stabilize joint; greatly limits ability to walk
Great and small saphenous	Large veins; usually easy to palpate and visualize	Higher incidence of complications related to impaired circulation; located close to perforating veins connecting to deep veins of the leg

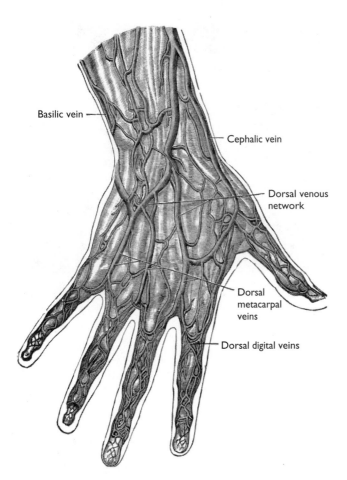

FIG. 6-16 *Superficial veins of the hand.* (From Williams PL et al, editors: *Gray's anatomy,* ed 37, New York, 1989, Churchill Livingstone, p. 806.)

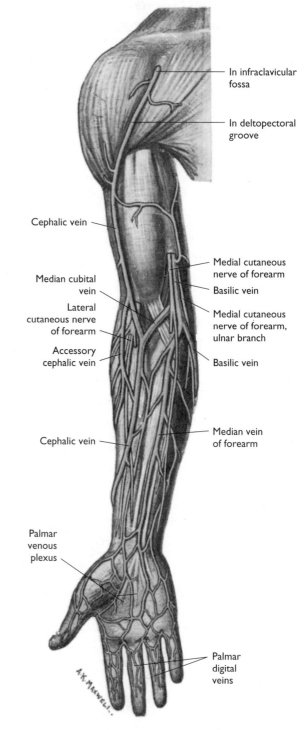

FIG. 6-17 *Superficial veins of the right upper extremity.* (From Williams PL et al, editors: *Gray's anatomy,* ed 37, New York, 1989, Churchill Livingstone, p. 806.)

veins, which pierce the deep fascia and connect the superficial veins with the deeper veins of the hand. The cephalic vein at this location is large enough for the insertion of a cannula, but there are several points to consider. The motion of the wrist may increase the patient's general discomfort, and irritation to the tunica intima results from movement of the cannula. Also, there are three long tendons that control the motion of the thumb. Although the vein is superficial to these tendons, slight movement of the thumb during the venipuncture procedure could easily obscure the vein.

The cephalic vein moves up the lateral aspect of the arm into the antecubital fossa. There may also be a network of veins on the lateral forearm that forms the accessory cephalic, joining the cephalic vein at or above the antecubital fossa (Fig. 6-17).

Moving medially across the palmar side of the forearm, the median vein ascends from the superficial palmar veins. In the wrist, these veins may appear to be suitable for venipuncture but are usually situated between two branches of the median nerve. This results in extremely painful venipuncture and should be avoided (see Fig. 6-17).

The basilic vein is on the posterior-medial aspect of the forearm. Although it is usually a large vein, it may have been overlooked, and venipuncture may be awkward. This vein can be easily palpated and punctured when the patient's arm is placed across the chest, with the nurse on the opposite side of the patient from the arm being examined (Fig. 6-18).

The radial and ulnar veins parallel the arteries of the same name in the venae comitantes. There is communication between the deep and superficial veins, and the muscle pump can be used to distend the superficial veins. Instructing the patient to open and close the hand helps force blood from the deep veins into

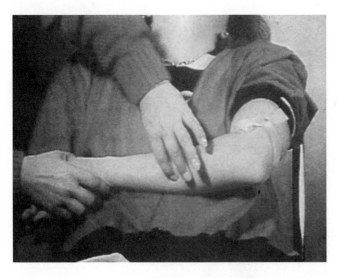

FIG. 6-18 *The basilic vein is easily palpated and punctured by placing the patient's arm across the chest toward the nurse, who is positioned on the side opposite the intended site.*

Table 6-5   Antecubital Cannula Insertion Sites for Children and Adults

SITE	ADVANTAGES	DISADVANTAGES
Basilic	Largest vein; straight pathway in upper arm and thorax	May be located too far to the posterior side for sterile procedure and routine care; may only be able to palpate a short segment
Median	Communicates with larger basilic; easily accessible for insertion and routine care	Median cubital
Median basilic	Joins with larger basilic; easily accessible for insertion and routine care	Valve may be located at junction with basilic, causing obstruction to cannula advancement
Median cephalic	Easily accessible	Valve may be located at junction with basilic, causing obstruction to cannula advancement; terminates in smaller cephalic; may not be present in some patients
Accessory cephalic	Easily accessible for insertion and routine care	Valve may be located at junction with cephalic, causing obstruction to cannula advancement; terminates in smaller cephalic; may not be present in some patients
Cephalic	Easily accessible for insertion and routine care; easy palpation and visualization above and below antecubital fossa	Smaller than basilic; pathway in upper arm and thorax is variable and unknown

the superficial veins, thus distending them for easier palpation and puncture.

The median vein joins the basilic vein slightly below the antecubital fossa on the medial aspect (see Fig. 6-17). The basilic vein at this level is the best insertion site for antecubital catheters. However, on some patients, this vein may be located too far to the posterior aspect of the elbow, making venipuncture difficult. Palpation of this vein should begin on the distal end in the forearm and the course of the vein followed to evaluate its location.

In the antecubital fossa, the cephalic vein communicates with the basilic vein by the median cubital vein (see Fig. 6-17). There is also communication with the deep veins where the median cubital vein enters the basilic vein. Variations in the median cubital vein may be seen. Some patients may have two branches of this vein, one angling toward the basilic, known as the *median basilic,* and the second one angling from the center of the fossa toward the cephalic, known as the *median cephalic vein.* Because of variations, careful evaluation and assessment of each patient is important when inserting an antecubital cannula (Table 6-5).

The upper part of the arm has three veins of importance. The cephalic vein continues upward lateral to the biceps muscle. The basilic vein is medial to the biceps and extends to the superior axilla, where it becomes the axillary vein (see Fig. 6-17). The brachial vein is located deep in the arm as a vena comitans in the sheath with the brachial artery.

The distal end of the axillary vein can be considered as the beginning of the veins in the shoulder area. The axillary vein is classified as a deep vein; it extends from the lateral aspect of the chest in the axilla to the lateral border of the first rib. The axillary vein receives the brachial vein at its midpoint and the cephalic vein near the border of the rib. The cephalic vein can also have variations in its path. It may only join the axillary vein, only connect with the external jugular in the neck, or branch into two smaller veins connecting with the axillary and external jugular veins (Fig. 6-19). There are three suprascapular veins and several other veins joining the axillary vein in this area, and as many as 40 valves can be documented in this region.[12] For this reason, antecubital catheters can take several wayward paths, and the actual tip location can be confirmed only by chest radiography.

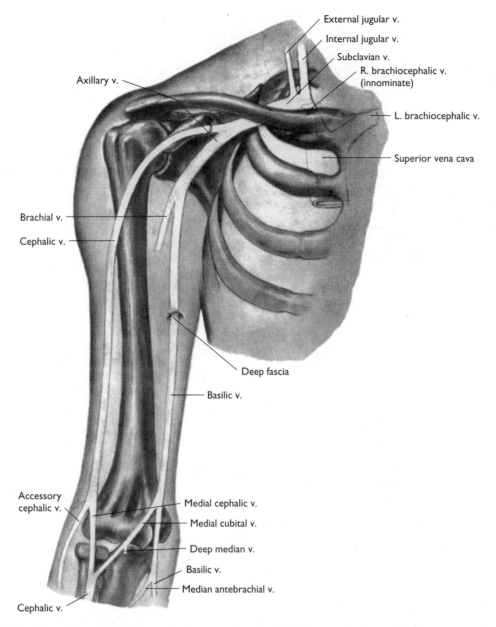

FIG. 6-19 *Veins of the right shoulder and upper arm.* (From Jacob SW, Francone CA: *Elements of anatomy and physiology,* ed 2, Philadelphia, 1989, WB Saunders, p. 192.)

There are four jugular veins draining the head and face, with three of them located superficially (Fig. 6-20). The external jugular vein is on the outer border of the neck. The posterior external jugular vein drains the occipital region and the anterior jugular vein drains the face, with both joining the external jugular at the base of the neck. The external jugular joins the subclavian vein at its midpoint. The internal jugular vein is a deep vein covered by the muscles of the neck. It joins the subclavian vein at its proximal end.

From the lateral edge of the first rib to the sternal edge of the clavicle, the continuation of the axillary vein is the subclavian vein. The vein angles upward as it arches over the first rib and passes under the clavicle, forming a narrow passage for the vein (see Fig. 6-19). The apex of the lungs is also extremely close to

the location of the subclavian vein, increasing the potential for pneumothorax when the subclavian is punctured (see Fig. 6-19). Table 6-6 lists locations for central venous cannulation.

At the top of the thoracic inlet, the internal jugular and subclavian veins join to create the brachiocephalic vein, also called the *innominate vein*. At this junction is the last venous valve before the heart. The left brachiocephalic vein, which is approximately 6 cm in length, is about twice as long as the right (Fig. 6-21).

There is another structure at this location, the thoracic duct, which is a large, deep lymphatic vessel that receives a large quantity of lymph from the entire body (Fig. 6-22). This large lymphatic vessel may be damaged during puncture of the large blood vessels in this area. Lymph is composed of various

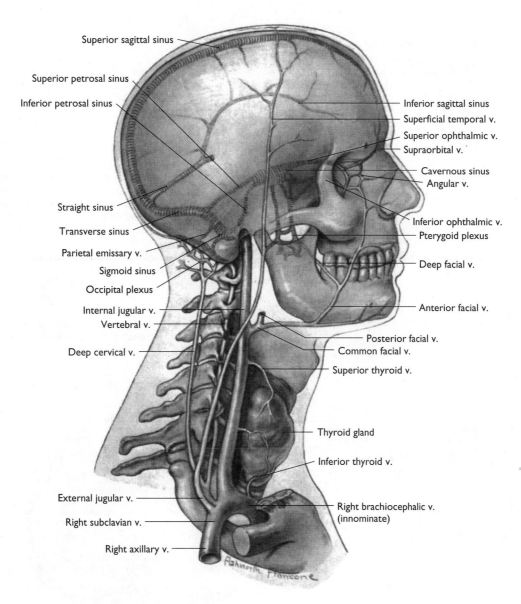

FIG. 6-20   *Venous drainage of the head and neck.* (From Jacob SW, Francone CA: *Elements of anatomy and physiology*, ed 2, Philadelphia, 1989, WB Saunders, p. 186.)

fluids and cells draining from capillary beds. Lymphatic vessels follow the path of other blood vessels throughout the body. The flow of fluid is aided by valves inside the vessels and is the result of muscular contraction and compression from the pulsation of neighboring arteries.

The two brachiocephalic veins unite at the lower border of the first rib to form the superior vena cava. About 7 cm long and 2 cm wide, it descends to the level of the third costal cartilage, where it joins the right atrium of the heart. On chest radiography, its location is seen in the right mediastinal border. At the second costal cartilage, the fibrous pericardium of the heart begins and encompasses the lower half of the superior vena cava.

Other tributaries unite with the great thoracic veins and have

been documented as aberrant locations for central venous cannulas.[6,13] The internal thoracic (mammary) vein joins the superior vena cava at the superior end. The left and right inferior thyroid veins join the respective brachiocephalic veins, draining the esophageal, tracheal, and laryngeal areas. The left superior intercostal vein joins the left brachiocephalic vein. The azygos vein drains the spinal column and enters the posterior side of the superior vena cava immediately above the beginning of the pericardium (Fig. 6-23).

In the lower extremity, the pattern of vascular distribution is similar to that of the upper extremity, with the superficial veins in the subcutaneous fascia and the deep veins accompanying the deeper arteries. The greatest difference is the presence of more valves in the lower extremity. The dorsal metatarsal veins form a

Table 6-6   Central Venous Insertion Sites in Children and Adults

SITE	ADVANTAGES	DISADVANTAGES
Subclavian		
Infraclavicular	Easily accessible for insertion; flatter surface to maintain occlusive dressing; more published studies using this site; some believe this site has better anatomic landmarks; preferred for children	Longer needle may be necessary to pass through skin and muscle compression of vein and cannula with possible fracture of cannula if insertion is made in a medial site
Supraclavicular	Shorter distance from skin to vein; easily accessible	Occlusive dressing may be difficult to achieve in hollow contour above clavicle
		Both sites associated with pneumothorax, hemothorax, hydrothorax, brachial nerve plexus injury, thoracic duct injury, and injury to other superior mediastinal structures
Jugular		May damage carotid arteries
Internal	Larger vein diameter; multiple insertion sites; easily accessible; straighter path to superior vena cava	
External	Superficial vein, usually visible and easy to palpate	Cannula tip location in superior vena cava not always as successful as internal jugular
	Both sites are associated with fewer complications than subclavian	Maintaining occlusive dressing on either is extremely difficult because of movement of neck and beard on male patients
Femoral	Alternative site in emergencies; tip location in large inferior vena cava	Occlusive dressing is extremely difficult with high infection rates associated with this site; associated with higher incidence of thrombosis and other serious complications

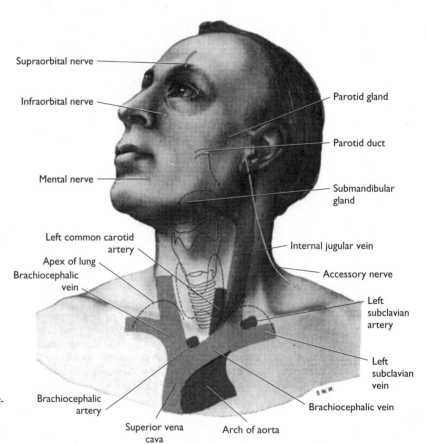

FIG. 6-21 *Surface projections of some important structures in the face, neck, and upper part of the thorax.*
(From Williams PL et al, editors: *Gray's anatomy*, ed 37, New York, 1989, Churchill Livingstone, p. 808.)

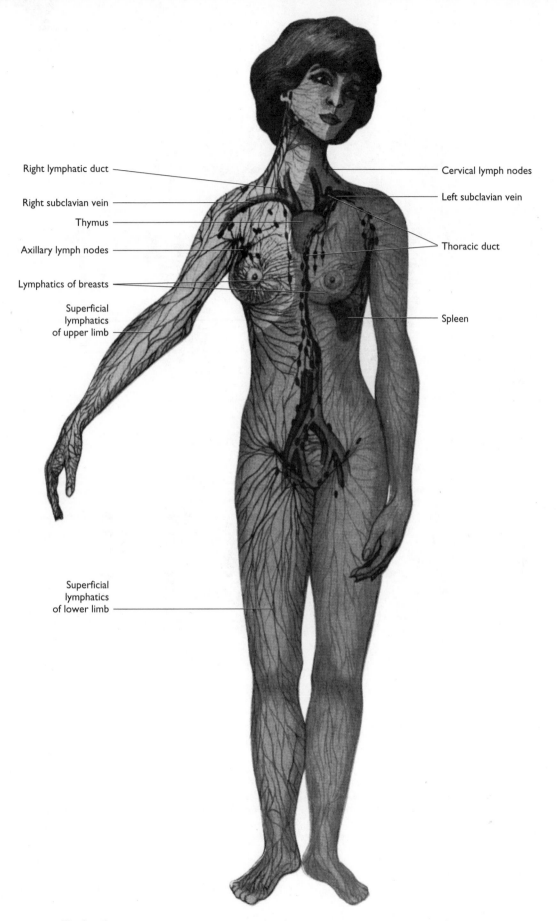

Right lymphatic duct

Right subclavian vein

Thymus

Axillary lymph nodes

Lymphatics of breasts

Superficial
lymphatics
of upper limb

Superficial
lymphatics
of lower limb

Cervical lymph nodes

Left subclavian vein

Thoracic duct

Spleen

FIG. 6-22 *The lymphatic system.* (From Solomon EP, Phillips GA: *Understanding human anatomy and physiology,* Philadelphia, 1989, WB Saunders, p. 240.)

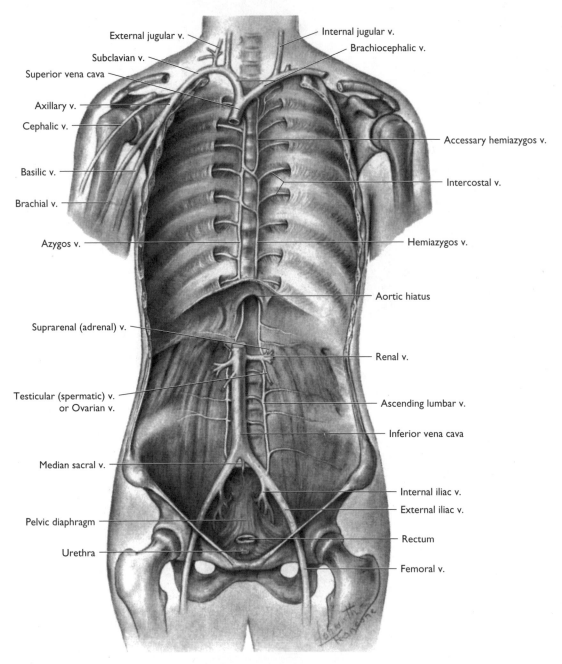

FIG. 6-23 *Vena cava and tributaries.* (From Jacob SW, Francone CA: *Elements of anatomy and physiology,* ed 2, Philadelphia, 1989, WB Saunders, p. 89.)

network across the top of the foot. On the border of each foot lie the medial and lateral marginal veins. The great saphenous vein, the longest vein in the body, extends from the medial marginal vein in the foot up the medial aspect of the leg to the femoral vein in the inguinal area. The small saphenous vein arises from the lateral marginal vein at the ankle to above the knee, where it joins the popliteal vein (Fig. 6-24).

The superficial veins are connected to the deep veins by perforating veins at the ankle, distal calf, and around the knee. These perforating veins have valves that prevent blood from flowing from the deep veins to the superficial veins. Muscular

action pumps blood toward the heart. However, if the valves are not functioning properly, or during periods of muscle relaxation or atrophy, blood can move into the superficial veins. The increased pressure in the superficial veins causes fluid to leak into the subcutaneous tissue, with edema seen on examination. This increased pressure leads to blood stagnation and results in enlarged and tortuous superficial veins called *varicosities.* Ulcerations can result from the damaged tissue and lack of circulation. Because of this process, the use of veins in the feet and ankles for the routine delivery of any IV therapy is not recommended.

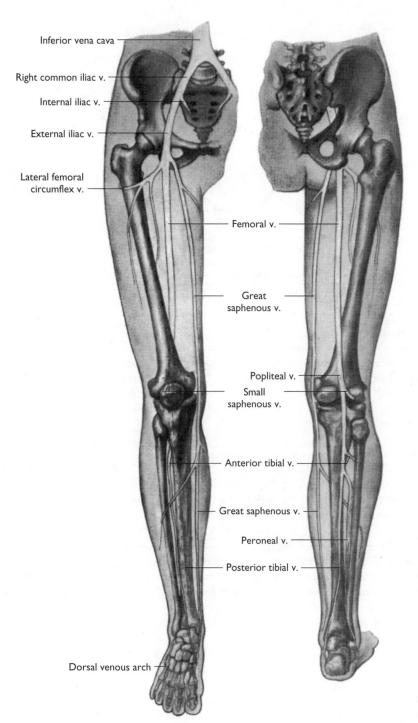

Inferior vena cava

Right common iliac v.

Internal iliac v.

External iliac v.

Lateral femoral
circumflex v.

Femoral v.

Great
saphenous v.

Popliteal v.
Small
saphenous v.

Anterior tibial v.

Great saphenous v.

Peroneal v.

Posterior tibial v.

Dorsal venous arch

FIG. 6-24   *Veins of the right pelvis and leg.* (From Jacob
SW, Francone CA: *Elements of anatomy and physiology,* ed 2, Philadelphia, 1989, WB Saunders, p. 196.)

SYSTEMIC BLOOD FLOW

Flow of any fluid is the amount of fluid that can pass a given
point in a given period. For instance, the cardiac output of
blood in an average resting adult is about 5 L/min. Blood
circulates in a closed system and depends on more factors than
the amount of blood pumped by the heart. These factors are the
same as those for fluid flowing through any other closed system:
the volume and properties of the fluid, pressures within the
system and the resistance to those pressures, velocity or speed of

flow, type of flow, and the ability of the system to comply with
changes in demand.

Blood volume and distribution

Precise regulation of blood volume is the result of a complex
interaction between cardiac output, excretion of excessive
amount of fluids and electrolytes by the kidneys, and hormonal
and nervous system factors. Inability of the heart to pump

strongly enough to perfuse the kidneys, an increase in red cell production (polycythemia), and the creation of additional space for blood, such as during pregnancy or with large varicose veins, can increase the total volume of the system.

Physical properties of blood

The viscosity of any fluid is defined as the degree of resistance to flow when pressure is applied. Two factors determine the viscosity of blood: the percentage of cells in blood (hematocrit) and the level of plasma proteins. The effect of the hematocrit is far greater than that of the plasma proteins. Friction from a high concentration of cells increases viscosity. Generally, the hematocrit ranges from 38% to 42%; its viscosity is about 3 times greater than water, the viscosity of plasma proteins is about 1.5 greater than water.[4] Many diseases, injuries, and fluid and nutritional imbalances can alter this normal value, with a corresponding increase in viscosity.

Viscosity is affected by vessel diameter. The most rapid flow in large vessels is found in the center of the vessel, with the flow closest to the vessel intima being the slowest. As the velocity of flow decreases, the viscosity increases; therefore blood flowing through small vessels and capillaries has a higher viscosity. Red blood cells can adhere to each other or to the vessel walls and form stacks, called *rouleaux*. Cells can become lodged in constricted places within small vessels as well. Offsetting the factors that increase viscosity is the fact that, in capillaries and small vessels, cells line up and pass through in a single file, decreasing the viscous properties of many cells moving randomly together. This is called the *Fahraeus-Lindqvist effect,* and it is found in vessels smaller than 1.5 mm wide.[4] Because of these contradicting factors, it is difficult to assess the total effect of the hematocrit on viscosity in small vessels and capillaries.

The presence of cannulas in vessels with a small lumen decreases the velocity of flow, which might have the same effect on the viscosity of blood. Therefore it is important to use the smallest cannula in the largest possible vessel. This allows room for blood to flow adequately between the wall of the vein and the wall of the cannula. Knowledge of the patient's hematocrit and careful attention to adequate hydration are also important.

Pressure and resistance to flow

Because of the pumping action of the heart, the greatest pressure, about 100 mm Hg, is found in the aorta. From this point, the pressure gradually decreases until it reaches the junction of the vena cavae and the right atrium, where it measures 0 mm Hg. In the capillary bed, the pressure ranges from 35 mm Hg on the arterial side to 100 mm Hg on the venous side, with a functional pressure in the capillary of about 17 mm Hg.[4] The difference in pressure causes the blood to flow.

Flow through a single vessel is most affected by the diameter of the vessel (Fig. 6-25). When the diameter doubles, the flow rate increases 16 times, and with a fourfold increase in lumen diameter, the flow rate dramatically increases 256 times.

Force from this pressure is met by resistance from the vessel wall or vasomotor tone. Resistance is controlled by the vasomo-

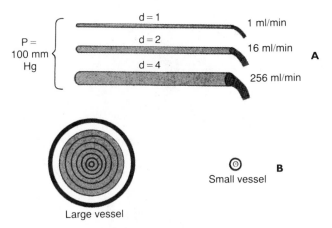

FIG. 6-25 A, *Demonstration of the effect of vessel diameter (d) on blood flow.* **B,** *Concentric rings of blood flowing at different velocities; the farther away from the vessel wall, the faster the flow.* (From Guyton AC: *Textbook of medical physiology,* ed 8, Philadelphia, 1991, WB Saunders, p. 156.)

tor center in the brainstem, which sends impulses to the sympathetic nerve endings located in all vessels except the metarterioles, precapillary sphincters, and capillaries.

Blood flow through the capillary bed is not constant, as in other vessels, but intermittent and is based on the needs of the tissue served. When the oxygen level in the tissue decreases, the precapillary sphincter opens, allowing flow to proceed. The primary purpose of the thin capillary membrane is allowing diffusion of substances through the membrane. Two opposing forces control the amount of molecular movement across the membrane: hydrostatic pressure and colloid osmotic pressure.

Hydrostatic pressure is created by fluid in the vessel and the interstitial space. Colloid osmotic pressure is the opposing force exerted by plasma proteins. Proteins do not pass through the capillary membrane easily, which results in a difference in protein concentration between the plasma and interstitial fluid, and this difference remains steady. The concentration of plasma proteins is normally about 7 g/dl, with the interstitial protein level about 2 to 3 g/dl.[4] Colloid osmotic pressure is also called *oncotic pressure* to distinguish it from the osmotic pressure of fluid moving from the interstitial space into each individual cell.

As blood enters the arterial side of the capillary, the hydrostatic pressure is greater, forcing fluid to move into the interstitial space. The smaller amount of fluid in the capillary decreases the hydrostatic pressure, causing the colloid osmotic pressure to force fluids back into the venous side.

Pressure in the peripheral veins is directly related to the pressure in the right atrium and to the heart's ability to pump blood out of the right atrium.

Normally, the right atrial pressure is 0 mm Hg, roughly equal to the atmospheric pressure around the body. In a variety of clinical conditions, this can range from as high as 30 mm Hg during cardiac failure or the transfusion of massive amounts of blood to as low as -5 mm Hg when the blood flow to the heart has been altered by hemorrhage or some other severe impediment.

Velocity and types of blood flow

Velocity is the distance blood moves in a specific period. Normally, blood moves through the aorta at a rate of 33 cm/sec, but in capillaries the velocity drops to 0.3 mm/sec.[4]

Flow can be in two types or patterns: laminar or turbulent. In laminar flow, the blood moves in layers or concentric circles through the vessels (see Fig. 6-25). As blood moves through the vessels, the layer touching the vessel wall is slowed because of adherence to the wall. The next layer slides easily over the outer one, and the innermost layer moves easiest.

Turbulent flow is in all directions, flowing crosswise and lengthwise along the vessel (see Fig. 6-25). This type of flow is created when the vessel's inner surface is rough, there is an obstruction or a sharp turn in the vessel, or the amount of flow has increased greatly.

Clotting process

The human body is normally quite efficient in hemostasis, or the prevention of blood loss. Hemostasis occurs in five stages: (1) vasoconstriction or vasospasm, (2) formation of a platelet plug, (3) activation of the clotting cascade, (4) formation of the clot, and (5) clot retraction and dissolution (Fig. 6-26).[3,4]

The first stage of the clotting process begins immediately after vessel injury when the vessel wall contracts and reduces the blood flow from the vessel opening. Nervous responses, smooth muscle spasm, and various factors released from the traumatized tissue and platelets cause this contraction. Vessels that have sustained greater trauma such as from crushing will bleed less than one that has received a sharp cut. The greater the degree of trauma, the greater the vasospasm.

The second step is the formation of a platelet plug. Platelets are round discs usually only about 2 to 4 μm wide.[4] Although they are not whole cells and cannot reproduce, they do contain several factors and enzyme systems that cause contraction. They also assist in the repair of damaged vessels by releasing a factor that causes growth of endothelial cells, smooth muscle cells, and fibroblasts. The platelet surface has a glycoprotein coat that prevents its adherence to intact endothelium, yet causes the platelet to adhere to damaged endothelial cells and the collagen in the other layers of the vessel wall. When platelets pass over a damaged portion of the vessel wall, they swell, change shapes, and release enzymes that increase their stickiness. These changes attract more platelets, forming a loose plug that is capable of stopping blood loss in a small vessel opening. Adhered platelets also release serotonin and histamine, causing additional smooth muscle contraction.

The third step is the activation of the complex clotting cascade that results in the formation of a blood clot. Fibrin threads form and attach to the platelet plug. This meshwork attracts red blood cells, phagocytes, and microorganisms that tightly fill the vessel hole.

Fibrin, the end result of the clotting cascade, is not normally found in circulating blood. Blood coagulation is a battle between the components that promote clotting, called *procoagulants,* and those that prevent clotting, called *anticoagulants.* These two groups comprise more than 50 substances found in the blood. Normally, the anticoagulants are dominant, but at

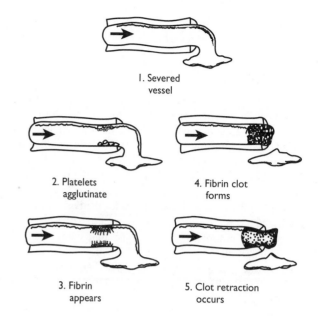

FIG. 6-26 *Clotting process in the traumatized blood vessel.* (From Guyton AC, Hall JG: *Textbook of medical physiology,* ed 9, Philadelphia, 1996, WB Saunders, p. 464.)

sites of vessel damage, the procoagulants become active and prevail over the anticoagulants.

The coagulation or clotting cascade acts in two different but interacting pathways: the extrinsic pathway, which starts with vessel or tissue damage, and the intrinsic pathway, which starts with the blood. The extrinsic pathway includes tissue factor released from damaged tissue; factor VII and tissue factor activate factor X, which combines with phospholipids and factor V to form prothrombin activator. When the blood is traumatized or when blood contacts collagen in the vascular wall, the intrinsic pathway begins by activating factor XII and platelet phospholipids. Through enzymatic actions, factor XII activates factor XI, then factor IX, and then factor X. With the help of factor V, platelets, and phospholipids, prothrombin activator is formed.

The end result of both pathways is the formation of prothrombin activator. With the help of calcium and prothrombin receptors on platelets, prothrombin activator converts prothrombin, a plasma protein, to thrombin.

The fourth stage is the formation of the clot. Thrombin, a protein enzyme, converts fibrinogen, a large protein made by the liver, to fibrin. Early in the formation, fibrin strands are loosely bound together and can be broken apart very easily. However, within minutes, fibrin-stabilizing factor is released from the platelets inside the clot to form a strongly bonded and cross-linked mesh of fibrin. Fibrin attaches to the vessel wall, closing the hole in the vascular wall. Within an hour, the clot retracts to force out serum with all the clotting factors removed. As the clot becomes smaller the vessel edges are pulled together.

A blood clot continues to produce thrombin and attract platelets, causing it to grow. Within a day or so later, the clot stops growing and begins to break down. Tissue plasminogen activator (t-PA) is released from the injured tissue and endothelium. Plasminogen is converted to plasmin, an enzyme with action similar to digestive enzymes. Plasmin digests the fibrin and other components of the clot.[4]

MECHANISMS OF DEFENSE

Intact skin, mucous membranes, and the biochemical barriers discussed earlier compose the first line of defense. During the delivery of all infusion therapy, skin is the first barrier to be breached. The second mechanism of defense is the inflammatory response, which clears the body of harmful chemicals, foreign bodies, and microorganisms. This process involves many types of cells and plasma proteins and begins within seconds after injury. Inflammation is not specific to the type of invader and proceeds with the same process regardless of the type of injury or the number of times cellular injury has occurred. The immune response is the third line of defense and involves only one type of serum protein, called *immunoglobulins*, and one type of cell, called *lymphocytes*. The immune system has a memory, providing long-lasting and often permanent protection.[3]

Inflammation

Cellular injury initiates the process of acute inflammation. Many aspects of infusion therapy begin with cellular injury. Venipuncture breaks the skin, subcutaneous tissue, and the vessel wall. The degree of cellular injury depends on the skill used to enter the vein and advance the cannula to the desired location. Using peripheral veins to insert midline and peripher-ally inserted central catheters increases the potential for inflammation because longer vein sections can be injured. Injury to the skin surface can result from repeated application and removal of dressings and tape, rigid pieces of tubing anchored tightly to the skin, cannula migration into or out of the insertion site, and use of antiseptic agents. Rapid infusion of large volumes and infusion of solutions with extremes in osmolarity and pH through veins with small amounts of blood flow can injure the vein wall. Invasion of microorganisms is always a distinct possiblity with any type of infusion therapy. Temperature changes and oxygen and nutrient deprivation also produce cellular injury.

Three systems of cellular components are set in motion when injury occurs: (1) mast cells degranulate; (2) complement, kinin, and clotting systems are activated; and (3) other cellular components, such as granulocytes and platelets, are released. Classic signs and symptoms of this activity include redness, heat, edema, pus formation, thrombus formation, and pain.

The sequence of events in the process of inflammation (Fig. 6-27) begins with contraction of the arterioles close to the injury followed by vasodilation, which increases blood flow to the area. Plasma and blood cells move into the tissue, causing swelling. Blood volume in the capillaries decreases and becomes more viscous. White blood cells move into the area and stick to vessel walls. Endothelial cells lining capillaries and venules retract, creating space between the cells for more fluid to leak into the tissue. Vascular permeability continues through the acute phase, allowing fluids and cells to move to the injured tissue, where they stimulate and control inflammation.

Neutrophils move into the area, followed by monocytes,

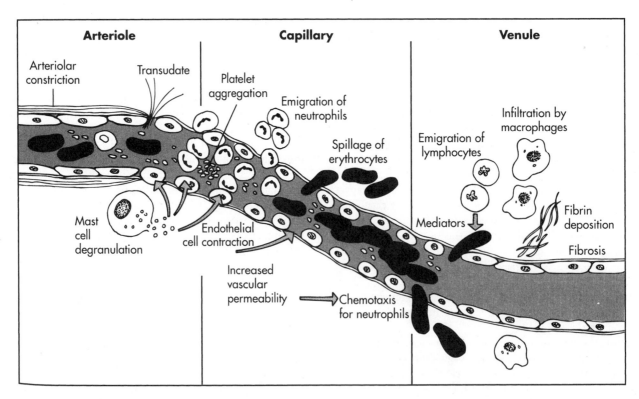

FIG. 6-27 *Sequence of events in the process of inflammation.* (From McCance KL, Huether SE: *Pathophysiology: the biological basis for disease in adults and children,* St Louis, 1998, Mosby, p. 207.)

macrophages, and basophils. These white blood cells ingest microorganisms, parasites, and cellular debris. Three plasma protein systems (complement, kinin, and clotting) and immunoglobulins help control inflammation and bleeding.

Mast cells exert the greatest impact on the inflammatory response. These cells are filled with granular substances and are located close to blood vessels in connective tissue of skin, lungs, and the gastrointestinal tract. Basophils are white blood cells that function similarly to the mast cell. When stimulated, mast cells release histamine, neutrophil chemotactic factor, and eosinophil chemotactic factor, causing an immediate reaction. At the time of injury, the mast cell wall also releases arachidonic acid, which produces leukotrienes and prostaglandins. These substances act in the later stages of the event and are responsible for the prolonged signs and symptoms.

Histamine causes smooth muscle constriction in large vessels but dilation of postcapillary venules. This results in greater circulation in the microcirculation and increased vascular permeability. Histamine's effects can be seen on neurons, glandular cells, blood cells, and cells of the immune system.[14]

Neutrophil and eosinophil chemotactic factors are biochemical mediators that attract a specific type of white blood cell to the injured site. Leukotrienes, previously known as the slow-reacting substance of anaphylaxis, act in a fashion similar to histamine. Prostaglandins increase vascular permeability; cause itching, pain, and platelet aggregation, and can inhibit inflammation by suppressing the release of more histamine. Aspirin and some nonsteroidal antiinflammatory drugs block the production of prostaglandins, thus inhibiting inflammation.

Physical injury, chemical injury, IgE-mediated mechanisms, and activation of the complement system all stimulate mast cells to release their granules (Fig. 6-28). Physical injury includes trauma by cannula advancement, heat, ultraviolet light, and x-rays. Chemical injury comes from toxins, snake and bee venom, and drugs such as vancomycin, morphine, barbiturates, and many muscle relaxants used during anesthesia. Neuropeptides and tissue enzymes can also cause chemical injury.

The human complement system consists of three groups of plasma proteins: the complement system, the clotting system (discussed earlier), and the kinin system. In the inflammatory response, the complement system is of prime importance. In this group, about 10 proteins account for approximately 10% of the proteins in circulation.[3] This system involves a cascading of enzyme activity that can be started in two ways. The classic pathway begins with the antigen-antibody complex containing IgG or IgM interacting with C1, the first protein in the system. The alternative pathway for activation of complement comes from polysaccharides, such as endotoxins on bacterial and fungal cell walls. The primary purpose of these proteins is to enhance inflammation by rendering bacteria capable of being killed, attracting leukocytes, and acting as anaplylotoxins, which cause mast cells to degranulate. The clotting proteins' purpose in inflammation is to form the mesh network that traps microorganisms and foreign bodies.

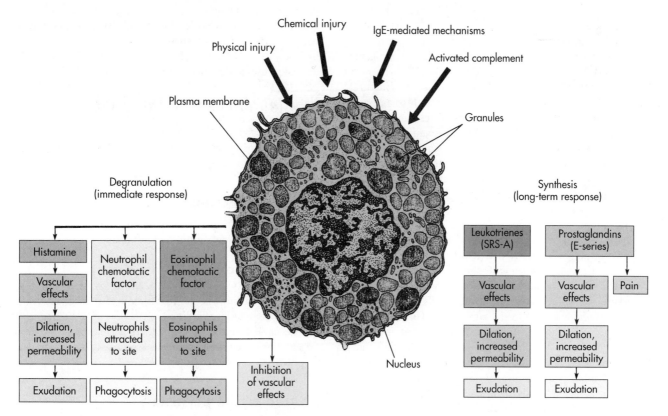

FIG. 6-28 *Effects of degranulation and synthesis of mast cells.* (From McCance KL, Huether SE: *Pathophysiology: the biological basis for disease in adults and children*, St Louis, 1998, Mosby, p. 208.)

The kinin system consists of three hormones, the most important of which is bradykinin. The function of all kinins is to cause smooth muscle contractility, vasodilation, and increased capillary blood flow. Bradykinin appears to be of the greatest importance in producing pain, especially when the pain is caused by tissue damage.[4] Small amounts of bradykinin injected intradermally can cause a large amount of edema by dramatically increasing the size of the openings in the capillary wall.[4]

Other cells involved in the inflammatory response are granulocytes and monocytes (immature cells) and macrophages (mature cells in tissue). Granulocytes include neutrophils, eosinophils, and basophils. Their purpose is to engulf and destroy microorganisms, dead cells, and other foreign matter.

Platelets act in the inflammatory process to release serotonin, which acts in a similar fashion to histamine.[3]

Immunity

The immune response begins when a foreign substance, known as an *antigen,* is introduced into the body. Antigens include bacteria, fungi, parasites, viruses, pollens, foods, venoms, drugs, vaccines, transfusions, and transplanted tissue. Once the body has been challenged by these invaders, certain physiologic and biochemical interactions lead to the maturation and activation of two types of immunocompetent cells—B and T lymphocytes. Antigens are incapacitated by the antibodies produced by B lymphocytes and are then attacked by T lymphocytes. Some B and T lymphocytes turn into memory cells, which remember the antigen and stand ready to attack it even faster on subsequent exposures.

Immunity can be manipulated in several ways. Natural immunity is present at birth and does not require antigenic stimulation. For instance, there are many animal diseases, such as cowpox, that humans cannot contract because of natural immunity. Acquired immunity can be either actively or passively obtained after birth as a result of the immune response. Immunization provides acquired immunity, for example, as does contracting a disease such as rubella. Passive acquired immunity comes from the infusion of preformed antibodies or T lymphocytes, such as emergency treatments for snake bite, tetanus, or rabies. Passage of maternal antibodies to the fetus is another example of passive acquired immunity.

The immune process has two distinct stages. Soon after exposure to an antigen, the B lymphocytes enter a latent period during which no antibodies can be detected. After 5 to 7 days, the primary stage begins when IgM, one class of antibodies, can be detected. The antibodies are broken down if no further antigens are introduced. However, memory cells have been left. When the second exposure to the same antigen occurs, IgG, a second type of antibody, is produced rapidly and in larger quantities than IgM. Vaccination is an example of active acquired immunity through this primary and secondary response.

Mature lymphocytes produce most of the immune response. These cells originate in the liver and spleen and migrate through two different pathways toward maturity. B lymphocytes mature in the liver and bone marrow, are held in the lymphoid tissue throughout the body, and produce humoral immunity. T lymphocytes mature by migrating through the thymus gland, are held in lymphoid tissue, and produce cell-mediated immunity.

Antigens are complex, large-molecule proteins that are foreign to the host and whose structures match receptor sites on lymphocytes or antibody molecules. The foreign nature of antigens is critical to the immune response because the body is able to distinguish self-antigens such as those found on red blood cells.

Antibodies are immunoglobulins possessing a specific receptor site for a specific antigen. There are five types of antibodies: IgG, IgA, IgM, IgE, and IgD. About 75% of the antibodies in a normal human are IgG. IgE is of particular importance because it mediates allergic reactions.[4]

Allergic reactions can be caused by either T lymphocytes or large amounts of IgE. Reactions caused by T lymphocytes are usually limited to skin eruptions in the area where the agent contacted the skin. Cosmetics, chemicals, and latex that produces contact dermatitis fall into this category. However, some people have a greater tendency to form IgE, increasing their risk of allergic and anaphylactic reactions. IgE has a strong attraction to mast cells and basophils, causing the release of preformed mediators such as histamine and the synthesis of leukotrienes and prostaglandins discussed earlier.

Other substances that aid in the processes of inflammation and immunity include cytokines, interleukins, and interferons. Cytokines are glycoproteins that function as messengers in the immune response. Because of their ability to communicate between cells, they have also been called the "hormones" of the immune system. Interleukins are biochemical messengers produced by macrophages that increase the number of neutrophils and other enzyme activities during inflammation and immune response. Interferons are small proteins produced and released by many types of cells whose primary purpose is protection against viruses and reduction of tumor growth.[3,4]

NURSING DIAGNOSES AND EXPECTED OUTCOMES

A partial list of appropriate nursing diagnoses is represented by the following.[15]

Risk for infection

The risk of infection is related to the effects of medications (antibiotics, steroids), chronic diseases, and to the presence of invasive lines.

Expected outcomes

1. The patient will not develop any signs or symptoms of infection during the administration of prescribed medications or use of invasive lines.
2. The patient and significant others will demonstrate understanding of the causes and risks associated with infection and practice precautionary measures.

Altered tissue perfusion

This diagnosis is related to exchange problems, as in the infusion of nephrotoxic antibiotics (aminoglycosides, vancomycin, antifungal agents), interruption of arterial or venous blood flow, hypovolemia, and hypervolemia.

Expected outcomes

1. The patient will have good fluid and electrolyte balance as evidenced by adequate urinary output and serum electrolyte results.
2. The patient will maintain safe serum levels of medications as evidenced by serum drug monitoring.
3. The patient will regain normal blood levels of nitrogenous waste products as evidenced by normal blood urea nitrogen and serum creatinine levels.

Risk for peripheral neurovascular dysfunction

The risk for peripheral neurovascular dysfunction is related to trauma to arteries from puncture for cannula insertion or blood sample withdrawal, interruption in venous flow, as in thrombosis or thrombophlebitis development, and decreased venous flow, as in the insertion of a large-gauge cannula in a vein.

Expected outcomes

1. The patient will regain warm, dry skin.
2. The patient will not have palpable venous cords or pain.
3. The patient will not have peripheral edema distal to cannula placement.

Risk for impaired skin integrity

The risk for impaired skin integrity is related to age; mechanical factors of dressing material, tape, or antiseptic solutions; decreased nutritional intake; and medications (steroids, hormones).

Expected outcomes

1. The patient's skin integrity will be maintained by the use of appropriate types of dressing materials and appropriate application and removal techniques.
2. The patient will maintain good hydration and nutritional status.

Impaired skin integrity

Impaired skin integrity is related to age; mechanical factors of dressing material, tape, or antiseptic solutions; decreased nutritional intake; and medications (steroids).

Expected outcome

1. The patient will have healing of skin lesions with return to intact skin.

Pain

Pain is related to injury by chemical agents (vesicant medications and solutions with extreme tonicity or pH ranges) and physical agents (insertion of any parenteral cannula).

Expected outcome

1. The patient will have an increasing comfort level as evidenced by decreasing complaints of pain, use of improved coping mechanisms, employment of pain relief measures, and decreased focus on pain.

REFERENCES

1. Williams P et al, editors: *Gray's anatomy*, ed 38, London, 1995, Churchill Livingstone.
2. Freedberg I et al, editors: *Fitzpatrick's dermatology in general medicine*, ed 5, vol 1, New York, 1998, McGraw-Hill.
3. McCance KL, Huether SE, editors: *Pathophysiology: the biological basis for disease in adults and children*, ed 3, St Louis, 1998, Mosby.
4. Guyton A: *Textbook of medical physiology*, ed 9, Philadelphia, 1996, WB Saunders.
5. Andris DA, Krzywda EA: Catheter pinch-off syndrome: recognition and management, *JIN* 20(5):233, 1997.
6. Hadaway LC: Thrombotic and nonthrombotic complications: loss of patency, *JIN* 21(5S):S143, 1998.
7. Tierney L, McPhee S, Papadakis M, editors: *Current medical diagnosis and treatment*, ed 37, Stamford, Conn, 1998, Appleton and Lange.
8. Drexler H: Endothlial dysfunction: clinical implications, *Prog Cardiovasc Dis* 39(4):287, 1997.
9. DeMeyer G, Herman A: Vascular endothelial dysfunction, *Prog Cardiovasc Dis* 39(4):325, 1997.
10. Schafer AI: Vascular endothelium: in defense of blood fluidity, *J Clin Invest* 99(6):1143, 1997.
11. Marx M: The management of the difficult peripherally inserted central venous catheter line removal, *JIN* 18(5):246, 1995.
12. Agur A: *Grant's atlas of anatomy*, ed 10, Baltimore, 1999, Williams & Wilkins.
13. Collin GR, Ahmadinejad AS, Misse E: Spontaneous migration of subcutaneous central venous catheters, *Am Surg* 63(4):322, 1997.
14. While M: Mediators of inflammation and the inflammatory process, *J Allergy Clin Immunol* 103(3, pt 2):S378, 1999.
15. Kim MJ, McFarland GK, McLane AM: *Pocket guide to nursing diagnosis*, ed 7, St Louis, 1997, Mosby.

*F*luids and *E*lectrolytes

Rose Anne Waldman Lonsway, BSN, MA, CRNI, Judy Hankins, BSN, CRNI

The study of fluids and electrolytes can be intimidating. With all its intricacies, the body relies on water, one of the simplest elemental forms, to sustain life. Water makes up almost two thirds of an adult's body weight. The relationship and balance of water with electrolytes among the body's compartments determine human health and well-being.

The continuous biochemical processes of the body maintain the body in a state of equilibrium. Water moves between various spaces and compartments. This movement depends on the types and amounts of solutes in the body. The body strives to match daily excretion with intake. Any alteration in intake or excretion results in an imbalance. Recognition and prevention of, or interventions to correct, these imbalances are among the most important roles the nurse has when caring for the patient requiring intravenous (IV) therapy.

It is important to understand the purpose that water serves in the human body. It does the following:

- Provides a medium for cellular metabolism
- Helps transport materials into and out of cells
- Is the solvent in which many of the solutes available for cell function are dissolved
- Helps regulate body temperature
- Maintains the physical and chemical consistency of intracellular and extracellular fluids
- Helps digest food through hydrolysis
- Provides a medium for excreting waste

It is estimated that a normal healthy person needs approximately 2600 ml of fluids daily to meet the body's water requirements. It has also been estimated that the absolute minimum amount of water required by that same healthy person is approximately 1500 ml/day. These facts demonstrate the importance of water in body function to prevent breakdown of the homeostatic regulating mechanisms. An alteration in the body's normal fluid and electrolyte balance not only affects functions within the fluid compartments but can eventually affect every body system. Therefore it is vital to understand how water and electrolytes work within the homeostatic framework.

Illness or disease states can easily disrupt the delicate balance of body fluid and its solutes, and treating these imbalances can lead to further complications. With proper knowledge of the IV fluids and electrolytes that are administered daily, it is possible to prevent further complications. It is therefore imperative that the nurse responsible for delivering fluids, electrolytes, and other medications have a thorough working knowledge of normal fluid and electrolyte balances and movements within the body. Understanding the physiologic effects of IV fluids and electrolytes in the presence of an imbalance is an important aspect of infusion therapy.

TRANSPORT MECHANISMS

Understanding fluid and electrolyte therapy begins with understanding the intake, output, and utilization of water and electrolytes. Regulating mechanisms include osmosis, diffusion, and filtration, all of which affect the movement of water and electrolytes within the body. Each cell is surrounded by a membrane, which is selectively permeable to some substances depending on the construction of the membrane and the ionic charge of particles or solutes attempting to move through it.

Regulating mechanisms

Osmosis. Osmosis is the movement of fluid through a semipermeable membrane. During osmosis, fluid moves in relation to the concentration of solutes; it moves through a membrane from an area of low solute concentration to an area of high solute concentration. This process continues until the solutions on both sides of the membrane are of equal concentration. The force of this movement depends on the concentration gradient—that is, the difference in concentration on either side of the membrane. The process of osmosis depends on how much of the membrane is involved and on certain characteristics of the solution—the temperature, solute solubility, and particularly the concentration. (One of the involved fluid compartments must contain a solute capable of moving through the membrane.)[1]

The number of solutes in a solution is expressed by a unit of measurement called the *osmol*. *Osmolality* describes the number of osmols per kilogram of water. The liter is the usual unit of measure for water volume. Osmolality can be expressed as a total volume of 1 L of water plus a small volume occupied by the solutes in that liter of fluid. *Osmolarity* refers to the number of osmols per liter of solution. Osmolality is expressed as Osm/kg water; osmolarity is expressed as Osm/L. Usually, there is little difference between these two measurements when expressed in clinical practice. The important thing to remember is that osmolality reflects the potential for water movement and water distribution between and within body fluid compartments.

Diffusion. Diffusion is the random movement of molecules and ions from an area of higher concentration to an area of lower concentration in a solution, such as the exchange of oxygen and carbon dioxide between the alveoli and capillaries in the lungs. Several factors influence how diffusion occurs: membrane permeability, the size of the diffusing molecule or ion, differences in electrical potential of the ions involved, and pressure gradients on either side of the membrane. Diffusion occurs through two processes: simple and facilitated. Simple diffusion occurs through either the lipid bilayer (for lipid-soluble substances) or the protein channels (for lipid-insoluble substances). Facilitated diffusion uses carrier proteins to move substances through a membrane.[2]

Filtration. Filtration is the movement of solutes and water through selectively permeable membranes, always moving from an area of higher pressure to an area of lower pressure. Filtration involves the movement of solutes and water in relation to

hydrostatic pressure. It differs from diffusion and osmosis in that diffusion and osmosis are a response to concentrations, and filtration is a response to pressure.

Pressure during filtration is hydrostatic. Hydrostatic pressure is generated by the pumping action of the heart and is opposed by oncotic pressure. Oncotic pressure is exerted mainly by plasma proteins, specifically albumin. The Donnan equilibrium effect is important to understanding oncotic pressure.[2] This principle states that electrolytes separated by a semipermeable membrane behave in predictable ways.[3,4] For example, if solutions containing different amounts of sodium and chloride are separated by a semipermeable membrane, water, sodium, and chloride will move across the membrane until equilibrium exists on both sides of that membrane (diffusion). If a nondiffusible protein is added to one side of the membrane, it changes the equilibrium. Equilibrium occurs, but if the protein is an anion, the concentration of cations is higher on the side of the membrane containing the protein (anion). This accounts for the difference in osmotic pressure between the two sides of the membrane and is called *oncotic pressure* (Fig. 7-1).[2,5]

The movement of fluid into or out of the capillaries depends on the balance between opposing forces. These forces are referred to as *Starling forces* when they relate to the movement of water and solutes through capillaries. Again, it is oncotic pressure that opposes capillary hydrostatic pressure.

The arteriolar side of a capillary has a hydrostatic pressure of approximately 32 mm Hg. This generally exceeds the plasma oncotic pressure, resulting in filtration, or the movement of fluid out of the capillary and into the interstitium.[2]

The venous (venule) side of the capillary has a pressure of approximately 15 mm Hg and, as such, is lower than the plasma oncotic pressure (approximately 22 mm Hg). In other words, the plasma oncotic pressure is greater than the hydrostatic

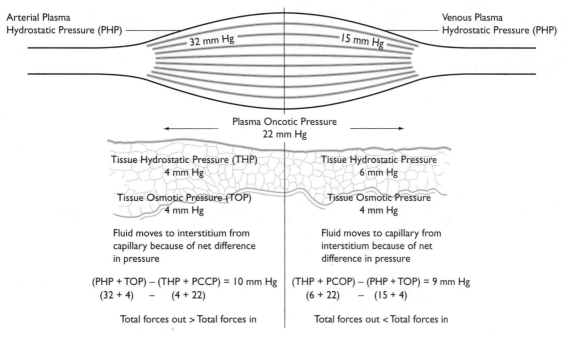

FIG. 7-1 *Oncotic pressure: differences in osmotic pressures between two sides of a membrane.*

pressure, resulting in fluid being pulled from the interstitium into the plasma in the vessel. This process is also known as *absorption.*

Capillary hydrostatic pressure and plasma oncotic pressure are influenced by tissue hydrostatic pressure and tissue osmotic pressure. The net effect of tissue and capillary hydrostatic and oncotic pressures determines movement between capillaries and the interstitium.

Interstitial fluid is formed at the arteriolar side of the capillary bed and plasma fluid is formed at the venule side of the capillary bed. This fluid formation is constantly occurring to maintain homeostasis.

Examples of filtration are glomerular filtration in the kidney, and the movement of fluids and electrolytes between the interstitium and capillary beds.

Active transport. Another way in which solutes and fluids move in the body is active transport, whereby molecules or ions move through a selectively permeable cell membrane. This movement is against the way these molecules naturally flow, or against the concentration gradient. In diffusion, substances move from areas of higher concentration to areas of lower concentration without expending energy. However, energy is required to move a molecule *against* its natural concentration gradient. This energy is provided by chemical reactions within the cell. Active transport, which may be primary or secondary, requires a pump, such as a sodium-potassium pump.

The sodium-potassium pump, an example of primary active transport, is present in all cell membranes and is fueled by adenosine triphosphate (ATP). Sodium and potassium ions can diffuse through cell membranes in small amounts. When they do, sodium and potassium concentrations eventually become equal inside and outside the cell. The sodium-potassium pump moves sodium to the outside of the cell and potassium back to the inside of the cell against the concentration gradient. This transfer is especially important for the transmission of impulses in nerve and muscle fibers. It also affects the glands, allowing the secretion of substances, and allows all body cells to assist in preventing cellular swelling. The importance of this active transport process can be seen when the metabolism of the cell stops and ATP is no longer available to keep the sodium-potassium pump working. In this event, the cell immediately begins to swell and can eventually burst.

Secondary active transport results when stored (or extra) energy from diffusion pulls another substance into a cell along with its primary target. When the movement is from outside of the cell to the inside of the cell, it is called *cotransport.* The reverse process is countertransport.[2]

Ionization. An important factor in the movement of fluid in the body is the electrical charge of the particles or solutes found in a particular fluid. Solutes are chemical compounds that act in one of two ways when in solution: they either remain whole or develop an electrical charge when dissolved. Compounds that develop an electrical charge break into particles, called *ions,* in a process called *ionization.* Such chemical compounds are commonly known as *electrolytes.* Some electrolytes have a positive charge when placed in water, whereas others develop a negative charge. Ions are dissociated particles of an electrolyte, and they too carry either a positive charge (a cation) or a negative charge (an anion). Cations are electrolytes such as

| Table 7-1 | Electrolyte Composition of Extracellular and Intracellular Fluid |

	FLUID CONCENTRATION (mEq/L)		
ELECTROLYTE	**INTRACELLULAR**	**EXTRACELLULAR (INTRAVASCULAR)**	**EXTRACELLULAR (INTERSTITIAL)**
CATION			
Na^+	−10	142	145
K^+	141	−5	−4
Ca^{2+}	−2	−5	−3
Mg^{2+}	−27	−2	−3
ANION			
Cl^-	−1	104	116
HCO_3^-	−10	−27	−30
HPO_4	100	−2	−2

sodium, potassium, calcium, and magnesium. Anions are chloride, bicarbonate, phosphate, and sulfate.

The number of electrically charged ions in a defined amount of fluid is measured as milliequivalents per liter (mEq/L) (*milliequivalent* refers to the chemical activity of an element). To achieve electrical balance, the number of cations and anions in a solution (expressed in milliequivalents) must always be equal. Milliequivalents are used as the measure of ions rather than milligrams because milligrams measure only the weight of the electrolyte. Weight gives no indication of the number of ions or the number of electrical charges contained in the ion. Therefore mEq is the more descriptive measure of a patient's electrolyte status (Table 7-1).[1]

Other substances important in the homeostasis of fluids and electrolytes are glucose, protein, organic acids, oxygen, and carbon dioxide. Although these are not necessarily considered charged particles, they are important in the body's state of balance.

Homeostatic mechanisms

There are many homeostatic mechanisms that help keep the volume and composition of body fluids within the narrow range defined as normal. Before discussing the regulating organs, there are two principles that are helpful to remember when considering homeostasis in the body.

The first principle states that the overall amount and composition of fluid within each compartment must remain stable and that each compartment must be electrically neutral—that is, the ions must be balanced between anions and cations. There should be no net electrical charge in any compartment at any given time. In addition to maintaining balance, the compartments are constantly exchanging and replacing individual ions. The work required to maintain this balance can use up to 20% of the body's ATP stores.

The second principle states that the osmolality among the intracellular, interstitial, and intravascular compartments needs to be equal. In osmosis, if there is a difference in the total number of active particles, the water moves into the compartment that contains the higher number of particles. A solution of higher osmolality has a lower water concentration (or higher particle concentration) than a solution of lesser osmolality.

Regulatory organs

Many organs, including the kidneys, heart and blood vessels, lungs, skin, adrenal glands, hypothalamus, pituitary gland, parathyroid gland, and gastrointestinal (GI) tract, are associated with maintaining the body's homeostasis.

The kidneys are considered the primary force in homeostasis because the kidneys' major function is to adjust the amount of water and electrolytes that leave the body to equal the amount that enters the body. The kidneys selectively excrete or maintain electrolytes as they monitor the body's feedback mechanisms, and thereby help maintain acid-base balance and fluid balance. Kidneys excrete waste and remove foreign substances from the blood. They produce bicarbonate to maintain the acid-base balance, and also erythropoietin, a hormone that stimulates the bone marrow to accelerate the production of red blood cells. The kidneys selectively retain or excrete hydrogen ions, which help maintain the pH of the extracellular fluid.

There are many hormonal and enzymatic influences on the kidney that assist in homeostasis. Renin is produced in and secreted by the juxtaglomerular apparatus of the kidney. Renin is a proteolytic enzyme that triggers the release of angiotensin I, angiotensin II, and thereby aldosterone. The renin-angiotensin-aldosterone system regulates sodium reabsorption in the renal tubules. Homeostasis depends on an appropriate circulating volume. Renin helps maintain appropriate circulating volume.[5]

Natriuretic factor, also known as *atriopeptin* or *atrial natriuretic peptide* (ANP), is classified as a hormone and is secreted from the cardiac atria. It influences fluid loss, electrolyte loss, and vascular tone changes. This factor can cause renal vasodilation and increased excretion of sodium. It is thought that it can interfere with the secretion of aldosterone and thereby interfere with sodium reabsorption in the kidney, specifically the distal tubules and collecting ducts. It is secreted in the atria when blood volume increases and increased central venous and right atrial pressures exist. Changes in levels of ANP may allow only very small changes in blood volume when, for example, sodium and water intake is increased abnormally.[2,3,5] All these influences work together to balance the excretion and reabsorption of fluids and electrolytes through and within the kidney. It is obvious why alterations in kidney function have a devastating effect on the system as a whole.

The heart and blood vessels also play a major role in fluid balance. The pumping action of the heart and the resulting circulation through the blood vessels allows blood to reach the kidneys in sufficient volume to regulate water and electrolytes. Circulation of blood through the kidneys also allows urine to form. Adequate renal perfusion is the foundation for adequate renal function. In addition, there are special stretch receptors in the blood vessels and atrium of the heart, whose purpose is to react to hypovolemic states by stimulating fluid retention.

The lungs also contribute to homeostasis through the ventilatory process. Under the control of the medulla oblongata and in response to hydrogen level changes in the blood, the lungs act rapidly to correct metabolic acid-base disturbances. The lungs also regulate oxygen and carbon dioxide levels.

The pituitary gland stores antidiuretic hormone (ADH). ADH is manufactured in the hypothalamus and causes the body to retain water. This water-conserving function has several effects. One is the maintenance of osmotic pressure by controlling water retention or excretion by the kidneys. ADH also plays a small role in the control of blood volume. When blood volume decreases, the ADH level increases and water is retained. When blood volume rises, ADH secretion is decreased and water is excreted through the kidneys.

The adrenal glands, positioned above the kidneys, consist of two different sections: the adrenal cortex and the adrenal medulla. The adrenal cortex secretes two mineralocorticoid hormones, aldosterone and cortisol, that affect homeostasis. Aldosterone acts on the kidney's tubular cells, is active in the reabsorption of sodium and water, and can decrease potassium excretion. An increase in the level of aldosterone results in the retention of sodium and the loss of potassium. When sodium is retained, water is also retained. A decreased secretion of aldosterone results in the excretion of sodium and water and the retention of potassium. Cortisol, among its many functions, helps regulate blood pressure by regulating the amount of vasoconstriction necessary to maintain a normal blood pressure. Aldosterone is considered the more powerful of the two hormones, but when cortisol is secreted in large quantities, it can also affect sodium and fluid retention and potassium excretion.

The parathyroid glands are attached to the lateral lobes of the thyroid gland. There are usually four to five glands, but the number varies among individuals. Parathyroid hormone (PTH), secreted from the parathyroid glands, has an effect on calcium and phosphate concentrations and influences the reabsorption of calcium. An increase in the PTH level increases the serum calcium concentration and lowers the serum phosphate concentration. The reverse is also true; a decreased secretion of PTH lowers the serum calcium and elevates the serum phosphate concentrations. Decreased serum calcium levels stimulate the release of PTH, which in turn increase the serum calcium level. The thyroid gland, which secretes calcitonin, also has an effect on calcium levels in the body. If there is an increase in the serum calcium level, this causes an increased secretion of calcitonin. The effect of calcitonin on calcium is opposite that of PTH.

Other organs that affect fluid and electrolyte balance in the body are the skin and the GI tract. Because the skin communicates with our environment, it allows water to escape from the body through perspiration. The GI tract also plays a role in water absorption and reabsorption.

All the organs of homeostasis can be likened to a symphony. To make music, each musician needs to play his or her part in harmony with the other musicians. When they play together, beautiful music can be made. So it is with the organs of homeostasis. Through their interdependencies and interaction, they all work together to meet a common goal: the maintenance of a balanced state in the human body.

FLUID AND WATER MOVEMENT
Fluid compartments

The internal environment of the human body is largely composed of fluid, with water being the most abundant component. Approximately 60% of body weight in an adult is water (Fig. 7-2). The amount of total body water as a percentage of body weight varies somewhat among individuals because of differences in the amount of adipose tissue, which contains little water.

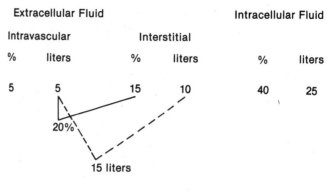

FIG. 7-2 *Distribution and amount of body fluids in an "average" adult.*

Body water is distributed between the intracellular, extracellular, and transcellular compartments. Intracellular fluid is the fluid content of all cells, and represents about two-thirds of total body weight.

Extracellular fluid constitutes about one third of total body weight. The extracellular fluid compartment is divided into two separate areas. Fluid found in tissue spaces between blood vessels and cells of the body, including lymph fluid, is referred to as *interstitial fluid.* The other type of extracellular fluid is plasma, which accounts for approximately 5% of total body weight. Extracellular fluid serves two functions in the body. First, it provides a relatively constant environment for the cells. Second, it helps transport substances to and from the cells. Plasma, sometimes referred to as *vessel fluid,* is a highly specialized fluid in the body and contains red blood cells and protein in large amounts. Protein helps retain the special nature of plasma because it provides osmotic pull and preserves vessel water composition. The protein content is what makes plasma highly specialized because protein is generally found only in a particular space or vessel. Any particle confined to a particular space pulls water into that space.[2,3,6]

Transcellular fluid is considered a component of the extracellular fluid compartment. The fluid that is contained in transcellular areas is specialized and is composed of cerebrospinal, pleural, peritoneal, or synovial fluid. GI fluid is also classified as transcellular. It is separated from the blood, but unlike the other fluid compartments, it is separated by capillary endothelial cells and epithelial tissue; therefore it is compartmentalized fluid.

Transcellular fluid is not usually considered when talking about fluid and electrolyte balance; however, because of the special attributes of transcellular fluids, physical symptoms are attributed to their loss.

Although intracellular and extracellular fluids contain the same types of anions and cations, the amounts in which they are found vary between the two compartments. The principal cation in intracellular fluid is potassium. Found in lesser amounts are magnesium, sodium, and calcium. The most prevalent anion in intracellular fluid is phosphate, with smaller amounts of bicarbonate and chloride. The fluid cation found in most abundance in extracellular fluid is sodium; present in much smaller amounts are potassium, calcium, and magnesium. The principal

anion of extracellular fluid is chloride, and bicarbonate and phosphate are found in smaller amounts.

Therefore major electrolytes in extracellular fluid are sodium as a cation and chloride as an anion. Sodium, chloride, and bicarbonate represent more than 90% of the total amount of solutes found in the extracellular space. Potassium is the major cation in cells, and magnesium is also found in high concentration. The anions in the intracellular compartment are phosphate, sulfate, bicarbonate, and proteinate (Fig. 7-3).

Movement of fluids and electrolytes

One way that water moves in the body is through osmotic pressure. The distribution of water in the body depends on electrolyte balance and on the distribution of electrolytes and fluids within the intracellular and extracellular compartments. Osmotic gradients are established and maintained by solutes. Although water is largely unconfined within the respective compartments, electrolytes are usually confined to their respective compartments.

Effects of body fluid concentration. If there is no water movement through a membrane because of an osmotic balance, the solutions on either side of the membrane are isotonic. That is, they exert the same amount of osmotic pressure on each side of the membrane, and they contain the same amount of osmotically active solutes. Isotonic osmolality is approximately 300 mOsm/L.[6] Fluid containing a large number of solutes is considered hypertonic when compared with water containing no solute particles. Conversely, water is considered hypotonic when compared with a fluid containing many solute particles. *Osmotic pressure* refers to how strongly water can be pulled across a membrane; the strength or pressure of that pull depends on the amount of solutes or molecules in the solution.

Colloids. Electrolytes and other low-molecular-weight substances exert a normal osmotic pressure. Colloids, such as protein and albumin, are nondiffusible substances that have a higher molecular weight. Therefore they exert a higher osmotic pressure, the colloid osmotic or oncotic pressure, which causes water to be pulled into the intravascular space.

Crystalloids. Diffusible substances are referred to as *crystalloids.* They are important in fluid balance because they can

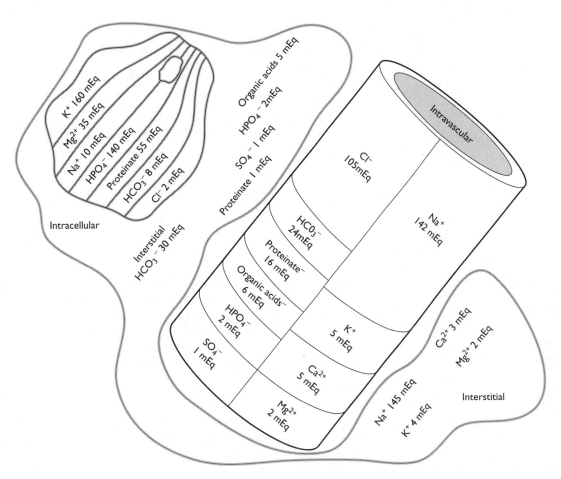

FIG. 7-3 *Anions and cations of intracellular, interstitial, and intravascular fluids.*

pass through capillary walls, which are the barriers between plasma and interstitial fluid. Crystalloids can expand both the intravascular and interstitial spaces. Usually, only about 25% of crystalloids administered remain in the intravascular space, with the rest moving to the interstitial space. Examples of crystalloids are dextrose in water, electrolytes in water, and sodium chloride solutions.

Plasma. Because it contains protein, the plasma component of extracellular fluid responds in a special way to fluid balance. Proteins pull water into the intravascular space.

Sodium. Fluid balance is also regulated by the sodium concentration in plasma and is also influenced by glucose and urea in plasma. Sodium contributes more than 90% of extracellular fluid solutes. The osmotic pressure produced by sodium determines the state of cellular hydration. Osmosis occurs when the extracellular fluid contains an electrolyte content lower or higher than normal. For example, if plain water with no electrolyte content were injected into the bloodstream, the red blood cells in the plasma would absorb the water. This would cause the cells to swell and burst. If a solution with a high sodium content were injected into the body, the red blood cells would lose water to the salt and the cells would shrink.

Solute concentration. Solute concentration and the associated osmotic force affect body water distribution. As stated

earlier, water moves from an area of lower solute concentration to an area of higher concentration, or an area of high osmolality. A change in the osmolality of one compartment always alters the osmolality of the other compartment; stated another way, a change in extracellular fluid compartment osmolality dictates a change in the osmolality of intracellular fluids. The body is striving for homeostasis, and there is water movement until the osmolality values of both compartments are relatively equal.

Fluid pressure. To understand the movement of fluids and solutes within the body, fluid pressures and the amounts of solutes and water in the various compartments must be considered. As water moves to achieve a state of equilibrium, so do pressures exerted on the fluids change to reach a state of equilibrium. There are four pressures to consider when studying water exchange between plasma and interstitial fluid. Movement is determined by blood hydrostatic and colloid osmotic pressures on one side of the capillary membrane and by interstitial fluid hydrostatic and colloid osmotic pressures on the other side. Blood hydrostatic pressure forces fluid out of the capillaries into the interstitial fluid on one side; however, blood colloid osmotic pressure draws it back into the capillaries. Interstitial fluid hydrostatic pressure forces fluids out of the interstitial space into the capillaries, and interstitial fluid colloid osmotic pressure moves fluid back out of the capillaries. The net effect is that two of these pressures exert a force in one direction, and two exert pressure in the opposite direction. The difference between these two sets of opposing pressures represents the net or effective filtration pressure. An increase in plasma volume causes an increase in hydrostatic pressure of the blood, which then affects the pressure gradient and the movement of fluid. This results in a condition known as *edema*.

Hydrostatic pressure is comparable to the principle of filtration, which is the transfer of water-soluble substances from an area of high pressure to an area of low pressure. Fluid and water-soluble substances are moved by hydrostatic pressure in the vessels. Hydrostatic pressure can be exerted by the pumping action of the heart. The difference in arterial and venous pressure also plays a role in the movement of fluids. Hydrostatic pressure is greater than colloid osmotic pressure at the arterial end of a capillary, which causes fluids to move out of the vessel. Conversely, the osmotic force is greater than the hydrostatic pressure on the venous end of a capillary, enabling fluid to reenter a capillary on the venous end.[2]

Vascular effects. For the body to function correctly, there must be enough circulating fluid to support osmosis, diffusion, and filtration. Baroreceptors, or stretch receptors, located in the carotid sinuses and the aortic arch, respond to the amount of stretch in the vessel wall. The stretch depends on the volume of blood flowing through it. If there is a drop in arterial pressure, these baroreceptors generate fewer impulses, which in turn causes an accelerated heart rate and an increase in blood pressure. The mechanism controlling water movement between fluid compartments is a rapid-response system. Its primary action is to maintain a normal blood volume, even at the expense of interstitial fluid volume. The interstitial space may expand by several liters over a long period without major changes in the intravascular or intracellular compartments.

Body fluid volume and composition. Age, gender, and the amount of adipose tissue all affect the amount of fluids in the human body. Women have less body fluid than men because men have less body fat. This gender difference in fluid amount is not seen until adolescence but remains throughout life. A newborn's fluid content is 70% to 80% of body weight. Premature infants have an even higher percentage of fluid, approximately 90% of their body weight. Infants are more susceptible to fluid volume deficit because their bodies have a higher fluid percentage and they have more extracellular fluid. More than half of the newborn's body fluid is extracellular fluid. In adults, extracellular fluid accounts for only one third of body fluid. Extracellular fluid is more readily lost from the body. By the end of the second year of life, the infant's total body fluid approaches that of the adult, or approximately 60%—36% cellular fluid and 24% extracellular fluid. The adult body composition of 40% cellular and 20% extracellular is reached by puberty. After the age of 40 years, the total fluid percentage of body weight begins to decrease for both men and women. After 60 years of age, the percentages decrease even more, because with aging there is a decrease of lean body mass and an increase in fat content. Therefore the body holds less water. Changes in fluid volume and composition throughout life are shown in Table 7-2.[6]

Table 7-2	**Body Fluid Volume and Composition**		
	APPROXIMATE PERCENTAGE BY GENDER		
AGE	**MALE**	**FEMALE**	**BOTH**
Premature infant			90
Term newborn			70–80
1 year			64
Puberty–39 years	60	52 (40 cellular, 20 extracellular)	
40–60 years	55	47	
>60 years	52	46	

Adapted from Metheny NM: *Fluid and electrolyte balance: nursing considerations,* ed 3, Philadelphia, 1996, JB Lippincott, p. 5.

Water regulation
Intake

Requirements. The goal is to maintain a state of equilibrium between fluid compartments and between the body's daily fluid intake and output. The average healthy adult requires from 2000 to 2800 ml of fluid a day. Usually, 1000 to 1500 ml of this total are taken into the body in liquid form. Another 800 to 1000 ml come from food eaten during the day. Oxidation in body tissues accounts for another 350 ml. Fluid loss amounts to approximately 2500 ml/day. When the body is functioning correctly, the intake is balanced by the output.

Mechanisms of intake. There are various ways to achieve intake and output of fluids and electrolytes. Water is taken into the body by food or drink. The liquid that is ingested is measured as part of intake. Liquid is also taken into the body through food. Water is formed by oxidation when food is broken down into energy by the body. Oxidation releases water for use in metabolism; approximately 350 ml of water comes from the oxidation process daily. Thirst is controlled by osmoreceptors found in the hypothalamus and by intravascular volume. Thirst is an even more important mechanism in supplying endogenous water to the body and is activated when the total body water content is decreased by about 2%. ADH plays an important role in preventing dehydration and therefore hypertonicity of body fluids.

Thirst mechanism. The thirst mechanism is activated when stimulated by osmoreceptors in the anterior hypothalamus. Plasma osmolality and sodium concentrations are usually kept within a narrow range. The upper limit of this range is determined by the osmotic threshold for thirst, referred to as the *threshold* for drinking.[2] When the sodium concentration increases by about 2 mEq/L above the normal level, the physical desire for water increases. The drinking mechanism is stimulated, causing the organism to desire water so that the extracellular fluid level returns toward normal as water is ingested.[2]

Output. The kidneys, in addition to excreting urine, can adjust the amount of water and electrolytes that leave the body so that it equals the amount of water and electrolytes that enter the body. They have a vital role in fluid and electrolyte balance and in acid-base balance. On average, the kidneys filter approximately 170 L of water in a 24-hour period. This amount varies according to the fluid intake. The usual amount of fluid output through the kidney is approximately 1 ml of urine/kg of body weight per hour in all age groups.

Perspiration. Water and electrolytes can be lost through the skin; these are referred to as *sensible losses*. Sensible losses, or perspiration, can account for up to 6 L of fluid in 24 hours under hot, dry conditions, with the average being 1.5 L lost in 24 hours. Perspiration is considered a hypotonic solution; it contains chiefly sodium and potassium. Losses by perspiration vary according to environmental temperature. Body temperature and ambient room temperature also affect the amount of perspiration. The skin also loses water by evaporation, which can be up to 600 ml/day. Evaporation is considered an *insensible loss.*

Respiration. Approximately 300 ml of water are lost through the lungs in any 24-hour period. This is considered insensible water loss, and the amount lost varies according to the rate and depth of respiration. In addition, the lungs play a role in homeostasis because of their ability to eliminate about 13,000 mEq of hydrogen ions in 24 hours, which is significantly more than the kidneys excrete.

Gastrointestinal tract. Although the GI tract is responsible for 100 to 200 ml of fluid loss daily, it can actually filter up to 8 L of fluid in 24 hours. Much of this fluid, however, is reabsorbed through the small intestine. Greater losses can occur from adverse conditions such as diarrhea, vomiting, or fistula development.

Other mechanisms. Water and electrolytes can be lost through other mechanisms, such as tears and through feces. Abnormal losses can occur from the use of strong diuretics, which deplete body fluids and electrolytes, or through wound drainage, fever, hyperventilation, mechanical ventilation, and GI tubes.

Antidiuretic hormone. The release of ADH in response to osmotic dehydration is affected by plasma osmolality. Osmoreceptors can detect very small changes in the concentration of sodium and other solutes in plasma. Sodium concentration is the driving force in ADH secretion.[7] With a normal plasma osmolality, the secretion of ADH is low enough to permit maximum urinary output. If plasma becomes hyperosmolar, ADH is secreted to maintain maximum water retention in the kidneys, and solutes continue to be excreted in an effort to bring osmolality back to normal. The reverse is also true—in a hypoosmolar state, ADH secretion is diminished, allowing the excretion of water while solutes are retained by the kidney. This process returns the plasma to a more normal osmolality.

Effects of age on intake and output. When considering the intake of fluid into the body and the output of that fluid and associated electrolytes, the affect of age on homeostatic mechanisms should be considered. The elderly may experience up to a 50% reduction in kidney function, which results from a decrease in blood flow to the kidneys. There is also an inability to concentrate urine when the fluid intake is reduced, so the glomerular filtration rate is also decreased. This indicates that the elderly are more susceptible to drug toxicities because of decreased renal function. Cardiac output and stroke volume of the heart are lowered in the elderly. Glands may atrophy, which reduces the ability to eliminate fluid through perspiration and causes some control of body temperature to be lost. There is

sometimes a loss of muscle tone of the intestinal tract. Thirst mechanisms may be diminished in the aging person, so the attempt to reach homeostasis based on thirst is then compromised.

Likewise, infants also require special consideration. There is proportionately more water in the extracellular compartment of an infant than in that of an adult. Therefore the infant is more vulnerable to fluid volume deficit. The infant may turn over half of its extracellular fluid daily, whereas adults may change only one sixth of their extracellular volume in the same 24-hour period. This means that the infant has less body fluid in reserve. Infants have a large amount of metabolic waste to excrete because their daily fluid exchange is up to two times greater per unit of body weight than that of an adult. Large volumes of urine are formed each day to excrete all the waste products. Infants have a proportionally higher body surface area than adults, so they have a greater fluid loss potential through their skin. Infants can also suffer greater losses from the GI tract in a relatively shorter period than adults.

Fluid disorders

Homeostatic mechanisms of the body are complex and delicate. Generally, this system has the ability to maintain equilibrium, but sometimes these mechanisms fail and the body can be in a state of fluid deficit or excess.

Fluid volume excess. An increase in extracellular fluid volume is known as *fluid volume excess* or *hypervolemia*. The increased volume may occur with the intravascular or interstitial fluids. Hypervolemia is generally the result of an increase in body sodium concentration, which in turn causes water retention. Hypervolemia may be classified as isotonic, hypotonic or hypertonic, or isoosmolar, hypoosmolar, or hyperosmolar. The concentration of sodium determines the classification. If the serum sodium is decreased, excess fluid is hypotonic and may be known as *water intoxication*. Hypertonic fluid volume excess is rare and is usually related to excessive sodium intake.[1-3] When both the sodium and water are retained, the relative serum sodium concentrations remain essentially normal.[8] Once an imbalance develops, the body attempts to compensate. This occurs through the release of atrial natriuretic factor, which causes the kidneys to increase the rate of filtration and excretion of sodium and water. There is also a decrease in the aldosterone and ADH levels.

Cause. Fluid volume excess is related to an increase in sodium, water, or a combination of the two, which can be caused by regulatory mechanisms.[6] The kidneys, which help regulate sodium and water, may be diseased, leading to sodium and water retention. This is particularly true in the presence of a decreased output. Increased secretion of ADH and aldosterone results in fluid retention.

Another major organ that is a part of the normal regulatory system is the heart. In conditions such as congestive heart failure, the diseased heart cannot circulate the intravascular fluids adequately. This pseudointravascular deficit signals the kidneys to conserve sodium and water, leading to a fluid volume excess.

A malfunctioning liver could lead to excessive fluid retention. In cirrhosis, for example, the retention is related to a decreased serum albumin level, which facilitates the loss of intravascular fluids into the interstitial space. Additional fluid may be lost into the peritoneal cavity because of hepatic venous obstruction. Again, this decreased intravascular volume signals the kidney to release more renin, which leads to an increase in the aldosterone level and results in sodium and water retention.

Hypervolemia may occur as a result of an excessive sodium and fluid intake. This is generally caused by the excessive administration of IV fluids, particularly those that contain sodium. Also, the excessive ingestion of sodium contained in food or medications may lead to fluid volume excess; this is especially true in those with a heart or kidney abnormality.

Other possible causes of hypervolemia are the administration of excessive doses of steroids and fluid volume shifts within the body. In the case of steroids, the increased fluid volume is related to sodium and water retention. A shift of interstitial fluid to plasma may occur with the treatment of burns. Often, initial burn treatment includes the administration of large amounts of IV fluids because of a fluid volume deficit. Several days later, there is a shift of fluid from the interstitial space back into the intravascular space, which could lead to hypervolemia.

Assessment. The signs and symptoms of hypervolemia are related to the location and degree of fluid volume excess and to the rate of onset. A sudden, rapid onset results in more pronounced problems.

Probably the most visible characteristic is edema, which is increased fluid volume in the interstitial space. When edema is present, it is usually most visible in dependent areas, as well as around the eyes. The degree of edema may be determined by applying finger pressure around the ankle and sacral areas. Removing the finger leaves a small indention or pit as the fluid excess becomes more severe.

Weight gain usually accompanies the increased fluid volume. This would not occur, however, if the increase were a shift from another compartment. Weight gain occurring over a short time frame is considered to indicate a mild fluid excess if the increase is 2%, a moderate excess if the increase is 5%, and a severe excess if the increase is 8%.[6]

Fluid may shift to another cavity in the body, primarily the abdominal cavity. Accumulation in the abdominal cavity, known as *ascites,* is often seen in patients with advanced renal or hepatic disease. It is noted by shortness of breath or decreased cardiac output caused by the increased pressure of the excessive fluid volume.

Another characteristic of hypervolemia is pulmonary edema, which can lead to moist rales, shortness of breath, and wheezing. There may be an increase in blood pressure, distension of the neck veins, slower emptying of the peripheral veins, and a more rapid and bounding pulse rate. Polyuria is present if the kidneys are functioning normally.

Laboratory findings reveal a decreased hematocrit resulting from hemodilution. If the excessive volume is caused by water retention, the serum sodium level and osmolality decrease. In most cases, the urine-specific gravity also decreases. Pulmonary congestion may be revealed on chest x-ray examination. Because of a decrease in oxygen transport capabilities with pulmonary edema, the arterial blood gases may show a decreased Pao_2 and $Paco_2$ and an increased pH.

Correction. Treatment of fluid volume excess depends on its cause. When the cause cannot be determined, it is necessary to treat the disorder symptomatically. This generally includes restriction of sodium and fluid intake, bed rest, and/or diuretic administration. There may be special requirements for some patients, such as paracentesis in the case of ascites. Dialysis may also be indicated in the presence of renal disease.

Sodium restriction may extend to the diet and to medications, particularly those containing a sodium salt. There are also a variety of over-the-counter preparations that contain sodium.

The use of diuretics is not always the answer but is helpful in most cases of edema. Severe hypervolemia may necessitate administration of diuretics by the IV route.

Nursing interventions should include monitoring vital signs and body weight. Any continued presence of edema should be noted. Intake and output records and electrolyte levels should be monitored, particularly after diuretic administration.

Observations should be clearly documented, including the response to diuretics. All abnormal observations should be communicated to the physician.

Fluid volume deficit. Fluid volume deficit, or hypovolemia, occurs as a result of excessive but relatively equal fluid and electrolyte depletion in the extracellular compartment. The body attempts to compensate for the losses by stimulating thirst, increasing the heart rate, and releasing ADH and aldosterone. If the deficit is severe and not corrected in a timely manner, it could lead to renal failure and death. As with fluid volume excess, a fluid volume deficit can be classified as isotonic, hypotonic, or hypertonic (or osmolar). With isotonic deficit, the loss of water and solutes is equal. In a hypertonic deficit, the loss of fluid is greater than solute loss. Hypotonic deficits, which occur less often than the other types, exhibit a decreased concentration of solute (usually sodium and potassium) in the extracellular fluid.[1-3]

Cause. Hypovolemia may result from an abnormal loss of body fluids or inadequate fluid intake, which affects the fluid and electrolyte content. Fluid deficit may be caused by the loss of GI fluids. This may occur through vomiting, diarrhea, suctioning, and fistulas.

The skin is another mechanism for fluid loss. Under normal conditions, fluid is lost through the skin as a means of regulating body temperature. In the presence of a fever, however, there are abnormal, insensible fluid losses. Any type of trauma related to the skin, such as burns and cuts, also facilitates the abnormal loss of fluids.

Excessive loss takes place through the renal system. This may be caused by polyuria related to administering osmotic diuretics or concentrated IV solutions and tube feedings. Polyuria may also occur with hyperglycemia and some renal disorders.

Trauma, surgery, and bleeding disorders may result in hemorrhage, which rapidly decreases the intravascular fluid volume. There may also be a decrease in the circulating volume because of *third spacing*. With this phenomenon, there is a shift of fluid from the circulating volume into a space where it cannot easily be exchanged with fluid in the extracellular space. Because third spacing is only a shifting of fluid, there is no actual fluid loss.

The fluid deficit in this case is the result of the decreased circulating volume.

Finally, hypovolemia may occur because of a decreased fluid intake, particularly in the infant and older adult population. Infants have a larger body surface area and tend to lose more fluid than adults. They depend on others to provide oral fluids. Older adults have a decreased sense of thirst and therefore are less likely to seek fluid replacement. The ability to replace fluid may be further complicated by decreased mobility. Patients who cannot respond to thirst (because they are confused or comatose, for example) are subject to fluid volume depletion.

Assessment. As with fluid volume excess, the signs and symptoms of hypovolemia are related to the degree of the deficit and how fast it occurs. There is a loss of weight as the fluid volume decreases, except in the case of third spacing.

Assessment reveals a decreased central venous pressure, flattened jugular vein while in the supine position, and slow filling of the hand veins. The lower circulating volume leads to decreased blood pressure and possibly postural hypotension. With less volume, there is decreased tissue perfusion, which creates a variety of problems, including muscle weakness, dizziness, lethargy, and confusion. As the body tries to maintain an adequate intravascular volume, the pulse rate increases and becomes weaker. The kidneys try to conserve fluid, so there is a decreased urine output.

Skin turgor should be checked by pinching the skin, which slowly returns to the normal position in the presence of hypovolemia. The tongue, which normally has one furrow, has several small furrows. The eyes appear sunken and the face has a pinched expression.

As fluid loss becomes more severe, the patient may go into shock. The extremities become cool and clammy, diaphoresis occurs, urinary output drops sharply, and the patient may become comatose.

Laboratory findings reveal an increased blood urea nitrogen (BUN) level. This is the result of the kidneys conserving water and urea, which follows the water. The hematocrit also increases except when the deficit is caused by hemorrhage. With blood loss, red blood cells and serum are lost in equal amounts. However, as the body attempts to compensate for the fluid deficit, interstitial fluid shifts into the intravascular space and the hematocrit decreases. There is an increase in the urinary specific gravity and osmolality. The electrolyte levels, serum osmolality, and acid-base balance vary according to the type of fluid lost and the causative factor.

Treatment. The treatment of hypovolemia includes correcting the cause of the deficit and returning the extracellular fluid to a normal level. If the deficit cannot be replaced by oral fluids, IV therapy should be initiated based on physician orders, patient assessment, and established procedures. An isotonic electrolyte solution such as lactated Ringer's is generally used to initiate therapy for hypovolemia. The severity of the deficit generally dictates the administration rate. As the fluid is replaced, the IV solution may be changed to one that provides free water. This helps the kidneys excrete wastes.

If the deficit is severe enough, oliguria may be present. In this case, it is important to determine whether the cause is fluid volume deficit or renal disease. This may be accomplished through a fluid challenge test, in which the patient is monitored closely as IV solutions are administered. If the kidneys respond by producing urine, then oliguria is probably the result of fluid volume deficit. When there is no increase in urinary output, the cause of the oliguria is most likely related to renal failure or decreased cardiac function.

During treatment for fluid volume deficit, the patient must be monitored closely. This includes monitoring the urinary output, vital signs, hemodynamic pressures, and body weight. Monitoring laboratory test results can help maintain normal fluid and electrolyte levels. The rate of administration for IV solutions should be monitored to prevent fluid overload. Assessment findings need to be clearly documented and the physician notified of abnormal results.

ACID-BASE BALANCE

The body's complexity and delicate balance is also seen in the principles of acid-base balance. It is imperative that this balance be maintained within a very narrow range, with a pH between 7.35 and 7.45. Any excess in either direction, without correction or intervention, can result in death. It is interesting to note that most byproducts of metabolism (waste products) tend to be acidic. To achieve homeostasis, the body attempts to excrete acidic substances in a way that balances the amount of acidic products generated through metabolism.

To understand pH, and therefore acids and bases, one must first understand the function of hydrogen in pH. Certain characteristics of a solution are measured by its pH, which is the hydrogen ion concentration of the solution. Because this concentration is very small, it is generally expressed as a logarithm. For example, water has a pH of 7, which can be expressed as a negative logarithm, or 0.0000001 (10^{-7}). The logarithm makes it much easier to work with and conceptualize the pH value.

The concentration of hydrogen ions in a solution determines its acidity or alkalinity. If a solution is acidic, it has a low pH. If a solution is alkaline, it has a high pH. The normal pH range is 1 to 14, with 7 being approximately neutral. Water, with its pH of 7, is considered neutral because of the balance between the concentration of hydrogen ions (H^+) and hydroxyl (OH^-) ions. Hydroxyl ions are released when a base breaks apart in water, and hydrogen ions are released when an acid dissociates in water.

Acids

An acid is a chemical substance that dissociates and donates hydrogen ions to a solution or in combination with another substance. Acids can be classified as strong or weak. Strong acids such as hydrochloric acid (HCl) release hydrogen ions into solution and tend to remain dissociated in that solution. Weak acids such as carbonic acid (H_2CO_3) also give up hydrogen ions in solution, but not completely, as does the strong acid. Weak acids are only partially dissociated in acidic solutions.

Volatile acids are acids that can form a gas and are eliminated from the body as a gas, so they therefore are excreted from the lungs. An example of a volatile acid is carbonic acid, which is a combination of carbon dioxide (CO_2) and water (H_2O). Nonvolatile or fixed acids cannot be converted into gas form. They are excreted by the kidneys in the urine and in small amounts in feces. Nonvolatile acids result from various metabolic processes. Some are produced in the form of uric acid, which is an organic acid. Some may be in the form of sulfuric and phosphoric acids. Nonvolatile acids and the hydrogen they release are eliminated by the kidneys. It is important to remember that any discussion of acids is a discussion of hydrogen ion concentration. To summarize, nonvolatile hydrogen ions are excreted through the renal system or the kidneys, and volatile hydrogen or acids are excreted through the lungs or respiratory system.[2-4]

Respiratory system influences. Most of the carbonic acid available in the body is found in conjunction with carbon dioxide gas. Therefore the pH of body fluids is affected by changes in the carbon dioxide concentration. When the concentration of carbon dioxide gas in body fluids is increased, the pH decreases. Conversely, when the concentration of carbon dioxide gas is decreased, the pH increases. The rate of alveolar ventilation is a major factor in the regulation of carbon dioxide concentration in the body. Alveolar hyperventilation causes carbon dioxide to be blown off through the lungs. In turn, the release of carbon dioxide through the lungs decreases its concentration in body fluids and increases the pH. On the other hand, alveolar hypoventilation causes the retention of carbon dioxide, which decreases the pH.

When hydrogen ion concentration is affected, pH is also affected. Therefore the rate of ventilation changes in conjunction with alterations in the rate and depth of breathing. The peripheral and central chemoreceptors found in the body respond to changes in carbon dioxide and hydrogen ion concentrations. The peripheral chemoreceptors found in the carotid and aortic bodies respond to carbon dioxide and hydrogen ion concentrations in circulating blood by stimulating networks in the medulla oblongata, increasing or decreasing respiration accordingly.

The central chemoreceptors in the medulla monitor hydrogen ion concentrations in the cerebral blood flow and brain interstitial fluid. They then signal the medulla to change the rate and depth of alveolar ventilation. An increase in hydrogen ion concentration and the subsequent drop in pH decrease the rate of alveolar ventilation. This feedback mechanism does have a limitation, however, in that the control of hydrogen ion concentration through the respiratory feedback system cannot always return the hydrogen ion concentration to its normal value. This is because, as the pH moves toward 7.4, the stimulus to increase or decrease ventilation is removed. Carbon dioxide gas exchange occurs through the lungs and excretes the bulk of acid formed in the body. More than 99.5% of the normal daily acid load and 100% of the CO_2 that results from metabolism are eliminated through the lungs.

The respiratory feedback system is a rapid-response system that can begin to correct changes in pH within minutes, although it may take several hours to achieve. Therefore it is necessary for a second system to take over when the respiratory feedback mechanisms are not sufficient by themselves.

Bases

A base is a chemical substance that, when dissociated in solution, can combine with a hydrogen ion. When the base takes on a hydrogen ion, it in effect removes the hydrogen from a solution. Examples of bases are bicarbonate and protein. Proteins can function as bases because they act as anions and easily bind or accept hydrogen ions. Bases may be strong or weak, just like acids. A strong base easily accepts hydrogen and removes it from solution. Hydroxyl ions (OH^{2-}) are strong bases. Weak bases do not have the same affinity for hydrogen ions as strong bases and are only partially dissociated in alkaline solutions. Bicarbonate is considered a weak base.

In the human body, most of the acids and bases required for life are weak acids and weak bases. Strong acids and bases would allow sudden and dangerous changes in the pH of body fluids, whereas weak acids and bases allow for a greater degree of stabilization of pH. Weak acids or bases can neutralize strong acids or bases.

For example, consider the following equation:

$NaHCO_3$ Sodium bicarbonate (weak base)	+	HCL Hydrochloric acid (strong acid)	→	H_2CO_3 Carbonic acid (weak acid)	+	NaCl Sodium chloride (salt)

By adding hydrochloric acid, which is a strong acid, to sodium bicarbonate, which is a weak base, they dissociate and combine to yield carbonic acid, which is a weak acid, and sodium chloride. By reacting this way, the weak base minimizes the change in pH by neutralizing the strong acid.

The same can be seen with a weak acid used to neutralize a strong base:

H_2CO_3 Carbonic acid (weak acid)	+	NaOH Sodium hydroxide (strong base)	→ (yields)	$NaHCO_3$ Sodium bicarbonate (weak base)	+	H_2O Water

When carbonic acid (weak acid) is added to sodium hydroxide (strong base), the chemical dissociation and combination yields sodium bicarbonate, which is a weak base, and water. Again, this minimizes a precipitous change in body pH. A strong acid or a strong base in each of these examples has been buffered by the addition of a weak acid or a weak base.

Renal system influences. Like the respiratory system, the renal system responds to changes in hydrogen ion concentration, *but* it responds more slowly. It may take up to several days for the renal system to fully achieve its purpose in pH correction. The kidneys work to regulate bicarbonate concentration in extracellular fluid and to excrete the acidic results of metabolism that the lungs cannot eliminate.

Metabolic or nonrespiratory acid-base imbalances may result from the excessive accumulation or loss of fixed or nonvolatile acids and their buffers. Several major processes are involved in the renal system's regulation of hydrogen. Hydrogen is secreted through the kidneys. There is a relationship between the amount of hydrogen secreted and the concentration of carbon dioxide in the extracellular fluid. When there is a higher concentration of carbon dioxide in the extracellular fluid, more hydrogen ions are secreted. Conversely, the lower the amount of carbon dioxide in extracellular fluid, the fewer hydrogen ions are secreted.

Because the respiratory system is responsible for the excretion of most hydrogen ions, there is only a small degree of hydrogen ion elimination through the kidneys. The kidneys, however, reabsorb bicarbonate in an amount that equals the remaining excess hydrogen ions. When hydrogen moves from the cells and tubules of the kidneys into the urine formed in the tubules, it can be exchanged for sodium ions and the hydrogen is excreted. Sodium ions are usually paired up with an anion, which preserves electrical neutrality between the positively and negatively charged ions. The sodium ions that are reabsorbed move into the plasma and then combine with HCO_3^- (bicarbonate ion) to form sodium bicarbonate. As a result of hydrogen-sodium exchange, bicarbonate is produced to maintain homeostasis.

The amount of exchange between hydrogen and sodium can be influenced by a deficiency in chloride, an increase in the level of plasma carbon dioxide, and aldosterone secretion, which alters the retention of sodium. These factors accelerate the exchange process, which can be slowed by a decrease in the carbon dioxide level or a decrease in aldosterone secretion. Urine pH also influences this exchange. When the urine pH reaches a value between 4.0 and 4.5, this halts the secretion of hydrogen. This, in turn, stops the exchange of hydrogen and sodium.

Hydrogen can also combine with ammonia (NH_3) in the distal tubules of the kidneys. When the NH_3 moves from the cells into the urine, it attaches to hydrogen in the urine and forms the ammonium ion (NH_4^+). Ammonium then combines with an anion (either chloride or sulfate), and they all are excreted in the urine. The purpose of this mechanism, again, is to increase the amount of bicarbonate and to balance the carbonic acid/sodium bicarbonate ratio by regulating and excreting hydrogen ions. Ammonium ions are substituted for bicarbonate ions, resulting in the excretion of ammonia. This allows for the preservation of bicarbonate, the excretion of excess hydrogen ions, and the maintenance of neutrality between positive and negative ions.

It is also possible for phosphates to combine with hydrogen ions, allowing the hydrogen to be excreted with the phosphate in urine. If all these mechanisms fail to restore the acid-base balance, it is possible for potassium and extracellular fluid volume changes to achieve this balance.[1,2]

Buffers

In addition to respiratory and renal system influences, there is a system of buffers that works to maintain acid-base balance. In the presence of an acid-base disturbance, there are three main mechanisms to regain homeostasis, and two have already been discussed. One is the increase in alveolar ventilation. This depends on the lungs and chemoreceptors and acts to reverse an alteration within 1 to 2 minutes. The second defense mechanism is hydrogen ion elimination coupled with increased bicarbonate reabsorption. This occurs in the kidneys and provides the strongest defense against acid-base disturbances. However, it takes several hours to several days for the renal system to try to reestablish equilibrium. The third defense is a system of buffers. The buffer system begins immediately to equilibrate the hydrogen ion concentration.

A buffer protects the body against hydrogen ion concentra-

tion fluctuations. Buffers can inactivate excess hydrogen ions and hydroxyl ions. By doing so, they can maintain the pH within the normal range.

Carbonic acid–sodium bicarbonate buffer system. Carbonic acid (H_2CO_3) and sodium bicarbonate ($NaCO_3$) work together as a buffer system that is affected by the lungs and the kidneys. Carbonic anhydrase, the enzyme that catalyzes the reaction, is found in the alveoli walls of the lungs and in epithelial cells in the renal tubules. The lungs excrete or retain carbonic acid or its component, carbon dioxide, and the kidneys excrete or retain sodium bicarbonate. This is the most important buffering system in the extracellular fluid. It can buffer up to 90% of the hydrogen ions contained in extracellular fluid, and has little affect on the cells.

Because of the effects of carbonic acid or sodium bicarbonate, the buffering must occur through the lungs or kidneys. This means that the pH can be moved up or down by the renal system, the respiratory system, or both, acting together. Carbonic acid and sodium bicarbonate are measured by their relative concentrations. The ratio between the two is 1:20, or 1 part of carbonic acid to every 20 parts of sodium bicarbonate. When monitoring acid-base balance, it is important to monitor this ratio. When it is disturbed, the hydrogen balance in the body is also disturbed.[2,5,6]

Phosphate buffer system. The phosphate buffer system operates at a slightly different pH than the carbonic acid–sodium bicarbonate buffer system. Phosphate buffer is more abundant in cells, so its role is more cellular than extracellular. It works mainly in the tubular fluid of the kidneys. This system can buffer strong acids and strong bases into weak acids and weak bases so that the weakened state of the acids or bases has little effect on the pH of the blood.

Protein buffer system. Proteins can act as both intracellular and extracellular buffers and as acids or bases, a property referred to as *amphoteric.* Their ability to behave as either acid or base depends on the pH of the solution and makes proteins a powerful buffering agent. Proteins tend to buffer carbon dioxide quickly and bicarbonate more slowly, over several hours.

In addition, hemoglobin and oxyhemoglobin can act as a buffer system. This system works because of a reaction that occurs between hemoglobin and hydrogen ions in red blood cells. The red blood cell is permeable to bicarbonate ions. Therefore, when a hydrogen ion is bound by hemoglobin, a bicarbonate ion diffuses out of the red blood cell into the plasma. The bicarbonate ion is then exchanged for a chloride ion to maintain electrical neutrality.

Compensatory mechanisms

Compensatory mechanisms are activated in the presence of a hydrogen imbalance. There are three basic compensatory mechanisms. The first is the dilution of hydrogen in the extracellular fluid and the buffering systems discussed earlier. The second compensatory mechanism is the respiratory system, and the third is the renal system.

The goal of compensation is to return the pH to normal without overcompensating or correcting the pH past the point of normal. The normal range for pH is from 7.35 to 7.45. The absolute normal value is considered 7.4. By definition, acidemia is a condition in which hydrogen ion concentration is elevated in the blood. Stated another way, the blood could have an acid excess or a base deficit, reflected by a pH of less than 7.35. Alkalemia is a condition in which hydrogen ion concentration is decreased. Stated differently, the blood could have an acid deficit or a base excess, indicated by a pH greater than 7.45. Acidosis and alkalosis are the processes that result in acidemia or alkalemia. These terms may be used interchangeably.

Blood values: measurement and interpretation

The evaluation of acid-base balance is based on various blood gas values. In addition to acid-base balance, these values are used to determine the level of oxygenation within the patient's body, both extracellularly and intracellularly. Usually, blood gases are measured from arterial blood, which provides information about the oxygenation status of the blood passing through the lungs. Occasionally, mixed venous blood is used rather than arterial blood to determine oxygen levels in the tissues. If the tissues are receiving adequate oxygen, this can mean that ventilation and circulation within the body are adequate to meet the patient's needs and establish acid-base balance.

The three variables monitored most often are the pH, $Paco_2$, and HCO_3^- levels. As stated earlier, pH measures the level of hydrogen ions present, which determines the alkalinity or acidity of the blood.

The $Paco_2$, or Pco_2, is a measure of the tension exerted by carbon dioxide in its gas form. The *P* represents the pressure or tension exerted by the carbon dioxide gas. The *a* designates arterial blood. If it were a venous sample, the letter *v* would be substituted for *a*. When there is no *P* preceding the CO_2 level, it refers to the total CO_2 rather than the amount of carbon dioxide in the blood as a gas. The total CO_2 content is the amount of CO_2 gas that can be obtained from plasma when a strong acid is added in a laboratory setting. The total CO_2 content consists of bicarbonate, carbonic acid, and dissolved carbon dioxide gas.

Because the total CO_2 content measures the sum of bicarbonate, carbonic acid, and dissolved CO_2, an elevation of the plasma CO_2 content indicates alkalosis. A decrease in plasma CO_2 content indicates acidosis.

By measuring the $Paco_2$, the presence of alkalosis and acidosis may be determined. When this value is lower than 35 mm Hg, hypocapnia is present, indicating respiratory alkalosis. Conversely, when this value is greater than 45 mm Hg, hypercapnia is said to be present, indicating respiratory acidosis.

When discussing blood gases, consideration must be given to CO_2 and oxygen (O_2) concentrations in the blood. Pao_2 is the amount of pressure exerted by oxygen dissolved in arterial blood. Most oxygen carried by the blood is carried by hemoglobin. A small amount of oxygen is dissolved in plasma. Therefore there are three ways to measure oxygen in the blood. The first is oxygen content, defined as the number of milliliters of oxygen carried in 100 ml of blood. The Po_2, or the pressure exerted by oxygen dissolved in plasma, is the second measurement. The third is the oxygen saturation of hemoglobin.

Table 7-3	Normal Blood Gas Values*	
PARAMETER	**ARTERIAL**	**VENOUS (MIXED)**
pH	7.35-7.45	7.33-7.43
O_2 saturation	≥95%	70%-75%
Pao_2	80-100 mm Hg	35-40 mm Hg
$Paco_2$	35-45 mm Hg	41-51 mm Hg ($Pvco_2$)
HCO_3^-	22-26 mEq/L	24-28 mEq/L
Base excess	−2-+2	0-+4

*May vary slightly with the institution and geographic location.

Oxygen saturation is a measure of the percentage of oxygen that is carried on the hemoglobin in relation to the total amount of oxygen that the hemoglobin is able to carry. Oxygen saturation provides the closest estimate of the total amount of oxygen carried in the blood. The Po_2 is only the pressure exerted by the small amount of oxygen that is dissolved in the plasma. There is a relationship between the Po_2 and the O_2 saturation of hemoglobin. An oxyhemoglobin dissociation curve shows this relationship. When the Po_2 in plasma is low, hemoglobin carries less oxygen. Conversely, when the Po_2 in plasma is high, the hemoglobin carries a great deal of oxygen.

The hemoglobin molecule has room to carry four molecules of oxygen. If all four oxygen receptor sites on the hemoglobin are filled, 100% O_2 saturation has been reached. If three oxygen receptor sites are filled and one is not, 75% O_2 saturation has been reached. When measuring the arterial oxygen content, it is the sum of the oxygen chemically bound to hemoglobin and the oxygen dissolved in plasma that equals the Po_2. A normal O_2 saturation level is considered 95% or higher. The normal Pao_2 level is from 80 to 100 mm Hg in arterial blood.

The bicarbonate level is the concentration of bicarbonate in plasma that has been specially manipulated with oxygen at a $Paco_2$ of 40 mm Hg. This is done in a laboratory to saturate the hemoglobin fully and is called the *standard bicarbonate measure*. When this equilibration is performed, any abnormality remaining in the standard bicarbonate level is known to have a metabolic cause. A normal bicarbonate level is between 22 and 26 mEq/L. Other values used to evaluate blood gas status are base excess and anion gap.

The interpretation of blood gas results begins with three basic steps (see Table 7-3 for a list of normal blood gas values). The first step in the process is to look at the value of the pH. As stated earlier, 7.35 to 7.45 is a normal pH, with 7.4 being a midpoint. If the pH is lower than 7.35, an acidotic state exists in the body. If the pH is greater than 7.45, an alkalotic state exists. The second value to assess is the $Paco_2$, which has a normal value between 35 and 45 mm Hg. If the value of $Paco_2$ is below 35 mm Hg, a state of respiratory alkalosis exists. If the value is greater than 45 mm Hg, a respiratory acidosis exists. This is true because the $Paco_2$ is considered a respiratory measurement, and CO_2 is considered to act as an acid.

The third value to examine is the bicarbonate level. Again, the normal bicarbonate level is 22 to 26 mEq/L. A value lower than 22 mEq/L indicates metabolic acidosis, and a value higher than 26 mEq/L indicates metabolic alkalosis. The bicarbonate

Table 7-4	Aid to Interpreting Blood Gas Values
RESPIRATORY ALTERATIONS	
• pH up	Pco_2 down
• pH down	Pco_2 up
METABOLIC ALTERATIONS	
• pH up	Pco_2 up
• pH down	Pco_2 down

Box 7-1   Causes of Respiratory Acidosis

- Depression of the respiratory center (medulla)
- Drug overdose
- Any medication or condition that causes respiratory depression
- Guillain-Barré syndrome
- Myasthenia gravis
- Chronic bronchitis
- Emphysema
- Pneumothorax
- Hemothorax
- Pulmonary fibrosis
- Acute alcoholism
- Burns of the respiratory tract
- Congestive heart failure
- Adult respiratory distress syndrome

level reflects a metabolic response, which can also be referred to as *nonrespiratory* or *renal*.

There are several helpful hints to remember when interpreting blood gas values. Although it has already been stated, it should be noted that if a change in pH is mainly caused by a change in the bicarbonate level, the cause of the alteration is nonrespiratory or metabolic. If the change in pH is caused by changes in the Pco_2, the driving force behind the alteration is respiratory in nature. When the pH and Pco_2 move in opposite directions, the primary effect on the acid-base imbalance is the respiratory system. If the change in pH and Pco_2 are in the same direction, there is a nonrespiratory or metabolic cause. Table 7-4 may be useful in making these determinations.

The body always tries to keep the ratio of bicarbonate to Pco_2 at 20:1. This indicates a ratio of alkali (bicarbonate) to acid (CO_2). When it remains at 20:1, the pH remains unchanged, or around the normal level. If the bicarbonate increases, alkalosis is present, which causes the pH to rise. If the bicarbonate (base) falls, there is an acidotic state and the pH falls. The change in this ratio is described as *base excess*.

Base excess is most descriptive of the concentration of bicarbonate in the blood and is generally only affected by metabolic processes. The normal base excess is between +2 and −2. A positive base excess value signifies that there is too much base present and not enough acid. A negative value indicates too little base and too much acid. Therefore a positive base excess value reflects a metabolic alkalosis and a negative value indicates metabolic acidosis. Plasma proteins and hemoglobin may also be considered bases and can influence base excess, although to a smaller degree.

Acid-base alterations

Respiratory acidemia occurs when an event causes the $Paco_2$ to rise above 45 mm Hg. This event is usually associated with a decreased ventilatory exchange, which results in the CO_2 of the blood increasing because of an increase in the hydrogen ion concentration. The pH of the blood then decreases to below 7.35. Because of alveolar hypoventilation, CO_2 is not eliminated through the lungs. Various disease states and alterations can cause this acidotic state (Box 7-1).

The causes of respiratory acidosis may be acute or chronic. The differentiation between acute and chronic states of acidosis is usually attributed to how long the carbon dioxide retention has lasted. In the chronic state, $Paco_2$ levels can increase slowly, or they may remain stable over time, but elevated. In the acute state, there is a rapid or sudden rise in the CO_2 level with a previously normal-acid base balance. Generally, chronicity re-

sults from a disease or condition that in some way decreases or prevents the gaseous exchange that normally occurs between the blood and alveolar air or that causes obstruction. Obstruction prevents the exhalation of carbon dioxide by decreasing the surface area of the lung.

Assessment. Patients experiencing respiratory acidosis may exhibit headache, fatigue, or drowsiness resulting from central nervous system depression. Confusion, disorientation, or coma may result, as well as fatigue, weakness, tremors, dyspnea, hypoventilation, cardiac arrhythmias, and possibly cyanosis. It is important to recognize that the clinical presentation between acute and chronic respiratory acidosis is slightly different. This is particularly noticeable in patients with chronic obstructive pulmonary disease (COPD).

Compensatory response. Patients with COPD gradually accumulate CO_2. Because the alteration occurs gradually, compensatory changes have already occurred when the $Paco_2$ level exceeds 50 mm Hg. The respiratory center and the medulla no longer use CO_2 to stimulate respiration. Hypoxia then becomes the major respiratory drive in place of the increased CO_2. In this chronic state, if a patient receives too much oxygen, the stimulus for respiration is then removed. The patient develops carbon dioxide narcosis because the lack of oxygen as the stimulus to breathe is compensated for by the delivery of oxygen from an external source. In addition, because of the compensated state of chronic respiratory acidosis, blood gas results will show an elevated bicarbonate level in a patient with chronic alterations. When a state of respiratory acidosis exists, the body responds in various ways (Table 7-5). The initial response includes the initiation of buffering by noncarbonate buffers. In other words, hemoglobin and proteins in the extracellular fluid and phosphates, proteins, and lactate in the intracellular fluid are activated in an attempt to regulate and overcome the increase in hydrogen ions. The respiratory rate increases to try to "blow off" excess hydrogen ions as a byproduct of the breakdown of carbonic acid into water and CO_2. If the alteration is not corrected by this mechanism, other buffer systems go into effect. The kidneys secrete hydrogen ions and retain bicarbonate. Sodium is reabsorbed to maintain ionic balance. The buffer also increases the chloride shift in the blood because red blood

Table 7-5   Blood Gas Alterations in Respiratory Acidosis*

PARAMETER	DIRECTION OF CHANGE
pH	Down (<7.35)
$Paco_2$	Up (>45 mm Hg)
HCO_3^-	Normal or up (>26 mEq/L)
Na^+	Normal (usually)
Cl^-	Down in compensation
K^+	Up

*Breathing pattern—hypoventilation.

cells give up a greater number of chloride ions and exchange them for bicarbonate. This results in excess carbonic acid being neutralized, and the normal 20:1 ratio between sodium bicarbonate and carbonic acid is reinstated.

Nursing diagnoses

Nursing assessment. In the patient with respiratory acidosis, nursing assessment and monitoring should include the following:

- Vital signs
- Skin color
- Skin temperature
- Moistness of mucous membranes
- Muscle strength
- Level of consciousness
- Monitoring of laboratory results

High-risk nursing diagnoses

- Ineffective airway clearance
- Ineffective breathing pattern, hypoventilation
- High risk for electrolyte imbalance
- Impaired gas exchange
- High risk for injury, cardiac arrhythmia
- Sensory-perceptual alteration, altered level of consciousness
- Alteration in thought process

Potential outcomes

- Patient's blood gas values and vital signs are improved.
- Patient has minimal or no signs/symptoms of impaired gas exchange.
- Patient demonstrates methods necessary to improve breathing pattern.

Respiratory alkalosis. Any disease process that reduces carbon dioxide in the blood or $Paco_2$ results in respiratory alkalemia. The hydrogen ion concentration is decreased, which causes the pH to rise to a level above 7.45. Because the problem is respiratory in nature, the $Paco_2$ is lower than 35 mm Hg. The respiratory alkalosis is caused by hyperventilation, which comes from the alveolar level. The hyperventilation decreases the hydrogen ion concentration, resulting in the increased pH. Respiratory alkalosis can arise from several disorders and may be classified as acute or chronic (Box 7-2).

Assessment. The patient with respiratory alkalosis presents with hyperventilation and dyspnea and may sigh frequently. Tachycardia, atrial arrhythmia, and possibly severe ventricular arrhythmia may follow respiratory alkalosis. Palpitations, syncope, substernal chest pain, and seizures have occurred after mechanical overventilation. Carpal-pedal spasm, paresthe-

Box 7-2   Causes of Respiratory Alkalosis

- Hyperventilation syndrome
- Trauma
- Infection, particularly encephalitis or meningitis
- Brain tumors (tumors may be malignant or nonmalignant)
- CVA (cerebrovascular accident)
- Pharmacologic agents (salicylate poisoning, nicotine, aminophylline-type drugs, some catecholamines)
- Heat stroke
- Fever
- Gram-negative septicemia
- Exercise beyond the person's normal capabilities
- Carbon monoxide poisoning
- Hypotension
- Severe anemia
- Pneumonia
- Pulmonary edema
- Pulmonary emboli
- Mechanical overventilation
- Chronic respiratory alkalosis
- Recovery phase of CVA
- Recovery phase of central nervous system infections
- Central nervous system malignancies
- Severe ongoing anemia
- Heart conditions that cause cyanotic conditions
- Pregnancy
- Hepatic disease
- Treatment for metabolic acidosis

Table 7-6   Blood Gas Alterations in Respiratory Alkalosis*

PARAMETER	DIRECTION OF CHANGE
pH	Up (>7.45)
$Paco_2$	Down (<35 mm Hg)
HCO_3^-	Normal until compensation
Na^+	Normal
Cl^-	Up with compensation
K^+	Down
Ca^{2+}	Down

*Breathing pattern—hyperventilation.

sia, tingling in the fingers and toes, and circumoral numbness may also be seen. Patients may state that they are light-headed, complain of weakness and muscle cramps, and exhibit hyperactive deep tendon reflexes. They may possibly convulse if hypocalcemia is present.

Compensatory response. When the pH of the extracellular fluid reaches/exceeds 7.45, hydrogen ions are released from the intracellular compartment (Table 7-6). These ions are usually exchanged for potassium. Production of lactate and other metabolic acid is increased to compensate for the alkalotic state. The body then initiates the same three compensatory mechanisms discussed earlier for respiratory acidosis.

The buffer system works in the plasma by increasing the plasma content of organic acids. These acids then combine with excess bicarbonate ions to provide neutralization and maintain the 1:20 ratio between carbonic acid and sodium bicarbonate.

The pulmonary system decreases the rate and depth of respiration to achieve an increase in the CO_2 level. This continues until the CO_2 reaches a level that again stimulates respiration in the medullary centers and the baroreceptors. The change in respiration also causes excess hydrogen ions to be secreted to compensate for the decrease of carbonic acid in the plasma.

Hydrogen ions secreted above the needs of the compensatory mechanisms are excreted through the kidney. This also decreases the amount of ammonia that is produced, which allows for the retention of hydrogen ions until the 1:20 ratio of carbonic acid–sodium bicarbonate is reinstated.

Nursing interventions attempt to alleviate the underlying cause of hyperventilation. The cardiac, pulmonary, and neurologic systems and fluid and electrolyte status must all be monitored.

Nursing diagnoses
Potential nursing diagnoses
- Anxiety
- Ineffective breathing pattern
- Hyperventilation
- High risk for electrolyte imbalance
- Knowledge deficit regarding the role of inducing altered breathing pattern
- High risk for injury, seizure activity, cardiac arrhythmia
- Sensory perceptual alteration, altered level of consciousness, impaired gas exchange
- Self-care deficit: bathing, hygiene, toileting

Potential outcomes
- Patient's blood gas values and vital signs are improved.
- Patient demonstrates effective breathing patterns as evidenced by blood gas values within normal limits, with no evidence of cyanosis.
- Patient verbalizes less fatigue and weakness by increased participation in self-care activities.

Metabolic acid-base alterations.
Metabolic acid-base alterations include any acid-base disturbance that is not caused by an alteration in the CO_2 level in the extracellular fluid. These metabolic alterations involve bicarbonate levels and base excesses. When metabolic processes lead to a buildup of acids or loss of bicarbonate, the bicarbonate values drop below the normal range, resulting in a negative base excess value. Conversely, when there is a loss of acid or an accumulation of excess bicarbonate, the bicarbonate levels rise, resulting in a positive base excess value. As stated earlier, base excess refers to bicarbonate. It may also include other bases in the blood such as plasma, protein, or hemoglobin. Metabolic alterations include metabolic alkalosis and metabolic acidosis.

Metabolic acidosis.
Metabolic acidosis results from an accumulation of metabolic acids. Metabolic acids are also referred to as *fixed* acids and include all acids except carbonic acid, which is a respiratory acid. Metabolic acidemia results when there is a decrease of bicarbonate concentration in the extracellular fluid to less than 22 mEq/L. A base deficit exists, and the pH is below 7.35. These values result from an increase in metabolic (fixed) acids (Table 7-7).

When discussing metabolic acidosis, it is important to understand the concept of the *anion gap*. An anion is a substance with a negative charge. Body fluids are essentially electrically

Table 7-7 Blood Gas Alterations in Metabolic Acidosis

Parameter	Direction of Change
pH	Down (<7.35)
$Paco_2$	Normal, until compensation occurs
HCO_3^-	Down (<20 mEq/L)
Na^+	Normal (unless diuresis)
K^+	Up or normal
Cl^-	Up, down, or normal

neutral. The number of cations (positively charged ions) equals the number of anions (negatively charged ions). Because sodium accounts for approximately 90% of the cations in extracellular fluid, it represents a large amount of the positively charged ions. To compensate, the sum of the chloride and bicarbonate ions approximates the number of sodium ions. When minor ions, such as sulfate, phosphate, and organic acids, are included in the measurement, the approximation is more accurate.

Because of their prevalence in the blood, sodium, chloride, and bicarbonate are easily measured and are referred to as *measured anions*. Minor ions, however, are difficult to account for and are referred to as *unmeasured ions,* or the *anion gap*. Metabolic acidemia can result from an increase of unmeasured anions, but it can also be caused by conditions that do not increase unmeasured ions. Therefore it is important to understand the difference to allow proper monitoring of the patient and anticipate potential problems.

The use of a formula helps determine the amount of anion gap, which indicates which process is occurring. The anion gap is calculated by using the values of the serum sodium, chloride, and bicarbonate levels. The serum chloride and bicarbonate ion concentrations are added together and subtracted from the serum sodium concentration:

$$[Na^+] - ([Cl^-] + [HCO_3^-])$$

If this difference is greater than 15 mEq/L, there is an increase in unmeasured ions, the anion gap. The normal range for the anion gap is 10 to 14 mEq/L.[3-5,7]

There are three major mechanisms that allow metabolic acidosis to occur: (1) loss of base from the body through the GI tract, (2) loss of base from the body through urine, and (3) an increase in metabolic acid production. An increase in acid production may overwhelm body buffer systems and pulmonary and renal mechanisms. This is considered an *extrarenal* cause of metabolic acidemia. A *renal* source of metabolic acidemia could result from a problem in the renal tubules, which would cause retention of acid.

Metabolic acidosis may be classified as high anion gap (normochloremic) or normal anion gap (hyperchloremic). Causes of metabolic acidemia with an increased anion gap (greater than 15 mEq/L) include normal chloremic ketoacidosis, diabetes, alcoholism, starvation, uremia, lactic acidosis, and toxins from salicylate, methanol, or ethylene glycol poisoning. Metabolic acidemia associated with a normal anion gap (10 to 14 mEq/L) is associated with hyperchloremia and potassium loss caused by diarrhea, renal tubular acidosis, nephritis, early renal failure, and urinary tract obstruction. It can also be drug induced;

amphotericin B or the infusion of hydrochloric acid can cause metabolic acidemia.

It is believed that diarrhea is probably the most common cause of normal anion gap metabolic acidemia. With diarrhea, it is possible to lose large amounts of bicarbonate through the intestines.

Assessment. Patients with an alteration toward metabolic acidosis have tachypnea, hyperpnea, Kussmaul's respiration (particularly when acidosis is severe), fatigue, weakness, malaise, nausea, vomiting, abdominal pain, stupor, and coma. Sometimes headache, drowsiness, confusion, cardiac arrhythmia, hypotension, shock, and pulmonary edema are also present.

Compensatory response. Hemoglobin and phosphate buffers are predominant in the compensation for metabolic acidemia because bicarbonate ions are used to lower hydrogen ion concentration. The lungs compensate by increasing alveolar ventilation—blowing off carbon dioxide to reduce hydrogen ion levels. Because the cause of the alteration is nonrespiratory, the lungs' response is explained by the increased hydrogen ion concentration in the cerebrospinal fluid. Because the lungs cannot excrete fixed acids, the kidneys are the primary compensatory mechanism for correcting the alteration. The urinary buffers of ammonia and ammonium and the phosphate buffer system are called on, but it may be 24 hours before the renal system can begin to move the pH in the proper direction. It is estimated that 4 or 5 days may be needed for the entire acid load to be excreted.

Monitoring. Monitoring required for this condition includes assessing vital signs, intake and output, weight, skin color, temperature, GI function, muscle strength, and laboratory values. It may be necessary to institute seizure precautions and maintain bed rest if the acidosis is severe. The patient may need assistance in maintaining conscious orientation.

Nursing diagnoses
- High risk for electrolyte imbalance
- High risk for infection
- High risk for injury: altered level of consciousness or cardiac arrhythmias, compromised protective reflexes
- Sensory perception alteration, altered level of consciousness
- Alteration in thought process

Potential outcomes
- Patient is oriented to time, place, and person or has a measurable decrease in signs and symptoms of an impaired thought process.
- The patient does not develop an infection, as evidenced by normal temperature and vital signs.
- The patient has no incidence of injury.
- The patient returns to acid-base balance as evidenced by a mental status usual or normal for the patient.
- Respirations are unlabored (between 16 and 20 breaths/min).
- Patient shows no signs of headache, nausea, or vomiting.
- Patient's blood gas values return to the normal range.

Metabolic alkalosis.
A metabolic alkalemic state results from a process that increases bicarbonate ion concentration or decreases hydrogen ion concentration. The result of this alteration increases the pH to a level greater than 7.45. Metabolic alkalosis tends to occur less often than metabolic acidosis. The exception to this is the patient with nasogastric suctioning or fluid loss from the upper GI tract, such as vomiting. The

Table 7-8	Blood Gas Alterations in Metabolic Alkalosis
PARAMETER	**DIRECTION OF CHANGE**
pH	Up (>7.45)
$Paco_2$	Normal (up when compensation occurs)
HCO_3^-	Up (>26-30 mEq/L)
Na^+	Normal
K^+	Down
Cl^-	Down

bicarbonate concentration can increase either because of loss of hydrogen ions from the extracellular fluid or by addition of bicarbonate to the extracellular fluid.

Metabolic alkalosis can develop from diuretic therapy, excessive ingestion of alkaline drugs, corticosteroid therapy, severe hypocalcemia, and in the patient with vomiting or continuous nasogastric suction without proper electrolyte replacement. These alterations result in hydrogen ion loss and excess sodium bicarbonate, which affects the 1:20 ratio between carbonic acid and sodium bicarbonate and causes a base alteration.

Assessment. The patient may exhibit signs of confusion, irritability, disorientation, muscle cramps, hyperactive tendon reflexes, tetany, carpal-pedal spasms, polyuria, polydipsia, nausea, vomiting, diarrhea, or hypoventilation. Laboratory tests reveal decreased serum potassium and serum chloride levels, although the sodium level generally remains unchanged (Table 7-8).

Compensatory responses. Intracellular phosphates and proteins shift to the extracellular compartment. The phosphate and protein buffering systems provide hydrogen ions, which buffer excess bicarbonate ions. Alveolar hypoventilation occurs in an effort to retain carbon dioxide, thereby increasing the $Paco_2$. During compensatory efforts, a secondary respiratory acidosis may occur because of the retention of carbon dioxide and decreased oxygen intake. This results in hypoxia. The $Paco_2$ attempts to rise in relation to the increase in pH. This is necessary to reestablish the 20:1 ratio, enabling the pH to move back toward the normal range. The kidneys can excrete bicarbonate rapidly and therefore attempt to restore normal bicarbonate levels in the extracellular fluid. If chloride ions are unavailable, the bicarbonate may be reabsorbed. This is because sodium reabsorption requires a negatively charged ion, either chloride or bicarbonate. When there is not enough chloride, the kidney reabsorbs bicarbonate in its place.

Monitoring. The patient should continue to be monitored for vital signs, intake and output, weight, level of consciousness, muscle strength, and ongoing laboratory values. Losses from the upper GI tract should be monitored, such as gastric suctioning or vomiting.

Nursing diagnoses
- Electrolyte imbalance: high risk for hypochloremia, hypokalemia, hypocalcemia
- High risk for injury: altered level of consciousness, cardiac arrhythmia, neuromuscular irritability, seizure activity, tetany, sensory-perceptual alteration

Potential outcomes
- Patient verbalizes fewer problems with sensory perception alteration deficit.

- Patient experiences no injury related to neuromuscular irritability, seizure activity, or tetany.

Mixed acid-base alterations.

The preceding acid-base alterations are considered primary acid-base alterations. It is possible for patients to undergo single imbalances, but there are clinical conditions in which a patient may exhibit two primary acid-base disturbances concurrently. When a patient has an acid-base alteration, it is important to remember that, as compensation occurs, more than one acid-base alteration may occur simultaneously. Mixed acid-base disorders can include combinations of respiratory acidosis, respiratory alkalosis, metabolic acidosis, or metabolic alkalosis. When the normal compensatory responses to one of these alterations fail, a mixed disturbance can occur. Mixed disturbances can also occur in various clinical circumstances. When dealing with mixed alterations, the arterial pH alone cannot give the total picture of the underlying pathophysiology. The pH provides information only on the current status of the hydrogen ion.

An example of a mixed acid-base alteration is metabolic acidosis and respiratory alkalosis. This condition can be associated with cardiac and pulmonary arrest, severe pulmonary edema, or poisoning. With this alteration the patient can exhibit a high, low, or normal blood pH. The pH level depends on the severity of the two primary disorders. The bicarbonate and $Paco_2$ values are usually low. The mixed alteration of metabolic acidosis and metabolic alkalosis is another condition in which there is little change in the blood pH. Conditions that may lead to metabolic acidosis and metabolic alkalosis are salicylate intoxication, sepsis, and severe liver disease. The mixed alteration of metabolic alkalosis and respiratory acidosis is usually evidenced by a high bicarbonate level and a high $Paco_2$. Conditions associated with this alteration are chronic pulmonary diseases such as COPD, particularly in a patient with chronic respiratory acidosis who has suddenly experienced improved ventilation.

The combination of metabolic alkalosis and respiratory alkalosis can result in severe alkalemia, which is associated with critical illness. Contributory conditions include severe liver disease coupled with vomiting, gastric suction, overinfusion of Ringer's lactate and bicarbonate, diuretics, steroids, and massive transfusion of citrated blood.

It may be difficult to recognize these mixed acid-base alterations without a systematic examination of the patient and laboratory data. It is helpful to follow the steps given earlier to evaluate blood gas results systematically. In mixed alterations, it is extremely important to apply the anion gap calculation and base excess measurements to understand both the primary and complicated disturbances.

Degree of compensation.

The last factor to consider in acid-base balance alterations is the degree of compensation present. Acid-base alterations can be uncompensated, compensated, fully compensated, or partially compensated. In some instances, they can also be considered corrected. An acid-base alteration is considered corrected when all the acid-base values (usually pH, $Paco_2$, bicarbonate) return to normal. This is accomplished by effecting a change in the acid-base component that is primarily affected (Table 7-9). Compensation occurs when the alteration in pH is returned toward normal by resolution of the component not primarily affected by the alteration.

Table 7-9   Direction of Compensation in Acid-Base Alterations

Disturbance	Primary Effect	Compensation	pH
Metabolic acidosis	Low HCO_3	Low $Paco_2$	Toward high alkaline
Metabolic alkalosis	High HCO_3^-	High $Paco_2$	Toward low alkaline
Respiratory acidosis	High $Paco_2$	High HCO_3^-	Toward high alkaline
Respiratory alkalosis	Low $Paco_2$	Low HCO_3^-	Toward low acid

In other words, if the primary alteration is of respiratory origin, the compensatory system is metabolic.

An acid-base alteration is acutely uncompensated when there is an abnormal pH and a change in one blood value, either the respiratory or metabolic. In partial compensation, the pH has moved toward normal but has not yet achieved normality. All three values (pH, $Paco_2$, and HCO_3^-) remain abnormal. Compensation occurs more slowly than changes credited to the buffering process. When an acid-base alteration is corrected, all values return to normal.[3]

Reaching an understanding of alterations in acid-base balance is complex and sometimes confusing. The material presented in this section is an overview. For more in-depth information, it is recommended that further study be undertaken to fully understand the more complex principles and their applications.[1,2]

PRINCIPLES OF ELECTROLYTE THERAPY
Electrolytes

As noted earlier, chemical compounds known as *electrolytes* dissociate in water to positive ions (cations) or negative ions (anions). Disorders of electrolytes can have profound effects on the body.

Sodium.

Sodium is found mainly in the extracellular fluid and has a positive charge (cation). The normal value for serum sodium level is 135 to 145 mEq/L. The most important role of sodium is in controlling water distribution and maintaining extracellular fluid volume. This control is accomplished through the kidneys' excretion and conservation of sodium, which is primarily determined by water intake and excretion. Excess sodium triggers the thirst mechanism and the resulting fluid intake stimulates ADH secretion, leading to fluid retention and normalization of the serum sodium concentration. On the other hand, a decreased serum sodium level inhibits the secretion of ADH and allows for water diuresis, which results in equalization of the water and sodium levels. When the intake and output do not balance or the internal control mechanism is not functioning properly, imbalances occur.

Hyponatremia.

Once the serum sodium level falls below 135 mEq/L, homeostasis no longer exists. The sodium deficit is referred to as *hyponatremia*.

Cause. Sodium deficit, or hyponatremia, may be related to water gain, sodium loss, shift of sodium into the cell, or shift of water from the cell.[6] Usually, when losses occur, there is an approximately equal proportion of water and sodium or a slightly larger amount of water lost. However, because deficits lead to thirst and greater intake, the amount of water may exceed the sodium. The continued use of certain diuretics, particularly thiazides, may lead to excessive losses of sodium.

An increased extracellular fluid volume may be related to increased production of ADH, as found in the syndrome of inappropriate antidiuretic hormone secretion (SIADH). SIADH can be caused by neoplasms, central nervous system disorders, medications, or pulmonary disease. As water is retained, serum sodium is diluted. Psychogenic polydipsia, a psychiatric disorder, may occasionally initiate an excessive intake of fluids that the normal kidney may not be able to excrete. Edema may lead to dilution of the sodium content. Sodium deficits resulting from water gain may be caused by continued or excessive hypotonic or sodium-free IV solutions. Hyponatremia can also occur postoperatively as a result of the release of vasopressin.

Finally, the laboratory may report an artificial hyponatremia. This occurs in the presence of elevated serum triglyceride levels and myeloma proteins.[9]

Assessment. Assessment findings vary according to the degree of the deficit and the rate of onset; a more rapid onset results in more severe symptoms. GI symptoms include anorexia, nausea, and vomiting. Many of these are caused by low serum sodium concentration, which allows water to be pulled into the cells. The major impact of this fluid shift is seen in the form of neurologic effects, including muscular weakness and spasms, personality changes, irritability, and possibly eventual seizures and coma. Women appear to be at higher risk for developing severe neurologic symptoms and irreversible brain damage.[6]

When the cause of hyponatremia is a decreased extracellular fluid volume, the symptoms are those of fluid volume deficit (elevated pulse rate, postural hypotension, decreased blood pressure). In contrast, when the causative factor is increased extracellular volume, the symptoms are those of fluid volume excess (increased blood pressure, edema, weight gain, distended neck veins).

Laboratory findings reveal decreased serum osmolality and serum and urine sodium levels, except in SIADH and adrenal insufficiency.

Correction. Hyponatremia is corrected by replacing the sodium, preferably by oral replacement. Sodium may also be replaced through gastric tube feedings and IV solutions (e.g., 0.9% sodium chloride solution). When IV replacement is deemed necessary, the delivery rate depends on the severity and duration of symptoms as well as the extracellular fluid volume. It is necessary to maintain a delicate balance between the reduction of edema of the brain, increasing the serum sodium, and preventing osmotic demyelination.[6]

Deficits related to fluid gain may be treated with diuretics to help excrete the excess fluid. With severe hyponatremia, hypertonic saline solutions (3% or 5% sodium chloride) may be used in addition to loop diuretics. Caution must be exercised when hypertonic saline solutions are being administered to prevent intravascular fluid overload.

The treatment plan for hyponatremia resulting from SIADH involves removing the cause. If this is not possible, fluids need to be restricted and diuretics administered. Additional medications to inhibit the action of ADH may be used for patients requiring long-term therapy.

Hypernatremia. Sodium excess, or hypernatremia, occurs when the serum sodium level exceeds 145 mEq/L.

Cause. Excessive amounts of sodium and an abnormal loss of water are causative factors for sodium excess. Excessive volume may result from an increased intake or decreased loss of sodium. As the sodium level increases, thirst also increases and leads to fluid intake that normalizes the concentration. This mechanism generally prevents hypernatremia. However, there are some situations in which this process fails and the hypernatremia is caused by an inability to respond to thirst. This can happen with infants, older adults, and comatose patients who cannot obtain replacement fluids or when there is a problem with the hypothalamus. It may also result from the administration of medications and sodium-containing IV solutions, particularly hypertonic saline.

Water loss may occur in many ways and for a number of reasons. Increased losses may occur through the skin because of fever or burns, in the lungs because of infections, and in the kidneys because of osmotic diuresis. Water may also be lost because of a lack of ADH or the kidneys' inability to respond to ADH, as in diabetes insipidus.

Assessment. Assessment of a patient with hypernatremia reveals thirst, dry and sticky mucous membranes, and a decrease in tears and saliva. The temperature is elevated, and the skin appears flushed. There may be problems with speech because the tongue is rough, red, dry, and swollen. The fluid status depends on the cause; water loss leads to symptoms of fluid volume deficit and sodium gain leads to those of fluid volume excess.

Many of the symptoms are related to alterations in intracellular volume as fluid is drawn from the cells in an attempt to decrease the intravascular sodium concentration. Restlessness, weakness, and fatigue are early signs of a moderate sodium imbalance. As the imbalance becomes more severe, with increased cellular dehydration, the signs become more apparent. Dehydration of brain cells leads to agitation, seizures, and coma.

Laboratory findings show an elevated serum sodium level and serum osmolality. If the hypernatremia is the result of fluid loss, the central venous pressure is low. There is also an increased urine specific gravity and osmolality, with the exception of diabetes insipidus or osmotic diuresis, in which there is a decrease.

Correction. Correction of hypernatremia depends on the cause and is directed toward decreasing the sodium to normal levels. When the excess levels are caused by sodium gain, initial treatment is restricting sodium intake.

An excess in sodium resulting from fluid loss necessitates the restoration of the fluid volume through oral or IV fluids. Dextrose 5% in water or hypotonic saline may be given to correct the sodium imbalance. Caution must be exercised to prevent too rapid a correction or overcorrection, which might cause a shift of fluid into the cells and lead to cerebral edema, seizures, permanent neurologic damage, or death.[6] Diuretics may be used in conjunction with IV solution to decrease the potential for overcorrection.

Treatment of diabetes insipidus depends on its type (see section on diabetes later in this chapter) and primary problem. Measures include replacing ADH, administering diuretics, and restricting sodium.

Nursing interventions vary according to the cause and may include restricting sodium intake or initiating IV therapy to improve the fluid volume deficit. Monitoring includes observing neurologic signs and providing a safe environment in the presence of confusion, delirium, and seizures. During fluid replacement, any signs of cerebral edema should be reported immediately to the physician.

Potassium. Potassium is the main cation in the intracellular compartment. There are approximately 2500 to 3000 mEq of potassium in the body, and all but approximately 2% are located in the cells.[6] The normal serum potassium level is 3.5 to 5.0 mEq/L. Potassium is important in influencing neuromuscular function and in cell metabolism. It is continually moving into and out of the cells. The potassium-sodium pump helps keep most of the potassium in the cell and the sodium outside the cell. Acid-base balance also plays a role in maintaining potassium levels. Potassium tends to be pulled out of cells in the presence of acidosis and shifted back into cells with alkalosis.

The majority of potassium is excreted through the kidneys. The amount excreted is related to the serum level, presence of aldosterone, and the rate of urine flow. The kidney does not control the excretion of potassium as closely as sodium.

Hypokalemia. Hypokalemia, or potassium deficit, occurs when the serum potassium level falls below 3.5 mEq/L.

Cause. The major cause of hypokalemia is potassium loss, which may occur for various reasons. The primary site for potassium loss is the renal system. Potassium loss is often associated with the use of diuretics, but GI disorders such as vomiting and diarrhea account for some depletion. Gastric suctioning and fistulas are also factors in developing potassium deficits. Losses may be excessive because of increased aldosterone levels, magnesium depletion, increased sweating, and osmotic diuresis.

The cause may stem from inadequate intake. As long as oral intake is not a problem, potassium levels are maintained easily through ingestion of a variety of foods. However, when intake by mouth is limited or not possible, the deficit can result from inadequate replacement in parenteral or total parenteral nutrition solutions.

The increased release of aldosterone and epinephrine may be triggered by physical or emotional stress. Aldosterone increases urinary excretion, taking potassium at the same time. Serum levels are decreased by additional epinephrine production, which increases the shift of potassium into the cells.

The temporary shifting of potassium from the extracellular compartment into the cells may also be related to alkalosis, increased glucose, insulin, and the process of tissue repair from burns and trauma.

Assessment. Minor potassium deficits are often asymptomatic. Symptoms are generally focused on neuromuscular changes. With more severe deficits, there is a slowing of impulses required for the muscles and nerves to transmit signals. As a result, there may be fatigue, muscle weakness, leg cramps, paresthesias, and diminished deep tendon reflexes. There is decreased bowel motility, nausea, and vomiting.

Cardiac abnormalities are common in the presence of hypokalemia. Various atrial and ventricular arrhythmias may occur. Electrocardiogram (ECG) changes may include flattened and inverted T waves, enlarged U waves, and ST-segment depression. With potassium deficits, patients become more sensitive to cardiac toxicity in the presence of digitalis preparations.[6]

Laboratory findings reveal a serum potassium level below 3.5 mEq/L. Arterial blood gas values often indicate metabolic alkalosis. Potassium is found in urine samples, with the amount depending on the cause of the deficit. The ECG shows abnormal tracings, as described earlier.

Correction. The goal of treatment is to replace the potassium. Diet or potassium supplements may be used to treat mild to moderate deficits. If oral intake is not possible or the deficit is severe, potassium is replaced through the IV route. IV preparations of potassium include potassium acetate, potassium phosphate, and potassium chloride, with the latter being the most frequently used. Because potassium is excreted by the kidneys, a non–potassium-containing solution may be used to provide hydration and determine renal function before administering any potassium preparations. Potassium must not be given by IV push and must be diluted and thoroughly mixed throughout the IV solution before it is administered. The final IV concentration should usually not exceed 40 mEq/L, with a flow rate not to exceed 20 mEq/hr except in cases of severe depletion, in which initial concentrations of 60 to 80 mEq/L may be used.[10] Premixed KCl boluses are available in single-use containers, which may decrease accidental overinfusion and ensure dispersion of the KCl throughout the solution. Caution should be exercised when administering high concentrations because of the potential for cardiac side effects. In these situations, cardiac monitoring is recommended. An IV solution containing additional potassium may prove to cause pain in the area where it first enters the vein. This may necessitate decreasing the concentration or the flow rate.

Nursing interventions include establishing IV access and administering a properly diluted potassium admixture, as ordered. Questionable orders or laboratory findings should be referred to the physician before initiating therapy. During the administration of potassium-containing solutions, the patient should be observed for possible vascular intolerance. ECG readings, urine output, and serum potassium levels should continue to be monitored. All procedures and assessments should be properly documented.

Hyperkalemia. Hyperkalemia, or potassium excess, occurs when the serum potassium level exceeds 5.0 mEq/L.

Cause. The cause of hyperkalemia is primarily related to decreased excretion, increased intake, or shift of potassium from the cells. It is most often associated with renal disease leading to inadequate excretion. Potassium-sparing diuretics may lead to excessive fluid loss, leaving high potassium levels. Adrenal insufficiency and any condition causing a decreased aldosterone level may increase fluid excretion, leading to hyperkalemia. The potassium excess may also result from the administration of certain medications, such as nonsteroidal antiinflammatory agents in association with renal disease. Medications creating potassium excess in the absence of underlying renal disease include indomethacin and piroxican.[6]

The administration of inappropriate amounts of potassium may lead to excesses. This may occur through oral intake as well as inadequate dilution or rapid infusion of potassium-containing solutions. Normally, the body can adapt to influxes of potassium, but factors affecting absorption or excretion may inhibit normalization of the levels.

Hyperkalemia may be caused by potassium shifting from the cells. This may result from cell breakdown, as in trauma, burns, or hemolysis; severe infections; or lysis of malignant cells (following chemotherapy). An excess may result when beta-adrenergic blockers interfere with potassium shifting into the cells. The conditions associated with cell breakdown often occur in conjunction with acidosis. Metabolic acidosis also enhances the movement of potassium from the cells as the positively charged hydrogen ion enters the cells. Hyperglycemia resulting from insulin deficiency may pull potassium from the cells as water moves out of the cells in an attempt to dilute the excessive intravascular glucose content. Because insulin forces potassium into the cells, insulin deficiency may lead to hyperkalemia.

When laboratory tests indicate a high serum potassium level without any clinical indicators, consideration should be given to the method of collecting the blood sample. Inaccurate high levels may occur because of the tourniquet being in place too long, hemolysis of blood cells, delayed separation of serum and cells, or drawing blood samples in close proximity to an infusing IV solution containing potassium.

Assessment. Assessment for hyperkalemia usually reveals altered cardiac or neuromuscular activity. Cardiac arrhythmias are probably the most prominent characteristics. With excessive levels, initially there are high, peaked T waves. Progressively, there is a prolonged PR interval, followed by disappearance of the P wave, widened QRS complex, ventricular fibrillation, and finally, possible cardiac standstill.

Excessive potassium levels alter the impulses needed to send messages to the nerves and muscles. This leads to paresthesias (of the face, tongue, hands, and feet), irritability, and GI hyperactivity, resulting in nausea, diarrhea, and abdominal cramping.

Diagnostic findings reveal a serum potassium level above 5.0 mEq/L. Values indicative of metabolic acidosis are often seen with arterial blood gas studies. ECGs indicate the abnormal findings described earlier.

Correction. The treatment goal for hyperkalemia is to eliminate the cause of the excess and return the potassium level to within normal limits. Mild excesses may be treated by eliminating the cause. Slower but more permanent forms of treatment include cation exchange resins, hemodialysis, and peritoneal dialysis. Treatment of more excessive amounts may include the use of hypertonic glucose IV infusions and insulin (particularly for insulin-deficient patients) to shift potassium into the cells. Insulin helps move potassium into the cells, whereas glucose helps prevent hypoglycemia. The effect lasts for several hours. Administering sodium bicarbonate intravenously also shifts potassium back into cells. This usually takes effect in approximately 5 to 10 minutes and lasts for several hours. Both therapies are temporary measures because they do not actually remove potassium from the body. An IV infusion of calcium

gluconate may be used. It acts within 1 to 2 minutes but lasts only 30 to 60 minutes. It is preferable not to use this form of therapy for digitalized patients. Again, the calcium is only a temporary measure, but it also helps counteract the adverse effects of potassium on the neuromuscular membranes.

Nursing interventions include monitoring the serum potassium level, cardiac function, intake and output, and signs and symptoms. IV access may be needed to administer solutions and medications. When sodium- or calcium-containing medications are used, it is important to observe for imbalances of these electrolytes. Patients receiving digitalis should be monitored for digitalis toxicity if calcium gluconate is the treatment of choice.

Calcium. The normal serum level of total calcium is 4.3 to 5.3 mEq/L, or 8.5 to 10.5 mg/dl. Calcium is important in the formation of teeth and bones. It is also necessary for muscle contraction and neural function, where it regulates contractions and transmission of nerve impulses and has a sedative effect on nerve cells. It is important for normal blood coagulation. Calcium is available in ionized and nonionized forms. The ionized component is considered free calcium and makes up slightly less than half of the total serum calcium. Most of the remaining nonionized calcium is bound to protein, and a small percentage is chelated to nonprotein anions, including phosphate, citrate, and carbonate.

Calcium is regulated by the PTH, which is released by the parathyroid gland, as well as by calcitonin from the thyroid gland. The PTH promotes the transfer of calcium from bone to plasma.

The action of shifting calcium from plasma to bone is produced by calcitonin. Calcium is eliminated through urine, the GI tract, bone deposition, and sweat. It has a reciprocal relationship with phosphorus.

Hypocalcemia. A calcium deficit, or hypocalcemia, occurs as the serum calcium level drops below 4.5 mEq/L (8.5 mg/dl).

Cause. Calcium deficits may be related to reduced intestinal absorption, increased loss, altered regulation, and albumin, phosphorus, and magnesium imbalances.

The decreased intestinal absorption of calcium may be related to vitamin D deficiency, small bowel disease (in which most of the dietary calcium is absorbed), and decreased intake. Intestinal surgery also affects calcium absorption.

Excessive losses of calcium may be caused by renal disease or the use of loop diuretics. Calcium may also be lost through fistulas or damaged skin, as might occur with burns.

Because the parathyroid glands produce PTH, any damage to or surgical removal of these glands may lead to hypocalcemia. Because slightly less than half of ionized calcium is bound to albumin, any decrease in these albumin levels affects calcium levels. Alkalosis may increase the amount of calcium bound to albumin.

Medications that may decrease calcium include anticonvulsants, phosphates, mithramycin, calcitonin, and disodium edetate. Any medication that lowers magnesium may decrease calcium mobilization from bone.

Other electrolytes play a role in maintaining balanced calcium levels. Because of the reciprocal relationship of calcium and phosphorus, as the serum level for one goes up the other level goes down. Therefore excessive phosphorus levels result in deficient calcium levels. This may occur with extensive tissue damage, hypothermia, or cell destruction caused by cancer chemotherapy. Hypomagnesemia is also associated with calcium deficits. This is the result of impaired PTH secretion and decreased response to the hormone.

Assessment. Many of the symptoms associated with hypocalcemia are related to neuromuscular activity, such as tetany, convulsions, and numbness and tingling of the fingers, toes, and circumoral region. There may be muscle cramps and hyperactive deep tendon reflexes. Chvostek's sign is positive and is presented as unilateral twitching of the facial muscles by tapping the facial nerve just in front of the ear. Trousseau's sign is also positive and is apparent through the development of carpal spasm following inflation of a blood pressure cuff on the upper arm. Mental changes may include depression and confusion. As the deficits increase in severity, there may be respiratory effects, including dyspnea and laryngeal muscle spasms. Cardiovascular findings may show arrhythmias and a prolonged QT interval as a result of elongation of the ST segment and may develop a form of ventricular tachycardia (torsades de pointes).[11]

Hypocalcemia may cause dry skin, brittle nails, and dry hair. It has also been reported that chronic deficits may lead to retarded growth and lower IQ scores in children.[6]

Laboratory test results show a decreased serum calcium level. There may also be other electrolyte imbalances, including excessively high phosphorus and abnormally low magnesium levels.

Correction. The goal of treatment should be to eliminate the cause of the deficit and return the serum calcium level to normal. Acute symptomatic hypocalcemia requires immediate treatment.

Calcium deficits necessitate the use of oral or, in emergency situations, IV administration of calcium. Calcium chloride (2% to 10% solution) and calcium gluconate (10% solution) may be used, with the latter being preferable. The initial calcium dose for emergency serum elevation is 7 to 14 mEq for adults, 1 to 7 mEq for children, and less than 1 mEq for infants, with additional doses as dictated by serum levels.[10] Caution should be exercised while administering calcium to patients taking digoxin because it sensitizes the heart to digoxin.[12]

Calcium chloride ionizes more readily and is therefore more potent and irritating to tissues than calcium gluconate. IV infusion of both medications should be given slowly to prevent sensations of heat, tingling, hypotension, bradycardia, cardiac arrhythmias, and cardiac arrest.[10] Both calcium preparations can cause tissue irritation and burning, and there may be necrosis and sloughing of tissue if IV extravasation occurs. Because of the potential side effects, a more diluted concentration of calcium gluconate is preferred to a direct IV injection.

Nursing interventions need to include ongoing monitoring of signs and symptoms, laboratory tests results, and ECG readings. Precautions related to respiratory problems and tetany should be exercised. Because of potential problems related to extravasation, the IV site should be monitored carefully.

Hypercalcemia. Hypercalcemia, or calcium excess, occurs when the serum calcium level exceeds 5.5 mEq/L.

Cause. The most common causes of hypercalcemia are malignancy and hyperparathyroidism, with other causes account-ing for only a small percentage of the hypercalcemia-related cases.[6] Malignancy-related excesses may be related to lysis of the bone or an indirect tumor-related mechanism such as prostaglandin activity; tumor release of PTH or PTH-related protein; osteoclastic-activating cytokines; growth factors; and vitamin D–like sterols released by the tumor.[6] Androgens, estrogens, and progestins, which are used to treat malignancies, may cause calcium excess.

When hyperparathyroidism is present, there is an increase in the PTH level. This higher concentration causes an excessive amount of calcium to shift from the bone, an increase in retention of calcium by the renal system, and increased GI absorption.

Other causes include excessive administration of IV calcium and oral intake of calcium through milk and antacids. There may be a decrease in urinary excretion because of thiazide diuretics or renal failure. Hypercalcemia may follow prolonged immobilization as a result of the lack of weight-bearing bone stress, which is important for bone resorption and deposition.[10] Finally, there may be an increase in the ionized portion of calcium because of acidosis.

Assessment. Assessment findings of hypercalcemia vary according to serum levels and rate of development. Symptoms are related to the effects of calcium on neuromuscular excitability and cell membrane permeability. This sedative action results in fatigue, muscular weakness, and depressed deep tendon reflexes. The neuromuscular effect also carries over to the GI tract, where there may be anorexia, nausea, vomiting, or constipation.

Excessive calcium levels can alter the kidneys' ability to concentrate urine, resulting in polyuria and fluid volume depletion. These adverse effects may lead to acute or chronic renal failure.

Cardiovascular findings include heart rate reduction and disturbances in the rhythm, myocardial muscle function, and systemic vasculature.

Hypercalcemia can produce mental changes, including confusion, depression, and memory impairment. If theses symptoms are not corrected, they may lead to acute psychosis.

Laboratory findings reveal an increased serum calcium level. The ECG demonstrates a shortened QT interval and ST segment. The PR interval can be prolonged. Radiologic findings may indicate bone changes and reduced bone density.

Correction. As with all imbalances, the treatment goal is directed at eliminating the cause and returning the calcium level to within normal limits. Mild hypercalcemia may be treated by decreasing or eliminating medications that might contribute to the excess, encouraging mobilization and increasing fluid intake.

Hypercalcemia may become life-threatening and necessitates immediate treatment. Patients with normal renal and cardiac function initially receive a 0.9% sodium chloride solution. The solution is given rapidly to provide sodium and intravascular volume, because patients often also have a fluid volume deficit. The saline solution helps dilute the calcium concentration and facilitates calcium excretion. Furosemide (Lasix) is usually given in conjunction with saline infusions to help prevent fluid overload and further increase calcium excretion. Once adequate fluid volume has been attained, slower infusions of 0.9% and/or

0.45% sodium chloride solutions may be given to increase calcium elimination.

Other measures include the administration of calcitonin, IV phosphate, and diphosphates, as well as peritoneal dialysis or hemodialysis. Mithramycin (Plicamycin), a cytotoxic antibiotic, may be used to decrease bone resorption. Corticosteroids may be used to reduce intestinal calcium absorption and to decrease reabsorption by the renal system. However, the long-term side effects of glucocorticoid therapy need to be considered.

Nursing interventions include ongoing monitoring of serum calcium levels, ECGs, and renal function. Following emergency treatment, caution should be taken to observe for signs of calcium, potassium, and magnesium deficits. The patient should be monitored for signs of fluid overload when large volumes of IV saline are being administered. All information should be documented clearly and precisely, and the physician notified of any abnormal findings.

Magnesium. Magnesium is a cation that is located primarily in the bones and teeth. The remainder of the magnesium in the body is located in the cells, where it is the second most abundant electrolyte, and approximately 1% is found in the extracellular fluid. Normal serum levels are 1.5 to 2.5 mEq/L. Like calcium, the serum levels do not accurately reflect the total amount of magnesium in the body. Because part of the magnesium is bound to protein, serum albumin levels should be considered when making decisions related to imbalances. Magnesium is controlled mainly through renal excretion and distal small bowel absorption.

The role of magnesium is multifaceted and includes the activation of enzymes related to carbohydrate and protein metabolism. It is important in activating the sodium-potassium pump. Magnesium acts directly on the myoneural junction, affecting neuromuscular irritability and contractility. It acts on the skeletal muscle by depressing acetylcholine release at the synaptic junction. The cardiovascular system is affected because magnesium contributes to vasodilation, resulting in changes in blood pressure and cardiac output.[12] Magnesium levels and activity are interdependent with those of calcium (antagonist) and potassium.

Hypomagnesemia. Hypomagnesemia, or magnesium deficit, occurs when the serum magnesium level falls below 1.5 mEq/L. The deficit is often found in the critically ill patient and may be mistaken for hypokalemia.

Cause. Magnesium deficit may result from decreased intake, abnormal absorption, increased output, or chronic alcoholism. A decreased intake may be related to prolonged malnutrition, prolonged administration of magnesium-deficient, sodium-rich IV or total parenteral nutrition solutions, and occasionally a diet deficient in magnesium.

Decreased uptake of magnesium may occur with any problem related to the lower GI tract because this is where most of the absorption takes place. This may occur in the presence of inflammatory bowel disease or following surgical procedures involving the lower GI tract.

Many consider the most common cause of hypomagnesemia in the United States to be chronic alcoholism.[8] Individuals suffering from alcoholism often suffer from semistarvation, leading to reduced intake of magnesium-containing foods. Im-

paired renal function allows for increased losses and intestinal malabsorption, which decreases the utilization of the electrolyte. In addition, there may be intermittent diarrhea, which increases the losses.

Other causes include refeeding following prolonged malnutrition because magnesium is pulled from intravascular fluid and deposited into new cells. Some medications, such as diuretics, laxatives, aminoglycosides, and cisplatin (Platinol), may cause deficits. Increased elimination through prolonged diarrhea, intestinal fistulas, vomiting, and prolonged nasogastric suctioning may lead to magnesium deficits. Magnesium deficits may also be caused by impaired renal reabsorption, pancreatitis, burns, and surgical procedures.

Assessment. Symptoms related to hypomagnesemia are most often manifested through neuromuscular changes, and their severity is directly related to the level of the deficit. Symptoms include increased reflexes, muscle weakness, tremors, convulsions, and tetany. Chvostek's and Trousseau's signs are positive. Paresthesias may be present. Increased nerve transmission may lead to mood changes ranging from apathy and depression to extreme agitation and hallucinations.

Hypomagnesemia may result in various cardiac arrhythmias, such as supraventricular tachycardia and ventricular fibrillation. This deficit may increase the potential for digitalis toxicity.

Laboratory findings include magnesium below 1.5 mEq/L and low levels of calcium and potassium. ECG changes include prolonged PR and QT intervals, widened QRS complex, depressed ST segment, and inverted T waves.

Correction. The goal of treatment is to eliminate the cause and correct the deficit. The aggressiveness of treatment is directly related to the severity of the deficit. Mild deficiencies may be treated with diet or oral supplements, whereas more severe deficits may necessitate intramuscular or IV administration of magnesium.

Magnesium sulfate is usually the drug of choice, particularly for more severe deficits. The onset of action is immediate, and the duration of action is approximately 30 minutes. Caution should be exercised because of the potential for overdose and for hypermagnesemia, which may lead to respiratory paralysis. Before administering magnesium, the nurse must check the knee-jerk reflexes. If these are absent, the dose should be withheld and the physician notified. The respiration rate should be at least 16 and the urinary output 100 ml over the 4 hours preceding IV administration of magnesium sulfate. The dosage, which varies according to the severity of the deficit, may be given intramuscularly or intravenously. Parenteral administration of magnesium is contraindicated for patients with heart block or myocardial damage. The suggested IV dose is 5 g in 5% dextrose in water or 5% dextrose in saline, to be infused over 3 hours.[10]

Nursing interventions should include monitoring of serum magnesium level and urinary output, because magnesium is eliminated by the kidneys. Calcium and phosphorus levels should also be checked. There should be periodic checks of the knee-jerk reflexes because these disappear before respiration becomes depressed. Vital signs should be monitored and preparations made to counteract depressed respirations in case of magnesium excess, including artificial ventilation and IV calcium administration. Seizure precautions should also be exercised. All procedures and responses to therapy should be clearly and precisely documented.

Hypermagnesemia.

Hypermagnesemia, or magnesium excess, usually occurs when the serum magnesium level exceeds 2.5 mEq/L.

Cause. Hypermagnesemia usually results from decreased output or increased intake. The major cause of decreased output is renal disease. However, even when there is decreased output, it is often also associated with additional intake, such as magnesium-containing medications or IV solutions. Patients with endocrine disturbances such as hypothyroidism or hyperparathyroidism may have excess magnesium.

Antacids and laxatives are examples of medications that, if used excessively, may lead to hypermagnesemia. The use of enemas and continuous or large doses of magnesium to treat eclampsia or delay delivery may also increase magnesium levels.

Assessment. Clinical indicators, which are primarily related to the nervous and cardiovascular systems, usually do not appear until severe levels are reached. A review of current literature reveals no consistency in the relationship of magnesium levels to clinical indicators. However, once the magnesium ions are excessive, they interfere with the transmission of neuromuscular impulses. This may lead to increased muscle weakness, paralysis, and depressed deep tendon reflexes. Respiratory muscles may be depressed, leading to respiratory arrest in the presence of excessively high levels.

As the serum levels increase, so do the cardiovascular indicators. Small increases may result in flushing and a sensation of skin warmth caused by peripheral vasodilatation. With more severe increases, the pulse rate may decrease, which could lead to complete heart block.

Laboratory findings reveal an increased serum magnesium level. ECG readings may show prolonged QT and QRS intervals. Tracings in the presence of excessively high levels may indicate heart block and cardiac arrest.

Correction. Treatment should be directed at eliminating the cause and returning magnesium levels to within normal limits. Magnesium-containing foods and medications should be eliminated, if possible. Moderate excesses may be treated by the IV administration of 0.45% sodium chloride solution and diuretics to help the kidneys excrete the excess magnesium. The kidneys need to be functioning properly before initiating this form of therapy.

For more severe excesses, calcium gluconate may be administered intravenously. This antagonizes the action of the magnesium but is only a temporary measure. Dialysis may be indicated in the presence of renal impairment.

Nursing interventions include monitoring serum magnesium levels, patellar reflexes, and vital signs. Precautions should be exercised, including having equipment and medication available in the event of respiratory or cardiac arrest. Patients and families should be instructed in regard to the excessive use of over-the-counter magnesium-containing medications. All procedures, including the administration of IV solutions and medications, and observations, particularly those related to the deep tendon reflexes and respirations, should be relayed to the physician and accurately documented.

Phosphorus.

Phosphorus is found in the intracellular and extracellular fluids and is the primary anion in the intracellular compartment. Most phosphorus is located in the teeth and bones, with only a small amount in the soft tissue. Like calcium and magnesium, serum levels do not necessarily reflect the true levels of the total body content. Most phosphorus is in the form of phosphate, and the two terms are often used interchangeably. Normal serum phosphorus levels range from 1.8 to 2.6 mEq/L, or 2.5 to 4.5 mg/dl, and vary according to gender, age, and diet.

The metabolism and homeostasis of phosphorus are related to those of calcium. They have an inversely proportional relationship, and both are controlled by the parathyroid glands. Both electrolytes need vitamin D for absorption from the GI tract.

Phosphorus is important in carbohydrate, protein, and fat metabolism. It is necessary for nerve and muscle function and for the maintenance of the acid-base balance, in which it is the primary urinary buffer. Phosphorus is used to form energy-storing substances such as ATP.[11] It is also essential in the functioning of red blood cells, utilization of vitamin B, and transmission of hereditary traits.

Hypophosphatemia.

Hypophosphatemia, or phosphorus deficit, results when the serum phosphorus level falls below 1.8 mEq/L.

Cause. Hypophosphatemia may result from increased losses or utilization, decreased intestinal absorption, or intracellular shifts. Increased losses of phosphorus may be the result of glycosuria, hypokalemia, or hypomagnesemia. The use of diuretics (thiazides) increases the elimination of phosphorus.

Problems related to the GI tract, such as diarrhea, vomiting, vitamin D deficiencies, and lack of absorption, lead to phosphorus deficits. Continuous use of antacids leads to phosphorus binding.

Transient intracellular shifts play a major role in phosphorus deficits. The administration of concentrated glucose solutions increases insulin production, which causes phosphorus to shift into the cells. Shifts may also be related to an increased intracellular pH, as with respiratory alkalosis.

Malnourished patients may develop phosphorus deficits as calories are provided for nourishment. Because of poor nourishment and GI problems such as diarrhea and vomiting, the alcoholic patient may also experience hypophosphatemia.

Assessment. As with most electrolyte imbalances, symptoms related to hypophosphatemia are related to the severity of the deficit and whether it is acute (sudden decrease) or chronic (gradual decrease). Symptoms include those related to the neurologic system, such as confusion, seizures, coma, paresthesias, weakness, numbness, and ataxia. Weakness may lead to difficulty speaking and breathing.

Cardiovascular findings are related to decreased respiratory function and include myocardial dysfunction and chest pain. If prolonged, arrhythmias may develop. Hematologically, the phosphorus deficit affects the structure and function of blood cells, which may lead to hemolytic anemia and a reduction in oxygen transport.[12] Platelet dysfunction may result in bruising and bleeding.

Diagnostic findings show a decreased serum phosphorus level, and perhaps decreased serum potassium and magnesium levels. Calcium and alkaline phosphatase will be elevated.

Correction. The treatment goal is to eliminate the cause of the deficit and help return the phosphorus level to within normal limits. The best treatment is preventing the imbalance by not using phosphorus-binding medications, such as antacids, particularly if there is increased potential for phosphorus deficits.

Mild to moderate deficits may be treated through diet and oral supplements. More severe deficits may necessitate IV supplements, such as sodium phosphate or potassium phosphate. The IV site should be monitored closely because potassium phosphate can cause necrosis and sloughing of tissue.

Hyperphosphatemia. Hyperphosphatemia, or phosphorus excess, occurs when the serum phosphorus level exceeds 2.6 mEq/L.

Cause. Hyperphosphatemia is most often related to renal disease (acute and chronic). It might also be caused by increased intake, destruction of cells, excessive losses from nonrenal causes, and shifts from cells to the extracellular fluid.

In renal failure, the diseased kidney cannot excrete phosphorus, which leads to excessive levels. Increased intake may be the result of laxatives containing phosphate, vitamin D excess, or phosphorus supplements.

Shifts may occur from cells being damaged, as with chemotherapy, and releasing phosphorus. Respiratory acidosis may also cause an intracellular to extracellular shift.

Assessment. Most symptoms of hyperphosphatemia are related to hypocalcemia. The Chvostek's and Trousseau's signs are positive. There may be anorexia, nausea, vomiting, tachycardia and muscle spasm, pain, or weakness. When excess levels of phosphorus are sustained for prolonged periods, precipitation of calcium phosphate may occur in areas other than the bones.

Laboratory findings reveal an increased serum phosphate level, above 2.6 mEq/L, and decreased calcium. Other tests, such as creatinine and PTH levels, may be performed to help determine the cause.

Correction. Treatment is directed toward alleviating the cause. Nursing interventions include monitoring serum phosphorus and calcium levels. Patient and family education is directed at avoiding foods and medications that contain high phosphorus levels. Precautions should be exercised in the event of hypocalcemic tetany, such as monitoring for seizures, confusion, and laryngeal muscle spasms. When kidney function is normal, IV saline infusions may be used to increase excretion. Phosphorus can be forced into the cells when used in conjunction with insulin. Dialysis may be necessary with abnormal renal function.

Chloride. Chloride is the major anion in the extracellular fluid. It is found in the blood in combination with sodium and in the stomach with hydrogen. Chloride helps maintain serum osmolarity, acid-base balance, and the balance of cations in the intracellular and extracellular fluids. The renal and GI systems are the major regulators of chloride, and normal values are 97 to 110 mEq/L.

Hypochloremia. Hypochloremia, a chloride deficit, occurs when the chloride level falls below 97 mEq/L.

Cause. Hypochloremia can occur following GI losses, including vomiting and nasogastric suctioning. Chloride can also be lost when diuretics are used. The deficit could be related to chloridorrhea or water in the body.

Assessment. The symptoms are related to changes in other electrolytes or pathophysiologic processes. Laboratory findings include a serum chloride level below 97 mEq/L and alterations in other electrolyte levels (depending on the cause) and acid-base balance.

Correction. Treatment should be directed toward eliminating the cause as well as monitoring and replacing the appropriate electrolytes.

Hyperchloremia. Hyperchloremia, chloride excess, occurs when the level exceeds 110 mEq/L.

Cause. The causative factors include sodium excess and bicarbonate deficit.

Assessment. Symptoms are related to the causative factor. Laboratory findings reveal a high serum chloride as well as alterations for other electrolytes or acid-base balance.

Correction. Elimination of the cause is the first priority. The intake/output of chlorides should be monitored along with the serum levels of chloride and other electrolytes. All pertinent information should be documented appropriately.

Application of principles to the postoperative patient

Preparation to prevent or minimize complications related to fluids and electrolytes should begin, if possible, before surgery. A thorough history and physical may indicate preexisting conditions, such as diabetes mellitus, renal disease, or cardiovascular disease. These conditions may also indicate that the patient has been unable to eat properly or has experienced prolonged nausea and vomiting. The history identifies recent medications. Of particular importance are corticosteroids, which could alter the response to surgery. Diagnostic tests reveal the fluid and electrolyte status. Physical assessment also provides helpful information related to such characteristics as edema, dry skin and membranes, and abnormal vital signs.

It is much easier to deal with many of these issues before surgery rather than during surgery or postoperatively. IV solutions may be given to correct fluid volume deficits and, depending on the type of solution, to provide calories and electrolytes. Diuretics may be given to eliminate excessive fluid volume. If known far enough in advance, the patient's nutritional state can be improved by administering total parenteral nutrition solutions.

During surgery there is always the danger of excessive loss of blood leading to fluid volume deficit. Depending on the volume lost, replacement may include the administration of IV fluids and blood and blood products. There may be third spacing of fluids, which could create a fluid volume deficit.

Postoperatively, there are imbalances in fluid volume, including fluid volume excess and fluid volume deficit. In addition to the neuroendocrine response from the anesthetic, there is also stress related to the pain and trauma of surgery. The response to these factors is an increased release of ADH and adrenocorticotropic hormone (ACTH). ADH leads to the retention of fluid, and ACTH increases the release of aldosterone and hydrocortisone, resulting in the retention of water and sodium and the elimination of potassium. The net result is increased fluid volume. The period of fluid retention lasts approximately 48 to 72 hours after surgery.[11] Other factors that may predispose the patient to excessive fluid volume include medications, possible fluid shifts, tissue catabolism, and the excessive administration of IV fluids.

Other factors that are not related to the stress response of surgery may also affect output. These may include hypovolemia caused by presurgery fluid status or loss of fluid during the surgical procedure. In addition, altered cardiovascular functions or renal failure may stimulate the body to retain water and sodium.

The surgical process may precipitate electrolyte imbalances. Electrolyte dilution may occur along with the fluid volume excess discussed earlier. A potassium deficit is the most common imbalance noted. However, caution should be exercised in administering supplements because some potassium is released because of surgical trauma to the cells. A sodium deficit may also occur, perhaps related to fluid volume excess, surgery-related stress, and medications received before and during surgery. Treatment is not generally indicated, but caution should be exercised to eliminate unnecessary free water to prevent water intoxication.

Electrolyte excess may occur in the presence of fluid volume deficit. Hyperkalemia may also result from the release of potassium from the cells during the surgical process.

There may be alterations in the acid-base balance. Pain, anesthetics, and narcotics may be responsible for shallow respirations, which could in turn cause respiratory acidosis. Patients who are on ventilators or hyperventilate for any reason may develop respiratory alkalosis. Metabolic acidosis may occur as a result of excess lactic acid in patients who are hypotensive.

Other states

Syndrome of inappropriate antidiuretic hormone secretion. The SIADH occurs when there is excessive release of ADH or a similar substance. Predisposing factors include medications, including nonsteroidal antiinflammatory drugs; tumors, especially oat cell carcinoma; and central nervous system disorders. Excessive ADH decreases the excretion of water. As this occurs, the serum sodium level and osmolality decrease. The increased extracellular fluid volume increases glomerular filtration and decreases aldosterone release, resulting in the increased elimination of sodium. Because the intracellular concentration is greater, extracellular fluid is pulled into the cells. This can be life-threatening, particularly if water is drawn into the brain cells.

Assessment reveals findings related to fluid volume excess with edema and to intake exceeding output. Depending on the severity of the sodium deficit, there may be neurologic indicators, such as lethargy, headaches, seizures, and finally, coma. Laboratory results reveal decreased serum sodium, BUN, and creatinine levels. Urine test findings show a low sodium level and increased specific gravity and osmolality.

Treatment is directed at correcting the cause. If this is not possible, treatment depends on the severity of the imbalance, ranging from fluid restriction to the IV administration of concentrated saline solutions and diuretics.

Burns. The skin is the largest organ of the body and serves a variety of functions. It acts as a protective barrier, regulates body temperature, and houses sensory receptors. The skin comprises the epidermis, the outer layer; the dermis, the inner layer; and a subcutaneous layer that binds to underlying organs. The severity of a burn depends on the total area involved, depth, and location; the patient's age; and any other injuries or preexisting medical problems. Burns may be classified as first-degree (partial thickness), second-degree (superficial), or third-degree burns (full thickness).

Burned skin can no longer provide a protective barrier, setting the stage for fluid and electrolyte imbalances. The injury to the cells and vascular system allows fluid to shift from the plasma into the interstitial space. This may result in fluid volume deficit and, depending on the level of severity, possible renal damage.

Proteins and electrolytes are lost at the same time that water is being lost. Damaged cells release potassium. This, in conjunction with hypovolemia and renal damage, leads to hyperkalemia. There are also abnormal losses of sodium, calcium, and phosphorus. Depending on the degree of pain, there may be hyperventilation, leading to respiratory alkalosis. The damaged cells may release acids, or there may be hypovolemia-induced lactic acid production, resulting in metabolic acidosis.

It is important to maintain fluid volume. Moderate to severe burns necessitate IV fluid replacement. It is important that fluids be delivered at a rate high enough (but no higher) to maintain the desired intravascular volume and urinary output. After the first 24 hours, the damaged capillaries usually start to seal and the fluid loss decreases. Mobilization of edema returning fluid to the vascular space starts at approximately 72 hours.[11] Fluid, electrolyte, and acid-base status should be monitored carefully at this time.

Fluid replacement therapy varies among physicians and according to the type of fluid and volume. Some regimens include lactated Ringer's solution, which is a balanced electrolyte solution that approximates components found in plasma. Others use 0.9% sodium chloride, but this may create an imbalance because of an excessive amount of chloride. Some physicians advocate the use of colloids to replace plasma. Nursing interventions should include initiating an IV line to deliver fluid replacement, monitoring the administration process, and evaluating vital signs. Equally important is checking output. Laboratory findings to monitor include serum electrolyte and blood gas levels. Preexisting conditions or other injuries may necessitate other laboratory tests. All information needs to be documented and the physician notified of any abnormal findings.

Diabetes. There are two forms of diabetes that affect fluid and electrolyte balance: diabetes insipidus and diabetes mellitus.

Diabetes insipidus. Diabetes insipidus is a disorder related to water imbalance caused by a lack of ADH (central/neurogenic) or by failure of the kidneys to respond to the ADH (nephrogenic/renal). Excessive water loss through the kidneys results in a decreased volume in the extracellular fluid compartment. Without proper treatment, dehydration (intracellular and extracellular), hypotension, and hypovolemic shock can occur.[10] Characteristics of diabetes insipidus include an intense thirst, weight loss, excessive urinary output, and neurologic symptoms such as confusion, irritability, and seizures. Laboratory findings reveal an increased serum sodium level and osmolality. The urine osmolality is decreased. It is important to determine the cause of the polyuria, which can be accomplished by vasopressin administration.

Diabetes insipidus is treated by ADH replacement (vasopressin) for the central type, and thiazide diuretic medications may be used to decrease the polyuria associated with both the central and nephrogenic forms of diabetes insipidious.[6] Initially, lost fluid may need to be replaced by IV solutions (hypotonic). Caution should be exercised during fluid replacement to prevent water intoxication.

Nursing interventions include monitoring intake and output, body weight, and serum sodium levels. An IV may need to be initiated to replace fluid. During vasopressin administration, the patient needs to be monitored for other complications, particularly water intoxication.

Diabetes mellitus. Diabetes mellitus is caused by a lack of insulin, which leads to an elevated blood sugar level and increased urinary output. Diabetes mellitus is related to decreased glucose utilization, increased fat mobilization, and protein utilization. The hyperglycemia related to diabetes mellitus can lead to diabetic ketoacidosis (DKA) or hyperosmolar hyperglycemia nonketotic syndrome (HHNS).

Causative factors of DKA include insufficient insulin secretion, inadequate insulin intake, and incidents that initiate steroid hormone secretion. The process begins with insulin deficiency, which decreases glucose utilization by the cells and results in an increased blood glucose level and glucose production by the liver. As this process continues, serum osmolality increases, thus pulling fluid from the cells into the extracellular fluid. This results in cellular dehydration and polyuria and, when prolonged, leads to fluid volume deficit.

The absence of insulin decreases the use of glucose, and the body must search for other sources of fuel. Fat stores are mobilized, leading to an increased serum lipid level. Increased fat metabolism increases ketone formation and causes a decrease in the pH of body fluids (metabolic acidosis). Ketones may be excreted in the urine or by the lungs.

The body tries to compensate for the acid through the lungs (rapid, deep breathing) or elimination through the kidneys or serum. The increased serum glucose results in osmotic diuresis, causing fluid and electrolyte imbalances.

Characteristics of DKA include polyuria, polydipsia, nausea, vomiting, and hyperventilation with acetone odor respirations. Because there is the potential for fluid volume deficit, characteristics ranging from weight loss to postural hypotension may be present. There may also be a variety of signs and symptoms related to electrolyte imbalances caused by electrolyte excesses or deficits.

Laboratory findings reveal hyperglycemia and increases in serum osmolality, BUN and creatinine levels, hemoglobin, hematocrit, and total protein. Serum bicarbonate level and pH decrease. Serum electrolyte imbalances, including those involving potassium, sodium, and phosphorus, may involve excesses or deficits, depending on the severity of the ketoacidosis and the treatment status. Causative factors of hyperosmolar hyperglycemic nonketotic syndrome include inadequate insulin secretion/action, inadequate insulin intake, or response to certain medications. The insulin level is not sufficient to prevent hyperglycemia but is adequate to prevent ketonuria. The hyperglycemia results in osmotic diuresis leading to fluid and electrolyte disturbances.

Polyuria and electrolyte losses result in dehydration of the extracellular and intracellular fluids. This dehydration results in neurologic changes. Thromboemboli may occur as the fluid volume deficit increases.

Laboratory findings may reveal metabolic acidosis and decreased serum sodium, potassium, phosphorus, and magnesium levels.

Treatment is similar for both DKA and HHNS. Fluids are replaced, initially with a 0.9% sodium chloride solution (although a 0.45% sodium chloride solution may be used depending on preexisting conditions related to fluid retention). Subsequent infusions may be changed to 0.45% sodium chloride solution to provide free water, which facilitates renal excretion and the normalization of serum osmolality. As intravascular dilution occurs, the serum glucose level drops, which may necessitate the use of a glucose-containing IV solution. Insulin may be given to help correct high glucose levels. An initial bolus may be given, supplemented with continued insulin in IV solution as needed. Only regular insulin should be given intravenously.

Nursing interventions include initiating and monitoring an IV line to help maintain homeostasis. Laboratory data, particularly serum glucose and electrolyte levels, need to be continually monitored. The patient should be observed for symptoms related to fluid volume deficit and electrolyte imbalances. Close monitoring should include observation for signs and symptoms of hypoglycemia to guard against overcorrection. All procedures and responses to therapy should be properly documented.

SUMMARY

Under normal conditions, the body maintains a state of equilibrium, or homeostasis. This balanced state is achieved through various checks and balances. The preceding information describes this delicate process and the imbalances that may occur when the body cannot function properly. Correction of the imbalance may be as simple as eliminating the cause or as complex as initiating life support measures, including the use of IV fluids and medications.

Part of the homeostatic mechanism involves the maintenance of fluid balance. Water travels throughout the various body compartments. Fluid shifts are an attempt to balance fluid intake and output and are affected by the solutes contained within the various compartments, preexisting medical conditions, intake volume, and the environment. The crucial role of water has been discussed in detail throughout this chapter. Alterations in this role can lead to imbalances and complications. Fluid volume also affects the concentration of solutes, and any imbalances may precipitate various side effects.

Equally important to fluid balance is electrolyte balance. Electrolytes have a direct impact on the movement of fluid and thus on the maintenance of fluid balance. These ions affect the functioning of all major systems, including the cardiovascular, renal, and neurologic systems. The body generally maintains the proper types and concentrations of electrolytes to ensure normal activity. Abnormal concentrations can lead to ill effects, with severe excesses and deficits possibly leading to death.

It is important that the nurse be knowledgeable about normal fluid and electrolyte levels and their importance to the overall maintenance of homeostasis. It is also important to recognize abnormal findings and to understand their impact on the body. When recognized and treated promptly, most imbalances can be resolved and the body returns to a normal state.

The nurse also needs to be familiar with proper treatment modalities, which help ensure that appropriate equipment and supplies are available. This familiarity allows the nurse to question possible incorrect treatment orders or laboratory findings. Knowledge of normal and abnormal findings related to fluid and electrolyte balance, along with expertise in IV therapy, help ensure prompt, quality patient care.

REFERENCES

1. Ignatavicius DD, Workman ML, Mishler MA: *Medical surgical nursing across the continuum,* Philadelphia, 1999, WB Saunders.
2. Guyton AC, Hall JE: *Textbook of medical physiology,* ed 9, Philadelphia, 1996, WB Saunders.
3. LeFever K, Poulanka BJ: *Handbook of fluid, electrolyte, and acid-base imbalances,* Albany, NY, 1999, Delmar.
4. Smith E, Kinsey M: *Fluids and electrolytes: a conceptual approach,* ed 2, New York, 1991, Churchill Livingston.
5. Kokko JP, Tannen RL: *Fluids and electrolytes,* ed 4, Philadelphia, 1996, WB Saunders.
6. Metheny NM: *Fluid and electrolyte balance: nursing considerations,* ed 3, Philadelphia, 1996, JB Lippincott.
7. Preston RA: *Acid-base, fluids and electrolytes made ridiculously simple,* Miami, 1997, MedMaster, Inc.
8. Braunwald E, ed: *Harrison's principles of internal medicine,* ed 11, New York, 1987, McGraw-Hill.
9. Cavanaugh, BM: *Nurses manual of diagnostic tests,* ed 3, Philadelphia, 1995, FA Davis.
10. McEvoy GK: *AHFS drug information 99,* Bethesda, Md, 1999, American Society of Hospital Pharmacists.
11. Horne MM, Heitz UE, Swearingen PL: *Fluid, electrolyte, and acid-base balance: pocket guide series,* ed 3, St Louis, 1997, Mosby.
12. Paradisco C: *Fluids and electrolytes,* ed 2, Philadelphia, 1999, JB Lippincott.

Chapter

8

Infection Control

Kathryn Carlson, BS, CRNI, Maxine B. Perdue, BSN, MHA, MBA, CRNI, CNAA, Judy Hankins, BSN, CRNI*

The actual number of device-related infections is probably greater because the intravascular device or infusate is often not cultured. Therefore the primary goal is not simply to identify and treat these infections, but to prevent them.[1] Easily preventable device-related infections greatly increase treatment costs and morbidity rates.

Nurses involved in maintaining vascular access devices must have the knowledge and competency to initiate appropriate care protocols, implement nursing actions that prevent complications, and make appropriate nursing interventions if complications occur. The principles of infection control provide the foundation for the delivery of IV therapy. Prevention begins with being knowledgeable about the risk factors that can predispose a patient to an intravascular device–related infection.

To understand the principles of infection control, it is important to understand some key concepts. The following infection control terms are briefly defined here and are discussed in greater detail later in this chapter:

A *nosocomial infection* is hospital acquired; that is, it was not present or incubating at the time of admission.

Colonization is the growth of microorganisms in a host without overt clinical expression or detected immune reaction. Microorganisms often colonize on the surface or in the inner lumens of intravascular devices. Colonization also refers to the persistent presence of microorganisms at a particular site. Certain species of bacteria form colonies on the surface of the skin or in certain regions of the body. For example, the colonization of *Staphylococcus aureus* in the nares or on the epidermal surface of the skin is considered normal.

A *bacteremia* is a bloodstream infection that is identified by positive blood cultures. Although there are many types of bacteremias, most are commonly classified as primary and secondary. A primary bacteremia has no identified underlying source but is usually associated with the use of IV devices. A secondary bacteremia arises from an existing infectious source. For example, patients with burns or intraabdominal wound infections are at risk for developing a secondary bacteremia. Signs and symptoms of bacteremia include fever, chills, hypotension, and a positive blood culture.

Sepsis, or *septicemia,* is a systemic infection in the circulating blood caused by pathogenic microorganisms or their toxins. Septicemia can occur when microorganisms migrate into the bloodstream and cause a profound systemic reaction. Signs and symptoms of septicemia are described later in this chapter.

The administration of intravenous (IV) therapy increases the risk of infectious complications. It is estimated that more than 30 million patients per year in the United States receive infusion therapy in hospitals, physician's offices, skilled nursing facilities, and ambulatory centers, as well as at home.[1] These patients receive a staggering array of diagnostic procedures and therapeutic regimens that bypass their natural host defenses and increase their risk for nosocomial infections. Even though fewer than 1% of infusions are identified as producing bloodstream infections, there are an estimated 50,000 to 100,000 bloodstream infections in U.S. hospitals each year. Of this total, approximately 55,000 are caused by central venous catheters (CVCs).[1]

*The author and editors wish to acknowledge the contributions made by Roxanne Perucca, Carolyn Hedrick, and Jim Johnson as authors of this chapter in the first edition of *Intravenous Nursing: Clinical Principles and Practice.*

Immune System and Susceptibility to Infection

When a venipuncture is performed, the body's first line of defense, the cutaneous barrier, is broken. Breaking the skin barrier provides an avenue for the entry of many microorganisms such as fungi, bacteria, and viruses. Because the immune system is a complex network of cells and organs, only an overview is provided here. (Note the values used in this chapter are for adults and may vary depending on the reference or health care facility.)

Leukocytes (white blood cells) are an important component of the immune system. The total leukocyte count of a newborn is at its highest level, and the reference range remains higher than the adult level into the teenage years.[2] The normal white blood cell (WBC) count ranges from 4.1 to 10.9×10^9/L.[2,3] Neutrophils and lymphocytes compose 80% to 90% of the total WBC count. A differential WBC count provides more specific information related to infections and disease processes (Table 8-1).[3]

Granulocytes and monocytes are the foundation of the body's nonspecific immune response. Neutrophils, referred to as *polymorphonuclear leukocytes,* are the body's first line of defense against infection. *Segments* are mature neutrophils. When infections occur, the bone marrow releases immature neutrophils (sometimes identified as bands) that, together with mature neutrophils, engulf and destroy bacteria. The phenomenon is referred to as a *shift to the left.* Polymorphonuclear leukocytes can destroy invading bacteria and remain in the peripheral blood for 6 to 10 hours before moving into tissue, performing their function, and dying.[3] Neutrophils are the first cells to appear in large numbers within exudates in the initial inflammation stages. *Neutropenia* refers to a decrease in the absolute neutrophil count. A neutrophil count of less than 1.75×10^9/L predisposes the individual to infection; counts under 0.5×10^9/L, known as *agranulocytosis,* predispose to serious, life-threatening infections.[3]

The next leukocyte in the line of defense is the monocyte cell, also referred to as a *macrophage.* Neutrophils and monocytes engulf and partially digest, or phagocytize, invading antigens. Monocytes are slower to respond to infections and inflammatory diseases, but once activated, they are stronger than neutrophils, ingesting larger particles of debris. Although monocytes respond late in the acute phase of infection, they continue to function during the chronic phase.

Lymphocytes have the ability to recognize specific antigens from any foreign living organism, such as viruses, fungi, and bacteria. An increase in the number of lymphocytes (lymphocytosis) occurs in viral infections. Lymphocytes can be divided into two main subgroups: T cells and B cells. B cells produce immunoglobulins, and T cells are responsible for effector and regulatory functions. Cell-mediated immunity is the responsibility of the effector T cells. This includes defense against intracellular bacterial or fungal infections, cytolysis of virus-infected cells, allograft rejection, graft-versus-host reaction, and certain types of tumor immunity.[3] Regulatory T cells moderate the functions of effector T cells and B cells by inducing or suppressing proliferation and differentiation of these cells.

There are four subsets within the T cell system. Helper/inducer T lymphocytes (CD4) induce other T cells and help B cells produce antibodies. Interleukin (IL)-2, a growth factor produced by T cells, stimulates the proliferation and differentiation of activated T cells.[3] A cytokine, IL-1, released by macrophages, stimulates CD4 cells to produce IL-2.[3] The second subset, delayed hypersensitivity T lymphocytes, produces chemotactic lymphokines in response to particulate and soluble antigens. One of the chemotactic lymphokines, macrophage-activating factor, induces membrane alterations that cause clumping and immobilization of cells. This factor, interferon, has several functions, including inhibiting tumor cell growth. Cytotoxic T lymphocytes, the third subgroup, destroys antigen-specific target cells on contact.[3] The final subgroup, suppressor T lymphocytes (CD8), comprises three cells—inducer, effector, and transducer—that regulate humoral and cell-mediated responses.[3]

Eosinophils and basophils are other types of WBCs. During allergic reactions and parasitic conditions, as well as after radiation exposure, the number of eosinophils increase. However, an increase in steroids, either during stress or administered parenterally, decreases the number of eosinophils and basophils.

Although the immune system is complex and dynamic, its components are interdependent. One missing element can cause the entire immune system to be ineffective. Patients who are immunocompromised are at greater risk for developing an intravascular device–related infection. Often, patients who require vascular access devices have a severe underlying illness, receive multiple infusions of solutions and medications, require extended hospitalization, and may be immunosuppressed.

There are many risk factors that increase a patient's susceptibility to developing an IV-related infection.[4] Because certain patient risk factors cannot be controlled (Box 8-1), it is especially important to eliminate those that can be controlled by implementing nursing protocols to prevent IV-related infection.

Table 8-1	**Leukocytes**
Cell Type	**Normal Range (cells/mm³)**
GRANULOCYTES	
Neutrophils (total)	$1.8-7.7 \times 10^9$/L
Eosinophils	$0-0.45 \times 10^9$/L
Basophils	$0-0.1 \times 10^9$/L
AGRANULAR (MONONUCLEAR)	
Lymphocytes	$1.0-4.8 \times 10^9$/L
Monocytes	$0-0.8 \times 10^9$/L

Box 8-1   Factors That Influence a Host's Defense Against Infection

- Leukopenia
- Diminished granulocyte function
- Immunosuppression and immunodeficiency
- Burns
- Presence of concurrent infection
- Severe underlying illness
- Age (<1 yr or >60 yr)

IV-RELATED INFECTIONS AND COMPLICATIONS

Source of microorganisms

Despite improved catheter technology, antibiotic-impregnated catheters, cuffs, and dressing materials, catheter-related infections continue to occur. IV-related infections can result when the IV infusion system becomes contaminated. Contamination can occur by intrinsic or extrinsic means. Microorganisms may be introduced into the IV system by IV fluids or additives, IV tubing, ointment, and IV cannulas or catheters. Contaminates can be introduced during container and administration set changes or when medications are added to the infusion system. Contamination can also occur because of inadequate handwashing, improper aseptic technique while inserting an IV device, incorrect preparation of the insertion site, or soiled, damp, or no-longer-intact dressing on the insertion site.

IV-related infection can result from an endogenous or exogenous source of microorganisms. An endogenous infection is caused by the patient's own flora. For example, the microorganisms from endotracheal secretions may colonize a central venous access device inserted into the subclavian or jugular vein of an intubated patient. Exogenous infection is an infection resulting from the transmission of organisms from a source other than the patient. Inadequate handwashing by health care personnel can spread transient flora from patient to patient and cause an exogenous infection.

Contamination of the infusate, the administration equipment, the insertion site, or the venipuncture device can lead to the growth of microorganisms.

Fluid-related contamination. Infections related to IV therapy vary from local to systemic, with outcomes ranging from localized pain to death. Fluid-related contamination is one of the main causes of IV-related infections and may have intrinsic or extrinsic causes. The fluids given by the IV route include fluids, medications, blood, and blood products. Contamination of infusate is the most common cause of epidemic device-related bloodstream infections.[1] In addition to the IV fluids and equipment, contaminated antiseptic solutions can also cause infections.

Causative organisms for fluid-related contamination include the following: Tribe Klebsielleae(*Enterobacter cloacae, Enterobacter agglomerans, Serratia marcescens,* and *Klebsiella* species); *Burkholderia cepacia, Burkholderia acidivorans,* and *Burkholderia pickettii; Citrobacter freundii* and *Flavobacterium* species; and *Candida tropicalis.*[1]

Fluid-related microorganisms may be present in large numbers and still not be visible to the naked eye. Therefore close scrutiny of the patient (for signs of infection), product container (for cracks or leakage), and fluid (for color and clarity) is vital. Microorganisms can be introduced into IV products before they arrive at the health care facility (intrinsic) or during the course of clinical use (extrinsic).

Intrinsic contamination. IV products can become contaminated before reaching the health care facility, and many articles have described worldwide occurrences. Probably the most well-known incident occurred in the United States between 1970 and 1971. It involved IV products manufactured by one company after changing the lining of the screw cap closures.

This change resulted in 378 patients in 25 hospitals developing *E. (Aerobacter) cloacae* or *E. agglomerans* septicemia.[1]

IV fluids can become contaminated at any time during the sterilization process. After the product has been sterilized, any damage to the IV fluid container provides an entry point for microorganisms. This can result from a damaged port seal, a crack in a bottle, or a hole in a plastic IV bag. Damage and contamination of the IV container can occur at the manufacturing site or at any point during storage or delivery to the health care facility. A defect in the fluid container may occur during the manufacturing or sterilization process. For example, if no seal is placed or if a seal is positioned incorrectly on the port of an IV bag, fluid contamination may result.

Although intrinsic contamination does not occur as often, when it does occur, its effects may be far-reaching because of the large volumes of product that are produced and processed at one time. Also, if a contaminant is introduced into the fluid at the manufacturing level, there is more time for the microorganism to proliferate before it actually reaches the patient.

Prevention is the best intervention. Close inspection of IV fluids and their containers is imperative. Bottles should be checked carefully for cracks, including cracks that may be hidden by the label. The neck of the bottle should be checked to ensure that all the closure components are intact. IV bags should be checked for puncture holes by squeezing the container and rotating the bag. Fluid containers should be observed for droplet formation on the bag surface. All protective coverings and seals of entry ports should be inspected to ensure proper fit. The clarity of the solution should be inspected and the manufacturer's expiration date should be noted. If there is any question about the sterility of the IV product, it should not be used. If intrinsic contamination is suspected, the IV nursing supervisor, pharmacist, manufacturer, and the U.S. Food and Drug Administration (FDA) should be notified immediately. Samples of the affected product with the same lot number should be made available for inspection and analysis.

Blood and blood products may also be contaminated at the collection site. The collection bag may have been contaminated during the manufacturing process or during transportation and storage of the product. The port may have been contaminated during the collection process or, in the case of components, during the separation process. The storage time and temperature are directly proportional to the increased growth level of microorganisms. The resulting transfusion reaction is most often related to the endotoxins produced by psychrophilic, gram-negative bacteria. The following endotoxins are associated with transfusion reactions: *Pseudomonas* species, *C. freundii, Escherichia coli,* and *Yersinia enterocolitica.*

Just as with IV fluids and medications, blood and blood products should be inspected carefully. The blood collection container needs to be checked for possible damage. Contaminated blood may appear normal, have a purple color, or show signs of hemolysis. In any case, it should not be used if the integrity of the product is suspect.

A patient experiencing a transfusion reaction related to contaminated blood may have a number of signs and symptoms, including high fever, diarrhea, vomiting, hemoglobinuria, renal failure, shock, generalized muscle pain, and disseminated intravascular coagulation. Even though contamination is rare, it can be fatal. Treatment with IV antibiotics and vasopressor medications or steroids should be initiated immediately. However, the best treatment is prevention through adherence to aseptic technique, administration of blood immediately after it is removed from controlled refrigeration, infusing within 4 hours, and replacing the IV administration set and filter following administration of the product.

Extrinsic contamination.
Extrinsic contamination occurs in the health care facility or in the patient's home. IV fluids or medications may be contaminated during the admixture procedure, which can result from the improper use of laminar flow hoods or by using malfunctioning hoods. Incorrect use of admixing equipment, such as needles, syringes, or calibrating devices, may lead to contaminated products. Because products may be prepared in large numbers in IV admixture programs, the potential for patient exposure to contamination is high. Admixed fluids that are not refrigerated for long periods have an increased rate of proliferation of microorganisms, thus increasing the risk and severity of infection. IV products, whether in the hospital or alternative care setting, may also be contaminated when adding medications to fluid containers already in use. Damage may occur during delivery and storage of the product, which allows microorganisms to enter the sterile container. Finally, the IV fluid may become contaminated by improper technique while administering intermittent medications or by the failure to maintain a sterile, closed infusion system.

Clinical indications of extrinsically contaminated IV fluids are rare. When there is a resulting septicemia, however, the signs and symptoms are indistinguishable from those of septicemia with an intrinsic cause.

Early detection and treatment are extremely important in achieving a positive outcome. The treatment of an extrinsically induced septicemia is the same as that of an intrinsic infection. As with all infections, prevention is preferable. Maintaining aseptic technique is important. This includes proper handwashing, correct use of sterile admixing equipment and supplies, and proper use of laminar flow hoods. Staff members involved in this admixing process should be required to demonstrate competencies on a routine basis, particularly the individuals staffing admixture programs.

Equipment-related contamination.
Equipment used to administer IV fluids, medications, and blood products should provide a sterile pathway from the container to the patient. Equipment may become contaminated during the manufacturing process, when therapy is initiated, or during therapy.

Intrinsic contamination.
On the manufacturing level, the product may be made improperly, with a missing or ill-fitting IV set port cover, for example. The product may become contaminated during sterilization or during storage and delivery. Contamination during storage can occur at the manufacturing site, the wholesaler, the health care facility, or an alternative care setting, including the patient's home. Products are delivered in a variety of ways and to numerous sites before reaching the patient, and product contamination can occur at any time along the way.

Extrinsic contamination.
Extrinsic contamination may occur when therapy is initiated or during the course of administration. The IV line may become contaminated when the administration set is added to the fluid container if the spike of the set comes in contact with the outside of the IV container port. Equipment may become contaminated when add-on devices are attached (e.g., filters, stopcocks, extension sets). Finally, the sterile pathway may become contaminated when the administration set is added to a vascular access device.

The venipuncture procedure offers opportunity for the contamination of equipment. Inadequate site preparation, touch contamination of the cannula, and improper application of the dressing are primary causes of extrinsic contamination.

During the course of therapy, the IV pathway may become contaminated at any point. This may occur when additional solutions or medications are connected or when air is removed from the line. Accidental separation of the line at any connection may result in contamination. If flushing is necessary, as with intermittent infusions, the line may become contaminated. Some equipment, such as intermittent administration sets or stopcocks, tends to be more susceptible to contamination because of an increased manipulation of the products. Soiled or damp dressings are also a source of contamination. Tubing that is left in place longer than the recommended time, including blood sets, provides a source for microorganisms to proliferate. Suppurative phlebitis and an intravascular thrombus can yield a large number of microorganisms that can circulate throughout the body.

Many extrinsic sources exist that can contaminate the IV system. Many catheter-related infections are caused by extrinsic contamination of the insertion site or the IV catheter. Both are considered crucial areas for the prevention of IV-related infections.

Contamination at the insertion site.
There is a consensus that microbes colonizing the skin surrounding the insertion site are the source of most catheter-related bloodstream infections.[5] Studies of a variety of catheters indicate that heavy cutaneous colonization of the insertion site is a powerful predictor of catheter-related infections.[1] Patients with burns having a large population of microorganisms on the skin surface also experience very high rates of catheter-related infections.[1]

Studies also indicate that the skin at the insertion site is the most common source of colonization and infection for vascular catheters that have been in place for less than 10 days.[6] The organisms migrate from the skin through the insertion site along the external catheter surface and colonize the distal intravascular tip of the catheter.[6] This colonization leads to bloodstream infection.

Skin related microorganisms causing catheter-related bloodstream infections include *Staphylococcus epidermidis, S. aureus, Bacillus* species, and *Corynebacterium* species. Organisms on the hands of medical personnel inserting or caring for catheters, including *Pseudomonas aeruginosa, Acinetobacter* species, *Stenotrophomonas maltophilia, Candida albicans,* and *Candida parapsilosis,* can cause infection.[6] Of the two types of flora, resident and transient, resident flora are not easily removed. Transient flora are loosely attached to the skin and can be readily removed with soap, water, and mechanical friction.

Skin temperature plays an important role in infection; the higher the temperature, the greater the occurrence of microbial growth. The skin on the upper and lower extremities has a lower temperature than that on the trunk and neck. Most CVCs are inserted into the trunk, which has a higher temperature and thus a greater potential for microbial growth. Peripheral sites rarely have more than 50 to 100 colony-forming units (CFUs) of bacteria per 10 cm² of skin, whereas the skin on the neck and chest has greater than 1000 to 10,000 CFUs/cm². This reduced amount of skin flora may play a role in the lower rates of catheter-related septicemia reported for peripherally inserted central catheters and midline catheters.

Skin surface moisture is another important property of infection control. Much controversy exists over what type of dressing material should be used with a CVC. Technology related to transparent semipermeable (TSM) dressings is evolving. Newer types of TSMs are available that allow for improved moisture vapor transmission and reduced microbial colonization by antiseptic bonding. Studies have concluded that the collection of moisture enhances the proliferation of microorganisms, so it is essential to maintain a dry, sterile, and intact IV site dressing.

Catheter-related contamination. The IV catheter is an extrinsic source for potential contamination of the IV system. There are two forms of microorganisms that may be located on catheter surfaces: broad based and free floating. Broad-based organisms are embedded in a biofilm (slime), whereas free-floating organisms disseminate over the catheter surface.[6] Studies show that most indwelling vascular catheters usually have microorganisms imbedded in a biofilm layer, and this can occur as early as 24 hours after insertion.[6]

Physical characteristics of the catheter surface, the surface characteristics of adherent bacteria, the presence of host-derived proteins, and the intrinsic phenotypic charges of adherent bacteria that form the biofilm determine the adherent nature of microorganisms (Fig. 8-1). For microorganisms to adhere to a catheter, there must be an interaction with the catheter's physical characteristics. Examples of catheter characteristics that allow for such interaction include irregular surfaces and charge differences. An example of bacteria surface characteristics is hydrophobicity. Hydrophobic staphylococcal organisms adhere well to some surfaces, such as polyvinyl chloride, silicone, and polyethylene, but not so well to polyurethane or Teflon polymers.[6]

Maki reports that the lowest infection rates occur when small peripheral, IV steel needles, Teflon, or polyurethane catheters are used.[1] During catheter insertion, the patient's proteins are deposited on the catheter surface. These proteins include fibronectin, thrombospondin, fibrinogen, vitronectin, and to a lesser extent, laminin.[6]

The microorganism *S. aureus* appears to be dependent on the presence of preabsorbed plasma or tissue. Other organisms, such as *S. epidermidis,* adhere only to fibronectin and not to other receptors of the patient's protein. Because many tissue proteins are an integral part of thrombus formation, the presence of thrombus on the catheter surface appears to promote microorganism adherence leading to catheter infections.[1] The adherence of organisms to catheter surfaces and the resulting biofilm formation are byproducts of intrinsic phenotypic changes of the colonizing bacteria.[6] The biofilm bacteria are resistant to antibiotics and to host defense agents. Although all catheters are colonized with organisms embedded in biofilm, only a small portion actually result in a bloodstream infection.[6] CVCs are associated with an increased risk of catheter-related infection.

Catheter design and composition contribute to the risk of

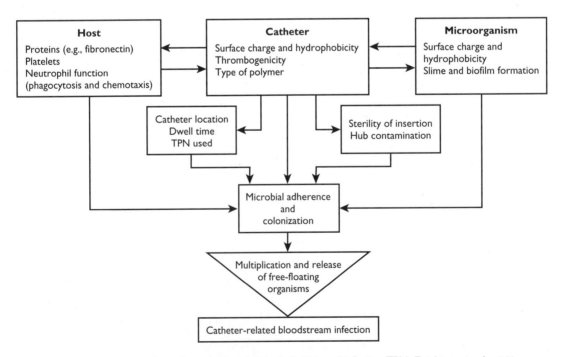

FIG. 8-1 *Pathogenesis of vascular catheter–related colonization and infection.* TPN, *Total parenteral nutrition.*

infectious complications. Catheter size has an obvious impact; the larger the catheter, the larger the venipuncture site through the skin and vessel and the greater the injury to tissue. With a larger catheter, it is more difficult to stabilize and maintain an intact dressing. It is recommended that the smallest gauge cannula of the shortest length possible be used to administer the prescribed therapy.

The relationship between the number of catheter lumens and the risk of a cannula-related infection is uncertain. Patients who require multilumen catheters are often critically ill, require total parenteral nutrition, may be immunocompromised, and have extended hospitalizations. When treating such patients, it is important to reduce the number of cannula manipulations as much as possible, to adhere to strict aseptic technique, to maintain a closed system, and to designate each lumen of a multilumen catheter for a specific purpose. Current data are inconclusive regarding the catheter hub as a potential source of contamination. Some investigators have shown that the colonization of microorganisms on the catheter hub is an important source of pathogens causing catheter-related infections.[1]

Catheter composition has also been suggested as a possible factor in IV-related infections. Most CVCs are composed of polyvinylchloride or a silicone elastomer. Both materials are soft and flexible. Polyvinylchloride, polyethylene, and silicone catheters have been reported to have a higher incidence of coagulase-negative staphylococcus colonization than polytetrafluoroethylene (Teflon) or polyurethane catheters.[1] Polyurethane and silicone elastomer catheters have been associated with decreased thrombogenicity.[7]

Microscopic examination of infected CVCs has shown heavy colonization on the external surface.[1] Studies have shown that coagulase-negative staphylococci, the predominant aerobic species on human skin, is the most common agent of catheter-related bacteremia.[1]

Hematogenous dissemination. Another causative factor of IV catheter–related infections is hematogenous seeding from a distant site of infection. Central venous and arterial catheters can be colonized from remote, unrelated sites of infection. Most fungal vascular-access infections appear to be the result of hematogenous seeding from another site of infection.

Phlebitis

One of the most common complications associated with IV therapy is phlebitis, an inflammation of the vein. Factors that may contribute to phlebitis include the following:

- Patient's history and present condition
- Cannula location and insertion technique
- Condition of the cannulated vein
- Cannula material, length, and gauge
- Cannula stabilization
- Duration of cannulation
- Compatibility of solutions
- Type and pH of medication or solution
- Skin preparation
- Frequency of dressing change
- Ineffective filtration

Signs and symptoms of phlebitis include pain, tenderness, redness (erythema), elevated skin temperature at the insertion site, palpable cord along the affected vein, reduction in the infusion rate, and elevated body temperature while the phlebitis progresses.[8]

The three major types of phlebitis are related to the causative factors: mechanical, chemical, or bacterial. *Mechanical phlebitis* is caused when the vein becomes irritated from the use of a cannula too large for the size of the vein, movement of the cannula within the vein, or repeated catheter manipulation. Unnecessary vein irritation can be avoided when the smallest-gauge and shortest-length cannula is used to administer the prescribed therapy. Proper cannula stabilization and adequate taping can eliminate any movement of the cannula within the vein. When manipulation of the cannula is reduced, the potential for venous irritation is decreased.

Chemical phlebitis occurs when acidic or alkaline solutions or medications are infused. The lower or higher the pH of a solution or medication, the greater the risk of developing phlebitis. Any additive that increases the tonicity of the solution increases the phlebitis risk. Particulate matter is another factor related to the development of chemical phlebitis. Particulates can be found in solutions, especially those containing medications, and may result from improperly mixed or diluted medications.

Bacterial phlebitis occurs when the IV system becomes contaminated, allowing bacteria to enter the solution and proliferate. Bacterial contamination of the infusion system can be caused by the compromise of aseptic technique during the admixture of fluids, inadequate skin preparation, failure to inspect containers for cracks or leaks, and improper cleansing of injection sites. Bacterial phlebitis is also referred to as *septic phlebitis*.[8]

Phlebitis may also be suppurative. This term is used when purulent drainage (pus) can be expressed from the cannula insertion site. Suppurative phlebitis, which increases the risk of systemic infection, is rare with peripheral IV cannulas; it more commonly occurs with the use of CVCs.[1]

The *Infusion Nursing Standards of Practice* recommends that a phlebitis scale be used to rate phlebitis according to the signs and symptoms exhibited.[9] This scale should be established in the institution's policy and procedure to provide a uniform measurement of the degree of phlebitis. (See Chapter 24 for a phlebitis scale.) The following practices help prevent phlebitis:

- Use of aseptic technique for fluid preparation and cannula insertion
- Infusion of hypertonic solutions through larger veins or CVCs
- Cannula site rotation according to *Infusion Nursing Standards of Practice*[9]
- Use of the smallest gauge cannula to administer the prescribed therapy
- Securement of catheter to promote maximum stabilization
- For non–lipid-containing solutions that require filtration: use of a 0.2-micron filter containing both a bacteria/particulate-retentive and an air-eliminating membrane
- For lipid infusions or total nutrient admixtures that require filtration: use of a 1.2-micron air-eliminating filter

Close monitoring of the insertion site and prompt intervention can prevent peripheral thrombophlebitis. This condition involves not only inflammation of the vein but also the formation of a blood clot within the vein. Signs and symptoms include a decreasing flow rate, tenderness along the vein, progressively cordlike condition of the vein, limb edema, redness above the venipuncture site, warmth along the vein, and an increase in the basal temperature.[8] Thrombophlebitis can cause an embolism if left untreated. The treatment of choice is removal of the IV catheter. The infusion should be restarted in the opposite extremity using new equipment and solution.

Septicemia

Septicemia, or sepsis, can occur when pathogenic microorganisms or their toxins migrate into the bloodstream and cause a systemic infection. Septicemia can result from any of the following conditions: localized infection at the insertion or exit site, catheter tunnel, or portal pocket; infusion of contaminated fluids; colonization of the patient's own cutaneous flora through the cutaneous tract during catheter insertion; and inadvertent contamination introduced during catheter manipulation. Intravascular device–related septicemia is often caused by staphylococci (especially coagulase-negative staphylococci), *Trichophyton beiglii*, *Corynebacterium* species, *Candida* species, *Fusarium* species, or *Malassezia furfur*.[1]

Catheter-related fungal infections are often associated with the administration of total parenteral nutrition and the long-term administration of broad-spectrum antibiotics.

A localized catheter-related infection is usually evidenced by redness, edema, or purulent drainage at the insertion or exit site, tunnel, or portal pocket; an elevated temperature; and elevated WBC counts. Signs and symptoms of an intravascular device–related septicemia include fever, chills, tremors, nausea, vomiting, abdominal pain, diarrhea, confusion, seizures, hyperventilation, respiratory failure, shock, vascular collapse, and death. Identifying septicemia in critically ill patients can be difficult. Nurses must be aware of the patient's history, possible risk factors, and the clinical signs and symptoms of septicemia, and must implement prompt interventions if septicemia is suspected.

APPROPRIATE ANTIMICROBIAL THERAPY FOR INFECTION

It is helpful to view therapy for infectious diseases, especially in hospitalized patients, in terms of the three stages described by Quintiliani and colleagues.[10] When an infection is diagnosed or suspected, broad-spectrum therapy, usually IV, is initiated. Broad-spectrum therapy will effectively treat most of the possible offending organisms. This "stage 1" therapy may be guided by a report of sample microscopy (e.g., morphology: bacilli, cocci, or other forms; Gram stain: positive or negative). Stage 1 patients are usually unstable from the infectious process. Attempts to isolate causative organisms by sampling suspected sites of infection are generally made before initiating antibiotics. Antimicrobials effective against several nosocomial pathogens are listed in Table 8-2.

Table 8-2   Antimicrobial Agents Effective Against Some Nosocomial Pathogens

ORGANISM	ANTIMICROBIAL AGENTS
GRAM-POSITIVE	
Staphylococci (methicillin-sensitive)	First-generation cephalosporin, nafcillin
Staphylococci (methicillin-resistant)	Vancomycin
Enterococci	Ampicillin or vancomycin with or without an aminoglycoside (gentamicin)
Clostridium difficile (diarrhea, colitis)	Oral vancomycin, oral metronidazole
GRAM-NEGATIVE	
Klebsiella spp., *Escherichia coli*	Cephalosporin, quinolone (e.g., ciprofloxacin)
Enteric bacilli (*Enterobacter, Citrobacter, Serratia*)	Imipenem or third-generation cephalosporin (not *Enterobacter*), with or without aminoglycoside, cefepime, ciprofloxacin
Pseudomonas aeruginosa	Ceftazidime, aztreonam, or extended spectrum penicillin (e.g., piperacillin) with or without aminoglycoside, ciprofloxacin, imipenem
ACINETOBACTER SPP.	Imipenem, ciprofloxacin, piperacillin
LEGIONELLA SPP.	Erythromycin with or without rifampin, levofloxacin, azithromycin
OTHER	
Candida spp.	Amphotericin B, fluconazole, ketoconazole
Aspergillus spp.	Amphotericin B, itraconazole
Anaerobes	Clindamycin, metronidazole, ticarcillin/clavulanate, ampicillin/sulbactam

In stage 2, therapy is adjusted to antimicrobials active against the isolated organisms. Results of antibiotic sensitivity testing, if available, are used to guide therapy. Using antimicrobials with a narrow spectrum of activity minimizes their effect on institutional and normal host bacterial flora, and these drugs are often less expensive. A final stage is reached when the patient shows signs of successful treatment and is converted to oral therapy before discharge.

Selecting antibiotics at any stage of therapy involves several considerations in addition to an assessment of the likely pathogens involved. Factors such as the patient's underlying disease states, renal and hepatic function, sites of infection, age, and immune status should be considered. In general, patients with compromised immune systems require more aggressive antimicrobial therapy and monitoring. Drug factors include toxicity, drug interactions and compatibilities, cost, and pharmacokinetics.

Pharmacokinetics describes how the body processes drugs physiologically, including absorption (not a factor with IV medications), distribution within the body, metabolism, and excretion. Dose, route, and frequency of administration are chosen with these factors in mind.

Monitoring antimicrobial therapy involves continued consideration of patient factors (signs and symptoms of infection), pathogen factors (isolation and testing of infecting organisms), and drug factors (dosage adjustment and toxicity monitoring).

Patient factors

Body temperature is maintained within narrow limits by the hypothalamic temperature regulatory centers in the brain. Fever (core body temperature elevated above normal) is often a sign of infection. When proper antibiotic therapy and host defenses work together to eradicate an infection, fever usually resolves; its response is therefore a good measure of the effectiveness of antibiotic therapy. Exogenous chemicals, including antimicrobials and other medications, can sometimes cause fever. Concurrent corticosteroids, acetaminophen, aspirin, or other nonsteroidal antiinflammatory drugs act as antipyretics; they may mask a fever and can complicate the monitoring of antimicrobial therapy. The predictability of fever as a response to infection in the elderly has also been questioned.[11]

Another indicator of infection and response to antimicrobial therapy is the peripheral leukocyte count (WBC count). The WBC count is typically elevated in response to an acute bacterial infection. Because of the short life span of leukocytes, it usually drops rapidly during successful treatment. Patients with low leukocyte counts (neutropenia) may respond poorly to therapy for infection. Similarly, patients with other defects in humoral or cellular immunity may have impaired neutrophil function and be at risk for bacterial and fungal infections despite normal leukocyte counts. Noninfectious causes of elevated leukocyte counts include myeloproliferative disorders, trauma, acute myocardial infarction, and corticosteroid or lithium therapy. The presence of immature granulocytes (band neutrophils) is an indicator of bone marrow response to the presence and treatment of infection. These are reported as *bands, stab cells,* or a *left shift.*

Pathogen factors

An important part of monitoring antimicrobial therapy is culturing the offending pathogens for identification and in vitro susceptibility testing. Many microorganisms are identified in the laboratory by growth pattern or biologic substrate use. An increasing number of organisms are identified using immunologic or genetic tests, some of which are rapid because they do not require the organism to grow for the purpose of the test (e.g., direct antigen tests for diagnosis of group A streptococcus).

If the IV catheter is implicated as a source of infection, it should be cultured. The recommended method for culturing a catheter, according to the *Infusion Nursing Standards of Practice,* is the semiquantitative culture technique.[9] To perform a semiquantitative culture, the area around the insertion site is thoroughly cleansed with alcohol and permitted to air dry. Alcohol is recommended because the residual antimicrobial activity of iodine-containing solutions may kill organisms on the catheter when it is removed. After the catheter is withdrawn, at least 5 cm of the tip and the catheter segment, beginning 1 to 2 mm inside the skin-catheter junction point, is clipped with sterile scissors and allowed to fall into a sterile specimen tube or cup. If present, purulent drainage should be cultured before cleaning the site. A positive, semiquantitative culture of 15 CFUs or more confirms a local cannula infection.[1] The semiquantitative culture technique may fail to detect bacteremia and significant colonization of the internal lumen of the catheter tip.[8] Another disadvantage of this method is that the catheter must be removed, even though it may not be the source of infection.

A helpful alternative to the semiquantitative culture technique is the use of quantitative blood cultures drawn through a peripheral vein and through the IV cannula. If the results of the catheter blood samples are greater than or equal to five times the peripheral blood sample, a catheter-related infection is suspected and the catheter should be removed. If a catheter has been replaced over a guidewire, the new catheter should be removed to prevent recurrence of the organism.

Once isolated and identified, organisms are tested for susceptibility to antimicrobial agents. Several testing methods have been developed and standardized. The multiple-tube dilution method involves growing the organisms in broth containing serial dilutions of the antibiotic being tested to determine the minimum inhibitory concentration (MIC). The MIC is the dilution that inhibits growth and is used as a measure of susceptibility. In the agar-plate-disk diffusion test (Kirby-Bauer), antibiotic-impregnated disks are placed on a surface on which the organism grows. After incubating for several hours, a zone of inhibition, in which no organisms grow because of the presence of antibiotic, is evident around each disk. The size of this zone defines susceptibility for that antibiotic agent. The broth dilution test has been automated through the use of microtube methods. Many automated systems combine identification of the organism with susceptibility testing, thus decreasing the time needed to make this information available to clinicians. In addition, slow-growing organisms or those difficult to culture may be tested for certain characteristics predictive of antimicrobial susceptibility. For example, *Hemophilus influenzae* is tested for the production of β-lactamase enzyme, rendering it resistant to ampicillin sodium.

Assessing patients' responses to antiinfective therapy also involves monitoring for resolution of the physical signs of infection. This monitoring can be direct (physical examination) or indirect (using imaging techniques).

Drug factors

For therapy to be successful, antimicrobial agents must reach sites of infection in concentrations sufficient to inhibit or kill the pathogen. Distribution volume, tissue penetration, plasma protein binding, elimination, and other pharmacokinetic characteristics determine the quantity of drug reaching the infected tissue. When given by intermittent infusion or injection, blood concentrations fluctuate. Maximum levels (peaks) are achieved just following a dose; the lowest levels or nadir concentrations (troughs) are determined just before administering a dose. The extent of bacterial killing for some agents (aminoglycosides, quinolones) depends on how high the peak level is above the MIC (concentration-dependent killing), whereas for others (e.g., penicillins, cephalosporins), the factor determining success appears to be the amount of time the drug concentrations remain above the MIC (time-dependent killing).[12]

Several antimicrobial agents require blood concentration monitoring and dosage adjustment to minimize toxicity while maintaining efficacy. These drugs have a narrow therapeutic window (index), meaning there is a very narrow margin between the dosage required to produce a therapeutic effect and the dosage that is toxic. In addition, individual patients handle drugs differently, so a standardized dosage might produce subtherapeutic levels in one patient and toxic concentrations in another. Pharmacokinetic principles are used to adjust dosing regimens to achieve desired blood concentrations.

Formerly, treating infections with IV antibiotics involved serious risks and the potential for adverse reactions. With the availability of infusion rate control devices and safer antibiotics, this is less true today. However, monitoring for toxicity remains an important component of successful antibiotic therapy. The toxicity of some commonly used IV antibiotics is shown in Table 8-3.

Persistent infection during antimicrobial therapy may be related to several causes. Organisms may be resistant to the antimicrobial being used. Alternatively, the antimicrobial may not be reaching the site of infection because of patient noncompliance, inadequate dose, or persistence of the infection in a site not penetrated by the drug (e.g., abscess, empyema). The antibiotics themselves may cause fever, as described earlier. Compromised host immune systems, as in the case of neutropenia after cytotoxic chemotherapy, may result in poor response to antimicrobial pharmacotherapy. Changing antibiotics may treat resistant organisms and "drug fever." Peripheral septic thrombophlebitis may necessitate surgical resection of the vein, with or without continued antibiotic therapy. Septic thrombosis of the central veins necessitates removal of the catheter and high-dose bactericidal antimicrobial therapy.

ANTIMICROBIAL RESISTANCE

Antibiotics have played an important role in drug therapy management for more than 50 years. Their use has significantly decreased morbidity and mortality rates of infectious diseases. However, their wide use has brought an evolution of resistance that seems to know no end. Rates of bacterial resistance are steadily increasing, and nearly all antibiotics have been associated with some degree of resistance.[13] Antibiotic resistance limits the choice of therapy for treating infections and significantly increases morbidity, mortality, and cost.

Antimicrobial function

The mechanisms by which antimicrobial agents develop resistance are linked to the very process by which these agents affect microorganisms.[13] To be effective, an antibiotic must gain entry to the bacterial cell and exert action by disrupting a specific function of the bacterium without itself being metabolized or inactivated.[14] The bacterium produces enzymes that attack the antibiotic in an attempt to destroy it. Once the antibiotic survives this process, it binds to the site where it is most effective. This process revolves around the antibiotic molecule's ability to bind to a sufficient number of binding sites within a microorganism to kill it, impair its maturation, or interfere with its replication mechanism.[13]

Resistance defined

Resistance is a complex phenomenon involving the microorganism, the antimicrobial drug, the environment, and the patient, separately and in their interaction. Transmission of drug-resistant organisms is an important component in this phenomenon. "*Microbial resistance* is defined as the ability of a specific microorganism to withstand a drug that interferes with its growth function. Resistance usually involves gradation, rather than being an 'all or none' phenomenon."[14]

Table 8-3 **Major Toxicities of Some Intravenous Antimicrobial Agents**

Drug Class	Dose/Infusion-Related Toxicity	Other Toxicity
Penicillins	Phlebitis, CNS (seizures rare)	Hypersensitivity
Cephalosporins	Phlebitis	Hypersensitivity, bleeding, hypoprothrombinemia
Imipenem/cilastatin	Phlebitis	Seizures
Erythromycin	Phlebitis, ototoxicity	
Tetracyclines	Nephrotoxicity, ototoxicity	
Vancomycin	Infusion-related histamine reaction—"red man syndrome," rash, hypotension	Additive—nephrotoxicity with aminoglycosides
Amphotericin B	Phlebitis, hyperkalemia, renal dysfunction, infusion-related hypokalemia, fever, shaking chills, hypomagnesemia	Anemia, electrolyte disturbances
Acyclovir	Phlebitis, obstructive renal toxicity	
Fluconazole	Hepatotoxicity	
Ciprofloxacin, ofloxacin	CNS toxicity (?)	
Metronidazole	Neuropathy	
Cotrimoxazole (Septra, Bactrim)	Bone marrow depression	Hypersensitivity

CNS, Central nervous system.

Phenomenon of resistance

In recent years, much has been learned about the phenomenon of resistance to bacterial agents. Antimicrobial resistance can occur because of natural selection, mutation, or a combination of these two major forces. Bacteria can be intrinsically resistant to certain classes of antibiotics or they can develop resistance genes. Resistance is categorized as natural or acquired. *Natural resistance,* also known as *inherited resistance,* indicates an organism has always been resistant to the particular antibiotic. *Acquired resistance* indicates an organism was sensitive to the antibiotic at one time and developed resistance after exposure to the antibiotic.[13]

Natural resistance

A microbial strain may be resistant to an antibiotic before coming in contact with it. This can happen because of inherent or intrinsic resistance, genetic mutation, or the transfer of genetic material.

Inherent, or *intrinsic, resistance* refers to the inherent possession of genes that confer resistance to an antibiotic by microorganisms. Such a gene may always be inactive, or it may become inactive from exposure to a specific antibiotic. A microbe may also be resistant because of an intrinsic characteristic, such as the lack of a binding site for a particular antibiotic. Examples are *Mycoplasma pneumoniae*, which does not have a peptidoglycan cell wall and is therefore resistant to the β-lactam inhibitors of cell wall synthesis, and the natural resistance of gram-negative bacteria to vancomycin because of the inability of vancomycin to penetrate their complicated outer membrane.[15-17]

Genetic mutation occurs during the course of rapid multiplication of the microbe and can lead to the emergence of an antibiotic-resistant mutant that multiplies.[18] It is not necessary that there be a previous exposure to an antimicrobial for this to occur. An example of this is the occurrence of resistance to tetracycline and streptomycin documented in 1960 among people in the Solomon Islands who had never used antibiotics.[14]

Transfer of genetic material occurs when bacteria acquire new genetic material producing resistance by transformation, transduction, or conjugation. Bacteria acquire free DNA containing resistance genes during transformation and incorporate this DNA into their own genomes. In transduction, a bacteriophage (bacterial virus) infects the bacterium, transmitting resistance genes. Conjugation is a type of horizontal transmission of elements conferring resistance. Resistance elements that are transmitted through conjugation include plasmids and transposons. *Plasmids* are extrachromosomal genetic elements and *transposons* are mobile segments of DNA.[17,19] They may be floating in body fluids with other organisms. Resistance elements or gene segments may be transferred between two bacterium of the same species or of different strains or species. This transfer is not limited to pathogenic bacteria. Normal body flora, or resident bacteria, may be reservoirs for resistant genes. These resident bacteria may transfer resistance genes to pathogenic bacteria within the body. Conjugation has been described as occurring within the bowel, vagina, and urine of catheterized patients.[14]

Acquired resistance

Acquired resistance occurs in one of two ways. In gram-positive organisms, naturally occurring resistant mutants can be selected from the surrounding susceptible population in response to antimicrobial pressure from excessive use of antibiotics. The second mechanism is the acquisition of exogenous material causing the bacteria to mutate. The exogenous materials are small pieces of circular DNA called *plasmids,* which become encoded with an R gene, signifying resistance to a particular antibiotic. Plasmids can carry R genes for several drugs and are capable of passing this resistance from strain to strain of one species and from one species to another. Vancomycin-resistant enterococcus, penicillin-resistant pneumococci, and methicillin-resistant *S. aureus* (MRSA) are examples of bacteria capable of passing resistance.[20]

Factors contributing to resistance

Microorganisms resist the action of antibiotics through several mechanisms. They can produce antibiotic-inactivating enzymes, change the permeability of the cell wall, and alter proteins to which the antibiotic binds. The excessive use of antibiotics increases the prevalence of resistant strains of bacteria. Using broad-spectrum antibiotics without changing to a more focused, narrow spectrum drug after culture and sensitivity reports are obtained also contributes to the development of resistant strains of bacteria. In addition, the prolonged use of a broad-spectrum antibiotic eliminates normal flora, possibly resulting in a secondary or "superinfection," colonization by drug resistant strains, or development of pseudomembranous colitis, caused by *Clostridium difficile. C. difficile* is often present in the gastrointestinal (GI) tract in small amounts, and when the bacteria that normally suppress its growth are eradicated, the bacteria grow and produce a toxin, resulting in colitis.

The greatest challenge in overcoming the phenomenon of bacterial resistance to antimicrobials is related to selective pressure, the process that is commonly referred to as *survival of the fittest.*[13] With the many advances in antibiotic therapy, countless microorganisms have been destroyed by antiinfective chemicals. While weaker members of microbial colonies are killed, survivors become stronger and more resistant.[13] This phenomenon is readily observed by the shift in organisms causing infectious disease in health care institutions.[13]

In the fight against infectious disease, much emphasis has been placed on patients in intensive care units (ICUs). More than 75% of patients in hospital ICUs now receive antibiotic therapy. This high use of antibiotic therapy suggests excessive use of broad-spectrum antibiotics, increasing the chance of resistance developing. In addition, ICU patients are sicker and have multiple opportunities for infection through CVCs, Foley catheters, and wounds.

Other potential causes for increased antimicrobial resistance include the following:

- An aging population with increased severity of illness
- Immune systems compromised by disease or procedures such as organ transplantation

- Advances in technology such as implanted ports and CVCs creating opportunities for infection
- An increase in antibiotic resistance in the community
- Ineffective infection control practices
- Increased patient demand for antibiotics
- Inappropriate prophylactic use
- Prolonged use of empiric antibiotic regimens
- International travel
- Use of antibiotic additives in animal feed

Methicillin-resistant organisms

Widespread dissemination of MRSA in hospitals occurred in the late 1970s.[14] Confirmed isolation of MRSA, or its suspected presence, has largely been responsible for the dramatic increase in the use of vancomycin. MRSA is characterized by the presence of a gene that alters the penicillin binding sites. This genetic alteration renders *S. aureus* resistant to other antibiotics, such as macrolides, aminoglycosides, and clindamycin, leaving few therapeutic alternatives to vancomycin. Currently, vancomycin is the drug of choice for treating MRSA. When methicillin-sensitive *S. aureus* is the offending pathogen, the β-lactamase–resistant penicillins are more effective than vancomycin. Two other antibiotic-resistant staphylococci of clinical importance are methicillin-resistant *S. epidermidis,* which is most often associated with prosthetic device infections, and vancomycin-intermediate and vancomycin-resistant *S. aureus.*

Vancomycin-resistant organisms

Another resistant pathogen is vancomycin-resistant enterococci (VRE). Enterococci are normally found in the GI tract. The normal flora in the GI tract are intrinsically resistant to most antibiotics. The development of acquired resistance to aminoglycosides and vancomycin is increasing dramatically. VRE occurs most often in debilitated patients in close confinement, such as in ICUs and nursing homes.[21,22] Of greater concern is that these resistant strains show no synergy when an aminoglycoside is combined with an antibiotic with cell wall activity, such as ampicillin or vancomycin, producing vancomycin/ampicillin-resistant enterococci (VAREC). The greatest threat comes from strains causing severe infections such as bacterial endocarditis, where bacteriocidal activity is paramount to a cure. VAREC is of major concern, because for the first time, certain infections are resistant to all known systemic antibiotics. Of even greater concern is the possibility that the genetic material responsible for resistance to vancomycin will become prevalent among *S. aureus.*

New drug therapy

Pharmaceutical manufacturers are looking diligently for drugs that can be used to treat the newer infections and infections that have developed resistance to presently available antibiotics. One of the latest drugs is gatifloxacin (Tequin), which is being marketed as a safe, highly effective antibiotic with few side effects and little chance of developing bacterial resistance. It is active against gram-positive organisms such as *S. aureus* (methicillin-susceptible strains only) and *Streptococcus pneumoniae,* gram-negative organisms such as *E. coli* and *H. influenzae,* and atypicals such as *Chlamydia pneumoniae, Legionella pneumophilia,* and *M. pneumoniae.*[23] Gatifloxacin is indicated for the treatment of bronchitis, sinusitis, community-acquired pneumonia, urinary tract infections, and gonorrhea. Clinical trials have shown good results,[23] and the drug bears watching as its use increases.

Hope for the future

Although new drug discoveries allow antibiotics to be one step ahead of bacterial pathogens, the rapid evolution of resistance limits the duration of the effectiveness of specific agents against certain pathogens. The best hope for the future is the development of a better understanding of how antimicrobial resistance spreads and the implementation of effective infection control strategies.[20] Informed infusion nurses can be the key to the future. Their role and experience allows them to consult with physicians regarding antibiotic use, to educate patients regarding infection control practices and the wise use of antibiotics, and to develop guidelines for prevention and control of nosocomial infections. They can effect changes by sharing information and being proactive. Infusion nurses should accept this challenge, as patient advocates and as consumers who may need effective antimicrobial therapy.

Effective strategies. Nurses can play a major role in controlling the spread of resistant organisms. Some effective nursing strategies are listed in Box 8-2.

The environment is an important source of resistant pathogens. Proper cleaning of bedside tables, rails, door handles, and other inanimate objects in the patient's environment is essential.

Box 8-2   Strategies for Controlling the Spread of Resistant Organisms

- Identify risk factors.
- Develop and implement isolation policies and procedures.
- Educate staff, patients, and families.
- Adhere to the *Infusion Nursing Standards of Practice.*
- Develop institutional guidelines outlining surveillance and nosocomial infection control.
- Use an antimicrobial soap for handwashing before and after all procedures, even when gloves are worn.
- Use barrier precautions such as gloves, masks, gowns, and goggles when caring for patients with resistant strains of bacteria.
- Use disposable patient care items or specially designated items for patients in protective isolation.
- Disinfect nondisposable items, or sterilize them when no longer needed and before returning to service.
- Educate patients and caregivers regarding the importance of handwashing before and after handling infectious waste, wearing gloves if contact with excreta is necessary or possible, and properly disposing of waste.
- Disinfect equipment used for multiple patients after each use (e.g., stethoscopes).

Home care nurses must keep their bags clean and uncontaminated. All equipment that has been used or is potentially contaminated should be cleaned before being placed back into the nurse's bag. Contaminated equipment that cannot be cleaned in the home should be placed in an impervious bag and transported to the cleaning site. All personnel and caregivers should comply with isolation precautions, especially those pertaining to patients who are colonized with resistant bacteria, particularly those patients with VRE. Isolation policies should be based on Centers for Disease Control and Prevention (CDC) and Hospital Infection Control Practices Advisory Committee guidelines. Standard precautions must be strictly followed.

Aggressive control of resistant outbreaks should be reinforced. Health care workers, caregivers, and support staff need to understand the importance of meticulous infection control practices. When indicated and practical, infected patients and caregivers should be isolated to reduce the potential for transmission to other patients. Surveillance of identified infections should be intensified through culture screening. When indicated, MRSA carriers may be decolonized with mupirocin or bacitracin ointment.

Careful discharge planning is an important aspect of nursing management. The patient's social situation and the health status of caregivers must be assessed. Protective isolation precautions are usually not necessary in the home unless someone with a chronic disease resides with the patient. If patients are discharged to skilled nursing facilities or other long-term care settings, the staff must be informed of the diagnosis of resistant bacteria so that the patient can be placed in protective isolation. Cohorting of patients with the same resistant organism is permissible. In the case of VRE, the CDC recommends three consecutive VRE-negative cultures at least 1 week apart from multiple body sites before discontinuing isolation.

Until scientists develop additional therapies against resistant pathogens, prevention of transmission relies on good, aseptic practices and compliance with strategies known to be effective.

CONTROL MEASURES
Principles of asepsis

Adhering to the principles of aseptic technique can decrease the risk of catheter-related infection. Asepsis begins with the proper use of topical antimicrobial agents. Topical antiseptics are used for handwashing, preparation and maintenance of the insertion site, and disinfection of equipment.

There is universal agreement regarding the value and importance of proper handwashing technique. Although most health care personnel are aware of the importance of handwashing, the recommendations are often ignored. Vigorous handwashing, preferably with an antiseptic containing product, should take place before inserting the catheter and handling the device or administration set.[1]

Before an antimicrobial solution is applied, any excess hair may be removed by clipping. Shaving is not recommended because of the increased potential for microabrasions. Clippers with disposable heads for single-patient use are suggested. The antimicrobial solutions recommended by the *Infusion Nursing*

Standards of Practice for cannula-site preparation are 2% tincture of iodine, 10% povidone-iodine, alcohol, and chlorhexidine, as single agents or in combination.[9] All site preparations are applied with friction, working outward from the insertion site in a circular pattern. An area equal to the size of the dressing should be prepared. Most catheter care protocols begin with the application of alcohol, which rapidly reduces microbial counts on the skin. Isopropyl alcohol 70% has instant kill by denaturing protein. After the alcohol preparation has been allowed to air dry, an application of tincture of iodine (1% to 2% iodine and potassium iodine in 70% alcohol) or povidone-iodine is applied if the patient is not allergic to iodine. Tincture of iodine has the combined effect of isopropyl alcohol and iodine and can cause skin irritation.

Povidone-iodine solutions are referred to as *iodophors* and consist of iodine and a carrier substance. The amount of free iodine is decreased, but the antimicrobial effects are similar to those of iodine. As a result of applying iodophors, less skin irritation occurs. Iodine and iodophors penetrate the cell wall and replace the microbial contents with free iodine.[24] Iodophors require approximately 2 minutes of skin contact time to allow for the release of free iodine. Povidone-iodine has the capability to kill gram-negative and gram-positive organisms, fungi, and yeast. However, povidone-iodine is rapidly neutralized in the presence of blood, serum, and other protein-rich materials.

Chlorhexidine-gluconate (Hibiclens) has been used for years as a handwashing agent and is now being promoted for use as a skin antiseptic. Unlike povidone-iodine or alcohol, application of a 2% chlorhexidine solution to the skin leads to a residual antibacterial activity that persists for 6 hours after application. Chlorhexidine bonds chemically to the protein in the bacterial cell wall. A study conducted by Maki concluded that a 2% chlorhexidine solution used for site preparation before insertion and for postinsertion site care could substantially reduce the incidence of device-related infection.[1]

In the past, acetone was used to remove fatty acids and microorganisms harbored on the skin. A study performed by Maki reports that cleansing with acetone increases local inflammation at the exit site, produces skin irritation, and does not improve microbial removal or reduce the incidence of catheter-related infection.[1]

Clinical trials conducted on the efficacy of antimicrobial ointments have not been conclusive. One large randomized trial found no benefit against infection with the application of topical povidone-iodine ointment to CVC insertion sites. However, a more recent comparative trial with subclavian hemodialysis catheters reports a fourfold reduction in catheter-related infection.[1] The application of an antimicrobial ointment is controversial, and its use should be defined in organizational policy and procedure.[9] Practice recommendations suggest that if an antimicrobial ointment is used, the dressing should be changed every 48 hours.

There has been considerable controversy about the level of barrier precautions necessary for the insertion of a CVC. Maki's study concluded that using maximal barrier protection (sterile gloves, long-sleeved sterile gown, surgical mask, and a large sterile sheet drape) resulted in a decreased risk of catheter-related bloodstream infection.[1]

Prevention

Catheter-related infections. The incidence of catheter-related infections can be decreased by policies and procedures that establish catheter care protocols. The administration of IV therapy should be based on established, professional, nursing standards of practice. Standardization of care is a critical component. Studies have validated that specialized nurses are most likely to maintain aseptic technique in the delivery of IV care and that their rate of catheter-related infections is substantially lower.[1]

The preventive strategy to reduce catheter-related infection begins with routine inspection of the insertion site. Early detection and treatment are extremely important. Institutional policies and procedures should state the method and frequency for monitoring and administering site care. Consideration should be given to the following when establishing those policies and procedures:

- Patient age
- Patient condition
- Therapy prescribed
- Practice setting

The information obtained from site inspections allows the nurse to implement immediate interventions if any signs or symptoms of a catheter-related infection become evident. Early nursing interventions minimize the severity of local complications.

Intrinsic and extrinsic equipment contamination can best be prevented by carefully inspecting all equipment before use and by practicing meticulous technique while performing procedures. Routine peripheral site changes also reduce the risk of developing phlebitis. The *Infusion Nursing Standards of Practice* recommends that short, peripheral catheter sites be rotated at least every 72 hours and immediately if contamination is suspected or there is a complication.[9] Ideally, at the time of recannulization, the administration set and the solution container should be changed. If the cannula is removed because of a complication, the administration set and fluid container should be discarded and a new system implemented. The new infusion system should be restarted in the opposite extremity, if possible.

Maintaining a closed system decreases the incidence of catheter-related complications and infection. The number of tubing connections is directly proportional to the potential for contamination. Therefore limiting the number of junctions within the infusion system lessens the risk of contamination. Administration sets with preattached in-line filters are recommended. If connections are necessary, Luer-Lok fittings are preferable. If this is not possible, the junctions should be secured. All add-on devices should be changed according to the institution's tubing change policy and procedures.

Quality control measures should be used to ensure the best possible IV care. Admixed solutions should be prepared using aseptic technique under a laminar flow hood. A program for sterility testing can be used in the admixing process to monitor aseptic technique and ensure product integrity.

Before therapy is initiated, all solution containers should be visually inspected for the presence of precipitates and cloudiness. Glass bottles should be free from cracks. Bags should be squeezed to ensure that there are no defects in the seams or tiny holes. The expiration date on the IV container and admixture label should be verified before the infusion is begun.

All administration sets and extensions should be examined before use. This inspection should include observation of the entire set and ensuring that the protective coverings over the proximal end (spike) and distal end are intact. If the product or package integrity is compromised, the product should not be used. Visual inspection of the venipuncture device also helps prevent the use of a defective product.

Guidelines are important in the selection and purchase of IV-related equipment. IV nurses should actively participate in the selection of these products. Before new products are considered, they should be evaluated to ensure that they fall within the standards of care and allow for the safe administration of IV therapy. Criteria for evaluating new products include the following:

- Connections should be able to withstand normal pressures of electronic infusion devices.
- Catheters should be radiopaque in case of catheter breakage.
- Equipment must be accurate and help prevent inadvertent contamination.
- Closed systems that do not require air are preferable because they decrease the chance for contamination.

In addition to regular monitoring and quality assurance measures, new products and strategies should be evaluated regularly to prevent or minimize catheter-related infections. Migration of skin flora through the skin opening down the transcutaneous tract is considered the most common cause of colonization leading to microorganisms in the blood and infections.[25]

Antimicrobial-impregnated catheters (chlorhexidine and silver sulfadiazine) have been shown to reduce the rate of central venous colonization.[25] Also, there were fewer removals or exchanges of these catheters, and the extending protective effects decreased patient risk and hospital cost. Thus far, no anaphylactic reactions to the chlorhexidine component have been reported to the FDA. Chlorhexidine and silver sulfadiazine-impregnated catheters should be considered if catheterization is expected to last less than 2 weeks or when there is a high rate of infection despite adherence to other strategies.[5]

Another study found that using coated triple-lumen catheters (chlorhexidine and silver sulfadiazine) reduces the incidence of significant growth on the tip or intradermal segments but has no effect on the incidence of catheter-related bacteremia.[26] A tissue interface barrier has been developed to help protect against extraluminal microbial migration. This device consists of a detachable cuff made of biodegradable collagen to which silver ions are chelated.[1] The cuff is attached to the CVC before insertion. After insertion, the subcutaneous tissue grows into the cuff, creating a physical and chemical barrier against pathogen migration.

Studies related to transparent polyurethane dressings show mixed results regarding their influence on the incidence of catheter-related infection. Using povidone-iodine in a transparent catheter dressing to decrease cutaneous colonization has not proven to be effective.[1] However, a dressing containing chlorhexidine may prove to be more effective. A nonrandomized clinical trial using historical controls has shown reduction of CVC bloodstream infection with the use of chlorhexidine-impregnated composite sponges.[1] Prospective, randomized studies are needed before determining the true value of this product.

The use of IV antimicrobial prophylaxis has been considered a preventive measure against catheter-related infections. Using vancomycin or teicoplanin during CVC insertion has not proven effective in decreasing infections.[5] Adding vancomycin to catheter flush solutions or total nutrient admixtures reduced the risk with coagulase-negative staphylococci in one study of neonates.[5]

Another study looked at heparin and vancomycin, which were instilled in the catheter lumen and allowed to dwell for 1 hour every 2 days in neutropenic cancer patients. The results of using the antibiotic-lock technique showed a decrease in the frequency of gram-positive catheter-related infections during chemotherapy-induced neutropenia.[27] However, the routine use of vancomycin or other therapeutic agents is not generally recommended because of the risk of antimicrobial resistance.

Several of the protein components of a thrombus have been shown to increase the adherence of *S. aureus, S. epidermidis,* and *Candida* species to CVCs.[5] In turn, thrombus formation is associated with catheter-related bloodstream infections. Prophylactic use of warfarin and heparin has reduced thrombus formation, but the reduction in catheter-related bloodstream infection varies by study.[5]

It has been thought that subcutaneous tunneling of catheters might help decrease the occurrence of catheter-related infections. Subcutaneous tunneling of short-term catheters inserted in the internal jugular vein showed a reduction, but tunneling for femoral veins failed to show a statistically significant difference.[5] One study of nontunneled catheters cared for by specialized IV nurses showed a low incidence of catheter-related bloodstream infection.[1] Findings vary from one study to another, and more research is needed to determine the value of catheter tunneling in reducing catheter-related bloodstream infections.

Quality assurance programs can significantly decrease the incidence of catheter-related complications. These tools evaluate the adherence to departmental policies and procedures. A quality control evaluation tool can be used to ensure that proper procedures are followed when performing venipunctures or delivering site care. A checklist can be used for peer review of the process and should include the following: standard precautions, selection of equipment, priming of the administration set, vein selection, prepping procedure, venipuncture technique, stabilization of the catheter, dressing procedure, and labeling of the site and set. A surveillance system is essential for all nursing personnel who maintain vascular access devices. Establishing a collaborative relationship with the epidemiology department can be an excellent resource for monitoring the delivery of quality IV care, understanding culture reports on vascular access devices, identifying nursing units that need education or intervention to improve the delivery of IV care, and acquiring the latest research and information regarding infection control practices.

Blood-borne pathogen transmission. The CDC, the Occupational Safety and Health Administration (OSHA), and the American Hospital Association recommend the application of standard precautions by health care workers at all times to prevent the transmission of blood-borne pathogens. OSHA's standard makes standard precautions an enforceable legal requirement and delineates what OSHA inspectors survey.[28] These rules instruct health care workers to use protective barriers such as gloves, masks, protective eyewear, and fluid-impervious gowns whenever there is a risk of exposure to blood or body fluids. Health care workers must treat blood and body fluids from all patients as being potentially infected with hepatitis B virus, human immunodeficiency virus, and other blood-borne pathogens.

Gloves can reduce the IV nurse's risk of infection, but they offer little protection from needlestick injuries. To protect against needlesticks, the use of needleless systems, safety syringes, and cannulas is recommended. Needles should never be recapped, bent, or broken. After use, needles and syringes should be disposed of in an impervious, puncture-resistant container located as close as possible to the patient's care area. When no puncture-resistant container is available or when no additional needles or syringes can be placed in the container, recapping needles using a one-handed method is permissible.

Employers are responsible for educating their employees regarding standard precautions; identifying hazardous wastes; supplying personal protective equipment such as goggles, gloves, needleless devices, and safety syringes; and monitoring workers' compliance with protective measures. Employees are responsible for recognizing hazardous wastes, reading material safety data sheets, and following recommendations for the safe handling and disposal of hazardous materials.

Infection control in the alternative care setting

Increasingly, vascular access devices are being used in alternative care settings such as skilled nursing facilities, physicians' offices, ambulatory infusion centers, and homes. The same basic principles for infection control and standards of practice apply in the home or alternative care setting. Few studies are available about vascular access device infection rates or catheter care protocols in alternative care settings. However, it is generally believed that the at-home risk factors for developing a catheter-related infection should be somewhat reduced. One study concluded that bloodstream infections were not often seen in outpatients receiving therapy via midline or CVCs.[29] Further research is needed to describe infection risks and the nursing management of vascular access devices in homes and alternative care settings.

In all health care environments, patient education is an important tool for preventing catheter-related complications. In the alternative care setting, thorough patient/family teaching regarding vascular access management is even more crucial. Information regarding catheter management should be individualized to meet the patient's needs but should remain consistent with the established policies and procedures of the infusion care company and the *Infusion Nursing Standards of Practice*. Patient education regarding IV therapy in an alternative care setting should address infection control principles such as handwashing, aseptic technique, sterility, and the proper method of handling equipment. Information regarding dressing changes, site assessments, and recognition of signs and symptoms of possible complications should also be provided. It is essential that the patient and family be provided adequate nursing support and follow-up to prevent catheter-related complications.

NURSING DIAGNOSIS
Potential nursing diagnoses

- High risk for infection
- Impaired skin integrity
- Anxiety
- Pain
- Knowledge deficit related to IV complications

Patient outcomes

Infection control is important in ensuring positive outcomes for IV therapy. The outcomes include the following:

- Patient shows no evidence (signs or symptoms) of infusion-related infections throughout the course of therapy.
- Patient experiences minimal anxiety related to IV therapy as evidenced by verbalization of concerns, lack of restlessness, normal vital signs, and appropriate sleep patterns.
- Patient experiences minimal pain as evidenced by responses of 1 on a pain scale of 1 to 5, with 1 being mild pain and 5 being severe pain.
- After initial teaching session, patient lists signs and symptoms to report to nurse and identifies ways to prevent infection of catheter site.

REFERENCES

1. Bennet JV, Brachman PS, editors: *Hospital infections,* Philadelphia, 1998, Lippincott-Raven.
2. Fischbach F: *Nurses quick guide to common laboratory and diagnostic tests,* ed 2, Philadelphia, 1998, Lippincott.
3. Stiene-Martin EA, Lotspeich-Steininger C, Koepke J: *Clinical hematology: principles, procedures, and practices,* ed 2, Philadelphia, 1998, Lippincott-Raven.
4. Nafziger DA, Wenzel RP: Catheter-related infections: reducing the risk—and the consequences, *J Crit Illness* 5(8):857, 1990.
5. Mermel LA: Prevention of intravascular catheter-related infections, *Ann Intern Med* 132:391, 2000.
6. Raad I: Intravascular-catheter-related infections, *Lancet* 351:893, 1998.
7. Linder LE, et al: Material thrombogenicity in central venous catheterization: a comparison between soft, antebrachial catheters of silicone elastomer and polyurethane, *J Parenter Enteral Nutr* 8:399, 1984.
8. Phillips LD: *Manual of IV therapeutics,* Philadelphia, 1997, FA Davis.
9. Intravenous Nurses Society: Infusion nursing standards of practice, *JIN* (suppl) 23(65), 2000.
10. Quintiliani R, et al: Economic impact of streamlining antibiotic administration, *Am J Med* 82(suppl A):391, 1987.
11. Gallo J, et al: *Reechels care of the elderly,* Philadelphia, 1999, Lippincott Williams & Wilkins.
12. Amsden GW, Ballow CH, Bertino JS: Pharmacokinetics and pharmacodynamics of anti-infective agents. In Mandell, GL, Bennett, JE, Dolin R, editors: *Principles and practice of infectious diseases,* Philadelphia, 2000, Churchill Livingston.
13. Antimicrobial resistance: evaluating the issue. White Paper in Antimicrobial Resistance: Optimizing Use in the Clinical Setting, Novation, The Supply Company of VHA & UHC. February 2000.
14. Cohen FL, Tartasky D: State of science: microbial resistance to drug therapy: a review, *Am J Infec Control* 25(1):51, 1997.
15. Felmingham D: Antibiotic resistance: do we need new therapeutic approaches? *Chest* 108(suppl):70S, 1995.
16. Burns JL: Mechanisms of bacterial resistance, *Pediatr Clin North Am* 42:497, 1995.
17. Fraimow HS, Abrutyn E: Pathogens resistant to antimicrobial agents, *Infect Dis Clin North Am* 9:497, 1995.
18. Berkowitz FE: Antibiotic resistance in bacteria, *South Medical J* 88:797, 1995.
19. New HC: Emergence and mechanisms of bacterial resistance in surgical infections, *Am J Surg* 169(suppl 5A):13S, 1995.
20. Opal SM, Mayer KH, Medeiros AA: Mechanisms of bacterial antibiotic resistance. In Mandell GL, Bennett JE, Dolin R, editors: *Principles and practice of infectious diseases,* Philadelphia, 2000, Churchill Livingston.
21. Hospital Infection Control Practices Advisory Committee: Recommendations for preventing the spread of vancomycin resistance, *Am J Infect Control* 23(2):87, 1995.
22. Lam S, et al: The challenge of vancomycin-resistant enterococci: a clinical and epidemiologic study, *Am J Infect Control* 24(3):170, 1996.
23. Bryan HB: Tequin (gatifloxacin): remarkable new antibiotic avoids bacterial resistance, *Adv Nurse* 2(10):24, 2000.
24. Larson E: Guidelines for use of topical antimicrobial agents, *Am J Infect Control* 16:253, 1988.
25. Collin GR: Decreasing catheter colonization through the use of an antiseptic-impregnated catheter, *Chest* 115:1632, 1999.
26. Heard S, et al: Influence of triple-lumen central venous catheters coated with chlorhexidine and silver sulfadiazine on the incidence of catheter-related bacteremia, *Arch Intern Med* 1(58):81, 1998.
27. Carratalo J, et al: Antibiotic-lock technique for the prevention of gram-positive central venous catheter-related infections in neutropenic cancer patients, *Cancer Weekly Plus* Oct 21:26, 1996.
28. Occupational Safety and Health Administration: *Occupational safe exposure to bloodborne pathogens: final rule,* Washington, DC, 1991, Department of Labor, Docket No. H-370.
29. Tokars JI, et al: Prospective evaluation of risk factors for bloodstream infection in patients receiving home infusion therapy, *Ann Intern Med* 131(5):340, 1999.

Chapter
9

Parenteral Fluids

Judy Hankins, BSN, CRNI, Carolyn Hedrick, BSN, CRNI

Fluids and electrolytes play an important role in maintaining homeostasis. When imbalances occur, parenteral fluids are the most common intravenous (IV) agents used for correction. IV solutions are also used to provide nutrients or act as a vehicle for medication administration.

To provide IV therapy safely, the IV nurse should be aware of the patient's physical status and clinical picture and understand the legal implications of treatment. Determination of the type of fluid needed is based on the nursing assessment, laboratory findings, and the purpose for which it is being prescribed. To act properly on the physician's order, the nurse must be familiar with the various IV solutions, including their uses, components, and potential complications.

This information should be incorporated into a plan of care or clinical pathway. This care plan should also include applicable nursing diagnoses with measurable outcomes. With careful organization and a strong database, the delivery of IV therapy should be a safe and effective treatment modality.

PATIENT SAFETY

The determination that a patient's treatment plan should include IV therapy brings with it responsibility for patient safety. This includes being cognizant of the patient's physical status, individual clinical considerations, and legal implications.

One of the first considerations should be the physical status of the patient. This includes knowing the patient's age and fluid and electrolyte requirements. Infants, adults, and older adults have different body compositions and means of monitoring homeostasis. Infants have higher rates of extracellular fluid exchange, metabolism, and fluid loss than average adults. There are also variables in the adult population; women and obese patients, for example, have a lower percentage of body fluid than men.

The percentage of body fluid generally continues to decrease as people age because fat content increases. In older adults, changes related to the renal system often result in a decreased concentrating ability, so fluid loss may increase. Respiratory changes can result in a decreased ability to remove secretions. Neurologic changes often lead to a lessened sense of thirst, which is an indicator of fluid needs. The ability to perspire may be diminished because of skin changes, so it is more difficult to use the standard test of skin turgor to determine fluid status. Additional information concerning the older adult can be found in Chapter 31, and concerning the infant in Chapter 30.

All body systems, regardless of age, are affected by fluid exchange, and this exchange can influence fluid and electrolyte status. This must be considered when planning and administering therapy to prevent dehydration or fluid overload.

Clinical considerations are important aspects of patient safety; these include the appropriate route of administration, product, and administration rate. In determining the proper route of administration, the concentration of the IV solution should be considered. Fluids with higher osmolality, such as total parenteral nutrition solutions, need to be given through a central line.

The patient's sensory deficits should be assessed. Special planning on an individual basis may be necessary to prevent physical injury and provide effective treatment, particularly for patients with sight or hearing impairment. For example, the plan of care could include a special visual alarm on a pump for someone who has a hearing impairment.

The patient's mobility should be considered when planning IV fluid therapy. Selecting a site in the nondominant extremity may ensure better compliance. Otherwise, when the patient moves about, it may be difficult to maintain a viable IV line, compromising delivery of the prescribed IV therapy. Specific problems include the patient's removing the access device, the tubing being pulled apart, and the IV set being dislodged from the IV solution container.

Site selection is equally important for the immobile patient. Extremities may require elevation or exercises to prevent stasis during fluid administration. Placement of the catheter should receive special consideration for those patients who require assistance for turning and getting out of bed. Advanced planning can eliminate the interruption of IV solution administration. The patient's orientation should be assessed. Caution should be exercised for those who are confused, disoriented, or agitated to prevent accidental dislodging of the access device and IV tubing. Control clamps should be placed out of reach, if possible, or mechanical infusion devices should be used to prevent deviation of the IV solution flow rate.

Ensuring that the correct product is provided to the patient is an area in which the potential for errors is high. Before administering an IV solution, the nurse should check it carefully against the order in the patient's medical record. The physician should be contacted if there is any doubt about what has been ordered. Often, the IV solution is used as a vehicle for administering IV medication. Caution should be taken to ensure stability and compatibility of medications. Pharmacists can help make this determination when questions arise. Verification of the product's expiration date is also an important component of providing a correct and safe IV solution. The potential for errors can be eliminated by comparing the type of solution, any additives, and the volume with the original order. The actual administration date should be verified.

The correct flow rate should also be determined during the order check. This is another situation in which errors often occur. The correct administration rate is important. Delivering a highly concentrated solution too rapidly could lead to fluid overload. Incorrect flow rates for electrolyte-containing solutions may lead to excesses or deficits in the body's electrolyte content.

Another area related to patient safety concerns the patient's legal rights. Before treatment begins, the patient has the right to refuse or consent to the planned course of therapy, unless decided otherwise by the courts. This is based on the patient's freedom of religion and right of privacy,[1] including the right to consent to any invasion of bodily integrity. The patient should be fully informed about the IV solution, any medications to be administered, and the process of delivering the fluids. Information related to possible complications or side effects should be provided to the patient before treatment.

In addition to freedom of choice, the patient has the right to expect that IV solutions and all related supplies and equipment are safe for use. IV solution containers should be checked for defects such as holes in a bag or cracks in a bottle. Clarity of the solution and the absence of particulate matter should be verified.

Proper aseptic technique should be used when admixtures are being prepared in laminar flow hoods by properly trained personnel. Access devices, IV tubing, and other related materials should be sterile and function as designed to prevent undue harm to the patient.

Intravenous Solution Administration and Monitoring: Nurse Qualifications

It is important that not only the products for IV solution administration but also the personnel involved meet required standards. Responsibilities related to IV solution administration may be delegated to the registered nurse (RN) or the licensed practical/vocational nurse (LPN/LVN). In some health care facilities, basic venipuncture procedures and monitoring may be shared by the RN and LPN/LVN, whereas the more specialized procedures are delegated only to the RN. This varies from one state to the next. However, a basic requirement is meeting state board standards, including licensure. A license granted by the State Board of Nursing signifies that a nurse has met the requirements for entry into practice.

Once a nurse has been hired to administer or monitor IV solutions, the health care agency has the responsibility to see that the employee is properly oriented. Continuing education programs should be provided regularly to review basic material and to provide information about new IV solutions and techniques for their delivery.

Today, with an increased emphasis on IV therapy and new, sophisticated technology, nurses are choosing to become certified in the specialty of IV therapy. This certification requires that a nurse master knowledge related to all areas of IV therapy, including IV solutions and the skills necessary to practice in the clinical setting. This process ensures continued competency through educational programs or the retesting required to maintain certification credentials, thus providing additional protection to the public.

Quality patient care in the specialty of IV therapy requires a nurse have a thorough knowledge of IV solutions and the medications administered in those solutions. First, the nurse must understand how the IV solution is to be used. It may be needed to provide free water, replace or maintain electrolytes, deliver medications, or supply calories. IV solutions can also be used to decrease certain electrolytes or fluids.

After determining how the solution is to be used, it is helpful to know the action of the solution. The IV solution may be used to dilute and therefore decrease the level of an electrolyte in the body. Some IV solutions containing one electrolyte may be used to counteract the action of another electrolyte. Understanding how the solution or electrolyte is eliminated is useful. For example, before giving potassium to a patient with a renal disease, it is important to know that this electrolyte is eliminated by the kidneys. Knowing how an IV solution works, what it contains, and how it is used helps determine whether the product is indicated to treat a specific disease or condition. If the IV solution contains potassium, for example, it is not indicated for treating hyperkalemia.

The nurse also needs to be familiar with the contraindications for, side effects of, and adverse reactions to IV solutions or medications. The body maintains a delicate balance of fluids and electrolytes. When IV solutions are administered, there is always the possibility that a fluid deficit or excess may occur. It is therefore important to know the signs and symptoms of these imbalances. Some products, such as 10% dextran, may produce an anaphylactoid reaction. Colloidal solutions, such as hetastarch, may interfere with platelet function because of hemodilution. A competent nurse who administers IV solutions should be aware of possible side effects and should alert other health care workers to potential problems and how they might be detected. There are times when a solution may be contraindicated because of an existing problem or condition. For example, because a possible side effect of 10% dextran is bleeding, it is not indicated for patients with severe bleeding disorders. The side effects and contraindications of certain commonly used IV solutions are presented in more detail later in this chapter.

The nurse should be adept at completing accurate physical assessments before initiating treatment. This is beneficial to the physician in determining the need for IV therapy. The need for physical assessment does not stop at this point. These skills should be used continually while monitoring therapy, and findings should be shared promptly with the physician and other appropriate health care workers.

The nurse, as the one who pulls all the pieces of the treatment plan together, is one of the best advocates for patient safety and well-being. To be an effective advocate, the nurse must know how to use information from the patient history, physical assessment, and laboratory findings and must have a thorough knowledge of IV solutions and their administration. With all these pieces in place, a determination about the appropriateness of the order can be made. The nurse should contact the physician if there are any discrepancies. Only in this way can the patient be assured of receiving appropriate IV therapy.

DETERMINATION OF FLUID NEEDS
Clinical status

The complex subject of fluid and electrolyte balance is the basis for parenteral fluid administration. This delicate balance (or homeostasis) is easily affected by normal changes (e.g., aging) and abnormal changes (e.g., disease processes) in the body. Chapter 7 presents more information on clinical status, including nursing assessment and monitoring.

Laboratory findings

The next important aspect of determining fluid needs is the review and interpretation of a patient's laboratory findings. The two systems that have the most direct impact on fluid and electrolyte balance are the renal and cardiovascular systems. Therefore tests that reflect the proper functioning of the kidneys and heart require consistent and close scrutiny.

Renal function tests start with determination of the blood urea nitrogen (BUN) level. Elevated levels are primarily caused by kidney disease of acute or chronic etiology or urinary tract obstructions. Variations above normal can also be caused by fluid volume deficit, protein intake in excess of body needs, or a catabolistic state (e.g., starvation). A decreased BUN level may mean decreased protein metabolism or overhydration.

Creatinine is the next indicator to evaluate. Every kidney disease that reduces renal function elevates the serum creatinine level. The higher the level, the greater the reduction in the rate of glomerular filtration. Severe fluid volume depletion may be indicated by a creatinine level that is only slightly elevated.[2]

Because BUN and creatinine levels indicate renal function, they should be evaluated together. In volume depletion, the BUN level is elevated, whereas the creatinine level is normal or slightly elevated.

Urine specific gravity measures urine concentration. In fluid volume deficit, the specific gravity is elevated because of water loss from such processes as third spacing of body fluid, burns, and gastrointestinal fluid loss. In fluid volume excess, the specific gravity is decreased, as with renal disease.

Urine osmolality is the final test to be evaluated when determining renal function. Fluid volume deficit elevates the urine osmolality, whereas fluid volume excess decreases it. Urine osmolality should be evaluated in conjunction with serum osmolality, and the specimens should be collected simultaneously.

Cardiovascular tests begin with an electrocardiogram. Fluid and electrolyte imbalances can often be detected and even diagnosed by the significant changes they cause in the P, QRS, and T waves of the tracing.

The next determination is serum electrolytes, including potassium, sodium, calcium, magnesium, chloride, and phosphorus. Each electrolyte has a normal range. Deviations from normal indicate specific conditions related to deficits and excesses in body fluid and in one or more of the electrolytes. (For further information on individual electrolytes, see Chapter 7.)

The complete blood count (CBC) should be evaluated. This screening test includes the following measurements: hemoglobin, hematocrit, red blood cell (RBC) count, white blood cell (WBC) count, differential RBC and WBC count, and a red cell examination with stain. Abnormalities in fluid and electrolyte balance cause fluctuations in CBC results. For example, severe dehydration caused by nausea, vomiting, and diarrhea results in an elevated hematocrit, whereas rapid administration of excessive amounts of intravenous fluid decreases the hematocrit.

Blood gases are important indicators because they determine the patient's acid-base status. These tests measure the hydrogen ion concentration, the partial pressure of oxygen, and the partial pressure of carbon dioxide in arterial blood. Acid-base disturbances may be caused by fluid- and electrolyte-related problems, such as vomiting, diarrhea, and kidney disorders.

Abnormal clotting test results indicate fluid needs. The activated partial thromboplastin time (aPTT) detects deficiencies in almost all the clotting factors. In acute hemorrhage, this indicator is decreased. The prothrombin time (PT) screens for defects in other areas of the clotting mechanism. Causes of a prolonged PT include medications, vitamin K deficiency, hepatic disease, and obstructive jaundice. Plasma volume expanders such as hetastarch and crystalloid solutions may cause the aPTT and PT to be prolonged. These fluids may be indicated in cases of fluid imbalance (e.g., burns, removal of ascitic fluid).

Serum amylase measures the enzyme amylase that is produced by the pancreas and salivary glands and helps with the digestion of carbohydrates. An elevation of this enzyme level is most commonly seen in pancreatitis. Fluid and electrolyte imbalances and infections are seen with the acute form of pancreatitis.

The serum glucose level should also be monitored. If this level is greatly elevated, osmotic diuresis occurs, resulting in a fluid volume deficit.

Bilirubin is an important determination because it indicates disease processes such as anemias, cirrhosis, hepatitis, and biliary tree obstruction. Bilirubin results from the destruction of old blood cells and produces an orange-yellow or jaundice color. The diseases associated with abnormal bilirubin levels each have the potential for causing fluid and electrolyte disturbances.

Lactate dehydrogenase is another cellular enzyme associated with carbohydrate metabolism. Tissue injury causes release of this enzyme, which is found in body organs, skeletal muscles, and RBCs. This test is especially useful in determining myocardial damage after an infarction, damage that could lead to fluid and electrolyte problems.

The last laboratory measurement to review is osmolality, which measures the concentrating ability of the renal system. Osmolality can be measured in serum and urine. Dehydration causes an increase in osmolality, whereas overhydration results in a decrease.[2]

Fluid requirements

When determining fluid needs, it is important to know the purpose for administering IV solutions. For example, is this fluid needed for replacement or maintenance? The purpose is important because it affects the type and amount of fluid that is ordered.

Replacement therapy has a twofold rationale. The first rationale is to restore fluid lost when the previous output exceeded intake. After kidney status has been considered, a hydrating solution (e.g., 5% dextrose in 0.2% sodium chloride) is administered. This restores an adequate output of urine and then allows electrolytes to be replaced. The other rationale for replacement therapy is to restore present fluid and electrolyte losses, such as loss of intestinal fluid through continuing diarrhea. A solution such as lactated Ringer's injection can be used to replace this type of loss. Replacing continuing losses prevents acidosis and alkalosis.

Maintenance therapy provides the ongoing nutrient needs of the patient, including water, electrolytes, dextrose, protein, and vitamins. Water is necessary for adequate kidney function and to replace insensible losses.

Water and electrolyte requirements can be provided by the administration of balanced solutions that contain a daily supply of electrolytes. Increased needs for particular electrolytes should be monitored through laboratory tests and strict measurement of intake and output. These measurements should be considered according to the patient's history, present condition, and ongoing nursing assessments. Electrolytes can be added to the IV solutions when deficiencies are identified. Solutions containing no electrolytes can be used when excesses exist.

Glucose (dextrose) improves liver function by being converted into glycogen; supplies calories for energy, thus sparing protein; and inhibits the development of ketosis, which is caused by the burning of fat stores for energy. Because of these vital functions, it is an important nutrient for body maintenance. Glucose can be provided by peripheral IV infusions in 5% and 10% concentrations. Total parenteral nutrition solutions provide glucose in 25% concentrations.

Protein is another nutrient necessary for maintenance. It is required when an illness extends over a long period. The body normally uses protein for cell repair, enzyme and vitamin synthesis, and wound healing. Amino acid solutions provide IV protein, and the daily requirement for a healthy adult is calculated at 0.80 g/kg of body weight per day.[3]

Vitamins enable the body to use other nutrients. Vitamin B complex, for example, is needed to metabolize carbohydrates and to maintain gastrointestinal function, and vitamin C pro-

motes wound healing. These two vitamins are often administered intravenously because they are water soluble. Water-soluble vitamins must be replaced because they are excreted in the urine. Fat-soluble vitamins, on the other hand, are retained by the body and do not have to be provided in maintenance therapy.

Calculating fluid needs

Having discussed the considerations for determining fluid needs, the next step is to review the basic calculations required for proper administration.

Body surface area (BSA) is a patient-specific measurement used to calculate fluid or fluid maintenance requirements. The BSA is determined in square meters by using a nomogram to correlate weight (in kilograms) and height (in inches). Because 1500 ml of fluid per day are required for each square meter of BSA,[2] then:

$$m^2 \times 1500 = \text{Maintenance requirements/day}$$

Weight is an important indicator of fluid balance. A 1-kg weight loss or gain is approximately equal to a 1-L loss or gain of fluid. For the sake of consistency, the patient should be weighed at the same time every day, using the same scale and wearing the same amount of clothing. A history of recent weight gain or loss is extremely helpful in determining the type and severity of fluid imbalances. For an adult weighing approximately 120 pounds, the severity of fluid volume excess or deficit in acute gains or losses of body weight is determined by the following scale: 2%, mild; 5%, moderate; 8% or greater, severe.[2]

An important point to remember is that there may be no change in body weight when third spacing is occurring. However, a severe volume deficit may be present because of this loss of usable body fluid.

Ongoing monitoring is vital to the well-being of the patient with potential fluid and electrolyte imbalances. A nursing physical assessment covering all areas previously discussed should be performed regularly and consistently. The intake and output record should be a standard nursing order on these patients. Accuracy is of utmost importance; therefore all liquids (intake or output) should be measured carefully and should be estimated when they cannot be measured. Laboratory tests should be repeated frequently and the results evaluated in view of the patient's clinical status.

Caloric need is another measurement that might be required when administering parenteral fluids. Maintenance requirements in a healthy individual may be calculated by using a basal metabolic rate (BMR) chart. The relevant value is found on the chart and is multiplied by the patient's BSA (obtained from a nomogram), as shown in the following equation:

$$BMR \times BSA = \text{Maintenance requirements}$$

As stated earlier, osmolality is the measurement of the concentrating ability of the renal system. Changes in osmolality affect water movement into and out of the cell. An increase in extracellular osmolality causes cells to shrink or shrivel, whereas a decrease causes cells to swell and burst. Because of the affects of these changes, intravenous preparations have a narrow osmolality range. Extracellular osmolality is primarily determined by the sodium level because it is the main solute found in extracellular fluid. A rough estimation of extracellular osmolality can be made by multiplying the plasma sodium concentration by 2. A more accurate estimate also takes into consideration glucose and urea. After dividing the weight per liter of glucose and urea by the molecular weight of each, the result is the osmolality concentration. This allows the equation to be expanded, and is a more accurate estimate. The formula for determining the osmolality of extracellular fluid (ECF) is as follows[4]:

$$\text{Osmolality of ECF} = 2[\text{plasma Na}^+] + \frac{\text{Plasma glucose}}{18} + \frac{\text{BUN}}{2.8}$$

where 18 and 2.8 are the molecular weights of the glucose and BUN.

For example,

$$\text{Osmolality of ECF} = 2(135) + \frac{90}{18} + \frac{28}{2.8}$$
$$= 270 + 5 + 10$$
$$= 285$$

Fluid order and preparation

The initiation of parenteral fluids begins with the fluid order. This order, written by the patient's physician or a prescriber authorized by the State Nurse Practice Act, contains the instructions necessary for the nurse to administer the solutions and medications required.

Fluid type and amount. The first component of the order is the fluid type and amount. The individual writing the order identifies the specific solution needed to treat the patient's condition. In doing this, the prescriber takes into consideration the present diagnosis, other existing conditions, the length of the current illness, body size and weight, the physical assessment findings, and laboratory data. The amount of the solution may be written as part of the order (e.g., 5% dextrose in water, 1000 ml) or may be determined by the rate prescribed (e.g., 200 ml/hr).

Medications and dosage. The second component of the fluid order is the type and dosage of any necessary medications. In parenteral therapy, the medication may be anything from an electrolyte to replace losses to a chemical or drug for treating a specific problem. The dosage is tailored to the patient's age, size, and acuity level. If the physician allows the pharmacy to make generic substitutions, this is also noted on the original order. Some institutions have standing order agreements with their medical community regarding medication substitutions.

Flow rate. The next vital component of the fluid order is the flow rate. This must be specified, and the nurse is responsible for calculating this rate if the physician orders an amount of solution to be infused over a certain period. The nurse is also responsible for recognizing signs and symptoms that may indicate an infusion rate is either too fast or too slow.

A fluid order that specifies a keep vein open (KVO) flow rate is incomplete, and the physician should be consulted for a definite hourly rate. (Make an exception if there is an institutional policy approved by the medical and surgical staffs regard-

ing the definition of a KVO rate [e.g., KVO = 20 ml/hr].) Otherwise, this notation for a rate is the decision of each nurse caring for the patient and has legal implications, in that each nurse's definition of KVO might be different and difficult to defend.

Orders also include the date and time for the infusion to be initiated. This may be stated as a definite time (e.g., 10 PM) or may be indicated by the date and time the order is written.

Route of administration. Another component of the fluid order is the route of administration. Parenteral fluids may be introduced into the body in several ways (i.e., intravenously, intraarterially, subcutaneously, or intraosseously). Factors such as the patient's disease process, vein condition, degree of hydration, and medications required for treatment play important roles in determining the best and most effective route.

Infusion device. The last component of the fluid order may be the use/implementation of an infusion device. Many facilities have protocols for the use of such devices, whereas other facilities have policies that allow for the routine use of infusion devices on all patients. In the latter case, the device would not need to be addressed in the order.

Solution preparation and labeling. After the order is written, the solution must be prepared. The fluid may be plain (containing no additives), premixed (medication is added during the manufacturing process), or admixed (medication is added by the facility using the product). Aseptic technique should be strictly followed when preparing all solutions, and they should be prepared in a laminar flow hood. Possible solution and medication incompatibilities should also be investigated. These precautions help ensure the most sterile product possible for delivery into the vascular system.

All solutions should be properly labeled for the patient. The label should provide the patient's name and room number (if applicable), date and time the solution is needed, medication name and amount, fluid name and amount, initials of the person performing the admixture, initials of the person who verifies the preparation to be correct, and expiration date. Any substitutions or special instructions should be noted. The prescribed flow rate may also be seen on the label.

Order verification. The nurse administering the solution is responsible for verifying the order. The original and complete order should be read and compared with the solution label to be certain that the fluid is correct.

Appropriateness of order. The last responsibility of the nurse is to consider the appropriateness of the solution prescribed for the patient's condition. Many disease processes influence the fluid and electrolyte balance. Thus renal function, cardiac function, clinical status, and maintenance requirements must be examined. A physical assessment and chart review provide valuable information for making this determination. They also assure the nurse that the fluid ordered, if delivered correctly, will not complicate the patient's clinical condition.

Patient identification. Patient identification is the next step in the process. Not only should the patient's name be stated by the patient, if able, and the nurse, but the arm band (if applicable) should be checked. If there is any question concerning any component of the order or the type of solution ordered in regard to the patient's condition, the physician should be contacted before therapy is initiated.

CHARACTERISTICS AND TYPES OF INTRAVENOUS FLUIDS

Various IV solutions are available for treating myriad medical needs. Containers are available in various sizes and volumes, from 25 to 3000 ml, and may be flexible or glass. The multiple components that make up IV solutions vary among the different types of solutions. Not only do the components vary, but the amount of each component may be different. These components and their characteristics must be considered when selecting the appropriate intravenous solution (Table 9-1).

Tonicity

Body fluids are continually moving from one compartment to another in an attempt to maintain homeostasis. This is accomplished through several processes, including osmosis, in which water moves from a less concentrated fluid to one that is more concentrated. This is controlled by the osmotic pressure. In describing solutions, the term *tonicity* is often used in place of osmotic pressure or tension, and it is usually related to the number of particles found in blood.

The term *osmolality* is also used in relation to particle content. It represents the number of particles (solute) per kilogram of solvent (water) and is expressed as milliosmoles (mOsm). When the particle count increases, the concentration also increases, resulting in changes in chemical behavior. The osmolality of body fluids is approximately 285 mOsm/L.[2]

Isotonic solution. A solution that is isotonic has the same tonicity as plasma. This means that the osmotic pressure is the same on the inside and outside of a living cell that is in contact with a solution. As a result, water neither enters nor leaves the cell. Examples of isotonic IV solutions include 0.9% sodium chloride, 5% dextrose in water, and lactated Ringer's. These solutions are used to expand the extracellular fluid and do not cause movement of fluid from or into the blood cells. The approximate osmolality of isotonic IV solutions is 280 to 300 mOsm/L.[4]

Hypotonic solution. Solutions that are considered hypotonic have an osmolality of less than 280 mOsm/L. Therefore these solutions exert less osmotic pressure than fluid in the extracellular compartment, allowing water to be drawn from the extracellular fluid. If blood cells are placed into a hypotonic solution, water is drawn from the solution into the blood cells. Depending on the degree of hypotonicity, the volume of fluid being pulled into the blood cells may cause them to swell and burst. An example of a hypotonic IV solution is 0.45% sodium chloride. A hypotonic solution may be used in the initial treatment of diseases such as diabetic ketoacidosis, where the patient may lose proportionally more water than electrolytes. Patients should be monitored closely when receiving hypotonic solutions. Sterile distilled water should never be used without additives because its high degree of hypotonicity can cause hemolysis.

Hypertonic solution. The osmolality of hypertonic solutions is greater than 300 mOsm/kg, so they exert more osmotic pressure than extracellular fluid. When hypertonic solutions are used, fluid is pulled into the vascular system. Blood cells placed into a hypertonic solution lose water to the solution, causing the cells to shrink. Patients receiving hypertonic solutions should be monitored to prevent fluid overload, particularly if the solutions are extremely concentrated and are being given at a rapid rate. Examples of hypertonic solutions include 3% and 5% sodium chloride, 20% dextrose in water, 50% dextrose in water, and 5% dextrose in lactated Ringer's.

Types of intravenous solutions

Various types of IV solutions may be administered; the appropriate fluid depends on the patient's condition and disease. IV solutions may cause adverse side effects, so precautionary measures should be followed (Table 9-2).

Dextrose intravenous solutions. Parenteral dextrose solutions are available in various concentrations, including 2.5%, 5%, 10%, 20%, 30%, 40%, 50%, 60%, and 70%. Dextrose is also available in combination with other types of solutions (e.g., 5% dextrose in lactated Ringer's, 5% dextrose in 0.9% sodium chloride). The 5% and 10% solutions can be given peripherally. Concentrations higher than 10% are diluted or given through central veins. A general exception is the administration of limited amounts of 50% dextrose given slowly through a peripheral vein for emergency treatment of hypoglycemia.

IV dextrose solutions contain water and dextrose, a monosaccharide (simple sugar) that is freely soluble in water. Dextrose provides calories (hydrous [hydrated] 3.4 calories/g and anhydrous [contains no water] 3.85 calories/g) and increases the level of glucose in the blood. The 5% dextrose in water solution provides 5 g of dextrose/100 ml (170 cal/L). The osmolarity of this solution (253 mOsm/L) is slightly less than normal but is still generally considered isotonic.

In addition to providing calories, 5% dextrose in water also provides free water in approximately the same volume. The dextrose is metabolized quickly to carbon dioxide and water. This leaves only water, which can cross all membranes and be distributed as needed in the appropriate fluid compartment.[5]

More-concentrated dextrose solutions, 20% to 70%, are hypertonic, and range from 1010 to 3530 mOsm/L. When these solutions are being administered, consideration should be given to the possibility that tolerance to glucose may be compromised by sepsis, stress, and hepatic and renal failure, and by some medications, such as steroids or diuretics. Hypertonic solutions can act as a diuretic and can reduce central nervous system edema.[6]

Major uses. The major use of dextrose solutions is for hydration and to provide calories, particularly the more-concentrated solutions. The higher concentrations are usually added to amino acid solutions and are given through a central line to help provide total parenteral nutrition. Hypertonic dextrose solutions, mainly 50%, are used to correct blood glucose levels related to hypoglycemia. Dextrose solutions may also be used as solvents for IV medication administration. Drug information should be reviewed to ensure compatibility between the IV fluid and medication.

Table 9-1   Characteristics of Intravenous Solutions

Manufacturer(s)/IV Solution*	Tonicity	Osmolarity (mOsm/L) A	B	M	Approximate pH A	B	M	Na+	K+	Ca+	Mg2+	Cl-	HCO3-	Lactate	Acetate	Citrate
DEXTROSE/SALINE SOLUTIONS																
A, B, M/dextrose 2.5% and 0.45% sodium chloride	Isotonic	280	280	280	4.3	4.5	4.6	77				77				
M/dextrose 5% and 0.11% sodium chloride	Isotonic			290			4.3	19				19				
A, B, M/dextrose 5% and 0.2% sodium chloride	Hypertonic	329	321	320	4.3	4.0	4.4	34 / 38.5*				34 / 38.5*				
A, B, M/dextrose 5% and 0.3% sodium chloride	Hypertonic	355	365	365	4.3	4.0	4.4	56 / 51*				56 / 51*				
A, B, M/dextrose 5% and 0.45% sodium chloride	Hypertonic	406	406	405	4.3	4.0	4.3	77				77				
A, B, M/dextrose 5% and 0.9% sodium chloride	Hypertonic	560	560	560	4.3	4.0	4.4	154				154				
M/dextrose 10% and 0.2% sodium chloride	Hypertonic			575			4.3	34				34				
M/dextrose 10% and 0.45% sodium chloride	Hypertonic			660			4.3	77				77				
A, B, M/dextrose 10% and 0.9% sodium chloride	Hypertonic	813	813	815	4.4	4.0	4.3	154				154				
SALINE SOLUTIONS																
A, B, M/0.45% sodium chloride	Hypotonic	154	154	155	5.6	5.0	5.6	77				77				
A, B, M/0.9% sodium chloride	Isotonic	308	308	310	5.6	5.5	5.6	154				154				
B, M/3% sodium chloride	Hypertonic		1027	1030		5.0	5.8	513				513				
A, B, M/5% sodium chloride	Hypertonic	1711	1711	1710	5.6	5.0	5.8	855 / 856§†				855 / 856§†				
DEXTROSE SOLUTIONS																
A, B, M/5% dextrose and water	Isotonic	253	252	253	5.0	5.0	4.5									
A, B/10% dextrose and water	Hypertonic	505	505		4.6	4.0										
A, B/50% dextrose and water	Hypertonic	2526	2520		4.9	4.5										

Data from Abbott, Baxter, B. Braun/McGaw.
A, Abbott; *B*, Baxter; *M*, B. Braun/McGaw.
*Abbott.
†Baxter.
§B. Braun/McGaw.

Continued

Table 9-1   Characteristics of Intravenous Solutions—cont'd

Manufacturer(s)/IV Solution*	Tonicity	Osmolarity (m)Osm/L — A	B	M	Approximate pH — A	B	M	Na+	K+	Ca+	Mg2+	Cl−	HCO3−	Lactate	Acetate	Citrate
ELECTROLYTE SOLUTIONS																
A/Normosol R	Isotonic	294			6.6			140	5			98	23‡		27	
B/Plasmalyte A	Isotonic		294			7.4		140	5		3	98	23‡		27	
B/Plasmalyte R	Isotonic		312			5.5		140	10	5	3	103		8	47	
M/Isolyte E	Isotonic			310			6.0	140	10	5	3	103			49	8
A, B, M/Ringer's	Isotonic	309	309	310	5.4	5.5	5.8	147	4	4		155				
A, B, M/lactated Ringer's	Isotonic	273	273	275	6.6	6.5	6.2	147.5† / 130	4 / 4	4.5§† / 2.7† / 3		156§† / 109† / 110§		28		
DEXTROSE/ELECTROLYTE SOLUTIONS																
A, B, M/dextrose 5% in Ringer's	Hypertonic	561	561	560	4.9	4.3	4†	147	4	4.5† / 4*§		156† / 155*§				
A, B, M/dextrose 5% in lactated Ringer's	Hypertonic	525	525	527		5.0	4.6	130	4	2.7† / 3.0		109† / 112§		28		
A, B, M/dextrose 2.5% in half-strength lactated Ringer's	Isotonic		263	263		5.0	5.0	65	2	1.4 / 1.5§		54 / 55†		14		
MISCELLANEOUS SOLUTIONS																
A, B/5% sodium bicarbonate injection	Hypertonic	1203	1190		7.8	8.0		595					595			
A, B/sodium lactate injection (1/6 M sodium lactate)	Hypertonic	334	334		6.7	6.5		167						167		
B/10% mannitol injection	Hypertonic		549			5.0										
B/15% mannitol injection	Hypertonic		823			5.0										
A, B/20% mannitol injection	Hypertonic		1098			5.0										
A, B/6% dextran and 0.9% sodium chloride	Isotonic	309	309		4.5	5.0		154				154				
A, B/10% dextran and 0.9% sodium chloride	Isotonic	310	311		4.7	5.0		154				154				
A, B/10% dextran and 5% dextrose injection	Slightly hypotonic	255	255		4.4	4.0										

Data from Abbott, Baxter, B. Braun/McGaw.
A, Abbott; B, Baxter; M, B. Braun/McGaw.
*Abbott.
†Baxter.
‡Gluconate.
§B. Braun/McGaw.

Table 9-2 **Summary of Intravenous Solutions**

IV SOLUTION	POTENTIAL USES	SIDE EFFECTS AND PRECAUTIONS
Dextrose	Provides calories; provides free water; diluent for IV medication administration	Tolerance to glucose may be compromised by stress, sepsis, hepatic and renal failure, steroids, and diuretics; vein irritation; water intoxication; possible agglomeration; hypertonic solutions: hyperglycemia, osmotic diuresis, hyperosmolar coma, hyperinsulinism
ELECTROLYTES		
Sodium	Sodium replacement; chloride replacement; treats hyperosmolar diabetes; metabolic alkalosis (with Na depletion and fluid loss); diluent for IV medication administration; initiation and discontinuation of blood transfusions	Hyponatremia (with continuous or excessive use of 0.45% NaCl); calorie depletion; hypernatremia; peripheral edema; depletion of other electrolytes; hyperchloremia
Multiple electrolytes	Provides calories (if contains dextrose); provides electrolytes; provides free water	Excessive electrolytes (with rapid administration/solution type); electrolyte deficit (with same solutions where there are abnormal losses or no intake); calorie deficit (if contains no dextrose); fluid overload (related to Na content); IV solution content should be considered in relation to preexisting conditions; metabolic alkalosis (excessive administration of lactated Ringer's)
Other electrolyte solutions	Same as above	Same as above
PLASMA EXPANDERS		
Dextran	Shock/anticipated shock related to trauma, surgery, burns, or hemorrhage; prevention of venous thrombosis and pulmonary embolism prophylactically during surgery	Anaphylactoid reactions; GI disturbances; interferes with laboratory testing: decreased hematocrit and plasma protein, temporary extended bleeding time; hypervolemia: electrolyte imbalances, tissue dehydration; preexisting conditions should be considered (e.g., renal or cardiac disease); use caution in presence of active hemorrhage
Mannitol	Promotes diuresis and excretion of toxic substances; for intracranial pressure and cerebral edema; reduces intraocular pressure	Hypervolemia: electrolyte imbalances, tissue dehydration; extravasation may lead to skin irritation and tissue necrosis; interferes with laboratory testing; preexisting conditions should be considered (e.g., renal or cardiac disease); use caution because of possible crystal formation
Hetastarch	Shock related to trauma, burns, hemorrhage, and surgery; increase granulocyte yield during leukapheresis	Hypervolemia: electrolyte imbalances, tissue dehydration; anaphylactoid reactions; interferes with laboratory testing: may increase bleeding times, platelet function, decreased hematocrit and plasma protein; preexisting conditions should be considered (e.g., renal or cardiac disease); hypervolemia: electrolyte imbalances, tissue dehydration

GI, Gastrointestinal.

Continued

Complications. There may be complications related to administering dextrose solutions intravenously. Vein irritation may occur because of the slightly acidic pH (3.4 to 4.0) of the solution. The use of 5% dextrose in water for hydration should be monitored closely, particularly if used past the initial stage of treatment. Because this solution does not contain electrolytes, continual administration may dilute the body's normal store of electrolytes and can lead to excess extracellular fluid, congestive conditions, or pulmonary edema. It can also lead to water intoxication, which may be signaled by rapid weight gain, thirst, diluted urine, nonpitting edema, arrhythmias, and low sodium levels. If this process is not corrected, symptoms of cerebral intracellular fluid excess, including seizures, coma, and death, will occur while water shifts into the brain cells.[6] Dextrose solutions should not be used in the same IV line with blood because of possible agglomeration (clustering).

There are other problems associated with the use of hypertonic dextrose solutions. If given rapidly, these solutions may cause hyperglycemia, which can lead to osmotic diuresis and result in a loss of fluids and electrolytes and possibly hyperosmolar coma. There may be a need to add insulin to total parenteral nutrition solutions containing dextrose to prevent adverse effects related to insulin production. Unless hypertonic solutions are diluted before peripheral administration, vein

Table 9-2   Summary of Intravenous Solutions—cont'd

IV SOLUTION	POTENTIAL USES	SIDE EFFECTS AND PRECAUTIONS
PLASMA EXPANDERS—cont'd		
Albumin	Shock/impending shock caused by hypovolemia; provide protein (hypoproteinemia); hyperbilirubinemia; erythroblastosis fetalis	Preexisting conditions should be considered (e.g., renal or cardiac disease); hypervolemia: electrolyte imbalances, tissue dehydration; interferes with laboratory testing: decreased hematocrit and plasma protein; anaphylactoid reactions; bleeding postoperatively and posttrauma
Plasma protein fraction	Shock related to burns, surgery, hemorrhage, etc; temporarily provides protein	Cardiac and GI symptoms; chills, fever, urticaria; back pain; hypervolemia; hypernatremia; bleeding postoperatively and post-trauma; preexisting conditions should be considered (e.g., cardiac or renal disease)
Sodium bicarbonate	Metabolic acidosis; severe hyperkalemia	Possible metabolic alkalosis, hypocalcemia, and hypokalemia (with rapid administration); hypernatremia; preexisting conditions should be considered (e.g., cardiac or renal disease); hypervolemia: electrolyte imbalances; extravasation may lead to skin irritation and tissue necrosis
Sodium lactate	Mild to moderate metabolic acidosis	Hypernatremia; hypervolemia: electrolyte imbalances; metabolic alkalosis and/or hypokalemia (with rapid administration); preexisting conditions should be considered (e.g., cardiac or renal disease)
Premixed solutions	Vary according to medication added	Vary according to medication added

irritation, vein damage, and thrombosis may result. Hypertonic solutions are contraindicated for patients with preexisting conditions such as anuria, intraspinal/intracranial hemorrhage, delirium tremens (in the presence of dehydration), diabetic coma, and known allergies to corn or corn products.

Before any medication is added to a dextrose solution, compatibility information should be checked. Dextrose may also affect the stability of admixtures (e.g., ampicillin sodium). A pharmacist should be contacted for additional information about questionable admixtures.

Sodium-containing intravenous solutions

Major uses. Because sodium controls water distribution and is the major cation found in extracellular fluid, it is important to replace it when it is lost. Various IV solutions are available to supplement sodium intake, with pH values ranging from 4.5 to 7. Their concentrations vary from 0.45% to 5%. The 0.45% sodium chloride solution is hypotonic, with 1000 ml containing 77 mEq of sodium and 77 mEq of chloride. It provides sodium, chloride, and free water and is used primarily as a hydrating solution. It may also be used to treat hyperosmolar diabetes or assess renal function status.

Sodium chloride also comes as an isotonic solution containing 154 mEq of sodium and 154 mEq of chloride per liter. This 0.9% sodium chloride solution closely approximates the osmotic pressure of body fluids. It does not enter the intracellular fluid compartment but does expand the extracellular fluid.

Continuous infusion of 0.45% sodium chloride may lead to dilution and depletion of electrolytes. Because of the small amount of sodium in this solution, continuous use or excessive

amounts may result in hyponatremia. Another complication that should be monitored is calorie depletion because there are no calories in the solution.

The 0.9% sodium chloride solution is used to replace sodium and chloride. It is used to treat metabolic alkalosis accompanied by sodium depletion and fluid loss.[5] This solution is often used to initiate or discontinue blood transfusions because it does not hemolyze erythrocytes. Some medications require this isotonic solution as a diluent to ensure stability.

There are two hypertonic sodium-containing solutions: 3% and 5%. The 3% sodium chloride solution contains 513 mEq/L of sodium and the same amount of chloride and has an osmolarity of approximately 1025 mOsm/L. The 5% solution has 855 mEq/L of sodium and an equal amount of chloride and has an approximate osmolarity of 1710 mOsm/L. More-concentrated solutions are used to prepare nutrition solutions.

Hypertonic sodium chloride solutions are used to treat severe hyponatremia, which can be caused by excessive sweating, vomiting, renal impairment, heart failure, surgery, or excessive water intake. These solutions are generally reserved to treat severe deficits or for patients who are symptomatic because of hyponatremia or hypochloremia.

Complications. The use of an isotonic saline solution may result in complications. Rapid infusion rates or continuous administration of only 0.9% sodium chloride solutions may lead to hypernatremia and fluid overload, potentially leading to all the problems associated with these conditions, including peripheral edema, acid-base imbalances, and electrolyte dilution. Other electrolytes, especially potassium, may be depleted by the continuous infusion of isotonic sodium chloride. Because there are no calories, there may be problems related to nutritional status.

In addition, the rapid or continuous use of hypertonic 3% or 5% sodium chloride IV solutions may result in hyperchloremia or hypernatremia. Excessive amounts of chloride may lead to the loss of bicarbonate with an acidifying effect.[5] Close monitoring of the flow rate and laboratory test results can eliminate many of the complications associated with sodium administration.

Multiple electrolyte intravenous solutions. A number of formulations provide electrolytes, some of which contain calories. The signs, symptoms, and laboratory test results of the patient should be used to determine the correct formulation. The electrolyte content of a specific solution varies among manufacturers.

Ringer's injection. Ringer's injection is an isotonic solution with a pH of 5.0 to 7.5. The electrolyte content of Ringer's injection approximates that of plasma and includes sodium, 147 mEq/L; potassium, 4 mEq/L; calcium, 4 mEq/L; and chloride, 155 mEq/L.

Major uses. Ringer's injection is used to replace electrolytes and to provide water for hydration. The solution is often used to replace extracellular fluid losses.

Complications. Even though the content is similar to that of plasma, continual delivery of only Ringer's injection may lead to complications. The solution contains potassium and calcium, but the amount is not adequate for maintenance or replacement if there is inadequate intake or abnormal loss of these electrolytes. Rapid administration may lead to excessive amounts of electrolytes. Administration of only this type of fluid could result in a calorie deficit. Ringer's injection may also cause fluid overload, which could dilute the electrolytes. As with any type of fluid, this could also cause a congestive disorder or pulmonary edema. Because Ringer's injection contains electrolytes, there is always the danger of delivering an excessive amount of one or all of the components.

Ringer's injection also is available with dextrose added (5% dextrose in Ringer's). It provides the same electrolytes as Ringer's injection plus 5 g of dextrose (170 calories per liter). The osmolality is 561 mOsm/L, making it a hypertonic solution, and the pH is approximately 4.3. It has the same applications as Ringer's injection, plus the ability to provide calories.

Before Ringer's injections are used, each solution component should be considered. For example, because the solution contains potassium, precautions need to be exercised when treating patients with cardiac or renal disorders. If the solution contains dextrose, caution should be exercised if the patient has diabetes mellitus.

Clinical evaluation and periodic laboratory tests are important to ascertain fluid balance, electrolyte levels, and acid-base status. The type and volume of fluid administered depends on the patient's age, weight, and condition.

Lactated Ringer's solution. Another solution that contains multiple electrolytes is lactated Ringer's. The electrolyte content is similar to that of plasma and includes sodium, potassium, calcium, and chloride. Lactate, an organic ion, has been added as a buffer and is metabolized to produce bicarbonate, which is normally found in extracellular fluid. Lactated Ringer's is an isotonic solution with a pH of about 6.6.

Major uses. Lactated Ringer's solution (Hartmann's solution) provides electrolytes and is used to treat hypovolemia. When oral intake is limited or absent or when losses are abnormally high, lactated Ringer's does not provide adequate electrolytes for maintenance therapy. Magnesium may have to be supplemented because lactated Ringer's does not provide it.

Complications. The complications produced by Ringer's injection are also applicable for lactated Ringer's solutions. These include overhydration, electrolyte excess (particularly sodium), electrolyte dilution, and calorie depletion. Excessive administration may lead to metabolic alkalosis.

Because lactate is metabolized in the liver, lactated Ringer's solution is contraindicated in patients with hepatic disorders. A different solution should be considered in the presence of lactic acidosis because the body's buffering system can be overloaded.

Some calories (170 cal/L) may be provided in addition to electrolytes by using 5% dextrose in lactated Ringer's. The inclusion of dextrose changes the concentration and makes it a hypertonic solution (527 mOsm/L) with a pH of about 4.9.

The same problems and contraindications are applicable for 5% dextrose in lactated Ringer's. Consideration should be given to conditions and diseases affected by dextrose administration.

Other electrolyte solutions. Other electrolyte solutions are available in addition to the group of Ringer's and lactated Ringer's solutions. The names and formulations differ, depending on the manufacturer (see Table 9-1). The use of the various electrolyte combinations often depends on the experience of the physician and on solution availability. The patient's clinical picture, including laboratory test results, should be assessed when selecting the appropriate solution. Electrolyte solutions are generally isotonic until dextrose is added and they become hypertonic. However, this may vary depending on the electrolyte content. All electrolyte formulations contain sodium, potassium, and chloride. Some may also contain calcium, magnesium, phosphate, and buffers, with the latter being provided as bicarbonate, gluconate, lactate, and acetate.

These solutions may be used for maintenance or replacement of electrolytes. Solutions containing dextrose provide calories. Depending on the formulation, the fluids may be used to treat hypovolemia and to provide free water.

Before any electrolyte solutions are used, the patient's history and physical and laboratory findings should be assessed. The solution should then be selected to meet the individual's electrolyte, caloric, and hydration needs.

Complications include fluid overload, electrolyte excess, electrolyte depletion, electrolyte dilution, and calorie depletion. Complications result from the administration rate, IV formulation, preexisting conditions and diseases, and current illness.

Plasma expanders. Solutions used to expand the intravascular space are known as *colloids,* or *plasma expanders.* The increase in volume is accomplished by these solutions pulling fluid from the interstitial spaces. Plasma expanders include dextran, mannitol, hetastarch, and albumin.

Dextran. Dextran solutions have effects similar to those of human albumin for expanding intravascular volume. There are two types of dextran: high molecular weight and low molecular weight.

High-molecular-weight dextrans. High-molecular-weight dextrans, dextran 70 and dextran 75, are available with average molecular weights of 70,000 and 75,000, respectively. These 6% solutions are diluted in either 5% dextrose injection or 0.9% sodium chloride solution. The intravascular volume is increased in excess of the volume infused. The maximum effect occurs approximately 1 hour after administration, and with normal renal function, the increased volume is excreted within 24 hours. The increased volume depends on the amount of solution administered, the preadministration fluid status, and renal status. After administration, the large dextran molecules (those with a molecular weight of 50,000 or more) are slowly broken down to glucose, which is then metabolized to carbon dioxide and water.[5]

Major uses. High-molecular-weight dextran is used to treat shock or impending shock related to trauma, surgery, burns, or hemorrhage.[7] Dextran solutions should not be used as substitutes for blood and blood products. However, they may be used on short notice if there is no time for crossmatching or if blood or blood products are unavailable.

Complications. High-molecular-weight dextran may cause wheezing, tightness in the chest, urticaria, nasal congestion, and gastrointestinal disturbances, including nausea, vomiting, and severe anaphylactoid reactions. Because dextran can interfere with laboratory testing, blood samples for typing, Rh determinations, and crossmatching should be drawn before dextran administration and a part of the sample should be retained if additional tests are needed. Dextran administration may result in a rouleau formation (stacking of erythrocytes). Also, dextran may yield high values of glucose. Because fluid is being drawn into the vascular system, patients should be monitored for circulatory overload. The increased fluid volume may result in a lowered hematocrit and plasma protein level. The hydration status needs to be monitored closely because overhydration leads to dilution of electrolytes and lack of adequate fluids may result in tissue dehydration. When larger volumes of dextran are administered, the bleeding time may be temporarily extended.

Dextran is contraindicated for patients with renal diseases, congestive cardiac failure, and bleeding disorders. It should not be used for patients with known hypersensitivity to dextran.

Low-molecular-weight dextran. Low-molecular-weight dextran is a polymer of glucose that has an average molecular weight of approximately 40,000. The 10% dextran 40 is available in 5% dextrose injection and 0.9% sodium chloride solution. The maximum volume expansion is attained shortly following completion of administration and is affected by the volume delivered, the preexisting plasma volume, and the excretion rate. Most of the dextran (70%) is excreted by the renal system within 24 hours. Like the higher-molecular-weight dextran, the larger molecules are degraded to glucose and metabolized to carbon dioxide and water. The fluid expansion improves circulatory status, including microcirculation, even though the exact mechanism is unknown.[5]

Major uses. Low-molecular-weight dextran is used for early fluid replacement and to treat shock related to vascular volume loss such as that produced by burns, hemorrhage, surgery,

and trauma.[7] Because of its action in preventing sludging of blood, low-molecular-weight dextran is used to help prevent venous thrombosis and pulmonary embolism during surgical procedures.

Complications. An anaphylactoid reaction is rare but may be fatal. Hydration status is important because limited intake may deplete tissue fluids and excessive fluids may dilute electrolytes. Circulatory overload may occur, leading to various congestive states. Dextran can have an adverse effect on hepatic function. Higher dosages may increase bleeding times. Because of the expansion of vascular volume, the hematocrit and plasma protein may be diluted. Blood should be drawn before dextran administration because dextran may interfere with laboratory testing, depending on the test method or the agent used in the testing process.

Low-molecular-weight dextran should not be given to patients with cardiac or renal disease caused by possible overload problems and is contraindicated in the presence of thrombocytopenia, hypofibrinogenemia, and hypersensitivity to dextran. Dehydrated patients should receive fluids before and during dextran infusion to prevent tissue dehydration. Caution should be used when active hemorrhage is present. Patients should be monitored for pulse, blood pressure, central venous pressure (if possible), and urine output. Rates may need to be slowed and the patient monitored for circulatory overload if the central venous pressure is not being monitored. Also, dextran administration may need to be slowed or discontinued depending on the status of the patient.

Mannitol. Mannitol is a hexahydroxy alcohol substance that is available in concentrations from 5% to 25%. This solution is limited to the extracellular space, where it draws fluid from the cells and eventually ends up in the plasma. A small percentage of mannitol is reabsorbed, and most of it is excreted by the kidney within 3 hours. It ranges from 275 to 1375 mOsm/L, depending on the concentration, and has a pH of 4.5 to 7.

Major uses. This colloid is used to promote diuresis in the oliguric phase of acute renal failure and to promote excretion of toxic substances. The treatment of intracranial pressure and cerebral edema may include the use of mannitol. When other forms of treatment have been unsuccessful, mannitol may be used to reduce high intraocular pressure. It does not penetrate the eye and may be used where irritation is present. Mannitol should be given 1 to 1.5 hours before eye (ocular) surgery to achieve the maximum pressure reduction.[5]

Complications. Fluid and electrolyte imbalances are the most common and severe complications encountered with mannitol administration. Fluid is drawn from the cells into the vascular system, which may lead to cell dehydration or fluid overload. The excess fluid may cause an increased loss or dilution of electrolytes, leaving a deficit. If dehydration occurs, there may be an electrolyte excess, with the greatest effect being on the sodium and potassium levels. There may be alteration of acid-base balance. Mannitol may have an adverse effect on the nervous system, including toxicity and interference with cerebrospinal fluid pH. Extravasation of mannitol may lead to skin irritation and tissue necrosis. Mannitol may interfere with laboratory tests, including mannitol-induced electrolyte changes, blood ethylene glycol concentration, and inorganic phosphorus blood concentrations.[5]

Mannitol should be used cautiously for patients with impaired cardiac or renal systems. It is contraindicated in the presence of anuria, severe pulmonary and cardiac congestion, severe dehydration, pregnancy, and intracranial bleeding (present other than during a craniotomy).

Mannitol should also be monitored for crystal formation. The use of an in-line filter is recommended during the administration.

Hetastarch. Hetastarch is a synthetic polymer with colloidal properties similar to those of human albumin. It has an approximate pH of 5.5 and an osmolarity of 310 mOsm/L. It is available in a 6% concentration in 0.9% sodium chloride. The colloidal osmotic effect pulls fluid from the cells into the intravascular space, thus increasing the volume in this area. Maximum volume expansion occurs shortly after completion of the infusion. The duration of effect depends on the preadministration plasma volume, distribution of the hetastarch in body water, and renal function status. The molecules in this solution vary in size. The smaller hetastarch molecules (hydroxyethylated glucose) are excreted rapidly, but it may take 2 weeks or longer for the larger molecules (starch) to be degraded sufficiently for elimination. Hetastarch does not interfere with blood typing and crossmatching, as do other colloidal solutions.

Major uses. This solution is used for early fluid replacement and to treat shock related to a decreased circulating volume resulting from trauma, burns, hemorrhage, and surgery. It is also used with leukapheresis to help increase the yield of granulocytes by centrifugal means.[5]

Complications. The administration of hetastarch may produce a severe anaphylactoid reaction. It may interfere with platelet function and increase bleeding times. As with any volume expander, the danger of fluid overload is always a possibility. This may lead to disorders related to congestion, dilution, or depletion of electrolytes; dehydration of peripheral tissue; electrolyte excess; and a decrease in the hematocrit, platelet counts, hemoglobin, and plasma protein levels.

Hetastarch is contraindicated in patients with liver disease and severe cardiac and renal disorders, particularly when oliguria or anuria is present. It also should not be used in the presence of bleeding disorders.

The patient should be evaluated clinically and laboratory tests monitored regularly. Partially used containers should be discarded because hetastarch does not contain preservatives.

Albumin. Albumin is a natural plasma protein prepared from human blood and blood-related products and is available in 5% and 25% concentrations. It contains 130 to 160 mEq of sodium per liter. It plays an important role in regulating plasma volume and tissue fluid balance. The administration of albumin causes fluid to be pulled from the interstitial space into the intravascular space. Because it is a plasma protein, there may be a slight increase in the plasma protein volume. The 5% solution is isotonic. The 25% solution is hypertonic, and in a well-hydrated patient, each volume (amount given) draws about 3.5 volumes of additional fluid into circulation within 15 minutes.[5]

Major uses. Albumin is used for plasma volume expansion in treating shock or impending shock related to a circulatory volume deficit. Albumin is used widely in the management of medical and surgical conditions. However, in most cases, there are problems related to the administration of albumin. The 5% solution is generally used to treat hypovolemia, and the 25% solution is usually reserved for treatment when there are fluid and sodium restrictions.

Complications. The potential for complications should be considered if cardiac, hepatic, or renal disease is present. These systems may be unable to handle the increased intravascular volume if they are impaired. The increased circulating volume may result in fluid overload and lead to further complications. Anemia may occur if large volumes of albumin alone are used to replace blood loss. The rapid influx and excretion of fluid may dilute or deplete electrolytes. The serum protein concentration and hematocrit should be monitored because these levels may be decreased. Symptoms of allergic reactions may be present. Bleeding may occur postoperatively or posttraumatically as the intravascular volume and pressure increase. Albumin is contraindicated in patients with severe anemia, cardiac failure, or known hypersensitivity. Angiotensin-converting enzyme inhibitors (ACE) should be withheld for at least 24 hours before administering large amounts of albumin because of an increased risk of atypical reactions (e.g., flushing, hypotension).[5]

Plasma protein fraction. Plasma protein fraction (PPF) is isotonic and is similar in action to human albumin in expanding intravascular volume. It is a 5% solution containing proteins, with approximately 83% to 90% being albumin derived from pooled blood, plasma, and serum. It is not blood group or Rh specific and contains no clotting factors. It is a transparent, nearly colorless to slightly brownish solution that contains 130 to 160 mEq of sodium per liter and no more than 2 mEq of potassium per liter.[5]

Major uses. PPF, which is used to expand plasma volume, causes fluid to shift from the interstitial spaces into the circulatory system. It is used to treat shock related to burns, surgery, hemorrhage, or any condition resulting in a volume deficit. When treating hypovolemia-related conditions, the initial dose is 250 to 500 ml (12.5 to 25 g of protein). Thereafter, the dose is related to the patient's condition and response. The flow rate should be adjusted according to the patient's response but should not exceed 10 ml/min.[5] PPF is not a substitute when whole blood, RBCs, or albumin is indicated.

PPF may also be used temporarily to provide protein in cases of hypoproteinemia. However, as with other indications, it does not offer advantages over albumin.

Complications. Adverse side effects include tachycardia, flushing, erythema, nausea, vomiting, headache, chills, fever, urticaria, back pain, and hypersalivation. These side effects are common.

As with any solution used for volume expansion, caution should be exercised to prevent vascular overload. Patients should be monitored for signs of hypervolemia, such as pulmonary edema. Because of the sodium content, sodium levels should be monitored. The patient should be observed for signs of bleeding as the intravascular volume and blood pressure increase. Caution should also be exercised in the presence of hepatic or renal failure. PPF is contraindicated with cardiopulmonary bypass procedures and may be contraindicated in patients with severe anemia or cardiac failure.

Alkalizing solutions

Sodium bicarbonate.
Sodium bicarbonate solution is an alkalizing agent and a sodium salt. The 5% sodium bicarbonate solution dissociates to provide the bicarbonate ion, which is the principal buffer in extracellular fluid. Bicarbonate helps maintain osmotic pressure and acid-base balance. It contains 0.595 mEq each of sodium and bicarbonate ions per milliliter and the osmolarity is 1190 to 1203 mOsm/L. Sodium bicarbonate is physically and/or chemically incompatible with many drugs, especially calcium, and compatibility information should be checked before admixing. The administration of sodium bicarbonate increases plasma bicarbonate concentration and may increase plasma pH until the body compensates and returns the level to a normal value.

Major uses. Sodium bicarbonate is used to treat metabolic acidosis associated with many diseases, including severe renal disease, uncontrolled diabetes, and cardiac/circulatory diseases. It is administered in the treatment of severe hyperkalemia, in which it alkalinizes the plasma and results in a temporary shift of potassium into the cells. The sodium in the solution also antagonizes the cardiac effects of the potassium. It can be administered by intraosseous injection in pediatric patients during cardiopulmonary resuscitation.[5]

Complications. Metabolic alkalosis, hypocalcemia, and hypokalemia may occur following the rapid or excessive administration of sodium bicarbonate. There may be water and sodium retention leading to hypernatremia, particularly when there is a preexisting condition such as renal or cardiac disease. The fluid overload may lead to electrolyte imbalances. Extravasation may cause chemical cellulitis, necrosis, ulceration, or sloughing.

Patients with metabolic and respiratory alkalosis are not good candidates for sodium bicarbonate therapy. It is also contraindicated in the presence of hypocalcemia or hypochloremia. Caution should be exercised when cardiac or renal problems exist.[5]

Sodium lactate.
Sodium lactate (one-sixth M lactate) is an alkalizing agent. It is a racemic salt with the *l-isomer* being oxidized in the liver to bicarbonate and the *d-isomer* converted to glycogen. It contains approximately 167 mEq each of sodium and lactate ions and 55 calories per liter.[5]

Major uses. When the production and use of lactic acid are normal, sodium lactate is used to treat mild to moderate metabolic acidosis. Because it takes 1 to 2 hours to convert lactate to bicarbonate, it is not recommended for treating severe acidosis.

Complications. Caution should be taken when using sodium lactate for patients with hypervolemia, congestive heart failure, or renal disorders causing oliguria or anuria. The sodium contained in the solution may lead to hypernatremia and hypervolemia. There may also be deficits or excesses of other electrolytes. Excessive amounts or rapid administration may lead to metabolic alkalosis or hypokalemia. It should not be used for patients having excessive lactate levels or impaired lactate utilization. Sodium lactate should not be used to treat lactic acidosis or in the presence of hypernatremia or respiratory alkalosis.

Premixed intravenous solutions.
A large number of premixed IV solutions are available. These solutions have many advantages over manually prepared admixtures. Premixed solutions have been sterilized after the admixture procedure and therefore have a longer shelf life. There is no difficulty in selecting the correct diluent, and the pH has been adjusted to improve stability. Finally, the correct amount of medication has been added to the proper volume and type of IV solution. Premixed solutions decrease the amount of time needed to get the fluid to the patient, which is particularly important in emergency situations.

There are also disadvantages in using premixed IV solutions. The wrong amount of medication may be used if a particular admixture comes in more than one dosage or if there are multiple types that are premixed and the wrong medication or solution is used. Premixed IV solutions can also cost more.

The number of premixed medications available is increasing. Potassium chloride comes in several concentrations and in various IV solutions. Its use depends on the patient's history, physical assessment, and laboratory findings. Before any of the potassium-containing solutions are administered, it is important to establish good renal function. Complications are related to the content of the particular fluid. Rapid infusion or continual administration may lead to hypervolemia, electrolyte excess (particularly potassium), or electrolyte dilution. Using only one type of solution over an extended period may result in electrolyte depletion and, if no source of nutrients is available, calorie depletion. The patient should be monitored carefully for electrolyte imbalances during the course of treatment.

Other medications premixed in IV solutions include heparin sodium, theophylline, lidocaine hydrochloride, nitroglycerin, dobutamine hydrochloride, and dopamine hydrochloride. There are also a variety of medications that are premixed in small volumes of IV solutions, including antibiotics and H_2 antagonists. In addition to premixed products, there are also products that allow the medication container to be attached directly to the IV solution. Just as for premixed potassium solutions, it is important to review the patient's history, physical assessment, and laboratory findings. The nurse should be familiar with complications related to the particular medication and the base IV solution to which it has been added. The pharmacy department should be contacted if information is unclear or unfamiliar.

In regard to the complications of IV fluid administration, there are metabolic and physical concerns. The metabolic issues have been discussed in detail as related to each solution. There are also physical complications involved with IV fluid administration. These include vascular tolerance, which depends on the patient's general health status, condition of the veins and pH and concentration of the IV solution or medication. Acidic solutions and hypertonic solutions may irritate the lining of the vessel and become painful for the patient. The infiltration of hypertonic solutions may cause irritation and subsequent necrosis and sloughing of subcutaneous tissue. Most complications can be corrected by slowing the infusion rate or by discontinuing the solution or admixture.

SUMMARY

Parenteral fluid administration has many facets in maintaining homeostasis and is not without its complexities and complications. These concerns challenge the nurse who is caring for the patient with potential imbalances. The nurse, by effectively evaluating the many nursing considerations involved in fluid administration, can help ensure positive outcomes for patients receiving parenteral fluids.

Patient outcomes

- The patient returns to a state of fluid and electrolyte equilibrium as evidenced by normal laboratory values, urinary output, and stable weight.
- The patient does not develop an infection as evidenced by normal vital signs and absence of inflammation.
- By the end of the first teaching session, the patient can verbalize the reasons for administering parenteral fluids, briefly describe the initiation procedure, and list two signs or symptoms that should be reported to the nurse.

REFERENCES

1. Miller RD: *Problems in health care law,* ed 7, Gaithersburg, Md, 1996, Aspen.
2. Metheny NM: *Fluid and electrolyte balance: nursing considerations,* ed 3, Philadelphia, 1996, Lippincott-Raven.
3. Weinstein SM: *Plummer's principles and practices of intravenous therapy,* ed 6, Philadelphia, 1997, Lippincott-Raven.
4. Horne MM, Heitz UE, Swearingen PL: *Pocket guide to fluid, electrolyte, and acid-base balance,* ed 3, St Louis, 1997, Mosby.
5. McEvoy GK: *AHFS drug information 1999,* Bethesda, Md, 1999, American Society of Health System Pharmacists.
6. Paradiso C: *Fluids and electrolytes,* ed 2, Philadelphia, 1999, JB Lippincott.
7. Gahart BL, Nazareno AR: *Intravenous medications,* ed 14, St Louis, 1998, Mosby.

Blood Component Therapy

Jane A. Weir, BA, BSN, CRNI

This chapter provides a foundation on which to construct a broader understanding of the more encompassing subject of transfusion therapy. The topics addressed here are not intended to be all-inclusive of the discipline of transfusion therapy, nor are they offered as a "how to" manual. They are intended to establish a firm theoretical footing and a practical framework upon which the practitioner may build.

It was fewer than 200 years ago that James Blundell performed the first blood transfusion to save a life. Since then, because of the incredible advances in knowledge and technology that have been made in blood group identification, collection, fractionation, storage, and transmissible disease testing, transfusion medicine has evolved into a specialty of its own. This specialty has made advances in new surgical procedures possible and has supported the ever-changing approaches to cancer chemotherapy.

Blood component therapy has advanced so far so fast and is so common in today's medicine that there could be a tendency to approach this familiar therapy with some complacency. Therefore it should be remembered that blood infusion is a "living transplant" that carries with it significant risks, only a few of which are avoidable. Consequently, this effective and readily accessible therapy should be used prudently; the potential benefit should always outweigh the potential for harm. Furthermore, it is the practitioner's duty in transfusion therapy to be knowledgeable in the application of this therapy and to be familiar with its possible untoward effects and their appropriate interventions.

DONOR TESTING

All blood donated for the purpose of homologous transfusion must be subjected to a number of tests (Table 10-1).

ABO and Rh typing (red cell antigens)

ABO forward typing is the process in which red blood cells are mixed with a known antibody (anti-A or anti-B). This process identifies the antigens present on the red blood cells by the visually apparent agglutination of the cells when an antibody combines with the corresponding antigen (e.g., anti-A with antigen A).

ABO reverse typing tests serum for the presence of predicted ABO antibodies by adding red blood cells of a known ABO type.

The Rh factor is the red cell antigen D. Rh typing is accomplished by testing red cells against anti-D serum. If agglutination occurs, the red cells possess the D antigen and the blood is Rh+. Some people demonstrate a weak expression of the D antigen (formerly referred to as D^U). In the past, laboratory testing to identify this weak D antigen included the indirect antiglobulin test. However, that test is no longer necessary in most cases because licensed anti-D reagents are sufficiently potent to identify patients with a weak expression of the D antigen as Rh positive. These individuals are considered Rh positive as donors and recipients.

Additional testing for red cell antigens is not recommended or encouraged by the American Association of Blood Banks (AABB).

Screening for unexpected antibodies

Unexpected antibodies are those other than anti-A or anti-B. Many blood banks screen all donated units for clinically significant antibodies rather than limiting their search to the donor group most likely to harbor them. The most likely donors of blood with unexpected antibodies are those with a history of pregnancy or previous transfusion. In general, clinically significant antibodies are those known to have caused hemolytic disease of the newborn, a frank hemolytic transfusion reaction, or unacceptably short survival of transfused red blood cells.[1]

Screening for transmissible disease

All donor blood must be tested to detect units that might transmit disease. Components and whole blood units must not be used for transfusion unless all tests are nonreactive, are negative, or have values within normal limits.

1. Test for syphilis using the serologic test for syphilis as required by the U.S. Food and Drug Administration (FDA).
2. Test for the presence of the hepatitis B surface antigen to identify hepatitis B infectivity.
3. Test for the presence of the antibody to hepatitis C virus (HCV).
4. Test for the presence of the hepatitis B core antibody. This component of the hepatitis B virus (HBV) testing may indicate an HBV carrier state.
5. Alanine aminotransaminase (ALT) is a serum enzyme that, if elevated, can signal liver malfunction. This test is no longer

required by the AABB, but many blood centers still perform it.

6. Test for the presence of the antibody to the human immunodeficiency viruses 1 and 2 (anti–HIV-1/2). A positive result using the standard screening methods necessitates a repeat standard screen and then a confirming screen using a more specific assay. In addition to this enzyme-linked immunosorbent assay (ELISA) to detect antibody, all blood must be tested for the presence of HIV (HIV-1 antigen test).
7. Test for the presence of the antibody to the human T-cell lymphotropic virus I (HTLS-1/2). (See Adverse Effects later in this chapter.)

BLOOD STORAGE AND PRESERVATION

Because blood is a living tissue at the time of its harvest from a donor and because it must remain healthy during its storage, substances are added to meet two conditions necessary for successful shelf life:

1. A food source must be provided to maintain adequate nutrition to the stored cells.
2. Anticoagulation must be achieved to ensure that the blood remains in its liquid cellular state for the duration of the storage period.

Several anticoagulants-preservatives are available from which to choose. All of them provide the aforementioned necessary conditions for shelf life, but they differ in the length of storage time that they provide (Table 10-2).

CPD (citrate-phosphate-dextrose) and CPDA-1 (citrate-phosphate-dextrose-adenine) differ in composition by just one substance—adenine. However, the addition of adenine extends the shelf life by 14 days and is of great significance to a blood transfusion service whose concern revolves around adequate blood reserves and their ability to supply upon demand. CPDA-1 is considered the anticoagulant-preservative of choice for whole blood and is also used when the donated unit may be processed into separate components.

The additive systems, commonly called *adenine-saline,* are approved by the FDA for the extended storage of red blood cells. These systems differ in composition by manufacturer. However, there is a limited menu from which these compounds are made. They contain various combinations of saline, adenine, dextrose, phosphate, citrate, and mannitol. These additives allow red cells to be stored for up to 42 days. The additive systems, which are secondary or "add-on" solutions, are used only with red cells that were harvested in a primary anticoagulant-preservative

Table 10-1   Testing of Donor Blood

TEST	TO DETERMINE
ABO—forward typing	Presence of antigen A or B on RBC
ABO—reverse typing	Presence of antibody A or antibody B in plasma
Rh typing:	
With anti-D sera	Presence of D antigen on RBC
With anti-D sera or with indirect antiglobulin test	Presence of the weak D antigen
Screen for unexpected antibodies	Presence of antibodies other than anti-A and anti-B
Screen for transmissible disease:	
Serologic test for syphilis	*Treponema* infection
Hepatitis B surface antigen	Infectivity for hepatitis B
Hepatitis C (anti-HCV)	Infectivity for hepatitis C
Hepatitis B core antibody	May indicate HBV carrier
Alanine aminotransferase*	Indicates liver damage
Human immunodeficiency virus (HIV):	
Enzyme-linked immunosorbent assay	Presence of antibody to HIV-1 and HIV-2
HIV-antigen	Presence of antibody to HIV virus
Human T-cell leukemia/lymphoma virus (HTLV-I)	Presence of antibody to HTLV-I/II

RBC, Red blood cell; *HBV,* hepatitis B virus.
*No longer required but included by many centers.

Table 10-2   Anticoagulants-Preservatives

ANTICOAGULANT-PRESERVATIVE	COMPOSITION	SHELF LIFE PROVIDED (DAYS)
CPD	Citrate, phosphate, and dextrose	21
CPDA-1	CPD plus adenine	35
Additive systems	CPD plus various preservative combinations	35-42

such as CPD. The red cells are then separated and mixed with the additive system.

Anticoagulants and preservatives

The following is a brief summary of the substances that help preserve blood.

Citrate. Sodium citrate by itself, or sometimes in combination with citric acid, achieves anticoagulation by inhibiting several calcium-dependent steps in the coagulation cascade. It also slows the process of glycolysis, which is the conversion of glucose to lactic acid and adenosine triphosphate (ATP) through various metabolic pathways (Embden-Meyerhof, Kreb's cycle, and the electron transport system). Slowing glycolysis allows adequate amounts of ATP to continue to be produced and the limited supply of sugar in the stored cells to be preserved.

Phosphate. Inorganic phosphate acts as a buffer that helps maintain the pH.

Dextrose. When sugars were first investigated as possible participants in blood preservation, red blood cells were thought to be impermeable to them. Therefore it was theorized that sugar would act as a colloid to protect the cells against hemolysis. It was soon recognized that red blood cells are permeable to dextrose and that this was an excellent food source for the stored cells.[2] Dextrose is a deterrent to hemolysis but not because of a colloidal action. It supplies the food from which ATP, the principal intracellular energy-storage compound, is formed. Adequate supplies of ATP are necessary for the continued integrity of the cell.

Adenine. Although other factors appear to be involved, the ATP content of stored red blood cells generally can be equated with their viability (i.e., their capacity to survive in the recipient's bloodstream after transfusion). In the 1950s, it was shown that the ATP content of stored cells could be restored by adding adenosine, which is made of adenine and the 5-carbon sugar, ribose.[2,3] However, because of its toxicity, adenosine was never used in transfusion practice. Later it was discovered that adding adenine by itself accomplishes the same positive result of restoring ATP levels in stored red cells.[2]

Mannitol. Mannitol, which appears to reduce hemolysis by its effect as an osmotic stabilizer, is found in at least one of the additive systems.

Rejuvenation of red cells

Red cells that have been stored up to 3 days beyond their expiration dates can be incubated (at 37° C for 1 hour) in FDA-approved solutions containing inosine, pyruvate, phosphate, adenine, and sometimes glucose. This incubation will increase the cellular levels of ATP and 2,3-DPG. These rejuvenated cells may be washed and used within 24 hours, or they may be glycerolized and frozen for extended storage.[1]

IMMUNOHEMATOLOGY

Immunology is the scientific discipline that deals with the immune system and immune response (antibody response to antigenic stimulus). Immunohematology narrows the view of immunology to focus specifically on the antigens and antibodies of the blood.

The antigens of the blood, called *agglutinogens,* are found as integrated parts of the red cell membrane, as components of the white cells, and as soluble substances in the plasma. The largest group of agglutinogens, which numbers more than 400 belonging to 24 known systems, is associated with red cells.

The first set of red cell antigens discovered, those of the ABO system, was identified by Landsteiner at the turn of the twentieth century. The ABO system is the most important of the known antigen systems and is the foundation for determining compatibilities in transfusion therapy.

The ABO system

There are four blood types in the ABO system: A, B, AB, and O. The name of the blood type is determined by the name of the antigen on the red cell. The type of antigen present on the red cell is an inherited characteristic; the A and B genes are equally dominant, and the O gene is recessive (Table 10-3).

The A and B genes dictate the presence of A and B antigenic determinant sites, respectively. Although the O gene is inactive and does not code for any of the erythrocyte alloantigens, blood group O erythrocytes do exhibit an antigenic glycoprotein on their surface—the H antigen. This glycoprotein is not the product of the O gene, as evidenced by its presence on red blood cells of all types.

The relationship between the A, B, and H antigens can be explained as follows. During the synthesis of the blood group molecules, the H antigen is synthesized first; thus the H antigen is present on all red cells. If the A gene is present, it will code for a transferase (enzyme), which will facilitate the attachment of the sugar *N*-acetylgalactosamine to the H antigen. This chemical complex is the antigenic determinant for the blood group A. Similarly, the B gene will code for a different transferase that will allow for the attachment of an alternate sugar group, D-galactose, which will complete the antigenic determinant for blood type B. Group O individuals do not possess either enzyme system, and thus group O erythrocytes possess only the unmodified H antigen on their surface.[1,4]

The antibodies of the ABO system occur naturally (i.e., without direct antigen stimulation) and are called *isohemagglutinins.* They are complete, and in the presence of red cells that exhibit the corresponding antigen, they can cause agglutination in a saline medium. The antibody that agglutinates type A is

POSSIBLE GENOTYPES	PHENOTYPE	BLOOD GROUP	RED BLOOD CELL ANTIGEN	PLASMA ANTIBODY
OO	O	O	Neither A nor B	A and B
AA or AO	A	A	A	B
BB or BO	B	B	B	A
AB	AB	AB	A and B	Neither A nor B

Table 10-3 ABO Blood Groups

called *antibody A* (anti-A), and the corresponding antibody for the antigen B is called *antibody B* (anti-B).

This adversarial relationship between antigen and the corresponding antibody is the basis for understanding compatibilities within the ABO system. The antigens are located on the cells, and the antibodies reside in the plasma. If a unit of red cells is to be administered it should be thought of as an antigen and should be given only to a recipient who does not exhibit the corresponding antibody. Conversely, plasma should not be given to a recipient who possesses the corresponding red cell antigen (Table 10-4).

The Rh system

The Rh system is complex and extensive. Because nearly 50 Rh antigens have been identified, a complete discussion of this system is not included here. Sufficient for the topic of routine transfusion therapy are the unmodified terms of Rh+ (Rh positive) and Rh– (Rh negative), which refer to the presence or absence of the red cell antigen D.

The blood recipient who carries the antigen D (Rh positive) may receive products that are either Rh+ or Rh–. However, a recipient who is Rh negative should receive only blood products that are Rh negative. This is especially true for Rh-negative women of childbearing age who might become sensitized to the D antigen, which could raise the potential for complications in subsequent pregnancies.

The HLA system

The HLA blood grouping system consists of a series of highly immunogenic antigens that can be found predominantly on the cells of the leukocyte family. These antigens exist on the surface of the lymphocytes, granulocytes, monocytes, and platelets. Although the HLA antigens and their precipitated antibodies are best known for their role in transplantation rejection, they also contribute to several of the complications of transfusion therapy, including the following:

1. Febrile nonhemolytic reaction (FNH)
2. Immune-mediated platelet refractoriness
3. Transfusion-related acute lung injury (TRALI)
4. Transfusion-associated graft-versus-host disease (TA-GVHD)

PREPARATION AND CLINICAL APPLICATION OF BLOOD COMPONENTS
Whole blood

Whole blood requires no processing beyond collection into an anticoagulated closed collection system and testing. It is stored at 1° to 6° C with the satellite pack attached. If packed cells are needed at any time during the shelf life of the blood, this satellite pack will allow for their separation within a closed system. However, because whole blood transfusions are rarely used except to treat massive blood loss, most homologous donations are not stored as whole blood but are separated into components soon after donation. Autologous donations, which are planned to be transfused back to the donor within the shelf life period for refrigerated blood, are stored whole. These units are often given as whole blood. They can be spun down and given as packed cells if the donor-recipient does not need or cannot tolerate the additional volume that the plasma represents.

Clinical applications for the administration of whole blood include the following:

- When increased oxygen-carrying capacity and volume expansion are needed
- When active bleeding has resulted in a 25% to 30% blood volume loss
- When exhange transfusion is performed

Although whole blood may be appropriate for the preceding clinical situations, it is not always readily available. Therefore the use of packed red cells in combination with plasma has become the standard when replacement therapy is needed in surgery or trauma cases.[1]

Packed red blood cells

Packed cells are prepared by separating the plasma from the cellular portion of a unit of whole blood. This can be done any time before the expiration date. Cells can be separated from plasma by centrifuge, which causes a rapid separation, or by sedimentation, in which cells will settle to the bottom of an upright container and the plasma will concentrate on top. Once separation has occurred, 200 to 250 ml of plasma can be manually expressed off into the attached satellite bag.

The shelf life of a unit of packed red blood cells (PRBCs) is the same as that for the unit of whole blood from which it was obtained, but it can be extended if an additive system is mixed with the cells at the time of their separation (see previous discussion, Anticoagulants and Preservatives). These additive

Table 10-4	**Summary of Compatibilities**	
COMPONENT	**COMPATIBILITIES**	
Whole blood	Give type-specific blood only	
Packed red cells (stored, washed, or frozen/washed)	**Donor**	**Recipient**
	O	O, A, B, AB
	A	A, AB
	B	B, AB
	AB	AB
Fresh-frozen plasma	**Donor**	**Recipient**
	O	O
	A	A, O
	B	B, O
	AB	AB, B, A, O
Platelets	RBC: ABO and Rh compatible *preferred*	
	Donor	**Recipient**
	O	O, A, B, AB
	A	A, AB
	B	B, AB
	AB	AB
Cryoprecipitate	Plasma: ABO compatible *preferred*	
	Donor	**Recipient**
	O	O
	A	A, O
	B	B, O
	AB	AB, B, A, O

systems, which must be used within 72 hours of the blood donation, extend the shelf life of the packed cells from 35 to 42 days.

PRBCs are used for routine blood replacement during surgery and to increase the oxygen-carrying capacity (i.e., the red blood cell mass) in patients with symptomatic anemia that cannot be treated with pharmaceuticals.

Modified packed red blood cells

Saline-washed red blood cells. Saline washing of red blood cells (RBCs) is carried out in the blood bank using automated or semiautomated equipment. The washed cells are suspended in sterile normal saline, and the processed product has a hematocrit of 70% to 80%. This process removes platelets and cellular debris, diminishes plasma to trace levels, and reduces the number of leukocytes. It should be noted that the leukocytes are not eliminated, so this component does contain viable lymphocytes and it can precipitate the graft-versus-host response. Stored packed cells may be washed at any time during the shelf life. However, because the washing is performed in an open system, their shelf life at 1° to 6° C is only 24 hours after washing. This limited shelf life is imposed because of concerns for bacterial contamination; washed red cells are not considered free from the risk of disease transmission.

Washed packed cells are used for patients with recurrent or severe allergic reactions thought to be related to one or more plasma proteins and for neonatal and intrauterine transfusions.

Frozen-deglycerolized packed cells. Two decades ago, there were many reasons for freezing blood, but they have diminished over time because of improved technologies. Today, blood is frozen for one reason: long-term storage. For autologous blood, this extended storage capacity means that blood can be stored well beyond the 42-day shelf life afforded by refrigeration. This permits scheduling of elective surgical procedures well in advance and allows the donatation of enough blood to provide for the safety of autologous transfusion.

In addition to its application in autologous transfusion, blood is frozen to maintain stores of rare blood types. AABB's *Standards for blood banks and transfusion services*[5] allows frozen blood intended for routine transfusion to be stored for up to 10 years. For blood of rare phenotype, this 10-year frame may be extended at the discretion of the blood bank director.

Blood that is to be frozen may be collected in CPD or CPDA-1 and stored as whole blood. It can also be stored as packed cells with or without an additive system. Most often, blood is glycerolized and frozen within the first 6 days after donation. Glycerol is added to the cells before freezing because it is a cryoprotective agent that prevents cell dehydration and mechanical damage from ice formation. Although the first 6 days after donation is the usual window in which to freeze blood, red cells nearing the end of their shelf life may be rejuvenated for up to 3 days after expiration and then frozen. PRBCs preserved in adenine-saline solutions may be frozen up to 42 days after donation. These options help eliminate unnecessary waste of valuable blood stores. Frozen blood is maintained at –65° C or colder.[1]

When a unit of frozen blood is needed, it is first thawed in a water bath (37° C) or a dry warmer (37° C). It is then washed to remove the glycerol, which is hypertonic to the blood. The washing process used to deglycerolize red cells is the same as that used to process washed red cells.

As with saline-washed packed cells, there are concerns for bacterial contamination with frozen-deglycerolized cells. This product must be infused within 24 hours of processing. Also, as is true with washed packed cells, frozen-deglycerolized cells are not considered free from the risk of disease transmission. Clinical applications for frozen-deglycerolized red blood cells are the same as those for washed PRBCs.

Leukocyte-filtered red blood cells. Leukocyte-filtered RBCs, also known as *leukocyte-reduced RBCs,* are indicated for patients who have experienced repeated febrile nonhemolytic reactions associated with the transfusion of red cells or platelets (see discussion in Adverse Effects: Immediate). They should also be used as prophylaxis against alloimmunization in selected patients who are expected to receive long-term blood component therapy and for recipients who are at risk for posttransfusion cytomegalovirus (CMV) infection.

Leukocyte-reduced packed cells can be prepared in the blood bank by centrifugation and filtration and by automated saline washing of liquid or previously frozen blood. In the past, frozen and washed packed cells, which have a 95% to 99% reduction in leukocytes, were considered the components of choice when white blood cell reduction was indicated. However, the newer generations of leukocyte filters, which are more efficient in terms of leukocyte reduction and less costly, have made leukocyte-filtered components the products of choice. The cells may be filtered during the initial processing of red cells before storage or during transfusion using an in-line filter. The AABB *Technical Manual*[1] states that in all clinical applications of leukocyte-reduced products, prestorage leukocyte-filtered components are recommended over those that are filtered during transfusion.

Clinical applications for leukocyte-reduced red blood cells include the following:

- Patients with repeated febrile nonhemolytic transfusion reactions
- Patients at risk for HLA alloimmunization who may face hemotherapy
- Patients at risk for posttransfusion CMV infections

Granulocytes

Granulocytes are usually prepared by leukopheresis. This preparation also contains other leukocytes, platelets, and some red cells in 200 to 300 ml of plasma. They should be transfused as soon as possible after collection but may be stored at 20° to 24° C without agitation for up to 24 hours.[1]

The use of granulocyte transfusion in adults is rare. When this therapy is used, the recipient is usually severely neutropenic with documented infection that is unresponsive to aggressive antibiotic therapy. According to the AABB,[1] the candidate for granulocyte transfusion should meet the following four conditions:

1. Neutropenia (granulocyte count less than 500/μl)

2. Fever for 24 to 48 hours, unresponsive to appropriate antibiotic therapy, or bacterial sepsis unresponsive to antibiotics or other modes of therapy
3. Myeloid hypoplasia
4. A reasonable chance for return of marrow function[1]

In the pediatric population, granulocyte transfusion has been used in conjunction with antibiotic therapy for severe bacterial neonatal sepsis. Although controversy surrounds this choice of therapy, there appear to be clinical situations in which granulocyte transfusion can supplement antibiotics. The AABB[1] states that pediatric candidates for granulocyte transfusion are infants with all of the following conditions:

1. Strong evidence of bacterial septicemia
2. An absolute neutrophil count below 3000/μl
3. A diminished marrow storage pool

Granulocytes should come from CMV-negative donors because they cannot be given though a leukocyte filter to reduce the risk of CMV transmission. Granulocytes should also be irradiated to reduce the risk of GVHD.

Fresh frozen plasma

Fresh-frozen plasma (FFP) is prepared by removing the plasma from a unit of whole blood and freezing it within 6 hours of collection. The storage time for FFP is 1 year at 18° C or colder. This component, if kept frozen and then thawed in a warm water bath (30° to 37° C) just before use, is an excellent source of all clotting factors, including the labile factors V and VIII and fibrinogen. The activity of these labile factors is lost when plasma is stored in the nonfrozen state.[1]

FFP is indicated when clotting factors are needed for which a concentrate is not available, in the presence of severe liver disease where limited synthesis of plasma coagulation factors may be suspected, and when needed to counteract the effects of warfarin therapy (Box 10-1).

Platelet concentrates

Platelet concentrates can be prepared by two methods: as single units from multiple donors or as multiple units from a single donor.

Multiple donors, single units

1. A donated unit of whole blood that is less than 6 hours old and stored at room temperature is centrifuged to separate off the platelet-rich plasma.

---

2. The platelet-rich plasma is then centrifuged at 20° C to separate the platelet concentrate from the now platelet-poor plasma. Fifty to seventy milliliters of plasma are allowed to remain with the platelet concentrate.
3. After this second centrifugation, that which remains is a single unit of random-donor platelet suspended in plasma. The plasma will ensure that the platelets are kept at a pH of 6 or higher to maintain their viability during the 5-day storage period at 20° to 24° C.

Single donor, multiple units. Plateletpheresis is the harvesting of multiple units of platelets from a single volunteer donor. The quantity taken from a single donor is equal to approximately 6 units of random-donor platelets. The platelets are harvested by automated machines called *cell separators*. These separators isolate the blood component to be harvested as a concentrate, and those components not needed are returned to the donor.

Although plateletpheresis is an efficient way to obtain supplies of platelets, there are two reasons why this method is not used exclusively. First, there are several risks to the donor, including allergic reactions, chills, syncope, and citrate toxicity. The citrate toxicity is related to the anticoagulation of the donor blood, which is necessary before the blood is processed through the cell separator.[2] This anticoagulation, in varying amounts, is ultimately infused along with the returned components to the donor. The second reason that plateletpheresis is limited in its use is concern over its cost-versus-benefit ratio.

Single-donor platelets have been used for patients who need repeated platelet infusions and who are at risk for alloimmunization to foreign leukocyte antigen (HLAs) that are present on leukocytes and platelets. It has been widely accepted that the risk for alloimmunization increases with the increasing number of donors to whom the recipient is exposed. Therefore the single-donor option reduces the recipient's exposure from six donors to one with each single-donor unit. It now appears that platelet alloimmunization and refractoriness are more closely aligned with exposure to leukocytes during transfusion than to the number of donor exposures, but the single-donor option for platelet replacement in the multitransfused patient remains desirable.[1]

Refractoriness is the state of being inadequately responsive to platelet transfusions. This occurs in about 20% to 70% of multitransfused thrombocytopenic patients and is more likely to be seen in patients being treated for malignant hematopoietic disorders.[1]

There are both nonimmune reasons and immune-response causes for refractoriness. Some of the nonimmune causes of platelet refractoriness are active bleeding, sepsis, splenomegaly, disseminated intravascular coagulation (DIC), and antibiotic therapy. Of the possible immune-response causes, the presence of antibodies in the recipient to multiple HLAs is the most common precipitating factor. As explained earlier, alloimmunization to HLA is a direct result from previous exposure to white blood cells through transfusions. Therefore it has been recommended that all blood components containing white blood cells that are to be used for recipients requiring long-term transfusion support should be leukocyte reduced by filtration.[6] This would limit exposure to foreign HLAs and reduce the risk for

---

Box 10-1   Clinical Applications for Fresh-Frozen Plasma

- For patients with active bleeding who have multiple coagulation factor deficiencies secondary to liver disease
- For patients with disseminated intravascular coagulation and evidence of demonstrated dilutional coagulopathy from large-volume replacement
- For patients with congenital factor deficiencies for which there are no concentrates (e.g., factors V and XI)
- For warfarin reversal

Table 10-5   Factor VIII Complex

FACTOR	ACTIVITY
VIII:C	Procoagulant
VIII:Ag	Immune reactant antigen
VIII:vWF	von Willebrand's factor: required for normal platelet function

Table 10-6   Inherited Coagulopathies

TYPE	ALSO KNOWN AS	FACTOR DEFICIENCY
Hemophilia A	Classic hemophilia	VIII:C
Hemophilia B	Christmas disease	IX
von Willebrand's disease	Vascular hemophilia or angiohemophilia	VIII:C VIII:Ag VIII:vWF

Box 10-2   Major Inherited Coagulopathies

HEMOPHILIA A (CLASSIC HEMOPHILIA)

This sex-linked inherited disorder is manifest in males but is transmitted by female carriers. The clotting factor deficiency in classic hemophilia is factor VIII:C. Commercial factor VIII concentrates provide factor VIII:C. In the past, cryoprecipitate was used to treat this deficiency. Today, it is used only if commercial virus-inactivated concentrates are unavailable.

VON WILLEBRAND'S DISEASE

This condition, the most common of the inherited coagulopathies (Table 10-6), is not sex linked and affects both sexes. All three of the measurable activities of the factor VIII complex are deficient in von Willebrand's disease. However, it is the deficiency of factor VIII:vWF that is responsible for the capillary defect seen in this coagulopathy. Von Willebrand factor is necessary for normal platelet function, and thus a diminished level of this factor will result in platelet dysfunction characterized by capillary defect.

Mild cases of von Willebrand's disease can be treated with DDAVP (desmopressin acetate), which is a synthetic analog of vasopressin. DDAVP appears to cause the release of endogenous stores of high-molecular-weight von Willebrand's factor from the vascular subendothelium.[1]

More severe cases of this disease are treated with virus-inactivated commercially prepared factor VIII concentrates. Although not all commercial concentrates contain therapeutic levels of vWF, there are a limited number that meet this need. If the appropriate commercially prepared product is unavailable, severe cases may be treated with cryoprecipitate or fresh-frozen plasma. In this situation, cryoprecipitate would be the component of choice because of its higher concentration of vWF.

HYPOFIBRINOGENEMIA

This deficiency may be inherited or acquired as part of the disseminated intravascular coagulation (DIC) syndrome. Cryoprecipitate is the only source currently available for concentrated fibrinogen.

FACTOR XIII DEFICIENCY

This clotting factor is also called the *fibrin stabilizing factor*. A deficiency of this factor leads to bleeding, poor wound healing, and an increased incidence of spontaneous abortion.[6] Intravenous supplementation of factor XIII is accomplished by the use of cryoprecipitate.

---

alloimmunization and the majority of immune-response refractoriness. When these antibodies are known to be present, one approach is to transfuse multiunit platelets from a single donor.

The most suitable single-donor platelet preparation in cases of known HLA sensitization is the HLA-matched product, obtained by plateletpheresis from a volunteer donor who is HLA-matched to the recipient. Although this is a limited match (the donor and recipient have only some HLA antigens in common), this product is the most appropriate for the patient who has demonstrated unresponsiveness to platelet concentrates. HLA-matched platelets should be irradiated to prevent TA-GVHD (see Adverse Effects later in this chapter).

In addition to the HLA-matching approach to providing platelets in refractoriness, a second option is pretransfusion platelet crossmatching. This approach is predictive and can therefore avoid subsequent platelet transfusion failures.[1] However, platelet crossmatching is not without shortcomings. When 70% or more of the donors are reactive to the recipient, finding enough compatible donors can be a problem. Both HLA matching and platelet crossmatching have their merits, and many facilities use a combination of these approaches for refractory patients.[1]

Cryoprecipitate (cryoprecipitated antihemolytic factor)

Cryoprecipitated antihemophilic factor is prepared by slowly thawing a unit of FFP at 4° to 6° C and recovering the cold precipitated protein by centrifugation. Once harvested, Cryo can be refrozen at –18° C or colder and stored for 1 year. This component is a rich source of the entire factor VIII complex (Table 10-5), factor XIII, fibronectin, and fibrinogen, and it is the only source of concentrated fibrinogen.

Cryoprecipitate is used to treat hypofibrinogenemia and factor XIII deficiency (Box 10-2).

ADMINISTRATION OF BLOOD COMPONENTS

Administering a blood component is the last step in the process of matching a donor component with a recipient. Remembering that the most common causes of fatal transfusion reactions are improperly labeled blood samples, mislabeled component units, and misidentified recipients, it is clear that most fatal transfusion errors are clerical rather than laboratory failures. The transfusionist is the last person in the administration process with the opportunity to note a clerical error. Therefore the transfusionist should be attentive to every detail of the administration procedure and guard against the relaxed approach that so often accompanies familiarity.

Policies and procedures for the administration of blood components vary greatly among providers of this therapy, but their purpose, which is to ensure precision and safety, is universal (Box 10-3). Therefore those who administer transfusion therapy should be knowledgeable of policy and adhere strictly to

Box 10-3   **Basic Guidelines for Blood Administration**

1. Gloves should be worn when handling blood products.
2. Blood should not be out of controlled refrigeration for longer than 30 minutes before being initiated as a transfusion.
3. Blood should not be stored in non–blood bank refrigerators because they are subject to vast fluctuations in temperature.
4. No intravenous solution other than isotonic saline (0.9%) should be added to or administered simultaneously with blood.
5. A blood administration set should not be affixed ("piggybacked") into a main line that has been used for any solution other than isotonic saline.
6. All blood components must be filtered using in-line or add-on filters that are appropriate for the component or specifically requested by a physician's order.
7. A new administration set and filter should be used for each transfusion. A blood filter should not be used for more than 4 hours.[1]

the procedures embraced by their particular institution or home care provider.

Table 10-7 presents a detailed summary of blood components, including their preparation, indications for use, blood type compatibility, administration, and special considerations.

SPECIAL EQUIPMENT
Blood warmers

Blood warming during transfusion is recommended in limited situations. Blood can be warmed by any of several commercial instruments that were designed for this purpose. Most of these instruments consist of dry heating blocks or controlled water baths that surround a portion of the infusion tubing downstream from the blood supply and immediately before the infusion site.

Blood warming should not be attempted with uncontrolled measures such as holding the unit of blood under hot water or warming it in a microwave oven. Such severe treatment of the blood cells can result in hemolysis or severe reactions. The AABB[1] states that warming devices must not raise the temperature of the blood to a level that causes hemolysis. These devices should have a visible thermometer and, ideally, an audible alarm that sounds before the manufacturer's designated temperature limit has been exceeded.[1] Hemolysis occurs at temperatures above 42° C.[6]

All blood warmers are designed to help transfer heat. The efficiency of this heat transfer depends on the following factors:

- The temperature of the heating element (flat bed or water bath)
- The surface area of the heating element
- The diameter and the surface area of the tubing being used to deliver the blood
- The length of time the blood being infused remains in contact with the heat source

If any of these factors (temperature, surface area, or contact time) are changed, the efficiency of the heat transfer is altered. Therefore, when rapid infusion is necessary, the transfusionist needs to be aware that increasing the infusion rate reduces the time in contact between the blood and the heating element and the efficiency of the heat transfer.

Indications for blood warming
Multiple trauma/massive blood loss. Hypothermia is a serious threat for the patient who has lost large quantities of blood and requires multiple transfusions of refrigerated blood. A decrease in body temperature at the sinoatrial (SA) node to 86° F (30° C) can precipitate cardiac arrhythmias and cardiac arrest.[1] Therefore, when large quantities are to be infused very rapidly, blood warming is indicated. This is especially true if the infusion is through a central catheter. However, the present generation of blood warmers has been criticized for slow heat transfer and suboptimal flow rates. This has led to the use of blood warmers that use higher temperatures and positive-pressure-pump administration. An alternative technique, called *rapid admixture*, has been reported.[7] This technique involves keeping 0.9% sodium chloride intravenous (IV) solution stored in a clinical incubator at 70° C. When needed, the warmed bag of 0.9% sodium chloride (250 ml) is connected directly to the unit of packed cells to be infused, and the saline is squeezed into the blood bag. This warms the blood to 37° C in less than a minute.

Cold agglutinin disease. Cold-loving autoantibodies correspond to the carbohydrate antigens I and i, which are found on red blood cells.[4] Many otherwise normal individuals have some anti-I in their serum, which can be demonstrated when tests are done at 4° C. This antibody, if present, is usually found at low titers and does not cause hemolysis. However, cold agglutinin hemolysis occurs both as a self-limited syndrome in association with certain infectious diseases and as a chronic illness, often without cause. Sometimes, however, it is seen to accompany lymphoma and other reticuloendothelial malignancies. The anti-I titers seen in cases of hemolysis are high, and red cell destruction can occur either extravascularly within the phagocytic cells or intravascularly, leading to hemoglobinemia.

The trigger for the activation of the anti-I to bind with the antigen on the red blood cell, and thus cause hemolysis, is exposure to cold temperatures. Therefore recipients of blood transfusion who are known to carry a significant titer of anti-I should be transfused using an in-line blood warmer.

Pediatric application for blood warming. In pediatrics, blood warming should be used for exchange transfusions in infants and for blood infusion rates exceeding 15 ml/kg/hr in children.[8]

Specialized blood filters

Blood filters are used to eliminate blood clots and cellular debris that occur during storage of the infusing blood component. The size of the particles being filtered out is determined by the micron pore size of the filter. A standard blood filter of 170 microns will trap particles that are 170 microns or larger. However, microaggregates, which consist of degenerating platelets, leukocytes, and fibrin strands, range in size from 20 to 160

Table 10-7 Summary of Blood Components

Component	Preparation/Composition	Use/Indications	ABO/Rh Compatibility		Administration	Special Consideration
			Donor	**Recipient**		
Whole blood	RBCs WBCs Plasma Platelets (WBCs, platelets, and some clotting factors not viable after 24 hr of storage)	Increase RBC mass Increase volume	O A B AB Rh+ Rh−	O A B AB Rh+ Rh−, Rh+	1. Transfuse through a blood filter. 2. Should infuse within 4 hr.	1. One unit of whole blood will increase Hct by 3%; will increase Hgb by 1 g/dl. 2. Availability of packed RBCs has made use of whole blood obsolete in most cases. 3. Never infuse blood with anything except 0.9% saline.
Red blood cells (RBCs): packed	RBCs WBCs Platelets Minimal plasma	Increase RBC mass and oxygen-carrying capacity	O A B AB Rh+ Rh−	O, A, B, AB A, AB B, AB AB Rh+ Rh−, Rh+	1. Transfuse through a blood filter. 2. Should infuse within 4 hr.	1. Hct of product is 60%-80%. 2. One unit of RBCs will increase Hct by 3%; will increase Hgb by 1 g/dl. 3. Never infuse packed RBCs with anything except 0.9% saline.
RBCs: leukocyte reduced	RBCs Negligible WBCs Minimal plasma and platelets	Same as packed RBCs plus: to decrease risk for alloimmunization (HLA) and disease transmission (CMV)	Same as packed RBCs		If not processed in blood bank, use in-line or add-on leukocyte reduction filter.	1. Leukocyte-reduction filter for RBCs is not interchangeable with a leukocyte-reduction filter for platelets. 2. Other considerations are the same as above for packed RBCs.
Red blood cells: saline washed	RBCs Minimal WBCs 99% plasma proteins removed No platelets	Same as for packed RBCs plus: Decrease risk for allo-immunization to leukocyte or HLA antigens; however, not component of choice for this purpose Reduce incidence of urticarial and anaphylactic reactions to plasma	Same as packed RBCs		Same as packed RBCs	1. Units must be given within 24 hr of saline washing. 2. Never infuse RBCs with any IV fluid or medications except 0.9% saline. 3. Does contain viable lymphocytes and can induce GVHD.
Red blood cells: frozen-deglycerolized	Same as washed RBCs	Same as packed RBCs plus: Prolonged blood storage Autologous blood Rare blood types	Same as packed RBCs		Same as packed RBCs	1. Blood may be frozen up to 10 yr. 2. Once blood has been thawed and deglycerolized, it must be transfused within 24 hr.

Product	Composition	Indications	Donor / Recipient	Administration	Special considerations
Fresh-frozen plasma	Plasma with all clotting factors	Treatment of some coagulation disorders. Reversal of warfarin in patients who require emergency invasive procedures	**Donor** — **Recipient** O — O A — A, O B — B, O AB — AB, O, A, B Rh+ — Rh+, Rh− Rh− — Rh−, Rh+	1. Transfuse through a blood filter.	1. Must be infused within 24 hr of thawing. 2. May be stored for up to 1 yr at −18°C.
Platelets: random donor	Platelets. Plasma. Small numbers of RBCs and WBCs	To control or prevent bleeding associated with deficiencies in platelet number or function. Not usually effective in conditions of rapid platelet destruction (i.e., ITP and DIC)	ABO/Rh compatibility is preferred (because of RBCs in product), but not mandatory; an Rh− female in childbearing years should receive Rh− platelets; if she receives Rh-positive plates, titers should be monitored and/or consideration given for administration of Rh immune globulin	1. Transfuse through a blood filter. 2. Once individual units are pooled, they should be infused within 6 hr. 3. Concentrates may be infused individually or pooled immediately before administration.	1. Prophylactic pretransfusion medications (i.e., an antihistamine and/or acetaminophen) may be given to decrease incidence of chills, fever, and allergic reactions. 2. Repeated transfusions may lead to alloimmunization to HLA and other antigens and result in the development of a "refractory" state manifested by unresponsiveness to platelet transfusion. 3. A leukocyte-reduction filter for platelets may be used. 4. One unit of platelets should increase platelet count of a 70-kg adult by 5000/μl.
Platelets: apheresed	Platelets (1 unit approximately equivalent to six random-donor units). Some RBCs, WBCs, and plasma	Same as random-donor platelets. May be used in nonrefractory patients to limit multiple random donor exposures, especially in long-term hemotherapy	Same as random-donor platelets	Same as random-donor platelets	1. Prophylactic pretransfusion medications may be given. 2. A leukocyte-reduction filter for platelets may be used.
Platelets: HLA-matched	Same as apheresed platelets but with some donor HLA antigens in common with the recipient	Same as random-donor platelets. Used for patients who are unresponsive to random-donor platelet concentrates as a result of HLA alloimmunization. May be used in patients being considered for future transplant	Same as random-donor platelets	Same as random-donor platelets	1. Prophylactic pretransfusion medications may be given. 2. A leukocyte-reduction filter for platelets may be used. 3. Advance scheduling to obtain HLA-matched platelets is usually required. 4. A blood sample for HLA typing should be done before immunosuppressive therapy is started. Leukopenia can make HLA typing difficult.

Continued

WBCs, White blood cells; *Hct*, hematocrit; *Hgb*, hemoglobulin; *CMV*, cytomegalovirus; *IV*, intravenous; *GVHD*, graft-versus-host disease; *ITP*, idiopathic thrombocytopenia; *DIC*, disseminated intravascular coagulation; *IM*, intramuscular.

Table 10-7 Summary of Blood Components—cont'd

Component	Preparation/Composition	Use/Indications	ABO/Rh Compatibility		Administration	Special Consideration
			Donor	**Recipient**		
Granulocytes	Granulocytes, varying amounts of leukocytes, platelets, and some RBCs in 200-300 ml of plasma Should come from CMV-negative donor Should be irradiated	Treatment of patients with severe neutropenia with serious infection unresponsive to antibiotic therapy Adults: rarely used Pediatrics: some applications	O A B AB Rh+ Rh–	O, A, B, AB A, AB B, AB AB Rh+ Rh–, Rh+	1. Transfuse through blood filter. 2. *Do not* use leukocyte-reduction filter. 3. Transfuse ASAP after collection.	1. Use of pretransfusion medication strongly urged (e.g., antihistamines, acetaminophen, steroids, meperidine). 2. Prophylactic use is *not* appropriate.
Cryoprecipitate	Factor VIII; von Willebrand's factor; factor XIII; fibrinogen (suspended in plasma and frozen)	Treatment of deficiencies in factor XIII and fibrinogen If factor VIII concentrates unavailable, may be used for hemophilia A and severe von Willebrand's disease	O A B AB Rh+ Rh– Cryoprecipitate contains a small amount of plasma and no RBCs; *plasma compatibilities are preferred but not required*	O A, O B, O AB, O, A, B Rh+, Rh– Rh–, Rh+	1. Transfuse through blood filter. 2. May be infused as single units or pooled.	1. Saline 0.9% may need to be added to each bag of cryoprecipitate to facilitate recovery of product. (There are only 10-15 ml of cryo/plasma in each bag.) 2. Cryoprecipitate must be infused within 6 hr of thawing or 4 hr of pooling.
Factor VIII concentrate	Lyophilized concentration of factor VIII, trace amount of other plasma proteins This product is virus inactivated	Factor VIII deficiency (hemophilia A) Some of the newer concentrates can be used in von Willebrand's disease	Not required		1. Quantity of factor VIII present in each vial noted as International Units (IU). 2. Reconstituted with sterile diluent. 3. IV injected using filter needle or given by IV drip using a component recipient set.	1. May be used prophylactically before therapeutic procedures. 2. Risk of transmission of infectious disease is reduced.
Factor IX concentrate	Lyophilized concentration of factor IX; virus inactivated	Factor IX deficiency (hemophilia B), also known as *Christmas disease*	Not required		1. Quantity of factor IX present in each vial noted as activity units. 2. Reconstituted with sterile diluent. 3. IV injected using filter needle or given IV drip using a component recipient set.	1. Risk of transmission of infectious disease is reduced.

Albumin	Available as a 5% or 25% solution.	Not required	5% is used for volume expansion when crystalloid solutions are not adequate	1. 5% solution is isotonic. 2. 25% solution is hypertonic, will increase circulating volume by 3-4 times infused volume. Infuse slowly.	1. Does not transmit viral diseases because of extended heating period during processing.
Immune serum globulin: nonspecific	IgG antibodies	Not required	Provide passive immune protection. Treatment of immunodeficiency disorders	1. May be given IM or IV, but various preparations are route of administration specific.	1. IM injections may be painful. Warm compresses may alleviate discomfort. 2. There is a possibility of hypersensitivity and anaphylactic reactions.
Immune serum globulin: Rh immune globulin	IgG anti-D	Not required	Administered to Rh− patients who have been exposed to Rh(D) antigens through transfusions or pregnancy. May be given antepartum to prevent sensitization to Rh(D) in Rh− woman carrying an Rh+ fetus. May be given before amniocentesis	Administered IM	1. Should be given within 72 hr of exposure for maximum effect. 2. IM injections may be painful. Warm compresses may alleviate discomfort. 3. Antepartum administration at 28 wk.
Immune serum globulin: hepatitis B immune globulin	High titers of hepatitis B antibody	Not required	Provides passive immunity following exposure to the hepatitis B virus	Administered IM	1. Should be given as soon as possible after exposure for maximum effect. 2. If given more than 7 days after exposure, its value is questionable. 3. IM injections may be painful. Warm compresses may alleviate discomfort.

microns.[1] Some of these microaggregates, which form in blood after 5 days or more of storage, can pass through standard blood filters without difficulty. Therefore, when it is deemed medically necessary to eliminate debris smaller than 80 to 170 microns, specialized filters have to be used.

Microaggregate filters. Microaggregate filters eliminate debris as small as 20 microns. They are used routinely during cardiopulmonary bypass[1] and often during large-volume replacement in massive trauma. The use of these specialized filters is not considered warranted in routine transfusion therapy.

Leukocyte-reduction filters. Leukocyte-reduction filters were first developed in Europe in the 1970s. The original filter material was cotton wool, which was later replaced by cellulose acetate fibers. Today, the most widely used leukocyte-reduction filters are of a flatbed, multilayered design and use polyester fibers to form the filter network. This latest generation of prestorage leukocyte-removing filters reliably reduces the number of leukocytes by 99.9%.[1]

One of the reasons for using leukocyte-reduction filters is to circumvent or prevent HLA alloimmunization. The minimum dose of white blood cells capable of stimulating antibody production is unknown. Although using leukocyte-filtered components will not completely eliminate the risk for alloimmunization, the filtered product nonetheless carries the lowest level of residual leukocytes. Another reason for using the filters is to reduce the risk for CMV transmission. Transfusion-associated CMV infections have been linked to the transfused peripheral blood leukocytes in which the virus established latent infection.

Prestorage filtration to reduce leukocytes has been advocated for the following reasons:

- To reduce the risk for transfusion-associated viral disease where the virus is known to have a latent phase in the white blood cells (some herpesviruses and some human T-cell lymphotropic viruses)
- To reduce the risk for febrile and allergic transfusion reactions; during storage, leukocytes degranulate and fragment, releasing substances that promote such reactions[1]
- To produce superior-quality packed cells that are leukocyte reduced and free of microaggregates.

ADVERSE EFFECTS

From the standpoint of disease transmission, blood component therapy has never been safer than it is today. With new technologies in filtration, cell separation, and cell salvaging for autotransfusion, never have so many options been available for hemotherapy, and never has the therapy been used as often as it is today. Widespread use, however, is a double-edged sword. Blood component therapy can deliver great therapeutic benefit, but it is also known to carry significant risks, not all of which are preventable. The balance between risk and benefit should always be weighted toward therapeutic benefit.

The adverse effects of blood transfusion can be classified as immunologic or nonimmunologic, depending on whether the immune system is triggered. These classifications may be further divided into categories of acute and delayed effects. Acute effects are those that happen within the first 24 hours of transfusion.

Delayed effects are those that appear beyond the acute time frame.

Acute effects

Acute adverse effects of blood transfusion can be immunologic or nonimmunologic (Table 10-8).

Immunologic classification

Intravascular hemolysis. The cause of intravascular hemolysis, a potentially fatal reaction, is ABO incompatibility. Because mortality has been associated with intravascular hemolysis, rapid recognition and immediate intervention can avoid the need for dialysis in the face of renal failure (see Table 10-8 for signs and symptoms).

The most common causes of ABO incompatibility are improperly labeled pretransfusion blood samples drawn for type and crossmatch, improperly identified donor units, and improperly identified recipients. Therefore the intravascular hemolytic reaction, which is the primary cause of transfusion-associated death, is also preventable. It cannot be overstated that every step of policy and procedure for identifying blood samples, recipients, and donor components for transfusion should be taken with strict attention to detail. Extra steps should be taken if a hemolytic reaction is suspected (Box 10-4).[1]

Extravascular hemolysis. Extravascular hemolysis is caused by the presence of antibodies to blood group systems other than ABO, such as Rh, Kidd, Kell, or Duffy. These antibodies do not cause immediate hemolysis within the vascular tree, but they bind with the corresponding antigen-carrying red cells. These cells are then seen as "defective" by the body and are destroyed extravascularly. This hemolysis is not as rapid as that seen in ABO incompatibility, and the symptoms are usually less dramatic. The posttransfusion direct antiglobulin test will be positive because the red cells are coated with antibodies in vivo.

Febrile nonhemolytic reaction. A *febrile nonhemolytic (FNH) reaction* is a temperature rise of 1° C or more occurring in association with transfusion and without any other explanation.[1] A common cause for this event is an antigen-antibody response involving HLA antigens on donor white cells in conflict with antibodies in the recipient. The outward appearance of this reaction, which can include significant temperature increases often accompanied with rigors, can be dramatic and unnerving to the blood recipient. However, the signs and symptoms of this reaction are usually self-limiting.

FNH reactions usually are seen in recipients who have a history of multiple transfusions or multiple pregnancies and who have developed a significant HLA antibody titer. For individuals who have experienced two or more of these reactions, leukocyte-filtered products should be considered for future transfusions.

Transfusion-related acute lung injury. Transfusion-related acute lung injury (TRALI), which is the most severe transfusion reaction, probably occurs more often than is reported. It is caused by acquired leukocyte antibodies (anti-HLA or neutrophil antibodies). The offending antibodies can be found in the donor plasma, and the donor group with the highest potential for harboring these leukocyte antibodies is multiparous women.

Table 10-8   Acute Adverse Effects[1]

REACTION/COMPLICATION	ETIOLOGY	SIGNS AND SYMPTOMS	TREATMENT
IMMUNOLOGIC RESPONSE			
Intravascular hemolysis	ABO incompatibility, red cell infusion	Fever Low back pain Pain at IV site Hypotension Renal failure	Support blood pressure Maintain urine output Dialyze for renal failure
Extravascular hemolysis	Non-ABO incompatibility (e.g., Rh, Kidd, Kell)	Fever Anemia Increased bilirubin Positive DAT	Geared to symptomology, which can resemble intravascular, but seldom as severe
Febrile nonhemolytic (FNH)	Antibody to donor leukocytes	Fever Chills Rigors	Antipyretics With history of FNH: pretreat with antipyretics
Transfusion-related acute lung injury (TRALI)	Anti-HLA antibodies, neutrophil antibodies	Acute respiratory insufficiency Chills Fever Cyanosis Hypotension	Respiratory support IV steroids
Urticaric/allergic	Antibodies against foreign plasma protein	Urticaria	Oral or intramuscular antihistamines Temporarily stop the infusion and resume after resolution of symptoms
Secondary response: anaphylaxis	Antibody to donor plasma, usually anti-IgA	Flushing Dyspnea Hypotension	Blood pressure support (low-dose dopamine) Epinephrine
NONIMMUNOLOGIC RESPONSE			
Bacterial contamination	Most severe: gram-negative psychrophilic organisms (endotoxin-producing)	Fever Shock DIC Renal failure	High-dose antibiotics Blood pressure support Steroids

IV, Intravenous; *DAT,* direct antiglobulin test; *DIC,* disseminated intravascular coagulation.

Box 10-4   If Hemolytic Reaction Is Suspected

1. STOP THE TRANSFUSION. Take down the blood and all tubing involved. Attach a new bag of saline (using all-new administration equipment) to the IV catheter and keep the IV open.
2. Notify the physician and the blood bank immediately.
3. Check the blood bag compatibility tag, label, and patient identification for clerical errors.
4. Send anticoagulated and clotted blood samples, a blood transfusion reaction form (if applicable), and the blood bag to the blood bank. The blood bank may also request a fresh urine sample.
5. The physician may order blood urea nitrogen, creatinine, and coagulation studies.

IV, Intravenous.

Although not completely understood, there appear to be two mechanisms by which this immune response precipitates symptoms of acute respiratory insufficiency disproportionate to the volume of blood infused and without evidence of heart failure:

1. The leukocyte antigen-antibody reaction produces white cell aggregates large enough to be trapped in the pulmonary microvasculature, producing transient changes in vascular permeability with resultant pulmonary edema.[1]
2. The immune response may activate complement, which ultimately leads to the release of histamine and serotonin. Both histamine and serotonin, which participate in smooth muscle constriction and increased vascular permeability, could be active contributors to respiratory distress and pulmonary edema.

In most cases, if TRALI is recognized early and treated promptly with vigorous respiratory support, this potentially disastrous posttransfusion event will recede within 2 to 4 days.[1] (See Table 10-8 for the signs, symptoms, and appropriate interventions.)

Urticaria. Urticaria, an acute hypersensitivity reaction, is usually seen after a transfusion with plasma or blood components that are accompanied by a large volume of plasma (whole blood or platelet concentrates). The cause of this reaction is thought to be a foreign plasma protein to which the recipient responds with an allergic display.

If the signs and symptoms do not broaden beyond simple urticaria, the physician may opt to interrupt the transfusion long enough to administer an antihistamine by IV injection, wait for the symptoms to recede, and proceed slowly with the transfusion. If a patient has a history of multiple allergic reactions to transfusions, pretreatment with an antihistamine may be appropriate.

Secondary response: anaphylaxis.
The secondary, or anamnestic, response almost always occurs in individuals who have been sensitized (carry an antibody titer) to a foreign protein. The anaphylactic reaction occurs quickly and can proceed to life-threatening shock. The following features of the anaphylactic reaction distinguish it from other acute responses:

- Occurs after the infusion of only a few milliliters of blood or plasma
- Occurs in the absence of fever

The array of symptoms that may accompany the secondary response includes respiratory distress, bronchospasm, abdominal cramps, nausea, vomiting, diarrhea, shock, and loss of consciousness.[1]

Some of these reactions occur in IgA-deficient recipients who, through previous transfusion or pregnancy, have developed an anti-IgA titer. When these individuals are given blood products that contain IgA, the secondary response may be precipitated.

It is possible to obtain blood components from donors who are IgA deficient. Most authorities recommend that these components be reserved for individuals in whom anti-IgA has been identified and who have had previous documented anaphylactic reactions.[1] If IgA-deficient donor blood is unavailable, frozen-deglycerolized or washed cells may be used.

Nonimmunologic classification
Marked fever with shock.
Marked fever with shock is caused by bacterial contamination of donated blood, which can occur at any time during harvesting and processing. Mesophilic (warm-loving) organisms proliferate best in components that are stored at room temperature, whereas psychrophils (cold-loving) multiply best in refrigerator temperatures. Gram-negative psychrophils are responsible for the most clinically dramatic and life-threatening septicemic transfusion reactions. These severe reactions are characterized by high fevers, hypotension, DIC, and renal failure. Averting a fatal outcome requires that these reactions receive immediate intervention with high-dose IV antibiotics combined with therapy for shock, including steroids and vasopressors.[1]

Nonimmune hemolysis.
Most cases of nonimmune hemolysis are related to improper handling of the blood product during processing, storage, or administration. Nonimmune hemolysis can result from the following:

- Red cell exposure to nonisotonic IV solutions
- Improper storage such as nonglycerolized freezing or overheating
- Mechanical stress resulting from the following:
  - Less-than-adequate gauge infusion catheter
  - Roller pump for infusion (cardiac bypass)
  - Improperly set psi on pressure infusion pump
  - Improperly inflated or positioned blood bag pressure cuff

Miscellaneous adverse effects
Circulatory overload.
Posttransfusion congestive heart failure usually is seen in individuals who are already cardiac or pulmonary decompensated. However, high infusion rates or large-volume replacement can precipitate decompensation in those who are borderline unstable.

Hypothermia.
Hypothermia is seen with rapid infusion of large volumes of refrigerated blood and can result in cardiac arrest (see Specialized Equipment: Blood Warmers).

Citrate overload (hypocalcemia).
Citrate is metabolized by the liver, and blood recipients with liver impairment may be unable to handle the high citrate load that accompanies large-volume transfusion. As the plasma level of citrate rises, it binds with free calcium and a secondary hypocalcemia results. Depending on the severity of the calcium deficit, the calcium may be replaced by oral supplement or intravenous infusion.

Delayed effects
Immunologic classification
Graft-versus-host disease.
A well-recognized but rare complication of transfusion therapy is TA-GVHD. It is most often caused by the infusion of immunocompetent lymphocytes into a severely immunosuppressed recipient. Historically, those who have been viewed at highest risk for GVHD are those whose immune systems are suppressed for one of the following reasons:

- Congenital immunodeficiency
- HIV infection
- Premature birth
- Immune suppression secondary to aggressive chemotherapy or radiation therapy in ongoing cancer treatments, or intentional immune suppression in transplantation

Once infused, the immunocompetent lymphocytes engraft, multiply, and turn against the "foreign tissues" of the recipient-host. The resulting clinical picture of this immune response is dramatic, including fever, hepatitis, bone marrow suppression, and overwhelming infection progressing to an often fatal outcome. TA-GVHD has a 90% to 100% mortality rate.

TA-GVHD can be prevented by pretransfusion irradiation of all blood products containing lymphocytes. This radiation does not kill the donor lymphocytes, but it renders them incapable of replication in the recipient and thus eliminates an essential step in the graft-versus-host response. Irradiation does not affect the function of the red blood cells, platelets, or granulocytes.[1]

When irradiation of red blood cells is indicated, it is usually carried out as close to the time of transfusion as possible. Any unit of cells that is properly typed and crossmatched to the recipient is appropriate for this purpose, without regard for its length of time in storage. Mature red blood cells are seen as relatively resistant to radiation damage.

Prestorage irradiation of packed cells has never been seen as optimal but has been recognized as necessary in situations in which immediate pretransfusion irradiation is not an option. There are two ways to accomplish the irradiation of PRBCs and their subsequent storage to meet the need for delayed infusion:

1. The cells can be irradiated and stored in their liquid state at 4° C. This preparation expires on the original expiration date for the component or 28 days from the date of irradiation, whichever comes first.
2. The red cells may be irradiated immediately after donation, stored in the liquid state for up to 6 days, and then frozen for future use.

A number of cases of TA-GVHD have been recognized in immunocompetent patients who received directed-donation transfusions from blood relatives. The cause of this immune response seems to be in the similar genetics shared by the donor and recipient. The donor lymphocytes are sufficiently similar not to be recognized as "foreign" by the recipient. However, with engraftment and proliferation of these donor cells, which are sufficiently dissimilar not to recognize the recipient as "self," the immune system is triggered and the natural cascade of events leads to the graft-versus-host response. For this reason, the AABB[1] recommends the irradiation of all directed-donations from blood relatives.

The AABB *Standards for blood banks and transfusion services*[5] recommends irradiation of cellular components in the following situations:

- For patients identified as at risk for TA-GVHD
- Transfusion of HLA-selected products
- Transfusion of cellular components between blood relatives
- Cellular component intrauterine transfusions

Posttransfusion thrombocytopenic purpura.
Posttransfusion thrombocytopenic purpura[1] is a rare event related to a platelet-specific antibody. It is seen almost exclusively in multiparous women. The development of this antibody is most likely a result of sensitization during pregnancy of an antigen-negative woman, producing a discernible antibody titer. This entity can also be seen in men and women who were sensitized by previous transfusion. Regardless of the method of sensitization, posttransfusion purpura is not common; 98% of the population carries the antigen, leaving only 2% of the population at risk.

When an antibody-positive individual is transfused with antigen-positive platelets, the donor platelets will be destroyed. In some recipients, their own antigen-negative platelets will also be destroyed, leading to a clinical picture of severe thrombocytopenia. Although this condition is usually self-limiting, it can be severe enough to warrant exchange plasmapheresis and/or treatment with intravenous immunoglobulin. Continued infusion of platelets appears to be an ineffective treatment because the transfused platelets are destroyed as rapidly as they are given. Following recovery, the AABB recommends that future transfusions be done with washed PRBCs or with components from antigen-negative donors.[1]

Nonimmunologic classification

Transmitted disease. A blood transfusion is not a benign procedure. Warnings concerning the "cookbook" approach of prescribing routine transfusions for all patients exhibiting a hematocrit below a predetermined level date back to at least the 1950s.[9] It is only rather recently, however, that we have seen a significant reduction in the number of transfusions. In the present atmosphere of heightened awareness surrounding the adverse effects of hemotherapy, this trend comes as no surprise.

Diseases transmitted through blood transfusion are not limited to those with a viral cause, although viruses seem to be the center of attention. Diseases caused by bacteria and protozoa are also transmitted by transfusion.

Bacterial infection. Bacterial contamination of a donated unit of blood can have several causes: (1) preexisting donor infection, (2) contamination during the phlebotomy procedure, or (3) contamination during processing.

An opportunity for contamination exists during the acquisition of the donor unit. A small percentage of percutaneously acquired blood samples are contaminated, primarily with components of the normal skin flora. These organisms belong to a group called *mesophiles,* which have an optimal growth temperature range of 30° to 44° C. They do not survive refrigerator temperatures (4° to 6° C) well and are therefore not associated with posttransfusion bacteremias traceable to refrigerated components.

Platelets that are stored at room temperature pose a higher risk for harboring and transmitting mesophiles. Although few in number, cases of posttransfusion septicemia resulting from platelet concentrates that have been contaminated with normal skin flora have been documented. *Staphylococcus epidermis* and diphtheroid bacilli are the most common isolates from platelet concentrates, but many other organisms have been linked to postplatelet transfusion septic incidents. However, bacterial counts are usually low in the contaminated units, and clinically recognized septicemia from platelet transfusion is rare.

Psychrophiles are the opposite of mesophiles. These organisms have optimal growth temperature around 29° C. However, they can tolerate low temperatures and will proliferate at a substantial rate even at 0° C. Psychrophilic organisms, which are primarily pseudomonads, present a challenge to blood banks and transfusion therapists. In addition to their ability to survive refrigerator temperatures, pseudomonads can use citrate as their carbon source. The combination of the citrate-based anticoagulant-preservative system and the refrigerator temperatures under which blood is stored provides a suitable environment for these gram-negative organisms to flourish.

Transfusion-associated gram-negative sepsis, although extremely rare, has a potentially fatal outcome. The rapidly progressing clinical picture demands immediate intervention and usually includes high fever, shock, DIC, and renal failure. Treatment may include high-dose antibiotics and therapy to combat shock, including high-dose steroids and vasopressors.[1]

Syphilis. At one time, because syphilis is blood-borne and sexually transmitted, it was a notable posttransfusion complication. However, syphilis is now rarely seen secondary to blood transfusion, for two reasons:

1. All donated units are serologically tested for syphilis (mandated by FDA).
2. *Treponema pallidum* is not likely to survive temperatures of 4° to 6° C for more than 72 hours.

Protozoal infection

Malaria. There are four species of malarial plasmodia in humans: *Plasmodium vivax, P. ovule, P. malariae,* and *P. falciparum.* The clinical presentation of the diseases produced and the incubation periods differ by species. However, all share a life cycle stage in which the parasites reside within the host erythrocytes. During this erythrocyte cycle, the disease can be transmitted through blood transfusion.

Malaria parasites survive for at least a week at room temperature or at 4° C. They can survive cryopreservation with glycerol and subsequent thawing. Any component that contains red cells can transmit infection.[1]

The known source of posttransfusion malaria is asymptomatic carriers who donate blood. Because there is no practical screening test to identify such donors, deferral of prospective donors is based on their medical and travel histories.[1] The

AABB *Standards for blood banks and transfusion services* defers donation of red cells from persons who have had malaria in the preceding 3 years. Casual travelers to areas in which malaria is endemic are deferred for 1 year.[5] The occurrence of posttransfusion malaria in the United States is estimated at 0.25 cases per million transfusions.[1]

Babesiosis. As with malaria, the causative agent of babesiosis is a protozoan, *Babesia microti*. This parasite, which is found mostly on the northeast coast of the United States with a concentration on Cape Cod and the islands of Massachusetts, has the northern deer tick as its vector. The clinical picture resulting from this infection can range from the mild febrile event seen in most cases, to a severe and even fatal outcome, which has occurred when the infection is superimposed on immunosuppression or splenectomy.

Although not common, babesiosis can be transmitted via blood transfusion for three reasons:

1. *Babesia microti* has an intraerythrocytic phase in its life cycle.
2. The parasite can survive up to 35 days at 4° C.
3. An individual infected with this parasite can be asymptomatic and donate blood.

Symptoms of transfusion-transmitted babesiosis are often so mild that the true nature of the infection goes undiagnosed; this may explain the small number of cases in the United States.[1] Persons with a history of babesiosis are indefinitely deferred from donating blood because lifelong parasitemia can follow recovery from symptomatic disease. No screening test to detect asymptomatic carriers is currently available for the *Babesia* species.

Chagas' disease. Chagas' disease—or American trypanosomiasis—is a life-threatening cardiac disease endemic to South and Central America. The agent of Chagas' disease is the protozoan *Trypanosoma cruzi*, which is a flagellate transmitted by blood-sucking insects. This parasite invades the macrophages of the host and spreads throughout the body. A small percentage of those infected develop symptoms of an acute illness, but most infected individuals remain asymptomatic. Chagas' disease is considered life-threatening throughout its three phases: acute, latent, and chronic. In the acute phase, mortality is most often secondary to congestive heart failure. In the chronic phase, death is often a result of lethal arrhythmias.

The characteristic of Chagas' disease that makes it a concern for transmission by blood transfusion is its high incidence of asymptomatic infection. This disturbing lack of symptoms is true during the acute and latent phases of the illness. There are screening tests for the antibody to *T. cruzi;* however, posttransfusion Chagas' disease is rare in the United States. There is no evidence to suggest that routine blood donor screening would significantly improve the safety of the blood supply.[1,10]

Viral infections. The identification of HIV and the recognition of its impact on hemotherapy has renewed interest in posttransfusion disease of viral cause. The three virus groups of greatest concern in blood component therapy are the primary hepatic viruses, herpesviruses, and human T-cell lymphotropic viruses.

Primary hepatic viruses. Posttransfusion disease linked to the primary hepatic viruses has not been eradicated. However, its incidence has been significantly reduced because of the following procedural changes in blood acquisition and screening:

- Routine serologic testing of donor units for hepatitis B viral markers (1972)
- Routine alanine aminotransferase and hepatitis B core antibody testing (1987)
- Routine testing for antibodies to HCV (1990)
- Reliance on an all-volunteer blood donor force (Paid donor groups were shown to be associated with a sevenfold increase in the incidence of posttransfusion hepatitis.[4])

With the additions to screening procedures and the more restrictive policies regarding blood donation, the estimated current risk of posttransfusion hepatitis (HBV and HCV) is 1 in 60,000 to 100,000/unit.[1]

The hepatitis virus family consists of six identified human pathogens: hepatitis A, hepatitis B, hepatitis C, hepatitis D (or delta agent), hepatitis E, and hepatitis G. Of these, only HBV and HCV are associated with posttransfusion disease.

HBV belongs to a group of viral agents called the *hepadnaviruses,* which are DNA viruses that attack liver cells. This intact virion has three areas of antigenic capability: (1) hepatitis B surface antigen, which is incorporated into the outer shell or envelope; (2) hepatitis B core antigen, which is the protein of the nucleocapsid; and (3) the poorly understood hepatitis B core-related antigen, which is thought to be part of the virion core. The host response to each of the hepatitis B antigens is to produce distinct antibodies to each.

Hepatitis B is acquired through exposure to infected blood or body secretions. Blood exposure usually is associated with percutaneous injury or blood transfusion. Infection acquired through body secretions is associated with sexual activity. Individuals infected with HBV usually experience liver damage, and 10% become chronically infected.[6] The chronically infected asymptomatic carrier of HBV is of concern in blood banking. Healthy-appearing individuals can be infected with and infectious for HBV. However, posttransfusion hepatitis B, which was once a common and greatly feared event with potentially fatal consequences, has been significantly reduced because of advancements in screening technology for detecting infectious donors. However, transfusion-related hepatitis B has not been eliminated.

HCV infection usually presents a significantly less dramatic clinical picture than HBV. Many HCV infections are detected only through liver function studies. Most individuals infected with HCV become chronic carriers, with approximately 85% having persistent serologic evidence of the presence of the virus for years. At least 50% of these carriers have evidence of liver disease, but most HCV-infected individuals remain asymptomatic.[1,11] As with hepatitis B infection, the asymptomatic chronic carrier is the primary concern in blood banking. HCV is responsible for 90% to 95% of all transfusion-related hepatitis.[6]

Routine screening for the antibody to hepatitis C (anti-HCV) was begun in 1990 for all donated bloods.

Herpesviruses. The human herpesvirus family includes herpes simplex 1 and 2, varicella-zoster virus, CMV, and Epstein-Barr virus. All members of this family are known to establish latent infection with the potential for reactivation after varying periods of time. The ability to establish latency categorizes the herpesviruses as persistent infections. The ability to establish persistence is the hallmark of most transfusion-transmitted viruses. However, although all members of this family show persistence, not all members are a risk for posttransfusion infection. The only herpesvirus of significant concern in transfusion therapy is CMV.

CMV has worldwide distribution. The prevalence of anti-CMV ranges from 40% to 90% among healthy blood donors.[1,12] Although most people infected with CMV are asymptomatic, this virus is known to be a common cause of congenital viral infection, an etiologic agent for a mononucleosis-like syndrome, and a significant pathogen in bone marrow, liver, and heart transplantation patients.

CMV is one of the infectious agents most often transmitted by blood transfusion. This is probably attributable to the fact that prospective blood donors can be infected with CMV and be infectious without knowing it. This lack of awareness is explained by the following facts about CMV:

- CMV infections, both primary and recurrent, are largely asymptomatic.
- Viremia occurs in both primary and recurrent infections.
- Most importantly, sites of latency for CMV include one or more of the peripheral blood leukocytes.

Despite CMV's high potential for involvement in posttransfusion infection, the transfusion of blood from a seropositive donor to a seronegative recipient does not result in an automatic posttransfusion infection. Studies of the transmissibility of CMV by blood transfusion consistently show that only some seropositive donors transmit the virus. Although approximately 50% of blood donors can be expected to be CMV seropositive, it is estimated that less than 1% of seropositive cellular components are able to transmit the virus.[1,13]

Asymptomatic infection with no known sequelae is the outcome of most transfusion-associated CMV infections. Therefore blood with a reduced risk for transmitting CMV is not necessary in the immunocompetent recipient, with one exception. Because cytomegalovirus can be transmitted perinatally, a seronegative expectant mother requiring a transfusion should be given CMV-negative blood.[1] Infants infected with CMV in utero may develop a variety of congenital abnormalities, including deafness and mental retardation.

The immunocompromised individual is at much greater risk for significant morbidity and even mortality from transfusion-associated CMV infection. Recipients who should be protected from the risk of CMV transmission include the following[1]:

- Low-birth-weight premature infants born to a seronegative mother
- Seronegative recipients of any organ transplant, including bone marrow, from a seronegative donor
- Recipients of intrauterine transfusions
- Seronegative individuals who are candidates for autologous or allogenic marrow transplant
- Those few patients with acquired immunodeficiency syndrome (AIDS) who are free from CMV infection

Blood components appropriate for transfusion to those at risk for posttransfusion CMV infection include blood and blood components from CMV-negative donors and leukocyte-filtered cellular blood components.

Human t-cell lymphotropic viruses. Human T-cell lymphotropic viruses (HTLVs) are retroviruses and can cause persistent, permanent infection. Because they appear to target the T lymphocyte, they are candidates for transmission by blood transfusion even when latent.

HTLV type I was the first of this virus family to be identified. It was isolated by Robert Gallo and associates in 1978 from an American man with T-cell leukemia, and it was the first human retrovirus found to have a causal association with malignant disease, adult T-cell lymphoma-leukemia.[1,14] In addition, HTLV-I is associated with the neurologic condition HTLV-associated myelopathy (HAM), also referred to as *tropical spastic paraparesis*. These conditions occur in a small minority of persons harboring the virus (no more than 2% to 4%).[1]

Donor screening for anti–HTLV-I in the United States began in 1988. At that time, the confirmed rate of positive tests was approximately 1 in 5000 units collected. A tenfold reduction in that rate has occurred since screening began and seropositive donors have been eliminated from the donor pool.[1,15]

HTLV type II was isolated in 1982 from a man with hairy cell leukemia. However, no causal relationship to that disease has ever been established. HTLV-II has a strong genetic sequence resemblance to HTLV-I[1,14]; antibodies to both show marked cross-reactivity in tests with viral lysates.[1] The only disease associated with HTLV-II is HAM, which is more often associated with HTLV-I.[1,16]

For both HTLV-I and HTLV-II, infection and seropositivity are lifelong. However, infection does not present as an acute event, and with the exception of the development of adult T-cell lymphoma-leukemia or HAM, most infected individuals are unaware of the infection.[1]

The current combined risk for transfusion-transmitted HTLV-I/II infection is approximately 1 in 500,000 units.[1,15]

Human immunodeficiency viruses. HIV type I (HIV-1) and type II (HIV-2) are the causative agents of AIDS. AIDS was recognized in 1981, and its causative organism was isolated in 1983/1984. The French group that claimed to have discovered this virus called it *lymphadenopathy I*, and the American group that made the same claim called it *human T-cell lymphotropic virus III* (HTLV-III). In the spring of 1985, routine testing for the antibody to HTLV-III was begun on all blood donations. In 1986, an international committee recommended the common name of human immunodeficiency virus. The subsequent discoveries of at least two types and multiple subtypes of HIV led to the current classification system of human immunodeficiency viruses.

HIV-II, which was isolated in 1985, was found to be endemic in many countries of West Africa but seldom seen elsewhere.[1,17] The first case of HIV-2 infection seen in the United States was in 1988 in a recent immigrant from West Africa. The diseases caused by HIV-1 and HIV-2 are very similar. However, HIV-2 appears to have a longer incubation period and a lower incidence of progression to AIDS.[1,18] In 1991, the combination antibody tests for HIV-1/HIV-2 were instituted in this country, providing a better surveillance of HIV-2.

AABB *Standards for blood banks and transfusion services*[5] requires that all units of blood and components be nonreactive for anti–HIV-1, anti–HIV-2, and HIV-1 antigens (HIV-1-Ag) before they are issued for transfusion. Today, with antibody and antigen testing procedures in place on all donated blood, the estimates for posttransfusion HIV risk in the United States range from approximately 1 in 450,000 to 1 in 660,000 transfusions.[1,15,19]

AUTOLOGOUS BLOOD TRANSFUSION

Autologous blood transfusion (also known as *autotransfusion*), is the collection and reinfusion of the patient's own blood for the purpose of intravascular volume replacement.[20] This procedure's historical roots can be traced to 1818, when an Englishman, James Blundell, salvaged vaginal blood from patients with postpartum hemorrhage. By swabbing the blood from the bleeding site and rinsing the swabs with saline, he found that he could reinfuse the result of the washings. This unsophisticated method resulted in a 75% mortality rate but marked the start of autologous blood transfusion.[21] In the early 1900s, others tried autotransfusion (during limb amputation, ruptured ectopic pregnancies, splenectomies, and neurosurgery) with varying degrees of success. The interest in autotransfusion dwindled during World War II because there was a large pool of donors. After the war, blood testing, typing, and crossmatching techniques were improved, making blood banks the answer to the increased demand for blood.[21] In 1970, Klebanoff brought modern credibility to the concept of autotransfusion with his report of a roller pump system for retrieving blood, a system that was used successfully in Vietnam.[22]

The National Blood Policy, published in 1974, provided for the increased use of autotransfusion throughout the country. Its four goals were to maintain the following: (1) an adequate blood supply; (2) availability of blood to all people; (3) efficient utilization of blood; and (4) the highest standards of transfusion therapy with the safest blood.[21]

In response to increasing public and professional awareness and concern about potential infectious disease complications of homologous blood transfusion, interest in alternative transfusion programs mushroomed in the early 1980s.[23] Autologous blood represents the safest possible blood for transfusion (Box 10-5).

There are four categories of autotransfusion available: (1) preoperative autologous blood donation, (2) perioperative isovolemic (normovolemic) hemodilution, (3) intraoperative cell salvage, and (4) postoperative blood salvage.

Preoperative autologous blood donation

The most widely available autologous option is the preoperative collection, storage, and reinfusion of donated blood, sometimes referred to as *predeposit donation*. Patients scheduled for elective surgical procedures who anticipated the need for blood replacement should be considered candidates for this option.

The ideal donor-patient is in good health, is afebrile, and has 4 to 6 weeks until surgery. The hemoglobin concentration should be no less than 110 g/L (11 g/dl). The packed cell volume, if substituted, should be no less than 0.33 (33%).[5] Patients with active infection or who may be bacteremic are not eligible because bacteria may proliferate while collected blood is stored.

An important aspect of patient management for those participating in predeposit programs is iron replacement. The requesting physician should prescribe supplemental iron as soon as surgery is scheduled. Insufficient iron is often the limiting factor in collecting multiple units of blood over a short time.[1]

The preferred phlebotomy schedule is weekly, with the last unit drawn no less than 72 hours before surgery. The amount of blood harvested at each session is determined by the donor's age, weight, and medical history. The donated blood is usually stored in the liquid state at 1° to 6° C for 35 to 42 days, depending on the anticoagulant-preservative system used. If a longer storage period is necessary, the blood may be frozen. In addition, autologous blood that has not been frozen at the time of donation can be rejuvenated and subsequently frozen when it reaches its expiration date. This practice prevents autologous blood from being discarded when surgery is delayed.

The FDA requires testing of all autologous donations for syphilis, HIV-1 antigen, HIV-2 antibodies, antibodies to hepatitis C, hepatitis B surface antigen, and hepatitis B core antibody. Because autologous donors may not meet the strict requirements for allogenic donors, the donated autologous units are discarded if they are not used by the donor.[1] The AABB *Standards for blood banks and transfusion services*[5] no longer permits the use of autologous blood for any recipient other than the donor.

Perioperative isovolemic (normovolemic) hemodilution

Hemodilution is an option for patients who can tolerate rapid withdrawal of blood before surgery. This procedure involves collecting up to 2 L of blood in CPD or CPDA-1 immediately before surgery, usually after anesthesia has been induced, and replacing the blood with a sufficient volume of crystalloid or colloid solution to attain normovolemic hemodilution. The blood collected at the start of the procedure is stored at room temperature in the operating room. Because the blood is fresh and kept at room temperature, the platelets and clotting factors remain viable. Blood stored at room temperature should be transfused within 8 hours. If the surgical procedure is expected to last longer than 8 hours, the blood should be stored in monitored refrigeration. Refrigerated blood should be transfused within 24 hours.[1]

The rationale for hemodilution is based on studies done in the early 1970s that demonstrated that isovolemic hemodilution, using dextran and crystalloid, lowers blood viscosity and that maximum oxygen delivery is attainable when the hematocrit is lower than 30%. The studies suggested that the viscosity-

---

Box 10-5   Advantages of Autologous Blood Transfusion

1. Reassures patients concerned about blood risk
2. Prevents transfusion-transmitted disease
3. Prevents red cell alloimmunization
4. Provides compatible blood for those with alloantibodies
5. Supplements the blood supply
6. Prevents some adverse transfusion reactions

lowering effect of hemodilution leads to an increase in cardiac output and perfusion and that this increase easily compensates for the lower oxygen-carrying capacity of the diminished supply of red blood cells.[23]

The application of this option has obvious limitations. First, the patient on whom this procedure is done must be able to tolerate a significant blood loss before the surgery is begun. Second, because the amount of blood that can safely be drawn off is limited, it may not be adequate to meet the volume replacement required. In such cases, homologous blood is used as a supplement. Therefore, like predeposit autologous transfusion, hemodilution may reduce but does not always eliminate the need for homologous blood use.

Intraoperative autotransfusion/intraoperative cell salvage

Intraoperative autotransfusion (IAT) is the collection of shed blood from the surgical field and its subsequent reinfusion to the patient. It can be used in cardiac, vascular, and selected trauma surgeries, and in liver transplants and orthopedic procedures. IAT is especially useful when preoperative donation is impossible or inadequate. The rule of thumb in IAT is that a return of 3 units makes it cost-effective. However, many argue that any cost using this method is offset by the reduced risk of autologous transfusion versus homologous transfusion.

Numerous blood-collection and cell-processing machines are available. The objective is the same for all: collect, in some cases process, and return the patient's blood. If processing machinery is used, the blood shed from the surgical field is suctioned off and anticoagulated through a dual-lumen catheter that terminates in a collection reservoir. When the volume in this reservoir reaches the optimal level for processing, the blood is washed, spun, and returned to the patient.

IAT should not be used in certain situations. Because neither filtration nor washing can completely remove bacteria from blood, salvage is not attempted if the operative field has gross bacterial contamination. In addition, IAT is not usually used if a collagen hemostatic agent has been placed in the wound. These powered agents, which activate the clotting cascade when in contact with red blood cells, have a molecular size similar to that of red cells and may not be eliminated by cell washing. Also, because malignant cells cannot be removed from salvaged blood, IAT is usually contraindicated in cancer resections. Returning salvaged blood could result in the seeding of malignant cells to other areas.

Postoperative blood salvage

Postoperative salvage is the collection of shed blood from the postoperative surgical wound for reinfusion to the patient. Continuous and intermittent techniques and equipment are available for salvaging blood lost after surgery. These methods are usually used to collect blood lost from chest tubes or joint cavities. Because anticoagulation is not used, this blood is defibrinated and contains high titers of fibrinogen-fibrin degradation products. Such collections may be processed using cell-washing techniques before reinfusion, or they may be reinfused

without processing. In either case, they must be filtered, and microaggregate filtration is preferred when cell washing has not been used. Because of the opportunity for contamination of these collections, it is recommended that shed blood collected under postoperative or posttraumatic conditions be reinfused within 6 hours of the initiation of the collection.

REFERENCES

1. Vengelen-Tyler V, editor: *Technical manual,* ed 13, Bethesda, Md, 1999, American Association of Blood Banks.
2. Mollison PL, Engelfriet CP, Contreras M: *Blood transfusion in clinical medicine,* ed 9, London, 1993, Blackwell Scientific.
3. Gabrio BW, Donohue DM, Finch CA: Relationship between chemical changes and viability of stored blood treated with adenosine, *J Clin Invest* 34:1509, 1955.
4. Kruskall MS: Blood transfusion. In Robinson SN, Reich PR, editors: *Hematology,* ed 3, Boston, 1993, Little, Brown.
5. Menitove J, editor: *Standards for blood banks and transfusion services,* ed 19, Bethesda, Md, 1999, American Association of Blood Banks.
6. Dailey JF: *Blood,* Arlington, Mass, 1998, Medical Consulting Group.
7. Judkins D, Iserson KV: Blood warming: avoid hypothermia, *J Emerg Nurs* 17:146, 1991.
8. Lane T, editor: *Blood transfusion therapy: a physicians handbook,* ed 5, Bethesda, Md, 1996, American Association of Blood Banks.
9. Crosby WH: Misuse of blood transfusion, *Blood* 13:1198, 1958.
10. Appleman MD, et al: Use of questionnaire to identify potential blood donors at risk for infection with *Trypanosoma cruzi. Transfusion* 33(1):61, 1993.
11. Alter HJ: To C or not to C: these are the questions, *Blood* 85:1681, 1995.
12. Gunter K, Luban N: Transfusion-transmitted cytomegalovirus and Epstein-Barr virus diseases. In Rossi EC, Simon TL, Moss GL, Gould SA, editors: *Principles of transfusion medicine,* ed 2, Baltimore, 1996, Williams & Wilkins.
13. Sayers M: Cytomegalovirus and other herpesviruses. In Peltz LD, et al, editors, *Clinical practice of transfusion medicine,* ed 3, New York, 1996, Churchill Livingstone.
14. Hjelle B: Transfusion-transmitted HTLV-I and HTLV-II. In Rossi EC, Simon TL, Moss GL, Gould SA, editors, *Principles of transfusion medicine,* ed 2, Baltimore, 1996, Williams & Wilkins.
15. Schreiber GB, Busch MP, Kleinman SH, Korelitz JJ: The risk of transfusion-transmitted viral infections: the retrovirus epidemiology donor study, *N Engl J Med* 334:1685, 1996.
16. Murphy EL, et al: HTLV-II infected blood donors: the REDS investigators, *Neurology* 48:315, 1997.
17. Busch M: Transfusion-associated AIDS. In Rossi EC, Simon TL, Moss GL, Gould SA, editors: *Principles of transfusion medicine,* ed 2, Baltimore, 1996, Williams & Wilkins.
18. O'Brien T, George JR, Holmberg SD: Human immunodeficiency virus type 2 infection in the United States: epidemiology, diagnosis, and public health implications, *JAMA* 267:2775, 1992.
19. Lackritz EM, et al: Estimated risk of transmission of the human immunodeficiency virus by screened blood in the United States, *N Engl J Med* 333:1721, 1995.
20. Martin E, Harris A, Johnson N: Autotransfusion systems (ATS), *Crit Care Nurse* 9(7):65, 1989.
21. Nicholson E: Autologous blood transfusion, *Nursing Times* 84(2):33, 1988.
22. Peterson K: Nursing management of autologous blood transfusion, *J Intrav Nurs* 15(3):128, 1992.
23. Silvergleid A: *Clinical practice of transfusion medicine,* ed 2, New York, 1989, Churchill Livingstone.

Pharmacology

Jean B. Douglas, BS, PharmD, FASHP, Carolyn Hedrick, BSN, CRNI*

administration and application of the nursing process. The second section discusses the various aspects of IV drug delivery. Commonly used equipment is described, as well as the different modes of IV drug administration. The greatest emphasis is placed on the final section, where the different classifications of IV drugs are presented and the drug most representative of each classification is examined in detail.

CONSIDERATIONS FOR INTRAVENOUS DRUG ADMINISTRATION

As nurses assume greater responsibility for IV drug administration, they require increased knowledge. Although nursing students are usually restricted from administering IV drugs (except under the close supervision of their instructor), nursing education has begun to place more emphasis on the pharmacology and administration of drugs by the IV route. Health care facilities supplement this educational base by providing specialized courses for nurses assigned to IV teams and critical care. However, the staff nurse in the hospital and home care settings may receive only limited orientation to infusion therapy. This is unfortunate because the responsibility for IV drug administration and patient monitoring often rests with the staff nurse.

The intravenous (IV) route is a common route of parenteral drug administration in many health care settings. IV drugs were once reserved for emergency situations or critically ill patients. They are now routinely used throughout the hospital, as well as in outpatient and home care settings. With the dramatic increase in the use of the IV route for drug delivery, nurses have assumed increased responsibility. Nurses administer IV drugs, monitor patients' responses to pharmacologic agents, and instruct patients regarding the prescribed drug therapy. Nurses must therefore have a thorough understanding of the principles of IV drug administration. This knowledge is necessary both for the safety of the patient and to ensure quality patient outcomes.

It is the intent of this chapter to broaden the nurse's knowledge regarding IV drug therapy. Because of the breadth of the subject, this chapter has been divided into three sections. In the first, the nurse's role in IV drug administration is reviewed. Specific consideration is given to legal aspects of IV drug

Nursing responsibilities

The determination of who may administer IV drugs is based on Nurse Practice Acts. Each state has such an act, but most only broadly define the scope of professional nursing responsibilities. This differs for a licensed practical nurse (LPN) in that several states have established boundaries in which the LPN may practice. These boundaries may include specific educational programs that the LPN must complete before administering IV drugs and restrictions on the drug administration procedures that may be performed.

In addition to Nurse Practice Acts, health care facilities have established policies regarding nursing responsibilities. Although these policies cannot exceed the limits established by the Nurse Practice Act, they may clarify or place further restrictions on nursing functions. For example, institutional guidelines for IV drug administration define who may administer certain drugs. Some hospitals also issue "IV push lists," which place restrictions on drugs administered by direct IV injection.

*The author and editors wish to acknowledge the contributions made by Donna R. Baldwin as author of this chapter in the first edition of *Intravenous Nursing: Clinical Principles and Practice.*

A third set of criteria regarding IV drug administration is contained in the *Infusion Nursing Standards of Practice.*[1] This document provides information to measure the quality of IV nursing care, including IV drug administration. Because the standards are meant to protect the public and define nursing accountability, they are the basis for the development of IV policies in all practice settings in which IV drugs are administered.

Legal considerations

To legally administer an IV drug, or any drug, the medication must be prescribed by a physician or appropriate licensed professional. However, it is the nurse's responsibility to ensure that the order is complete, correct, appropriate, and valid. A complete order must contain the name of the drug, dosage, route of administration, frequency or time of administration, date and time the order was written, and signature. Problems arise when any of these components are missing or are unclear.

A correct and appropriate order is one that is indicated and proper for the patient's condition. Indications for each drug classification and specific drugs are discussed later in this chapter. Determination of the appropriateness of the order is based on the nursing assessment of the patient and requires knowledge of pharmacokinetics and pharmacodynamics. Pharmacokinetics focuses on the effects of the body on the drug; pharmacodynamics involves the effects of the drug on the body.

A valid medication order requires that the order be written and signed by the physician or other authorized health care professional. Although verbal orders are acceptable in some situations, the order is not legally finalized until it is countersigned by a licensed physician or appropriate licensed professional.

There are additional legal considerations regarding controlled substances. Controlled substances are prescription drugs that, because of their high potential for drug dependence or abuse, are covered by the Controlled Substances Act of 1970. The act established five categories of controlled substances, known as *schedules,* based on potential for abuse and dependence and the medical indications for the drug's use. Many of the IV drugs administered for pain control are Schedule II drugs, which have specific prescription and record keeping requirements.[2]

Another area that has legal implications is the administration of investigational drugs. Informed consent must be obtained from all patients and/or families participating in clinical drug trials. This means that the patient must be supplied information by the principal investigator regarding the risks, benefits, expected effects on the disease process, and alternatives to the investigational therapy before consenting to participate in the trial. In addition, the clinical trial must be approved by the appropriate institutional committee, and drug information must be readily available for the nurse administering the drug.

Legal consideration must also be given to the occurrence of medication errors. Errors may be associated with prescribing and dispensing the drug, but they more commonly occur because of failure to follow safe administration procedures. The five rights of medication administration specify that the *right* dose of the *right* drug must be administered to the *right* patient at the *right* time by the *right* route. Errors have resulted because of the "look alike" generic names (e.g., the cephalosporin antibiotics), failure to identify the patient appropriately, administration of the drug by an incorrect route, and the physician's failure to specify the route. Documentation of errors as part of a risk management program can help identify trends and prevent these errors. Such documentation should be initiated by the person discovering the error.

Nursing process

The administration of IV drugs requires proper application of the nursing process. The patient must be assessed, the drug therapy planned and implemented, the patient outcomes evaluated, and the plan of care reviewed and revised based on the evaluation. These basic steps are interrelated and are essential to ensure that drug therapy results in the desired patient outcomes.

Assessment. Patient assessment begins with a review of the patient's health history. The following are pertinent questions:

What is the current disease?

What other medications are being used?

What medications were used in the past?

Did the previous medications have any unexpected effect?

During the questioning, it is particularly important to obtain information about known allergies to drugs, foods, and environmental factors. There are cross-sensitivities between many drugs, so an allergy to one may result in similar effects with another. A primary example is the possible cross-sensitivity between penicillins and cephalosporins.

A second area to be assessed is the patient's lifestyle and resources. This is particularly important in home care and should include the family or other caregiver as well as the patient. Specific factors to consider are the patient's and family's daily schedules and the physical and human resources available. How will the drug therapy schedule affect the daily schedule? Will the caregiver be available at the scheduled administration times? Are there material resources available to enable safe and appropriate use of the drug and equipment required for administration?

The third area to assess is the patient's and family's knowledge level and desire for information. This factor may significantly influence adherence to the drug regimen. Because the desire for information and the ability to comprehend it vary among patients, assessing these factors aids in allotting adequate time for patient and family education.

The last area to be assessed is patient-related factors that may alter the patient's response to the drug. These include genetic factors, preexisting conditions, and age. Genetic factors, such as the absence of a specific enzyme, may affect the drug's action within the body. Preexisting renal, liver, and cardiovascular disease may impair the metabolism or elimination of the drug. Age is also a predictor of drug response. For example, children do not have the mature physiologic mechanisms needed for adult dosages, whereas physiologic changes in older adults tend to extend the effects of drugs within the body. In addition, drug interactions and incompatibilities with other medications and body fat may negatively affect the drug response.

Planning. A comprehensive assessment helps identify the nursing diagnosis specific to the patient and the drug therapy. Examples of nursing diagnoses are "fluid volume deficit related to drug-induced diuresis," perhaps for a patient on furosemide, and "knowledge deficit related to the drug regimen," which can apply to any patient.[2] Nursing diagnoses are instrumental in defining and communicating patient problems related to drug therapy. Several textbooks are available to help the nurse determine the appropriate nursing diagnoses.

Once the pertinent nursing diagnoses have been identified, the patient's plan of care may be established. The care plan should include short- and long-term goals, and it should focus on actions to achieve the desired patient outcomes.

An important feature to consider when planning care for the patient is the time-response nature of drug action. Although the drug may be administered as a single dose, it is more common for it to be administered repeatedly. Repeated administration at regular intervals causes the plasma concentration of most drugs to reach a constant concentration in the blood. If plans are not made to administer the drug at the scheduled times, the plateau may not be reached, seriously affecting the effectiveness of the drug therapy.

Another time-response factor to consider when planning the patient's care is the therapeutic drug concentration range. Whereas a plateau is achieved with a fixed dosing schedule, there are still peaks and troughs in the drug plasma concentration. The peak concentration occurs immediately after IV administration, and the trough level is the minimum concentration present immediately before administration of the next scheduled dose. Several drugs have a relatively narrow margin of safety, meaning that there is little difference between concentrations that produce therapeutic responses and those that cause serious adverse effects. When such drugs are prescribed, arrangements must be made to determine whether the drug levels are within a therapeutic range. The most important aspect of this planning is ensuring that blood samples are drawn appropriately in conjunction with a scheduled dose. For example, the administration of gentamicin requires that a trough specimen be drawn before the scheduled dose and a peak specimen following infusion.

A third time-response aspect to consider is the plasma half-life of the drug. *Half-life* refers to the amount of time required for the elimination processes to reduce the blood concentration of the drug by 50%.[3] For example, many IV drugs are eliminated by the kidneys. Because renal impairment may increase the half-life of such drugs, planning should include verification that reduced dosages have been prescribed.

Implementation. The three important facets of implementing drug therapy are patient education, drug administration, and documentation. Because of differences among health care settings, these facets may not receive equal attention. In home care, greater emphasis is placed on patient education to prepare the patient for the self-administration of medication. This differs from the hospital setting, in which IV drugs are usually administered by the nurse. Regardless of the setting, documentation plays a vital role because it validates that the actions have been implemented.

Evaluation. Evaluation of the drug therapy determines the drug's effectiveness and may suggest beneficial modifications

of the patient's plan of care. A therapeutic response is desired because it signifies that the intended effects of the drug have been produced. However, there may be an ineffective or toxic response. An ineffective response may indicate that less than the minimum required dose has been administered or that other factors have interfered with the action of the drug. For example, a patient who experiences only slight relief from pain after the administration of morphine has an ineffective response. In contrast, a toxic response is an exaggeration of the usual pharmacologic actions of the drug or the appearance of signs and symptoms related to drug toxicity. For example, the toxic response to digoxin is typically evidenced by the clinical symptoms of anorexia, nausea, and vomiting.

The patient should also be evaluated for unexpected and undesired effects of the drug. Although these responses are often called *side effects,* this term is misleading. Side effects are therapeutically undesirable but are a consequence of the normal action of the drug. An example is the loss of potassium from the body after the administration of furosemide. *Untoward drug responses,* also known as *adverse effects,* are undesired and unexpected responses. Table 11-1 describes several potential untoward drug responses.

Untoward effects may be caused by the interaction of the drug with other drugs within the body. Drug-drug interactions may be *potentiative,* meaning one drug intensifies the effects of the other drug, or *inhibitory,* meaning one drug reduces the effects of the other drug; or the drug combination may produce a new response that neither drug used alone would produce. Potentiative and inhibitory interactions may be beneficial or detrimental. Sulbactam and ampicillin illustrate a beneficial potentiative interaction that increases ampicillin's therapeutic action. A detrimental potentiative interaction occurs with warfarin and aspirin, which increases the risk of bleeding. A beneficial inhibitory interaction occurs between morphine and naloxone when treating overdoses, reversing the toxicity of the opioid analgesic. A detrimental inhibitory interaction occurs between terbutaline and propranolol, which causes a reduction in bronchial dilation. An example of a drug-drug interaction resulting in a new response is the combination of disulfiram (Antabuse) and alcohol, which causes hazardous effects that do not occur when either drug is used alone.[2]

DRUG ADMINISTRATION

The nurse's role in IV drug administration is determined by the health care setting. In the inpatient setting, the nurse may be responsible for drug preparation and administration, whereas home care usually requires the nurse to educate the patient or family in self-administration techniques.

Drug preparation

Generally, IV drugs and admixtures are prepared in a centralized pharmacy, where there is greater assurance of accuracy and sterility. Although a pharmacist typically prepares the admixtures, this may be performed by nurses or technicians employed by the pharmacy and working under the direction of the pharmacist. In emergencies or when medication must be prepared immediately before administration, nurses may also prepare IV drugs.

Table 11-1	**Untoward Drug Responses**	
RESPONSE	**EFFECTS**	**EXAMPLE**
Tolerance	Increasing amounts of drug needed to produce same therapeutic response	Patient receiving morphine infusion over 2 wk has decreasing relief from pain
Tachyphylaxis	A rapidly developing tolerance occurring after very few doses	Has been reported with sodium nitroprusside
Accumulation	Amount of a drug builds up in the body, resulting from input exceeding output	May occur when the usual adult dosage of gentamicin is administered to a patient with renal impairment
Idiosyncrasy	Unpredictable response that differs in quality from expected response but not caused by hypersensitivity	Aplastic anemia develops in 1 in 40,000 patients who receive chloramphenicol
Drug allergy	Adverse response to a drug resulting from previous exposure to that or a related drug and mediated by an antigen-antibody reaction; hypersensitivity	Reaction that occurs when penicillin is given to patient with penicillin allergy
Dependence	Continued administration of the drug required to prevent withdrawal syndrome	Patient receiving hydromorphone for cancer pain has visible tremors, restlessness, and profuse perspiration when a dose is withheld

Laminar flow hood. When IV drugs are prepared in the pharmacy, they are usually prepared under a laminar flow hood. The design of the laminar flow hood decreases the possibility of airborne contaminants entering the IV solution. Air enters the back of the hood and is circulated through filters before it is directed into the work area in uniform, parallel streams. Either a horizontal or vertical laminar flow hood may be used; however, vertical models are recommended for preparing cytotoxic agents.

Drug containers. IV drugs are available in various containers, including ampules, vials, partially filled solution containers, additive piggyback vials, and premixed admixtures. Ampules pose the greatest risk because of the possibility of particulate contamination. Glass fragments may enter the ampule when it is broken open; the related risks are reduced when the drug is drawn up with a filter needle. Vials pose another risk of particulate contamination because of the potential risk of *coring;* when the needle is introduced through the rubber stopper of the vial, the needle bevel may cut away fragments of the rubber seal.

Partially filled containers and additive piggyback vials, often referred to as *minibags* or *minibottles,* are potential sources of particulate matter. This may be the result of incomplete reconstitution of the powdered drug or precipitates formed by the physical incompatibility of the admixture. Partially filled containers of 50 to 100 ml of 0.9% sodium chloride or 5% dextrose in water (D_5W) require that a liquid form of the drug be added to the container. In an additive piggyback vial, the drug is in powdered form, which must be reconstituted with a small volume of diluent. Because these containers are used to infuse the drug into the patient, an in-line filter should be used after preparation to remove any particulate matter.

Premixed admixtures are prepared by the manufacturer and require no further preparation. However, they are sometimes available in frozen form, which must be restored to room temperature before administration. Cefazolin (Ancef) is an example of an admixture available in frozen form. It is generally recommended that frozen admixtures not be warmed by placing them in a water bath or exposing them to microwave radiation.[4] Special units are available for rapidly thawing premixed frozen minibags, but the preferred method is to allow the admixture to thaw at room temperature.

Diluents. Another consideration for the preparation of IV drugs is the diluent used to reconstitute the drug. Diluents with bacteriostatic properties, such as bacteriostatic sodium chloride, contain benzyl alcohol as a preservative. Although this bacteriostatic agent is desirable in most situations, it is contraindicated for neonates and for the administration of intraspinal or epidural drugs.[4] In addition, certain drugs, such as amphotericin B (Amphotec/AmBisome), are incompatible with preservatives and must be reconstituted with sterile water for injection.[5]

Drug compatibility and stability. The preparation of IV drugs is accompanied by the risks of incompatibility and instability. *Incompatibility* is an undesirable reaction that occurs between the drug and the solution, container, or another drug. The three types of incompatibilities associated with IV drugs are physical, chemical, and therapeutic. *Stability,* on the other hand, refers to the length of time the drug retains its original properties and characteristics.

Drug incompatibilities. A *physical incompatibility* refers to a visible reaction, such as a color change, haze, turbidity, precipitate, or gas formation, occurring within the drug.[3] The largest number of physical incompatibilities involve precipitate formation, such as that seen when diazepam is added to D_5W.

Chemical incompatibility involves the chemical degradation of the drug and is the result of hydrolysis, reduction, oxidation, or decomposition. It differs from physical incompatibility in that the reaction may not be visible.[3] Such a reaction may occur when penicillin is added to a very acidic or alkaline solution.

Therapeutic incompatibility, which occurs within the patient, is the result of the overlapping effects of two drugs administered concurrently.[3] Although the effects may not be evident until the patient's response to the drug therapy has been evaluated, knowledge of potential incompatibilities may prevent their occurrence. Examples of therapeutic incompatibility were previously discussed as part of the evaluation of drug interactions.

Drug stability. One of the most important factors in drug stability is the solution's hydrogen ion concentration, or pH. Most drugs are stable over a narrow range of pH values.

Table 11-2   Factors That Affect Drug Stability

FACTOR	EFFECT	EXAMPLE
Number of additives	The greater the number of drugs contained in the admixture, the greater the chance of one of the drugs becoming unstable	Multiple additives in TPN solution
Dilution	Limited amounts of a drug are stable in the solution, whereas large doses may be unstable	Only limited amounts of heparin and hydrocortisone are stable in amphotericin solution
Time	The length of time the drug is in solution may affect stability	Ampicillin is stable for only 4 hours when added to D_5W
Light	Some drugs are sensitive to light and exposure may result in degradation of the drug	Exposure of levarterenol may result in degradation of drug
Temperature	Lower temperatures usually extend the stability of the drug	Cephalothin is stable for only 6 hr at room temperature, but up to 48 hr when refrigerated
Order of additives	The order in which drugs are added to a solution affect compatibility and stability	Addition of lipids to TPN solution
Container	The composition of the container may affect the stability of the drug	Potency of insulin reduced by at least 20% when added to a plastic container

TPN, Total parenteral nutrition; D_5W, 5% dextrose in water.

This means that they are unstable in either very acidic (pH below 4) or alkaline (pH above 8) solutions. The concept of stability is best characterized by penicillin. This drug is most stable in a slightly acidic environment (pH of 6.5) but deteriorates if added to a very acidic or alkaline solution. Additional factors that affect drug stability are listed in Table 11-2.

Modes of IV drug administration

The mode of IV drug administration depends on the drug used, the patient's condition, and the desired effects of the drug. Generally, it is specified by the physician or other qualified provider. Each of the four primary modes of administration—continuous infusion, intermittent infusion, direct injection, and patient-controlled analgesia—has advantages and disadvantages.

Continuous infusion. *Continuous infusion* refers to the admixture of the drug in a large volume of solution that is infused continuously over several hours to several days. The solution container is connected to an administration set, and the drug (in solution) is infused through the venous access device. Depending on the potency, an electronic infusion control device may be used to deliver the drug accurately at the prescribed rate of flow.

Continuous infusion is used when the drug must be highly diluted, constant plasma concentrations of the drug must be maintained, or large volumes of fluids and electrolytes must be replaced. Examples are infusions of nitroprusside or potassium chloride. Disadvantages associated with continuous infusion are possible fluid overload and potential incompatibilities between the infusion and other IV drugs administered through the same venous access device. Patient comfort issues and mobility should also be considered.

Intermittent infusion. For an intermittent infusion, the drug is added to a small volume of fluid (25 to 250 ml) and infused over 15 to 90 minutes at intervals. Advantages of the intermittent mode are the ability of the drug to produce peak blood concentrations at periodic intervals, decreased risk of

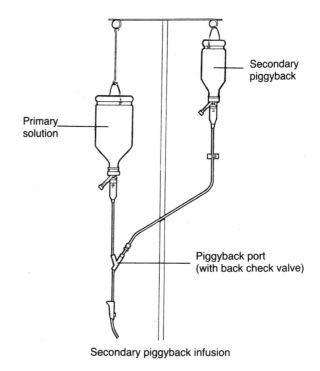

FIG. 11-1 *Secondary piggyback.* (Redrawn with permission from Baptist Memorial Hospital: *I.V. procedure manual*, Memphis, 1991, Baptist Memorial Hospital.)

fluid overload, and greater convenience for the patient. However, there are disadvantages. The increased concentration of the drug in the intermittent solution may cause venous irritation, the drug may be less effective than if administered by continuous infusion, and additional equipment is required. IV antibiotics are generally administered using this mode.

Intermittent infusions may be administered in various ways. One of the most common methods is for the drug to be given as a piggyback infusion through the established pathway of the primary solution (Fig. 11-1). Although the primary infusion is interrupted during the piggyback infusion, the drug from the intermittent infusion container mixes with the primary solution below the piggyback injection port. Hence, if this method is used, the drug and the primary solution should be compatible.

A second way to administer intermittent infusions is simultaneous infusion. With this method, the drug is administered as a secondary infusion concurrently with the primary infusion (Fig. 11-2). Rather than connecting the intermittent infusion at the piggyback port, it is attached to the lower secondary port. One of the major disadvantages of this method is the tendency for blood to back up into the tubing once the secondary infusion has been completed, possibly occluding the venous access device. This does not occur with the piggyback method because hydrostatic pressure closes the back check valve (incorporated into the administration set) once the intermittent infusion is completed. Although drug incompatibility is a possibility with both methods, it is a greater risk with a simultaneous infusion.

A third method is the use of a volume control set. Although it was originally designed to control the fluid volume delivered to the patient, a drug may be added to a small amount of solution in the volume control set and infused at the desired rate (Fig. 11-3). This method shares many of the disadvantages previously discussed. However, it is still used in some pediatric settings because it limits the amount of fluid the child receives.

The fourth method for administering intermittent infusions is directly into the venous access device. The device must be one that is intended for intermittent administration, such as a peripheral heparin or saline lock or a long-term, centrally placed catheter. The drug is added to a minibag or minibottle and infused intermittently. Between doses, the drug container and tubing are eliminated. This method is generally preferred because it decreases the risk of fluid overload and affords greater freedom of movement for the ambulatory patient. However, failure to promptly remove the empty drug container and tubing and flush the venous access device may result in occlusion of the venous access device.

Technologic developments have produced alternatives for the administration of intermittent doses. One manufacturer has introduced a system whereby the drug is supplied in a powdered form that is attached between the primary solution and the infusion set. Once the drug vial is connected, the solution flows from the primary container through the drug vial and to the patient. Although the use of this system eliminates the costs associated with preparing and administering the traditional piggyback, it is applicable only to situations in which the drug and primary solution are compatible.

A second innovation has been the introduction of intermittent doses of drugs that are activated at the time of use. Rather than preparing and refrigerating the drug before administration, the pharmacy simply dispenses the drug vial attached to a small container of solution. Immediately before administering the drug, the nurse activates the system by removing the barrier between the drug and the solution. Although this has proven cost-effective, errors have been reported because of failure to remove the barrier and activate the system.

The third major innovation is the result of the space program and is based on elastomeric technology. The system consists of an elastomeric drug container that is specially designed to establish a set delivery rate. Once the pharmacist fills the system

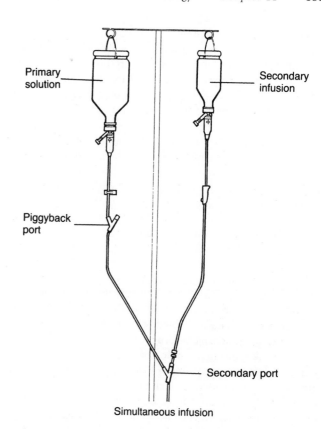

FIG. 11-2 *Simultaneous infusion.* (Redrawn with permission from Baptist Memorial Hospital: *I.V. procedure manual,* Memphis, 1991, Baptist Memorial Hospital.)

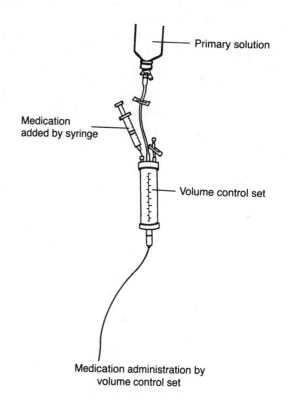

FIG. 11-3 *Volume control set.* (Redrawn with permission from Baptist Memorial Hospital: *I.V. procedure manual,* Memphis, 1991, Baptist Memorial Hospital.)

with the drug, it may be infused at the preset rate by opening the slide clamp on the tubing attached to the container. An advantage of this system is that neither gravity nor electronic assistance is required for precise delivery of the drug. However, not all drugs may be administered with an elastomeric container. Because of the expense, it is usually reserved for the home setting.

Direct injection. *Direct injection,* also known as *IV push* or *bolus,* is the administration of a drug directly into the venous access device or through the proximal injection port on a continuous infusion set. The purpose is to achieve rapid serum concentrations, but this may be accompanied by a greater risk of adverse effects. Instead of regulating the rate of administration by the infusion rate, direct injection requires only the time it takes to push the plunger of the syringe. Many drugs have maximum rates at which they may be administered, so the rate of the injection must be timed and the drug injected in increments. Because the drug may be incompatible with the infusing solution or heparin may be present in the intermittent device, the vascular access device should be flushed with normal saline before and after injecting the drug.

Direct injections may require that the drug be drawn into a syringe before administration or that the drug be available in a prefilled syringe. A needle 1 inch or shorter should be used to administer the medication because longer needles may puncture the IV tubing or the vascular access device. Another alternative is a needleless system, which also prevents inadvertent puncture of the tubing or device.

Patient-controlled analgesia. A fourth mode of administration is patient-controlled analgesia (PCA), which promotes patient comfort through the self-administration of analgesic agents. With this method, an electronic pump (PCA pump) is programmed to administer a small bolus of the drug when activated by the patient. The bolus amount and the time between doses (lock-out interval) are predetermined by the physician and programmed into the pump by the nurse. Technologic advances have added features to the pump, permitting both continuous infusion and patient-controlled doses.

DRUG CLASSIFICATIONS

Drug reference books generally list medications alphabetically, even when a classification system is used. Such a system aids the nurse in clinical practice, but it is not conducive to learning. To help the nurse understand the wide array of IV drugs discussed in this chapter, a prototype approach is used. The drugs are divided into different categories: antibiotics, other antiinfective drugs, central nervous system (CNS) drugs, cardiovascular drugs, hematologic agents, agents for electrolyte and water balance, gastrointestinal (GI) drugs, hormones and synthetic substitutes, immune modulators, respiratory smooth muscle relaxants, and vitamins. The drug most representative of each classification is examined in detail. Additional drugs related to the prototype, including antidotes, are then discussed in terms of their differences and similarities or their relationship to the prototype.

Drug dosages vary widely, even among the prototype and its related drugs. To include dosing information on all the drugs discussed would require more pages than are allotted for this chapter. Therefore drug dosing is discussed only when pertinent to understanding administration of the drugs and their potential side effects. Information on dosing schedules for each drug is available in the *American Hospital Formulary Service Drug Information* and *Drug Facts and Comparisons.*[4,6] These were the primary references consulted for specific drug information, although additional references may be cited to explain the various drug classifications.

Antibiotics

Antibiotics are used to treat infection and represent the largest category of commonly used IV medications. Antibiotics may be categorized as either bactericidal or bacteriostatic. Bactericidal agents can destroy the organism by lysis of the cell wall or by prevention of its intact formation. Bacteriostatic agents inhibit growth of the organism by inhibiting protein synthesis. Although bacteriostatics may eliminate the organism in high concentrations, they usually depend on the patient's immune system to eradicate the organism once its growth has been inhibited. Theoretically, the bacteriostatic agent inhibits bacterial growth, making administration of a bactericidal agent ineffective because its primary action is against growing cells. Actually, both types of agents may be used in combination to enhance the effectiveness of each.

The primary contraindication for antibiotics is a known sensitivity to the drug. A patient with a history of hypersensitivity reactions to a certain antibiotic should be considered allergic to all antibiotics within the same class. For example, a patient who has a known sensitivity to penicillin is also considered allergic to aminopenicillins. In addition, there is evidence of a cross-sensitivity among some antibiotics, such as penicillins and cephalosporins. Therefore cephalosporins are used cautiously in patients who are sensitive to penicillin.

One of the major disadvantages of antibiotics is that their prolonged use may result in a bacterial or fungal superinfection. A superinfection occurs when the normal flora of the body is altered by an antibiotic, allowing the proliferation of bacteria or fungi that are resistant to the antibiotic.

Because antibiotics have been overused for decades, some are proving ineffective against resistant strains of bacteria. The clinician should check sensitivity data prepared by the clinical laboratory before selecting a specific antibiotic.

Penicillins. The penicillins include natural and semisynthetic antibiotics produced or derived by the fermentation of certain strains of the fungus *Penicillium.* Because of their relatively low cost, low toxicity, and good clinical efficacy in the treatment of many infections, penicillins are still some of the most important antibiotics.

Natural penicillins. The mechanism of action of the natural penicillins is bactericidal. These agents disrupt the synthesis of the bacterial cell wall, making the organism osmotically unstable. Instability of the cell wall causes it to lyse, and the organism is destroyed. Because the cell walls of gram-positive bacteria are relatively permeable to most penicillins, these drugs are generally effective against such organisms. However, gramnegative bacteria have an outer membrane around the cell wall that decreases accessibility to the natural penicillins.

Prototype: penicillin G potassium. Penicillin G is indicated for the treatment of severe infections caused by some gram-positive and anaerobic organisms. Because it exerts specific antibiotic action against these organisms and is relatively non-toxic to the host, penicillin G is generally considered the drug of choice for streptococcal, pneumococcal, and spirochetal infections. Specifically, penicillin is indicated in the treatment of meningitis, pericarditis, endocarditis, septicemia, and severe pneumonia.

Penicillin G may be administered as a continuous or intermittent infusion, and it has a relatively wide margin of safety. Adverse reactions are rare and are usually limited to hypersensitivity reactions. Although the manifestations of a hypersensitivity reaction may be only fever, chills, or eosinophilia, these reactions can be divided into four basic types.

The most common hypersensitivity reactions are dermatologic reactions. Symptoms include urticarial, erythematous, or maculopapular rash accompanied by pruritus. These reactions are delayed, occurring 48 hours or more after the administration of penicillin G.

The second type of hypersensitivity reaction is serum sickness–like reactions. These reactions are usually evident 6 to 10 days after the initiation of therapy and are characterized by fever, malaise, urticaria, arthralgia, myalgia, lymphadenopathy, and splenomegaly. Although the reaction may be severe, it is usually short lived and disappears within days or weeks after discontinuing the drug.

The third type of reaction includes hematologic reactions, such as hemolytic anemia, agranulocytosis, and leukopenia. Typically, this type of reaction is associated with large doses of penicillin G. A positive direct antiglobulin (Coombs') test occurs in up to 3% of patients receiving large doses, and a small number of these patients develop hemolytic anemia during or after penicillin therapy. Once the drug is discontinued, the hemoglobin concentration and reticulocyte count return to pretherapy levels, although the Coombs' test may not revert to negative for 3 months or longer.

The fourth and most serious type of hypersensitivity reaction is anaphylaxis. Although anaphylaxis is reported in fewer than 0.05% of patients receiving penicillin, it has been fatal in 5% to 10% of reported cases. Anaphylactic reactions to penicillin typically occur within 30 minutes of administration. They are characterized by laryngeal edema, bronchospasm, stridor, cyanosis, and circulatory collapse. Treatment includes immediate discontinuation of the drug and emergency measures such as maintaining a patent airway and administering epinephrine, oxygen therapy, and corticosteroids.

Penicillin interacts with several other antibiotics. Aminoglycosides are physically and chemically incompatible with penicillin and are inactivated if administered in the same IV container or administration set. Bacteriostatic antibiotics, such as chloramphenicol and erythromycin, may reduce the bactericidal action of penicillin, so concurrent use of these drugs is not recommended except in select situations.

Related drug. Penicillin G is commercially available as a potassium or sodium salt. Both are readily soluble in water and are considered aqueous, crystalline penicillins, but penicillin G potassium is usually preferred. The administration of either form requires special consideration because every 1 million units of penicillin G potassium contains 1.7 mEq of potassium and every 1 million units of penicillin G sodium contains 2 mEq of sodium.

Penicillinase-resistant penicillins. The critical component of the natural penicillins is the beta-lactam ring incorporated into the penicillin molecule. Some strains of bacteria produce an enzyme known as *penicillinase,* which destroys the ring. Thus the organism is considered penicillin resistant. To overcome this resistance, the penicillinase-resistant penicillins have been developed. These antibiotics are used exclusively to treat penicillinase-resistant organisms such as *Staphylococcus aureus* and *S. epidermidis.* Their mechanism of action, contraindications, and precautions are similar to those of the natural penicillins.

Prototype: methicillin sodium. Methicillin sodium (Staphcillin) is mainly indicated for the treatment of infections caused by penicillinase-producing staphylococci. It is also used preoperatively to reduce the incidence of staphylococcal infections associated with certain surgical procedures. Although methicillin may be administered as a direct injection, it is more commonly given as an intermittent infusion.

Some bacteria have been labeled as "methicillin resistant," but this is misleading. Certain strains of staphylococci are resistant to all penicillinase-resistant penicillins, not just methicillin. These resistant strains are prevalent in both the hospital and community and are being reported with increasing frequency.

The side effects of methicillin are similar to those associated with the use of penicillin G. Methicillin may cause transient asymptomatic elevations of serum alkaline phosphatase, alanine aminotransferase, and aspartate aminotransferase levels. In rare instances, transient neutropenia, leukopenia, granulocytopenia, and thrombocytopenia have been reported. Generally, these hematologic effects are not evident until more than 10 days after the initiation of therapy and resolve within 2 to 7 days once the drug is discontinued. There is also a 15% to 20% incidence of acute interstitial nephritis with the use of methicillin.

Related drugs. Two additional penicillinase-resistant penicillins are nafcillin sodium (Unipen) and oxacillin sodium (Bactocill). Both drugs are similar to methicillin, but nafcillin is more likely to cause phlebitis than other penicillinase-resistant penicillins. However, because it is less likely to cause acute interstitial nephritis, nafcillin may be prescribed more often than methicillin.

Aminopenicillins. Aminopenicillins have a free amino group added to the penicillin nucleus, which increases their bactericidal effectiveness against gram-negative bacteria. However, they are deactivated by penicillinase-producing organisms.

Prototype: ampicillin sodium. Ampicillin sodium (Omnipen-N) is highly effective in the treatment of severe infections caused by *Salmonella, Shigella, Proteus mirabilis,* and *Escherichia coli.* Although ampicillin may be administered by direct injection, it is generally administered as an intermittent infusion. Concentrated doses of ampicillin are stable for 4 hours in 5% dextrose in water and 5% dextrose in 0.45% sodium chloride, but potency is extended to 8 hours when added to isotonic sodium chloride without dextrose. When the drug is further diluted in a minibag or minibottle, stability may be extended up to 48 hours.

Adverse reactions to ampicillin are similar to those of penicillin G. Ampicillin sodium may also produce a distinct, nonimmunologic reaction characterized by a generalized erythematous, maculopapular rash similar to measles. The rash typically occurs 3 to 14 days after the initiation of therapy and generally disappears despite the continuation of therapy. It is more common in patients with mononucleosis and is not indicative of a hypersensitivity to penicillin. Hematologic effects such as neutropenia, agranulocytosis, and thrombocytopenia have also been reported, but these are usually reversible once the drug is discontinued.

Because of the probability of patients with infectious mononucleosis developing a rash during therapy, ampicillin is generally not prescribed to patients with this disease. In addition, the potential for ampicillin rash is increased for patients receiving allopurinol and ampicillin concomitantly.

Related drug. Ampicillin sodium–sulbactam sodium (Unasyn) is a combination of ampicillin and sulbactam that prevents inactivation of the drug by penicillinase-producing organisms. It is primarily indicated in the treatment of intraabdominal and gynecologic infections.

Extended-spectrum penicillins.
Because of structural differences in the side chains of the extended-spectrum antibiotics, they have a wider spectrum of activity than the other penicillins. Specifically, the extended-spectrum penicillins are effective against gram-negative organisms, including *Pseudomonas.* Like the natural penicillins, the extended-spectrum penicillins are ineffective against penicillinase-producing organisms.

Prototype: ticarcillin disodium. Ticarcillin disodium (Ticar) is bactericidal for several gram-negative, gram-positive, and anaerobic organisms. It is indicated for bacterial septicemia and infections of the respiratory, genital, and urinary tracts.

Ticarcillin may be administered by direct injection, intermittent infusion, or continuous infusion. However, administration should not exceed the recommended rates. Too rapid infusion of ticarcillin and higher-than-normal dosages have resulted in seizures. Other side effects of ticarcillin are similar to those of penicillin G and include dermatologic and hematologic reactions, thrombophlebitis, and anaphylaxis.

Drug interactions associated with ticarcillin are similar to those of the other penicillins. There may also be an increased risk of bleeding in patients who are receiving anticoagulants.

Related drugs. Other extended-spectrum penicillins include mezlocillin sodium (Mezlin), piperacillin sodium (Pipracil), piperacillin-tazobactam (Zosyn), and ticarcillin disodium–clavulanate potassium (Timentin). These drugs are usually selected based on laboratory sensitivity data and availability.

Cephalosporins.
Cephalosporins are bactericidal antibiotics that share a close structural similarity with the penicillins. Because of this, they have similar mechanisms of action, side effects, and contraindications. Cephalosporins are classified by their spectrum of activity, or *generation.*

First-generation cephalosporins.
First-generation cephalosporins are active against susceptible gram-positive bacteria, such as *S. aureus* and *S. epidermidis,* and some gram-negative organisms. Because of their low cost, they are the preferred drugs for most gram-positive infections.

Prototype: cefazolin sodium. Cefazolin sodium (Kefzol) is effective in the treatment of serious infections of the respiratory tract, genitourinary tract, cardiovascular system, and soft tissue. It may be administered as a direct injection or as an intermittent infusion. Because the primary route of elimination for cefazolin is the kidneys, renal impairment requires a reduced dosage.

Although cefazolin is considered relatively nontoxic, allergic reactions have been reported in up to 5% of patients receiving the drug. These reactions are similar to those associated with penicillin G and range from a mild rash to anaphylaxis. Nephrotoxicity has been reported, but it is rare and more likely to occur in geriatric patients or in those with renal impairment.

There are few reported drug interactions involving cefazolin. However, the concurrent use of nephrotoxic drugs such as aminoglycosides and cefazolin may increase the risk of renal toxicity.

Related drugs. Other first-generation cephalosporins are cephradine (Velosef), cephalothin sodium (Keflin), and cephapirin (Cefadyl). Of these agents, cephalothin has the greatest risk of nephrotoxicity and venous irritation.

Second-generation cephalosporins.
The second-generation cephalosporins have greater gram-negative activity than the first-generation drugs, but they are less effective against gram-positive organisms. Their mechanism of action, side effects, contraindications, and precautions are similar to those of cefazolin.

Prototype: cefoxitin sodium. Cefoxitin sodium (Mefoxin) is indicated for the treatment of serious infections of the respiratory and genitourinary tracts, gynecologic infections, and septicemia. The increased activity of cefoxitin against anaerobic bacteria also increases its usefulness in intraabdominal infections. Because it is excreted by the kidneys, a reduced dosage of cefoxitin is indicated in patients with renal impairment.

Related drugs. Additional second-generation cephalosporins are cefamandole nafate (Mandol), cefonicid sodium (Monocid), cefparanide (Precef), cefotetan disodium (Cefotan), and cefuroxime sodium (Zinacef). Cefamandole may increase bleeding tendencies because it eliminates intestinal bacteria that normally synthesize vitamin K and it inhibits clotting factor synthesis independent of vitamin K.

Third-generation cephalosporins.
Third-generation cephalosporins are more active against gram-negative organisms, including *Pseudomonas,* but are less effective against gram-positive organisms. An important characteristic of this category of drugs is their ability to cross the blood-brain barrier when the meninges are inflamed. Third-generation cephalosporins share many of the characteristics of the first- and second-generation drugs.

Prototype: cefotaxime sodium. Cefotaxime sodium (Claforan) is indicated for the treatment of bacteremia, septicemia, meningitis, and serious infections of the respiratory and genitourinary tracts. It is usually administered by intermittent infusion but may also be given by direct injection.

Related drugs. Related third-generation drugs include cefoperazone sodium (Cefobid), ceftazidime (Fortaz), ceftizoxime sodium (Cefizox), and ceftriaxone sodium (Rocephin). Ceftriaxone is generally preferred for home care because it requires only a single daily dose.

Fourth-generation cephalosporin. The fourth-generation cephalosporin, like the third generation's, has an expanded spectrum of activity against gram-negative bacteria compared with the first- and second-generation drugs. Activity is improved in vitro against *Pseudomonas aeruginosa* and certain Enterobacteriaceae, as well as gram-positive bacteria.

Prototype: cefepime. Cefepime (Maxipime) is used for the treatment of uncomplicated and complicated urinary tract infections, uncomplicated skin and skin structure infections, and moderate to severe pneumonia caused by susceptible organisms.

Aminoglycosides. Aminoglycosides are bactericidal antibiotics that are effective against several gram-negative organisms. Their name is derived from the amino sugars contained within their chemical structure.

Prototype: gentamicin sulfate. Gentamicin sulfate (Garamycin) is well distributed throughout all body fluids, achieves peak plasma concentrations within 30 minutes to 2 hours of administration, and maintains serum levels for up to 12 hours. It is often administered concurrently with penicillin because the two drugs have synergistic bactericidal effects. Gentamicin is effective in the treatment of serious infections of the respiratory, urinary, and GI tracts; septicemia; and infections of the skin and soft tissue.

The most significant side effects associated with gentamicin are ototoxicity (associated with high peak plasma levels) and nephrotoxicity (associated with high trough levels). It has been suggested that this is the result of accumulation of the drug intracellularly in the inner ear and kidneys. Otic effects are manifested by vestibular symptoms, such as dizziness, nystagmus, vertigo, and ataxia, or auditory symptoms, such as tinnitus and hearing impairment. Nephrotoxicity is evidenced by increased blood urea nitrogen and serum creatinine levels and decreased creatinine clearance and urine-specific gravity. Both ototoxicity and nephrotoxicity are more likely to occur in geriatric patients, patients with renal impairment, patients receiving high dosages or extended therapy, and patients receiving other ototoxic or nephrotoxic drugs. However, symptoms are usually reversible once the drug is discontinued.

Gentamicin may produce dose-related and self-limiting neuromuscular blockade. Symptoms range from general muscular weakness to seizures and a myasthenia gravis–like syndrome. Gentamicin may also provoke hypersensitivity reactions such as rash, urticaria, stomatitis, pruritus, fever, and eosinophilia.

There is a narrow margin between therapeutic and toxic levels of gentamicin. A therapeutic level of 4 to 8 μg/ml should be maintained and serum concentrations monitored to avoid peak levels greater than 12 μg/ml and trough levels above 2 μg/ml. Monitoring of gentamicin serum levels requires that the trough sample be drawn 30 minutes before a scheduled dose, the dose be administered as scheduled, and the peak sample be drawn 30 to 60 minutes after completion of the scheduled dose.

Once-daily dosing of aminoglycosides has been recommended for patients without serious infections, severe renal dysfunction (creatinine clearance below 40 ml/min), or impaired host defenses. This dosing regimen achieves therapeutic effects using the postantibiotic effect (the drug continues to eradicate bacteria for some time after it is discontinued) and reduces adverse effects. Higher concentrations are associated with increased bacteriocidal effects and reduction in resistance.

Reduced toxicity is seen with a single larger dose instead of multiple daily dosing or continuous infusion. Because of the larger total daily dosage, the infusion time should be extended to 60 minutes.

For certain microorganisms, such as *Serratia, P. aeruginosa, Acinetobacter* or indole-positive *Proteus, Citrobacter* species, and *Enterobacter,* an aminoglycoside antibiotic is added to the beta-lactam antibiotic to eradicate the infection. These microorganisms can develop resistance to the beta-lactam drug when it is administered alone. Using the aminoglycoside adds synergy and decreases mortality.

Related drugs. Aminoglycosides similar to gentamicin include amikacin sulfate (Amikin), kanamycin sulfate (Kantrex), netilmicin sulfate (Netromycin), and tobramycin sulfate (Nebcin). These drugs are usually reserved for the treatment of gentamicin-resistant infections.

Tetracyclines. Tetracyclines were the first broad-spectrum antibiotics developed. They are considered bacteriostatic but may have bactericidal activity in high concentrations. Although IV tetracycline is no longer available commercially, there are other tetracycline antibiotics that may be administered intravenously.

Prototype: doxycycline hyclate. Doxycycline hyclate (Vibramycin) is indicated for infections caused by susceptible organisms such as *Rickettsiae, Chlamydia,* and viruses, and as a substitute when penicillin therapy is contraindicated. Doxycycline is usually administered by intermittent infusion in 100 to 200 ml of fluid over 1 to 4 hours.

The most common side effects of doxycycline are dose-related effects on the GI tract. Manifestations include nausea, vomiting, diarrhea, and anorexia. Other adverse effects include hypersensitivity reactions and blood dyscrasias. In addition, the administration of doxycycline may cause venous irritation and thrombophlebitis, requiring that the IV site be rotated more frequently than every 48 hours. Photosensitivity reactions may occur, resulting in exaggerated sunburn on areas of the body exposed to the sun. Although it is not a significant risk for hospitalized patients, home patients should be alerted to this potential reaction.

Doxycycline is potentiated by alcohol and hepatotoxic drugs but is inhibited by cimetidine and alkalizing agents. In addition, doxycycline potentiates the effects of anticoagulants and digoxin.

Related drug. A related tetracycline is minocycline hydrochloride (Minocin). It is similar to doxycycline in its mechanism of action, side effects, and precautions. However, minocycline is less likely to cause venous irritation.

Macrolides. Like the tetracyclines, the macrolides are generally bacteriostatic but may have bactericidal activity when administered in high concentrations. The only erythromycin administered intravenously is erythromycin lactobionate, but a macrolide subclass of azalide antibiotics have experienced increased use because of better patient tolerance. A new antibiotic in this class is streptogramin.

Prototype: erythromycin lactobionate. Erythromycin lactobionate (Erythrocin) is primarily indicated for staphylococcal, pneumococcal, and streptococcal infections and in the treatment of legionnaires' disease. It may also be used as an alternative for patients allergic to penicillin. Although erythromycin may be administered as a continuous infusion, it is generally given as an intermittent infusion in 100 to 250 ml of fluid over 20 to 60 minutes. The infusion time may be extended if the patient experiences venous discomfort during administration.

Erythromycin is relatively free from serious side effects. However, the patient must be monitored for hearing loss secondary to IV erythromycin. The most common complaint is localized venous irritation during administration, which may be minimized by slowing the infusion rate, further diluting the medication, and rotating the site more often. Mild allergic reactions such as urticaria and rash have also been reported.

Because erythromycin is unstable if the pH is lower than 5.5, 1 ml sodium bicarbonate (e.g., Neut) may be added to acidic solutions such as D_5W to increase its stability. When erythromycin is in solution for only a short period, as with an intermittent infusion activated at the time of use, such buffering is considered unnecessary.

Increased serum levels of cyclosporine, digoxin, methylprednisolone, theophylline, and warfarin may occur with the administration of erythromycin. Therefore, if serum levels of these drugs are tested, the results must be interpreted accordingly.

Azalide subclass

Prototype: azithromycin. Like erythromycin, azithromycin (Zithromax) is indicated against gram-negative organisms, such as *Haemophilus influenzae, Chlamydiae, Mycoplasma,* and legionella. This drug may be used if the patient is known to be allergic to penicillin. This drug is administered by IV infusion in 250 to 500 ml of solution to give a concentration of 1 to 2 μg/ml over 1 hour. Azithromycin is well tolerated, but hypersensitivity reactions have been reported. Caution in liver-impaired patients is encouraged, and there is also concern for patients with ventricular arrhythmias. Few drug interactions have been reported, but they should be watched for, especially when used with digoxin, ergotamine, triazolam, and drugs metabolized by the P450 system.

Quinupristin/dalfopristin. Quinupristin/dalfopristin (Synercid) is a streptogramin antibacterial agent. It is a combination of two semisynthetic pristinamycin derivatives: quinupristin and dalfopristin in a ratio of 30:70 (weight.weight [w.w]). Synercid inhibits protein synthesis in the ribosomes and is converted to several major active metabolites in the body. Synercid has shown activity against *Enterococcus faecium, S. aureus,* and *Streptococcus pyrogenes.* Because the drug has a postantibiotic effect against certain organisms, dosing regimens of every 8 to 12 hours may be used for 7 days. The drug is compatible only with D_5W. Because D_5W flushes are not commercially available, a bag of D_5W must be used to flush the line. Stability is known to be a problem, so the drug must be prepared just before it is administered. Major side effects reported are inflammation, edema, pain at the infusion site, arthralgias, and the development of superinfections. It has been reported that if the dose is reduced, the arthralgias will improve. Because of the 25% incidence of venous intolerance, it is recommended that a central line or a peripherally inserted central catheter be used to administer this drug. The use of hydrocortisone or diphenhydramine does not decrease the phlebitis.[7]

Chloramphenicol. Chloramphenicol is a bacteriostatic antibiotic that may be bactericidal when used in high concentrations. Although different forms of the drug are available for oral and topical administration, only the sodium succinate salt of chloramphenicol may be administered intravenously.

Prototype: chloramphenicol sodium succinate. Chloramphenicol sodium succinate (Chloromycetin) is reserved for serious infections caused by susceptible organisms such as *H. influenzae, Rickettsia* species, and *Salmonella typhi.* It is often used in conjunction with penicillin G to treat anaerobic infections of the CNS. Regardless of the indication, the preferred method of administration is by intermittent infusion.

Although chloramphenicol is associated with fewer minor side effects than other antibiotics, it is more likely to cause serious and potentially fatal adverse reactions. Most notable are its hematologic effects, and chloramphenicol may cause two types of bone marrow depression. The first is irreversible, not dose related, and results in aplastic anemia, with a mortality rate that exceeds 50%. It is relatively rare. The second and more common type is dose related; it is usually reversible once the drug is discontinued. Symptoms include reticulocytopenia, anemia, leukopenia, and thrombocytopenia. Because of the possibility of hematologic effects, a serum level should not exceed 5 to 20 μg/ml, and laboratory values should be monitored carefully.

Chloramphenicol potentiates chlorpropamide, phenytoin, cyclophosphamide, oral anticoagulants, and hypoglycemic drugs. It inhibits iron dextran but is inhibited by rifampin. When administered concurrently with penicillin, chloramphenicol extends its own half-life and inhibits the action of penicillin.

Fluoroquinolones. A relatively new class of antibiotics, the fluoroquinolones, are usually bactericidal in action. These antibiotics contain a fluorine molecule, which increases the drug's potency against gram-negative and gram-positive organisms, and a piperazine, which is responsible for antipseudomonal activity. High concentrations of the drug are required for most anaerobic bacteria. Resistant strains of *Pseudomonas* have emerged where fluoroquinolones have been used excessively.

Prototype: ciprofloxacin. Ciprofloxacin (Cipro) should be diluted to a concentration of 1 to 2 μg/ml and infused over 60 minutes. Hydration is recommended to prevent crystalluria, and these drugs should be used cautiously in suspected CNS disorders. For patients with renal or hepatic impairment, dosages should be adjusted and monitored through the course of treatment. Photosensitivity has been reported, and the physician should be advised if joint or tendon pain occurs. Other adverse side effects include convulsions and hypersensitivity reactions.

Related drugs. Levofloxacin (Levaquin) is another fluoroquinolone that is used in ambulatory settings and hospitals because of its once-daily administration regimen and ability to penetrate soft tissues. Dosage adjustment in those with renal impairment is necessary. Ofloxacin (Floxin) and alatrofloxacin (Trovan) are also available. Alatrofloxacin use has been limited to hospitals because of reports of liver failure requiring transplantation. Gatifloxacin (Tequin) is the newest fluoroquinolone and is administered by IV infusion over 60 minutes. The usual dosage is 400 mg/200 ml daily. In patients with reduced renal function or in those undergoing dialysis, the dosage is 200 mg/100 ml daily. Close monitoring for prolongation of the QT interval of the electrocardiogram (ECG) is encouraged. This drug should be avoided in patients with known QT prolongation or uncorrected hypokalemia and in patients receiving antiarrhythmic agents of the quinidine and amiodarone types.[8]

Miscellaneous antibiotics. Some antibiotics do not belong to a specific classification. Because they share common properties with all antibiotics, only their unique characteristics are discussed here.

Aztreonam. Aztreonam (Azactam) is the first drug in a new class of antibiotics known as *monobactams.* Although monobactams differ structurally from beta-lactams, such as penicillins and cephalosporins, cross-sensitivity between the two classes of drugs may exist. However, because the probability of cross-sensitivity is not as great and does not typically result in a serious, life-threatening allergic reaction, aztreonam may still be indicated for patients with a beta-lactam allergy.

Clindamycin phosphate. Clindamycin phosphate (Cleocin) is a bacteriostatic antibiotic that is effective against anaerobic and aerobic organisms. It is chemically unrelated to penicillin, so it is useful in penicillin-sensitive patients. Side effects associated with clindamycin are diarrhea, pseudomembranous colitis, and a generalized rash. Because hypotension and cardiopulmonary arrest have been reported following too rapid administration of the drug, it is recommended that clindamycin be administered by intermittent infusion over a minimum of 10 minutes.

Imipenem-cilastatin sodium. Imipenem-cilastatin sodium (Primaxin) is a beta-lactam–antibiotic that has been structurally altered to increase its antibacterial activity. Because of its wide spectrum of activity, imipenem-cilastatin is effective in the treatment of polymicrobial bacterial infections, including *Pseudomonas* and many beta–lactamase-producing strains of bacteria.

Meropenem. Meropenem (Merrem) is a synthetic carbapenem antibiotic with the broad spectrum of activity of imipenem, with more activity against Enterobacteriaceae and less activity to gram-positive bacteria. It is indicated for intraabdominal infections and bacterial meningitis.

Vancomycin hydrochloride. Vancomycin hydrochloride (Vancocin) is a bactericidal antibiotic. It is considered the drug of choice for methicillin-resistant staphylococcal infections and for staphylococcal infections in patients who are allergic to penicillin. The two most serious side effects of vancomycin are ototoxicity and nephrotoxicity. In addition, rapid administration results in hypotension and a transient reddish blotching caused by histamine release. This reaction can be avoided if vancomycin is administered over a minimum of 60 minutes.

Other antiinfective agents

Because antibiotics are primarily effective against bacterial organisms, other agents are required to treat infections caused by fungi, viruses, and protozoa. Categories of drugs discussed in this section include antifungal agents, antiviral agents, and antiprotozoal drugs. Although sulfonamide combination products have antibacterial activity, they have been included in this section because of their unique properties.

Antifungal agents. Systemic fungal infections, although rare, are difficult to treat and are more common in immunosuppressed patients. Such infections may be treated with antifungal agents that act by binding to sterols in the membrane of the fungal cell. Once the drug binds to the cell membrane, the cell no longer has a protective barrier, the cellular constituents are lost, and the cell destroyed. Because bacteria do not contain sterols in their cell membranes, antifungal agents are not active against these organisms.

Prototype: amphotericin B. Amphotericin B (Fungizone) is the drug of choice for treating progressive and potentially fatal infections such as aspergillosis, blastomycosis, candidiasis, coccidioidomycosis, cryptococcus, and histoplasmosis. Because the drug is effective only against susceptible organisms, diagnosis of the organism must be confirmed by histologic studies before initiating treatment.

Before initiating amphotericin therapy, a test dose is administered to assess the patient's ability to tolerate the drug. Typically, 0.25 mg/kg of amphotericin in D_5W is infused over 4 to 6 hours, and the patient's pulse, respirations, temperature, and blood pressure are monitored every 30 minutes. The daily dose may be gradually increased up to 1 mg/kg or up to 1.5 mg/kg administered on alternate days. Because the maximum daily dose is 1.5 mg/kg, most fungal infections require months of therapy to achieve the total cumulative dose of 2 to 4 g.

Common dose-related side effects of amphotericin include headache, chills, fever, malaise, anorexia, nausea, and vomiting. Antipyretics, antihistamines, and antiemetics may provide symptomatic relief when administered before or during therapy, and hydrocortisone may be added to the infusion to decrease the severity of febrile reactions. Another expected reaction to amphotericin is thrombophlebitis at the injection site, but the incidence may be decreased by the addition of 1200 to 1600 units of heparin to the infusion.

The selective binding of amphotericin to sterols accounts for the toxicity of the drug. Some body cells, such as kidney cells, contain sterols that bind to the drug, making the cell subject to alterations in cellular permeability. Some degree of nephrotoxicity occurs in more than 80% of patients receiving amphotericin and may be manifested by elevated blood urea nitrogen and creatinine levels, hypokalemia, and hypomagnesemia. To decrease these nephrotoxic effects, sodium loading by direct IV 0.9% sodium chloride may be administered intravenously immediately before and after each dose of amphotericin.

Amphotericin may also bind with sterols in the cellular membrane of erythrocytes. Consequently, a reversible, normocytic, normochromic anemia occurs in most patients receiving amphotericin. Cardiovascular toxicities such as hypotension, ventricular fibrillation, and cardiac arrest are rare but may occur with rapid infusion of the drug.

Precautions regarding the administration of amphotericin may include infusing the drug over a minimum of 4 hours to reduce the incidence of side effects and monitoring the injection site for signs of phlebitis. However, more rapid infusion rates are now recommended if the patient's renal function is normal. Throughout therapy, the patient's serum electrolyte levels and renal function require monitoring, and the patient should be assessed for symptoms of electrolyte imbalance.

Amphotericin interacts with a number of drugs. For example, it produces additive nephrotoxic effects when administered with aminoglycosides, and it enhances potassium depletion when given with corticosteroids, diuretics, and cardiac glycosides.

Related drugs. Amphotericin B lipid complex (Abelcet), amphotericin B liposomal (AmBisome), and amphotericin B cholesteryl sulfate (ABCD) are newer agents that may be infused more quickly than amphotericin B (Fungizone) (over 2 hours initially and shorter for the next therapy, if tolerated). These agents have been reported to be less nephrotoxic but are generally reserved for patients who cannot tolerate amphotericin B. The newer agents are much more expensive than amphotericin B.

Another alternative to amphotericin is fluconazole (Diflucan), which is indicated for the treatment of serious systemic candidal infections and cryptococcal meningitis. Although adverse reactions may occur in patients receiving fluconazole, such reactions are more common in patients infected with human immunodeficiency virus (HIV). Nausea and vomiting, headache, and abdominal pain are among the adverse reactions that have been reported. Serious hepatic reactions and exfoliative skin disorders may also occur but are less likely in HIV-infected patients. In the ICU, patients are usually given a loading dose to get the serum levels to steady state sooner.

Antiviral agents.
Treatment for viral diseases is generally less effective than for bacterial infections. Because agents capable of killing the virus can also kill the host cells, antiviral therapy is limited to inhibiting the viral replication process. In addition, viral infections often progress without clinical signs or symptoms early in the course of illness, when the drugs might be most effective.

Prototype: acyclovir sodium. Acyclovir (Zovirax), indicated in the treatment of herpes simplex, varicella-zoster, Epstein-Barr virus, and cytomegalovirus infections, is one of the most common and useful antiviral agents. The activation of acyclovir by an enzyme produced by the virus causes the drug to inhibit DNA production within the virus, thus preventing viral replication.

Because of the risk of renal tubular damage with rapid administration of acyclovir, each dose is administered over at least 1 hour. Acyclovir crystals may occlude the renal tubules; therefore adequate hydration and urine output must be maintained before and during the infusion. The more common side effects associated with acyclovir are headache and thrombophlebitis.

Other antiviral agents. Other antiviral agents include ganciclovir sodium (Cytovene), vidarabine (Vira-A), zidovudine (AZT), foscarnet (Foscavir), and ribavirin (Virazole). Ganciclovir is structurally and pharmacologically related to acyclovir and is indicated in the treatment of cytomegalovirus in immunosuppressed patients, particularly those infected with HIV. Because of its mutagenic potential, guidelines for handling cytotoxic agents must be followed when preparing and administering ganciclovir. Vidarabine, on the other hand, is used specifically for the treatment of herpes simplex encephalitis. One of the newest antiviral agents is zidovudine, which is primarily used to decrease the severity of symptoms in patients with HIV and a confirmed history of *Pneumocystis carinii* pneumonia. The most serious side effects of zidovudine are hematologic effects, nausea, and headache.

Antiprotozoal drugs. The two drugs identified for their antiprotozoal activity, metronidazole and pentamidine, also have properties that make them effective against certain other organisms.

Prototype: metronidazole. Metronidazole (Flagyl) is a bactericidal agent that is effective against protozoa and specific anaerobic bacteria. Indications include serious intraabdominal, gynecologic, and lower respiratory tract infections; Crohn's disease; and antibiotic-related pseudomembranous colitis. Although metronidazole may be given as a continuous infusion, it is typically administered as an intermittent infusion over a minimum of 1 hour.

The most common side effects of metronidazole are nausea, anorexia, headache, and an unpleasant metallic taste. Peripheral neuropathy, characterized by tingling, numbness, or paresthesia of the extremity, has been reported but is reversible once the drug is discontinued. If alcohol is ingested while receiving metronidazole, disulfiram-like reactions, such as flushing, headache, nausea, sweating, and abdominal cramps, may occur. Patients with hepatic dysfunction require a lower dosage.

Related drug. Another antiprotozoal agent is pentamidine isethionate (Pentam). It is specifically indicated in the treatment of *P. carinii* pneumonia if the patient does not respond to trimethoprim-sulfamethoxazole. Severe hypotensive reactions may occur, particularly if pentamidine is administered over less than 60 minutes. Other adverse reactions include hypoglycemia and diabetogenic effects.

Trimetrexate. Trimetrexate (Neutrexin) is used to treat moderate to severe *P. carinii* pneumonia in immunosuppressed patients, including those with HIV. Patients should be monitored for pulmonary manifestations of concurrent bacterial, viral, fungal, or mycobacterial infections associated with immunosuppression or progression of the infection. Leucovorin should be administered concomitantly and for 72 hours after the last dose of trimetrexate. Trimetrexate should be given for 21 days, and leucovorin is given for 24 days.

Sulfonamide combination products.
Sulfonamides are broad-spectrum antimicrobial agents that have been used for more than 50 years. Although their general use has declined with the introduction of penicillins and cephalosporins, they remain an inexpensive and effective antibacterial therapy. Sulfonamides are usually bacteriostatic; they act by depriving the bacteria of folate products required for DNA synthesis. This inhibits the growth and reproduction of the microorganism. Body cells, unlike bacterial cells, do not synthesize their own folic acid and are unaffected by the drugs.

Sulfonamides are associated with numerous adverse reactions that involve nearly every body system. Because sulfonamide combination products contain a sulfonamide in addition to another drug, all precautions applicable to sulfonamides apply to the combination products.

Prototype: trimethoprim-sulfamethoxazole. Trimethoprim-sulfamethoxazole (Bactrim, Septra) is a combination of sulfamethoxazole and trimethoprim at a fixed 5:1 ratio. Because of its bactericidal properties, it is indicated in the treatment of severe urinary tract infections, *P. carinii* pneumonia, and shigellosis.

Because it contains a sulfonamide, trimethoprim-sulfamethoxazole is associated with three major types of side effects. First are hypersensitivity reactions, which range from rash to anaphylaxis. These reactions tend to be more common in HIV-infected patients receiving trimethoprim-sulfamethoxazole. Second, sulfonamides may crystallize in the renal tubules, causing renal damage. The risk is reduced by maintaining adequate hydration and urinary output or by reducing the dosage. Third, sulfonamides may have a toxic effect on the bone marrow, resulting in aplastic anemia, thrombocytopenia, and agranulocytosis. Overall, the most common side effects of trimethoprim-sulfamethoxazole are nausea, vomiting, and rash.

Sulfonamides bind to the plasma proteins, either displacing or being displaced by other protein-bound drugs. They potentiate the effects of warfarin and phenytoin but are inhibited by alkalinizing agents and thiopental. In addition, sulfonamides can be cross-sensitized with other drugs containing a sulfa structure, such as thiazide diuretics and oral hypoglycemics. Dosages must be reduced for patients with moderate to severe renal dysfunction.

Central nervous system drugs

The CNS is biologically complex and susceptible to interference by many pharmacologic agents. Because the CNS controls multiple physiologic functions, drugs that act centrally may have secondary effects on other body systems. There are many ways of classifying CNS drugs, but one of the most useful is according to their mechanism of action.

Analgesics. Analgesics are administered to relieve pain. Narcotic agonist analgesics may cause stupor or insensibility, also known as *narcosis*. These drugs are often referred to as *opiate agonists* because they are chemically related to morphine, which is derived from the opium poppy. Another category of analgesics is the mixed narcotic agonist-antagonists. When these drugs are administered to a patient who has received no other narcotic, they produce a morphinelike analgesia and respiratory depression. However, if mixed narcotic agonist-antagonists are administered to a patient who has received a narcotic, they partly antagonize the analgesia and respiratory depression.[2]

Narcotic analgesics. Although the narcotic analgesics vary in potency, they share several common properties. In addition to pain relief, narcotic analgesics act as agonists on specific opiate receptors, share the major side effect of respiratory depression, and cause drowsiness. Repeated administration may produce tolerance to the drug or the phenomenon of cross-tolerance. *Cross-tolerance* means that, once a tolerance to the action of one narcotic develops, the patient may also be tolerant to the action of other narcotics.

Prototype: morphine sulfate. The prototype of all narcotic analgesics is morphine sulfate. By binding to the opiate receptors, morphine relieves severe pain and inhibits the perception of pain. It may also alter the patient's mood, producing a feeling of euphoria. The primary indications for morphine are severe pain and apprehension associated with coronary occlusion or pulmonary edema, chronic pain associated with malignancies, and postoperative pain.

Although morphine may be administered by slow, direct injection or continuous infusion, it may also be administered as PCA. Using a PCA pump, the patient may self-administer frequent, small doses based on requirements for pain relief and the program prescribed for the PCA device.

The major side effect of morphine is respiratory depression. Patients with impaired respiratory function or those receiving morphine by rapid injection are at greatest risk. Other severe adverse effects of morphine include tachycardia, hypotension, myocardial depression, pinpoint pupils, excitation, and coma. Minor side effects such as nausea, vomiting, and constipation are more common.

The contraindications for morphine are based on its pharmacologic effects. Because morphine may produce respiratory depression, it is generally contraindicated in patients with poor pulmonary function, such as those with emphysema and asthma, and in patients with closed head injuries. Morphine also produces spasmogenic effects on the smooth muscle of the GI and genitourinary tracts. It is therefore contraindicated for benign prostatic hypertrophy, biliary tract surgery, and diarrhea caused by poisoning.

Morphine is potentiated by several drugs, so a reduced dosage of both drugs may be indicated. Potentiating drug categories include phenothiazines, monoamine oxidase inhibitors, neuromuscular blockers, and adrenergic blocking agents. CNS depressants, such as alcohol, barbiturates, hypnotics, and sedatives, also potentiate the effects of morphine. Cimetidine, in particular, may prolong or intensify the effects of morphine, causing disorientation, respiratory depression, apnea, and seizures, but these reactions are generally not associated with cimetidine alternatives.

Related drugs. The other narcotic analgesics are related to morphine but differ in terms of analgesic potency. Hydromorphone hydrochloride (Dilaudid) is approximately 5 to 10 times as potent as morphine, whereas meperidine hydrochloride (Demerol) has an analgesic potency equivalent to 20% that of morphine and a shorter duration of action.

Antagonists. Naloxone (Narcan) is a narcotic antagonist that blocks the opiate receptors, thus inhibiting or reversing the narcotic effects. Narcan is specifically used to counteract opiate-induced respiratory depression and narcotic overdose. The usual dosage is 0.4 to 2.0 mg administered as a direct injection. Potential adverse reactions include nausea, vomiting, hypotension or hypertension, tachycardia, and fibrillation.

Nalmefene (Revex) is the longest-acting commercially available parenteral opiate antagonist. Lower dosages should be used in patients at risk for experiencing cardiac side effects. If no response is seen after 21.43 μg/kg (1.5 mg/kg), another agent should be used.

Mixed opiate agonist-antagonists. Mixed opiate agonist-antagonists behave as agonists when administered to a patient who has not previously received a narcotic analgesic. In this manner, the drugs interact with the receptors and alter the function of the cells to produce effects similar to those of the narcotic analgesics. However, when mixed opiate agonist-antagonists are administered to a patient who is receiving a narcotic analgesic, they produce an antagonistic effect and inhibit the response to the narcotic analgesic. Mixed narcotic agonist-antagonists are also called *opiate partial agonists* because their actions are similar to those of opiate agonists, but only under specific conditions.

Prototype: buprenorphine hydrochloride. The prototype of the mixed opiate agonist-antagonists is buprenorphine hydrochloride (Buprenex). When administered as a narcotic agonist, buprenorphine is 30 times more potent than morphine. It is therefore indicated for the relief of moderate to severe pain, especially in patients with a hypersensitivity to narcotic analgesics. Although buprenorphine produces an antagonistic effect approximately three times greater than that of naloxone, it is rarely used clinically to reverse the effects of opiates.

The major side effect associated with buprenorphine is excessive sedation. Other effects on the nervous system include dizziness, vertigo, headache, confusion, euphoria, and insomnia. Nausea, vomiting, hypotension or hypertension, tachycardia or bradycardia, and respiratory depression have also been reported after buprenorphine administration.

Buprenorphine may potentiate the effects of CNS depressants, such as tranquilizers and sedatives. The concomitant administration of IV buprenorphine and oral diazepam has resulted in respiratory and cardiovascular collapse.

Related drugs. Two related mixed narcotic agonist-antagonists are nalbuphine hydrochloride (Nubain) and pentazocine lactate (Talwin). The mechanism of action, indications, and side effects of both drugs are similar to those of buprenorphine. However, respiratory depression associated with nalbuphine does not increase with increasing doses, as occurs with buprenorphine.

Butorphanol (Stadol) is a synthetic partial opiate agonist analgesic. It is structurally related to morphine but pharmacologically similar to nalbuphine and pentazocine.

Sedatives, hypnotics, and anxiolytics.
Several CNS depressants cause drowsiness (sedatives), induce sleep (hypnotics), or relieve anxiety (anxiolytics). These drugs may be chemically classified as barbiturates, which produce CNS depression ranging from sedation to anesthesia; benzodiazepines, which relieve anxiety without causing ataxia or sleep; and miscellaneous CNS agents that produce antiemetic and sedative or anxiolytic effects.

Barbiturates.
Barbiturates make up the traditional group of CNS depressants. They can produce varying levels of CNS depression ranging from mild sedation and hypnosis to coma and death. Generally, barbiturates share the same pharmacologic effects, side effects, contraindications, and drug interactions.

Prototype: phenobarbital sodium. Phenobarbital sodium (Luminal) may be used as a sedative because of its slow onset of action and its prolonged effect. However, it may produce a hypnotic effect at higher dosages. IV phenobarbital is primarily used as an anticonvulsant in pediatric patients. It inhibits abnormal electrical activity in the brain without producing marked sedation and is therefore indicated in the management of tonic-clonic (grand mal) and partial seizures.

Phenobarbital is administered by direct injection; too rapid administration of phenobarbital may cause respiratory depression, apnea, laryngospasm, and hypotension. The most common side effects of phenobarbital are excessive sedation and ataxia; facial edema, fever, and thrombocytopenia purpura may also occur. In addition, phenobarbital may cause pain or thrombophlebitis at the injection site.

Phenobarbital is contraindicated in patients who have a history of porphyria, which is characterized by excessive formation of porphyrins in the liver. Barbiturates such as phenobarbital stimulate porphyrin synthesis, which causes dermatologic reactions and peripheral nerve damage.

Phenobarbital may potentiate the effects of other CNS depressants and the adverse effects of antidepressants. Because phenobarbital stimulates the hepatic metabolizing enzymes, it increases the metabolism of corticosteroids and digitoxin, so increased dosages of these drugs may be required. It also inhibits the effectiveness of doxycycline, propranolol, oral anticoagulants, and theophylline.

Related drugs. Other barbiturates that may be administered intravenously are amobarbital sodium (Amytal), pentobarbital sodium (Nembutal), secobarbital sodium (Seconal), and thiopental sodium (Pentothal). These drugs differ primarily in their onset and duration of action. Thiopental and methohexital sodium (Brevital) are ultrashort-acting barbiturates used primarily for their anesthetic effects. Pentobarbital and secobarbital are short-acting barbiturates used for preanesthetic sedation. Amobarbital has a longer duration of action than pentobarbital and secobarbital and is used to control seizures caused by eclampsia, poisoning, meningitis, or tetanus.

Benzodiazepines.
Benzodiazepines differ from barbiturates chemically but share many of the same indications. Often, benzodiazepines are preferred to barbiturates because they have a greater margin of safety and are less likely to interact with other drugs and to cause physical dependence. Benzodiazepines have four basic actions: they reduce anxiety, produce sedation, relax muscle spasticity, and act as anticonvulsants.

Prototype: diazepam. Diazepam (Valium) depresses the autonomic, central, and peripheral nervous systems. For this reason, IV diazepam is indicated for the management of acute alcohol withdrawal, the emergency treatment of status epilepticus or recurrent seizures, the treatment of skeletal muscle spasm, and the relief of apprehension before electric cardioversion, endoscopy, or surgery.

Because of several reports of precipitation or absorption of the drug into plastic tubing, the preferred method of diazepam injection is by direct injection into the vein. When direct IV injection is not feasible, diazepam should be injected into the IV tubing as close to the vein site as possible. If this alternative method is used, the IV cannula should be flushed with normal saline before and after the administration of diazepam. The manufacturers state that diazepam may form a precipitate when mixed with other solutions, including sodium chloride, so the possibility of precipitate formation still exists when flushing the cannula. Nonetheless, most clinicians agree that this risk of precipitation is lower than if diazepam is mixed with other medications in the IV line.

The most common adverse reactions to diazepam are the results of CNS depression and are similar to the side effects associated with barbiturates. They include drowsiness, ataxia, confusion, syncope, and vertigo. Anticholinergic side effects, or atropine-like reactions, may also occur and result in blurred vision, mydriasis, and dry mouth. Other adverse reactions, such as apnea, hypotension, bradycardia, or cardiac arrest, are rare and are generally associated with rapid administration of the drug.

Because of the possibility of anticholinergic effects, diazepam is contraindicated in patients with acute narrow-angle glaucoma. It is also contraindicated for patients with acute alcohol intoxication whose vital signs are depressed and for patients with known hypersensitivity to the benzodiazepines.

Diazepam is potentiated by other drugs that produce similar CNS depression and by cimetidine. In addition, diazepam potentiates the effects of narcotics, barbiturates, antihistamines, and phenothiazines. When diazepam is administered concurrently with levodopa, the antiparkinsonian effects of levodopa may be inhibited.

Related drugs. The three other benzodiazepines that are most commonly administered by the IV route are chlordiazepoxide hydrochloride (Librium), lorazepam (Ativan), and midazolam hydrochloride (Versed). Chlordiazepoxide is primarily used for acute or severe agitation and acute alcoholism withdrawal, and lorazepam is used as a preanesthetic medication for adult patients. Midazolam is a short-acting benzodiazepine that has been effective in producing conscious sedation for endoscopic and cardiovascular procedures in healthy adults younger than 60 years of age. Because hypoxia or cardiac arrest may occur after midazolam is given, administration of the drug should be limited to settings in which respiratory and cardiac function may be monitored continuously.

Antagonist. Flumazenil (Romazicon) is a benzodiazepine receptor antagonist indicated for the reversal of the sedative effects of benzodiazepines. The duration and degree of reversal correspond with the dose of flumazenil administered and the resultant plasma concentration. The usual initial dosage is 0.2 mg administered by direct injection over 15 minutes; additional doses may be administered at 60-minute intervals. The onset of action is usually evident within 1 to 2 minutes after the injection is completed. Adverse effects include cutaneous vasodilation, dizziness, visual disturbances, cardiac arrhythmias, bradycardia or tachycardia, rigors, and pain at the injection site.

Miscellaneous central nervous system agents.
Two other CNS drugs, droperidol and promethazine hydrochloride, are often administered intravenously. Rather than reviewing their drug classifications, only information specific to these drugs is discussed here.

Droperidol. Droperidol (Inapsine) is classified as a tranquilizer. The primary indications of this drug are for preoperative sedation and for reduction of the incidence of nausea and vomiting during surgical and diagnostic procedures. Because of the cardiovascular side effects associated with droperidol, it is generally reserved for use under the direction of an anesthesiologist.

Promethazine hydrochloride. Promethazine hydrochloride (Phenergan) is a phenothiazine derivative with potent sedative properties; it produces antihistamine, antiemetic, anti–motion sickness, and anticholinergic effects, and it is often used as an adjunct for pain control in terminal cancer patients. The most common side effects of promethazine are venous irritation and phlebitis, suggesting that the peripheral IV site be rotated often or a central venous catheter be used.

Anticonvulsants. Epilepsy is a neurologic disorder characterized by a recurrent pattern of abnormal neuron discharges within the brain. The result is a sudden loss of consciousness, inappropriate behavior, and/or involuntary body movements. Seizures may be classified as partial, with electroencephalogram (EEG) changes confined to one area of the brain, or generalized, involving the symmetric distribution of abnormal brain discharges. Status epilepticus results when several generalized seizures with convulsions occur successively without intervals of restored consciousness or normal muscle activity. Although anticonvulsants suppress the start or reduce the spread of seizures, they do not treat the underlying cause of the seizures. Therefore the type of seizure, not the underlying cause, determines the drug of choice.[2]

Many of the drugs previously discussed have anticonvulsant properties. Phenobarbital is indicated for the treatment of generalized and partial seizures, and diazepam is the drug of choice for status epilepticus. Two additional categories of drugs, hydantoins and magnesium sulfate, are also indicated in the management of seizure activity.

Hydantoins. Hydantoins are used to treat clonic-tonic and complex partial seizures. Their principle feature is the ability to control seizures without causing sedation.

Prototype: phenytoin sodium. Phenytoin sodium (Dilantin) is a hydantoin derivative. Although it is used primarily for its anticonvulsant features, it also has antiarrhythmic properties similar to those of procainamide. The primary indications for phenytoin are the control of clonic-tonic and psychomotor seizures.

The preferred method for administering phenytoin is by direct IV injection at a rate not exceeding 50 mg/min. Because phenytoin precipitates if the pH is altered, the IV tubing and cannula must be cleared by flushing with normal saline before and after administration. This prevents phenytoin from mixing with other drugs. Solutions of 0.9% sodium chloride can be used to infuse phenytoin in concentrations of 100 mg in 25 to 50 ml of diluent. Higher concentrations have also been administered, but the maximum amount of diluent is 100 ml. When this alternative mode of administration is used, the drug infusion must be prepared immediately before use, administered within 1 hour, and infused above the filter.

When phenytoin is administered as an anticonvulsant, the most common side effects involve the CNS. Sluggishness, ataxia, nystagmus, confusion, slurred speech, dizziness, nervousness, and fatigue may occur. Gingival hyperplasia and excessive growth of the gums may also occur with extended therapy. Because of its antiarrhythmic properties, phenytoin is associated with adverse cardiovascular effects. Hypotension may occur with too rapid administration of the drug, whereas phenytoin toxicity may result in cardiovascular collapse. In addition, status epilepticus may result from abrupt withdrawal of the drug.

There is a narrow therapeutic margin associated with phenytoin. Acceptable plasma levels range from 5 to 20 µg/ml, and signs of toxicity occur once plasma levels exceed 20 µg. Symptoms of toxicity include nystagmus, ataxia, dysarthria, tremors, slurred speech, and nausea and vomiting.

The major contraindication for phenytoin is hypersensitivity to hydantoins. Because of its effects on cardiac electrical activity, phenytoin should not be administered to patients with sinus bradycardia, sinoatrial block, second- or third-degree heart block, or Stokes-Adams syndrome.

Phenytoin interacts with several other drugs to increase or decrease their effectiveness. Phenytoin is potentiated by anticoagulants, antidepressants, cimetidine, and phenothiazines, but it potentiates CNS depressants and muscle relaxants. Barbiturates and theophylline inhibit phenytoin, whereas phenytoin inhibits corticosteroids and digitalis. In addition, the concomitant administration of phenytoin and sympathomimetic antihypertensive drugs such as dopamine may result in severe hypotension and bradycardia.

Related drug. Fosphenytoin (Cerebyx), a prodrug of phenytoin, can be administered by IV infusion to achieve a more rapid effect.

Magnesium. Magnesium sulfate is a CNS depressant that exhibits anticonvulsant properties when administered parenterally. As such, magnesium sulfate is indicated for the prevention and control of seizures associated with severe preeclampsia or eclampsia. The onset of action is usually immediate and lasts for approximately 30 minutes. Other indications for the drug include the treatment of hypomagnesemia and as an additive in total parenteral nutrition solutions.

The primary adverse reaction associated with magnesium sulfate is magnesium intoxication. Symptoms of hypermagnesemia begin at serum magnesium concentrations of 4 mEq/L and include the absence of the knee-jerk reflex, hypotension with signs of tetany, hyperthermia, circulatory collapse, and depression of CNS and cardiac function. Because it is considered a CNS depressant, high dosages of magnesium sulfate may potentiate the effects of other CNS depressants.

Cardiovascular drugs

Drugs that alter cardiovascular function have a variety of actions. They can affect cardiac strength and rhythm, counteract hypotension, control hypertension, and improve blood flow. Because a comprehensive discussion of these agents is beyond our scope here, the focus is on the major categories of cardiovascular agents. The sympathetic nervous system plays a major role in cardiovascular function, and drugs acting on the CNS are discussed in this section. Table 11-3 summarizes the cardiovascular drugs typically used in cardiac resuscitation.

Drugs acting through adrenergic receptors.
Adrenergic receptors on the target cells within the sympathetic nervous system mediate the response of the neurotransmitters (norepinephrine and epinephrine). Drugs that elicit biologic responses similar to those produced by activation of the sympathetic nervous system are known as *sympathomimetics;* drugs that inhibit the effects of sympathetic stimulation are called *sympatholytics.* Because sympathomimetics mimic the sympathetic nervous system and provoke a response in the adrenergic receptors, they are also known as *adrenergic agonists.* In contrast, sympatholytics block the sympathetic nervous system and inhibit the adrenergic response, so they are referred to as *adrenergic blocking agents.*[2]

Cardiovascular drugs that elicit or inhibit the adrenergic response are also classified according to the subtype of adrenergic receptor site stimulated. There are four major subtypes of adrenergic receptors: alpha$_1$, alpha$_2$, beta$_1$, and beta$_2$. Alpha$_1$-adrenergic receptors mediate the typical sympathetic responses

Table 11-3	New Recommendations for Drugs Used in Cardiac Resuscitation[12]	
DRUG	**INDICATIONS**	**CONSIDERATIONS**
Lidocaine or	Ventricular arrhythmia	Evidence is weak for this agent as front line, but not listed as harmful
Amiodarone or Procainamide		Evidence supports use as first-line agent
Epinephrine or Vasopressin	Asystole; to elevate perfusion pressure	High dosage (0.1 mg/kg) not recommended Strong evidence with lower incidence of adverse effects
Atropine	Sinus bradycardia; high-degree AV block	Repeat until heart rate >60 bpm
Dopamine	Shock syndrome Hemodynamic imbalances	Renal perfusion varies with dosage Titrate to BP

AV, Atrioventricular; *bpm,* beats per minute; *BP,* blood pressure.

such as mydriasis and vasoconstriction, whereas alpha$_2$-adrenergic receptors provide a negative feedback to inhibit release of norepinephrine. Beta$_1$-adrenergic receptors mediate cardiac stimulation, but beta$_2$-adrenergic receptors mediate noncardiac responses, such as bronchodilation and vasodilation. Cardiovascular drugs that stimulate (or inhibit) both alpha- and beta-adrenergic receptors are considered totally nonselective; the drugs are highly selective if they stimulate (or inhibit) only one subtype of alpha- or beta-adrenergic receptor.

Alpha-beta-adrenergic agonists.
The alpha-beta-adrenergic agonists act on the alpha- and beta-adrenergic receptors. Because these drugs are nonselective, they imitate almost all actions of the sympathetic nervous system.

Prototype: epinephrine hydrochloride. Epinephrine hydrochloride (Adrenalin) is the least selective adrenergic agonist and is identical to the epinephrine synthesized within the body. It acts on the cardiovascular system by strengthening the force of cardiac contraction, increasing the contraction rate, and usually increasing cardiac output. Epinephrine elevates the systolic blood pressure and decreases the diastolic blood pressure, resulting in a widened pulse pressure. Because of its actions, epinephrine is considered the drug of choice for anaphylactic shock and is used in cardiac resuscitation. It is also the antidote of choice for histamine overdose and allergic reactions. The usual dosage for cardiac resuscitation is 0.5 to 1.0 mg of a 1:10,000 solution by direct injection; this may be repeated every 3 to 5 minutes, as required.

Because epinephrine stimulates both the alpha- and beta-adrenergic receptors, it may produce side effects in any patient receiving the drug. These are often transitory and include anxiety, dizziness, dyspnea, pallor, and palpitations. More serious side effects, such as cerebrovascular hemorrhage, fibrillation, severe headache, hypotension, pulmonary edema, and tachycardia, are associated with overdose or too rapid injection of the drug.

Epinephrine interacts with many drugs. It is potentiated by anesthetics and antihistamines but antagonized by adrenergic blockers. Epinephrine may be used alternately with isoproterenol, but the two drugs should not be used together because they are both cardiac stimulants.

Related drugs. Norepinephrine bitartrate (Levophed) is pharmacologically equivalent to the sympathetic neurotransmitter norepinephrine. It is an agonist for the alpha- and beta$_1$-adrenergic receptors but has almost no effect on beta$_2$-adrenergic receptors. Because it is more selective, the actions of norepinephrine are more limited than those of epinephrine. Norepinephrine is primarily used as a vasopressor agent to raise the blood pressure in acute hypotensive states. Because it is a potent vasoconstrictor, severe tissue necrosis can result from extravasation of this drug into the surrounding tissue.

Alpha-adrenergic agonists.
The alpha-adrenergic agonists mimic the action of naturally occurring norepinephrine on the alpha-adrenergic receptors but may also stimulate beta-adrenergic receptors of the heart (beta$_1$-adrenergic receptors). The primary effects of these drugs are vasoconstriction and cardiac stimulation.

Prototype: metaraminol bitartrate. Metaraminol bitartrate (Aramine) produces vasoconstriction, which results in elevation of the systolic and diastolic blood pressure. It also strengthens cardiac contractility and increases coronary, cerebral, and renal blood flow. Because of these actions, metaraminol is indicated for acute hypotensive states.

Metaraminol is less potent than norepinephrine, but it has similar side effects and precautions. In addition, metaraminol may cause increased arterial pressure, resulting in bradycardia. Although metaraminol may be administered by direct injection at the rate of 5 mg over 1 minute in emergency situations, it is usually administered as a continuous infusion by means of an electronic infusion device. During the infusion, the patient's blood pressure should be monitored every 5 minutes until the desired effect is achieved and every 15 minutes thereafter. As with norepinephrine, infiltration of metaraminol may result in tissue necrosis and sloughing.

Related drug. Methoxamine hydrochloride (Vasoxyl) is a potent vasopressor, but it does not produce undesired cardiac or CNS stimulation. IV administration is limited to emergencies in which the systolic blood pressure is lower than 60 mm Hg.

Beta-adrenergic agonists.
Drugs that act only on the beta-adrenergic receptors are used primarily to stimulate the heart or dilate the bronchi. When the mechanism of action is limited to only the beta$_1$-adrenergic receptors, the primary effect is cardiac stimulation. If the drugs act on the beta$_2$-adrenergic receptors, bronchodilation and vasodilation result.

Prototype: dopamine hydrochloride. Dopamine hydrochloride (Intropin) is a selective beta$_1$-adrenergic agonist indicated for the correction of hemodynamic imbalances. It produces a positive inotropic effect by stimulating cardiac contractile force and is sometimes classified as an inotropic agent. Because dopamine increases cardiac output, blood pressure, and urine output, it is administered as an adjunct in the treatment of shock. The patient's response must be monitored

carefully based on these effects, and the administration rate must be adjusted accordingly.

Dopamine is administered by continuous infusion using an electronic infusion device. The usual initial dosage is 2 to 5 µg/kg body weight. The dosage is then gradually increased by 5 to 10 µg/kg/min in 10- to 30-minute increments and titrated based on the patient's response to treatment. Blood pressure should be monitored every 2 minutes until the patient has been stabilized at the desired level and every 5 minutes thereafter. As with norepinephrine, there is a risk of tissue necrosis if the drug infiltrates into surrounding tissue.

The side effects of dopamine are associated with its cardiac effects. Bradycardia, tachycardia, hypertension, hypotension, vasoconstriction, and a widened QRS complex may occur. Other side effects include nausea, vomiting, headache, and dyspnea. The rate of infusion should be immediately decreased and the physician notified if there is a disproportionate rise in diastolic blood pressure, an increasing degree of tachycardia, or a decreased urinary output.

Related drugs. Dobutamine hydrochloride (Dobutrex) is a selective beta$_1$-adrenergic agonist that stimulates cardiac contractile force (positive inotropic effect), with less alteration in heart rate than dopamine. Following stabilization of the patient in the hospital, dobutamine can be continued in the home under closely supervised conditions.

Isoproterenol hydrochloride (Isuprel) differs from dopamine in that it stimulates both beta$_1$- and beta$_2$-adrenergic receptors to produce cardiac and bronchial effects. The primary indications for isoproterenol are the treatment of atrioventricular (AV) heart block, cardiac standstill, and bronchospasm.

Beta-adrenergic blockers.
Beta-adrenergic blockers bind with the beta-adrenergic receptors to prevent the action of the naturally occurring beta-adrenergic receptor agonists (norepinephrine and epinephrine). Most beta-blockers are nonselective in that they do not differentiate between beta$_1$- and beta$_2$-adrenergic receptors. In contrast, cardioselective beta-blockers produce their antiarrhythmic and antihypertensive effects by inhibiting only the beta$_1$-adrenergic receptors. Because the cardioselective blockers have no effect on the beta$_2$-adrenergic receptors that mediate bronchial dilation, they are generally safer for patients who have accompanying respiratory disease.

Prototype: propranolol hydrochloride. Propranolol hydrochloride (Inderal) is a nonselective beta-adrenergic blocker that acts on both beta$_1$- and beta$_2$-adrenergic receptors. Because it produces antiarrhythmic effects, propranolol is indicated in the management of life-threatening cardiac arrhythmias such as paroxysmal atrial tachycardia, atrial flutter, and atrial fibrillation. Cardiac function and blood pressure should be monitored continuously during administration.

Because of the nonselective beta blocking, propranolol may cause cardiovascular, respiratory, and metabolic side effects, especially in patients with severe cardiac disease, respiratory disease, or diabetes mellitus. Other side effects include syncope, vertigo, visual disturbances, and paresthesia of the hands.

Related drugs. Esmolol hydrochloride (Brevibloc) is a fast-acting nonselective beta-blocker indicated for the treatment of acute episodes of supraventricular or sinus tachycardia and atrial flutter or fibrillation. In contrast, metoprolol tartrate

(Lopressor) is a cardioselective beta-blocker. Although the exact mechanism of action is unknown, metoprolol has been effective in reducing cardiac mortality in patients with suspected or diagnosed myocardial infarction.

Alpha-adrenergic blockers. The alpha-adrenergic blockers prevent the naturally occurring alpha-adrenergic receptor agonists (epinephrine and norepinephrine) from binding to the alpha-adrenergic receptor sites.

Labetalol hydrochloride. Because of its effects on the alpha-receptors, labetalol hydrochloride (Normodyne) reduces peripheral vascular resistance, resulting in decreased blood pressure. It also blocks the beta-adrenergic receptors to produce propranolol-like depression of cardiac contractility. As a result of these alpha- and beta-adrenergic effects, labetalol is indicated for the management of blood pressure in patients with severe hypertension.

Phentolamine mesylate. Phentolamine mesylate (Regitine) blocks the alpha-adrenergic receptors and antagonizes responses to epinephrine and norepinephrine. Because of its ability to reduce blood pressure, phentolamine is primarily indicated for the treatment of hypertensive episodes associated with pheochromocytoma. It may also be added to solutions of norepinephrine or dopamine to prevent dermal necrosis in event of extravasation of the solution, or it may be administered subcutaneously into the tissue if extravasation does occur.

Drugs affecting cardiac strength and rhythm.

When the heart loses its ability to contract with normal strength, drugs are administered to strengthen the cardiac contraction. Such drugs include the beta-adrenergic receptor agonists (see previous discussion), cardiac glycosides, and miscellaneous inotropic agents. In contrast, alterations in cardiac rate or rhythm require the administration of antiarrhythmics.

Cardiac glycosides. Cardiac glycosides act directly on the myocardium to increase cardiac contractility and alter electrical impulse generation and conduction. This results in slower, stronger contractions, with increased cardiac output.

Prototype: digoxin. Digoxin (Lanoxin) is indicated in the treatment of congestive heart failure, atrial fibrillation and flutter, paroxysmal tachycardia, and cardiogenic shock. Effects begin within 5 to 30 minutes of administration and last up to 3 days.

Digoxin has a narrow margin of safety. Dosages must be individualized because a therapeutic dose for one patient may be toxic to another. Whereas the first signs of toxicity may be detected on ECG monitoring, the most common clinical symptoms are nausea, vomiting, and anorexia. Patients may also experience blurred vision, disturbed color vision, headache, confusion, and diarrhea.

Many drugs interact with digoxin:

1. Drugs that alter serum electrolyte levels, such as potassium-sparing diuretics, can affect the intensity of the response to digoxin.
2. Autonomic agents can alter the effects of digoxin on cardiac conductivity.
3. Drugs that affect the metabolism or excretion of digoxin, such as phenytoin, quinidine, or verapamil, may require adjustment of the digoxin dosage to maintain therapeutic effects.

Antidote. Digoxin immune Fab (Digibind) contains anti-digoxin antibodies that bind to the digoxin molecules, rendering them unable to exert their toxic effects. Because it is obtained from sheep serum, digoxin immune Fab is potentially allergenic.

Miscellaneous inotropic agents. Other inotropic agents enhance the strength of cardiac contraction but differ from cardiac glycosides and beta-adrenergic receptor agonists in their mechanism of action.

Prototype: amrinone lactate. Amrinone lactate (Inocor) produces inotropic and vasodilator effects. It is mainly indicated for the short-term management of congestive heart failure in patients who have been unresponsive to conventional therapies.

Antiarrhythmics. Cardiac arrhythmias occur when there is a deviation from the normal sinus rhythm. Under normal circumstances, there are changes in cardiac electrical activity that occur in a constant sequence. The normal heartbeat originates in the sinoatrial (SA) node at a rate of 60 to 80 beats per minute (bpm). If the heart rate is greater than 100 bpm, it is classified as tachycardia; rates lower than 60 bpm are classified as bradycardias. If the impulse originates in the SA node and only the rate is altered, the arrhythmia may be classified as sinus tachycardia or sinus bradycardia.

Impulses are transmitted from the SA node to the atrial muscle, causing the atria to contract. On ECG monitoring, this electrical activity is reflected by the P wave. The impulse is then passed from the atria to the ventricles through the AV node. Because the atria must complete their contractions before the ventricles are activated, there is a brief delay, demonstrated by the PR interval on the ECG. From the AV node, impulses pass through the bundle of His, bundle branches, and Purkinje fibers to activate the ventricles. This phase is the QRS complex on the ECG.

If the impulse is not delivered to the ventricles from the AV node, the ventricles attempt to beat at their own rate. Such a condition is known as *heart block,* and it may be partial or complete. The degree of partial heart block is classified in a manner that reflects the number of atrial contractions for each ventricular contraction. In complete heart block, no impulses pass from the atria to the ventricles.

With the normal heartbeat, there is a spontaneous depolarization of the SA node and a sequential conduction of the impulse along specific pathways within the heart. In abnormal conditions, however, a region of the heart other than the SA node may initiate its own impulse. Such an ectopic impulse causes the heartbeat to become unsynchronized, resulting in a serious arrhythmia.

To maintain the normal heartbeat, the myocardial cells have four unique properties. First, the cells have the ability to initiate their own activity by spontaneous depolarization, known as *automaticity.* Second, the cells depolarize at a regular rate, called *rhythmicity.* Third, the cells have the ability to transmit impulses at an appropriate rate, known as *conduction.* Last, the cells have *refractoriness,* meaning that they are resistant to further stimulation during repolarization.

Cardiac arrhythmias are usually classified according to their site of origin. If there is abnormal conduction above the ventricles, they are categorized as *supraventricular arrhythmias.* Examples of such arrhythmias are sinus bradycardia and atrial fibrillation or flutter. Sometimes, arrhythmias originating in the atria, such as atrial fibrillation or flutter, are further classified as *atrial arrhythmias.* When there is abnormal conduction in the ventricles, they are referred to as *ventricular arrhythmias.* Premature ventricular contractions (PVCs) and ventricular tachycardia are examples of ventricular arrhythmias.

Antiarrhythmics are administered to prevent or stop an irregular heart rate or rhythm. Because there is no universal antiarrhythmic, no single prototype can be identified. For purposes here, antiarrhythmics are grouped according to their mechanism of action and the most common drugs for each group are discussed. Because of the cardiac effects of these drugs, IV administration requires continuous ECG and blood pressure monitoring.

Group A. Some antiarrhythmics decrease the transport of sodium through the cardiac tissue and slow conduction through the AV node. Because this prolongs the refractory period and decreases the automaticity of the heart, these drugs are indicated for the treatment of supraventricular arrhythmias, such as atrial fibrillation and flutter. Examples of such drugs are quinidine gluconate and procainamide hydrochloride (Pronestyl).

Quinidine gluconate. Quinidine is indicated for the management of atrial fibrillation and flutter. It has also been used to treat Wolff-Parkinson-White syndrome, which is characterized by supraventricular tachycardia. Because quinidine acts by decreasing AV node conduction, adverse effects include AV block, decreased cardiac output, and cardiac standstill. Other adverse reactions include acute hypotension, diaphoresis, tinnitus, and visual disturbances. In rare instances, ventricular tachycardia and fibrillation have occurred. Caution should be exercised in patients who need digoxin. Although this drug interaction can vary among patients, digoxin dosage should be reduced if quinidine is added.

Procainamide hydrochloride. Procainamide hydrochloride (Pronestyl) is similar to quinidine but has a more rapid onset of action and is less likely to cause hypotension or cardiac depression. Procainamide acts by slowing the heart rate and conduction, decreasing myocardial irritability, and prolonging the refractory period, and it is indicated for the emergency treatment of ventricular and supraventricular arrhythmias. Side effects of procainamide are usually dose related and are similar to those associated with quinidine. Caution should be used in patients requiring amiodarone because high procainamide levels may result.

Group B. Group B antiarrhythmics decrease the refractory period, especially in the Purkinje fibers and the ventricular myocardium. By acting preferentially on areas of the myocardium in which impulse conduction rates and automaticity are abnormal, these drugs promote uniform conduction rates throughout the heart. As a result, ventricular excitability is reduced without a reduction in the force of the ventricular contractions. The best-known example of this group is lidocaine. Phenytoin, an anticonvulsant, also belongs in this group.

Lidocaine hydrochloride. Lidocaine hydrochloride (Xylocaine) is the drug of choice for the treatment of ventricular arrhythmias and ventricular tachycardias, especially following a myocardial infarction. The usual bolus dose is 50 to 100 mg administered at a rate not exceeding 25 mg/min. If the desired response is not achieved, a second dose (e.g., 25 to 50 mg) may be given 5 to 10 minutes later. Patients should not receive more than 200 to 300 mg within the first hour. After the bolus dose is administered, a continuous infusion of 1 to 4 mg/min is initiated to maintain a therapeutic serum level between 1.5 and 5 µg/ml. Dosage should be reduced for patients with congestive heart failure or liver disease. Greater-than-recommended doses and too rapid administration rates are likely to cause excessive cardiac depression and CNS stimulation.

Lidocaine has a relatively low margin of safety. Serum levels above 6 µg/ml are usually toxic and may suppress AV transmission, resulting in partial or complete heart block. In addition, high serum levels may produce adverse CNS effects. Sedation and drowsiness are associated with therapeutic blood levels. Higher levels may cause unconsciousness, generalized convulsions, and respiratory arrest. However, more common side effects (even at therapeutic blood levels) include apprehension, blurred vision, light-headedness, tinnitus, and numbness.

Lidocaine is potentiated by beta-adrenergic blockers and phenytoin. The concomitant administration of these drugs with lidocaine may result in cardiac depression and an increased likelihood of excessive CNS effects.

Phenytoin sodium. Phenytoin sodium (Dilantin) is chemically unrelated to lidocaine, but the two drugs are similar in their antiarrhythmic actions. As discussed earlier, phenytoin is an effective anticonvulsant. However, it is also indicated for the treatment of digitalis-induced arrhythmias because it normalizes AV conduction and suppresses ectopic pacemakers. Adverse reactions and side effects of phenytoin are similar to those of lidocaine. Too rapid administration or toxic serum levels may cause severe depression of cardiac contractility, severe hypotension, and excessive CNS effects.

Group C. Antiarrhythmic effects are also produced by the beta-adrenergic receptor blockers. As discussed earlier, beta-adrenergic blockers inhibit the cardiac response from sympathetic nerve stimulation. They slow the heart rate by inhibiting AV conduction, reduce the force of cardiac contractility, and decrease arterial pressure and cardiac output. Beta-adrenergic blockers are particularly effective in the management of arrhythmias caused by excessive sympathetic cardiac stimulation or sympathomimetic drugs. Propranolol hydrochloride (Inderal) and esmolol hydrochloride (Brevibloc) are beta-adrenergic blockers used to manage arrhythmias involving increased sympathetic cardiac stimulation.

Group D. Antiarrhythmics in this group prolong the action potential, increasing the cellular refractory period and producing an antifibrillatory effect. Although the drugs of this group are chemically unrelated, they share the ability to suppress ventricular tachycardia and prevent ventricular fibrillation. An example of this group of antiarrhythmics is bretylium tosylate (Bretylol).

Bretylium tosylate. Bretylium tosylate (Bretylol) increases the refractory period without increasing the heart rate and is effective in the treatment of life-threatening ventricular arrhythmias. Because it increases the ventricular fibrillation threshold, bretylium is indicated for the prophylaxis and treatment of ventricular fibrillation. Therefore bretylium is sometimes classified as an antifibrillatory agent.

The administration of bretylium is associated with adverse effects; however, reactions associated with initial doses differ from those related to subsequent administration. With initial administration, the patient may experience hypertension, tachycardia, or worsening of the arrhythmia. Because bretylium blocks the release of norepinephrine from the sympathetic nerves, its subsequent administration is often associated with postural hypotension. Other adverse effects include syncope, transient hypertension, substernal pressure, and bradycardia.

Group E. Calcium channel blockers slow electrical impulse conduction rates and increase the cellular refractory period by blocking the influx of calcium into the cells. This action reduces conduction of the impulse through the SA and AV nodes, prolongs the refractory period in the AV node, and reduces ventricular rates. A common calcium channel blocker is verapamil hydrochloride (Isoptin).

Verapamil hydrochloride. Verapamil hydrochloride (Isoptin) is effective in the treatment of supraventricular tachyarrhythmias and temporary management of a rapid ventricular rate in atrial flutter or fibrillation. Verapamil acts by decreasing the myocardial contractility, afterload, arterial pressure, vascular tone, and oxygen demand within 5 minutes of administration. Potential side effects include dizziness, headache, abdominal discomfort, bradycardia or tachycardia, hypotension, and PVCs.

When verapamil is administered, potential drug interactions must be considered. Because digoxin is potentiated by verapamil, lower dosages of digoxin may be required. The concomitant administration of verapamil and beta-adrenergic drugs must be avoided because both drugs depress myocardial contractility and conduction through the AV node. Excessive hypotension may result from the administration of antihypertensive drugs and verapamil. Diltiazem (Cardizem) is also in this group and inhibits the cardiac conduction system primarily at the AV node. Heart rate should be monitored.

Group F. Atropine sulfate is not usually classified as an antiarrhythmic, but it has antiarrhythmic effects. It is an anticholinergic drug that blocks the action of acetylcholine (ACh) on the SA node. Because ACh slows the heart rate, atropine blocks the action and restores the heart rate to a more normal level. Therefore atropine is indicated in the treatment of sinus bradycardia, syncope associated with Stokes-Adams syndrome, and AV block with profound bradycardia.

Group G. A newer antiarrhythmic that is different from other antiarrhythmic agents is amiodarone (Cordarone). The primary effect is to delay repolarization by prolonging the action potential and effective refractory period of the atria, ventricles, His-Purkinje system, sinus node, AV node, and accessory pathways, if present. Following a single IV dose, the major effect is on the AV node, whereas following chronic oral therapy, the effect is on the atria, ventricles, and AV nodal tissue.

Amiodarone will inhibit alpha- and beta-adrenergic responses to sympathetic stimulation and catecholamine administration, such as epinephrine, norepinephrine, and isoproterenol. It also relaxes cardiac and vascular smooth muscle, thereby dilating both systemic and coronary arteries. Following IV administration of 150 mg IV bolus, systemic blood pressure, systemic vascular resistance, coronary vascular resistance, and left ventricular end-diastolic pressure are decreased, while cardiac index may increase slightly. Amiodarone has also been reported to be highly effective in nonsustained ventricular tachycardia and frequent PVCs.

The most common adverse effect observed with IV amiodarone is hypotension. The drug has worsened existing arrhythmias or caused new arrhythmias in 2% to 5% of patients. Few data are available on drug interactions with parenteral amiodarone therapy. Because this drug has a long half-life, the potential exists for drug interactions not only with concomitantly administered drugs, but also with drugs administered after amiodarone has been discontinued.

Group H. Ibutilide (Corvert) prolongs repolarization of cardiac tissue by prolonging the action potential and effective refractory period in both atrial and ventricular cardiac tissue. The drug has negligible effects on heart rate, cardiac contractility, or blood pressure. Ibutilide is used IV for rapid conversion of recent-onset atrial flutter or fibrillation to sinus rhythm. However, like other agents, it can cause potentially fatal arrhythmias. In addition, concomitant administration of other antiarrhythmics can cause prolonged refractoriness of cardiac tissue.

Vasodilating agents. Nitroglycerin is used to control blood pressure in cardiovascular procedures; to treat ischemic pain, congestive heart failure, or pulmonary edema associated with acute myocardial infarction; and to control blood pressure during surgical procedures.

Prototype: nitroglycerin. Nitroglycerin (Nitroglycerin in 5% dextrose injection) is used during severe hypertension or hypertensive emergencies. An IV infusion dosage of up to 100 μg/min may be required, with effective dosages ranging from 5 to 100 μg/min. Hypotensive effect is usually seen within 2 to 5 minutes. Because nitroglycerin readily migrates into many plastics, manufacturers' instructions for dilution, dosage, and administration must be followed carefully. Headache, the most common adverse effect, is relieved by reducing the dosage or adding analgesics. Nitrate ions released during metabolism of nitroglycerin can oxidize hemoglobin to methemoglobin. Patients without cytochrome-b_5 reductase activity require about 1 mg/kg of nitroglycerin before they manifest clinically important methemoglobinemia. Tolerance has developed following high or sustained plasma drug concentrations but does not occur in all patients. Careful laboratory monitoring is required to avoid inadequate anticoagulation in patients receiving IV nitroglycerin and heparin.

Antihypertensives. The treatment of hypertension involves using drugs in a logical sequence. This generally accepted plan, known as the *stepped-care* approach, is presented in Table 11-4. The approach begins with the lowest effective dose of a single drug. If the drug fails to control the hypertension, small doses of additional drugs are used rather than markedly increasing the dosage of the initial drug. Step 1 drugs are often continued in the subsequent steps, and some step 2 drugs may be indicated for step 1 therapy when diuretics or beta-adrenergic blockers are inappropriate for a particular patient. (The beta-adrenergic blockers were reviewed earlier and thiazide diuretics are discussed in the subsection Agents for Electrolyte and Water Balance.) The latest guidelines for treating hypertension, developed by a national panel of experts, were published in 1997. The guidelines continued to support the stepped care

Table 11-4	**Stepped-Care Approach to Managing Essential Hypertension**
Step	
1	Lifestyle modifications
2	Initial drug choices based on the following:
	▪ Uncomplicated hypertension
	▪ Compelling indications
	▪ Specific indications for certain drugs
3	Evaluate for side effects and response
	—select another drug from a different class
4	Continue adding agents from other classes

approach, with the initial treatment using either diuretics or beta-blockers in otherwise healthy patients. However, additional importance was placed on other therapies in patients with compelling comorbid conditions. New blood pressure classification guidelines were printed, along with risk stratification and treatment specifics.[9]

To manage essential hypertension, these drugs are usually administered orally. IV administration is typically reserved for subacute or acute hypertensive emergencies. Discussion of antihypertensive agents in this section focuses on drugs used to treat severe and abrupt increases in blood pressure and is limited to those not previously discussed.

Methyldopate hydrochloride. Methyldopate hydrochloride (Aldomet) is a centrally acting antihypertensive that depresses sympathetic nervous system activity through an action in the CNS. IV methyldopate is indicated for the treatment of hypertensive crises, especially for patients with renal or coronary insufficiency.

The usual dosage of methyldopate is 250 to 500 mg administered over 30 to 60 minutes as an intermittent infusion every 6 hours. The patient's blood pressure needs to be monitored carefully throughout the therapy and the dosage withheld if the blood pressure is not within the limits established by the physician. Potential side effects include dizziness, dry mouth, sedation, postural hypotension or paradoxic hypertension, and apprehension.

Hydralazine hydrochloride. Hydralazine hydrochloride (Apresoline) is a potent antihypertensive drug that lowers the blood pressure by relaxing the smooth muscle of the arteries and arterioles. For this reason, it is sometimes classified as a vasodilator. The primary uses of hydralazine are for the treatment of severe essential hypertension and to promote vasodilation in cardiovascular shock.

Hydralazine is administered as a direct injection at a rate not exceeding 10 mg/min. The usual dosage is 10 to 40 mg, but the dosage may be increased gradually as required to a maximum dosage of 300 to 400 mg/24 hr.

As with methyldopate, the patient's blood pressure must be monitored carefully. Potential side effects include anxiety, paresthesia, dry mouth, unpleasant taste, tachycardia, palpitations, and postural hypotension. The peripheral vasodilation produced by hydralazine may stimulate the carotid sinus reflex, thus increasing the heart rate and cardiac output.

Nitroprusside sodium. Nitroprusside sodium (Nipride) is a vasodilator that produces effects similar to those of hydralazine. Because the most common side effects are reflex tachycardia and reduced arterial pressure, nitroprusside may be contraindicated for patients with ischemic heart disease.

Nitroprusside is administered as a continuous infusion by an electronic infusion device. The dose is based on body weight but is usually 3 µg/kg/min. Because nitroprusside is converted to thiocyanate before it is excreted in the urine, cyanide poisoning may occur if the recommended maximum dose of 10 µg/kg/min is exceeded. Other potential side effects include abdominal pain, dyspnea, diaphoresis, palpitations, headache, and muscle twitching.

The potency of nitroprusside can be affected by exposure to light, so the solution container (and sometimes the administration set) should be covered with aluminum foil or an opaque material to protect the drug from light.

Diazoxide. Another potent vasodilator, diazoxide (Hyperstat), acts by relaxing the smooth muscle of the peripheral arterioles. Because the drug is administered as a single dose, it is preferred when an infusion pump and titration monitoring are not immediately available.

Enalapril maleate. Enalapril maleate (Vasotec) lowers the blood pressure by interrupting the renin-angiotensin-aldosterone system. It acts by inhibiting the angiotensin-converting enzyme, which inhibits formation of the vasoconstrictor angiotensin II, and by indirectly reducing the blood levels of aldosterone. As a result, the peripheral arterial resistance is reduced and the blood pressure is lowered. Enalapril is administered as a direct injection over 5 minutes. Adverse reactions include dizziness, dyspnea, paraesthesia, and abdominal pain.

Trimethaphan. Trimethaphan (Arfonad) is used in hypertensive emergencies in which immediate blood pressure reduction is necessary to prevent or limit target organ damage. Because of the nonselective blockage on the autonomic nervous system and potential for significant adverse effects, only highly trained clinicians equipped with appropriate infusion pump and microdrip regulation should use this agent.

Nicardipine. Nicardipine (Cardene) is a calcium channel blocker that can be given intravenously to manage hypertensive crises in the perioperative setting. Headache is the most common adverse effect. Because this drug has a negative inotropic effect, caution should be used when administering beta-blockers to patients with congestive heart failure.

Hematologic agents

When a blood vessel wall is injured or severed, the body activates processes to maintain hemostasis. This protective mechanism is accomplished by means of a clotting cascade that is activated through a series of intrinsic and extrinsic factors. Although coagulation is usually the desired reaction, there are several clinical situations in which hemostasis must be inhibited or the coagulation process reversed. Hematologic agents such as anticoagulants and thrombolytics, respectively, are the drugs indicated for such situations.

Anticoagulants. Anticoagulants interfere with the coagulation pathways to prevent clot formation. They are effective in decreasing the risk of clot formation and preventing the enlargement or fragmentation of blood clots; however, anticoagulants cannot dissolve existing clots.

Prototype: heparin sodium. The prototype for parenteral anticoagulants is heparin sodium. Small doses of heparin inhibit the conversion of prothrombin to thrombin, and larger doses inactivate thrombin and prevent the conversion of fibrinogen to fibrin. Heparin therapy is indicated for the prophylaxis and treatment of venous thrombosis and pulmonary emboli; diagnosis and treatment of disseminated intravascular coagulation; prevention of coagulation during arterial and cardiac surgery, hemodialysis, and blood transfusions; prevention of embolism associated with mitral valve diseases and atrial fibrillation; and treatment of acute myocardial infarction, unstable angina, and cerebral embolism.

To achieve a constant degree of anticoagulation, the preferred mode of IV administration of heparin is by continuous infusion. However, heparin may be administered by intermittent injection with the dosage adjusted according to coagulation times. The most common laboratory test for monitoring heparin action is the activated partial thromboplastin time (aPTT). A baseline aPTT is measured before heparin therapy is initiated. Because heparin prolongs the aPTT in a dose-dependent manner, the therapeutic range for the aPTT during heparin therapy is 1.5 to 2.5 times the control value. Anti-Xa levels can also be used to keep heparin therapeutic between 0.3 and 0.7 units/ml.

As a result of the pharmacologic action of heparin, the major adverse effects are bleeding and hemorrhage. The frequency and severity of these effects may be minimized with careful monitoring of the aPTT during therapy. Whereas bleeding may occur at any site, the most common locations are the GI and urinary tracts and mucosal surfaces such as the nasal passages and gums. Epistaxis, hematuria, or tarry stools may be the first signs of overdosage.

A more uncommon adverse reaction to heparin is thrombocytopenia. The patient's platelet count must be monitored closely because a paradoxic reaction resulting in platelet aggregation, or white clot syndrome, may occur. Other side effects related to heparin therapy are rare but include hypersensitivity reactions, alopecia, and osteoporosis.

Heparin is contraindicated in patients with active bleeding, blood dyscrasias, history of bleeding disorder, or known hypersensitivity to the drug. In disease states in which there is a risk of hemorrhage, such as arterial sclerosis, aneurysm, hemophilia, and ulcerative colitis, heparin should be used with extreme caution. If heparin is administered with thrombolytic agents and platelet-activated drugs, the risk of hemorrhage may be increased.

Heparin interacts with a number of drugs. Antihistamines, barbiturates, digitalis, phenothiazines, and tetracyclines may chemically neutralize heparin, reducing its anticoagulant action. Conversely, heparin may be potentiated by chloramphenicol, dextran, ibuprofen, indomethacin, and penicillin.

Heparin may also be used to maintain the patency of venous access devices designed for intermittent use. The usual concentration of the heparin flush is 10 or 100 units of heparin per 1 ml 0.9% sodium chloride. The amount of solution depends on the device to be flushed but should be enough to reach the tip of the cannula or implanted port. The intervals between flushes are determined by the type of device and the frequency of use. Generally, a heparin flush is administered immediately following each IV medication or every 8 to 24 hours. Because heparin is incompatible with several other medications, the SASH technique should be used to instill the heparin flush. With this technique, the device is flushed with 0.9% sodium chloride (S), the medication is administered (A), the device is again flushed with 0.9% sodium chloride (S), and a heparin flush is administered (H).

Note: Low-molecular-weight heparins, such as enoxaparin (Lovenox), dalteparin (Fragmin), and ardeparin (Normiflo), are smaller compounds with significant antithrombotic effect. These agents are administered subcutaneously only and should not be confused with other heparin preparations.

Antidote. In the event of heparin overdose, protamine sulfate is administered to neutralize the heparin's anticoagulant activity. Protamine molecules that have positive electrostatic charges combine with the negatively charged heparin molecules to form the protamine-heparin complex, which has no anticoagulant activity. The dosage of protamine is determined by the heparin dosage, and approximately 100 units of heparin are neutralized by 1 mg of protamine. Because blood concentrations of heparin decrease rapidly after administration, the dosage of protamine required also decreases as time elapses.

Side effects associated with the rapid administration of protamine include acute hypotension, bradycardia, dyspnea, transient flushing, and pulmonary hypertension. These effects are minimized when protamine is administered slowly and the total dosage for any 10-minute period does not exceed 50 mg. Hypersensitivity reactions are rare but have been reported in persons allergic to fish.

Thrombolytic agents. In contrast to anticoagulants, which prevent the formation of clots or thrombi, thrombolytic agents promote thrombolysis. When a thrombosis or embolism obstructs blood flow in organs such as the heart, lungs, or brain, thrombolytic agents act by dissolving the obstruction and preventing ischemic tissue damage in the organ involved.

Prototype: streptokinase. The prototype of the thrombolytic agents is streptokinase (Streptase). Streptokinase, a nonenzymatic protein, works in a complex manner to combine with plasminogen found in the thrombi and convert it to plasmin. The plasmin in turn degrades fibrinogen and fibrin clots. Indications for streptokinase include lysis of coronary artery thrombosis, acute massive pulmonary embolism, and deep vein and arterial thrombosis. Streptokinase has also been used to clear totally or partially occluded AV cannulas.

Because streptokinase prolongs the normal coagulation process, particularly the thrombin time, the major side effect is hemorrhage. The administration of streptokinase is intended to lyse thrombi, and this may result in bleeding at injection sites. Geriatric women, especially those with diabetes mellitus, are at particular risk for bleeding complications during streptokinase therapy. Other adverse reactions include febrile and sensitivity reactions, ranging from urticaria to anaphylaxis. When the drug is used to lyse coronary artery thrombi, a reperfusion-induced arrhythmia may result. Phlebitis may occur at the streptokinase infusion site; this can be managed by further dilution of the drug.

Major contraindications for streptokinase are active internal bleeding, intracranial or intraspinal surgery, a recent cerebrovascular accident, severe uncontrolled hypertension, intracranial neoplasm, or a history of hypersensitivity to the drug. Streptokinase is also contraindicated after recent major surgery and for patients with subacute bacterial endocarditis. Because of the risk of hemorrhage, streptokinase should not be administered concurrently with anticoagulants or platelet-activating drugs.

Related drugs. There are three other thrombolytic agents that are similar to streptokinase. Anistreplase (Eminase), made from streptokinase and human plasminogen, exhibits an action similar to that of streptokinase. Alteplase (Activase) is a biosynthetic form of the enzyme human tissue–type plasminogen activator. Because alteplase binds only to the fibrin in the thrombus, it may be associated with a decreased risk of hemorrhage. The efficacy of using alteplase for treating occluded venous access devices has been evaluated with positive results. Both anistreplase and alteplase are used to lyse thrombi that are obstructing coronary arteries in the management of acute myocardial infarction.

Hemostatics. Hemostatics are indicated for the control of unexpected hemorrhagic episodes. Although all the drugs in this category arrest bleeding, each has a specific indication in clotting.

Prototype: aminocaproic acid. Aminocaproic acid (Amicar) is indicated in the treatment of excessive bleeding caused by overactivity of the fibrolytic system. It inhibits plasminogen activator substances and increases fibrinogen activity in clot formation. The primary indication for aminocaproic acid is systemic hyperfibrinolysis associated with heart surgery, aplastic anemia, or carcinoma of the lung, prostate, cervix, or stomach. It has also been effective in the treatment of overdosage of thrombolytic agents.

Adverse effects of aminocaproic acid are generally mild and disappear once the drug has been discontinued. They include nausea, cramping, diarrhea, dizziness, tinnitus, nasal stuffiness, headache, and rash. Bradycardia, hypotension, and cardiac arrhythmias are associated with rapid infusion of the drug but may be prevented if aminocaproic acid is administered as recommended.

Aminocaproic acid is contraindicated in those with disseminated intravascular coagulation unless the patient is receiving heparin concomitantly. It is also contraindicated in patients with active intravascular clotting and possible active fibrinolysis, as well as in patients with cardiac, renal, or hepatic disease.

Related drugs. The two related hemostatics, antihemophilic factor (factor VIII) and factor IX complex (Konyne 80), differ from aminocaproic acid in that they are used for the treatment of hemophilia. Antihemophilic factor is indicated in the treatment of a congenital deficiency of factor VIII associated with hemophilia A, whereas factor IX complex is used to prevent and control bleeding caused by hemophilia B. Both drugs are prepared from pooled plasma. Various processes are used in the manufacture of these products to reduce the viral infectious potential of these agents.

A third hemostatic is desmopressin acetate (DDAVP), which is used to manage spontaneous or trauma-induced bleeding in patients with hemophilia A. Desmopressin is a synthetic polypeptide that causes a dose-dependent increase in plasma factor VIII and plasminogen activator. Because of the risks associated with antihemophilic factors prepared from pooled plasma, this synthetic product is used for patients with mild to moderate hemophilia A. Although donor units are screened, products prepared from pooled plasma may contain infectious material.

Aprotinin. Aprotinin (Trasylol) is an orphan drug used prophylactically to reduce perioperative blood loss and the need for blood transfusions in patients undergoing cardiopulmonary bypass during repeat coronary artery bypass graft (CABG) surgery. It is also used in high-risk CABG surgery. Aprotinin has reduced blood loss and transfusion requirements in these patients. Following a test dose, a loading dose, and a priming dose to the pump, a continuous IV infusion is initiated and administered until the surgical procedure is completed.

Agents for electrolyte and water balance

Fluid and electrolyte balance may be disturbed in many medical conditions and require intervention to restore equilibrium. To maintain homeostasis, drugs may be required to correct acid-base imbalances, mobilize fluid for excretion from the body, expand plasma volume, or replace or maintain electrolyte or fluid levels.

Agents used for acid-base imbalances. To preserve normal physiologic processes, the pH of the body must be maintained within a narrow range. The body works to maintain the pH of the extracellular fluid by means of various homeostatic buffering mechanisms. When these mechanisms fail, acidosis or alkalosis occurs.

Acidifying agents. Metabolic alkalosis may be caused by vomiting, excessive nasogastric suction, steroid administration, and Cushing's syndrome. The cause of the alkalotic condition must be identified and treated, and acidifying agents may be administered to counteract the alkalosis.

Prototype: ammonium chloride. Ammonium chloride is indicated for the treatment of hypochloremia and metabolic alkalosis. In metabolic alkalosis, hypochloremia is usually present, resulting in a bicarbonate excess. Once ammonium chloride is administered, it dissociates into an ammonium cation and a chloride anion. In the liver, the ammonium ions are converted to urea, freeing the hydrogen and chloride ions. The hydrogen ions then react with the excess bicarbonate to form water and carbon dioxide, which is excreted by the lungs. The chloride ions combine primarily with the sodium bases in the body, thus correcting the hypochloremic state.[10]

The major side effects associated with ammonium chloride are caused by ammonia toxicity. These include bradycardia, disorientation, headache, pallor, sweating, irregular respirations, coma, metabolic acidosis, and calcium deficit resulting in tetany.

Venous irritation and phlebitis may also occur after administration of the drug at a rate exceeding 5 ml/min.

Alkalinizing agents.
Acidosis occurs when the serum pH is lower than 7.35. The blood is acidic because of excess carbonic acid, which alters the bicarbonate to carbonic acid ratio. In this situation, alkalinizing agents are administered to buffer the excess acid and help return this ratio to normal.

Prototype: sodium bicarbonate. Sodium bicarbonate is indicated for the treatment of metabolic acidosis caused by circulatory insufficiency. It may also be used to treat hyperkalemia, hyponatremia, salicylate or barbiturate poisoning, and bronchospasm associated with status asthmaticus. Calculation of the appropriate dosage is determined by the pH, $Paco_2$, calculated base deficit, and clinical response. Although dosages may be prepared from solutions of sodium bicarbonate of varying percentages, the rate of administration of the final concentration should never exceed 50 mEq/hr. In addition, the incompatibility of the drug with other drugs necessitates flushing the IV line with 0.9% sodium chloride before and after the administration of sodium bicarbonate.

Several side effects are associated with sodium bicarbonate. Because of the hypertonicity of the drug, extravasation may result in chemical cellulitis, tissue necrosis, ulceration, or sloughing at the injection site. Rapid administration may cause alkalosis, hypokalemia, hypocalcemia, or cardiac arrhythmias resulting from an intracellular shift of potassium. Excessive doses or doses administered too rapidly have been associated with intracranial hemorrhage or hypernatremia.

Sodium bicarbonate may potentiate or inhibit several other drugs. For example, ephedrine and quinidine are potentiated by sodium bicarbonate, whereas tetracyclines, chlorpropamide, and salicylates are inhibited.

Diuretics.
Diuretics increase the amount of water eliminated through the kidneys, thus decreasing the total volume of water in the body. This occurs primarily because of a natriuretic effect whereby diuretics increase the renal excretion of sodium. There are different classifications of diuretics, but the main types administered intravenously are the loop, thiazide, and osmotic diuretics.

Loop diuretics.
Loop diuretics are so named because their primary site of renal action is in the ascending limb of the loop of Henle in the kidney. They inhibit the active reabsorption of sodium chloride so that it is excreted in the urine, along with body water.

Prototype: furosemide. The prototype for the loop diuretics is furosemide (Lasix). Because furosemide is extremely potent and has a rapid onset of action, it is indicated in the treatment of edema associated with congestive heart failure. Typically, the onset of action occurs within 5 minutes, and the effects last for approximately 6 hours. Other indications for furosemide include patients with end-stage renal disease, acute pulmonary edema, or nephrotic syndrome.

Because furosemide acts by inhibiting the reabsorption of water and electrolytes, major side effects are hyponatremia, potassium depletion, and hypovolemia, with resulting hypotension and circulatory collapse. Other side effects include tinnitus and hearing impairment if the drug is administered too rapidly or administered in conjunction with other ototoxic drugs. It is recommended that large doses of furosemide be administered by slow IV infusion rather than direct injection to reduce the ototoxic effects. Large doses should be infused at a rate not exceeding 4 mg/min; direct injections of 20 to 40 mg should be administered over 1 to 2 minutes.

The primary contraindications for furosemide are hypotension and anuria. Because it may decrease the plasma volume and produce a hypotensive effect, administration of the drug to a hypotensive patient may provoke an excessive reaction. Furosemide is chemically related to sulfonamide antibiotics and is therefore contraindicated in patients with a known allergy to sulfonamide antibiotics.

Furosemide interacts with a number of other drugs, primarily because of its ability to reduce blood volume indirectly. Examples are the increased risk of nephrotoxicity from cephalosporins, ototoxicity from aminoglycosides, and excessive hypotensive effects with some antihypertensives.

Related drugs. Three additional loop diuretics, bumetanide (Bumex), ethacrynic acid (Edecrin), and torsemide (Demadex), are similar to furosemide except in action. Approximately 1 mg of bumetanide is equal to 40 mg of furosemide. Ethacrynic acid is similar in potency to furosemide and is usually administered as a single dose of 100 mg. Because ethacrynic acid is not chemically related to the sulfonamides, it may be substituted for furosemide in patients with a known allergy to sulfonamide antibiotics. Torsemide (Demadex) may be helpful in patients with hepatic or renal disease.

Thiazide diuretics.
Thiazide diuretics enhance the excretion of sodium, chloride, and water by interfering with the reabsorption of sodium in the distal convoluted tubule in the kidney. Compared with loop diuretics, thiazides produce only modest diuresis.

Prototype: chlorothiazide sodium. Chlorothiazide sodium (Diuril) is indicated for the management of edema, toxemia of pregnancy, and diabetes insipidus. Volume and electrolyte depletion may result from the administration of this drug, so many of the precautions discussed for the loop diuretics are pertinent to chlorothiazide. Because of the potency of chlorothiazide, oral administration is preferable to the IV route. However, chlorothiazide is the only nonloop diuretic available for IV use and as such is often used in combination with loop diuretics when loop diuretics alone have failed. The purpose of this combination therapy is to produce a diuretic synergy. Because chlorothiazide is structurally related to the sulfonamides, cross-sensitivity may occur when both drugs are used.

Osmotic diuretics.
Unlike loop diuretics and thiazides, osmotic diuretics do not inhibit the reabsorption of ions through the renal tubules. Rather, they work by the mechanism of osmosis.

Prototype: mannitol. Mannitol (Osmitrol) is a sugar alcohol that induces diuresis by elevating the osmotic pressure in the renal tubules to hinder the reabsorption of water and electrolytes. It is primarily indicated for the prophylaxis of acute renal failure following cardiovascular procedures, severe trauma, and hemolytic transfusion reactions. Mannitol may also be used to reduce intracranial pressure, high intraocular pressure, and generalized edema and ascites.

The major side effects and contraindications for mannitol are the conditions for which loop diuretics and thiazides are indicated. Mannitol may increase blood volume and pressure, causing acute heart failure, pulmonary edema, or hypertensive crisis. Minor side effects are limited to chills, headache, and dizziness. Because of the osmolarity of the mannitol, thrombophlebitis may occur at the injection site.

Drug interactions with mannitol are rare. However, the therapeutic effect of drugs eliminated by the kidneys may be reduced as a result of increased diuresis.

Replacement solutions.
Replacement solutions are indicated for specific fluid or electrolyte deficiencies. Because replacement solutions were discussed earlier with parenteral fluids, this section is limited to electrolyte supplements and volume expanders.

Electrolyte supplements.
Electrolyte supplements are usually contained in electrolyte solutions and solutions of total parenteral nutrition. However, there are situations in which additional supplements must be administered as a result of an electrolyte deficiency. Because calcium and potassium are the two most common electrolytes administered in this manner, both are discussed as prototypes.

Prototype: calcium gluconate.
Calcium is a salt that is naturally present in the body. When there is a deficiency of calcium, tetany may ensue and a calcium supplement may be indicated. Other indications for calcium are as an antidote to magnesium intoxication (because an increase in calcium provokes a reciprocal decrease in magnesium), as adjunctive treatment in cardiac resuscitation, and following blood transfusions to maintain the calcium to potassium ratio.

Calcium gluconate may be administered by continuous infusion or by direct injection at a rate of 0.5 ml over 1 minute. Side effects associated with calcium administration include flushing, bradycardia, tingling, and depressed neuromuscular function.

Although calcium gluconate (Kalcinate) is the most common form of calcium salt used, two other forms are available. Calcium gluceptate has a calcium content equal to that of calcium gluconate, whereas calcium chloride is three times as potent.

Prototype: potassium chloride.
Hypokalemia may be caused by diuretic therapy, digitalis intoxication, vomiting, diarrhea, diabetic acidosis, and metabolic acidosis. In these situations, the administration of potassium may be warranted. However, IV administration of potassium is not without risks. Potassium should not be adminstered until kidney function has been determined by urine output. Precise measurement of the potassium deficiency is not possible; therefore too much potassium may be administered, resulting in hyperkalemia.

The IV administration of potassium requires that the drug be diluted in an appropriate volume of solution. Under no circumstances should potassium be administered undiluted as an IV injection; such administration results in cardiac arrest. The usual concentration of potassium chloride is 40 mEq/L, although higher concentrations may be prescribed. Because of the venous irritation associated with the IV administration of po-

tassium, it is recommended that the maximum peripheral concentration not exceed 80 mEq/L. If a central venous catheter is used, the concentration may be increased, up to 240 mEq/250 ml. However, continuous cardiac monitoring is recommended for infusions given at a rate greater than 10 mEq of potassium in 1 hour.

Other potassium supplements are potassium acetate and potassium phosphate. Potassium acetate is generally preferred for potassium deficiencies in patients with renal tubular acidosis because hyperchloremia is probably present. Potassium phosphate is indicated for specific intracellular deficiency not caused by alkalosis because phosphate is the ion usually attached to potassium in the body.

Volume expanders.
Volume expanders increase the plasma volume and provide fluid replacement. These drugs produce a colloidal osmotic effect that draws water from the interstitial to the intravascular spaces.

Prototype: dextran 40.
The primary indication for dextran 40 is as an adjunctive therapy in the management of shock resulting from hemorrhage, burns, trauma, and surgery. Dextran 40 is a low-molecular-weight polymer of glucose that increases plasma volume by one to two times its own weight. This means that each gram of dextran 40 holds 25 ml of water in the intravascular space.

Although the initial 500 ml of dextran 40 may be administered over 15 to 30 minutes, the remainder of the initial dose and subsequent daily doses should be evenly distributed over 8 to 24 hours. The patient's pulse, blood pressure, central venous pressure, and urine output should be monitored frequently during the first hour of the infusion and hourly thereafter. Because of the antigenic properties of dextran 40, allergic reactions ranging from mild urticaria to anaphylaxis may occur. Severe anaphylactoid reactions have been reported during the first minutes of the infusion.

Related drugs.
Whereas dextran 40 has a low molecular weight, the colloidal properties of dextran 70 and hetastarch (Hespan) are approximately equal to those of human albumin. However, the indications, precautions, and side effects of dextran 70 and hetastarch are similar to those of dextran 40.

Gastrointestinal drugs

Common disorders of the GI tract are nausea, vomiting, and peptic ulcers. The IV medications administered for these disorders are directed at controlling the symptoms rather than eliminating the underlying cause.

Antiemetics.
Vomiting is a complex reflex initiated by the vomiting center in the medulla and affecting the smooth muscle of the upper alimentary tract. IV antiemetics act centrally to control or prevent this process. Although the three antiemetics selected for discussion differ in their mechanisms of action and classification, they all control nausea and vomiting.

Prototype: metoclopramide hydrochloride.
Metoclopramide hydrochloride (Reglan) is a dopamine antagonist that blocks receptors in the vomiting center in the medulla. It is primarily indicated for the prevention of nausea and vomiting associated with cancer chemotherapy. A single dose is adminis-

tered 30 minutes before the administration of the cancer chemotherapy, and doses are repeated every 2 hours for two doses or every 3 hours for three doses. Metoclopramide may be administered either as an infusion over 15 minutes or by injection at a rate not exceeding 10 mg over 2 minutes. If it is administered too rapidly, metoclopramide causes intense anxiety, restlessness, and then drowsiness.

Adverse reactions associated with metoclopramide usually involve the CNS and include headache, restlessness, insomnia, and fatigue. Extrapyramidal reactions may also occur, especially in children or when large doses are administered, such as those used to prevent chemotherapy-induced emesis. Once the drug is discontinued, the side effects usually disappear.

Metoclopramide interacts with a number of other drugs. It is antagonized by anticholinergics and narcotics but potentiated by sedatives, hypnotics, and tranquilizers. Because it stimulates motility of the GI tract, metoclopramide may alter the absorption of oral medications and diminish their action.

Other antiemetics. Two other antiemetics that may be administered by the IV route are diphenhydramine (Benadryl) and prochlorperazine edisylate (Compazine). Diphenhydramine is an antihistamine indicated for the control of nausea and vomiting and the treatment of allergic reactions to blood products and other agents. Prochlorperazine is a phenothiazine derivative with potent antiemetic properties. As with other phenothiazines, the major side effects include orthostatic hypotension and extrapyramidal effects.

Newer therapeutic agents to alleviate nausea and vomiting are the 5-HT$_3$ inhibitors of serotonin. These agents are used in conjunction with chemotherapy and postoperative nausea.

Prototype: ondansetron. Ondansetron (Zofran) is used with emetogenic cancer chemotherapy and for postoperative nausea. This drug is well tolerated and reported to be more successful than metoclopramide. Dexamethasone (Decadron) may be added in those patients who are refractory to monotherapy. Headache is the most common side effect, along with dizziness.

Related drugs. Granisetron (Kytril) and dolasetron mesylate (Anzemet) have been used with varying success. Most oncology centers identify only one of the 5-HT$_3$ agents as their drug of choice. In addition, these newer agents may be restricted to be used after the more established antinausea drugs have failed.

Histamine antagonists. Histamine stimulates gastric acid secretion by stimulating the H$_2$ receptors. H$_2$ antagonists block the receptors and decrease acid secretion.

Prototype: cimetidine hydrochloride. Cimetidine (Tagamet) was the first H$_2$ antagonist introduced. Because it inhibits gastric acid secretion, cimetidine is indicated for the short-term treatment of active duodenal ulcers, active benign gastric ulcers, and hypersecretory conditions. The usual dose is 300 mg every 6 hours, administered as a direct injection in 20 ml 0.9% sodium chloride or as an intermittent infusion. When the prescribed dose is ineffective, the frequency of administration, not the amount, is increased. Continuous infusions of cimetidine have been recommended because they produce pH control.

Because of its chemical structure, cimetidine produces more side effects than the other H$_2$ blockers. With average doses, bradycardia, confusion, dizziness, delirium, hallucinations, diarrhea, muscular pain, or rash may occur. The rapid administration or overdosage of cimetidine may cause cardiac arrhythmia, hypotension, respiratory failure, or tachycardia. Therefore cimetidine should be administered over at least 2 minutes as a direct injection or over 15 minutes as an infusion.

Cimetidine interacts with a number of drugs because it reduces hepatic blood flow and inhibits the drug-metabolizing enzyme system in the liver. Increased plasma concentrations of warfarin, phenytoin, propranolol, lidocaine, metronidazole, and theophylline may occur if any of these drugs is administered concurrently with cimetidine therapy.

Related drugs. The related H$_2$ blockers are similar to cimetidine in that they share the same mechanism of action. However, they are more potent, have a longer duration of action, and are associated with a lower incidence of side effects. Ranitidine hydrochloride (Zantac) is twice as potent as cimetidine and its effects last for 6 to 8 hours. Famotidine (Pepcid) has been shown to be up to 20 times as potent as cimetidine and is effective for 10 to 12 hours.

Hormones and synthetic substitutes

The endocrine system controls homeostasis by releasing hormones. When there is hypoactivity of an endocrine gland, replacement therapy with a hormone or its synthetic analog is required.

Corticosteroids. Corticosteroids are hormones that are secreted by the adrenal cortex, or their synthetic analogs. In physiologic doses, they replace deficient endogenous hormones; pharmacologic doses may be used to decrease inflammation.

Prototype: hydrocortisone sodium succinate. Hydrocortisone sodium succinate (Solu-Cortef) is the drug of choice for replacement therapy in patients with adrenocortical insufficiency. Because of its antiinflammatory effects, hydrocortisone is also indicated for acute hypersensitivity reactions, aspiration pneumonitis, and systemic lupus erythematosus relapse. In the treatment of neoplastic disease, hydrocortisone may be used alone as palliative treatment or in combination with cytotoxic and immunosuppressive drugs.

The adverse effects of hydrocortisone are generally associated with massive doses or long-term therapy. These include hyperglycemia caused by the drug's effects on glucose metabolism; cushingoid symptoms, characterized by a moon face and buffalo hump; and sodium retention with resultant edema. In addition, hydrocortisone depresses the immune response, increasing the susceptibility to infection. Because the usual signs of inflammation are masked, infections may be widely disseminated before they are recognized.

Hydrocortisone interacts with several drugs. It inhibits anticoagulants but is inhibited by anticonvulsants and barbiturates. Concomitant administration with theophylline may potentiate its pharmacologic effects.

Related drugs. Two additional corticosteroids are administered for their antiinflammatory effects. Dexamethasone sodium phosphate (Decadron) is 20 to 30 times as potent as hydrocortisone, whereas methylprednisolone sodium succinate (Solu-Medrol) is 5 times as potent.

Estrogens. Estrogens are potent female hormones capable of producing widespread effects on the body. Although they may be given as replacement therapy, IV administration is generally used for the palliative treatment of cancer.

Prototype: diethylstilbestrol diphosphate. Diethylstilbestrol diphosphate (Stilphostrol) is used in the palliative treatment of prostatic or breast carcinoma, particularly in advanced stages of these diseases. Usually, 0.5 g is administered the first day, 1.0 g the second through fifth days, and then 0.25 to 0.5 g once or twice weekly as a maintenance dose. Each daily dose is diluted in 300 ml of solution and infused at a rate of 1 to 2 ml/min for the first 15 minutes. The rate is then increased so that the entire infusion is completed within 1 hour.

Because diethylstilbestrol is a female hormone, feminization in the male and uterine bleeding in postmenopausal women are expected. In addition, sodium and water retention may occur.

Insulin. Insulin acts as a catalyst in carbohydrate metabolism by facilitating the transport of glucose and promoting glucose utilization in the peripheral tissues. It also stimulates protein synthesis and inhibits the release of fatty acids from adipose cells. Although a number of forms of insulin are available, only regular insulin is administered intravenously.

Prototype: regular insulin. Regular insulin is indicated for the emergency management of acute diabetic acidosis and diabetic coma and as an additive in solutions of total parenteral nutrition. The dosage varies greatly based on the condition and response of the patient, but it generally ranges from 2 to 100 units/hr. Insulin may be administered by direct injection or continuous infusion. However, the potency of an insulin infusion may be reduced because of adsorption of the drug onto plastic IV solution containers or tubing. The percentage of adsorption is inversely proportional to the concentration of insulin; the greater the concentration, the lower the percentage of adsorption.

Regular insulin may also be administered in combination with glucose for the treatment of hyperkalemia. This is done to facilitate a shift of potassium into the cells, thus lowering the plasma potassium level.

Because insulin is a hypoglycemic agent, the most common adverse reaction is hypoglycemia associated with overdosage. Symptoms range from clammy skin, drowsiness, and headache to disorientation, convulsions, and coma. In addition, the hypoglycemic effects of insulin are potentiated by anticoagulants, salicylates, sulfonamides, and tetracyclines.

Related drugs. Human insulin (Humulin R, Novolin R) may be given intravenously in emergencies and in hospitals. Insulin Lispro (Humalog) is not recommended for IV use because clinical trials have not been completed.

Antidote. The antidote for an insulin overdose is glucagon hydrochloride. Glucagon acts by converting glycogen to glucose in the liver. The action of the drug is prompt, with the patient awakening within 5 to 20 minutes.

Pituitary agents. The posterior pituitary gland synthesizes and releases two hormones: vasopressin and oxytocin. Vasopressin promotes water retention by the kidney and constriction of the peripheral vasculature; oxytocin stimulates the myometrium. The synthetic analogs of these hormones produce similar effects.

Vasopressin. Vasopressin (Pitressin) elicits all of the antidiuretic responses produced by endogenous vasopressin. The primary indication is in the treatment of diabetes insipidus to control polyuria and dehydration. Vasopressin has also been used as adjunctive therapy in the treatment of acute, massive hemorrhage caused by esophageal varices and peptic ulcer disease. Adverse effects are usually associated with large doses and include increased blood pressure, bradycardia, heart block, and coronary insufficiency. It is recommended that vasopressin be administered as a continuous infusion at a rate of 0.2 to 0.4 units/min; the rate may be progressively increased up to 0.9 units/min.

Oxytocin. Oxytocin (Pitocin) is a synthetic posterior pituitary hormone that produces rhythmic contraction of the uterine muscle. Because of this, oxytocin is used to induce labor or control postpartum bleeding. It is administered as an infusion with the rate precisely controlled by an electronic infusion device. Initial administration rates for the induction of labor are 1 to 2 mU/min, whereas control of postpartum bleeding requires an initial rate of 10 to 20 mU/min. Once the infusion is initiated, the rate may be increased or decreased in increments, as necessary. Adverse effects for the mother include anaphylaxis, cardiac arrhythmias, uterine rupture, and subarachnoid hemorrhage; bradycardia and death are possible fetal reactions.

Corticotropin. Corticotropin (Acthar) is used mainly as an aid in the diagnosis of adrenocortical insufficiency. Glucocorticoids are preferred as antiinflammatory and immunosuppressant agents because their effectiveness does not depend on adrenocortical responsiveness.

Immune modulators

The immune system protects the body against foreign invaders. By distinguishing the body's own proteins from foreign proteins, it selectively attacks and destroys foreign substances that enter the body. This is known as the *immune response.* However, there are certain situations in which the immune system may need to be enhanced or suppressed. Drugs that elicit such responses are classified as *immune modulators.*[5]

Immunostimulants. *Immunostimulants* enhance the function of the immune system by producing immunity against certain diseases. Those administered intravenously accomplish this by transferring antibodies to the person who lacks endogenous active immunity. The result is a passive immunity against the infection.

Prototype: immune globulin IV. When immune globulin IV (Sandoglobulin) is used for patients unable to produce adequate amounts of IgG antibodies, it provides immediate antibody levels for up to 3 weeks. Immune globulin is also used to temporarily increase platelet counts in patients with idiopathic thrombocytopenic purpura or for those who have received bone marrow transplants. Because the drug is obtained from biologic sources, a wide range of allergic reactions is associated with immune globulin.

Immune globulin is administered as a continuous infusion. Although the recommended administration rate is determined by the commercial product used, manufacturer recommendations must be followed. Too rapid injection of the drug may result in a hypotensive reaction.

Immunosuppressants. An active immune system is desirable for protection against infections and neoplasms. However, in situations such as organ transplants and autoimmune disorders, the immune response needs to be suppressed. Because immunosuppressants are relatively new drugs, each is discussed separately.

Lymphocyte immune globulin. Lymphocyte immune globulin (Atgam) is a leukocyte-selective immunosuppressant used to delay or reduce the intensity of renal transplant rejection. A total of 21 doses is administered over 4 weeks, with each dose infused over at least 4 hours. Adverse effects are mainly flulike symptoms, allergic reactions, thrombophlebitis, and thrombocytopenia.

Azathioprine sodium. Azathioprine sodium (Imuran) is an immunosuppressant used to prevent the rejection of a renal transplant. Administration is begun within 24 hours of the transplant, and each dose is infused over 30 to 60 minutes. Side effects associated with azathioprine include leukopenia, thrombocytopenia, arthralgia, nausea, and vomiting.

Cyclosporine. Cyclosporine (Sandimmune) is a potent immunosuppressant used to prevent organ rejection in patients who have received heart, kidney, or liver transplants. Within 4 to 12 hours before transplantation, cyclosporine is administered as a continuous infusion over 2 to 6 hours. Possible adverse reactions include nephrotoxicity, hepatotoxicity, and hypertension.

Respiratory smooth muscle relaxants

The smooth muscles of the trachea and bronchi are sensitive to various stimuli and may contract, causing a narrowing of the airways. When bronchospasm occurs, the patient experiences wheezing, coughing, dyspnea, and tightness of the chest. In such situations, drugs that relax the smooth muscles of the respiratory tract are indicated.

Prototype: theophylline. Theophylline may be classified as a bronchodilator because of its ability to open the bronchial passages or as a xanthine derivative because of its chemical structure. It is primarily indicated for the management of bronchial asthma and reversible bronchospasm associated with chronic bronchitis or emphysema.

The initial loading dose of theophylline is usually 4.7 mg/kg lean body weight infused over 20 to 30 minutes. This is immediately followed by a continuous infusion of 0.5 to 0.7 mg/kg/hr for the first 12 hours, and then 0.1 to 0.5 mg/kg/hr for as long as prescribed. Because theophylline has a low therapeutic index, an electronic infusion device is recommended to infuse the solution and maintain a serum level between 10 and 20 $\mu g/ml$. Rapid infusion of theophylline or serum levels in excess of 20 $\mu g/ml$ may produce toxic reactions, such as anxiety, convulsions, ventricular fibrillation, and cardiac arrest.

Theophylline interacts with several other drugs. By altering the hepatic clearance of theophylline, cimetidine, propranolol, erythromycin, and ciprofloxacin increase serum theophylline concentrations, whereas rifampin and phenytoin decrease serum theophylline concentrations. In addition, the concomitant administration of theophylline with ephedrine and other sympathomimetics may predispose the patient to the development of cardiac arrhythmia.

Related drug. Theophylline ethylenediamine (Aminophylline) contains 79% theophylline and requires a minimum dilution of 25 mg/ml for administration.

Vitamins

Vitamins may be administered in IV solutions to maintain optimal vitamin uptake following surgery, extensive burns, trauma, or severe infections. Examples of vitamin additives are beta carotene (Aquasol A) for vitamin A, thiamine hydrochloride (Betaline S) for vitamin B_1, pyridoxine hydrochloride (Hexa-Betalin) for vitamin B_6, folic acid (Folvite) as part of the vitamin B complex, ascorbic acid (Cevalin) for vitamin C, and calcitriol (Calcijex) for vitamin D. These vitamins may also be administered as a multivitamin preparation (MVI-12), which contains vitamins A, D, and E and the B-complex vitamins.

Phytonadione (AquaMephyton) contains vitamin K_1 and is used to treat an overdose of warfarin. Because vitamin K_1 is essential for the production of prothrombin in the liver, the dosage and effects of phytonadione are determined by the patient's prothrombin levels. It is recommended that the infusion rate of phytonadione not exceed 1 mg/min; higher rates are associated with the risk of anaphylaxis.

Iron replacement therapy. Iron may be replaced intravenously when the target markers, such as hemoglobin and hematocrit, are reduced, showing a significant deficit in iron stores in the body. Iron is a hematinic used to replace the total body content of iron. Iron is needed for hemoglobin synthesis, oxygen transport, metabolism and synthesis of DNA, and various enzymatic processes. Iron loss in hemodialysis patients can occur because of increased iron utilization and blood loss. Hematologic response to parenterally administered iron is no more rapid than that seen with orally administered iron, if absorption problems are absent.

Prototype: iron dextran. Iron Dextran (INFeD) may be injected intravenously, undiluted, at a rate not exceeding 50 mg of iron per minute. If no adverse reactions occur from the test dose, up to 100 mg of iron per day may be given until the total calculated dose to replace iron stores has been given. Large doses, such as total dose infusions of iron in 250 to 1000 ml of 0.9% sodium chloride, may be associated with a higher incidence of adverse effects, including arthralgia, myalgia, and fever. Dilution with D_5W has caused more local pain and phlebitis than 0.9% sodium chloride.[4]

Related drug: sodium ferric gluconate complex in sucrose injection (ferrlecit). Sodium ferric gluconate complex in sucrose injection (Ferrlecit) is used to replace iron in patients who cannot tolerate the iron dextran product. Each 5-ml ampule contains 62.5 mg of elemental iron (125 mg/ml). A test dose of 25 mg/50 ml 0.9% sodium chloride over 60 minutes should be given before initiating iron replacement therapy. Hemodialysis patients usually require 125 mg in 100 ml 0.9% sodium chloride administered by IV infusion over 1 hour. Eight doses over eight dialysis treatments may be required to achieve a

Table 11-5   **Summary of IV Drugs**

CATEGORY	TYPE	PROTOTYPE	RELATED DRUGS
ANTIBIOTICS			
Penicillins	Natural	Penicillin G potassium	Penicillin G sodium
	Penicillinase resistant	Methicillin sodium (Staphcillin)	Nafcillin sodium (Unipen)
			Oxacillin sodium (Prostaphlin)
	Aminopenicillins	Ampicillin sodium (Omnipen-n)	Ampicillin sodium/sulbactrim sodium (Unasyn)
	Extended spectrum	Ticarcillin disodium (Ticar)	Mezlocillin sodium (Mezlin)
			Piperacillin sodium (Pipracil)
			Piperacillin-tazobactam (Zosyn)
			Ticarcillin disodium/clavulate potassium (Timentin)
Cephalosporins	First generation	Cefazolin sodium (Kefzol)	Cephadine (Velosef)
			Cephalothin sodium (Keflin)
			Cephapirin sodium (Cefadyl)
	Second generation	Cefoxitin sodium (Mefoxin)	Cefamandole naftate (Mandol)
			Cefonicid sodium (Monocid)
			Ceforanide (Precef)
			Cefotetan disodium (Cefotan)
			Cefuroxime sodium (Zinacef)
	Third generation	Cefotaxime sodium (Claforan)	Cefoperazone sodium (Cefobid)
			Ceftaxidime (Fortaz)
			Ceftizoxime sodium (Cefizox)
			Ceftriaxone sodium (Rocephin)
	Fourth generation	Cefapime (Maxipime)	
Aminoglycosides		Gentamicin sulfate (Garamycin)	Amikacin sulfate (Amikin)
			Kanamycin sulfate (Kantrex)
			Netilmycin sulfate (Netromycin)
			Tobramycin sulfate (Nebcin)
Tetracyclines		Doxycycline hyclate (Vibramycin)	Minocycline (Minocin)
Macrolides	Erythromycin	Erythromycin lactobionate (Erythrocin)	
	Azalide	Azithromycin (Zithromax)	
		Quinupristin/dalfopristin (Synercid)	
Chloramphenicol		Chloramphenicol sodium succinate (Chloromycetin)	
Fluroquinolones		Ciprofloxacin (Cipro)	Levofloxacin (Levaquin)
			Ofloxacin (Floxin)
			Alatrofloxacin (Trovan)
			Gatifloxacin (Tequin)
Miscellaneous	Monobactams	Aztreonam (Azactam)	
		Clindamycin phosphate (Cleocin)	
		Imipenem/cilastatin sodium (Primaxin)	
	Carbopenem	Meropenem (Merrem)	
		Vancomycin HCl (Vancocin)	
OTHER ANTIINFECTIVES			
Antifungals		Amphotericin B (Fungizone)	Amphotericin B Lipid complex (Abelecet)
			Amphotericin B Liposomal (AmBisome)
			Amphotericin B Cholesteryl sulfate (ABCD)
			Fluconazole (Diflucan)
Antivirals		Acyclovir sodium (Zovirax)	Ganciclovir sodium (Cytovene)
			Vidarabine (Vira-A)
			Zidovudine (AZT)
			Foscarnet (Foscavir)
			Ribavirin (Virazole)
Antiprotozoals		Metronidazole (Flagyl)	Pentamidine isethionate (Pentam)
		Trimetrexate (Neutrexin)	
Sulfonamide combination products		Trimethoprim-sulfamethoxazole (Bactrim, Septra)	

Continued

Table 11-5   **Summary of IV Drugs—cont'd**

CATEGORY	TYPE	PROTOTYPE	RELATED DRUGS
CENTRAL NERVOUS SYSTEM DRUGS			
Analgesic	Narcotics	Morphine sulfate	Hydromorphone HCl (Dilaudid)
			Meperidine HCl (Demerol)
			Antagonist: naloxone (Narcan)
			Nalmefene (Revex)
	Mixed narcotic agonist-antagonists	Buprenorphine HCl (Buprenex)	Nalbuphine HCl (Nubain)
			Pentazocine lactate (Talwin)
			Butorphanol (Stadol)
Sedatives, hypnotics, and anxiolytics	Barbiturates	Phenobarbital sodium (Luminal)	Amobarbital sodium (Amytal)
			Pentobarbital sodium (Nembutal)
			Secobarbital sodium (Seconal)
			Thiopental sodium (Pentothal)
			Methohexital sodium (Brevital)
	Benzodiazepines	Diazepam (Valium)	Chlordiazepoxide HCl (Librium)
			Lorazepam (Ativan)
			Midazolam HCl (Versed)
			Antagonist: flumazenil (Romazicon)
	Miscellaneous	Droperidol (Inapsine)	
		Promethazine HCl (Phenergan)	
Anticonvulsants	Hydantoins	Phenytoin sodium (Dilantin)	Fosphenytoin (Cerebyx)
	Magnesium sulfate	Magnesium sulfate	
CARDIOVASCULAR DRUGS			
Drugs acting through adrenergic receptors	α-β-adrenergic receptors	Epinephrine HCl (Adrenalin)	Norepinephrine bitartrate (Levophed)
	α-adrenergic agonists	Metaraminol bitartrate (Aramine)	Methoxamine HCl (Vasoxyl)
	β-adrenergic agonists	Dopamine HCl (Intropin)	Dobutamine HCl (Dobutrex)
			Isoproterenol HCl (Isuprel)
	β-adrenergic blockers	Propranolol HCl (Inderal)	Esmolol HCl (Brevibloc)
			Metoprolol tartrate (Lopressor)
	α-adrenergic blockers	Labetalol HCl (Normodyne)	
		Phentolamine mesylate (Regitine)	
Drugs affecting cardiac strength and rhythm	Cardiac glycosides	Digoxin (Lanoxin)	Antidote: digoxin immune Fab (Digibind)
	Miscellaneous inotropic agents	Amrinone lactate (Inocor)	
	Antiarrhythmics	Group A	Quinidine gluconate
			Procainamide HCl (Pronestyl)
		Group B	Lidocaine HCl (Xylocaine)
			Phenytoin sodium (Dilantin)
		Group C	β-adrenergic blockers
			Propranolol (Inderal)
			Esmolol (Bravibloc)
		Group D	Bretylium tosylate (Bretylol)
		Group E	Verapamil HCl (Isoptin)
			Diltiazem (Cardizem)
		Group F	Atropine sulfate
		Group G	Amiodarone (Cardarone)
		Group H	Ibutilide (Corvert)
Vasodilating agents		Nitroglycerin (nitroglycerin in 5% dextrose)	
Antihypertensives		Methyldopate HCl (Aldomet)	
		Hydralazine HCl (Apresoline)	
		Nitroprusside sodium (Nipride)	
		Diazoxide (Hyperstat)	
		Enalapril maleate (Vasotec)	
		Trimethaphan (Arfonad)	
		Nicardipine (Cardene)	

Table 11-5   **Summary of IV Drugs—cont'd**

CATEGORY	TYPE	PROTOTYPE	RELATED DRUGS
HEMATOLOGIC AGENTS			
Anticoagulants		Heparin sodium	Antidote: protamine sulfate
Thrombolytic agents		Streptokinase (Streptase)	Anistreplase (Eminase)
			Alteplase (Activase)
Hemostatics		Aminocaproic acid (Amicar)	Antihemophilic factor (Factor VIII)
		Aprotinin (Trasylol)	Factor IX complex (Konyne 80)
			Desmopressin acetate (DDAVP)
AGENTS FOR ELECTROLYTE AND WATER BALANCE			
Agents for acid-base balance	Acidifying agents	Ammonium chloride	
	Alkalating agents	Sodium bicarbonate	
Diuretics	Loop diuretics	Furosemide (Lasix)	Bumetanide (Bumex)
			Ethacrynate sodium (Edecrin)
			Torsemide (Demadex)
	Thiazide diuretics	Chlorothiazide sodium (Diuril)	
	Osmotic diuretics	Mannitol (Osmitrol)	
Electrolyte supplements	Calcium	Calcium gluconate (Kalcinate)	Calcium chloride
			Calcium gluceptate
	Potassium	Potassium chloride	Potassium acetate
			Potassium phosphate
Volume expanders		Dextran 40	Dextran 70
			Hetastarch (Hespan)
GASTROINTESTINAL DRUGS			
Antiemetics		Metoclopramide HCl (Reglan)	Diphenhydramine (Benadryl)
			Prochlorperazine edisylate (Compazine)
	5-HT$_3$	Ondansetron (Zofran)	Granisetron (Kytril)
			Dolesetron (Anzemet)
Histamine (H$_2$) antagonists		Cimetidine HCl (Tagamet)	Famotidine (Zantac)
			Ranitidine HCl (Pepcid)
HORMONES AND SYNTHETIC SUBSTITUTES			
Corticosteroids		Hydrocortisone sodium succinate (Solu-Cortef)	Dexamethasone sodium phosphate (Decadron)
			Methylprednisone sodium succinate (Solu-Medrol)
Estrogens		Diethylstilbestrol diphosphate (Stilphostrol)	
Insulin		Regular insulin	Antidote: glucagon HCl
Pituitary agents		Vasopressin (Pitressin)	
		Oxytocin (Pitocin)	
		Corticotropin (Acthar)	
IMMUNE MODULATORS			
Immunostimulants		Immunoglobulin IV (Sandoglobulin)	
Immunosuppressants		Lymphocyte immune globulin (Atgam)	
		Azthioprine sodium (Imuran)	
		Cyclosporine (Sandimmune)	
RESPIRATORY AGENTS			
Smooth muscle relaxant		Theophylline	Theophylline ethylenediamine (Aminophylline)
VITAMINS			
Multivitamin preparations (MVI-12)	Vit A beta carotene (Aquasol A)		
	Vit B thiamine (Betaline 5)		
	Vit B$_6$ pyridoxine (Hexa-Betalin)		
Phytonadione (Aquamephyton)	Folic acid (Folvite)		
	Ascorbic acid (Cebalin)		
	Calcitrol (Calcijex)		
Iron	Iron replacement therapy	Iron dextran (Infed)	Sodium ferrie gluconate complex in sucrose injection (Ferrlecit)

favorable hemoglobin response. Doses should be continued to maintain target levels of iron storage within acceptable limits. This product should not be mixed in other fluids or with other medications.[11]

SUMMARY

Table 11-5 presents a summary of the classifications of IV drugs discussed in this section.

REFERENCES

1. Intravenous Nurses Society: Infusion nursing standards of practice, *JIN* (suppl) 23(6S), 2000.
2. Lehne RA: *Pharmacology for nursing care,* ed 3, Philadelphia, 1998, WB Saunders.
3. Weinstein SM: *Plumer's principles and practice of intravenous therapy,* ed 6, Philadelphia, 1997, Lippincott-Raven.
4. McEvoy GK: *AHFS drug information,* Bethesda, Md, 2000, American Society of Health System Pharmacists.
5. Gahart BL, Nazareno AR: *Intravenous medications,* ed 14, St Louis, 2000, Mosby.
6. Kastrup EK, editor: *Drug facts and comparisons,* St Louis, 1999, Facts and Comparisons.
7. Package insert for Synercid, Aventis, 1999.
8. Package insert for Tequin, Bristol Myers Squibb, 1999.
9. Joint National Committee on Prevention, Detection, Evaluation and Treatment of High Blood Pressure: The sixth report of the Joint National Committee on Prevention, Detection, Evaluation, and Treatment of High Blood Pressure (JNC VI), *Arch Intern Med* 157:2413, 1997.
10. Metheny NM: *Fluid and electrolyte balance: Nursing considerations,* ed 4, Philadelphia, 2000, Lippincott Williams & Wilkins.
11. Package insert for Ferrlecit, Schein, 1999.
12. Guidelines 2000 for Cardiopulmonary Resuscitation and Emergency Cardiovascular Care: International consensus on science, *Circulation* 102(suppl I):I86, 2000.

Chapter

12

Parenteral Nutrition

Jeanne M. Wilson, RN, BSN, CRNI, Nancy L. Jordan RN, BS*

The administration of parenteral nutrition solutions has become a valuable treatment modality for patients with diseases that result in an impaired ability to ingest or absorb adequate nutrients through the gastrointestinal (GI) tract to satisfy nutritional requirements. However, as demonstrated throughout this chapter, the provision of parenteral nutritional support has become increasingly complex. To ensure safe, effective delivery, the nurse involved in the administration of parenteral nutrition must demonstrate competency in nutrition assessment, parenteral nutrition solution-related pharmacologic considerations, administration delivery systems and regimens, and patient teaching.

*The authors and editors wish to acknowledge the contributions made by Carolyn D. Ford and Cora Vizcarra as coauthors of this chapter in the first edition of *Intravenous Nursing: Principles and Practice.*

Protein-calorie malnutrition is common in critical illness, in severe stress and as a result of a prolonged NPO (nothing by mouth) status. This results in catabolism, which is the breakdown of body tissue and protein to use for energy. Protein catabolism for energy affects organ function throughout the body. Parenteral nutrition is administered to provide and maintain essential nutrients.[1]

Initially, parenteral nutrition was safely administered only in the hospital setting. Technologic advances, research, economics, and the refinement of delivery systems and techniques have enabled, if not driven, the administration of parenteral nutrition in other health care settings. Nurses in all care settings need to be proficient in recognizing malnutrition and caring for patients receiving parenteral nutrition, and they must integrate new technologies into patient care and apply research findings to clinical practice.

HISTORICAL PERSPECTIVE

The injection of substances intravenously began shortly after the description of blood circulation by William Harvey in 1628. Trial, error, and knowledge led to the development of protein hydrolysates in the 1930's. Peripheral infusions of amino acids were used in patients who could not tolerate enteral feedings.[2] However, solutions that could be tolerated by peripheral veins provided insufficient nonprotein calories. A 5% or 10% glucose solution providing 3.4 kcal/g (170 to 340 kcal/L) did not provide sufficient calories in volumes tolerated by the patient.

Aubaniac's description of percutaneous subclavian vein cannulation provided the means for hypertonic infusions of glucose, amino acids, and fats into the central circulation. Stanley Dudrick and colleagues demonstrated normal growth and development of beagle puppies supported only by intravenous (IV) nutrients.[3] In 1968, members of this group demonstrated normal growth, development, and positive nitrogen balance in a baby girl with intestinal atresia.[4] Using the central venous catheter (CVC), they were able to infuse highly concentrated solutions of glucose (ranging from 20% to 70%) and amino acids. Adequate calories could now be provided using concentrated solutions in volumes tolerated by the compromised patient. Since then, technologic advances and refinement of delivery systems have made infusion of parenteral nutrition solutions safe and effective in the treatment of malnutrition secondary to disease pathology.

CONCEPTS OF NUTRITION

The body is composed of adipose tissue and lean body mass. Adipose tissue consists of all body lipids and is relatively anhydrous. Lean body mass consists of the extracellular mass (extracellular fluid and supporting structures such as skeleton, tendons, and cartilage) and body cell mass (skeletal muscle, viscera, and body cells).[5] Nutritional balance is achieved when nutrients are provided in sufficient quantities for the maintenance of body function and renewal of these components. This balance depends on adequate intake of nutrients and the appropriate absorption, utilization, and excretion of nutrients.

NUTRITIONAL REQUIREMENTS
Fluids

The average healthy adult requires 2 to 3 L of fluid per day, or approximately 30 ml/kg/day. Fluids are lost through the kidneys, lungs, bowel, and skin. Fluid balance depends on a balance between fluid intake and output, so gains in fluid intake must equal losses in body fluid. Insensible losses are not measurable and can only be estimated. Insensible fluid losses include losses from perspiration, respiration, third spacing, hemorrhage into soft tissue or the abdominal cavity, ascites, and drainage from burns and wounds. Individual fluid requirements vary greatly and can fluctuate daily; therefore, accurate patient intake and output records are invaluable in determining fluid requirements. Estimates of fluid maintenance requirements can be obtained from body weight or body surface area (BSA). However, determinations made from body weight overestimate fluid requirements of obese patients and underestimate requirements of thin patients. In these instances, BSA in which both height and weight are considered is more accurate. Both methods provide adequate fluid for normal urinary excretion (1200 to 1500 ml/day) and for replacement of normal insensible losses (500 to 1000 ml/day).[6]

Protein

Protein is essential for body growth, maintenance, and repair of tissue. When proteins are digested, they are absorbed as amino acids, the basic structural unit of protein. Approximately 22 different amino acids are commonly found in proteins. Protein and amino acids are the only sources of nitrogen. Nonessential amino acids can be synthesized and are precursors for the synthesis of carbohydrates, fats, and other amino acids. Amino acids that the body cannot synthesize, called *essential amino acids,* must be obtained from the diet. If a nonessential amino acid is used faster than it is made, it becomes essential for that condition. For example, histidine is essential in infants but not necessarily in healthy children or adults. Glutamine is another example of a nonessential amino acid that becomes essential in certain disease conditions. Thus essentiality can be the result of a total inability to make the amino acid or the inability to make an adequate amount. In either case, the body does not store excess amino acids. Excess amino acids are used for energy, and excess nitrogen is excreted in the urine as urea.[7]

Amino acids are metabolized primarily in the liver, which monitors amino acid uptake and regulates its release. Specific essential amino acids (e.g., phenylalanine, tryptophan, methionine, threonine, lysine) and all of the nonessential amino acids are catabolized in the liver. The liver is also the site for urea synthesis, where nitrogenous wastes must be converted to urea before being transported to the kidneys for excretion.

Each amino acid has a distinct metabolic pathway that leads to oxidation and its conversion to carbon dioxide, water, and urea. Urea contains two amino acid groups: oxygen and one-carbon. Incomplete oxidation yields only a portion of the energy available from protein. Protein yields approximately 4 kcal/g of available energy. In addition, when some amino acids are split, they yield carbon structures that can produce glucose

Table 12-1   **Classifications of Amino Acids**

ESSENTIAL AMINO ACIDS	NONESSENTIAL AMINO ACIDS
Isoleucine	Alanine
Leucine	Arginine
Lysine	Asparagine
Methionine	Aspartic acid
Phenylalanine	Cysteine*
Threonine	Cystine
Tryptophan	Glutamic acid
Valine	Glutamine*
	Glycine
	Histidine*
	Hydroxyproline
	Proline
	Serine
	Taurine*
	Tyrosine*

*Conditionally essential.

through gluconeogenesis. In gluconeogenesis, the carbon structures fit into the glycolytic pathway and are either metabolized as if they were carbohydrate, producing energy, or resynthesized to form glucose. Other amino acids are ketogenic, in which the carbon structures fit into the lipid metabolic pathways and can form ketone bodies. Ketogenic amino acids cannot contribute to the formation of glucose. Other amino acids have branched chains, meaning that a portion of their carbon structure is glucogenic and a portion is ketogenic. These branched chain amino acids have an important role in the parenteral feeding of some hypermetabolic patients.[8,9] Table 12-1 presents the classifications of amino acids.

Body proteins are constantly undergoing catabolism and anabolism, and approximately 40% of the body's resting energy expenditure is used for these processes. During growth and in pregnancy, the body is making more protein than it is breaking down. Therefore the body is in a state of positive nitrogen balance, as described earlier. Under other conditions, such as restricted food intake, disease, or trauma, the body might be in negative nitrogen balance. Clinically, the balance between protein synthesis and degradation can be estimated by measuring the nitrogen balance.

Carbohydrates

Carbohydrates are compounds of carbon, hydrogen, and oxygen. Carbohydrates in the diet are classified as complex carbohydrates or simple sugars. The simple sugars are monosaccharides, meaning one-sugar, or disaccharides, a carbohydrate composed of two monosaccharides. The major monosaccharides are glucose and fructose; the others are galactose and mannose. The disaccharides include sucrose, maltose, and lactose.

The metabolism of carbohydrates involves a number of intricate chemical processes that depend on the presence of insulin, glucagon, and to a lesser extent, hormones such as epinephrine and norepinephrine. Carbohydrate metabolism, like all forms of metabolism, has a constructive phase called *anabolism* and a destructive phase called *catabolism*. Carbohy-

drate catabolism is the process whereby the body breaks carbohydrates down into smaller molecules and uses the energy that is released in the process. The three major processes involved in carbohydrate catabolism are glycolysis, the Kreb's cycle, and glycogenolysis. The initial process in carbohydrate catabolism is glycolysis, in which sugar is broken down into simpler compounds. This results in a split of the glucose molecule and a partial release of energy. The Kreb's cycle completes carbohydrate catabolism, which results in the total breakdown of glucose into carbon dioxide, water, and energy. When the blood glucose level is abnormally low, glycogen stores are converted to glucose by *glycogenolysis*.

Carbohydrate anabolism is a process whereby catabolic products of carbohydrates, fat, or protein are chemically converted into glycogen and stored principally in the liver. Unlike catabolism, this process does not release energy, but instead uses the body's energy. Two major processes are involved in carbohydrate anabolism: glycogenesis and glyconeogenesis. *Glycogenesis* is the process whereby glucose is converted to glycogen. It is the reverse of glycogenolysis and depends on the release of insulin. *Glyconeogenesis* is the transformation of fats and proteins into glucose or glycogen for use by cells as fuel. This process occurs when carbohydrates are not available.

Fats

Fats, organic substances that are insoluble in water, are responsible for a wide range of metabolic and structural functions. Fats are a particularly efficient form of energy because they are calorically dense (9 kcal/g) and are stored in the anhydrous state. Along with carbohydrates, fats are burned for energy in protein sparing. Fats function to support and pad critical organs, such as the kidneys, and to insulate the body against heat loss. Fats are an important component of cell membranes and are precursors of the regulatory compounds, such as the prostaglandins, glucocorticoids, mineralocorticoids, estrogens, androgens, and bile acids. Fat in food serves as a vehicle for fat-soluble vitamins (vitamins A, D, E, and K), which are essential to body metabolism. The major classes of lipids found in plasma include triglycerides, phospholipids, cholesterol, and free fatty acids.

The two essential fatty acids for humans are linoleic and α-linolenic acids. These fatty acids are necessary for cell membrane structure and stability and are precursors of prostaglandins.[7] The primary fatty acid in the diet is linoleic acid, a precursor to arachidonic acid. Linoleic is considered essential because the body cannot synthesize it, and it must therefore be supplied from an exogenous source, such as diet or parenteral feedings. The role of linolenic acid in adults is unclear, and its essentiality is controversial. Arachidonic acid can be synthesized from linoleic acid if there is an adequate supply.

Fats in the form of long-chain fatty acids must be administered to prevent essential fatty acid deficiency (EFAD). Approximately 2% to 4% of daily calories must be provided as essential fats to prevent deficiency states, although this amount remains controversial.

Long-term inadequate intake or malabsorption can cause EFAD. The clinical signs and symptoms of EFAD are dry, thick, desquamating skin; coarseness of the hair or alopecia; brittle nails; increased capillary fragility; diminished wound healing; enhanced platelet aggregation caused by decreased prostaglandin synthesis; thrombocytopenia; increased susceptibility to infection; hepatic dysfunction secondary to fatty liver; and growth retardation in infants. An increase in the lipid triene/tetraene ratio (greater than 0.1) will confirm the diagnosis.[9,10]

Ingested fat is emulsified by the action of gastric lipase and bile salts in the small intestine. As with carbohydrate and protein, lipid metabolism is influenced by various hormones (insulin and epinephrine) and vitamins (niacin, riboflavin, and pantothenic acid). Disease or drugs may alter lipid metabolism by increasing or decreasing fat digestion, absorption, mobilization, and utilization.

Patients receiving a seemingly appropriate amount of essential fats in the diet or from IV lipid emulsion who continue to demonstrate clinical signs and symptoms of EFAD may have a carnitine deficiency. Carnitine is a naturally occurring substance that transports long-chain fats into the mitochondria, where they are converted into energy. Serum carnitine levels are used to determine carnitine deficiency. If serum levels are normal and carnitine deficiency is still strongly suspected, a muscle biopsy may be indicated. Carnitine is available as an IV additive, oral solution, and tablets.

Electrolytes

Electrolytes play a critical role in almost all of the body's physiologic functions. Disorders of electrolyte homeostasis are associated with many disease states. In the patient requiring nutritional support, abnormal electrolyte concentrations reflect the primary disease, its complications, or its treatment. Electrolytes commonly used in a parenteral nutrition formula include sodium, potassium, calcium, magnesium, chloride, and phosphorus. Electrolytes are included in the formula to meet daily requirements and to correct deficits. The management of electrolytes for these patients can be one of the most time-consuming aspects of monitoring and managing nutritional support. The important points for minimizing electrolyte complications associated with nutritional support are close monitoring, awareness of preexisting deficits and factors that predispose a patient to electrolyte imbalance, and the recognition of signs and symptoms of deficiency.

Sodium. Together with chloride and bicarbonate, sodium is the major osmotic force in the extracellular fluid. Sodium is actively involved in the absorption of sugars and amino acids. It is the most abundant cation and contributes to the osmolarity of the extracellular fluid.

Potassium. Potassium is the main intracellular cation. It plays a role in cell metabolism, participating in such processes as protein and glycogen synthesis. Potassium absorption in the ileum is a passive process and depends on the concentration gradient. Potassium loss may be increased by diarrhea and the chronic use of laxatives.

Calcium. Calcium is responsible for the preservation and function of cell membranes, propagation of neuromuscular activity, regulation of endocrine and exocrine secretory functions, blood coagulation cascade, platelet adhesion process, bone metabolism, muscle cell excitation-contraction coupling, and mediation of the electrophysiologic slow-channel response in cardiac and smooth muscle tissue. In malnourished patients, serum calcium levels may be low because of decreased levels of albumin, to which half of calcium is bound, whereas ionized calcium levels remain normal.

Magnesium. Sixty percent of magnesium is bound to bone and unavailable for metabolism. The remaining magnesium is largely intracellular.[6] Serum magnesium concentrations do not accurately reflect total body magnesium. Magnesium is necessary for the control of neuromuscular irritability. Most of the absorption of magnesium takes place in the ileum. Resected ileum and excessive diarrhea can cause magnesium deficiency.

Chloride. Chloride is the principle anion of the extracellular fluid. It is essential for the diagnosis and maintenance of appropriate acid-base balance. Along with sodium, chloride contributes to the total osmolarity in blood and urine and plays a major role in water balance and extracellular fluid volume control. Chloride is generally excreted with sodium.

Phosphorus. Phosphorus is the major intracellular anion. It is the essential element in phospholipid cell membranes, nucleic acids, and phosphoproteins required for mitochondrial function. It regulates the intermediary metabolism of carbohydrates, fats, and proteins and regulates enzymatic reactions, including glycolysis. Phosphorus is a source of high-energy bonds of adenosine triphosphate, and is therefore important in muscle contractility, electrolyte transport, and neurologic function.

Vitamins

Vitamins are diverse organic compounds essential to normal tissue growth, maintenance, and function. They are involved in enzymatic processes that are important to energy and macronutrient (protein, carbohydrate, and fat) metabolism. Vitamins function primarily as coenzymes of energy-yielding nutrients, and as cofactors in the storage and utilization of energy. Based on their chemical properties, vitamins are classified as fat soluble or water soluble. Fat-soluble vitamins are stored in fatty tissues, but water-soluble vitamins have limited storage options. Because they can be stored, fat-soluble vitamins possess the potential for serious toxicity. Table 12-2 lists the fat- and water-soluble vitamins.

Because the body cannot synthesize vitamins, they must be

Table 12-2   Fat- and Water-Soluble Vitamins

FAT-SOLUBLE VITAMINS	WATER-SOLUBLE VITAMINS
Vitamin A (retinol)	Vitamin B_1 (thiamine)
Vitamin D	Vitamin B_2 (riboflavin)
Vitamin E (tocopherol)	Pantothenic acid
Vitamin K	Vitamin B_6 (pyridoxine)
	Vitamin B_{12} (cyanocobalamin)
	Biotin
	Vitamin C (ascorbic acid)
	Folic acid
	Niacin

obtained from dietary sources. Vitamin deficiencies can occur as a result of inappropriate or decreased food intake, diminished absorption, or increased requirements. Deficiencies may occur as a result of fad diets, in anorexia nervosa, and in conditions such as malabsorption, chronic illness, malignancy, immunosuppression, alcoholism, infectious disease treated with prolonged broad-spectrum antibiotics; deficiencies may also be seen in the elderly. Table 12-3 presents the clinical signs of malnutrition.

Vitamins are essential during nutrition support. Their key role in numerous metabolic processes makes their inclusion critical to the appropriate and efficient use of other nutrients.

Table 12-3	**Clinical Signs of Malnutrition**	
AREA OF EXAMINATION	**SIGNS ASSOCIATED WITH MALNUTRITION**	**NUTRIENT DEFICIENCY**
Hair	Dull, dry, sparse, lackluster, easily plucked (inspect comb, pillow, bed for hair), changes in pigmentation	Protein, calorie, zinc, linoleic acid
Eyes	Pale, red conjunctiva	Vitamin A
	Bitot's spots—dry, grayish, yellow or white foamy spots on whites of eyes	
	Xerophthalmia	
	Conjunctival—dull, roughened, pigmented whites and inner lids	
	Corneal—dull, milky, hazy, or opaque	
	Keratomalacia	
	Cornea becomes soft	
	Eyes become a gelatinous mass	
	Conjunctiva	
	Pale	Iron
	Red	Riboflavin
	Angular blepharitis—red, cracked, inflamed corners of eyes	Riboflavin, niacin
Lips	Cheilosis—vertical cracks of lips usually at the center	Riboflavin, niacin
	Angular stomatitis—cracks, redness at corners of mouth	Riboflavin, iron, niacin, pyridoxine
	May result in scars when healed	
Tongue	Magenta (purplish red)	Riboflavin
	Glossitis—beefy red	Folate, niacin
	May be painful, hypertensive, burn with fissures	
	Atrophic papillae—may appear smooth, pale	Riboflavin, iron, B_{12}
Teeth	Mottled enamel—white or brownish patches	Fluorine excess
Gums	Spongy, bleeding	Vitamin C
Glands	Enlarged thyroid	Iodine
	Enlarged parotid	Protein
Skin	Xerosis—dryness, flakiness	Vitamin A
	Follicular hyperkeratosis—looks like "goose flesh" that does not disappear with rubbing or warming	Essential fatty acid
	Petechiae—hemorrhagic spots on skin at pressure points	Vitamin C
	Pellagrous dermatosis—hyperpigmentation on body parts exposed to sun	Niacin
	Casal's necklace—hyperpigmentation along neck where exposed to sun	
Nails	Spoon-shaped, thin, concave	Iron
Musculoskeletal	Osteoporosis—loss of bone mass; bones become brittle and sparse	Malnutrition
	Distance between long trabeculae increases with decrease in transverse trabeculae	Vitamin C, D
	Fractures and deformities result, most often crush fractures of spine	
	May be nonnutritional (postmenopausal, congenital defects, endocrine disorders)	
	Osteomalacia—adult form of rickets	
	Mineral deficiencies lead to soft, brittle bones that bend rather than fracture	
	Usually results from malabsorption from gastrointestinal losses such as in sprue, pancreatic insufficiency, inflammatory bowel disease	
	Rachitic rosary—small lumps (beading) on ribs	
	Pidgeon chest	
	Epiphyseal enlargement—enlargement of ends of long bones	
Organ	Hepatomegaly	Protein
	Splenomegaly	
	Tachycardia	Iron, thiamine
Neurologic	Confusion, listlessness	Protein
	Sensory-motor, vibratory	Thiamine, B_{12}

From Curtas S: Nutrition assessment of the adult. In Hennessy KA, Orr ME, editors: *Nutrition support nursing,* ed 3, Silver Springs, Md, 1996, ASPEN.

Standard parenteral maintenance doses of all vitamins should be provided as additives to the total parenteral solution, unless the patient's condition necessitates the limitation or exclusion of selected vitamins.

Fat-soluble vitamins

Vitamin A. Vitamin A (retinol) is required for many body functions, most prominently the visual process. Retinol is found in the visual pigments of the eye for dim light vision and color vision. In addition, vitamin A is required for the synthesis of certain polysaccharides and is essential in the formation of many membranes. Vitamin A is necessary for proper immune function, particularly antigen recognition, and is essential for the integrity of epithelial surfaces.

Vitamin D. Vitamin D is converted to hormones that are directly involved in the regulation of calcium and phosphorus. This regulation includes the absorption of calcium, the deposition and release of calcium from the bones and teeth, and the entrance of calcium into certain cells or cell nuclei.

Vitamin E. Vitamin E (tocopherol) is an antioxidant that protects other organic compounds from being oxidized, thus protecting cell membrane integrity during normal metabolic processes. In particular, it prevents the oxidation and destruction of vitamin A and polyunsaturated fatty acids. Because oxidation products from unsaturated lipids may be carcinogenic, vitamin E may play a role in inhibiting the development of neoplasms by decreasing the oxidation of unsaturated fatty acids. Epidemiologic evidence suggests that low serum vitamin E concentrations are related to increased incidence of certain types of cancer.[11,12] Vitamin E also plays a role in the metabolism of selenium.

Vitamin K. Vitamin K is involved in blood clotting and the formation of certain dicarboxylic amino acids that bind calcium. Deficiency of this vitamin is usually manifested by a prolonged prothrombin time. Vitamin K is not usually included in commercial parenteral vitamin preparations because of stability issues, potential anaphylactic reactions, and interference with anticoagulant therapy. When indicated, it must be added separately to parenteral nutrition solutions.

Water-soluble vitamins

B vitamins. Vitamin B_1 (thiamine) is an important vitamin in the oxidation conversion of pyruvic acid and therefore in the Kreb's cycle. Thiamine is also part of certain nerve cells and is required for the proper transmission of nerve impulses.

Vitamin B_2 (riboflavin) is necessary for cellular growth and repair. It is also an integral part of several oxidative enzyme systems necessary for electron transport and thus for the efficient production of cellular energy.

Pantothenic acid is a constituent of coenzyme A and is the prosthetic group on an acyl carrier protein. It is necessary for the metabolism of glucose, protein, and fat.

Vitamin B_6 (pyridoxine) is intimately involved in amino acid metabolism, acting as a cofactor for numerous enzymes. It is essential for the synthesis of heme and for glycogen phosphorylase activity. Vitamin B_{12} (cyanocobalamin) is a coenzyme involved in the synthesis of DNA nucleotides and in lipid and amino acid metabolism. Biotin is required for the normal activity of the numerous enzyme systems involved in carbohydrate, fat, and protein metabolism.

Folate (folic acid) is transformed to numerous compounds (folates) that serve as coenzymes in a variety of one-carbon transfer reactions involved in purine biosynthesis and amino acid metabolism.

Niacin (nicotinic acid) is a component of nicotinamide adenine dinucleotide and nicotinamide adenine dinucleotide phosphate. These coenzymes are involved in many oxidation-reduction reactions occurring in cell respiration, glycolysis, and fat synthesis.

Vitamin C. Vitamin C (ascorbic acid) is required for normal amino acid metabolism and for the synthesis of collagen, adrenal hormones, vasoactive amines, and carnitine. It is important in cholesterol and folacin metabolism and leukocyte function.

Trace elements

Trace elements are inorganic compounds that constitute less than 0.01% of total body weight. Not all trace elements have been confirmed as essential nutrients. A trace element is considered essential if there is evidence for its physiologic role in metabolism; if it is present in healthy tissue in constant concentration; if its absence causes physical, structural, or biochemical abnormalities; and if its provision prevents or corrects the abnormality. The trace elements that have been identified as essential in humans perform many biologic functions, primarily as components of metalloenzymes. As such, they participate in carbohydrate, lipid, and protein metabolism; immune function; cell membrane integrity; oxygen transport; and hormonal activity.

Trace element requirements vary by age, sex, and clinical and metabolic status. Deficiencies result from decreased intake, increased losses, excessive metabolic requirements, or impaired GI absorption. The trace elements for which human deficiency states have been identified are copper, chromium, iodine, iron, manganese, molybdenum, selenium, and zinc. Others that are essential but for which deficiency states have not been recognized are cobalt, nickel, silicon, and vanadium.

Excessive intake of certain trace elements will cause toxicity. Careful monitoring and serum testing will help determine deficiency and replenishment status. Table 12-4 presents the clinical signs of trace element deficiency and toxicity.

Copper. Copper is a component of cuproenzymes, which primarily participate in oxygen utilization. Copper is involved in energy, cholesterol, and catecholamine metabolism; erythropoiesis; leukopoiesis; skeletal mineralization; phospholipid, elastin, and collagen synthesis; and iron metabolism. The most commonly reported abnormality related to copper deficiency is microcytic, hypochromic anemia and neutropenia. Clinical symptoms include skin pallor and depigmentation of the hair. Thermal injury, malignancy, small bowel fistula, diarrhea, and unsupplemented long-term parenteral nutrition predispose to copper deficiency.[13,14]

Chromium. Chromium participates in glucose metabolism as a key component of the "glucose tolerance factor," which potentiates the action of insulin. Deficiency may present as hyperglycemia not controlled by insulin and is the result of unsupplemented long-term parenteral nutrition.[13]

Table 12-4   Clinical Signs of Trace Element Deficiency and Toxicity

| TRACE ELEMENT | DEFICIENCY | | TOXICITY |
	CLINICAL SYMPTOMS	PREDISPOSING FACTORS	
Iron	Related to anemia: dyspnea on exertion, fatigue, listlessness, pallor, irritability, headache, increased susceptibility to infection	Gastrectomy, blood loss, malabsorption, chronic disease, pregnancy, menstruation	Lethargy, coma, vomiting, abdominal cramps Caused by excessive oral or parenteral intake
Zinc	Dermatitis, alopecia, diarrhea, apathy, depression, impaired taste, impaired wound healing	Malnutrition, pancreatic disease, malabsorption syndromes, HIV/AIDS, alcoholism, parenteral nutrition, increased losses; nasogastric suction, diarrhea, small bowel fistula	Headache, nausea, vomiting, abdominal cramps
Copper	Neutropenia, skin pallor, depigmentation of hair, microcytic hypochromic anemia	Rare: long-term parenteral nutrition, thermal injury, malignancies, diarrhea, small bowel fistula	Nausea, vomiting, diarrhea Caused by excessive parenteral intake or decreased levels of ceruloplasmin
Manganese	No definitive clinical symptoms	Unsupplemented long-term TPN	Not nutritionally related
Selenium	Myositis, white fingernails, cardiomyopathy, proximal muscle weakness	Unsupplemented long-term TPN, vitamin E deficiency	Rare: dental defects, dermatitis Toxic and therapeutic levels close
Chromium	Hyperglycemia not controlled by insulin, hypercholesterolemia	Unsupplemented long-term TPN	None reported
Iodine	Hyperthroid goiter, hypothyroidism, decreased basal metabolic rate, mental sluggishness		Acnelike lesions, "iodine goiter" or "toxic goiter" due to inhibition of thyroid hormone synthesis
Molybdenum	Rarely seen; tachycardia, tachypnea, mental status changes, visual changes, headache, nausea, vomiting, intolerance to sulfur-containing amino acids	Unsupplemented long-term TPN, short bowel syndrome	None reported

From reference 13.
TPN, Total parenteral nutrition.

Iodine. Iodine is required in much smaller quantities and is primarily a constituent of thyroid hormones. These hormones help regulate metabolic activity. Iodine deficiency presents as hyperthyroidism (goiter) or hypothyroidism, with decreased basal metabolic rate and mental sluggishness.[13]

Iron. The principal function of iron is the transport, storage, and utilization of oxygen. Iron deficiency is the most common nutritional deficiency in the United States, largely because of the needs of women and children. Iron deficiency causes anemia, resulting in dyspnea on exertion, fatigue, listlessness, pallor, irritability, headache, and increased susceptibility to infection.[13]

Manganese. Manganese functions in energy metabolism and antioxidant protection and is necessary for the action of vitamin K, which is responsible for clotting. It is a soluble cofactor in a number of enzymatic reactions. There are no definitive symptoms of deficiency.

Molybdenum. Molybdenum is required as a cofactor of three metalloenzymes: xanthine oxidase, sulfite oxidase, and aldehyde oxidase. It is therefore involved in oxidation-reduction reactions. Molybdenum deficiency is rare and occurs predominantly in patients with short bowel syndrome and those receiving unsupplemented long-term parenteral nutrition. Signs and symptoms of deficiency include mental and visual alteration,

tachycardia, tachypnea, nausea, vomiting, and intolerance of sulfur-containing amino acids.[13]

Selenium. Selenium is a constituent of glutathione peroxidase, which catalyzes the reduction of hydrogen peroxide to water. As an antioxidant, it protects the cell membrane and hemoglobin from oxidative damage and hemolysis. Selenium deficiency causes an incapacitating muscle myopathy and is linked to Keshan disease, a juvenile cardiomyopathy.

Zinc. Zinc is the most abundant of all the trace elements, second only to iron in body content. It is an integral part of more than 200 enzymes. It functions in numerous important processes such as amino acid metabolism, protein synthesis, acid-base balance, and folate availability. Zinc is important for normal functioning of the immune and reproductive systems, and the development and functioning of the nervous system.[14] Clinical situations and diseases that predispose to zinc deficiency include malabsorptive syndromes (e.g., celiac, Crohn's disease, short-bowel syndrome, jejunoileal bypass), pancreatic insufficiency, alcoholism, pregnancy, and prematurity. Increased GI losses (diarrhea, fistula, and nasogastric suction) predispose patients to zinc deficiency. Clinically, zinc deficiency presents as alopecia, skin rashes, diarrhea, night blindness, impaired taste, and poor wound healing.[13] In children, growth retardation and delayed sexual maturation are signs of zinc deficiency.

NUTRITIONAL DEFICIENCY

When nutrient utilization is insufficient to meet the body's requirements, a nutritional deficiency develops. It can be primary, in which there is a deficiency of specific nutrients, or secondary, resulting from impairment of digestion, absorption, or utilization of nutrients. When nutritional deficiency exists, the body's components are used to provide energy for essential metabolic processes. Body stores of carbohydrates, fats, and proteins are metabolized to provide energy. Carbohydrate is stored in muscle and the liver as glycogen, a short-term energy reserve. Fat is stored in adipose tissue, a long-term energy reserve. Body protein is divided into somatic and visceral compartments. The *somatic* compartment refers to muscle protein, and the *visceral* compartment refers to all other body proteins, including solid viscera and secretory proteins. Because protein is not stored in excess of the body's needs, the utilization of protein as an energy source without replacement adversely affects total body function.

MALNUTRITION

Malnutrition is any disorder of nutrition status, including disorders resulting from a deficiency of nutrient intake, impaired nutrient metabolism, or overnutrition.[14] Malnutrition is associated with an increased risk of morbidity and mortality and results from starvation and added stress of illness.

Starvation alters the distribution of carbohydrate, fat, and protein substrates. Brief starvation (24 to 72 hours) rapidly depletes glycogen stores and uses protein to produce glucose (gluconeogenesis) for glucose-dependent tissue, such as the central nervous system. Prolonged starvation (greater than 72 hours) is associated with an increased mobilization of fat as the principal source of energy, reduction in the breakdown of protein, and an increased use of ketones for central nervous tissue fuel.

Stress in the form of pain, shock, injury, and sepsis intensifies the metabolic changes seen in brief and prolonged starvation. The hormonal release of catecholamines, glucagon, and cortisol increases the metabolic rate and impairs the body's use of fuel.[15] Amino acids serve as the primary energy source and fatty acids serve as the secondary energy source. As a result of increases in protein breakdown and hepatic protein synthesis, lean body mass is wasted.[15] Nutritional support should be initiated before significant protein and calorie deficits occur. It is easier to maintain nutritional status than to replace nutritional deficits.

Three types of malnutrition have been defined and classified in the International Classification of Diseases (ICD) diagnostic code (Table 12-5).[6] The outcome of nutritional assessment determines the category to which an undernourished individual is assigned.

Types of malnutrition

Marasmus: protein-calorie malnutrition. *Marasmus* is a gradual wasting of body fat and somatic muscle with preservation of visceral proteins. This condition occurs as a result of a diet deficient in protein and calories but adequate in water and electrolytes.[16] Patients with marasmus appear starved, suffering from weight loss, decreased fat, depleted glycogen stores, loss of muscle mass, and usually dehydration. However, these patients will have a relatively normal visceral protein level. Therefore this type of malnutrition is sometimes referred to as

---

Table 12-5   ICD-9-CM Codes for Classification of Malnutrition

ICD-9-CM CODE	DESCRIPTION	CRITERIA*
260	Kwashiorkor	1. >90% of IBW 2. Transferrin <200 mg/dl, or albumin <3.5 g/dl 3. Decreased oral intake >2 wk 4. Anorexia, nausea, vomiting for >2 wk 5. 3+ for any one physical trait
261	Marasmus	1. <90% of IBW and/or <90% of UBW 2. Transferrin >200 mg/dl, or albumin >3.5 g/dl 3. Weight loss >10% in 6 mo 4. Decreased oral intake >2 wk 5. Anorexia, nausea, vomiting, diarrhea >2 wk 6. 3+ for any one physical trait
263.8	Hypoalbuminemic malnutrition	1. >90% of IBW 2. Albumin <3.5 g/dl 3. New onset of stress
262, 263.9	Mixed protein-calorie malnutrition	Any combination of the criteria listed for kwashiorkor and marasmus
263, 263.1	Malnutrition of mild to moderate degree	1. 60%-90% IBW and/or 60%-90% UBW 2. Transferrin of 100-200 mg/dl, or albumin 3.0-3.5 g/dl 3. Weight loss of 5%-10% in 6 mo 4. Decreased oral intake for 5-14 days 5. Anorexia, nausea, vomiting, diarrhea for 5-14 days 6. 1+ or 2+ for any one physical trait

From Grant JP: *Handbook of parenteral nutrition*, ed 2, Philadelphia, 1992, WB Saunders.
IBW, Ideal body weight; *UBW*, usual body weight.
*A minimum of three must be present.

adaptive starvation. Marasmus is clinically evident during prolonged starvation, chronic illness, and anorexia.[16] Marasmus is not limited to any age but is most common in children younger than 1 year and in the elderly.[17] If starvation continues long enough, the somatic and gut mass are exhausted, compromising visceral protein stores and decreasing cell-mediated immunity.

Kwashiorkor: protein malnutrition. Kwashiorkor is visceral protein wasting with preservation of fat and somatic (skeletal) muscle. With this type of malnutrition, the caloric intake is adequate or excessive, but the diet consists predominantly of carbohydrates, with little or no protein. It is characterized by a well-nourished or obese appearance, with increased extracellular water, pitting edema, growth retardation, changes in skin and hair pigmentation, and fatty liver. The distinction between marasmus and kwashiorkor is significant because the individual with kwashiorkor may appear well nourished but is clinically at a greater risk for infection and death.[16] Kwashiorkor is usually associated with trauma or physiologic stress and the long-term use of routine or standard IV infusions.

Mixed marasmus-kwashiorkor. Individuals with mixed marasmus-kwashiorkor malnutrition share some aspects of both conditions. Clinical findings include muscle wasting and visceral protein depletion, decreased fat stores, and immune incompetence. These individuals experience acute catabolism, appear cachectic, and are at an extreme risk of morbidity and mortality.

Effects of malnutrition

Protein-calorie malnutrition has a great impact on the morbidity and mortality of the patient, especially in the presence of the added stress of illness. An article published as early as 1936 described the interrelationship between malnutrition and increased morbidity and mortality.[18] Malnutrition affects every organ of the body. Protein breakdown occurs during periods of inadequate, reduced, or negative intake, causing muscle mass reduction in vital organs such as the heart, liver, GI tract, kidneys, and lungs.[19] Because the body does not store protein for future use, a deficiency in the intake, digestion, or absorption of protein leads to decreased strength and endurance (loss of muscle mass) and ultimately to decreased cardiac and respiratory muscle function. Hypoalbuminemia results in abnormal distribution of total body water and delayed wound healing.

Disease States Affecting Nutrition

Many disease states have an impact on nutritional status secondary to factors related to the disease process and associated treatments.

Esophageal dysfunction

Dysfunction of the esophagus disrupts the entrance of nutrients into the digestive process. Disorders affecting adequate propulsion of food to the stomach include the following:

- Gastroesophageal reflux, a disorder of esophageal motility with relaxation of the lower esophageal sphincter
- Chronic central nervous system disorders such as myasthenia gravis, Parkinson's disease, amyotrophic lateral sclerosis, multiple sclerosis, muscular dystropy, and Alzheimer's disease
- Bilateral or unilateral paralysis or dysphagia caused by cerebrovascular accidents
- Esophageal tumors, strictures, or varices that affect motility or cause obstruction
- Fistulas
- Trauma—direct or erosive

Esophageal dysfunction usually does not involve the rest of the GI tract and, unless contraindicated, can be supported with enteral nutritional intervention by nasogastric tube, gastrostomy, or jejunostomy. If the patient has severe protein-calorie malnutrition or requires surgery to correct the dysfunction, parenteral nutrition may be used.[20]

Gastric dysfunction

Dysfunction of the stomach may cause an inability to ingest food orally (because of nausea and vomiting) or to mechanically pass food on to the small intestine. Disorders of the stomach affecting nutrition include the following:

- Delayed gastric emptying, related to mechanical obstruction caused by lesions, tumors, or strictures blocking the gastric outlet; gastroparesis; or vagotomy and gastric surgery
- Rapid gastric emptying, often referred to as the *dumping syndrome;* may result from gastric resection, antrectomy, or vagotomy
- Peptic ulcer disease; lesions of the gastric mucosa cause bleeding and pain and often lead to gastric surgery
- Gastric cancer, which causes obstructive lesions
- Fistulas

Nutrition support is delivered by the enteral route to the small intestine unless the intestinal tract is involved. Special formulations such as elemental formulas may be used, or parenteral nutrition may be necessary.

Intestinal dysfunction

Inflammatory bowel disease. Inflammatory bowel disease (IBD) describes two chronic inflammatory intestinal conditions—Crohn's disease and ulcerative colitis—that affect nutrient intake and absorption.[21,22] Crohn's disease presents as an inflammation of any part of the GI tract. The inflammatory process is transmural, often involving the lymph nodes and mesentery. It is characterized by fistulas, abscesses, and bowel wall thickening with stenosis. Symptoms include pain, cramping, diarrhea, fever, nausea, and rectal bleeding.

Ulcerative colitis is primarily limited to the colon and affects the mucosa by producing congestion and edema. Ulcerations can produce abscesses, fistulas, and fibrous thickening of the GI wall. Symptoms include recurrent, bloody diarrhea with pus and mucus; colicky lower abdominal pain; weight loss; weakness; anorexia; nausea; and vomiting.

Malnutrition in patients with IBD is caused by several factors. The first and most important factor is decreased oral intake. Maintaining sufficient nutritional intake can be complicated by the nausea and vomiting associated with IBD, the pain and cramping that can follow eating, and the side effects of medication. The second factor in the development of malnutrition in IBD patients is the excessive loss of protein that occurs during acute diarrhea. The third factor is the malabsorption of vitamins and minerals that almost always accompanies IBD.

Parenteral nutrition may be used during the course of either type of IBD, although patients with Crohn's disease may benefit more with this intervention. When total parenteral nutrition (TPN) is used as the primary therapy in Crohn's disease, 40% to 80% of patients achieve remission within 14 to 21 days. TPN and bowel rest are of little benefit, however, in managing acute complicated cases of ulcerative colitis (toxic megacolon) and can actually increase morbidity in patients who need surgery urgently.[22]

Short bowel syndrome.
Short bowel syndrome (SBS) is characterized by severe diarrhea and malnutrition. Extensive surgical resection of the small intestine is the most prevalent cause of SBS. Common conditions requiring resection of the small intestine include Crohn's disease, congenital atresia, mesentery artery infarct, strangulated hernia, volvulus, and trauma. Surgical gastric bypass and intrinsic gut disease (sprue, Crohn's disease, cystic fibrosis, enteritis, scleroderma, pseudo-obstruction, Whipple's disease) can significantly reduce the absorptive capacity of the bowel, resulting in clinical manifestations of SBS without actual intestinal resection. In general, resection of 50% or more of the small bowel results in significant malabsorption. Resection of 70% of the small bowel is associated with severe metabolic disorders requiring intensive nutritional support. Factors affecting the severity of SBS include (1) the extent of the resection, (2) the site of the resection, (3) the presence or absence of the ileocecal valve, (4) the functional ability of the remaining bowel, and (5) the time elapsed since resection.[23] Because intestinal adaptation occurs up to 2 years after resection, functional improvement of the bowel can be observed and is evidenced by a gradual decrease in diarrhea and increased absorption of water, electrolytes, and nutrients. There is some evidence to suggest that anabolic therapy (recombinant growth hormone), glutamine, and dietary modifications may improve the absorption and integrity of the bowel.[24,25] Technologic advances have made it possible to add glutamine to parenteral nutrition solutions. The addition of H_2-receptor antagonists to parenteral nutrition solutions can indirectly reduce stool output, thereby decreasing fluid requirements. Maintaining nutrition and hydration requirements enterally in this patient population is particularly challenging, requiring, if not necessitating, parenteral support.

Pancreatic disease

The pancreas plays a vital role in the digestion and absorption of nutrients, providing both endocrine and exocrine functions. The pancreas is responsible for carbohydrate digestion and homeostasis, fat and protein hydrolyzation, and neutralization of gastric acid and is a catalyst in the activation of other enzymes needed for digestion. The pancreas secretes insulin and glucagon, which is responsible for energy metabolism, utilization, and storage.

Acute or chronic inflammation of the pancreas can lead to malabsorption, maldigestion, weight loss, and malnutrition. Pancreatitis may be acute or chronic, with symptoms ranging from mild to severe, and can be complicated by sepsis and multiorgan failure resulting in death. Acute pancreatitis may be caused by obstruction (choledocholithiasis, tumors), toxins (alcoholism), drugs, trauma, vascular accidents, infection, and metabolic aberrations (hypertriglyceridemia, hypercalcemia). Chronic pancreatitis is caused by gradual destruction of pancreatic tissue resulting in calcification and fibrosis. The most common cause of chronic pancreatitis is alcoholism.

Patients with pancreatitis may present with nausea, vomiting, fever, weight loss, abdominal pain radiating to the back, jaundice, diabetes mellitus, steatorrhea, GI bleeding, and elevated serum amylase and lipase levels. Interventions include avoidance of oral intake, possible nasogastric decompression, electrolyte and mineral maintenance, antibiotic administration, pain control, and when indicated, surgery.

The goal of nutritional support in pancreatitis is to minimize the stimulation of pancreatic secretions. Parenteral nutrition is indicated if bowel rest necessary to subdue symptoms exceeds 7 days. Disease severity is also a consideration.

Provision of parenteral nutrition to patients with pancreatitis is challenging because they may be hypermetabolic and glucose intolerant and may have hyperlipidemia. Parenteral nutrition formulations with decreased glucose loads and insulin supplementation may be required. The use of IV lipids in pancreatitis has been controversial. However, the current theory is that IV lipids may be used if serum triglyceride levels remain below 400 to 500 mg/dl during infusion and lipid dosage does not exceed 1 g lipid per kilogram of body weight.[26,27] Management of patients with pancreatitis includes frequent monitoring of serum glucose and triglyceride levels and intervention as needed.

Hepatic failure

The liver is a complex organ with myriad different known functions. It plays an essential role in nutrition equilibrium, uniquely the digestion, absorption, and storage of nutrients. The primary diseases of the liver include hepatitis (inflammation of the liver), steatosis (fatty liver infiltration), cirrhosis (fibrotic tissue formation), and primary liver tumors. Manifestations of liver disease include malaise, fever, nausea, vomiting, headache, jaundice, anorexia, ascites, clay-colored stools, dark urine, altered liver function tests, coagulopathy and hemorrhage, hepatic encephalopathy, and hepatorenal syndrome.

Metabolic changes include glucose intolerance, alteration in fat metabolism, protein intolerance, and an increase in nitrogen demand as a result of hepatocellular destruction. The combination of protein intolerance and increased nitrogen demand presents an extreme challenge for nutritional management.

Goals of nutritional intervention include providing sufficient protein to encourage hepatic regeneration and normalization of liver function without precipitating hepatic encephalopathy.[28] Both parenteral and enteral support may be used. Enterally, oral protein intake may be decreased to minimize ammonia production. Parenteral nutrition may be necessary to maintain adequate nutrition when complications prevent or restrict the use of the GI tract. Protein should be restricted to 0.5 to 1.0 g/kg body weight and titrated upward while closely monitoring mental status, serum blood urea nitrogen, and ammonia levels. Protein is better tolerated when administered parenterally because it avoids the ammonia produced by enteric bacteria following oral protein intake.[6] Because they are excreted via the biliary tree, copper and manganese should be omitted. Zinc, magnesium, and vitamin B complex should be supplemented, especially in alcoholic liver disease. Fluid and sodium restrictions may be indicated if ascites is present.[29]

Renal dysfunction

The kidneys maintain fluid and electrolyte balance through glomerular filtration of plasma and tubular reabsorption and secretion of water and metabolites. The entire plasma volume passes through the kidneys about 60 times daily, producing between 1 and 2 L of urine per day. The normal kidney regulates fluid, sodium, potassium, calcium, and acid-base balance. Renal dysfunction may occur because of decreased blood flow to the kidney or actual damage to the functional parts of the organ.

Acute renal failure (ARF), a sudden cessation of renal function, may occur after surgery, trauma, or burns and can be caused by hypotension, shock, and sepsis. It may also be related to adverse reactions to medications. ARF may resolve itself or necessitate renal dialysis. The use of enteral feeding in ARF is usually not feasible. The administration of parenteral nutrition slightly reduces mortality rates. Protein restriction is enforced to reduce urea accumulation; however, adequate nutrients must be provided to decrease protein breakdown and maintain positive or neutral nitrogen balance. Parenteral nutrition is associated with increased blood urea nitrogen concentrations, but these are not significant unless concentrations exceed 100 to 150 mg/100 ml.[6]

Chronic renal failure (CRF), resulting from a gradual, progressive loss of renal function, is related to specific diseases of the kidneys such as chronic glomerulonephritis, pyelonephritis, and polycystic disease. CRF results in constant fluid, electrolyte, and protein imbalance. Unlike ARF, dietary manipulations and enteral feedings are usually adequate in CRF.[6] Routine renal dialysis is usually needed in later stages of CRF. Malnutrition is common in patients with advanced renal failure or those receiving long-term dialysis. Once dialysis is begun, protein and water-soluble vitamin needs increase because of losses during dialysis.[30] Electrolytes and minerals should be monitored closely.

The goal of nutritional therapy depends on the stage of the disease. The goal of therapy for early renal failure is to preserve remaining renal function while attempting to improve nutritional status. The goal of therapy for advanced renal failure is to maintain metabolic status as near normal as possible while relieving uremic symptoms until dialysis begins or transplantation occurs.[30]

Cardiovascular dysfunction

Cardiac dysfunction can impair the perfusion of tissue involved in the digestive process. Cardiac failure results from severe coronary artery disease, cardiomyopathy, and valvular heart disease. Nearly all patients with cardiac disease demonstrate wasting of skeletal muscle and body fat because of poor cardiac output. Patients experience fatigue and shortness of breath associated with diminished cardiac reserves. Patient weight may increase because of fluid retention, but other signs of a malnourished state may also be evident. Cardiac cachexia often results from long-term congestive heart failure, most commonly in patients with chronic valvular disease. Starvation results in the wasting of cardiac muscle, thus depressing cardiac function. There are several possible causes of cardiac cachexia; it may be related to anorexia, malabsorption, hypermetabolism, and impaired delivery of nutrients and oxygen at the cellular level. Enteral nutrition must be monitored carefully in patients on the verge of congestive heart failure because the slight increase in metabolic rate may be enough to aggravate the symptoms of cardiac failure.

Nutrition support is usually indicated for malnourished patients who require surgery. The route of administration may be enteral or parenteral, and TPN should be continued postoperatively until adequate oral nutrition is possible. The TPN formula for the cardiac patient contains limited sodium, and the total fluid volume can be reduced by using a higher dextrose concentration. Nutritional intervention in cardiac disease is usually related to sodium and sometimes fluid restriction, potassium repletion, fat modification, and weight reduction.

Respiratory dysfunction

Diseases of the respiratory system interfere with oxygenation of blood and elimination of carbon dioxide. Acute episodes in patients with adult respiratory distress syndrome (ARDS), chronic obstructive pulmonary disease, and pneumonia may require intubation and mechanical ventilation. Ventilator-dependent patients who are malnourished are at higher risk for infection, pulmonary edema, hypophosphatemia, decreased ventilatory drive, respiratory weakness, and atelectasis.[31] These patients may be supported nutritionally by either the enteral or parenteral route. Formulas may need to be modified to prevent increased carbon dioxide production caused by high carbohydrate intake. Fat emulsions can be used to increase caloric density without increasing dextrose concentration. Providing calories in excess of actual needs can stimulate the ventilatory drive and complicate weaning attempts. Providing adequate but not excessive amounts of nutrients increases the success of weaning attempts in these patients.

Cancer

Cancer-associated malnutrition is manifested by weight loss, cachexia, depressed serum protein levels, and impaired immune function. Cachexia has many possible causes, including: (1) inadequate intake resulting from anorexia or tumor obstruction, (2) the side effects of chemotherapy or radiotherapy, (3) the catabolic effects of tumors, and (4) abnormal nutrient metabolism.

A meta-analysis of clinical trials of nutritional support for cancer patients has concluded that there generally is no increase in favorable clinical outcome, but rather an increase in potentially harmful side effects in oncology patients receiving TPN.[32] One exception appears in patients who have received bone marrow transplants, in whom early intervention has shown improved response and survival. Other exceptions include patients who have the following conditions: (1) long-term inability to receive nutrition orally, (2) cachexia caused by inadequate nutrient intake, (3) adequate clinical supervision to decrease complications, and (4) presence of a tumor expected to respond to chemotherapy or radiotherapy. Enteral intervention may be beneficial by improving the oncology patient's sense of well-being.

Acquired immunodeficiency syndrome

An estimated 90% to 100% of people affected by acquired immunodeficiency syndrome (AIDS) lose weight, resulting in malnutrition in most of these patients. *Wasting syndrome* is defined by the Centers for Disease Control and Prevention (CDC) as profound involuntary weight loss (more than 10% of baseline body weight), plus either chronic diarrhea or chronic weakness, and fever with absence of concurrent illness that could explain the symptoms.[33] By definition, a person infected with human immunodeficiency virus (HIV) is one who has developed any one of a series of AIDS-related illnesses or whose CD4 cell count is 200/mm[3] or less. There are multiple causes of nutritional depletion. Poor oral intake is common in AIDS patients, a result of pain, dysphagia, dysgeusia, anorexia, nausea, vomiting, bowel obstruction, fatigue, or depression. Malabsorption may be caused by infectious diarrheal disorders and functional changes in the GI tract, lactose intolerance, medications, and chemotherapeutic agents. HIV infection alone promotes hypermetabolism. However, when opportunistic systemic infections are present, hypermetabolism increases at approximately 20% to 60% above predicted hypermetabolic rates.[34]

Specific nutritional alterations have been noted in persons with HIV/AIDS. These alterations include a decrease in lean body mass, decreased circulating proteins (serum albumin, retinol-binding protein, prealbumin, and total iron-binding capacity), and circulating lipid changes (decreased cholesterol and increased triglycerides). Vitamins A, B_6, and B_{12}, and E; riboflavin; folate; zinc; copper; selenium; and iron are depleted.[34,35] There may be malabsorption of essential fatty acids.[36]

Generally, the GI tract is functional in patients with AIDS, allowing for oral and enteral feedings.[6] In patients with inadequate oral intake, providing that simple appetite-enhancing measures have been tried and deemed less than successful, appetite stimulants such as megestrol acetate or dronabinol may be useful.

If oral intake and appetite stimulation are not successful, the placement of a gastrostomy or jejunal access for enteral feeding should be considered. Today, there are many enteral products that meet the specific nutritional needs of patients affected with AIDS.

Parenteral nutrition is indicated for patients with GI failure, bowel obstruction caused by Kaposi's sarcoma or lymphoma, severe refractory diarrhea, intractable vomiting, esophageal candidiasis, or gallbladder cryptosporidiosis, as well as for those who do not benefit from enteral feedings.[6] In patients whose major problem is malabsorption, repletion of body cell mass is possible. However, it is less successful in patients with ongoing systemic infections.[37] Peripheral parenteral nutrition should be limited to short-term use in fairly well-nourished HIV patients. Because patients with AIDS demonstrate hypertriglyceridemia, lipids should be used with caution and monitored carefully. If intolerance is observed, lipids should be withheld. HIV patients who do not replete lean body mass when provided with nutrients may require anabolic therapy. Recombinant growth hormone therapy is currently the most effective intervention for increasing lean body mass in patients with AIDS, particularly those with adequate food intake and metabolic abnormalities.[38]

Hypercatabolic states

Hypercatabolic states result from trauma, burns, and sepsis. Patients with these conditions require aggressive nutritional support as soon as hemodynamic stability has been achieved. The nature and duration of the hypercatabolic state depend on the severity of injury or stress.

Metabolic changes that occur in the response to stress are neurohormonal and are mediated by the sympathetic nervous system. These changes support central anabolism and peripheral catabolism and result in negative nitrogen balance.[15,39] General responses include increased metabolic and catabolic rate; changes in body temperature; increased hormonal secretion affecting carbohydrate, fat, and protein metabolism; hyperglycemia with decreased insulin levels; and fluid and electrolyte imbalance. The stress response has two phases. The initial, or *ebb*, phase lasts 5 to 7 days and is followed by the *flow* phase. Nutritional support during the ebb phase is generally contraindicated. Nutritional repletion in the flow phase is used initially to maintain nutritional status and then to promote repletion of muscle and visceral protein. In critically ill patients, the goal of parenteral nutrition is to support the accelerated energy requirements and nitrogen flux of catabolism in an attempt to minimize body nitrogen losses, thus improving chances for a full recovery.[6]

NUTRITIONAL SCREEN

Nutritional screening can be a simple, quick, and inexpensive method for evaluating the patient's actual or potential nutritional risk. The Joint Commission on Accreditation of Healthcare Organizations requires the establishment of objective or subjective screening criteria to identify patients who are nutritionally at risk. Patients who are deemed at-risk should have a comprehensive nutritional assessment.

NUTRITIONAL ASSESSMENT

Nutritional assessment is a systematic review of the body systems combined with physical, anthropometric, and biochemical measurements that provide the information necessary to determine nutritional health.

Following are the goals of nutritional assessment:
- To establish baseline subjective and objective nutrition measurements
- To identify specific nutritional deficits

- To determine nutrition risk factors
- To establish nutritional needs
- To identify medical and psychosocial factors that may influence nutrition support

Nutritional assessment is used to determine the patient's nutritional status, to monitor therapy, and to evaluate outcomes. Nutritional assessment is best performed by members of a multidisciplinary team in consultation with a nutritional support team. Understanding the components of a nutritional assessment and their relevance to determining and monitoring the patient's nutritional status enables the nurse to provide optimal nursing care and seek appropriate consultation with those in other disciplines involved in nutritional support.

Physical assessment

Physical assessment is an essential part of a standard nutritional assessment. Special emphasis is placed on signs and symptoms relating to nutritional deficiencies. Signs of nutritional deficiencies are observed most commonly in the skin, hair, eyes, and mouth. Less commonly affected are the glands and nervous system. It is important to relate the findings of the physical examination to the patient's diet and medical history. Knowledge of specific nutrient functions is also helpful in recognizing nutritional deficiencies. Physical signs of nutritional deficiencies may not appear until there has been significant nutritional depletion. Detection of these signs by the health care team should prompt consultation with the nutritional support experts so that early intervention can be initiated.

Dietary history

To identify any possible dietary deficiencies, a thorough dietary history can delineate eating patterns (e.g., dietary intake, frequency, quantity and types of foods); identify possible food allergies, preferences, and intolerances; and consider socioeconomic, ethnic, and religious influences. Actual observation of the patient's eating patterns at mealtimes can be helpful in illuminating improper nutrition habits, including overconsumption and underconsumption. The patient's usual and current intake should be assessed by a 24-hour intake report, food records, or food frequency questionnaire. The 24-hour intake report is a simple documentation of what the patient recalls eating for the past 24 hours and is a rough estimation of the patient's usual eating patterns. For patients suspected of having poor oral consumption, a dietary intake record for 3 to 7 days is valuable. Questionnaires are also available to analyze dietary intake. From data collected, the dietitian can evaluate nutrient intake to define specific nutrient deficiencies and develop a plan of care.

Anthropometric measurements

Anthropometrics is the physical measurement of subcutaneous fat and muscle mass (somatic protein stores) in an attempt to estimate the energy stores of the body. The most common anthropometric measurements include weight, height, limb circumference, and skin fold thickness at various sites. Anthropometrics can be an unreliable indicator of nutritional gains for several reasons. Peripheral edema can inflate measurements, for example. Measurements repeated over time can vary for no other reason than differences in the measuring techniques used. Finally, benefits from nutritional repletion primarily affect cellular function and cannot be readily detected through increases in somatic mass. The validity of anthropometry is greatly enhanced when the measurements are obtained by a single skilled health care worker. Serial measurements over long periods (e.g., a month or longer) have the most value in determining changes in nutritional status.[39,40]

Height and weight indices

Height and body weight are the most used, noninvasive, and easily attainable anthropometric measurements. In assessing the importance of weight loss, current body weight is compared with the usual and ideal body weights. Usual weight is the patient's preillness weight. Ideal body weight is determined by using standard tables of age, height, and sex, such as the Metropolitan Life Insurance Table. The percentage of usual weight and percentage of weight loss are clinical expressions of weight change. A loss of 10% of the usual weight, or a current weight less than 90% of ideal, is considered a risk factor for nutrition-related complications. Weight loss over time is important to determine. Rapid weight loss over a short period increases the risks. The magnitude of weight loss cannot necessarily be correlated to the severity of malnutrition. Similarly, the lack of significant weight loss does not preclude malnutrition. The use of body weight and height indices alone in nutritional assessment is not totally reliable. Other factors must be considered, such as body composition and the rate and cause of weight loss. Patients should be weighed at standard intervals while wearing the same amount of clothing, at the same time of day, and on the same scale. Serial weight determinations or trending provide the most reliable and clinically relevant information for nutritional assessment.

Total body fat

Skin fold measurements are used to determine and assess body fat stores by estimating the thickness of subcutaneous adipose tissue. The use of calipers to assess skin fold thickness as a measure of subcutaneous fat is an easy, noninvasive, and inexpensive test. Various body sites may be used. However, the most common and easiest to measure is the triceps skin fold thickness, which is compared with percentile standards or serial measurements. It is important to remember that normal values and ranges vary greatly by population. To enhance validity, serial measurements should be done by the same clinician using the same body landmarks. Today, most experts value anthropometric measurements in determining the long-term patient's progress.

Bioelectrical impedance analysis (BIA) is an alternative tool for studying body composition by measuring electrical conductivity (resistance and reactance). BIA is formulated on the simple concept that tissue rich in water and electrolytes offers considerably less resistance to passage of an electrical current than does lipid-rich adipose tissue. The plethysmograph is used to pass an undetectable, painless electrical current (50 kHz) delivered through electrodes attached to the patient's hand and foot. Impedance is measured in ohms and expressed in terms of reactance and resistance. In healthy individuals, the measurements can be used to calculate body composition. Interpretations are based on the patient's own baseline and evaluated through serial measurements. A decrease from baseline indicates a gain in total body water and/or extracellular body water. Although BIA can be done at the bedside, specific conditions such as ascites, anasarca, severe peripheral edema, and massive overhydration may limit its accuracy as a method of assessing body composition, especially in critical illness. It is sensitive to detecting day to day fluctuation in body water.[41]

Alternative methods for determining body composition include the use of radiographic and ultrasound techniques, isotope dilution assays, dual-energy x-ray absorptiometry, neutron activation analysis, and total body electrical conductivity.[6] However, these may be costly and potentially nonreimbursable. In addition, some of these procedures cannot be performed at the bedside and are not accurate in certain disease states.

Skeletal muscle stores

Skeletal muscle represents 60% of the total body protein pool and is the major source of amino acids during times of stress and starvation. The anthropometric evaluation of skeletal muscle mass is predominantly performed using the upper extremities. Anthropometric measurement of muscle mass is accomplished by using midarm circumference and skin fold thickness to calculate midarm muscle circumference and midarm muscle area. The midarm circumference is measured using a tape measure at the same level as the triceps skin fold thickness. These measurements are compared with a nomogram and weight percentile chart to estimate the degree of marasmus-type malnutrition. If the point of measurement on the arm varies only slightly, wide variations in results can occur. This potential for error can make serial comparisons ineffective for evaluating nutritional change.[6] Despite these challenges, anthropometric measurements will best reflect change over time and are commonly used to evaluate the status of long-term patients.

Creatinine-height index

Creatinine excretion is used as an indirect measurement of body muscle mass. The amount of urinary creatinine excreted is an indicator of muscle mass and total body nitrogen. The creatinine-height index (CHI) is a ratio of a patient's 24-hour urine creatinine excretion compared with the height of matched controls of the same sex, expressed as a percentage. Therefore an index of 100% indicates a normal muscle mass, provided creatinine excretion is normal. Skeletal muscle depletion is defined by an index of less than 80% of normal. Although the CHI is based on a sound scientific concept and has been applied widely in clinical practice, there are several major problems with this determination that should curtail its further use. Potential errors can occur with the accuracy of a 24-hour collection period, which then greatly affect the results. Second, expected excretion tables have been derived from measurements in healthy young adults. Last, creatinine excretion decreases with age, and these standard tables do not apply to those older than 45 years of age.[6]

Laboratory data measurements

Routine laboratory tests may be helpful in detecting nutritional status from a biochemical standpoint. Several laboratory tests reveal certain aspects of nutritional deficiencies. Determinations of serum total protein, albumin, and transferrin were the first biochemical tests included in nutritional assessment. Serum total protein is of little value as a nutritional index because it is not specific; nonnutritional factors such as state of hydration, clinical condition, and hypermetabolism affect the serum total protein and complicate interpretation of this test. Other visceral proteins with shorter half-lives, such as retinol-binding protein and prealbumin, are significantly more accurate indicators of nutritional status. Changes in the levels of these proteins should be evaluated together because they reflect different body processes. Although the visceral proteins with shorter half-lives are better indicators of nutritional status, they too are affected by changing fluid balance, sepsis, medications, and stressful insult. Therefore all visceral protein measurements should be interpreted in the context of the patient's clinical condition.

Serum albumin. Albumin is the major protein synthesized by the liver and has a half-life of approximately 20 days. This important visceral protein maintains plasma oncotic pressure and functions as a carrier for substances such as metabolites, enzymes, drugs, hormones, and metals in the circulation. The serum albumin is considered the best single nutritional test for predicting outcome. However, its long half-life limits its value for detecting acute nutritional changes. Values are affected by level of hydration, immune status, and certain disease conditions that can lower serum albumin levels, such as draining wounds, fistulae, burns, liver dysfunction, renal failure, and proteinuria. Serum albumin levels are considered normal if they are greater than 3.5 g/dl. An albumin level of 3.0 to 3.5 g/dl indicates mild depletion, 2.4 to 2.9 g/dl reflects moderate depletion, and less than 2.4 g/dl is significant for severe depletion.[16]

Serum transferrin. Serum transferrin is a β-globulin synthesized predominantly in the liver that transports iron in the plasma. It has a serum half-life of 8 to 10 days and appears to be less significantly altered by hydration than albumin. Because of its shorter half-life and smaller body pool, serum transferrin levels are believed to more accurately reflect protein malnutrition in its initial stages and during refeeding. Transferrin is present in the serum at a concentration of 250 to 300 mg/dl.[6]

Transferrin can be measured directly by radial immunodiffusion and indirectly by using the total iron-binding capacity (TIBC) in the following equation:

$$\text{Transferrin} = (0.8 \text{ TIBC}) - 4.3$$

Levels measured directly are consistently lower than those measured indirectly. Transferrin levels can also be affected by nonnutritional conditions such as liver disease and protein-losing states. Pregnancy, birth control pill use, iron deficiency, and acute hepatitis can increase transferrin levels. Mild depletion is defined as serum levels between 150 and 200 mg/dl, those between 100 and 150 mg/dl reflect moderate depletion, and those less than 100 mg/dl indicate severe depletion.[6]

Prealbumin and retinol-binding protein. Prealbumin functions in thyroxine transport and as a carrier for retinol-binding protein. It has a half-life of 2 to 3 days and is therefore sensitive to acute changes in protein status. Increases in serum prealbumin concentrations most accurately reflect improvements in nutritional status. Sudden demands for protein synthesis, as in trauma or acute infection, can result in a rapid fall in protein levels; therefore results must be interpreted with caution. Normal serum concentrations range from 15.7 to 29.6 mg/dl. Mild depletion is reflected in levels of 10 to 15 mg/dl, 5 to 9.9 mg/dl reflects moderate depletion, and a level lower than 5 mg/dl indicates severe depletion.[6]

Retinol-binding protein is synthesized by the liver and is normally present in the serum at a concentration of 3 to 5 mEq/dl. Retinol-binding protein transports retinol in the plasma and circulates in a 1:1 molar ratio with prealbumin. It has a half-life of 12 hours, making it extremely sensitive to protein synthesis. As with prealbumin, this relatively short half-life allows for a more accurate assessment of acute depletion and repletion phases of nutritional change.[42] However, the half-life may be too short for clinical usefulness.

Immune competence

Among many factors influencing the immune response is the patient's nutritional state. Immune competence can be adversely affected by malnutrition, stress, and disease. The most commonly used method for assessing immunocompetence is the total lymphocyte count (TLC).

The TLC is derived from the routine complete blood count with differential. The following formula is used to determine the total lymphocyte count:

$$TLC = \% \text{ lymph} \times WBC/100$$

Usually, a TLC between 1200 and 2000/mm^3 indicates mild depletion, a TLC between 800 and 1199/mm^3 indicates moderate depletion, and a TLC lower than 800/mm^3 indicates severe depletion.[6] The TLC must be interpreted with caution because many nonnutritional factors may contribute to decreased lymphocyte counts.

Nitrogen balance

Nitrogen balance is a measure of daily nitrogen intake minus excretion. It is the most common clinical method for assessing protein turnover. Nitrogen intake is determined from calorie-protein intake records by dividing protein intake by 6.25. Nitrogen excretion consists of measured urinary nitrogen from a 24-hour urine collection plus a factor for other nitrogen losses through insensible (5 mg/kg body weight) and GI (12 mg/kg body weight) losses. Thus nitrogen balance is determined by the following formula:

$$\text{Nitrogen balance} = \text{Nitrogen intake} - \text{Total urinary nitrogen} -$$
$$\text{Insensible losses} - \text{GI losses}$$

A positive nitrogen balance indicates an anabolic state with an overall gain in body protein for the day, whereas a negative nitrogen balance indicates a catabolic state with a net loss of protein.

Measurement of energy requirements

Provision of adequate caloric intake depends on accurately measuring or predicting the energy requirements of the patient. Careful attention to calorie requirements is important to prevent overfeeding and underfeeding, both of which may have deleterious effects on recovery.[43]

A method of measuring energy requirements that is flexible enough to reflect changes in the clinical state of the patient is the energy balance technique. Energy balance is the difference between energy intake and expenditure. A positive energy balance (food intake exceeds expenditure) results in glycogen and fat synthesis. Negative energy balance results in weight loss as the body uses its own energy stores to meet requirements.[44]

Energy expenditure can be measured directly or indirectly. The direct method measures the actual heat produced by the body or the rate of heat loss. This method involves placing the subject in a sealed insulated chamber with an oxygen supply. A known volume of water is circulated through pipes at the top of the chamber. The production of heat from the subject changes the temperature of the circulating water, reflecting metabolic energy release. Studies done in the 1920s using direct calorimetry demonstrated that energy expenditure was almost directly related to the consumption of oxygen. However, the complexity of the procedure and the use of cumbersome equipment make direct calorimetry virtually impractical for routine clinical practice. These early studies allowed for the development of methods and formulas to determine energy requirements using indirect means.[43]

Total daily energy requirements in the healthy individual are divided into three components. The first component of energy expenditure is the resting energy expenditure (REE). The REE is the amount of energy required to maintain daily metabolic processes. The energy expenditure of physical activity is the second component. Obviously, a sedentary individual expends less energy than one who engages in intense physical activity. The third component of energy expenditure is the thermic effect of food, which is the energy required to process ingested food.[43,45]

Values used to determine REE are most commonly obtained from the Harris-Benedict equation, which calculates basal metabolic rate (BMR). The BMR is the approximate energy cost of maintaining basic physiologic activities, including heartbeat, respiration, kidney function, osmotic balance, brain activity, and body temperature.[43] Factors that affect the BMR are body size, age, sex, sleep, and climate. Energy requirements imposed by activity, metabolism, and stress are factored with the REE to calculate energy requirements. A limitation of the Harris-Benedict formula is that it is derived from healthy patients and has been criticized as potentially overestimating energy requirements for critically ill patients.[10] Despite this, the Harris-Benedict is still most commonly used. The Harris-Benedict equation and stress factors added to correct for the disease process are given in Table 12-6.

Estimates of energy requirements for weight maintenance in the clinical setting can be made using a formula proposed by Apelgren and Wilmore: REE × 1.25 × stress factor.[45] The REE is calculated by using the Harris-Benedict equation and adding an additional 10% for the thermic effect of food utilization. A 25% increase (a factor of 1.25) is allowed for physical activity and the

Table 12-6 Harris-Benedict Equation and Stress Factors Used to Correct for the Disease Process

Harris-Benedict Equation

BMR (male) $= 66.5 + (13.75 \times W) + (5.0 \times H) - (6.8 \times A)$
BMR (female) $= 665 + (9.56 \times W) + (1.7 \times H) - (4.68 \times A)$

CONDITION	STRESS FACTOR
Mild starvation	0.85-1.00
Postoperative recovery	1.00-1.05
Cancer	1.10-1.45
Peritonitis	1.05-1.25
Severe infection or multiple trauma	1.30-1.55

W, Weight in kilograms; *H,* height in centimeters; *A,* age in years.

stress of hospitalization. An additional 500 kcal/day is added for a weight gain of approximately 1 kg/wk.

Indirect measurements of energy expenditure more commonly used today include actual measurement of the rate at which oxygen is consumed and carbon dioxide is produced or estimates of the expenditure using nomograms and equations. The measured gas exchange reflects actual caloric expenditure under conditions present at the time of the test. Indirect calorimetry is the technique used in the measurement of REE based on oxygen consumption and carbon dioxide production. The instrument used for the determination of indirect calorimetry in the clinical setting is the metabolic measurement cart (MMC). The MMC is a portable system that estimates energy expenditure at the bedside in nonintubated patients and those requiring ventilatory support. Most metabolic measurement carts have a canopy system for long-term continuous measurements, along with a fully automatic calibration and computerized data system. Values obtained are approximately 10% greater than basal energy expenditure (BEE). REE values are influenced by activity, body size, medications, fever, environment, and disease state. Measurement of REE with an MMC is technically difficult, expensive, and time-consuming. However, the MMC may be indicated for patients who fail to gain weight despite receiving caloric loads estimated by the Harris-Benedict calculation. In addition, the MMC is used to determine appropriate substrate utilization as determined by the respiratory quotient (RQ).

INDICATIONS FOR PARENTERAL NUTRITION

Current accepted standards for nutrition support have been formulated by the American Society for Parenteral and Enteral Nutrition (ASPEN).[46] Parenteral nutrition support is used to nourish patients who are already malnourished or have the potential for developing malnutrition and who are not candidates for enteral support. It is important to note that when possible, the GI tract should be used for nutritional support to prevent atrophy and dysfunction of the gut. The autopsy records of severely cachectic patients in the Warsaw Ghetto Hospital described paper-thin bowels through which newsprint could be read. Although a patient can calorically and nutritionally be maintained on TPN over time, attempts to restore GI mass or

function intravenously have for the most part been unsuccessful.[6] It has also been suggested that the lack of glutamine, a conditionally essential amino acid that is the primary nutrient for the cells that line the GI tract, may also be an important factor related to gut atrophy and function. Researchers have reported that glutamine-enriched TPN solutions have restored and maintained mucosal anatomy and function in experimental animals.[47,48]

In the last 20 years, enteral nutritional therapy has greatly progressed. Today, myriad enteral products, including disease-specific formulas, are commercially available. Enteral therapy is indicated for patients who will not, should not, or cannot eat but who have a fairly functional GI tract.[42] When indicated, enteral therapy should be the first line of nutritional therapy because of its ability to maintain the mucosal barrier, structure, and function of the GI tract. Enteral therapy is an inexpensive means of nutrition support that poses fewer complications than parenteral nutrition.

TPN may be indicated as supportive therapy in other disease states as well. There are also conditions in which the efficacy of parenteral nutrition has not been clearly demonstrated. In some situations, TPN may be contraindicated. TPN is unlikely to benefit patients with advanced cancer whose malignancy is documented as unresponsive to chemotherapy or radiation. The use of TPN in sepsis, trauma, and general perioperative support may be appropriate in selected situations. Parenteral nutrition is an expensive intervention and can pose additional risk to the patient in the form of metabolic and septic complications, so the benefits of TPN support should outweigh the risks. The decision to use peripheral parenteral nutrition (PPN) versus TPN is determined by the extent of nutritional depletion as determined by degree of weight loss and serum albumin level, duration of illness, and clinical course before initiating parenteral nutrition. An algorithm that outlines the selection process for choosing the route of nutrition support in adult patients is presented in Fig. 12-1.

PPN solutions contain carbohydrate, protein, lipids, vitamins (except vitamin K), minerals, and trace elements. However, carbohydrate and lipid requirements usually cannot be completely met with PPN solutions. Therefore PPN is considered short-term or supplemental nutrition support.

TPN, which can provide all of a patient's nutritional requirements, is indicated when attempts with enteral nutrition or PPN have been unsuccessful, when gut dysfunction is anticipated for greater than 14 days, or when the patient is unable to tolerate the large volumes of fluid required to deliver sufficient calories via PPN solutions. The risk of infection and metabolic complications increases with the use of TPN versus PPN because of the differences in dextrose and electrolyte concentration. The goals of nutritional therapy depend on the patient's status (Box 12-1). In addition, there are a number of considerations for parenteral nutrition support (Box 12-2).[49-52]

PARENTERAL NUTRITION SOLUTIONS

Conventional IV solutions are low in calories; that is, 1 L of 5% dextrose provides 170 kcal and contains only small amounts of trace elements or electrolytes. Parenteral nutrition solutions, on

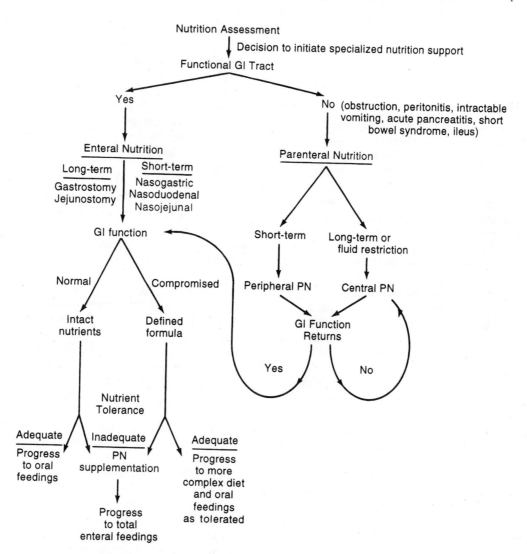

FIG. 12-1 *Clinical decision algorithm: route of nutrition support.* (Reprinted from ASPEN Board of Directors: Guidelines for the use of parenteral and enteral nutrition in adult and pediatric patients, *JPEN* 17[suppl]:7SA, 1993.)

Box 12-1   Goals of Parenteral Nutrition

1. To provide all essential nutrients in adequate amounts to sustain nutritional balance during periods when oral or enteral routes of feedings are not possible or are insufficient to meet the caloric needs of the patient
2. To preserve or restore the body's protein metabolism and prevent protein and calorie malnutrition
3. To diminish the rate of weight loss and maintain or increase body weight
4. To promote wound healing
5. To repair nutritional deficits

Box 12-2   Considerations for Parenteral Nutrition

Patient evaluation for parenteral nutrition is based on various objective measurements:

1. Any patient who is unable to ingest sufficient nutrients through the gastrointestinal (GI) tract is a potential candidate for parenteral nutrition.
2. The least invasive, least expensive means of supporting a patient's nutritional status must be considered.
3. The GI route should always be used, if appropriate. There can be serious adverse effects associated with a totally resting GI tract. Enteral nutrition preserves intestinal mass and structures, as well as hormonal, enzymatic, and immunologic function, better than intravenous nutrition.
4. Generally, nourished patients unable to eat for as long as 7 to 10 days do not require parenteral nutrition. However, the general rule is that whenever 5 to 7 days have passed with insufficient enteral intake, parenteral nutrition should be considered.
5. The indications and disease states for which parenteral nutrition is clearly beneficial are continually being established and reassessed.

the other hand, are complex solutions that provide all the known essential nutrients in quantities that promote weight gain, wound healing, anabolism, and growth.

Components

Parenteral nutrition solutions contain essential nutrients, including protein, carbohydrate, fat, electrolytes, vitamins, trace elements, and water. The proportions of these ingredients and the total calories provided must be carefully individualized to meet the patient's needs and clinical condition.

Protein. Protein, in the form of crystalline amino acid solutions for parenteral nutrition, is an essential component of every nutrition support regimen. A patient's estimated protein requirement depends on age, level of activity, nutritional status, renal function, hepatic function, and presence or absence of hypermetabolism. Aside from these quantitative differences, there may also be differences in the requirements for specific amino acids. Certain amino acids perform unique physiologic functions that may have a therapeutic or damaging effect on a particular patient. Thus the optimal provision of amino acids during parenteral nutrition depends on the total quantity provided *and* the specific amino acid composition.

Normal protein requirements depend on utilization and losses. Any condition that decreases normal utilization or increases nitrogen losses increases dietary protein requirements. The recommended dietary allowance for protein is based on the amount of protein needed to maintain nitrogen equilibrium and the fact that energy needs are met by nonprotein sources. A protein intake of 0.8 g/kg body weight per day is recommended for healthy adults; 2.5 to 3.0 g/kg body weight per day parenterally is recommended for neonates and infants.[53-55] Infant protein requirements gradually decrease to 1.5 to 2.0 g/kg body weight per day by 12 months of age. This decline continues until the growth cycle is complete.

Illness can dramatically influence the body's protein needs. During periods of stress, injury, or infection, patients may require as much as 1.5 to 2.0 g/kg body weight per day.[10,15,56] Burn patients may require up to 2.5 g/kg body weight per day.[10,15]

Currently available amino acid solutions differ in composition. Based on the specific amino acid profile, standard or specialized solutions are available. Standard amino acid solutions are a balanced profile of essential, semiessential, and nonessential amino acids. Specialized amino acid solutions have a modified amino acid profile to meet age- or disease-specific amino acid requirements. Amino acid solutions also differ in their nitrogen content per gram, electrolyte composition, osmolarity, pH, and available concentration. Amino acid solutions with preadded electrolytes usually contain amounts of the most common electrolytes needed to meet an adult's requirements. Specialized amino acid preparations have been developed for use in specific disorders such as renal and hepatic failure. Disease-specific amino acids are discussed later in this chapter.

An interaction exists between calorie and nitrogen substrates. Increasing the caloric support reduces the nitrogen required to achieve nitrogen balance, and increasing the nitrogen intake reduces the calories required to achieve nitrogen balance. The optimal calorie/nitrogen ratio in the patient requiring nutritional support remains individualized. The currently used calorie/nitrogen ratio ranges from 100:1 to 200:1. This means that for each gram of nitrogen, 100 to 200 calories must be provided for protein sparing. It is logical that patients under severe stress are likely to have a different optimal ratio than those who are chronically malnourished. A lower calorie/nitrogen ratio results in greater nitrogen retention, increased plasma transferrin, and a lower respiratory quotient when a patient is hypermetabolic.[56]

Carbohydrates. To ensure that the protein content of parenteral nutrition solutions is used for tissue synthesis rather than for energy, nonprotein calories must be administered. Carbohydrates are the body's preferred fuel, as well as its immediate source of energy. One carbohydrate molecule yields 4 kcal of energy for each gram of carbohydrate. The body burns carbohydrates rather than fats or protein, provided the carbohydrate intake is adequate, sufficient insulin is available to allow passage of glucose into the cells, and glycogen is present.

There are no specific minimum requirements for carbohydrates during parenteral nutrition, but they are an important component of most parenteral nutrition regimens. Dextrose is used almost exclusively in parenteral nutrition solutions as the source of carbohydrate calories. Other sources of parenteral carbohydrate and carbohydrate-like substances, such as fructose, galactose, glycerol, invert sugar, maltose, sorbitol, and xylitol, have also been used. However, with the exception of glycerol, most of these substances are no longer commercially available because of the high potential for adverse effects.[57]

Dextrose has a low caloric density, providing 3.4 kcal/g, and is available in concentrations ranging from 5% to 70%. Higher concentrations of dextrose are usually used in parenteral nutrition solutions to minimize the volume of dextrose in the overall admixture, thus allowing greater volume for amino acids, electrolytes, and micronutrients. Dextrose solutions with concentrations exceeding 5% are increasingly hypertonic. The normal serum osmolarity is approximately 310 mOsm/L. Parenteral solutions with an osmolarity of up to 900 mOsm/L may be administered peripherally. However, tolerance of solutions with 900 mOsm/L or less varies greatly by patient and vein condition. In general, parenteral solutions with a final dextrose concentration greater than 10%, or more than 900 mOsm/L, should be administered through a central vein.[58]

The optimal dose of dextrose differs for infants, children, and adults. In general, for balanced parenteral nutrition, dextrose is used to provide 40% to 60% of the total caloric intake. In adults, the optimal dose for maximal suppression of gluconeogenesis and glucose oxidation is 2 to 5 mg/kg/min.[58] This represents a parenteral nutrition regimen that contains 150 to 200 g of dextrose per liter administered centrally at a rate of 1.5 to 2.5 L/day. Overfeeding by supplying glucose in excess of this rate does not accentuate nitrogen retention and produces adverse effects such as fatty liver and increased carbon dioxide production, which may aggravate preexisting respiratory distress. Because of the higher resting energy expenditure and greater energy demands of growth and development in infants and children, their overall energy requirements are greater than those of adults.[59,60]

Glycerol, a sugar alcohol, is available as an IV carbohydrate-like solution used in parenteral nutrition. Glycerol is commercially available as a premixed solution, Procalamine, which is ready for infusion after vitamins and trace elements are added. Procalamine contains 3% amino acids and 3% glycerol premixed in 1-L bottles. It has a caloric density of 250 kcal/L and a solution osmolarity of 735 mOsm/L, and can therefore be administered peripherally. Because it is a partial nutritional solution, Procalamine is used only for patients whose nutritional requirements can be met by the nutrients and electrolytes present.[58]

Fats. Fat, in the form of lipid emulsions, serves two purposes in parenteral nutrition. It is a source of calories and of essential fatty acids needed to prevent essential fatty acid deficiency. Fat is the most calorically dense substrate available, with more than twice the caloric density of carbohydrate and protein, and provides approximately 9 kcal/g. Fat emulsions provide varying amounts of linoleic and linolenic acids sufficient to prevent or treat essential fatty acid deficiency.

The recommended dietary allowance for fat remains controversial. In parenteral nutrition, lipid emulsions should be provided in quantities sufficient to prevent essential fatty acid deficiency. Essential fatty acid deficiency can occur in as little as 5 days without fat supplementation. The minimum human requirement needed to prevent essential fatty acid deficiency should represent 2% to 4% of the total caloric intake, or at least 2.4 g linoleic acid per 2000 kcal of nutrient intake. Fats also provide calories for meeting energy requirements to optimize protein utilization and, when needed, to decrease the carbohydrate load. The optimal dose of lipid for the provision of calories is unknown. However, the maximum safe dose is no more than 60% (most patients receive 10% to 40%) of the daily caloric intake and should not exceed 2.5 g/kg for adults or 3 g/kg for pediatric patients.[58,60]

The parenteral lipid emulsions currently in use, which became commercially available in the United States in 1976, are emulsions of soybean oil or a combination of soybean and safflower oils. The other components of these fat emulsions include egg phosphatides, which act as an emulsifier, and glycerol, which adjusts the osmolarity to make the emulsion iso-osmolar. Lipid emulsions are available in concentrations of 10% and 20%. Ten percent lipid emulsion provides 1.1 kcal/ml, and 20% lipid emulsion provides 2.0 kcal/ml.

Adverse reactions to IV fat emulsions have been reported in various clinical settings, particularly when cottonseed oil emulsions were still commercially available. These reactions include syndrome of platelet dysfunction, hemolysis, and even death. Since soybean and safflower oil emulsions became available, these adverse reactions have not been reported, although acute reactions such as allergic reactions (including fever, chills, dyspnea, vomiting, headache, pressure over the eyes, and chest or back pain) have been reported. These reactions are associated with a preexisting allergic reaction to the source of lipid, the egg used as an emulsifier, or too-rapid infusion.[6]

Fat emulsions must be administered with caution to patients with liver disease, compromised pulmonary function, coagulation disorders, or pancreatitis. The administration of lipids to infants with elevated bilirubin levels may cause increased kernicterus. The serum triglyceride concentration must be measured and monitored, and the lipid intake may be adjusted accordingly.

Electrolytes. Because electrolytes play a critical role in almost all of the body's physiologic functions, they are included in the administration of parenteral nutrition to meet daily requirements and to prevent or correct preexisting deficits. Electrolytes commonly added to parenteral nutrition formulas include sodium, potassium, calcium, chloride, and phosphorus. Although general guidelines for electrolyte requirements during parenteral nutrition exist for adults and pediatric patients, individual needs must be considered to maintain electrolyte balance. An initial assessment of electrolyte status may indicate whether a patient has an altered electrolyte requirement. Patients with preexisting conditions, such as long-term diuretic use or ongoing losses of electrolytes such as with fistulas or diarrhea, can be anticipated to have increased electrolyte requirements. It may be necessary to restrict electrolyte intake in patients with severe renal dysfunction, edema, or congestive heart failure.

Electrolytes may be added to parenteral solutions singly or in combination; electrolyte mixtures are available in concentrations designed to meet the standard adult electrolyte requirement. Several amino acid products contain electrolytes in amounts designed to meet adult requirements if 2 L/day are given. The use of these products in parenteral nutrition is usually limited to stable adult patients whose electrolyte balance can be achieved by the contents of these products. The patient's acid-base status will determine whether a chloride or acetate salt should be used when admixing electrolytes in parenteral solutions.

Vitamins. Vitamins play an essential role in metabolism and cellular function; therefore a multiple-vitamin preparation is added to each day's parenteral nutrition solution. Pediatric and adult vitamin mixtures containing fat- and water-soluble vitamins are available. Most commercial vitamin products now contain folic acid and vitamin B_{12}. However, because of stability issues, potential anaphylactic reactions, and interference with anticoagulant therapy, they do not include vitamin K. When vitamin K is indicated, it can be added to parenteral nutrition solutions weekly or may be administered intramuscularly. Parenteral vitamin requirements generally are significantly lower than dietary vitamin requirements because the parenteral route bypasses the digestive and absorptive functions of the GI tract. Guidelines for parenteral vitamin intake in adults have been established by the Nutrition Advisory Group of the American Medical Association (AMA) Department of Foods and Nutrition.[61] Specific disease states and certain drugs may alter vitamin requirements, but specific needs can easily be met by adding to the parenteral solutions. Caution must be taken when administering additional fat-soluble vitamins because overadministration can lead to toxicity.

Trace elements. The efficient use of substrates for energy production and protein synthesis depends on the availability of trace elements for the numerous facilitative functions they perform. To ensure adequate amounts and prevent deficiency states, trace elements such as zinc, copper, chromium, and manganese are routinely added to parenteral nutrition solutions. It is particularly important to assess individual trace mineral requirements in malnourished patients who may have preexisting micronutrient deficiencies and in neonates who have limited body stores of trace elements and whose needs are critical for growth. Monitoring trace element status is based on regular clinical assessment for the presence of the signs and symptoms of deficiency.

Trace elements are inefficiently absorbed through the GI tract from dietary sources, so there are substantial differences between amounts required when nutrition is delivered enterally rather than parenterally. The AMA's Nutrition Advisory Group has recommended IV administration of chromium, copper, manganese, and zinc.[62] The Subcommittee on Pediatric Parenteral Nutrient Requirements (from the Committee on Clinical Practice Issues of the American Society of Clinical Nutrition) has also published guidelines for trace element intake in infants and children. There are no formal recommendations for selenium and molybdenum for adults, but clinical practice suggests inclusion of these trace elements during the parenteral nutrition of select patient groups, including long-term TPN patients and those with preexisting deficiencies. Recommendations for iron and iodine for adult patients have been made by individual practitioners. Parenteral iron, available as iron dextran, may be administered intravenously, which is the preferred route, or intramuscularly for iron deficiency.

Several commercial products meet guidelines for the daily intake of chromium, copper, manganese, and zinc for adults, children, and neonates. These products range from those that contain a single trace element to those that provide multiple trace elements and also contain selenium, molybdenum, and/or iodine.

Water. Maintenance fluid requirements for the adult are estimated by using one of two formulas. The first formula calculates 30 to 35 ml/kg/day. The second formula calculates 1500 ml for the first 20 kg of body weight, adding an additional 20 ml/kg for actual weight beyond the initial 20 kg.[57] This second formula can also be used for pediatric patients weighing 20 kg or greater. Calculations used to determine fluid requirements in pediatric patients weighing less than 20 kg are as follows: 100 ml/kg for children weighing 1 to 10 kg of body weight; and 1000 ml + 50 ml/kg for each kilogram over 10 kg for children weighing 11 to 20 kg.[63]

It is important to consider the patient's cardiac, respiratory, and renal status, as well as his or her preexisting hydration status. Critically ill patients may become fluid overloaded if calculations used to determine fluid requirements do not incorporate fluids yielded during oxidation of nutrient substances (approximately 500 ml water daily in typical TPN regimens), fluid liberated from muscle catabolism (500 ml daily during severe catabolism), and other exogenous sources such as IV fluids and medications.

Normal fluid losses include renal losses (30 to 120 ml/hr) and insensible losses (800 to 1000 ml/day in the adult). Increased fluid losses occur during fever, diarrhea, vomiting, GI suction or drainage, high respiratory rates, burns, wounds, or osmotic diuresis. These increased losses may indicate the need for additional fluid replacement.[64]

Care must be taken to continually assess the patient's hydration status during TPN therapy. This includes accurate daily intake and output; assessing for signs of cardiac, respiratory, and renal compromise; observing for rapid weight changes and peripheral edema; and managing serum electrolyte status.

Drug compatibility considerations. The compatibility of drugs in parenteral nutrition solutions is often in question and is difficult to answer because of the many factors that affect compatibility, such as the solubility, stability, and pharmacokinetics of drugs. However, a number of drugs have been added to parenteral nutrition solutions without any apparent incompatibility reactions.

The complex composition of parenteral nutrition solutions renders them highly susceptible to compatibility and stability problems. Adding drugs to parenteral nutrition admixtures poses an increased risk of physical and chemical incompatibility and solution contamination. Consequently, the clinician should be cautious when considering the addition of any drug in a concentration that varies from published guidelines. The pharmacist must consider the physical and chemical properties of all components of parenteral admixtures and ensure that adequate documentation exists to support the inclusion of various additives, particularly drugs.

Insulin. Patients with limited capability for producing insulin may require exogenous insulin when dextrose is administered. Although insulin can be administered subcutaneously to treat TPN-induced hyperglycemia, it may be more effective to add insulin to the parenteral nutrition solution. When handled in this manner, the insulin dose is changed as the rate of infusion is adjusted.[6] Blood sugar levels less than 200 mg/dl can be achieved in most patients. If the blood sugar concentration cannot be controlled by exogenous insulin, the amount of dextrose may need to be reduced and additional calories provided from lipids.

Heparin. Heparin in small doses (1000 to 3000 units/L) is sometimes added to parenteral nutrition solutions to decrease the likelihood of a fibrin sleeve, which may lead to venous thrombosis. However, concerns related to the possibility of heparin-induced thrombocytopenia have decreased this practice.[6]

H_2-receptor antagonists. H_2-receptor antagonists inhibit gastric acid secretion and are used during parenteral nutrition to prevent stress ulceration. They are effective in counteracting metabolic alkalosis induced by nasogastric suctioning or use of crystalline amino acid solutions that contain large amounts of acetate.[7]

In general, the only drugs that should be considered for inclusion in a parenteral nutrition admixture are those with stable dosage regimens supported by published guidelines and having appropriate therapeutic efficacy when given as a continuous infusion. Medications that may be added to parenteral nutrition solutions include the following: heparin, H_2-receptor antagonists (cimetidine, famotidine, ranitidine), hydrochloric acid (in lipid-free TPN), metoclopramide, narcotics (morphine sulfate, meperidine, hydromorphone, levorphanol), and regular insulin. Less commonly used but still compatible medication admixtures include albumin, furosemide, and aminophylline (stable dose regimen). Although albumin is compatible, it is expensive and has little or no clinical efficacy in increasing and maintaining the serum albumin level. Conflicting research exists on the compatibility of somatostatin in TPN solutions. Iron dextran is best given orally; however, it may be administered intravenously if GI absorption is inadequate. If peripheral access is unavailable, maintenance infusions of iron dextran (100 mg/day) can be added to nutrient solutions without great risk of anaphylactic reaction.[6] The use of iron dextran in TPN solutions remains controversial and the American Medical Association makes no recommendation for iron intake. TPN patients are at high risk for infection and circulating free iron is a risk factor for infection.[12] The use of iron dextran in 3-in-1 formulas is not recommended, particularly in large amounts or when the formula will not be administered within 24 hours of preparation.[6]

Most antibiotics are not administered continuously and therefore are not suitable for addition to parenteral nutrition solutions. Antibiotic compatibility information is limited for 3-in-1 solutions.[6] The CVC used for parenteral nutrition is considered inviolate. However, in extraordinary situations, patients with severely limited venous access may require that antibiotics be infused via the parenteral nutrition catheter. If antibiotic therapy is indicated in a person who is also receiving parenteral nutrition, providing that the antibiotic is compatible, the antibiotic should be administered via a piggyback infusion at the catheter hub rather than direct mixing with the parenteral nutrition solution. Reports describe short-term stability of antibiotics such as aminoglycosides, cephalosporins, penicillins, and vancomycin.[65] In addition, drug therapies in which the dosage fluctuates in relation to the patient's clinical status, such as vasopressor agents, are not practical additions. Such inclusions may reduce drug efficacy, lead to administration errors, or cause significant waste of the parenteral nutrition solution.

Using parenteral solutions to deliver drugs has some advantages, such as consolidation of dosage units and improved pharmacotherapy for certain drugs. It also conserves fluids in volume-restricted patients, eliminates multiple entries for drug administration into the vascular access device, and provides the economic benefits of reduced personnel time and material savings.

Standard solutions

Peripheral parenteral nutrition. PPN is used most effectively for weight maintenance of nonhypermetabolic patients, as a preliminary mode before central infusion, and as a supplement to enteral feedings. It is associated with fewer hazards and complications related to central venous access. The limitations of peripheral parenteral nutrition are the high tonicity and volume of infusate required to meet caloric demands. Because of their lower concentration (less than 900 mOsm/L), PPN solution can be infused into peripheral veins but will provide fewer calories and less protein per volume. The availability of fat emulsions has made PPN an attractive means for providing parenteral nutrition. Isotonic, high-calorie lipid emulsions help meet the nutritional needs of many patients by the use of PPN alone. Unfortunately, PPN is usually more difficult to maintain because of frequent episodes of phlebitis in superficial veins and the infiltration of solutions into subcutaneous tissue.

A typical standard PPN solution may contain 50 g dextrose with 35 g amino acids per liter. Final concentrations typically range from 1.75% to 3.5% amino acids and from 5% to 10% dextrose, electrolytes, trace elements, and vitamins, along with 500 ml of 10% or 20% lipids. No greater than a 10% final concentration of dextrose should be infused peripherally.[1]

Total parenteral nutrition. TPN formulations vary somewhat, depending on the patient's condition and the institution's preference. An example of a standard formulation is 42.5 g amino acids and 250 g dextrose per liter (500 ml of an 8.5% amino acid solution and 500 ml of 50% dextrose). This formula will provide 1000 calories/L and a nonprotein-calorie/nitrogen ratio of 150:1. IV lipid is usually provided separately twice weekly to prevent essential fatty acid deficiency.

Total nutrient admixture. *Total nutrient admixture (TNA), trisubstrate system, all-in-one system,* and *3-in-1 system* are all terms used to describe the combination of dextrose, amino acids, fat emulsion, electrolytes, trace elements, and multivitamins in one container. The addition of fat emulsion is the unique part of these admixtures. The components are mixed in one bag with a volume of up to 3 L, and the resulting solution provides a total nutrient supply for a 24-hour period.

Many advantages are associated with the use of TNAs. Because they decrease the amount of calories provided from glucose, they may be clinically useful for patients with diabetes or compromised respiratory function. The use of a TNA might reduce the risk of microbial contamination because it requires fewer manipulations of the solution container and tubing. There are also economic advantages associated with time and material savings for both nursing and pharmacy. TNA systems simplify the administration of parenteral nutrition for the home TPN patient.[66]

A number of considerations are associated with the use of TNAs. Because fat droplets have a mean particle size of 0.4 to 0.5 microns, they clog the standard 0.22-micron filter. However, TNA solutions can be administered through a 1.2-micron particulate filter. The extended use of lipid emulsions imposes limits on the quantity of lipid infused daily secondary to the potential for cholestasis. There is also the potential for fat emulsions that contain long-chain triglycerides to depress the immune system, although further study regarding this phenomenon appears to be warranted.[9,67] In addition, there is a potential for increased waste if this system is used in patients who are clinically unstable, with changing metabolic needs. Catheter occlusion resulting from fat deposits has been reported with long-term use of this therapy. Finally, there are only limited data regarding the compatibility and stability of this system with various products and concentrations.

The variable stability of many amino acids, lipid solutions, and electrolyte and mineral additives must be considered when preparing a TNA. The most fragile component of a TNA system is the fat emulsion. The destabilization of fat emulsions in the presence of a low pH value or high electrolyte concentration affects the methods used to prepare the TNA.[67] Dual-chamber parenteral nutrition bags, now in use in home care, keep lipids separate from the parenteral nutrition solution by means of a removable divider (Fig. 12-2). Although these dual-chamber bags decrease the amount of interface time between parenteral nutrition and lipid emulsions, the potential for instability still exists after the divider is removed and the two solutions are

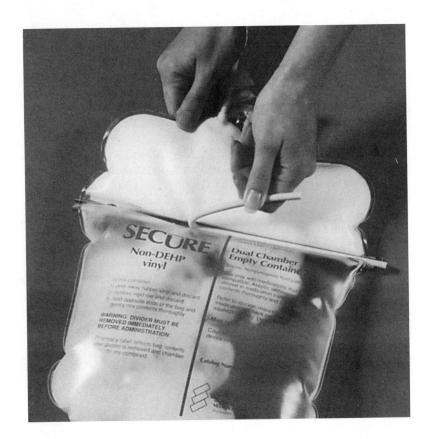

FIG. 12-2 *Dual chamber bag.* (Photo courtesy Metrix Company.)

mixed. All TNAs need to be visually inspected before administration for evidence of deterioration or cracking of the emulsion. When this occurs, there is a change in droplet size and dispersion of the emulsion, and the infusion of undispersed fat aggregates may be toxic. Emulsion stability is influenced by several factors, such as pH, electrolyte charge, temperature, and time. The pH and compounding sequence must be considered by the pharmacist when admixing this system. As with all IV admixtures, TNA solutions must be mixed in an aseptic environment because fat emulsions are an excellent microbial growth medium and should not hang or be at room temperature for longer than 24 hours. When refrigerated, TNA solutions will remain physically stable for up to 14 days.

Formulations for infants and young children.
Amino acids such as histidine, tyrosine, cysteine, and taurine, which are nonessential in adults, may be essential for infants and young children. Special amino acid formulations are available to meet these needs.

Disease-specific solutions

A number of disease-specific formulas, both parenteral and enteral, have been marketed for patients with renal or hepatic disease, respiratory failure, and stress. These products are briefly discussed here.

Renal failure.
Amino acid formulas high in essential amino acids are formulated with specific indications for patients with renal failure. Essential amino acids are converted to nonessential amino acids in vivo as needed and minimize ureagenesis.

Although there may be certain clinical advantages to using formulas high in essential amino acids, the practice remains controversial. It is believed that nonessential amino acids may be needed to optimize protein synthesis and achieve positive nitrogen balance.[68] During dialysis, all amino acids, essential and nonessential, are removed; therefore standard amino acid solutions containing both essential and nonessential amino acids are recommended to meet the protein requirements of dialyzed patients.

Hepatic failure.
Patients with hepatic failure have abnormal plasma amino acid profiles, characterized by high levels of aromatic amino acids and low levels of branched-chain amino acids. It has been theorized that this abnormal profile contributes to "false neurotransmitter" synthesis and the development of encephalopathy. Hepatic failure formulas contain little or no aromatic acids and high concentrations of branched-chain amino acids. These formulas were developed in an attempt to minimize hepatic encephalopathy in patients with liver failure. However, despite initial promising results using these modified amino acid solutions, it has not been clearly demonstrated that they are any more helpful than standard amino acid infusions in managing hepatic encephalopathy.[69] As a result, these solutions are not routinely recommended or used.

Stress formula.
Patients become hypercatabolic secondary to the metabolic state created by trauma, sepsis, and burns. Altered protein metabolism is a hallmark of the stressed patient. Protein catabolism with a resultant increase in nitrogen excretion and altered plasma amino acid concentrations has been observed in both adults and children with sepsis, trauma, and

major burn injury. Managing altered protein metabolism in the stressed patient requires quantitative and qualitative modifications in nutrition support. To offset the increased rate of nitrogen excretion, protein intake should be increased. Modified amino acid solutions, having an increased content of branched-chain amino acids in an otherwise balanced amino acid solution, can be used.

Respiratory insufficiency. Because of its large carbohydrate load, the standard parenteral nutrition formula administered to a critically ill patient can adversely affect the respiratory quotient. Fat emulsions can be used as an alternative source of calories, allowing for a reduction of the carbohydrate load. The production of CO_2 increases as the amount of infused glucose increases. In a patient with normal ventilatory function, the effect of the infusion on the respiratory quotient is not a major consideration. However, in the patient with compromised ventilation, increasing CO_2 production may precipitate respiratory failure or may delay or prevent weaning from a ventilator. Therefore, in patients with respiratory insufficiency, maintenance caloric requirements must be defined more precisely. When a patient is being weaned from a ventilator, the caloric intake is stabilized at maintenance levels. If weaning is hindered by CO_2 retention, the carbohydrate load is reduced to provide about 60% to 70% of the maintenance caloric requirements as glucose, and 30% to 40% of requirements as lipid emulsion.[70]

Administration of parenteral nutrition

Parenteral nutrition solutions should be compounded in a pharmacy using a laminar flow hood to ensure sterility. The solutions should be used immediately after preparation or refrigerated and removed 60 minutes before administration. To reduce the risk of bacterial contamination, parenteral nutrition solutions must be infused or discarded within 24 hours after hanging.

Initiation. The catheter tip location must be confirmed before initiating TPN. Before PPN is initiated, the peripheral site must be assessed carefully. Solution labels should always be compared with the physician's order. The solution and container should be checked for leaks, cracks, clarity, and expiration date, and TNA solutions should also be checked for discoloration or separation of oils.

TPN solutions are usually initiated gradually and increased as the patient's fluid and glucose tolerance allows. Changes in the rate of administration should be gradual because fluctuations in glucose levels can occur if the infusion is interrupted or irregular in rate. Initial glucose infusions should not exceed 250 g over 24 hours to allow for adequate endogenous insulin secretion. Solution administration may then be advanced to the required nutritional level, increasing by 1000 kcal/day. To avoid potential complications, TPN must be administered at a constant rate and not discontinued abruptly. PPN does not require a gradual introduction but may be initiated at the desired rate. To maintain a consistent and accurate flow rate, an electronic infusion device should be used.[1]

Discontinuation. PPN solutions containing less than 10% dextrose concentration usually can be discontinued safely without a tapering regimen because of the decreased risk of

Table 12-7	**Cyclic Parenteral Nutrition: Benefits and Indications**

BENEFITS

1. Improved quality of life through resumption of normal daily activities; allows the patient freedom from pumps during daytime hours, increased psychologic well-being
2. Allows for increased mobility, which maintains somatic muscle
3. Allows for more physiologic hormonal responses and stimulation of appetite
4. Prevention or treatment of hepatotoxicities induced by continuous TPN; reversal of fatty liver and enzyme level elevations and faster albumin level recovery
5. Prevention or treatment of essential fatty acid deficiency in patients on fat-free TPN; reduced insulin levels during TPN-free periods allows for lipolysis and release of essential linoleic acid

INDICATIONS

1. Patients who have been stable on continuous TPN and require long-term parenteral nutrition
2. Patients who are receiving home TPN
3. Patients who can handle the total infusion volume in a shortened time period
4. Patients who require TPN for only a portion of their nutritional needs
5. Patients who have hepatic steatosis or for its prevention

TPN, Total parenteral nutrition.

rebound hypoglycemia. The discontinuation of TPN solutions, however, requires a logical approach. Oral or enteral intake should provide two thirds to three fourths of the daily nutritional requirements before TPN is discontinued.[7] There are several techniques for discontinuing TPN therapy[15]:

1. *Transition feeding:* Initiate oral or enteral feeding while tapering parenteral nutrition concomitantly.
2. *Replacement with a peripheral IV:* Used when a central catheter must be removed suddenly. Dextrose 5% or 10% may be initiated at the same rate of infusion.
3. *Tapering technique:* Tapering the rate over 2 to 3 days may be required to reduce the incidence of rebound hypoglycemia if the patient is receiving more than 1000 kcal/day. The diagnosis, patient's condition, and length of therapy must be considered to evaluate whether tapering is necessary. The appropriate protocol for discontinuing TPN has been controversial and practice patterns vary among institutions.[6] The patient may have complicating conditions that predispose him or her to hypoglycemia following the rapid tapering of TPN, such as concurrent insulin administration or existing renal or hepatic disease. In the unstressed patient, rapid tapering can be accomplished by reducing the rate by 50% during the first hour and by 50% during the second hour.[71]

Cyclic regimens. Cyclic administration regimens involve the infusion of TPN on a cyclic basis over 8 to 16 hours rather than the standard continuous infusion over a 24-hour period. Indications and benefits of cyclic infusions are presented in Table 12-7. TPN can be transitioned to cyclic administration once tolerance to 24-hour continuous infusion has been obtained. The switch to cyclic infusion is accomplished by a gradual reduction in the hours of infusion, usually 1 to 4 hours a day. The hourly rate is determined by dividing the total required volume of TPN by the number of hours the TPN is to be infused. Cyclic TPN is usually administered at a rate no higher than 200 ml/hr. The ability to tolerate the glucose and fluid volume determines how rapidly the solution can be infused. With the average patient receiving 2 to 3 L, this usually requires 12 to 16 hours to complete. Patients receiving 2 L of fluid may tolerate 8-hour infusions to maximize freedom. Cyclic infusions are generally infused at night and turned off during daytime hours.

Fat emulsions. Before fat emulsions are administered, the solution should be inspected for frothiness, separation, or oily appearance. The low osmolarity of fat emulsions permits delivery by peripheral veins. Fat emulsions may be administered through a separate site or given through a lower Y connector in the existing TPN administration set. Fat emulsions may or may not require filtration depending on manufacturers directions and individual institutional policy. In cases in which filtration is required, a 1.2-micron filter may be used. Fat emulsion as part of the TNA solution also requires a 1.2-micron filter.[1]

Delivery time for a single container of fat emulsion varies from 4 to 12 hours depending on the patient's condition. However, solutions may hang up to 24 hours. An initial dose of a fat emulsion should be given slowly to test for possible allergic reactions. To administer a test dose for an adult, a 10% fat emulsion should be infused at a rate of 1 ml/min for the first 15 to 30 minutes, and a 20% fat emulsion should be infused at a rate of 0.5 ml/min for the first 15 to 30 minutes. Symptoms of adverse reactions include nausea, fever, chills, muscle aches, pain in the chest or back, and urticaria.[6] Fat emulsions should be given with caution to patients with hyperlipidemia. A baseline fasting triglyceride level may be obtained and monitored weekly; the weekly serum sample should be drawn 8 hours after infusion.[70]

Vascular access

Vascular access systems include subcutaneous venous ports, tunneled catheters, nontunneled catheters, and peripherally inserted central catheters. They may be single, double, or triple lumen, depending on the types of infusions needed. Generally speaking, subcutaneous venous ports and tunneled catheters are used for long-term IV therapy. Nontunneled catheters and peripherally inserted central catheters are used for short-term therapy.

Guidelines for vascular access and catheter care are basically the same for parenteral nutrition as for any other infusion. However, it is generally recommended that access devices be dedicated solely to the use of parenteral nutrition to decrease potential contamination.

As discussed earlier, peripheral venous access for PPN, a lower osmolar solution, should be limited to short-term or supplemental therapy especially if PPN does not provide the patient's nutrient requirements. TPN solutions require access into a central vein to allow rapid dilution of the solution to prevent phlebitis, pain, and thrombosis. Central access generally involves insertion into one of the major veins of the upper neck or chest, with the tip located in the superior vena cava. Because the subclavian area is flat, immobile, and relatively free of secretions, it is the ideal site for long-term IV access. The subclavian approach is more comfortable for the patient and the maintenance of an occlusive dressing is more easily achieved. Patients who require long-term access and have thrombosed subclavian access may necessitate less-than-ideal access measures. Other areas of vascular access are the femoral, ovarian, portal, azygos, or renal veins. Access can also be established through an arteriovenous fistula or shunt. These measures are extreme and should be considered only when subclavian access is impossible. Tunneled catheters and totally implanted venous ports are generally used for long-term parenteral support, but nontunneled catheters may also be used in certain circumstances. The system should be comfortable for the patient, must not limit mobility, and should be accessible enough to allow maintenance procedures by the patient, if possible. Patient preference, lifestyle, and manual dexterity are important when making decisions on the type of catheter to be used (Fig. 12-3). Because there is no external segment, implanted ports may be more acceptable to patients who have periods without parenteral nutrition during the remission phases of their disease. The needle usually remains in place for several days for continuous or cyclic therapy that is limited to several hours daily.

Perhaps the most critical aspect of the nursing management of TPN patients involves the care of the CVC before, during, and after insertion. Numerous studies have shown that adherence to strict protocols regarding insertion and care of the CVC reduces complications.[72] The type of catheter and regimen for catheter site maintenance is determined by the prescribed therapy, insertion site, patient's condition, age, and practice setting. Observation of the catheter access site should be documented every 8 hours in the hospital setting. Patency should be established before initiating infusates and periodically throughout the infusion period. Peripheral catheter sites should be rotated every 48 or 72 hours (dependent on documented phlebitis rate), and immediately for suspected contamination or complication.[1]

Dressing procedures vary depending on the condition of the patient (including immunocompetency factors), type of dressing, and policies set by the organization. Patients with tunneled catheters may be able to eliminate the need for sterile dressing procedures after the exit site is well healed. With peripheral and CVCs, occlusive gauze dressings should be changed every 48 hours in conjunction with administration set. Transparent semipermeable membrane (TSM) dressings may also be used and should be changed at established intervals. TSM dressings should be changed on peripheral short catheters whenever the site is rotated or sooner if the integrity is compromised. TSM dressings placed on central catheters, implanted ports, and PICCS are changed at least every 3 to 7 days. When TSM is placed over gauze, the dressing should be changed every 48 hours. The use of antimicrobial barriers or other dressing materials is established in organizational policy and procedure. The optimal time for these materials is unknown, however, they are typically changed weekly. Regardless of the type of dressing material selected, any dressing should be changed immediately if it is even suspected that its integrity is compromised. Aseptic technique should be maintained. Consideration should be given to the use of sterile gloves and a mask when changing the dressing.[1]

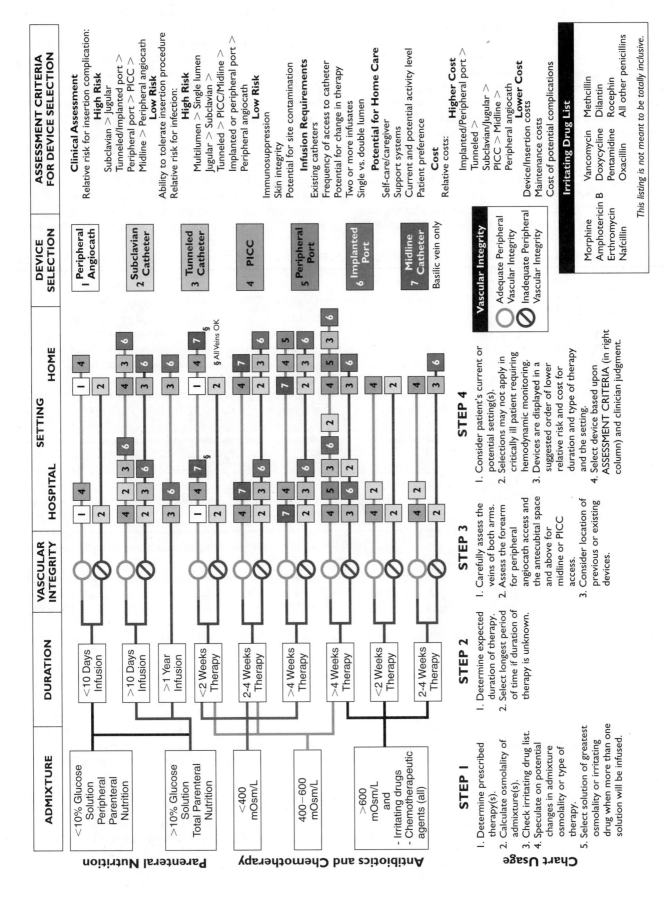

FIG. 12-3 *Vascular access device selection.* (Courtesy Marcia Ryder, PhDc, MS, RN.)

Equipment

All administration sets used to deliver parenteral solutions should be changed immediately using aseptic technique for suspected contamination or when the integrity of the product has been compromised. Administration sets used for parenteral nutrition or lipid emulsion are changed every 24 hours.[1] If these solutions are administered in a cyclic regimen, the administration set should be discarded immediately after each unit. In comparison with standard IV solutions, administration sets for parenteral nutrition are changed more frequently because of the dextrose and protein content of TPN solutions, which provide a greater potential for bacterial growth and contamination. All parenteral nutrition solutions should be filtered with a 0.2-micron filter and TNAs with a 1.2-micron filter. A filter should not be used with only-lipid emulsion infusions.[1] Fat emulsions may or may not require filtration, depending on manufacturer's directions and institutional policy. In cases in which filtration is required, a 1.2-micron filter should be used.

Nursing assessment

Using the nursing process, the nurse's care of the patient receiving nutritional support begins with assessment. Daily physical assessment and observation of the signs and symptoms of a catabolic state provide valuable information (Box 12-3).

During the physical assessment, the nurse should focus particularly on the GI tract but should also include the neurologic, cardiopulmonary, and renal systems. Assessment of the GI tract may be difficult if the patient's primary disease has involved this system. It is important to identify patients at risk for metabolic complications during parenteral nutrition. Candidates for complications include the very young and the elderly; those with glucose intolerance, renal dysfunction, neurologic damage, or excessive fluid loss such as fistula output or secretions; and patients who are intubated or receiving steroids or diuretics.

The nurse assesses the patient's weight daily, at the same time of morning, using the same scale, and with the patient wearing the same amount of clothing. Weighing is often an unpopular task, but the patient's weight provides a means of assessing whether calorie and fluid needs are being met or exceeded. If the patient continues to lose weight after several days of nutritional support, discussion with other members of the health team,

such as the dietitian and pharmacist, can be beneficial, particularly if the formula needs to be adjusted.

The nurse should also assess other factors that indicate fluid balance, such as intake and output, vital signs, peripheral or dependent edema, lung sounds, mucous membranes, skin turgor, and jugular vein distension. Measuring intake and output and vital signs should not be considered routine. These important activities have a meaningful relationship to the metabolic monitoring of the patient receiving nutrition support.

Baseline laboratory values are obtained early in the patient's course of therapy. Daily determinations are necessary to guide the concentration and formulation of the parenteral nutrition solution until the patient is stable. The nurse collaborates with the physician to ensure that tests are ordered and evaluated regularly to assess the objective status of nutrition and endocrine function. Laboratory tests measure total proteins, albumin, blood urea nitrogen, electrolytes, minerals, and vitamins. Additional laboratory tests include the serum magnesium level, complete blood count, prothrombin time, and liver function tests.

All patients receiving nutrition support should have frequent assessments of blood glucose levels because hyperglycemia can precipitate osmotic diuresis and hyperosmolar dehydration and can herald impending sepsis. Capillary blood sugar tests are often used to monitor glucose levels. Urine testing for the presence of glucose and ketones may be done, but the availability of capillary sugar tests has decreased its use. The accuracy of urine testing may be altered by drugs, the freshness of the testing materials and the urine, or the patient's renal function. When possible, testing should be performed with a double-voided urine specimen. An initial correlation of blood glucose and urine glucose levels may be needed to determine the patient's renal threshold for glucose. Patients with a high renal threshold may require frequent capillary sugar testing and sliding-scale insulin coverage. This allows better monitoring and tighter control of glucose levels, thereby deterring chronic microvascular and macrovascular complications associated with long-term hyperglycemia.

Although parenteral nutrition is viewed by medical personnel as a lifesaving procedure, patients are often unable to separate the procedure from the disease as the cause of hospitalization. Parenteral nutrition is a constant reminder of the disease and the limitation it imposes. These feelings can produce anger until the person resolves the conflict and regains some measure of autonomy. Thus nurses should not be surprised if patients resent the very procedures that are keeping them alive. It is important to assess negative responses and help the patient and his or her family identify coping mechanisms. The information obtained in the nursing assessment can help the nurse provide this assistance and to plan other aspects of care.

Patients receiving parenteral nutrition for long periods may need a great deal of emotional support. Nutrition is normally associated with food and eating; not eating can have a major psychologic effect on some people. Patients initially may have hunger pains and food cravings, even though their physiologic requirements are being met. Eventually, however, appetites are suppressed by parenteral nutrition, and the patient needs to be assured that appetite and bowel activity gradually return to normal when the parenteral feedings are discontinued.

Box 12-3	**Signs and Symptoms of a Catabolic State**

- Increased temperature, pulse, and respirations
- Decreased level of consciousness
- Poor skin turgor
- Lesions of skin and mucous membranes
- Dehydration
- Changes in bowel activity (number and character of stools)
- Decreasing body weight
- Tissue edema
- Eczema

Nursing diagnosis

Establishing a nursing diagnosis provides an important framework for identifying problems, setting goals, initiating interventions, and evaluating outcomes. Individual patient circumstances require additional diagnoses to be formulated. The North American Nursing Diagnosis Association's (NANDA) nursing diagnosis list is helpful in identifying an acceptable nursing diagnosis. Box 12-4 is an example of a nursing care plan for a patient receiving nutritional support.

Documentation remains an important nursing function. Documentation of information regarding the patient's status and response is critical to the success of nutrition therapy. Standardized forms may be used to record information pertinent to the patient's clinical progress, nutrition support regimen, fluid intake and output, and laboratory data, facilitating communication and documenting patient progress. Thorough documentation and evaluation of the plan of care also is important in substantiating the appropriateness of services provided and securing proper reimbursement.

Complications

Perhaps the most important complication of nutritional support is the failure to achieve the desired goals of therapy because of inadequate monitoring. The general goals of nutritional intervention are to support the lean body mass; support the structure and function of the organs to prevent nutrient deficiencies; and, perhaps most important, to do no harm. The nurse plays an important role in monitoring patients receiving nutritional support therapy. Measuring vital signs, recording intake and output, monitoring laboratory values, understanding the parenteral nutrition prescription, and observing, interpreting, and accurately reporting changes in the patient's condition and physiologic responses are vital for the successful management and care of the patient.

The complications of parenteral nutrition may be divided into three areas: metabolic, technical, and septic. The causes, treatment, prevention, and monitoring of these types of complications are summarized in Table 12-8.

PARENTERAL NUTRITION IN THE PEDIATRIC PATIENT

TPN must be modified in pediatric patients to meet the special demands of growth and development. Compared with adults, children have a higher basal metabolic rate per unit of body weight, an increased evaporative fluid loss, and immature kidneys with decreased water clearance.[73,74] Growth failure in children manifests itself as poor weight gain, below-normal height, and delayed appearance of secondary sex characteristics. In the newborn, the ratio of the metabolic rate to body weight is three times that of the adult. Neonates exhibit deficiencies of enzymes essential for the synthesis of certain amino acids (e.g., cysteine, taurine, tyrosine, histidine), so these are considered essential amino acids for this age group. Calcium and phosphorus requirements are greater for normal bone growth. Thus the tolerance period of starvation for a neonate ranges from 1 to 5 days, compared with 7 to 10 days in the older child or adult.[74]

A complete nutritional assessment of the pediatric patient is indicated in cases of recent weight loss greater than 10% (excluding dehydration), weight/height ratio below the 5th percentile, serum albumin less than 3.5 g/dl, and a diagnosis associated with the development of protein-calorie malnutrition.[63] Similar to the adult, nutritional assessment of the pediatric patient includes medical and dietary history and physical examination. In addition, nutritional assessment includes standard growth curves. The ratio of weight to height is used to determine wasting, and the ratio of height to age is used to determine stunting of growth. Anthropometric measurements are used to gauge somatic protein and fat stores. In addition, head circumference measurements are used. Serious malnutrition during critical stages of brain development may cause diminished brain growth and impairment of normal head growth.[63] Visceral protein stores are evaluated by determining serum albumin, serum transferrin, prealbumin, and retinol-binding protein levels.[73] Biochemical measurements may also include urinary excretion of creatinine (used to evaluate the status of skeletal muscle), skin testing for cellular immunity, and a determination of the percentage of lymphocytes. A decrease in lymphocytes or changes in lymphocyte response is an indication of poor nutritional status.[63]

Indications

Most pediatric patients requiring parenteral nutrition fall into two major categories: (1) patients with congenital or acquired anomalies of the GI tract and (2) patients with intractable diarrhea syndromes. A list of conditions that may require parenteral nutrition is provided in Table 12-9.

Nutritional requirements

Nutritional requirements for the pediatric patient are presented in Tables 12-10 and 12-11. Fluid requirement calculations should take into account the existing hydration status, body

Text continued on p. 240

Box 12-4   Example of Nursing Care Plan

NURSING DIAGNOSIS
Alteration in nutrition, less than body requirements
GOAL
Stabilize weight and gradually increase to 10% of ideal.
INTERVENTIONS
1. Work with patient to establish a scale of weight outcomes from most desirable to least desirable.
2. Weigh patient daily and record until the desired weight is reached.
3. Administer nutrition solution as prescribed. Monitor and record intake and output.
4. Collaborate with nutrition support team to monitor and evaluate patient's nutritional status.
EXPECTED OUTCOMES
1. Weight is stabilized (immediate outcome).
2. Weight gain of 1 pound every 3 weeks, increasing to 1 pound every 2 weeks (most desirable outcome).

Table 12-8 **Complications of Parenteral Nutrition**

CAUSE	SYMPTOMS/SIGNS	TREATMENT	PREVENTION	MONITORING
I. METABOLIC				
A. FLUID AND ELECTROLYTE IMBALANCE	Refer to Chapter 7, Fluid and Electrolytes			
1. Overhydration Excess fluid administration, particularly for renal insufficiency or immediately after trauma		Reduce fluid administration, provide diuretics.	Initiate parenteral nutrition (PN) only after fluid balance is stable, careful intake and output (I/O) monitoring with calculation of fluid needs and intake from other sources.	I/O, daily weights, blood urea nitrogen (BUN), serum sodium (Na) levels, and hematocrit.
2. Dehydration Inadequate fluid administration over-diuresis, excessive unreplaced fluid loss		Increase fluid administration.	Same as overhydration.	Same as overhydration.
3. Hyperkalemia Renal insufficiency or excessive potassium (K) administration		Reduce K or K binders provided.	Careful laboratory monitoring and calculation of K levels.	Serum K levels.
4. Hypokalemia Inadequate amounts provided; increased loss from diarrhea, fistulas, and burns; increased needs related to anabolism		Adjust amount of supplement provided.	Same as hyperkalemia.	Same as hyperkalemia.
5. Hypernatremia Excessive water loss		Reduce Na in infusion and fluid replacement.	Avoid excessive intake and careful fluid replacement.	Serum and urinary Na levels, I/O.
6. Hyponatremia Depletion of fluid through sweating or excessive gastrointestinal (GI) losses, excessive diuretic therapy, dilutional states, including congestive heart failure (CHF) and syndrome of inappropriate antidiuretic hormone secretion (SIADH)		Adjust fluid and Na intake as condition indicates.	Provide Na replacement unless contraindicated by cardiac, renal, or fluid status.	Same as hypernatremia.
B. GLUCOSE METABOLISM				
1. Hyperglycemia Rapid infusion of concentrated dextrose solution; high-risk conditions include diabetes, sepsis, and steroid medication		Provide insulin and/or part of nonprotein calories as lipid.	Slow initial administration of dextrose, reduce dextrose provided, provide insulin as needed.	Frequent blood and urine determinations.
2. Hypoglycemia Rapid discontinuation (DC) of PN		Administer dextrose.	Taper PN solution; if abrupt DC occurs, hang 10% dextrose to prevent rebound hypoglycemia.	Frequent blood or urine determinations especially during DC.

C. MINERAL IMBALANCE

Condition / Cause	Signs and Symptoms	Treatment	Action	Monitoring
1. Hyperphosphatemia Seen in long-term PN with phosphorus-containing solutions; also seen in decreased renal excretion	Paresthesia of the extremities, flaccid paralysis, listlessness, mental confusion, weakness, hypertension, cardiac arrhythmias, prolonged elevated phosphorus levels, which may result in tissue calcification	DC phosphorus (P); provide serum calcium (Ca) repletion.	Reduce P as indicated by serum levels.	Serum levels 1-2× weekly.
2. Hypophosphatemia Often seen in malnutrition. Predisposing factors include alcohol abuse, diabetes mellitus, antacid ingestion, and increased phosphorus requirements of anabolism	May include respiratory distress	Administer intravenous phosphate (PO_4) or add PO_4 to solution.	Use P in PN, 13.6 mmol/day; has been shown to prevent PO_4 depletion in most patients.	Serum level 1-2× weekly; more frequently with replacement.
3. Hypermagnesemia Excess magnesium (Mg) administration; inability to excrete Mg because of renal insufficiency	Sharp drop in blood pressure and respiratory paralysis; cardiac toxicity progressing from increased conduction time, hypotension, and premature ventricular contractions to cardiac arrest	Remove or decrease Mg in PN; severe cases may require mechanical ventilation, dialysis, correction of fluid deficit, and administration of calcium gluconate.	Restrict as appropriate.	Plasma levels 1-2× weekly; or more frequently as indicated.
4. Hypomagnesemia Risk factors include diuretic use, diabetic ketoacidosis, GI disease, aminoglycoside use, alcoholism, and chemotherapy	Nonspecific symptoms; GI and neurologic changes; neuromuscular hyperactivity, convulsions, and cardiac arrhythmia	Administer peripheral magnesium. Add Mg.	Provide Mg in PN solution.	Serum levels 1-2× weekly during initiation of PN and weekly thereafter; more frequent monitoring may be necessary during hypomagnesemia, repletion, and chemotherapy.
5. Hypercalcemia Neoplasia, excess vitamin D administration, prolonged immobilization, and stress	Thirst, polyuria, muscle weakness, loss of appetite; nausea, vomiting, constipation, itching	Administer isotonic saline, provide inorganic PO_4 supplement, mithramycin, corticosteroids.	Restrict as appropriate.	Plasma Ca levels 1-2× weekly.
6. Hypocalcemia Decreased vitamin D intake; hypoparathyroidism; reduced Ca intake, increased GI losses, decreased PO_4 intake	Paresthesia; tetany	Provide additional amounts of Ca.	Administer approximately 15 mEq daily to achieve Ca balance.	Plasma Ca levels 1-2× weekly; if serum albumin level is depressed, obtain ionized Ca level.

Continued

The authors wish to thank Ms. Karen Carrasco, RN, for her assistance in the preparation of this table.

Table 12-8 Complications of Parenteral Nutrition—cont'd

CAUSE	SYMPTOMS/SIGNS	TREATMENT	PREVENTION	MONITORING
I. METABOLIC—cont'd **D. NUTRITIONAL** **1. Carbohydrate Overfeeding** Rapid increase of feedings above requirements, particularly in patients with compromised pulmonary or cardiac function	CO_2 retention, cardiac tamponade	Decrease infusion to acceptable level.	Carefully calculate nutrient requirements; ensure appropriate distribution of energy substrate.	Respiratory quotients may help determine the proper energy substrate mix.
2. Protein Overfeeding Continued infusion of protein in excess of requirements	Elevated BUN levels; excess nitrogen excretion	Reduce amino acid content.	Carefully calculate protein requirements; provide adequate calories from carbohydrate and/or fat.	Serum BUN levels 1-2× weekly; nitrogen balance weekly.
3. Essential Fatty Acid Deficiency Inadequate fat intake; biochemical signs appear 1-2 weeks on a fat-free regime	Dermatitis; alopecia; changes in pulmonary, neurologic, and red cell membranes	Provide lipid emulsion at least 2× weekly.	Provide 2% to 4% of caloric needs as linoleic acid, or 8% to 10% of calories from fat; fat intake achieved by 500 ml of 10% fat emulsion 2 to 3× weekly.	Physical examination for symptoms.
4. Thiamine Deficiency Concentrated glucose infusion without adequate thiamine	Elevated blood and urine lactate and pyruvate levels, abnormal electrocardiogram (ECG), cardiomegaly, and dyspnea	Adequate thiamine intake per intravenous RDA.	Provide thiamine daily in PN.	Blood and urine lactate and pyruvate levels 2× weekly in patients at risk.
E. HEPATIC **1. Fatty Liver** Presumed to be infusion of carbohydrate in excess of hepatic oxidative capacity; overfeeding of calories and/or fat	Moderate elevation shown in liver function tests	Reduce the amount of carbohydrate administration; cycling of PN has been tried, but results are inconclusive. Rule out (R/O) other causes.	Balanced nutrient solutions containing energy from carbohydrate and fat; avoid overfeeding.	Liver function tests at least 1× weekly.
2. Cholestasis Unknown	Progressive increases in total serum bilirubin; elevated serum alkaline phosphatase	Prevent overfeeding; known to resolve at DC of PN and return to normal diet; R/O other cause.	Use the GI tract if possible.	Liver function tests at least 1× weekly.

Complication / Cause	Signs and Symptoms	Treatment	Prevention	Monitoring
F. REFEEDING SYNDROME — Initiation of PN, especially in severely malnourished patients	Acute fluxes: fluid-dependent edema, CHF, pulmonary edema; Electrolytes—decreased serum K, P, Mg, as a result of intracellular shift; water-soluble vitamin deficiency, glucose intolerance as lethargy, weakness, and confusion	Adjust electrolytes, minerals, and vitamins as needed. Administer diuretics as needed.	Careful initiation and slow advancement of PN. Careful monitoring during first 24-48 hours of PN therapy.	Serum electrolyte monitoring daily and more frequently as indicated during PN initiation.
II. TECHNICAL **A. PNEUMOTHORAX** — Venous anomalies; inexperience with catheter placement technique		A small pneumothorax may resolve untreated. A larger pneumothorax may require chest tube placement.	Experience with catheter placement is necessary; some institutions ensure this by restricting privileges for central line insertion.	Chest x-ray is performed and line placement is confirmed before line is used.
B. AIR EMBOLISM — Central line interrupted and the patient inspires air while the line is open	Dyspnea, cyanosis, chest pain, tachycardia, elevated central venous pressure, disorientation, shock, coma, cardiac arrest	High mortality rate if immediate action not taken. Place patient in reverse Trendelenburg position on left side immediately.	Proper dressing and catheter care techniques; proper training of patient and caregivers.	Observe for signs and symptoms.
C. CATHETER EMBOLIZATION — Pulling the catheter back through the needle used for insertion		Catheter snare technique or surgical removal of the catheter tip.	Remove needle and catheter at the same time.	Ensure catheter is intact when removed; if not obtain chest x-ray.
D. VENOUS THROMBOSIS — Mechanical trauma to vein; hypotension; infection; solution osmolality or precipitates		Urokinase, streptokinase, catheter change.	Proper selection of catheter material; addition of heparin to PN.	Observe corresponding arm for swelling.
E. CATHETER OCCLUSION — Hypotension; failure to flush catheter with heparin; fibrin sheath formation		Urokinase, streptokinase, catheter change	Proper catheter care.	Observe for inability to infuse.
III. SEPTIC **A. CATHETER-RELATED SEPSIS** — Improper technique in catheter insertion; infusion of contaminated solution; multiple-line violation and manipulation; skin colonization adjacent to catheter site; hematogenous seeding of the catheter by bloodborne organisms from other distant infections	Unexplained fever, chills, red, indurated area, or purulent discharge around the catheter site; a positive catheter tip culture and a positive blood culture to confirm infection	Removal of catheter and replacement at another site and concurrent antibiotic therapy.	Strict adherence to aseptic technique during line insertion, line manipulation, and catheter care.	Monitor for signs and symptoms. Assess for glucose intolerance as possible early warning sign of impending sepsis.

The authors wish to thank Ms. Karen Carrasco, RN, for her assistance in the preparation of this table.

Table 12-9   **Indications for Pediatric Total Parenteral Nutrition**

Disorder	Features
Short bowel syndrome	Necrotizing enterocolitis, intestinal atresias, midgut volvulus, complicated meconium ileus
Abdominal wall defects	Gastroschisis, omphalocele, cloacal exstrophy
Inflammatory bowel diseases	Ulcerative colitis, Crohn's disease
Other	Tracheoesophageal fistula, malignancy, trauma, burns, sepsis, hepatic or renal disease, cardiac cachexia, chylothorax

Table 12-10   **Nutrient Requirements**

Category	Age or Weight	Amount Per 24 Hours
Fluid	0-10 kg	100 ml/kg
	11-20 kg	1000 + 50 ml/kg over 10 kg
	>20 kg	1500 + 20 ml/kg over 20 kg
Calories	Infants (0-1)	90-120 kcal/kg
	Children (1-7)	75-90 kcal/kg
	Children (7-12)	60-75 kcal/kg
	Adolescents (12-18)	30-60 kcal/kg
Fats	Infants	0.5-3.0 g/kg
	Children	0.5-3.0 g/kg
Protein	Infants	2.5-3.0 g/kg
	Children	2.0-3.0 g/kg

Adapted from Taylor L, O'Neill JA: Total parenteral nutrition in the pediatric patient, *Surg Clin North Am* 71:477, 1991; and Warner B: Parenteral nutrition in the pediatric patient. In Fischer J, editor: *Total parenteral nutrition,* ed 2, Boston, 1991, Little, Brown.

weight and surface area, environmental conditions, temperature, and abnormal losses.

Energy requirements can be estimated by referring to the Harris-Benedict Equation (see Table 12-6) and applying the following formula[75]:

$$BEE\ (infants) = 22.10 + 31.05W\ (in\ kg) + 1.16H\ (in\ cm)$$

Energy requirements may also be estimated using standard tables based on body weight and age. Current recommendations for the caloric components in pediatric nutritional supplementation are that carbohydrates make up 50% of total calories, protein 15%, and fat 35%.[73] Peripheral parenteral nutrition uses 10% to 12.5% glucose and 2.5% protein. Central parenteral nutrition may use up to 30% glucose and 3.5% protein.[63]

Fats are necessary to prevent essential fatty acid deficiency (EFAD). Children require approximately 1% to 2% essential fatty acids in their diet. EFAD develops more rapidly in children than in adults, in as little as 1 week using fat-free solutions. The use of lipids may be harmful in the infant with jaundice. Fatty acids displace bilirubin from albumin and produce unbound bilirubin, which increases the risk of kernicterus.[54] To prevent ketonemia, no more than 60% of nonprotein calories should be

Table 12-11   **Nutritional Requirements for the Pediatric Patient**

Requirements	Term Infants and Children (dose/day)
VITAMINS; LIPID SOLUBLE	
A (mg)	700
E (mg)	7
K (mg)	200
D (IU)	400
WATER SOLUBLE	
Ascorbic acid (mg)	80
Thiamin (mg)	1.2
Riboflavin (mg)	1.4
Pyridoxine (mg)	1.0
Niacin (mg)	17
Pantothenate (mg)	5
Biotin (mg)	20
Folate (mg)	140
Vitamin B_{12}	1.0
ELECTROLYTES AND MINERALS	
Sodium	2-4 mEq/kg
Potassium	2-3 mEq/kg
Chloride	2-3 mEq/kg
Magnesium	0.25-0.50 mEq/kg
Calcium gluconate	100-500 mg/kg
Phosphorus	1-2 mmol/kg

Adapted from Warner B: Parenteral nutrition in the pediatric patient. In Fischer J, editor: *Total parenteral nutrition,* ed 2, Boston, 1991, Little, Brown.

from fats. A positive nitrogen balance usually requires 200 kcal/g nitrogen in children. Carbohydrates must be infused simultaneously with the amino acids to maximize utilization and prevent azotemia.

Vitamins are essential in the pediatric formula. Separate recommendations for adult and pediatric formulations were accepted in 1981 and revised in 1988 by the AMA's Nutrition Advisory Group and the American Society of Clinical Nutrition.[61,76] Requirements for electrolytes and minerals depend on such factors as diuretic administration, electrolyte losses, hydration, and renal function. As stated earlier, a greater need for these minerals exists in early infancy. Trace elements are considered essential only if parenteral nutrition continues for more than 4 weeks. The exception to this is zinc, whose requirements are determined by infant growth rates. The addition of zinc may be necessary after only 1 to 2 weeks on parenteral nutrition.

Formulations

Standard pediatric formulations contain mixtures of essential and nonessential amino acids. Amino acids such as histidine, tyrosine, cysteine, and taurine, which are nonessential in adults, may be essential for infants and young children. Special amino acid formulations are available to meet these needs.

EFAD can be prevented with 0.5 mg/kg/day of IV lipid administration. IV lipids can be advanced to 3.0 g/kg/day with careful monitoring of serum triglyceride levels to ensure serum clearance.[63] Fats should be administered continuously in infants over a 24-hour period to prevent wide fluctuations in plasma lipid fractions.

The American Society of Clinical Nutrition has developed recommendations for parenteral multivitamins in children.[76]

Administration

Vascular access. The basic principles of vascular access and catheter care for adults also apply to pediatric patients. A major responsibility is maintaining asepsis and preventing technical problems with the catheter, which is the most common complication requiring interruption of therapy in children.[54]

Monitoring. Data collection during the initiation of parenteral nutrition include daily weights, strict measurement of intake and output, and daily electrolytes until stabilized (then weekly). In addition to urine glucose measurements, serum glucose measurements may be done every 8 to 12 hours initially. Serum triglyceride and free fatty acid levels are measured weekly. Liver function tests are performed biweekly. Growth determinations include routine measurements of weight, height, head circumference, and anthropometric measurements for the duration of therapy. Many children require long-term support at home. Parents accept responsibility for routine catheter care and infusion procedures. Infusions are usually cycled over 10 to 12 hours at night to permit normal activities during the day. Technologic advancements have enabled some patients to receive home therapy for more than 7 years.[73]

Metabolic complications. As in the adult patient, metabolic complications in the pediatric patient are generally related either to disorders of glucose metabolism or to deficiencies or toxicities of specific components in the solution. Hepatobiliary dysfunction is one of the more common complications, second only to technical complications of the catheter. A pattern of cholestasis is seen with conjugated hyperbilirubinemia and elevation of other hepatic enzyme levels.[54] Management includes decreasing protein intake, cycling the infusion, and adding even minimal enteral feeding if possible.

HOME PARENTERAL NUTRITION

Home parenteral nutrition (HPN) therapy was first attempted in 1967 by Shils and colleagues.[77] Although the patient survived only a few months, a new conceptual advance was established, extending hospital care into the home setting. In the early 1970s, reimbursement for HPN was negotiated with third-party payers on a case-by-case basis. In 1976, Medicare approved reimbursement for HPN under the Part B prosthetic device benefit. Consequently, most private insurers and state Medicaid programs followed suit, recognizing the quality of rehabilitation achieved by HPN patients and the cost reduction of parenteral nutrition administration in the home versus in the hospital setting. Since the transition of parenteral nutrition to the home setting, many technologic advances in nutrition support and delivery systems have occurred.

Candidate identification

Four major factors in successful HPN have been identified.[78] The first factor is patient acceptance of this therapy in the home environment. Without the desire and dedication to make the necessary changes in lifestyle required by HPN, patient compliance and the therapy outcome will suffer. Adaptation to HPN may initially involve depression, alteration in body image, anxiety, and fear. Long-term psychosocial adaptation has been enhanced through close coordination by the health care team and the inclusion of psychologic counseling, when indicated.[79] Patients with chronic illness have shown greater adaptation to HPN than those who had been well and suffered an acute episode requiring this therapy.[65]

Second, the financial impact must be considered. Although less expensive than hospitalization, the cost is considerable. Coverage and limitations of the patient's insurance should be thoroughly understood. Guidelines vary among regional providers and are changing with the current concerns over health care costs and reforms. Declaration of disability or application for medical assistance may be necessary. Case management strategies may be implemented to help the patient and family meet the financial burden.

Third, the patient and/or caregiver must have adequate intelligence to understand and be willing to participate in the program at home. They must possess adequate eyesight and dexterity to manipulate the equipment and maintain catheter care.

Fourth, there must be adequate long-term IV access for infusion of the solution. Peripheral venous access is not suitable for HPN.

In addition, the home environment should be assessed for safety and suitability. Table 12-12 is an example of a home safety assessment tool.

Indications

HPN may be required for as little as 1 month or for a lifetime. The purpose may be temporary nutrition support during bowel rest, lifelong supplementation to maintain life, or supplementation to improve quality of life for certain incurable diseases.[79] Disease states in which HPN may be indicated include the following:

- Short bowel syndrome
- Functional, mechanical, or pseudo-obstruction
- Fistulas
- Chronic radiation enteritis
- Inflammatory bowel disease
- Congenital bowel defects
- Carefully selected malignancy patients
- Disorders of malabsorption, including sprue, pancreatitis, and cystic fibrosis
- Acquired immunodeficiency syndrome
- Dysmotility disorders

Administration considerations

Infusion devices used for HPN range from the larger devices commonly seen in the hospital setting to small, compact, battery-operated devices suitable for the totally ambulatory patient. Devices for the home patient should be user-friendly and should have various safety features, including sophisticated alarm systems, variable pressure settings, and tapering features

Table 12-12   Assessment of Home Environment for Home Nutrition Therapy

Patient name:	Therapy:	Date:
DISCUSSION	**REVIEWED**	**ACTION/COMMENTS**
SUPPLIES/STORAGE		
Stored appropriately		
Out of reach of children/pets		
Refrigerator clean, with adequate space for separation of solutions and medications from food		
ENVIRONMENT		
Removable hazards—throw rugs, furniture, obstructions, etc.		
Stairs—check lighting, handrail, difficulty in negotiating with equipment or physical limitation		
Electrical outlet—availability, convenience, adequacy		
Easy access to bathroom		
FIRE HAZARDS		
Smoker in house—caution on oxygen use and smoking in bed		
Discussion of smoke detectors		
Discussion of exit plan		
Caution to turn off oxygen if fire occurs		
MISCELLANEOUS		
Telephone availability		
Written instructions left in home		
Discussion of nearest emergency facility		
Discussion of telephone numbers		
Emergency numbers (physician, clinic, ambulance, etc.)		
On-call provider numbers		
Fire department number		
Police department number		
Patient demonstrates ability to use thermometer		
Disposal/spills		
Chemical and controlled substances into large biohazard containers		
Review of chemical spill kit		
Needles/syringes in sharps container		
All used tubing, bags, etc. bagged before placing in regular trash		
Any medication/blood spill cleaned using gloves and 1:10 bleach/water solution		
If spill occurs, clean with gloves on, using paper towels, etc. and double-bag technique		
Clothes or linens stained from spill—wash separately, use regular detergent with hot water and hot dryer		

Patient or caregiver:

Nurse clinician: Date:

From Furloines-Lynn S, Viall C: Home care. In Hennessy KA, Orr ME, editors: *Nutrition support nursing*, ed 3, Silver Spring, Md, 1996, Aspen.

that allow programmed rate changes during the infusion. Tapering programmability allows patients receiving cyclic therapy to taper infusion rates automatically within a given time and volume at the beginning and end of their daily infusion. Tapering at the beginning and end of infusions allows for gradual increase and decrease in insulin production to prevent hyperglycemia and hypoglycemia.

HPN solutions are highly individualized. Fats may be included daily or intermittently, as needed, and are usually admixed with the daily solution as a TNA. The solutions have a stability that usually allows a week's supply to be delivered and stored in the home refrigerator. Parenteral nutrition solutions that do not contain lipids may have a longer shelf life. Dual-chamber parenteral nutrition bags that keep lipids separated from the rest of the solution by means of a removable divider also increase shelf life and may make the solution viable for up to 2 weeks (see Fig. 12-2). Parenteral nutrition solutions should be taken out of refrigeration and left at room temperature approximately 1 hour before infusion to decrease hypothermic infusion effects. Multivitamins and any medications are added just before infusion and must be infused within 24 hours.

Continuous infusions are the least desirable in the home care setting but may be required because of caloric need, glucose fluctuations, or fluid intolerance. Cyclic infusions given over a portion of a 24-hour period allow the patient free time away from the therapy and foster return to normal life patterns.

Patient and family education

The most critical factor in the success of HPN may be the adequate preparation of the patient and caregiver by the clinician. Teaching is initiated using an individualized plan before discharge from the hospital and is a collaborative effort among all members of the health care team, including staff from the home care agency. Teaching methods may involve audiovisuals, mannequins, and written procedures. The patient and/or caregiver should be able to verbalize and/or demonstrate the care of a central line, simple IV troubleshooting, infection control practices (handwashing, sterile technique), and emergent procedures. In the first phase of education, the patient and caregiver observe the procedure being performed by the nurse. In the second phase, the patient or caregiver performs the procedure under nursing supervision. The goal is for the learner to demonstrate proficiency in each phase of the procedure. Each training session should be adequately documented. Table 12-13 is an example of a skills checklist for HPN.

Patient monitoring

Home care monitoring begins on the day of discharge from the hospital. The home care nurse should be in attendance for starting the infusion, assessing the home environment, evaluating the storage and work areas, and assessing the patient's and caregiver's response to discharge. Reiteration of the procedures is often necessary during the first week at home and may require frequent visits by the home care staff. Clinical self-monitoring is documented in a diary, including weight, temperature, urine or glucometer testing for glucose levels, and changes in urinary

volume. Laboratory monitoring of various blood levels is performed once or twice weekly at first, then less frequently as the patient becomes stable. Twenty-four-hour availability of the home care agency is required to handle unexpected problems. Periodic visits may be scheduled for continued monitoring, including the effectiveness of therapy, complications, laboratory analysis, adequate safety precautions, and coping skills.

Complications

No matter which type of system is used, the complications of long-term venous access remain the same. The major complication continues to be catheter-related sepsis. The best treatment is prevention through adequate teaching, reinforcement of technique, and prompt recognition of problems. Although some catheter infections can be treated successfully with antibiotics, catheter sepsis remains the main reason for catheter removal or hospitalization.[79] Catheter occlusion may occur because of improper flushing, resulting in blood clots in the catheter lumen. Thrombolytic agents have been successful in restoring patency to this type of occluded catheter. Catheter occlusion may also occur as a result of medication precipitates, calcium phosphate crystal precipitate, or lipid residue. Medication precipitates with a low pH can be cleared with hydrochloric (HCl) acid (0.1 N). High pH drug precipitates can be cleared using sodium bicarbonate. Ethanol 70% or sodium hydroxide (0.1 N) can be used to clear lipid residue.[80,81] Depending on the location of damage, broken catheters can sometimes be repaired.

The use of long-term TPN at home has been observed to produce biochemical and morphologic evidence of hepatic insult. Elevations in liver function tests and occasionally bilirubin occur. The changes are typically transient and are decreased by a mixed-fuel solution and cyclic TPN administration. Progressive liver failure is rare.

Metabolic complications include disorders of glucose metabolism, as in hospitalized patients. Complications unique to long-term HPN patients include vitamin, trace element, and essential fatty acid deficiencies. These can be avoided by laboratory testing and adequate supplementation in the TPN solution. Metabolic bone disease has been reported in long-term HPN patients and is characterized by increased serum calcium levels, excessive losses of calcium and phosphorus in the urine, low plasma levels of vitamin D, and low-normal plasma levels of parathyroid hormone. The disease results in osteopenia, mild to moderate bone pain, and fractures. The cause is unclear and likely has several contributing factors. Some factors that have been implicated are excess infusions of aluminum (thought to be a contaminant of parenteral nutrition solutions), calcium, protein, or glucose; cyclic versus continuous TPN administration; and the patient's previous nutritional state.[79,82,83] The treatment of metabolic bone disease is unclear. Some have reported a reversal of bone disease with the cessation of TPN or withdrawal of vitamin D supplementation. Further research continues in this area.

Generally, HPN has been found a safe and efficient method for the continuation of parenteral nutrition outside the hospital setting. Life itself can be prolonged while allowing the patient to return to the home environment.

Table 12-13   **Skills Checklist for Home Nutrition Therapy**

DEMONSTRATION/DISCUSSION	RETURN DEMONSTRATION	INDEPENDENT WITH SUPERVISION
PURPOSE OF THERAPY		
Patient verbalizes understanding		
INFECTION CONTROL		
Handwashing		
Preparing work surface		
Clean versus sterile		
CATHETER CARE		
Flushing		
Dressing change		
Clamp		
SOLUTIONS		
Storage		
Label/expiration date		
Inspection/appearance		
Preparation—additives		
ADMINISTRATION		
Method (pump)		
Filter		
Sequence		
WASTE MANAGEMENT		
Sharps container		
Hazardous materials chemotherapy		
Double bag		
SELF-MONITORING		
Temperature/weight		
Intake/output		
Other		
COMPLICATIONS		
Use of on-call system		
When to call physician		
GRIEVANCES		
Contact quality assurance		

Patient signature:

Instructing registered nurse:

Caregiver signature:

From Furloines-Lynn S, Viall C: Home care. In Hennessy KA, Orr ME, editors: *Nutrition support nursing*, ed 3, Silver Spring, Md, 1996, Aspen.

ETHICAL CONSIDERATIONS

TPN has been termed a marvel of modern medicine providing the medical community with the ability to support and sustain life, sometimes for long periods. As with other life-sustaining therapies, decisions to provide, withhold, or withdraw nutritional support can also provide dilemmas. The dilemma of withholding versus withdrawing therapy has been a topic of much debate and many publications. The distinction between withholding and withdrawing may lead to undertreatment if treatment is withheld to avoid having to withdraw it later. Withholding denies patients a therapeutic trial. Patients may also be overtreated because physicians believe that they cannot withdraw treatment that has been started.[84] However, there is no ethical requirement that a treatment must be continued once started, especially if the treatment is against the patient's wishes. It is admittedly more difficult to withdraw a treatment once started, especially if that action results in the patient's death. Establishing goals at the beginning of therapy and repeatedly evaluating the goals and outcomes throughout the course of therapy has been proposed as a means of guiding decision makers.[85]

Questions about ethics continue to loom large in the health care arena, as the paradigm of physician-driven health care shifts to health care team- and patient-driven care.[84] Since December of 1991, health care institutions that participate in Medicare and Medicaid have been required to provide patients with educational materials about the patient's right to terminate treatment. Today, patients are encouraged to choose a "health care proxy" or "health care agent" to act in their stead regarding health care should they become incapable of making their own decisions. Advance directives help guide the health care team and health care proxy or surrogate in determining the patient's wishes, goals, and values in the decision-making process. Because of the emotional nature of these decisions, many institutions have created ethics committees, multidisciplinary teams that consult with and assist the health care team.

The most widely accepted principles of medical ethics can be applied to these difficult situations:

- *Beneficence:* acting to benefit the patient
- *Nonmaleficence:* to do no harm
- *Autonomy:* respecting the privacy of the patient's or surrogate's rights
- *Disclosure:* providing adequate, intelligible, and truthful information for making medical decisions
- *Social justice:* allocating medical resources justly and equitably according to medical need, exercising reasonable economic stewardship, and with social sensitivity.[85]

As with all ongoing debates regarding end-of-life issues, the ideal scenario is that decisions be made by the patient or proxy and health care team, with the assistance of the ethics committee. With nutritional support experts armed with research demonstrating clear clinical efficacy, knowledgeable patients and surrogates, a health care team comfortable with their own end-of-life issues, and a supportive ethics committee all working in unison, decisions can be made in a respectful, peaceful, and dignified atmosphere.

REFERENCES

1. Intravenous Nurses Society: Infusion nursing standards of practice, *JIN* (suppl) 23(6S), 2000.
2. Elman R, Weiner DO: Intravenous alimentation with special reference to protein (amino acid) metabolism, *JAMA* 122:796, 1939.
3. Dudrick SJ, Wilmore DW, Vars HM, Rhoads JE: Long-term total parenteral nutrition with growth, development, and positive nitrogen balance, *Surgery* 64:134, 1968.
4. Wilmore DW, Dudrick SJ: Growth and development of an infant receiving all nutrients exclusively by vein, *JAMA* 203:860, 1968.
5. Paskin DL: Fluid, electrolyte, and acid-base balance. In Skipper A, editor: *Dietitian's handbook of enteral and parenteral nutrition,* ed 2, Gaithersburg, Md, 1998, Aspen.
6. Grant JP: *Handbook of parenteral nutrition,* ed 2, Philadelphia, 1992, WB Saunders.
7. Krzywda EA: Substrate metabolism-carbohydrate, lipid, and protein. In Hennessy KA, Orr ME, editors: *Nutrition support nursing,* ed 3, Silver Spring, Md, 1996, ASPEN.
8. Grant J, Kennedy-Caldwell C, editors. *Nutritional support in nursing,* Orlando, 1988, Grune & Stratton.
9. Sax H: Complications of total parenteral nutrition and their prevention. In Rombeau JL, Caldwell MD, editors: *Clinical nutrition, vol II, total parenteral nutrition,* Philadelphia, 1993, WB Saunders.
10. Howell WH: Macronutrient requirements. In Skipper A, editor: *Dietitian's handbook of enteral and parenteral nutrition,* ed 2, Gaithersburg, Md, 1998, Aspen.
11. Sitren SS: Vitamin E. In Baumgartner TG, editor: *Clinical guide to parenteral micronutrition,* ed 3, Melrose Park, Ill, 1997, Fujisawa USA.
12. Gottschlich MM, Mayes T: Micronutrients. In Skipper A, editor: *Dietitian's handbook of enteral and parenteral nutrition,* ed 2, Gaithersburg, Md, 1998, Aspen.
13. Andris DA: Substrate metabolism—micronutrients. In Hennessy KA, Orr ME, editors: *Nutrition support nursing,* ed 3, Silver Spring, Md, 1996, ASPEN.
14. Misra S, Kirby DF: Micronutrient and trace element monitoring in adult nutrition support. *Nutr Clin Pract* 15:120, 2000.
15. Leupold-DeCicco C, Monturo CA: Stress states: trauma, burns and sepsis. In Hennessy KA, Orr ME, editors: *Nutrition support nursing,* ed 3, Silver Spring, Md, 1996, ASPEN.
16. Curtas S: Nutrition assessment of the adult. In Hennessy KA, Orr ME, editors: *Nutrition support nursing,* ed 3, Silver Spring, Md, 1996, ASPEN.
17. Morrison G, Hark L: *Medical nutrition and disease,* Malden, Mass, 1996, Blackwell Science.
18. Studley HO: Relationship between nutrition status, infection and poor wound healing, *JAMA* 106:458, 1936.
19. Wilson JM: Nutritional assessment and its application, *JIN* 19:307, 1996.
20. Dragonescu JM, Lipshutz WH: Esophagus, stomach, and intestines. In Skipper A, editor: *Dietitian's handbook of enteral and parenteral nutrition,* ed 2, Gaithersburg, Md, 1998, Aspen.
21. Hannuer SB: Therapy for inflammatory bowel disease. In Wolfe MM, editor: *Therapy of digestive disorders,* Philadelphia, 2000, WB Saunders.
22. Englert DM, Lyon HD: Gastrointestinal disorders. In Hennessy KA, Orr ME, editors: *Nutrition support nursing,* ed 3, Silver Spring, Md, 1996, ASPEN.
23. Hiyama DT, Rolandelli MD: Short bowel syndrome. In Rombeau JL, Caldwell MD, editors: *Clinical nutrition, vol II, total parenteral nutrition,* Philadelphia, 1993, WB Saunders.
24. Byrne TA, et al: A new treatment for patients with short bowel syndrome—growth hormone, glutamine, and a modified diet, *Ann Surg* 222:243, 1995.
25. Wilmore DW, Byrne TA, Persinger RL: Short bowel syndrome: new therapeutic approaches. *Curr Probl Surg* 4:389, 1997.
26. Furman JA: Pancreatic function. In Skipper A, editor: *Dietitian's handbook of enteral and parenteral nutrition,* ed 2, Gaithersburg, Md, 1998, Aspen.
27. Steinberg WM: Management of Acute pancreatitis. In Wolfe MM, editor: *Therapy of digestive disorders.* Philadelphia, 2000, WB Saunders.
28. McCullough AJ: Nutritional therapy in liver disease. In Wolfe MM, editor: *Therapy of digestive disorders,* Philadelphia, 2000, WB Saunders.
29. McCutcheon KL, Harple KA: Nutritional alterations in hepatic and pancreatic disease. In Hennessy KA, Orr ME, editors: *Nutrition support nursing,* ed 3, Silver Spring, Md, 1996, ASPEN.
30. Liftman C: Renal function. In Skipper A, editor: *Dietitian's handbook of enteral and parenteral nutrition,* ed 2, Gaithersburg, Md, 1998, Aspen.
31. Schwartz DB: Respiratory disease and mechanical ventilation. In Skipper A, editor: *Dietitian's handbook of enteral and parenteral nutrition,* ed 2, Gaithersburg, Md, 1998, Aspen.
32. Lipman T: Clinical trials of nutritional support in cancer, *Hematol Oncol Clin North Am* 5:91, 1991.

33. Centers for Disease Control and Prevention: Revision of the CDC Surveillance case definition for acquired immunodeficiency syndrome, *MMWR* 36(15):5s, 1987.

34. Guenter P: HIV/AIDS. In Hennessy KA, Orr ME, editors: *Nutrition support nursing*, ed 3, Silver Spring, Md, 1996, ASPEN.

35. Holt DR, Barbul A: Parenteral nutrition and acquired immunodeficiency syndrome. In Rombeau JL, Caldwell MD, editors: *Clinical nutrition, vol II, total parenteral nutrition*, Philadelphia, 1993, WB Saunders.

36. Hecker LM, Kotler DP: Malnutrition in patients with AIDS, *Nutr Rev* 11:393, 1990.

37. Kotler DP, et al: Effect of home parenteral nutrition on body composition in patients with acquired immunodeficiency syndrome, *JPEN* 14:454, 1990.

38. Mulligan K, et al. Anabolic effects of recombinant growth hormone in patients with weight loss associated with HIV infection, *J Clin Endocrinol Metab* 77:956, 1993.

39. Leupold C: Nutritional alterations in illness: critical care-stress, trauma, burns, and sepsis. In Kennedy-Caldwell C, Guenter P, editors: *Nutritional support in nursing*, ed 2, Baltimore, 1988, ASPEN.

40. Charney PJ: Nutritional screening and assessment. In Skipper A, editor: *Dietitian's handbook of enteral and parenteral nutrition*, Gaithersburg, Md, 1998, Aspen.

41. Jacobs DO: Bioelectrical impedance analysis in nutrition and metabolism, *Nutr Clin Pract* 12:204, 1997.

42. ASPEN: Guidelines for the use of parenteral and enteral nutrition in adult and pediatric patients, *JPEN* (suppl) 17:1SA, 1993.

43. Ireton-Jones CS: Indirect calorimetry. In Skipper A, editor: *Dietitian's handbook of enteral and parenteral nutrition*, Gaithersburg, Md, 1998, Aspen.

44. Kennedy-Caldwell C, Guenter P: Nutrition support nursing: core curriculum, ed 3, Baltimore, 1996, ASPEN.

45. Barbul A. Measurements of relevant nutrition data for determining efficacy of nutritional support. In Fischer JE, editor: *Total parenteral nutrition*, ed 2, Boston, 1991, Little, Brown.

46. ASPEN: Standards for nutrition support, *Nutr Clin Pract* 10:208, 1995.

47. O'Dwyer ST, Smith RJ, Hwang TL, Wilmore DW: Maintenance of small bowel mucosa with glutamine-enriched parenteral nutrition, *JPEN* 13:579, 1989.

48. Hwang TL, O'Dwyer ST, Smith RJ, Wilmore DW: Preservation of the small bowel mucosa using glutamine-enriched parenteral nutrition, *Surg Forum* 37:56, 1986.

49. Bernard MA, Jacobs DO, Robeau JL: *Nutritional and metabolic support of hospitalized patients*, Philadelphia, 1986, WB Saunders.

50. Ebbert-Sauer ML: Adult parenteral nutrition. In Koda-Kimble, Young LY, editors: *Applied therapeutics: the clinical use of drugs*, ed 6, Vancouver, Wash, 1995, Applied Therapeutics.

51. Sax HC, Hasselgren PO: Indications. In Fischer JE, editor: *Total parenteral nutrition*, ed 2, Boston, 1991, Little, Brown.

52. Fleming RC, Nelson J: Nutritional options. In Kinney JM, Jeejeebhoy KN, Hill GL, Owen OE, editors: *Nutrition and metabolism in patient care*, Philadelphia, 1985, WB Saunders.

53. Cochran EB, Phelps SJ, Helms RA: Parenteral nutrition in pediatric patients, *Clin Pharm* 7:351, 1988.

54. Warner B: Parenteral nutrition in the pediatric patient. In Fischer JE, editor: *Total parenteral nutrition*, ed 2, Boston, 1991, Little, Brown.

55. Hoagland R, Stewart B, Storm H: Neonates. In Hennessy KA, Orr ME, editors: *Nutrition support nursing*, Silver Spring, Md, ed 3, 1996, ASPEN.

56. Hutchins AM, Shronts EP: Metabolic stress and immune function. In Skipper A, editor: *Dietitian's handbook of enteral and parenteral nutrition*, Gaithersburg, Md, 1998, Aspen.

57. Holcombe BJ: Adult parenteral nutrition. In Young LY, Koda-Kimble MA, editors: *Applied therapeutics: the clinical use of drugs*, ed 6, Vancouver, Wash, 1995, Applied Therapeutics.

58. Dickerson RN, Brown RO, White KG: Parenteral nutrition solutions. In Rombeau JL, Caldwell MD, editors: *Clinical nutrition: parenteral nutrition*, ed 2, Philadelphia, 1993, WB Saunders.

59. Okada A, Imura K: Parenteral nutrition in neonates. In Rombeau JL, Caldwell MD, editors: *Clinical nutrition: parenteral nutrition*, ed 2, Philadelphia, 1993, WB Saunders.

60. Hill ID, Madrozo de la Garza JA, Lebenthal E: Parenteral nutrition in pediatric patients. In Rombeau JL, Caldwell MD, editors: *Clinical nutrition: parenteral nutrition*, ed 2, Philadelphia, 1993, WB Saunders.

61. AMA Department of Food and Nutrition: Multivitamin preparations for parenteral use: a statement by the Nutrition Advisory Group, *JPEN* 3:258, 1979.

62. AMA Department of Food and Nutrition: Guidelines for essential trace element preparations for parenteral use: a statement by an expert panel, *JAMA* 241:2051, 1979.

63. Hennies GA, et al: Pediatrics. In Hennessy KA, Orr ME, editors: *Nutrition support nursing*, ed 3, 1996, ASPEN.

64. Lenssen P: Management of total parenteral nutrition. In Skipper A, editor: *Dietitian's handbook of enteral and parenteral nutrition*, ed 2, Gaithersburg, Md, 1998, Aspen.

65. Howard L, et al: Home parenteral nutrition in adults. In Rombeau JL, Caldwell MD, editors: *Clinical nutrition, vol II, total parenteral nutrition*, Philadelphia, 1993, WB Saunders.

66. Driscoll DF: Clinical issues regarding the use of total nutrient admixtures, *DICP* 24:296, 1990.

67. Warshawsky KY: Intravenous fat emulsions, *Nutr Clin Pract* 7:187, 1992.

68. Sculer CL, Wolfson M: Nutrition in acute renal failure. In Rombeau JL, Caldwell MD, editors: *Clinical nutrition: parenteral nutrition*, ed 2, Philadelphia, 1993, WB Saunders.

69. O'Keefe SJD: Parenteral nutrition and liver disease. In Rombeau JL, Caldwell MD, editors: *Clinical nutrition, vol II, total parenteral nutrition*, Philadelphia, 1993, WB Saunders.

70. Wilmore DW, Van Woert JH: Enteral and parenteral nutrition in hospital patients. In Rubenstein E, Federman DD, editors: *Scientific American medicine*, vol 4, New York, 1992, Scientific American.

71. Zibrida J, Carlson S: Nutrition support dietetics, *ASPEN Core Curriculum* 1993, 461-469.

72. Worthington PH, Wagner BA: Total parenteral nutrition, *Nurs Clin North Am* 24:355, 1989.

73. Taylor L, O'Neill JA: Total parenteral nutrition in the pediatric patient, *Surg Clin North Am* 71:477, 1991.

74. Testerman EJ: Current trends in pediatric total parenteral nutrition, *JIN* 12:152, 1989.

75. Pfeifer JA: Pediatric clinical nutrition. In Kennedy-Caldwell C, Guenter P, editors: *Nutrition support nursing*, ed 2, Baltimore, 1988, ASPEN.

76. Greene HL, et al. Guidelines for the use of vitamins, trace elements, calcium, manganese, and phosphorus in infants and children receiving total parenteral nutrition. Report of the Subcommittee on Pediatric Parenteral Nutrient Requirements from the Committee on Clinical Practice Issues of the American Society for Clinical Nutrition, *Am J Clin Nutr* 48:1324, 1988.

77. Shils ME, et al. Long term parenteral nutrition through external arteriovenous shunt, *N Engl J Med* 283:341, 1970.

78. Lin EM: Nutrition support: making the difficult decisions, *Cancer Nurs* 14:261, 1991.

79. Bower RH: Home parenteral nutrition. In Fischer J, editor: *Total parenteral nutrition*, ed 2, Boston, 1991, Little, Brown.

80. Breaux CW, et al. Calcium phosphate crystal occlusion of central venous catheters used for total parenteral nutrition in infants and children: prevention and treatment, *J Pediatr Surg* 22:829, 1987.

81. Intravenous Nurses Society: *Policies and procedures for infusion nursing*, 2000.

82. McCullough ML, Hsu N: Metabolic bone disease in home total parenteral nutrition, *J Am Diet Assoc* 87(7):915, 1987.

83. Seidner DL, Licata A: Parenteral nutrition-associated metabolic bone disease: pathophysiology, evaluation, and treatment, *Nutr Clin Pract* 15:163, 2000.

84. Burck R: Feeding, withdrawing, and withholding: ethical perspectives, *Nutr Clin Pract* 11:243, 1996.

85. Capron AM: The implications of the Cruzan decision for clinical nutrition teams, *Nutr Clin Pract* 6:89, 1991.

86. Young EA, Perkins HS, McCamish MA: Ethical dimensions and clinical decisions for parenteral nutrition: in dying as in living. In Rombeau JL, Caldwell MD, editors: *Clinical nutrition, vol II, total parenteral nutrition,* Philadelphia, 1993, WB Saunders.

Chapter 13

Oncologic Therapy

Katherine V. Vandegrift, CRNI, OCN*

Cancer is a chronic condition that consists of a large group of diseases characterized by uncontrolled growth and spread of abnormal cells. It remains the second leading cause of death in the United States, claiming more than 500,000 lives each year and affecting thousands more. Whereas 20 years ago most cancers were incurable, today about 50% of all cancer patients will survive. The key is early detection and treatment that focuses on cure and complete remission, when possible. Disease control and symptom management are the therapeutic goals when cure is not feasible. Treatment modalities include surgery, radiation therapy, chemotherapy, and more recently, immunotherapy, biologic therapy, hyperthermia, and genetic markers.[1-3]

The practice of oncology nursing is a specialty in itself, just as is intravenous (IV) therapy. This chapter focuses on a general overview of current commonly used antineoplastics, management of symptoms from side effects, and related patient education for the nurse administering IV chemotherapy. Because dosages and drug protocols change often and vary regionally, dosages are not presented here.

PATIENT ASSESSMENT AND HISTORY

It is advantageous for the nurse to understand the different classifications of cancer, presenting symptoms, and natural course of the disease. In addition to the usual medical history, the nurse needs to be particularly alert to prior organ impairment or any secondary diagnosis that might influence toxicities, side effects, and treatment modalities. This is especially true when drugs are contraindicated in the presence of specific preexisting conditions.

It is important to know whether the patient has had radiation therapy, including the dose and number of treatments. This information may provide a clue to potential complications from chemotherapy-associated recall. If the patient has had surgery, it is necessary to know whether the tumor was resected, what the size of the tumor was, whether the margins were clear, and how many (if any) nodes were positive.

Some chemotherapeutic agents have lifetime dosage limits. It is necessary to know exactly what drugs and doses the patient has received. A careful history of the toxicities the patient has experienced in the past and a summary of the management of these symptoms are helpful in determining the best approach to ensure patient comfort with subsequent treatments.

Physical findings, nutritional status, laboratory and diagnostic imaging studies, and the patient's psychosocial and spiritual state all help define the patient's needs and assist in the decision-making process to determine appropriate intervention.[1,2,4-7]

*The author and editors wish to acknowledge the contributions made by Mary Ann Doyle, as author of this chapter in the first edition of *Intravenous Nursing: Clinical Principles and Practice.*

PATIENT EDUCATION

The patient's right to information includes the option to refuse treatment and an explanation of the ramifications of this decision. The patient needs to know whether there is a realistic chance for cure or whether the focus of therapy is control or palliation. It is sometimes difficult to understand the patient who elects no treatment as an option, but health care professionals have an obligation to respect the patient's wishes. It is the responsibility of health care providers to help furnish patients with sufficient information to enable them to make informed, intelligent decisions related to their moral, religious, and ethical values.

The teaching method for the patient depends on his or her readiness to learn and learning style. Teaching should begin with initial patient contact and continue throughout the course of the disease. The nurse needs to tailor the education plan to the patient. Some patients require volumes of information, whereas others are overwhelmed with only a few facts. Learning is enhanced when all the senses are used and efforts should be made to supplement verbal information with visual aids. Charts, videos, printed material, and audio tapes are beneficial. Information relayed in the first 10 minutes is usually what is remembered. Retention drops off after that; therefore it is wise to address the most critical areas first. Retention improves with repetition. The physician is responsible for providing the patient with information so that the patient may give informed consent, but the nurse is in the unique role of reinforcing and expanding on that knowledge base. Written information should be easy to read and contain important and pertinent information. For the patient who requires more detailed information, supplemental reading can be provided. It is essential to find a balance between adequate information and overload. There is a difference between information that the patient "needs to know" and that which would be "nice to know."[1,2,4-8]

Patient education should include an explanation of the treatment goals and their rationale. The informed patient knows the names of the drugs that are administered, the long- and short-term side effects, symptom management, and lifestyle effects. Many institutions give patients written material on the medications ordered. The information should be easy to read, be in the appropriate language, describe side effects and any drug and food interactions, and provide other pertinent information. If the patient is receiving multiple medications, especially for a comorbid condition, a pharmacy consult can provide additional and useful recommendations.

Cancer patients have a need and a right to function at their maximum level and to participate in their usual activities of daily living. Therefore it is important that the patient know the treatment plan and schedule. A calendar or appointment card is helpful in ensuring that the patient understands the importance of timely treatments and coordinates these with personal agendas.

Patients and families should be encouraged to formulate realistic short- and long-term plans around the chemotherapy schedules. Patients should be encouraged to be as active as possible based on their physical capabilities. Rest periods and activities should be planned to maximize patient tolerance and enjoyment.

Because chemotherapy is a new experience for most people, many have a tendency to think that one dose can cure their cancer. Therefore they need to be psychologically prepared for a long-term commitment to treatment, and they also need to know the end point. In an adjuvant setting, the end point may be 3 months or as long as 1 year, depending on the histology and initial tumor burden. If the patient has active residual disease, the usual rule of thumb is that chemotherapy is continued for 6 to 12 months after a complete remission has been achieved. Treatment is specific to the disease, the stage of the disease, and the patient. Whatever the length of treatment, patient education improves patient compliance.

Information about the therapeutic goals and expected outcomes can be encouraging and supportive to the patient and family. A brief explanation of the action of chemotherapy fosters a better understanding of potential side effects.

The patient has a right to know the potential long- and short-term side effects and appropriate interventions. The patient needs to be able to determine whether the symptoms experienced are a result of the treatments, and thus self-limited, or whether there is a problem that requires medical intervention. For example, the asymptomatic patient should take infection precautions but should not be alarmed over an expected low white blood cell (WBC) count following chemotherapy administration. However, the patient should notify the physician if he or she develops an oral temperature of 101° F, regardless of the WBC count.

Educational information may influence the method of administration of the chemotherapy. For example, if the treatments are going to be continued for many months, the patient may consent to a central venous access device rather than have repeated venipunctures. Providing the patient with opportunities to make decisions regarding symptom management, scheduling activities, and personal agendas reestablishes control and brings independence back into the patient's life.

Patients also need to know what kind of monitoring is used to follow their progress. Periodic restaging evaluations are completed to determine tumor status and response to therapy. The patient needs to know what tests are included. The testing is specific to the patient and depends on tumor type and natural history of the disease. Restaging could include blood work for tumor markers, immune panels, chemistry, and blood counts. Other procedures such as imaging scans, barium enema, magnetic resonance imaging (MRI), computerized tomography (CT) scans, mammography, and an IV pyelogram may also be appropriate. In addition, procedures such as colonoscopy, cystoscopy, spinal tap, bone marrow aspiration, and biopsy are commonly used to monitor disease status.

The treatment modality that has the worst reputation is chemotherapy. Two out of three cancer patients are candidates for chemotherapy at some point in their disease process. Many patients have heard stories about the nightmare side effects of chemotherapy, but it is the most effective treatment currently available for nonlocalized cancer. Chemotherapy is also useful when there is concern of a recurrence from microscopic disease. It is estimated that 50% to 70% of all patients who have been newly diagnosed with cancer have micrometastasis. Only 30% to 40% of patients can achieve a complete remission with surgery alone.

There is a fine line between the dose that is therapeutic and the one that is toxic. Needless to say, chemotherapy should be given only under the supervision of a physician who has experience using antineoplastic drugs. Because of the potential life-threatening toxicities of cancer therapy, nursing staff and ancillary systems *must* be available to support and monitor the patient.

There are many misconceptions about cancer drugs. A lack of accurate information concerning chemotherapy contributes to the fear and anxiety seen in many patients and family members. A common myth is that the side effects of chemotherapy are worse than the disease itself. It is true that chemotherapy has side effects and, at times, life-threatening toxicities, but many of these problems can be prevented, managed, or controlled.

Chemotherapeutic agents can be administered by the oral, subcutaneous, IV, intraarterial, intrathecal, intraperitoneal, intrapleural, intravesicular, and even intralesional routes.[1-6,8,9] However, the primary focus in this chapter is on the IV administration of antineoplastics.

TREATMENT GOALS

The treatment goal of chemotherapy depends on the situation. Chemotherapy can be curative when given as primary treatment. For example, patients with acute lymphocytic leukemia, Hodgkin's disease, and testicular cancer have the potential for achieving a complete remission with chemotherapy.

The therapeutic goal is also curative when chemotherapy is given in an adjuvant setting for tumors such as primary breast, ovary, or colon cancer. Adjuvant therapy means treatment in addition to primary treatment, which usually consists of surgery or radiation.

The advantages of neoadjuvant chemotherapy before surgery have become evident in recent years. This therapy reduces the tumor size to provide the surgeon with a better chance of achieving complete resection and prevents the spread of dislodged cells during surgery. Micrometastasis distal to the resection site can be eradicated with chemotherapy before surgery. Neoadjuvant chemotherapy is geared toward improving the potential for a complete resection.

The choice between primary treatment and adjuvant treatment is determined by the amount of disease present. With primary treatment the tumor is macroscopic, and there is measurable disease that can be documented by physical examination, radiograph, CT scan, MRI, or blood tests. In the adjuvant setting, the patient is said to be *NED* (no evaluable disease), and treatment is given to eradicate the microscopic cells known to be present based on historic data.

Chemotherapy can also be given to control the disease when cure is not realistic but it may be possible to retard tumor growth, thereby increasing life expectancy and the quality of life. These situations include patients with advanced stages of breast or prostate cancer and multiple myeloma.

Chemotherapy given for palliation is aimed at comfort. It can decrease pain caused by a tumor by relieving pressure on nerves, decreasing lymphatic congestion, and relieving organ obstruction.

Rapidly dividing cells are the most sensitive to antineoplastic agents. Chemotherapy disrupts the reproduction of cells by altering the essential biochemical processes. Because not all cells will be killed with the first treatment, chemotherapy must be given a number of times, with each course killing a percentage of the cells. Because it affects cancer cells in various stages of the cell cycle, combination chemotherapy has proven superior to single-agent therapy; it kills more cells with each course and produces fewer side effects. There are several benefits of combination chemotherapy; it suppresses drug resistance, increases cancer cell kill, and causes less injury to normal cells.

There are few absolute rules concerning chemotherapy, but there are some basic considerations. In general, the smaller the tumor burden, the easier the tumor is to treat. Surgical debulking decreases the tumor burden and recruits resting malignant cells to start dividing, therefore increasing the sensitivity to chemotherapy. In most situations, the higher the chemotherapy dose, the better the chance for a tumor response. However, there must be a balance to prevent patient death while eradicating the tumor. Adjustments in supportive measures may need to be considered with dose escalation. Doses of chemotherapeutic agents are altered based on the degree of toxicity the patient experiences. The therapeutic margin is the difference between the dose producing the desired benefit and the dose resulting in unacceptable toxicity. The therapeutic margin of antineoplastics is rather narrow compared with other types of drugs.

The therapeutic index may be improved by several methods. The first is to increase the dose administered to the patient. If the dose-limiting factor is the severity of the toxicity, then better management of the side effects allows higher doses of chemotherapy without compromise to the patient. If the efficacy of the chemotherapeutic agents can be increased, there is a better tumor response with a lower chemotherapy dose.[1-6,8-10]

CELL CYCLE

To understand chemotherapy, it is necessary to understand the unique biochemical properties of the antineoplastic agents and their relationship to the cell cycle. Cell division is the same for cancer cells as it is for normal cells. The initial phase is the resting phase, designated as G_0. The cell performs its specific function during this part of the cycle. In other words, renal cells filter the blood and make urine and gastric cells digest food. Many enzymes are needed for DNA synthesis and are produced in this phase. G_0 is commonly referred to as the *resting phase* of the cell, but it can also be called the *postmitotic* or *presynthetic* phase.

When a cell is ready to divide, it enters into the next phase, designated as G_1. Synthesis of the proteins for RNA occurs during the G_1 phase. The duration of this phase varies greatly among the different cells, more than in any other phase. If a cell is in the G_1 phase for prolonged periods, it is sometimes referred to as G_0.

Enzymes necessary for synthesis of DNA are activated in the S phase. The length of time that the cancer cell is in this phase usually differs from that of normal cells.

The second gap phase is designated as G_2. At this time, the synthesis of DNA stops, and RNA and protein synthesis continue while the cell gets ready for mitosis.

Mitosis occurs during the final stage, the M phase, and usually lasts 30 to 90 minutes. This phase is subdivided into four steps. In *prophase,* the nuclear membrane is broken down and the chromosomes clump. In *metaphase,* the chromosomes line up in the middle of the cell. During *anaphase,* the chromosomes segregate into centrioles. In *telephase,* the final step, there is chromosome replication and cell division, which produces two daughter cells. These cells then go into the resting phase, G_0.

Several terms are connected with cellular kinetics. The *generation time* of a cell is usually measured by the time it takes the cell to replicate from midmitosis of the parent cell to midmitosis of the daughter cell. The *growth fraction* refers to the percentage of tumor cells that are actively dividing. This is measured by flow cytometry and has prognostic significance. The *doubling time* is the time it takes for the tumor to double in size. A cell divides and replicates, and with each division, the number of cells doubles, so one cell becomes two and two cells become four and so on. After 20 doublings, the tumor contains 1 million cells and is the size of a pinhead. After 30 doublings, the tumor is about 1 cm wide and contains 1 billion cells. As the tumor size increases, the doubling time decreases; this is known as the *Gompertzian growth curve.* As a tumor expands, its growth rate slows because of crowding with other structures, decreased blood supply, and decreased nutrients. The *loss fraction* is the rate at which the cells die.[1-6,10]

CHEMOTHERAPY CLASSIFICATIONS

Chemotherapeutic agents can be classified in several ways. They can be categorized according to their relationship to the cell-cycle activity, their pharmacologic or chemical structure, their potential to cause necrosis if extravasated, and their emetic potential.

The cell life cycle classification has two categories, cell-cycle–specific drugs and cell-cycle–nonspecific drugs. Antineoplastics can also be classified according to their chemical structure, such as antimetabolites, vinca or plant alkaloids, alkylating agents, antitumor antibiotics, liposomal anthracyclines, topoisomerase inhibitors, or miscellaneous agents.

Antineoplastic agents are most effective while the cell is dividing. Agents that have a specific action on a particular stage of the cell cycle are called *cell-cycle specific.* These drugs are most effective when large numbers of cells are actively dividing.

Chemotherapeutic agents that will destroy the cancer cell regardless of the activity of the cell are *cell-cycle nonspecific.* These drugs are effective against resting and dividing cells. Their cytotoxic effect takes place during the cell cycle and is expressed when the cell tries to divide or repair itself. The number of cancer cells affected is related to the amount of drug given.

There is a paradoxic relationship in the rate of cell growth and responsiveness to chemotherapy. Most neoplastic agents modify or interfere with DNA synthesis and therefore are most effective in cells that are preparing for or are in the process of cell division. The more aggressive the tumor, the greater the chance of a response to chemotherapy. Consequently, the greatest successes with chemotherapy are in hematologic malignancies that are diagnosed early. These malignancies, which have a short doubling time, include leukemia, lymphoma, Hodgkin's disease, and multiple myeloma.

Chemotherapeutic agents can also be classified by their potential to cause local tissue reactions. The potential for local toxic effects from drugs ranges from transient local discomfort during administration to severe tissue necrosis with potential damage to tendons and nerves. There is a lack of uniformity in the literature classifying drugs according to this toxic potential. Many drugs are listed as both vesicants and irritants.[1-6,8,10]

CHEMOTHERAPY DOSING

Chemotherapy doses are calculated using body surface area (BSA) to ensure that patients of various sizes and shapes receive the same amount of drug per the BSA. Clinical trials have provided a formula to determine the amount of each drug to be used in a particular regimen.

The first step in calculating the BSA is to determine the patient's height and weight. Using a nomogram, one draws a line connecting the two. The point at which the line crosses the center is the BSA. There is ongoing debate as to whether the actual body weight or the ideal body weight should be used because there is a difference in drug metabolism in the presence of fat. Most oncologists round off the BSA. A 10-lb (22-kg) change in weight changes the BSA. Therefore it is necessary to weigh the patient before each course of chemotherapy to determine whether the dose should be changed to avoid overdosing or underdosing.

The basic formula for determining the chemotherapy dose is as follows:

$$BSA \times mg/m^2 = Total\ dose$$

If doxorubicin is ordered at 50 mg/m^2, 50 $mg/m^2 \times 1.6$ BSA = 80 mg. Therefore 80 mg is the dose for that treatment. If another patient had a 1.4 m^2 BSA, the formula would not change: 50 $mg/m^2 \times 1.4$ BSA = 70 mg. Both these patients would be receiving the same dose in milligrams per square meter, but their total number of milligrams would differ.

This concept is particularly important with drugs that have an accumulated lifetime dose. Lifetime dosage is always calculated in milligrams per square meter. It is determined by adding the administered x mg/m^2 of the drug for each course of chemotherapy that the patient has received. It is necessary to know whether the BSA was determined based on ideal body weight or actual weight.[1-6,8-10]

SYMPTOM MANAGEMENT
Nausea and vomiting

Nausea and vomiting are two of the most common side effects of chemotherapy. Of the patients receiving antineoplastics, 70% to 80% experience nausea. Three distinct patterns of emesis are associated with chemotherapy administration. Acute emesis occurs in the first 24 hours and is the most severe. Delayed emesis begins 18 to 24 hours after treatment and may continue for several days. Anticipatory emesis is a conditioned response by patients who have experienced poor control of nausea and vomiting with previous courses of chemotherapy. It is important that antiemetics be administered as soon as possible before the treatment is started because just the sight of IV tubing or the nurse can precipitate nausea and vomiting. Prevention is the major goal.

Uncontrolled nausea and vomiting can lead to fluid and electrolyte imbalances, nutritional problems, and poor patient compliance and can have a great impact on the patient's quality of life. Management of nausea and vomiting has greatly improved with the introduction of the new class of selective serotonin $5HT_3$ receptor antagonists, ondansetron (Zofran), granisetron (Kytril), and dolasetron (Anzemet). These agents are highly effective in the treatment of chemotherapy-induced nausea and vomiting, with complete response rates up to 90% in the first 24 hours after treatment. The mechanism of action is the blocking activity of the serotonin receptors, which prevent serotonin from stimulating the vomiting reflex. All may be given orally or intravenously. The makers of Zofran are the first to introduce an orally disintegrating tablet that rapidly dissolves on the tongue without water. The serotonin antagonists do not cause the extrapyramidal reactions associated with metoclopramide (Reglan). The major side effects of these antiemetics are headache, diarrhea, fatigue, fever, and drowsiness. They are usually combined with a corticosteroid such as dexamethasone and have become the standard of care.

Not all chemotherapeutic agents cause nausea, and the severity of the symptoms is different for each drug. Chemotherapy can be classified by its emetogenic capacity, which can range from little or no nausea to as high as a 90% rate of vomiting. Some chemotherapeutic agents stimulate delayed nausea and vomiting, which needs to be considered in prescribing antiemetics for use after discharge.

Newer antiemetics that will have fewer side effects and even greater potential to control nausea and vomiting are being developed. It is easier to control nausea than vomiting, and it is better to have the patient sleep through chemotherapy than to be awake and nauseated. Patients often fear losing control or have an aversion to taking medications, and consequently, they delay asking for an antiemetic. The nurse has to use judgment and educate the patient who refuses to be medicated with an antiemetic.

Nausea intervention is an area in which the nurse has a fair degree of latitude and an opportunity to be creative. It is helpful to obtain a nausea history and institute any intervention that may have been helpful in the past. Patients should avoid eating or drinking 1 to 2 hours after chemotherapy treatments. Many patients find that cold food or foods served at room temperature taste better and do not have as strong an odor as hot foods. Dry toast or crackers may help settle the patient's stomach, especially first thing in the morning. Bland foods rather than spicy or strongly flavored foods are better tolerated. Clear liquids such as gelatin, juice, ginger ale or other carbonated beverages, and herbal tea provide fluids to prevent dehydration. Sport drinks also furnish limited amounts of electrolytes. Liquids should be sipped slowly. Tart foods such as sour hard candy, dill pickles, or lemons are helpful. Foods that are known to increase nausea, such as fried fatty foods or foods with a strong odor, should be avoided.

Efforts should be made to control the environment. Soft, relaxing music; low lights; and a quiet atmosphere can be helpful. Some patients respond well to diversions such as card games, movies, or crafts. Relaxation tapes, hypnosis, and biofeedback have become more popular with good results.

The patient should be instructed to eat in a relaxed environment. Strong odors of food and perfume can trigger nausea. Opening covers on the food tray before entering the room allows the steam to escape in the hall, avoiding the sudden aroma of food near the patient. Antiemetics should be administered before meals.

Other nonpharmacologic interventions include having the patient suck on ice chips or a popsicle. Rinsing the mouth often with water, mouthwash, baking soda or saline solution, or lemon- or mint-flavored water helps decrease nausea. Frequent cleansing of the teeth with a soft brush or gauze is also helpful, especially after an episode of emesis. Acupressure, acupuncture, behavior modification, biofeedback, hypnosis, massage therapy, and guided imagery have also been used.[1,2,4-6,8,10-16]

Myelosuppression

Myelosuppression is the most common dose-limiting factor in chemotherapy administration. All chemotherapeutic agents have some effect on blood counts, but certain agents or dose escalation can result in severe myelosuppression. Management of this potentially life-threatening side effect is paramount to patient care. Death in the myelosuppressed patient is usually the result of infection or bleeding. Patients need to be instructed on the importance of weekly blood counts so that appropriate intervention can be instituted as soon as possible. Patients also need to be aware that a drop in blood counts, especially WBCs, is expected and wanted. Doses of chemotherapy are escalated until myelosuppression is achieved.

Patients who are most likely to develop severe or prolonged myelosuppression are those who have bone marrow involvement, have received radiation to the flat bones, or have been heavily pretreated with chemotherapy, as well as elderly patients with aplastic marrow. These patients are particularly prone to hematologic problems. Patients who have diseased marrow with neoplastic infiltrates often experience pancytopenias until the marrow has been purged of the malignant cells.

Leukopenia and, more specifically, neutropenia predispose the patient to infection. An absolute granulocyte count (AGC) of 1500 to 2000/mm^3 puts the patient at a moderate risk for infection. Patients are sometimes placed on prophylactic antibiotics. An AGC lower than 500/mm^3 places the patient at a severe risk of infection. These patients should be started on broad-spectrum antibiotics within 12 hours of a drop in the WBC count. In the neutropenic patient, an elevated temperature may be the only sign of an infection. Antipyretics should be used with caution in these patients so as not to mask an infection. The use of vaccines should be avoided because of the increased risk of infection.

Many of the necessary precautions may seem obvious to the health care professional but may be foreign to the patient and family. Simple things like washing the hands after using the bathroom and staying away from crowds or other sources of infection can decrease the likelihood of complications. The patient should be instructed to always report fever, sore throat, and new onset of fatigue. The nurse should always be on the alert for sepsis, which in the neutropenic patient is an oncology emergency.

The use of colony-stimulating factors (CSFs) such as filgrastim (Neupogen), which acts on bone marrow to enhance granulocyte production, have had an impact on the management of leukopenia. When used, these biologic agents shorten the nadir and facilitate timely chemotherapy treatments. The nadir is the expected lowest WBC count after chemotherapy administration. The most common side effect of CSFs is a flulike syndrome, which can include muscle and joint aches and sometimes an elevated temperature. Administering the CSF just before the patient retires for the night and premedicating the patient with acetaminophen and/or diphenhydramine can help reduce these side effects. It is important to determine whether the temperature is produced by an infection or by the biologic preparation.[17,18]

Biologic response modifiers boost the function of the immune system or attack cells directly. Interleukin (IL)-2 promotes natural killer cell function, and IL-3 increases bone marrow production. Their most common toxic responses are hypotension, ascites, pulmonary edema, and weight gain. Interferons are proteins that boost the immune system. Their toxicities are dose related, with the most common side effect being flulike symptoms.[1,3,5,10,18-20]

Normally, the platelet count ranges between 150,000 and 400,000/mm^3. There is concern for the potential of bleeding when the count is below 100,000/mm^3, and necessary precautions need to be taken. Presenting signs of a potential problem include bleeding gums, petechiae, nosebleeds, and multiple bruises. Spontaneous, frank bleeding usually does not occur until the platelet count is below 20,000/mm^3. Thrombocytopenia places the patient at risk for central nervous system (CNS) and gastrointestinal (GI) bleeding. The patient is usually transfused with platelets if actively bleeding or if platelet counts are below 20,000/mm^3.

Oprelvekin (Neumega), a thrombopoietic growth factor, can be given by subcutaneous injection to prevent severe thrombocytopenia and to reduce the need for platelet transfusions. The most common side effects are edema (which can be severe), dyspnea, headache, atrial flutter or fibrillation, syncope, nausea, vomiting, and rash.[17,21,22]

The patient should be protected from unnecessary bleeding risks. Pressure should be applied to all venipuncture sites for 3 to 5 minutes after the cannula is removed. Shaving should be done with an electric razor rather than a blade. Tampons should be avoided to decrease the potential for vaginal bleeding. Hazardous activities that may cause injury, such as contact sports and working with sharp instruments, should be avoided. Vaginal and anal intercourse may cause bleeding, so other forms of intimacy should be explored during times of thrombocytopenia. Rectal temperatures should be avoided. Stool softeners can help prevent bleeding that results from hardened stool and the Valsalva maneuver. Patients should be cautioned against using aspirin, ibuprofen, indomethacin, warfarin, quinidine, and other drugs that may interfere with clotting. Patients should be instructed to report easy bruising, nosebleeds, bleeding gums, and bloody stools.

A differential diagnosis needs to be made in patients experiencing anemia because many GI tumors bleed. Anemic patients may be asymptomatic or present with headache, dizziness, light-headedness, shortness of breath, fatigue, pallor, hypothermia, and pale nail beds and conjunctiva. A patient is considered anemic if the hemoglobin level is lower than 8 g/dl. Many physicians do not transfuse if the patient is asymptomatic. One unit of red blood cells (RBCs) can be expected to raise the hemoglobin level by 1 g/dl.

In patients experiencing chronic anemia, without acute bleeding as the cause, erythropoietin (Procrit) can be effective in stimulating RBC production. Erythropoietin mimics the natural hormone produced in the kidneys, stimulating and increasing the rate of RBC production. It may be given intravenously or subcutaneously three times weekly until the target hemoglobin level is reached. Common side effects are headache, fever, fatigue, nausea and vomiting, diarrhea, shortness of breath, rash, and injection site reactions. Pain in the long bones and pelvis with cold sweats may occur for several hours after the injection. Blood pressure should be monitored often because hypertension resulting from a rapid hematocrit rise may precipitate seizures and vascular accidents.[17,23,24]

Weekly complete blood counts are needed to adjust the dosage, depending on the nadir. The nadir is the point at which the blood counts are the lowest, and it usually occurs 7 to 14 days after day 1 of chemotherapy. Patients with bone marrow involvement from primary tumor burden or metastatic disease may have prolonged myelosuppression. As a rule, cell-cycle–specific drugs have a swift nadir and a rapid recovery. Cell-cycle–nonspecific drugs have a late nadir and a delayed recovery. Mitomycin, cytarabine, and carmustine often cause a second drop in the blood count, and the patient needs to be aware of this possibility.

Blood counts are particularly important just before administering chemotherapy because bone marrow depression is the most significant dose-limiting factor. Chemotherapy may have to be delayed if adequate marrow recovery has not occurred. Subsequent doses of chemotherapy may be reduced if the drop in blood counts has been severe. Chemotherapy affects the stem cells in the bone marrow, which are rapidly dividing, rather than the cells in the circulation, which have already reached maturity. Most protocols require the WBC count to be at least 3000/mm^3 cells with an absolute granulocyte count of 1500.[1-6,8,10,17,19,23,25]

Anorexia and taste alterations

Anorexia and taste alterations are common among patients receiving chemotherapy. Lack of interest or an aversion to food can lead to anorexia, inadequate nutritional intake, and poor patient compliance, which can effect the patient's overall quality of life.

Many of the treatments that the patient receives result in taste alterations. *Dysgeusia,* which is also referred to as *taste blindness,* is a condition in which the gustatory sense is impaired. This results in familiar foods tasting entirely different and in some circumstances unpleasant. Patients receiving cisplatin, cyclophosphamide, vincristine, or 5-fluorouracil often complain that nothing tastes right. Some patients experience a bitter or metallic taste or no taste at all. Most patients prefer to have their food served on glass dishes, and many use a plastic fork if they have a metallic taste in their mouth.

The nurse can do many things to help the patient and family members deal with this distressing symptom (Box 13-1). The patient should be advised that gum and hard candy, especially the sour types, are beneficial between meals. The patient should also be instructed to brush his or her teeth often to help eliminate unpleasant tastes. Rinsing the mouth with a nonirritating mouthwash is often refreshing.

The patient and caregiver should be encouraged to experiment with different spices and flavorings. This is particularly important because the taste buds have changed and need to be stimulated. Most patients find they have an aversion to meats, especially red meats, which usually have a bitter taste. Many foods have an exaggerated sweetness that can increase the patient's nausea. Patients should be made aware that the food is not spoiled; rather their sense of taste has been affected by the chemotherapy. Cold foods or foods served at room temperature are usually better tolerated than hot foods. Cold fruits and cheeses are often a better alternative to a hot meal. Many patients tolerate multiple small meals better than three large meals. Patients should be encouraged to eat, but never nagged or forced to eat. Antiemetics and radiation to the head and neck cause the patient to experience xerostomia (dry mouth). Artificial saliva or water sprayed in the mouth can help moisten the mucous membranes. Hard, dry food can cause discomfort and is difficult to swallow, whereas soft, moist foods are more pleasing to the palate. Commercial mouthwashes, smoking, and alcohol should be avoided because these products can irritate the mucous membranes.

Depending on the patient's condition and severity of the symptoms, the patient may be a candidate for enteral or parenteral nutrition. Nutritional assessment, including a daily calorie count, indirect calorimetry, weight loss history, and measurement of visceral protein stores should be considered when contemplating intervention.[1,2,4-6,8-10,26,27]

Box 13-1 Nursing Suggestions to Help the Patient and Family Deal with Taste Alterations

1. Provide oral hygiene before meals.
2. Arrange food attractively.
3. Avoid strong cooking odors, such as cabbage or broccoli.
4. Eat in a pleasant, relaxed environment.
5. Use pleasant odors, such as cloves.
6. Avoid noxious odors, such as fish.
7. Enhance food flavors with herbs, spices, or marinade.
8. Serve cold foods rather than hot foods.
9. Eat frequent, small meals.
10. Administer antiemetics before meals.
11. Drink high-energy shakes.
12. Serve food on glass dishes and use plastic silverware.
13. Avoid gas-forming foods.
14. Obtain adequate rest before meals.
15. Take a short walk or get some fresh air to stimulate appetite.

Constipation

It is important for patients to know their particular bowel pattern. What is normal for one person may indicate a problem for another. Constipation is the difficult, and sometimes painful, passage of hard, dry stool. The severity of the problem can vary from mild discomfort to an ileus occurring in less than 96 hours. Appropriate intervention should be implemented if 2 days have elapsed since the last bowel movement.

There are many causes for constipation other than chemotherapy, including anxiety, depression, narcotics, muscle relaxants, hypercalcemia, immobility, dehydration, dietary deficiencies, and tumor involvement resulting in intrinsic or extrinsic compression. Intervention in part depends on the underlying cause, which also must be addressed. Patients taking narcotics often require prophylactic stool softeners, as do those receiving vinca alkaloids.

Management of the oncology patient is not the same as for the medical-surgical patient. Enemas should be used with caution in the myelosuppressed patient because they can irritate the mucous membranes and can cause microscopic tears in the mucous membranes of the bowel. This can result in bleeding, a low platelet count, and infection in the neutropenic patient. If impaction occurs, there may be no alternative except to administer an enema. Usually, an oil retention enema or a phosphate enema is ordered to hydrate the stool. If an enema is used, care should be taken to be as gentle as possible.

Prophylactic intervention leads to greater patient comfort. Patients at risk for constipation should be instructed to increase their dietary intake of fresh fruits, vegetables, and fiber. Unless contraindicated, the patient should have at least 2 to 3 L of fluids daily. Cheese, eggs, refined starches, chocolate, candy, and foods known to be constipating should be avoided. Eating at the same time each day helps regulate the patient. Because physical activity and exercise stimulate peristalsis, patients should be encouraged to be as active as possible. Patients should be instructed to respond to the urge to defecate immediately and not wait.

Laxatives, which facilitate the evacuation of feces from the colon, include stool softeners, cathartics, bulk laxatives, and lubricants. Bulk laxatives keep the stool soft and have been found helpful and gentle; they are a good choice for the oncology patient. Stool softeners cause fluid to shift into the colon, thereby preventing the stool from becoming dry and hard. Laxatives and cathartics stimulate peristalsis and move the waste through the intestinal system. Lubricants such as mineral oil and castor oil lubricate the colon and facilitate evacuation.[1,2,4-6,9,10]

Diarrhea

Diarrhea is the abnormal passage of five or more loose or watery stools in a 24-hour period. Diarrhea might be accompanied by abdominal cramps and flatus. The GI tract produces up to 8 L of fluid per day, and the colon reabsorbs the fluid and produces formed or semiformed stool.

As with constipation, there are many causes of diarrhea. Postoperative intestinal resection, inflammatory bowel syndrome, *Clostridium difficile* and other intestinal infections, malabsorption syndrome, and cancer-related treatments of chemotherapy, radiation, and biologic therapy can cause diarrhea. The epithelial cells lining the GI tract can be destroyed by the antimetabolites (e.g., 5-fluorouracil), which causes inadequate absorption and digestion of nutrients resulting in diarrhea.

Patients with six or more diarrhea stools a day are at risk for dehydration and electrolyte imbalance. Diarrhea has psychosocial ramifications and can be a source of embarrassment for the patient.

Nursing management of diarrhea includes instructing the patient on the importance of early intervention to avoid complications. Patients should be instructed to increase their intake of constipating foods such as cheese and eggs. Many patients have a lactose intolerance, which results in diarrhea; consequently, these patients need to use caution with dairy products. Buttermilk and yogurt contain *Lactobacillus* and can usually be tolerated by lactose-intolerant patients. Foods high in pectin, bulk, and fiber help slow peristalsis. Fluid replacement prevents dehydration. Patients should avoid spicy foods, which irritate the GI tract. Fatty or greasy foods stimulate evacuation of the colon. Raw fruits and vegetables, nuts, caffeine, seeds, popcorn, and alcohol should also be avoided. Foods and liquids should be served at room temperature.

Nursing interventions also include accurately recording intake and output. The stool should be measured, if possible. The consistency and number of stools should be noted. Three or more stools a day is an indication for intervention. Patients need to have at least 2 L of fluid per day. Because electrolytes are lost through the diarrhea, an electrolyte solution is recommended. Potassium is one of the major electrolytes lost; therefore fluids and foods high in this element should be used. Pharmacologic intervention should be started as soon as possible to avoid complications of fluid and electrolyte loss. Several prescription and over-the-counter medications are designed to control diarrhea. In cases of severe diarrhea, IV support is necessary.

Many agents once used to manage diarrhea, such as absorbents (e.g., psyllium derivatives, mucilloid preparations), anticholinergics (e.g., atropine sulfate, belladonna preparations), and opium derivatives (e.g., paregoric, codeine), are being replaced by drugs that have limited or minimal side effects. The current standards in the treatment of cancer-related diarrhea are loperamide (Imodium), diphenoxylate (Lomotil), or the new agent octreotide (Sandostatin).[1,2,4-6,8-10,26,28]

Alopecia

For most patients, especially women, the fear of alopecia is second only to nausea and vomiting. Alopecia is closely tied to self-image. Hair loss is traumatic, and many patients experience depression when their hair is falling out in large bunches. Patients should be reminded that hair loss associated with chemotherapy is temporary. However, postradiation alopecia may be permanent in doses exceeding 4000 rads. Many patients find that their hair is easier to manage if it is cut short. Others shave their heads when the hair starts to fall out. New growth occurs at a rate of about 0.25 inch/month. Often, the new hair has a different texture, color, or thickness.

Many patients are concerned that hair loss will occur immediately, with the first drop of medication, but this is not the case. Not all chemotherapeutic agents cause total alopecia, but the use of combination drugs increases the chance of at least some thinning.

Rapidly dividing cells such as hair follicles are easily affected by chemotherapy. Hair loss may be thinning, partial or complete, and involve not only the scalp but also eyebrows and eyelashes and facial, axillary, pubic, nasal, and body hair. Hair loss may begin in 7 to 10 days and is usually complete in 1 to 2 months. Regrowth usually occurs 3 to 6 months after the last chemotherapy treatment, but it sometimes happens before treatments are completed. Patients should have an opportunity to obtain a wig, hat, or scarf before hair loss occurs. Purchasing a wig before losing hair allows a closer match of color and style to the natural hair. Wigs are available in many shades, styles, sizes, lengths, and amounts of hair. The most affordable and easiest to care for are the synthetics. Human hair and synthetic blends that are machine made are now less expensive. The synthetic fibers of today are as fine as natural hair, soft, and very manageable.

Care of the scalp should be the same as for any area of exposed skin (Box 13-2). Patients should be instructed to use a gentle soap. Lotion or a moisturizer helps keep the scalp from becoming dry but should not be used during radiation treatments to the head. The skin on the scalp is tender and burns if exposed to bright sun. Scarves, turbans, or hats provide comfort, protect against the sun, and preserve body heat in the winter.[1-6,9,10]

Fatigue

Cancer-related fatigue is a common side effect (89%) that remains poorly understood and until recently received little attention. Fatigue is highly individualized and should be evaluated according to the patient's perception of how it effects his or her lifestyle. It is particularly distressing because it usually lasts through all treatments. Fatigue can affect health in general and have a great impact on the patient's quality of life, such as the ability to work and participate in family and social activities. This can result in depression, loss of hope, and diminished self-esteem, often resulting in patient noncompliance.

The patient should be encouraged to rest often, maintain good nutrition, and participate in exercise such as walking

---

Box 13-2   Recommendations for Thinning Hair

1. Use mild shampoo and conditioner and avoid excessive shampooing.
2. Avoid using such appliances as curling irons, hot combs, and blow dryers.
3. Avoid hair styles that place tension on the hair, such as pony tails and braids.
4. Use a wide-tooth comb to groom hair rather than a brush.
5. Avoid chemicals, such as permanents, coloring, or hair spray.

several times a week. The patient should also be encouraged to conserve energy for the most important tasks and ask assistance from family and friends.[1,2,4-6,9,10,29-31]

Stomatitis and mucositis

The mucous membranes of the GI tract, especially those of the mouth, can become red, irritated, and inflamed. Stomatitis can range from a mild irritation and sensitivity when eating acidic or spicy foods to full-blown sores, with difficulty swallowing. Chemotherapy-related stomatitis usually begins 5 to 7 days after treatment and lasts about 10 days.

Good oral hygiene is imperative in reducing the amount of bacteria in the mouth and decreasing the potential for infection (Box 13-3). A soft toothbrush or gauze prevents further irritation to the delicate tissue. When the mouth is particularly tender, it is advisable for patients to remove their dentures or partial plate at night and as much as possible during the day.

Patients find that rinsing the mouth with a baking soda or saline solution is soothing to the mucous membranes. Sodium bicarbonate is a mucolytic agent that breaks up mucous secretions. Many different formulas are available for a stomatitis cocktail. Most formulas contain diphenhydramine, an antacid, and a local anesthetic. An antifungal such as nystatin is also sometimes included. A stomatitis cocktail is generally taken as a swish, swirl, and swallow, ordered before meals, at bedtime, and as needed. Most commercial mouthwashes contain alcohol, which can burn the delicate mucous membranes, and should be avoided.

The patient should be instructed to eat soft foods with a smooth consistency. Usually, cold, wet foods are soothing to the irritated mucous membranes. Special attention should also be given to the lips to prevent cracking and drying. Applying lip balm, aloe vera, or a petroleum-based gel keeps the lips moist and promotes comfort and healing. Care should be taken to provide adequate nutrition and hydration. In cases of severe stomatitis, the patient may need to be hospitalized for fluid support and pain management.[1,2,4-6,8-10,26]

Cardiotoxicity

The side effect that causes the patient the greatest amount of psychologic distress is the cardiotoxicity that can result with many of the antineoplastics, such as paclitaxel, mitoxantrone, idarubicin, cyclophosphamide, 5-fluorouracil, floxuridine, and particularly doxorubicin. It is a dilemma for patients to be told that an effective drug for their cancer can damage their heart.

Early signs of cardiotoxicity are difficult to detect. An electrocardiogram may show a decrease in voltage of the QRS complex or nonspecific ST- or T-wave changes. The anthracyclines can damage the myocytes, weakening the cardiac muscle. This results in decreased cardiac output, with progression to congestive heart failure. The patient usually is asymptomatic until signs and symptoms of congestive heart failure appear. Patients complain of shortness of breath, especially on exertion, and a nonproductive cough. The physical examination shows neck vein distension, tachycardia, gallop rhythm, and edema.

A drop in the baseline ejection fraction signals a decrease in left ventricular function. In these situations, the risk of cardiac damage and complications must be weighed against a meaningful tumor response. Most physicians obtain a baseline MUGA scan or an echocardiogram with an ejection fraction and repeat these tests at the halfway point of the total accumulated lifetime dose and at the end of therapy. Frequent electrocardiogram monitoring to detect changes in the voltage of the QRS helps identify early signs of impending toxicity (Box 13-4). In selected patients, a percutaneous endomyocardial biopsy is indicated to determine the degree of myocyte damage.

Dexrazoxane (Zinecard) is a new cardiac-protective iron chelating agent given to prevent doxorubicin-induced cardiotoxicity when cumulative doses are reached. Dexrazoxane is not recommended for use with initial therapy but is indicated in patients who have received an accumulative dose of $300mg/m^2$ of doxorubicin and would benefit from continued therapy.

Common side effects are nausea, vomiting, fatigue, anorexia, stomatitis, and pain at the injection site. Dexrazoxane may increase myelosuppression when used with a regimen of fluorouracil, doxorubicin, and cyclophosphamide.[1-6,9,10,32,33]

Neurotoxicity

Neurotoxicity can be seen as either central or peripheral. CNS toxicity can be encephalopathy, seizures, cerebellar dysfunction, mental status changes, ophthalmic toxicities, and ototoxicities.

Box 13-3   **Predisposing Factors for Development of Stomatitis**
1. Poor-fitting dentures
2. Poor nutritional status
3. Head and neck radiation
4. Concurrent steroid therapy
5. High-dose chemotherapy
6. Advanced age
7. Antimetabolites, especially 5-fluorouracil and methotrexate
8. Antitumor antibiotics
9. Continuous infusion of chemotherapy versus short infusions
10. Hematologic malignancies

Box 13-4   **Risk Factors for Cardiotoxicity**
1. Prior radiation to the mediastinum or left chest wall
2. Hypertension
3. History of smoking
4. Advanced age
5. Cardiac disease
6. Multiple cardiac drugs
7. High-dose therapy and doses over recommended lifetime dosage

Peripheral toxicity causes axonal degeneration or demyelination involving sensory and motor dysfunction.

Paclitaxel, cisplatin, carboplatin, and the vinca alkaloids are the agents most likely to cause neurotoxicity. Peripheral toxicity usually does not occur until after five or more treatments. The exception to this is paclitaxel, which can produce paresthesia within 5 days of administration. When cisplatin is used concurrently with paclitaxel, the patient has an increased potential for neurotoxicity. Patients usually complain of numbness and tingling of the hands and feet. As the toxicity increases, the patient begins to complain of muscle pain, weakness, and disturbances in depth perception, particularly with ambulation. This can result in safety issues. Patients need to be cautioned about loose rugs, steps, and articles lying on the floor that may cause the patient to trip. Because there is a decrease in sensation, the patient needs to exercise caution with temperature changes. Hot water, heating pads, electric blankets, hot stoves, and radiators are more likely to cause burns with decreased perception of temperature. Exposure to cold is also a concern because these patients are less likely to realize the severity of the temperature. Patients should be adequately dressed for the weather, with special protection for the hands and feet.

Constipation and paralytic ileus are other concerns in this patient population. Symptoms can be manifested within 2 days, and this is particularly true in patients receiving vinca alkaloids. Vincristine has good tissue-binding capacity, which results in prolonged exposure of the neural tissue. The patient should be observed for abdominal distension and active bowel sounds, and the diet should be regulated according to the patient's needs, adding fresh fruits and vegetables, fiber, and fluids. Constipation can be compounded in the patient who is also receiving concurrent narcotics. Prophylactic stool softeners can assist in maintaining regularity, and suppositories, oral laxatives, or lubricants may be used. Enemas should be used with caution in the neutropenic patient. Depending on the severity, symptoms of neuropathy usually disappear in a few weeks. If treatment continues, deep tendon reflexes may not return, and muscle weakness may be a problem for many months. In severe cases, motor function may never return to normal.[1-6,8-10,34,35]

Renal toxicity

Renal toxicity is an elevation of the blood urea nitrogen (BUN) and creatinine levels. The chemotherapeutic agents most notorious for causing renal damage are cisplatin, carmustine, streptozocin, methotrexate, mitomycin-C, and to a lesser degree, carboplatin. Caution needs to be taken to protect the patient from this potentially life-threatening complication. Baseline laboratory values of the BUN and creatinine levels need to be obtained before administration of these nephrotoxic agents.

In the presence of renal compromise, the risk-versus-benefit ratio must be weighed carefully. Chemotherapy doses that could produce a meaningful tumor response may need to be reduced to protect the patient from further renal damage and to compensate for the longer half-life resulting from poor renal function.

Before these nephrotoxic chemotherapeutic agents are administered, vigorous hydration is often ordered. Mannitol and furosemide (Lasix) may also be ordered in an effort to flush out the kidneys. Accurate intake and output with frequent weights must be recorded. Signs of fluid retention or imbalance should be reported to the physician.

Mesna (Mesnex) is a cytoprotectant effective in reducing the incidence of ifosfamide-induced hemorrhagic cystitis. Mesna does not prevent hemorrhagic cystitis in all patients; therefore a morning urine sample should be checked for hematuria after ifosfamide administration. Common side effects are diarrhea (83%), headache (50%), fatigue (33%), nausea (33%), allergy (17%), and hypotension (17%).

Methotrexate precipitates in an acid solution, plugging the renal tubules. Raising the urinary pH can be accomplished by administering an alkylating agent to the patient before giving high-dose methotrexate in the form of bicarbonate, orally or intravenously. Measurement of the urinary pH is often ordered to ensure that the pH is greater than 7. If the pH drops below 7, additional bicarbonate is given.

The risk of hyperuricemia from tumor lysis syndrome is another factor that needs to be considered when administering nephrotoxic drugs. Alkalizing the urine prevents the precipitation of uric acid crystals in the renal tubules, and the administration of allopurinol helps prevent the formation of uric acid crystals. These prophylactic measures usually begin 12 to 24 hours before chemotherapy.

The nurse needs to be aware of any concurrent nephrotoxic drugs that the patient may be receiving. Amphotericin, the aminoglycoside antibiotics, and vitamin C all have the potential of potentiating nephrotoxicity.[1-6,8,10,26]

Pulmonary toxicity

Pulmonary toxicity is damage to the endothelial cells of the lung and results in pneumonitis and interstitial fibrosis. Bleomycin at dosages exceeding 250 units/m^2 or 400 units total dose and carmustine in total doses of 1500 mg/m^2 predispose the patient to pulmonary toxicity. Toxicity appears to be increased with the concurrent use of cyclophosphamide. Other antineoplastics known to be responsible for pulmonary toxicity include mitomycin and methotrexate.

Pulmonary toxicity usually develops over weeks to months but can develop within hours. The patient usually presents with dyspnea, a nonproductive cough, fatigue, and fever. Auscultation of the lungs reveals end-inspiratory basilar rales. The chest radiograph is nonspecific or has streaky infiltrates and consolidation. Elderly patients and patients with a smoking history, current or past radiation therapy to the lungs, or a preexisting pulmonary condition appear to be at greater risk for pulmonary toxicity.[1-6,8-10,32]

Sexual dysfunction

Rapidly dividing cells, such as in the ovaries and testicles, are most sensitive to chemotherapy. This is particularly true of the alkylating agents that may potentiate dysfunction when combined with the antimetabolites and antitumor antibiotics.

The sperm count is often reduced, resulting in infertility that can be temporary or permanent. It is recommended that the option of sperm or egg banking be presented to the patient before initiating chemotherapy. Many men have difficulty achieving an erection while receiving chemotherapy, which can interfere with a sense of well-being and self-esteem because the sexual drive remains intact.

Chemotherapy can suppress ovarian function. Within 6 months of starting chemotherapy, women often experience amenorrhea or changes in their menstrual cycle during treatment. Many women have symptoms of a medical menopause, including hot flashes, irritability, insomnia, and vaginal dryness. The use of a water-soluble lubricant relieves some of the symptoms of vaginal dryness. Women who are older than 40 often do not have return of their menstrual cycle on completion of their chemotherapy. The use of estrogen replacement or estrogen-containing vaginal creams is controversial, especially in hormone-dependent tumors such as breast cancer.

Medical literature has documented healthy live births to couples who have had chemotherapy. There does not seem to be an increase in birth defects, chromosomal abnormalities, or spontaneous miscarriages in couples when one partner has been exposed to chemotherapy.[1-6,8-10]

Extravasation

The terms *extravasation* and *infiltration* are often used interchangeably. An *infiltration* is an inadvertent administration of a nonvesicant into the surrounding tissue. *Extravasation* is an inadvertent delivery of a vesicant into the tissues. Vesicants cause blistering, severe tissue damage, and even necrosis if extravasated.

An irritant can cause local sensitivity and should not be confused with an extravasation. Chemotherapeutic agents can be irritants. A vesicant is also an irritant, but the intensity of the irritating action of a vesicant is so severe that plasma escapes from the extracellular space and blisters are formed. When fluid leaks into the tissue, the tissue is compressed because of restriction of the blood flow, which decreases the amount of oxygen to the site and thus lowers the cellular pH. There is a loss of capillary wall integrity, an increase in edema, and, depending on severity, eventual cell death. The box above presents precautionary measures to prevent extravasation.

An oversimplification of the chemistry of an extravasation divides drugs into two categories: those that bind to DNA and those that do not. Drugs that do not bind to DNA cause immediate damage but are quickly metabolized or inactivated. This type of injury is similar to a burn, in which the damage is immediate, followed by repair using the normal healing process. For a small extravasation, conservative treatment is indicated. Large extravasations may lead to contractures, the need for debridement and grafting, and, in severe cases, amputation. The box on p. 259 provides guidelines for extravasation management.

The vinca alkaloids do not bind to DNA but inhibit mitosis. Ulceration from these drugs is usually less severe than from the binding drugs. Ulcers from the vinca alkaloids are similar to those from the anthracyclines, but they do not tend to erode to

Extravasation Precautions

1. All peripherally administered chemotherapy should be given via a new IV site.
2. Educate the patient to report any sensation change. Monitor closely for signs of pain, especially in patients who cannot verbalize discomfort. Be particularly alert for complaints of stinging or burning, which are usually the first sign of an extravasation.
3. Assess the venipuncture site. Check for signs of edema or bleb formation.
4. Look for signs of infiltration, including slowing or cessation of drops or flow from the intravenous solution, increased resistance when administering the drug, and poor blood return when rechecking needle placement.
5. When in doubt, stop the infusion and restart the IV.
6. Notify the physician of the extravasation.

deeper structures; healing usually occurs in 3 to 5 weeks without surgical intervention.

The instillation of hyaluronidase (Wydase) intradermally or subcutaneously with a 25-gauge needle around the infiltrated site is the treatment of choice for a vinca alkaloid, paclitaxel, or etoposide extravasation. Hyaluronidase is a protein enzyme obtained from testicular tissue and is used to increase the absorption of fluids administered as hypodermoclysis. Hyaluronidase destroys tissue cement, which helps decrease or prevent injury by allowing for the rapid diffusion of extravasated fluid and rapid reabsorption. Although the drug is spread over a larger area, the injury is minimized.

The second category of drugs, those that bind to DNA, cause immediate damage and also lodge in the tissue, producing a prolonged effect. Because of this binding effect, the cells lose their ability to heal spontaneously. One of the drugs that bind to DNA is the alkylating agent nitrogen mustard, which rapidly fixes to tissue and causes immediate injury. The vein irritation can progress over several days to a dark bluish gray. Applying cold compresses for 6 to 12 hours is recommended, and sodium thiosulfate injected into the infiltration site is the suggested treatment.

Other chemotherapeutic agents that bind to DNA are in the antibiotic family. Because doxorubicin is one of the most widely used chemotherapeutic agents, it has the largest database of information concerning extravasation. Animal studies have shown a relationship between the doxorubicin concentration and the degree of ulceration. Surgical intervention is recommended, especially with doxorubicin, when the lesion is greater than 2 cm or if there is significant residual pain 1 to 2 weeks after extravasation. If no ulceration has occurred, there is no benefit in surgical excision unless there is persistent, severe pain. Once necrosis appears, surgical debridement is necessary. If the lesion is not debrided, it can progress to a thick, leathery eschar surrounded by a 2- to 3-cm rim of red, painful skin. The amount of blood in the tissue determines the degree of ulceration.

The eschar usually does not slough spontaneously, and when it is removed, deep subcutaneous, necrotic tissue is found.

1. If an extravasation is suspected, stop the infusion immediately and evaluate for swelling and blood return. If there is any doubt about the patency of the vein, restart IV at a new site.
2. Aspirate before removing the catheter. Studies have shown that there is a decrease in the size of the lesion with aspiration alone.
3. Apply ice, not heat, for 24 to 48 hours (use heat for vinblastine, vincristine, or vinorelbine) for 20 minutes at least four times a day. Ice causes vasoconstriction, decreases local drug uptake (especially with doxorubicin), decreases edema, and slows the metabolic rate of cells. Decreased local blood supply and the cooling effect may decrease local pain. Heat causes vasodilation, facilitates fluid absorption, and may enhance drug absorption, but it also increases metabolic demand of the tissue. Treating extravasations from the vinca alkaloids is the only time when heat is recommended rather than cold.
4. Elevate the extremity.
5. Administer the antidote with the needle in place or remove the needle and inject around the infiltration site. Health care facilities should have a policy that specifies the administration of a specific antidote.
6. Encourage the patient to resume normal activity with the arm to prevent stiffness and discomfort.
7. Notify the physician and obtain specific orders for an antidote.
8. Record the episode. Documentation should include the date and time of extravasation, the needle size, and the type of cannula used. Describe the site location. Describe the appearance of the site. Note whether it is pale, reddened, streaked, or edematous. The drug sequence is important. Sometimes, there is a delayed reaction, and it is important to know the order in which the drugs were given. Note the drug administration technique and whether it was a continuous infusion, a sidearm technique, or a push dose. The amount of extravasation is particularly important with drugs that bind to DNA. Note the intervention that was used.
9. Document that the physician was notified. In many institutions, a plastic surgeon is called by the primary physician at the time of a doxorubicin extravasation to start immediate planning for management of the injury and early assessment of the surgical potential.
10. Notify the risk manager or other appropriate individuals.

Depending on the location, tendons may also be necrotic, resulting in deformities, extensive joint stiffness, neuropathy, and causalgia. A wide excision of the entire necrotic and reddened area can salvage deep structures and retain function. It is wiser to sacrifice tendons and accept some degree of functional deficit in exchange for improved wound healing and resolution of pain. Active drug has been isolated from the wound as long as 3 months after an extravasation and up to 5 months after a doxorubicin infiltration. An ulceration containing doxorubicin glows a dull red under ultraviolet light. Mitomycin ulcers are typically deep and expansive and require a wide excision with split-thickness grafting.

It is important not to confuse a flare reaction with an extravasation. A *flare reaction* is a localized release of histamine that appears as a sudden streak along the vein. It is often associated with doxorubicin. Slowing the infusion will lessen or eliminate the symptoms, which should disappear in 30 to 60 minutes. Morphine is a common nonvesicant drug often associated with a flare reaction.[1-6,8-10,19,23,35-37]

CHEMOTHERAPEUTIC AGENTS
Antimetabolites

Most antimetabolites are cell-cycle specific, with their major activity occurring in the S phase of the cell cycle. They are structurally similar to vitamins and coenzymes and inhibit protein synthesis by deceiving cells with erroneous metabolites of a structural analog. Their major toxicities are hematopoietic and gastrointestinal. Other common side effects are elevated liver function tests, photosensitivity, and alopecia.[1,3,5,10]

Gemcitabine HCl. Gemcitabine (Gemzar), an antimetabolite, inhibits DNA synthesis and is cell-cycle specific in the S phase. It is indicated for first-line treatment in pancreas, non–small cell lung and colon cancers. Myelosuppression is the dose-limiting toxicity. Mild to moderate nausea and vomiting are very common (69%). Diarrhea, stomatitis, and constipation also occur. Other common side effects are fever, flulike symptoms, and mild to moderate rashes involving the trunk and extremities. Alopecia is minimal, involving about 15% of patients. Dyspnea and bronchospasm may occur in patients with previous lung conditions.[9,17,19,23,35-39]

Methotrexate. Methotrexate (MTX, Amethopterin, Mexate, Folex) is a folic acid antagonist that interferes with the synthesis of purine and thymidylate. It is cell-cycle specific in the S phase, and it is used in combination with other drugs or as a single agent. Methotrexate is active against acute lymphocytic leukemia, lymphomas, sarcomas, mycosis fungoids, gestational trophoblastic carcinomas, and breast, lung, head, and neck cancers. Methotrexate can crystallize and precipitate in acidic solution and can cause renal damage in the presence of urine with a low pH. This is particularly true with high-dose methotrexate.

Several precautionary steps should be taken before, and sometimes after, administering methotrexate. Because of the potential for renal toxicity, the BUN and creatinine levels should be checked to ensure adequate kidney function before administration. Antiemetics should be given beforehand to control the dose-related nausea associated with this drug. Slowing the rate of infusion and using large volumes of fluid to dilute the drug can also be helpful in managing nausea. Hydrating fluid is usually given before and after methotrexate dosing. The patient needs to be encouraged to increase oral fluids, and the fluid balance should be monitored.

Before administering high dosages of methotrexate, sodium bicarbonate should be given orally or intravenously to neutralize the urine and keep the urinary pH higher than 7. Following high doses, leucovorin (folinic acid) is usually given as a rescue agent within 24 to 36 hours. The BUN, creatinine, and serum methotrexate levels determine the dosage and frequency of leucovorin. The purpose of the leucovorin is to stop the action of the methotrexate, thereby preventing severe bone marrow toxicity.

The nadir usually occurs 5 to 14 days after treatment. Stomatitis and esophagitis can range from mild irritation and tenderness with a sensitivity to spicy or acidic foods to full-blown, painful sores. The stomatitis can interfere with eating and swallowing. GI ulceration and bleeding may occur. Nausea, vomiting, and anorexia are common. With prolonged use of methotrexate, an elevation in liver function tests, hepatic fibrosis, and occasionally cirrhosis can occur. Pneumonitis may develop and is not always reversible. Sudden death has been reported with methotrexate use.

Methotrexate can cause photosensitivity, with the patient's skin having an increased tendency to burn if exposed to bright, intense sunlight. It is recommended that the patient cover the exposed skin or use a sunscreen of a sun protection factor (SPF) of 15 or more. Radiation recall has been seen with this drug.

Methotrexate interacts with many drugs, including 5-fluorouracil, asparaginase, and vincristine. The patient should be instructed to avoid the use of aspirin, nonsteroidal antiinflammatory drugs, folic acid preparations, vaccines, and alcohol during treatment with methotrexate.[1,4-6,9,10,17,19,23,35-37]

5-Fluorouracil. Another antimetabolite, 5-fluorouracil (fluorouracil, Adrucil, 5-FU) inhibits the synthesis of DNA and RNA and is cell-cycle specific for the S phase. It is indicated in the treatment of GI malignancies, especially colorectal, pancreas, head, neck, breast, prostate, skin (topically), and liver (intraarterially) cancers.

The dose-limiting toxicities are stomatitis and diarrhea. Toxicity may be delayed 1 to 3 weeks. Nausea and vomiting are common, with severity being dose related. The patient should be premedicated with antiemetics. GI ulceration can lead to hemorrhage.

Myelosuppression is usually moderate, with a nadir of 7 to 14 days. Other side effects are anorexia, fatigue, alopecia, and photosensitivity. The patient should be instructed to avoid the sun between 10 AM and 2 PM, to wear long sleeves and pants when in the sun, and to use a sunscreen with an SPF of 15 or higher. Hyperpigmentation of the nail beds and peripheral veins is common. Hand-foot syndrome may occur, involving painful, erythematous desquamation of palms and soles. Leucovorin calcium has been given to potentiate the action of 5-fluorouracil but may enhance its toxicities.[3,9,17,19,23,35-37,40]

Floxuridine. Floxuridine (FUDR) is similar to the structure and action of 5-fluorouracil. It interferes with cell replication and inhibits DNA synthesis. It is cell-cycle specific for the S phase and is indicated in the treatment of liver, biliary, pancreatic, oral cavity, and breast cancers.

Nausea, vomiting, anorexia, and abdominal pain are common, with the dose-limiting toxicities being stomatitis and diarrhea. Myelosuppression is mild. Alopecia and dermatitis are common. Plantar-palmar syndrome may occur and is characterized by painful swelling and peeling of the hands and feet. Hyperpigmentation of the veins occurs with peripheral infusions. For liver tumors, floxuridine is usually administered intraarterially by infusion pump via a catheter implanted in the hepatic artery.[9,17,19,23,35-37]

Fludarabine. Fludarabine (Fludara, fludarabine phosphate) interferes with and inhibits DNA function. It is indicated in chronic B-cell lymphocytic leukemia that has not responded to standard treatment, low-grade lymphomas, and mycosis fungoides.

Common side effects are nausea, vomiting, anorexia, diarrhea, fever, chills, rash, myalgia, fatigue, weakness, GI bleeding, visual disturbances, and urinary infections. Cardiac problems such as arrhythmias, congestive heart failure, and myocardial infarction have occurred. Common respiratory side effects are cough, dyspnea, pneumonia, and upper respiratory infections. The concurrent use of pentostatin is not recommended because of severe risk of pulmonary toxicity. Because myelosuppression can be severe, fludarabine should not be administered with other severe myelosuppressants such as 5-fluorouracil or methotrexate. The nadir usually occurs on day 13 but has a range of 3 to 25 days. Confusion, coma, and death have been reported with very high dosages. Tumor lysis syndrome is common and usually begins with flank pain and hematuria. Most toxic effects are dose dependent and increase with advanced age, bone marrow impairment, and renal insufficiency.[9,17,19,23,35-37]

Cytarabine. Cytarabine (Ara-C, Cytosar-U, cytosine, arabinoside) is a cell-cycle–specific antimetabolite, with its action in the S phase, that inhibits DNA synthesis. It is indicated in the treatment of acute nonlymphocytic leukemia, acute lymphocytic leukemia, acute myelogenous leukemia, chronic myelocytic leukemia, and meningeal leukemia (intrathecally).

Myelosuppression is the dose-limiting toxicity, with a nadir at 7 to 9 days and a second nadir at 15 to 24 days. Anemia with megaloblastic changes in the bone marrow is common. Nausea and vomiting, with severity related to infusion rate, anorexia, diarrhea, and anal ulceration, are common. Alopecia is common, as are rashes, especially hand-foot syndrome (i.e., a rash on the palms and soles followed by blisters and desquamation). Tumor lysis syndrome may occur if the patient has a large tumor bulk. Corticosteroid eyedrops are usually started before cytarabine administration to prevent conjunctivitis, which is often seen. Cytarabine is incompatible with 5-fluorouracil and heparin in the same line.[3,9,17,19,23,35-37]

Pentostatin. Pentostatin (Nipent) is an antimetabolite that interferes with DNA replication and disrupts RNA processing. It is cell-cycle nonspecific and is indicated primarily in the treatment of refractory hairy cell leukemia and other leukemias unresponsive to therapy.

Anorexia, nausea, vomiting, stomatitis, abdominal pain, diarrhea, headache, fatigue, rashes, chills, fever, pain, depression, and nervousness are common. Leukopenia and thrombocytopenia are severe with a granulocyte nadir of 15 days. Pulmonary complications such as pulmonary edema can be life-threatening. Infections and hypersensitivity reactions are common and severe. Myocardial infarctions, arrhythmias, heart failure, and death have occurred. Coma has been reported in more than half of patients.[3,9,17,19,23,35-37]

Vinca and plant alkaloids

The vinca alkaloids, derived from the periwinkle plant, inhibit mitosis and are cell-cycle specific for the M phase. They are vesicants, and the major toxicities occur in the hematopoietic, integumentary, neurologic, and reproductive systems. The vinca alkaloids are for IV administration only and are fatal if given intrathecally.[1,3,5,10,35-37]

Vinblastine. Vinblastine (Velban) is cell-cycle specific for the M phase and blocks cellular division. It is indicated in Hodgkin's disease (stages 3 and 4); lymphoma; acquired immunodeficiency syndrome (AIDS)-related Kaposi's sarcoma; mycosis fungoides; histocytosis; testicular, bladder, renal cell, and non–small cell lung cancers; and choriocarcinoma.

The major toxicity is dose-related bone marrow depression, with a nadir of 5 to 10 days. CNS toxicity is common but occurs less often than with vincristine. Because of the neurotoxicity, it is recommended there be at least 7 days between doses. Symptoms include jaw pain, paresthesias, loss of deep tendon reflexes, and peripheral neuropathy. The patient should be monitored for foot drop and difficulty fastening buttons. Acute bronchospasm and shortness of breath may occur, especially if the patient is also receiving mitomycin. Constipation is common, and the prophylactic use of stool softeners is recommended. Nausea, vomiting, and alopecia are mild.

Vinblastine is a vesicant, and if extravasated, severe local tissue necrosis can occur. Treatment consists of immediately stopping the infusion, aspirating any residual drug before removing the cannula, and giving intradermal injections of hyaluronidase around the infiltrated area followed with warm compresses. The vinca alkaloids are the only drugs for which heat is recommended as treatment for an extravasation.[3,9,17,19,23,35-37]

Vincristine. Vincristine sulfate (Oncovin) is cell-cycle specific for the M and S phases and blocks cell division during the metaphase. It is indicated in the treatment of acute leukemia, Hodgkin's disease, non-Hodgkin's lymphoma, Rhabdomyosarcomas, neuroblastoma, Wilms' tumor, multiple myeloma, and breast carcinoma.

Vincristine has the same neurotoxicities as vinblastine, but they are usually more severe and may be permanent. Fine motor movements such as the ability to pick up and handle small objects should be monitored. The patient's gait should also be monitored for difficulty in walking, especially for a slapping gait, which indicates foot drop.

It is recommended that vincristine not be administered more often than every 7 days. Other side effects of vincristine are much the same as for vinblastine, except myelosuppression is mild, with a nadir of 10 to 14 days. The maximum dose for one treatment is 2 mg. Vincristine is a vesicant, and extravasations are treated the same as those of vinblastine.[3,9,17,19,23,35-37]

Vinorelbine. Vinorelbine tartrate (Navelbine) is a semisynthetic vinca alkaloid that inhibits mitosis. It is indicated in the treatment of nonresectable advanced non–small cell lung cancer as a single agent or in combination with cisplatin; it is used in combination with cisplatin for stage III non–small cell lung cancer. It has also been used in Hodgkin's disease and metastatic breast and advanced ovarian cancers.

Granulocytopenia is the dose-limiting toxicity, with a nadir of 7 to 10 days. There is increased risk of bone marrow suppression when used in combination with cisplatin. Acute shortness of breath and severe bronchospasm have been noted, especially when administered with mitomycin. Mild to moderate nausea and vomiting, stomatitis, anorexia, and diarrhea are common. As with other vinca alkaloids, constipation is common, as is peripheral neuropathy that may be first noted by loss of deep tendon reflexes. Transient elevations in liver enzymes, alopecia, and fatigue are common.

Vinorelbine is a contact irritant and gloves should be worn during administration. Extravasation should be avoided because this drug can cause severe local tissue necrosis.[3,9,17,19,23,35-37]

Etoposide. Etoposide (VP 16, Vepesid), another plant alkaloid, is indicated in the treatment of small cell lung, testicular, and ovarian cancers; relapsed Hodgkin's and non-Hodgkin's lymphoma; gestational trophoblastic tumors; and Ewing's sarcoma. Etoposide is cell-cycle specific, with activity in the G_2 and S phase and inhibition of DNA synthesis.

Myelosuppression is dose limiting, with a nadir of 7 to 14 days. Patients experience mild to moderate nausea and vomiting, anorexia, and diarrhea. Alopecia is seen in about 66% of patients, with thinning of the hair in the remainder.

Etoposide can cause severe hypotension if administered too rapidly. It should be administered in no less than 30 minutes, with a usual administration time of 1 to 2 hours. A baseline blood pressure should be obtained and the patient monitored at least every 15 minutes during the first treatment. If the systolic blood pressure falls below 90 mm Hg, the infusion is stopped and the physician notified.

Anaphylactic reactions have been reported and are more common in the initial infusion. Corticosteroids, antihistamines, pressor agents, volume expanders, and a crash cart should be available.

A metallic aftertaste may occur during the infusion and can sometimes be relieved by having the patient suck on hard candy. Radiation recall has also been reported. Extravasation should be avoided because etoposide is considered an irritant.[3,9,17,19,23,35-37]

Paclitaxel. Paclitaxel (Taxol) is a natural product obtained by a semisynthetic process from the needles and bark of the Western Yew tree. It inhibits the normal organization of the cellular process, and the cell-cycle specificity is unknown.

Paclitaxel is indicated as the second-line therapy in ovarian and breast cancers and AIDS-related Kaposi's sarcoma. It has also been used in the treatment of cervical, endometrial, non–small cell lung, gastric, head, and neck cancers, as well as metastatic melanoma.

Bone marrow suppression, especially neutropenia (90%), is dose related and is the major dose-limiting toxicity. If paclitaxel and cisplatin are being administered in the same treatment, paclitaxel should be given first; studies have shown that myelosuppression is profound if it is given after cisplatin. The nadir is 11 days.

Mild to moderate nausea and vomiting (52%), mucositis (31%), and diarrhea (38%) are common and occur more often with 24-hour infusions versus 3-hour infusions. Alopecia is very common, occurring in about 82% of patients.

Hypersensitivity reactions, which are common and can be severe, usually occur in the first 15 to 60 minutes of the infusion. All patients should be premedicated with corticosteroids, diphenhydramine, and H_2 antagonists before administration. The patient should be monitored for severe hypersensitivity reactions such as symptomatic hypotension, chest pain, and dyspnea with bronchospasm and angioedema. Minor reactions include flushing, rashes, tachycardia, asymptomatic dyspnea, and hypotension, which usually require no treatment.

Peripheral neuropathy has been observed in 62% of patients, and the occurrence increases with cumulative doses. This is usually manifested by numbness, tingling, and pain in the hands and feet. There may be loss of deep tendon reflexes and fine motor skills such as fastening buttons.

A baseline electrocardiogram with cardiac assessment should be performed before administering the first dose because of the potential cardiac side effects of the drug. Severe conduction abnormalities have been documented. If this occurs, the patient should receive cardiac monitoring with subsequent doses.

Paclitaxel must be mixed in a glass container and infused via a paclitaxel-compatible administration set to prevent leaching of DEHP (diethylhexylphthalate) found in most polyvinylchloride IV administration sets. An in-line 0.2-micron filter must be used to remove particulate matter that forms in the solution.

Paclitaxel is contraindicated in patients with a hypersensitivity to polyoxyethylated castor oil, which is a vehicle often used to transport drugs in solution.[3,9,17,19,23,35-37,41,42]

Alkylating agents

Government studies in biologic warfare after World War II led to the development of alkylating agents, the first antineoplastic drugs. Most alkylating agents are cell-cycle nonspecific, with the major toxicities being hematopoietic, gastrointestinal, and reproductive. They interfere with normal DNA replication.[1,3,5,10,35-37]

Mechlorethamine HCl.

The first nonhormonal chemotherapeutic agent was mechlorethamine hydrochloride (nitrogen mustard, Mustargen), and it is still widely used in the treatment of Hodgkin's disease, non-Hodgkin's lymphoma, chronic lymphocytic leukemia, bronchogenic carcinoma, and polycythemia vera. Nitrogen mustard is effective in the topical treatment of mycosis fungoides and has been used successfully as a sclerosing agent in malignant pleural effusions. It is a cell-cycle–specific alkylating drug. Its multiple mechanisms of action result in DNA miscoding, breakage, and failure of the cell to replicate.

Nitrogen mustard is unstable and rapidly undergoes chemical transformation and decomposition. Because of these properties, nitrogen mustard should not be mixed until ready to administer. It should be infused over 3 minutes and within 15 minutes of preparation.

If inadvertent contact with skin occurs, the area should be washed with copious amounts of water, followed by a rinse of 2.5% sodium thiosulfate solution.

Nitrogen mustard is a vesicant and can cause severe tissue necrosis and sloughing in the event of an extravasation. A dilute solution of sodium thiosulfate injected into the area helps neutralize the infiltration. The application of ice for 6 to 12 hours after the insult occurred helps reduce tissue damage.

The most common side effects seen with nitrogen mustard use are severe nausea and vomiting, which usually start within 30 minutes of administration and can last up to 36 hours. Anorexia and diarrhea are also common. The patient may note a metallic taste immediately after administration. Leukopenia

may last up to 21 days, with the nadir in 6 to 14 days. Bone marrow suppression can be profound when nitrogen mustard is given with radiation therapy. Thinning of the hair without complete alopecia is seen. Patients receiving this form of chemotherapy not uncommonly develop menstrual irregularities or impaired spermatogenesis.[3,5,9,17,19,23,35-37]

Dacarbazine.

Dacarbazine (DTIC-Dome, imidazole, carboxamide) is cell-cycle nonspecific and inhibits DNA, RNA, and protein synthesis. It possesses limited ability to cross the blood-brain barrier.

Dacarbazine is active against Hodgkin's disease, malignant melanoma, neuroblastoma, and soft-tissue sarcomas.

Patients usually experience pain at the IV site. Adequately diluting the drug and slowing the infusion may decrease the burning sensation and vasospasm that many patients experience. Slowing the infusion and applying ice above the injection site can also be helpful. Dacarbazine is a vesicant, and extravasation can cause tissue necrosis.

The nadir of dacarbazine is 7 to 14 days. Nausea, vomiting, myelosuppression, and flulike symptoms are the most common side effects; 90% of patients experience an onset of nausea and vomiting within 1 to 3 hours of administration, lasting up to 12 hours after treatment. The flulike syndrome can last for several days, with primary symptoms of fever and myalgias. Many patients complain of a metallic taste, which may interfere with nutritional intake. Skin reactions of pruritus, erythema, and photosensitivity have occurred. Exposure to the sun during the first 48 hours can cause facial flushing, paresthesia, and dizziness.

Dacarbazine is incompatible in the same tubing with heparin.[3,9,17,19,23,35-37]

Cyclophosphamide.

Cyclophosphamide (Cytoxan, Endoxan, Neosar, CTX) is one of the most widely used alkylating agents. It is cell-cycle nonspecific and causes cell death by cross-linking with DNA and interfering with RNA transcription. It is active in the treatment of lymphomas, leukemias, multiple myeloma, mycosis fungoides, neuroblastoma, retinoblastoma, sarcomas, and breast, ovary, testis, lung, and bladder malignancies.

Hemorrhagic cystitis is the most serious side effect; it can be severe and fatal. Vigorous hydration with 2 to 3 L of fluid a day is necessary before and after administration. The patient should be encouraged to void frequently to lessen the time the drug spends in the bladder. Mesna may be given to lessen the incidence and severity of cystitis.

Leukopenia is the dose-limiting toxicity, with a nadir of 8 to 14 days. Thrombocytopenia and pulmonary fibrosis may occur with high dosages. Cardiotoxicity can occur with high dosages and in combination with doxorubicin. Other common side effects are nausea and vomiting (with rapid infusions), hypersensitivity reactions, and alopecia.[3,9,17,19,23,35-37,43,44]

Ifosfamide.

Ifosfamide (IFEX) is cell-cycle nonspecific and inhibits DNA synthesis. It is indicated in the treatment of third-line germ-cell testicular cancer; pancreatic, bone, and soft-tissue sarcomas; non-Hodgkin's lymphoma; and lung cancer.

Myelosuppression is dose related, with a nadir of 10 to 14 days. Common side effects are dose-dependent nausea and vomiting (50%), alopecia (83%), and somnolence. Confusion (12%) has occurred, and coma and seizures have been reported.

The most serious and dose-limiting side effect is hemorrhagic cystitis. Vigorous hydration is recommended before, during, and after administration. The patient should be instructed to void frequently. Scheduled doses of mesna should always be administered with ifosfamide to prevent or lessen the severity of bladder toxicity.[3,9,17,19,23,35-37,43-45]

Cisplatin. Cisplatin (cis-diamminedichloroplatinum, platinum, CDDP, DDP, Platinol) is a heavy metal that is cell-cycle nonspecific and that inhibits DNA synthesis. It is indicated in the treatment of testicular, ovarian, bladder, head, neck, non–small cell lung, small cell lung, esophageal, cervical, breast, gastric, thyroid, and neurologic cancers, as well as in Hodgkin's and non-Hodgkin's lymphoma, sarcomas, melanoma, and advanced prostatic carcinoma.

Antiemetics should be administered before infusion because nausea and vomiting are usually severe, starting 1 to 4 hours after infusion and lasting up to 5 days. Persistent anorexia and taste alterations often occur. Myelosuppression is dose dependent, with a nadir of 18 to 23 days. Ototoxicity occurs in 31% of patients and is usually manifested by tinnitus and high-frequency hearing loss. Peripheral neuropathy occurs and has a cumulative effect. Although rare, anaphylactic reactions have occurred within minutes of the start of the infusion.

Renal toxicity is common, severe, and dose dependent. Vigorous hydration before and after treatment is necessary, with mannitol or furosemide given to maintain output. Renal function should be monitored during treatment.

Amifostine (Ethyol) reduces the toxic effects of cisplatin and protects the renal cells without interfering with the action of cisplatin. The most common adverse effects of this cytoprotectant are transient hypertension, nausea, and vomiting, which can be severe. The patient should be well hydrated before administration and should not be hypotensive or receiving antihypertensive therapy within 24 hours of administration. A baseline blood pressure should be taken, with blood pressure monitoring every 5 minutes. The drug is given intravenously for no more than 15 minutes with the patient in a supine position. Potassium and magnesium are usually added to the prehydration fluids to prevent hypokalemia and hypomagnesemia.

Cisplatin reacts chemically with aluminum and forms a precipitate, so only stainless steel needles should be used in preparation and administration.[3,9,14,17,19,23,35-37,43,46]

Carboplatin. Carboplatin (Paraplatin) is an analog of cisplatin. It is not cell-cycle specific. Its method of action is thought to be cross-linking of DNA strands. Carboplatin is indicated in the treatment of advanced ovarian cancer, endometrial carcinoma, non–small cell lung cancer, metastatic seminomas, recurrent brain tumors in children, relapsed and refractory acute leukemia, and head and neck cancers.

Nausea and vomiting can be moderate to severe and lasts about 24 hours. Mild anorexia and taste changes may occur. Myelosuppression is severe and dose related, with a nadir of 14 to 21 days. Hypersensitivity reactions are common and can occur within minutes of administration. Epinephrine, corticosteroids, and antihistamines must be available. Cardiac failure,

embolism, and cerebrovascular accident have been reported. Alopecia occurs in about 50% of patients.

Needles or IV administration sets containing aluminum should not be used because aluminum reacts with carboplatin, causing precipitate formation and loss of potency.

Carboplatin is contraindicated in patients with a history of allergies to cisplatin, platinum-containing compounds, or mannitol, as well as in those with severe bone marrow depression or bleeding. The patient should be instructed to avoid using products containing aspirin.[3,9,17,19,23,35-37]

Thiotepa. Thiotepa (triethylene-thiophosphoramide, TESPA, Thioplex) is cell-cycle nonspecific and causes cross-linking of DNA. Thiotepa is indicated in the treatment of breast and ovarian cancer, Hodgkin's disease, chronic granulocytic and lymphocytic leukemia, bronchogenic carcinoma, and superficial bladder cancer.

Nausea and vomiting are dose dependent. Myelosuppression is the dose-limiting toxic effect. The nadir is 7 to 10 days but can be as long as 28 days for thrombocytopenia. The patient should be instructed to avoid use of aspirin-containing products. Allergic reactions with hives, rash, and bronchospasm have been reported. The patient may experience pain at the IV site, which may be relieved by diluting the drug, slowing the infusion, or placing an ice pack above the site.[3,9,17,19,23,35-37]

Nitrosoureas. The nitrosoureas are lipid-soluble alkylating agents, most of which can cross the blood-brain barrier because of their lipid solubility. They interfere with DNA replication and repair and are cell-cycle nonspecific. Their major toxicities are hematopoietic and gastrointestinal.[1,3,5,10]

Carmustine. Carmustine (BiCNU, BCNU) is a nitrosourea that acts as an alkylating agent by interfering with DNA and RNA synthesis through alkylation. It is cell-cycle nonspecific and is indicated in the treatment of brain tumors, Hodgkin's disease, non-Hodgkin's lymphoma, and malignant melanoma.

Severe nausea and vomiting may occur 1 to 2 hours after infusion and last 6 to 8 hours. Stomatitis is common. Cumulative bone marrow suppression, which is delayed 4 to 6 weeks, is the major dose-limiting toxicity. Concomitant use of cimetidine is avoided because it may increase bone marrow toxicity. Pulmonary fibrosis has been reported with cumulative doses and may be progressive and fatal. Delayed onset has occurred from 9 days to 15 years after treatment. Nephrotoxicity progressing to renal failure and reversible hepatotoxicity have been reported.

Carmustine is an irritant causing intense pain at the infusion site. To decrease pain, the infusion can be slowed and ice placed above the IV site. Contact with skin causes brown staining.[3,9,17,19,23,35-37]

Streptozocin. Streptozocin (Zanosar, streptozotocin) is a cell-cycle nonspecific drug that inhibits DNA synthesis through cross-linking. It is indicated in the treatment of insulinomas, carcinoid tumors, non–small cell lung and colon cancers, hepatoma, and squamous cell carcinoma of the oral cavity.

Renal toxicity, which is severe and often fatal, is dose related and cumulative. Proteinuria is an early sign of nephrotoxicity. Renal function should be evaluated before and after treatment. In patients with preexisting renal disease, the potential benefit of streptozocin must be weighed against the risk of further renal damage. The use of other nephrotoxic drugs, such as the aminoglycosides, should be avoided. Liver dysfunction and hypoglycemia caused by sudden insulin release have been reported. Myelosuppression is mild, with a nadir of 1 to 2 weeks. Severe nausea and vomiting is common, particularly with daily treatments.

Streptozocin is an irritant and commonly causes pain and burning at the IV site. Slowing the infusion, diluting the concentration of the drug, and applying ice above the site may decrease the symptoms.[1,3,9,17,19,23,35-37]

Antitumor antibiotics

Although the antitumor antibiotics have some antiinfective qualities, their major action is cytotoxic. They interfere with nucleic acid synthesis and inhibit RNA synthesis by intercalation. They react with or bind to DNA and therefore inhibit DNA synthesis. Most are cell-cycle nonspecific. Their major toxicities are cardiac, hematopoietic, gastrointestinal, and reproductive. All of the antibiotics except bleomycin are vesicants.

The largest category of the antibiotics is the anthracyclines, including doxorubicin, dactinomycin, daunorubicin, mitoxantrone, and idarubicin. In addition to myelosuppression, the anthracyclines can cause alopecia, nausea, vomiting, and stomatitis.[1,3,5,10]

Doxorubicin HCl. Doxorubicin hydrochloride (Adriamycin, Rubex) inhibits DNA and RNA synthesis and is cell-cycle nonspecific. It is indicated in the treatment of acute lymphoblastic and myeloblastic leukemia, soft-tissue and bone sarcomas, neuroblastoma, Wilms' tumor, Hodgkin's and non-Hodgkin's lymphoma, and breast, bladder, thyroid, lung, gastric, and ovarian cancers.

Cardiotoxicity is the major dose-limiting toxicity, presenting as arrhythmias (which can be life-threatening), left ventricular heart failure, and irreversible cardiomyopathy. An electrocardiogram should be obtained as a baseline before administering doxorubicin, and cardiac function should be monitored periodically throughout the course of treatments.

Myelosuppression is severe, with a nadir of 10 to 14 days. Severe nausea and vomiting are dose dependent and occur 1 to 2 hours after the start of therapy. Common side effects are stomatitis, photosensitivity, radiation recall, hyperpigmentation, and flare reaction. Complete alopecia occurs in 3 to 4 weeks. The patient should be informed that the urine turns red-orange for 1 to 2 days.

The recommended lifetime cumulative dose is 550 mg/m^2. Doxorubicin is physically incompatible in the same line with 5-fluorouracil and heparin. It is recommended that continuous infusions be administered via central line because of the severe vesicant potential of doxorubicin. This drug causes very severe tissue damage and necrosis if extravasated.[3,9,17,19,23,35-37]

Idarubicin HCl. Idarubicin hydrochloride (Idamycin) is a synthetic anthracycline. It is cell-cycle specific for the S phase and acts by inhibiting DNA synthesis. It is indicated in the treatment of acute myeloid leukemia, chronic myelogenous leukemia, and acute lymphocytic leukemia.

Cardiotoxicity is the dose-limiting toxicity and can be fatal. Baseline cardiac function should be determined before the initial treatment and monitored throughout the course of treatment. Congestive heart failure, myocardial infarction, arrhythmias, electrocardiogram changes, and cardiomyopathy may occur. The maximum safe dose is unknown. Risk increases with preexisting cardiac conditions, radiation to the mediastinal area, and prior treatment with anthracyclines.

Myelosuppression is severe and dose related, with a nadir of 10 to 14 days. Other common side effects are severe nausea and vomiting, cramps, diarrhea, and mucositis. Although rare, severe enterocolitis with perforation has occurred. Alopecia, generalized rash, urticaria, and bulbous erythrodermatous rash on the palms and soles are common. Radiation recall and flare reaction may occur.

The patient should be informed that the urine may be red for several days. Idarubicin is a vesicant capable of severe tissue necrosis if extravasated. Idarubicin should not be mixed with heparin in an IV tubing or central access device as the drug will precipitate.[3,9,17,19,23,35-37]

Dactinomycin. Dactinomycin (actinomycin D, Cosmegen) is cell-cycle nonspecific and inhibits DNA replication and RNA synthesis. It is indicated in the treatment of Wilms' tumor, rhabdomyosarcoma, carcinoma of the testes and uterus, Ewing's sarcoma, gestational choriocarcinoma, and melanoma.

Nausea and vomiting are severe and usually occur within the first 1 to 2 hours after the start of treatment. Other common adverse reactions are anorexia, diarrhea, erythema, alopecia, and radiation recall. Myelosuppression is severe, with a nadir of about 10 days. Hepatotoxicity and anaphylaxis may occur. Dactinomycin is contraindicated in patients with existing or recent exposure to chicken pox or herpes zoster because death may occur.

Dactinomycin is a vesicant that can cause severe tissue necrosis if extravasated.[3,9,17,19,23,35-37]

Mitoxantrone. Mitoxantrone (Novantrone, DHAD) is similar to the anthracyclines daunorubicin and doxorubicin. It is probably cell-cycle nonspecific and exerts its antitumor effect by interfering with DNA and RNA synthesis. It is indicated in combination therapy in acute and chronic leukemias, advanced or recurrent breast cancer, ovarian cancer, and advanced hormone-refractory prostate cancer pain.

Myelosuppression is the dose-limiting toxicity, with a nadir of 10 to 14 days. Common adverse effects are mild nausea and vomiting, mucositis, diarrhea, abdominal pain, headache, fever, rash, dyspnea, and alopecia. Seizures, heart failure, arrhythmias, and a decrease in left ventricular ejection fraction have been reported. Cardiac toxicity may be more common in patients with a history of heart disease, radiation to the mediastinum, or prior anthracycline therapy. Hydration before and after administration is necessary to prevent uric acid nephropathy. Mitoxantrone will turn the urine blue-green within 24 hours and may cause a bluish discoloration of the sclera.

Mitoxantrone is an irritant with vesicant potential. If extravasation occurs, ulceration is rare unless a concentrated dose infiltrates. The skin in the involved area will turn blue.

Mitoxantrone is incompatible in the same tubing with heparin.[3,9,17,19,23,35-37]

Daunorubin HCl. Daunoruban hydrochloride (Daunomycin hydrochloride, Cerubidine) interferes with DNA synthesis and is cell-cycle nonspecific. It is indicated for the remission induction in acute nonlymphocytic and lymphocytic leukemia.

Chronic cardiotoxicity is dose related and presents as congestive heart failure, with a mortality rate of 50%. Acute cardiotoxicity may occur within minutes of administration and presents as supraventricular arrhythmias. Preexisting cardiac disease or exposure to other anthracyclines or cardiotoxic drugs increases the risk for cardiotoxicity. The recommended cumulative lifetime dose is 500 to 600 mg/m^2.

Bone marrow suppression occurs, with a nadir of 10 to 14 days. Common side effects are mild to moderate nausea and vomiting, diarrhea, mucositis, hepatotoxicity, complete alopecia (3 to 4 weeks), radiation recall, flare reaction, and photosensitivity. Extravasation will cause severe soft-tissue necrosis. Mixing daunorubicin hydrochloride with dexamethasone or heparin in the same line will result in precipitation.[3,9,17,19,23,35-37]

Mitomycin. Mitomycin (mitomycin-C, Mutamycin) inhibits DNA and RNA synthesis and is cell-cycle nonspecific. It is indicated in the treatment of adenocarcinoma of the stomach, pancreas, and colon and in advanced breast, non–small cell lung, ovarian, uterine, cervical, head, and neck cancers.

Myelosuppression is delayed 4 to 8 weeks and is cumulative. Mild nausea and vomiting may occur within 30 to 60 minutes and last up to 3 days. Anorexia, diarrhea, alopecia, purple bands on the nails, and pain at the infusion site are common. Interstitial pneumonitis may occur, with a nonproductive cough and fever as the presenting symptoms. When administered with vinca alkaloids, mitomycin may cause acute respiratory distress.

Mitomycin is a vesicant, and extravasation should be avoided.[3,9,17,19,23,35-37]

Bleomycin sulfate. Bleomycin sulfate (Blenoxane) is cell-cycle specific in the G$_2$ phase and inhibits DNA synthesis. It is indicated in the treatment of testicular carcinoma, lymphoma, malignant pleural effusions, and squamous cell carcinoma of the head, neck, skin, cervix, vulva, and penis.

The most significant toxicity of bleomycin is pulmonary. The earliest symptoms are dyspnea and rales, followed by pneumonitis and progressing to pulmonary fibrosis. This occurs in about 10% of patients and is fatal in 1%. Increased risk includes age older than 70 years, total cumulative dosage greater than 400 units, previous lung disease, history of radiation to the thoracic area, and concomitant use with other antineoplastics, especially methotrexate. Respiratory effort and lung sounds should be monitored frequently.

Nausea, vomiting, anorexia, and stomatitis are common but mild. Myelosuppression, if it occurs, is mild, with a nadir of 10 days. Febrile reactions, which may be delayed for 3 to 6 hours, are very common, especially in patients with lymphoma. Premedicating with diphenhydramine and acetaminophen may lessen the fever and chills. Hyperpigmentation, photosensitivity, nail changes, erythema, rash, skin tenderness, and alopecia occur in nearly half the patients. A test dose of 1 to 2 units is recommended because anaphylaxis may occur, especially in patients with lymphoma.

Bleomycin is the only antitumor antibiotic that is not a vesicant.[3,9,17,19,23,35-37]

Liposomal anthracyclines

Daunorubicin citrate liposome (DaunoXome) and doxorubicin hydrochloride liposome (Doxil) are two traditional drugs encapsulated with a polyethylene coating that allows the drug to evade detection by the immune system, thereby increasing the amount of drug reaching the tumor cell. The benefits of this new drug delivery system are increased circulation time, decreased side effects, and the ability to penetrate altered vasculature. Toxicities are similar to daunorubicin and doxorubicin but are less severe. They do not discolor the urine, and alopecia, nausea, and vomiting are rare. Their most common side effects are myelosuppression, cardiac events, stomatitis, skin reactions (e.g., hand-foot syndrome), and hypersensitivity reactions. Mild to moderate cardiac events may occur, presenting as chest pain, palpitations, and tachycardia. Allergic reactions have been reported (7%) in the first 5 minutes, with presenting symptoms of back pain, facial flushing, chest tightness, headache, chills, or hypotension.

Doxil and DaunoXome are approved for use in the treatment of advanced human immunodeficiency virus (HIV)-related Kaposi's sarcoma. Clinical trials are under way for treatment of other cancers, as single agents and in combination with other antineoplastics.

Doxil and DaunoXome should never be administered through an in-line filter because this will rupture the encapsulating coating. Liposomal anthracyclines are classed as irritants, not vesicants.

Extravasations should be treated by applying ice. Although maximum lifetime dosage does not appear to be a factor, a baseline cardiac assessment should be done before treatment. Neither drug should be mixed with saline, bacteriostatic agents (benzyl alcohol), or any other solution.[9,17,19,23,35-37,47,48]

Miscellaneous drugs

Asparaginase. Asparaginase (l-asparaginase, Elspar) is an enzyme that destroys asparagine, an amino acid necessary for protein synthesis. It is indicated in the treatment of acute lymphocytic leukemia and acute and chronic myelocytic leukemia.

Nausea and vomiting are mild but common. Mild bone marrow suppression occurs, with a nadir of 7 to 10 days. Prolongation of clotting factors may occur, and disseminated intravascular coagulation may develop. Renal failure, hepatotoxicity, hemorrhagic pancreatitis, fatal hyperthermia, depression, fatigue, coma, confusion, and death have been reported.

Hypersensitivity reactions are common. Intradermal skin testing with 2 IU of asparaginase is recommended before the first dose and should be repeated if doses are 7 days or more apart. The chance of a reaction increases with repeated doses and is more likely to occur in adults than in children. The site should be observed for at least 1 hour. A wheal indicates a positive response and is a contraindication to therapy.[3,9,17,19,23,35-37]

Docetaxel. Docetaxel (Taxotere) inhibits cancer cell growth by preventing cellular mitosis. It is indicated in the treatment of locally advanced or metastatic breast cancer that progressed during or after treatment with first-line antineoplastics.

Bone marrow suppression is the most common and dose-limiting toxicity, with a nadir of 7 days. Other common adverse reactions are mild to moderate nausea and vomiting, stomatitis, diarrhea, weakness, fluid retention, alopecia (80%), and severe hypersensitivity reactions. All patients should be premedicated with corticosteroids before and during administration of docetaxel to reduce the incidence and severity of fluid retention and hypersensitivity reactions. Docetaxel is contraindicated in patients with a known allergy to polysorbate 80, a sorbitol ester used in drug manufacture.[3,9,17,19,23,25,35-37,49,50]

Denileukin diftitox. Denileukin diftitox (ONTAK) is a cytotoxic protein that interacts with the IL-2 receptor on the malignant cell surface and inhibits cellular protein synthesis, resulting in cell death. Clinical studies have shown an overall response rate of 38% in the treatment of persistent or recurrent T-cell lymphoma whose malignant cells express the CD25 component of the IL-2 receptor. Acute hypersensitivity reactions are common (69%) and present primarily as hypotension, back pain, dyspnea, vasodilation, rash, chest pain, and tachycardia. Antihistamines, corticosteroids, epinephrine, and resuscitative equipment should be available during administration.

The dose-limiting toxicities are nausea and vomiting (64%), a flulike syndrome involving fever (81%), asthenia (66%), and digestive problems. In the clinical trials, 83% of patients experienced moderate to severe hypoalbuminemia 7 to 14 days after administration. Clinical trials also demonstrated that 27% of patients experienced vascular leak syndrome characterized by hypotension, edema, and hypoalbuminemia. The onset of symptoms was delayed; the syndrome appeared self-limited and did not require treatment. Weight, edema, blood pressure, and serum albumin levels should be monitored between treatments.

Because of the risk of absorption, denileukin diftitox must not be prepared or administered in a glass container or given through an in-line filter.[35-37,51]

Topoisomerase I inhibitors

Topoisomerase I inhibitors are a new class of semisynthetic antineoplastic agents extracted from the Chinese tree *Campotheca acuminator*. Topotecan and irinotecan are currently the only drugs approved for use.[1,3,5,9,52]

Irinotecan HCl. Irinotecan hydrochloride (Camptosar) is a topoisomerase I inhibitor that prevents the production of the enzyme topoisomerase I, which is necessary to DNA replication. It is indicated in the treatment of metastatic carcinoma of the colon or rectum that has reoccurred or progressed after 5-fluorouracil therapy.

Irinotecan hydrochloride can cause severe diarrhea, acute (within 24 hours) or late onset (3 to 11 days after treatment). Severe sweating and orthostatic hypotension may occur. The patient's fluid status and serum electrolytes must be monitored to prevent dehydration and electrolyte imbalances, which can be life-threatening. The patient should be informed about the potential for severe diarrhea and instructed to avoid use of laxatives.

Myelosuppression is severe, with a nadir of 14 to 21 days. Other common side effects are nausea, vomiting, anorexia, abdominal enlargement, flatulence, constipation, flushing, shortness of breath, and alopecia. Insomnia, dizziness, headache, back pain, and muscular weakness are common CNS side effects.

Irinotecan hydrochloride is an irritant and should not be allowed to come into contact with skin. If contact does occur, the skin should be washed thoroughly with soap and water. If extravasation occurs, the infusion should be stopped immediately, the site flushed with sterile water, ice applied, and the physician notified.[3,9,17,19,23,35-37,52-54]

Topotecan HCl. Topotecan hydrochloride (Hycamtin) is a topoisomerase I inhibitor that prevents the production of the enzyme topoisomerase I, which is essential to DNA replication. It is indicated in the treatment of metastatic carcinoma of the ovary after failure of initial or subsequent chemotherapy and small cell lung cancer after failure of first-line chemotherapy. Bone marrow suppression, primarily neutropenia, is the dose-limiting toxicity, with a nadir of 11 to 15 days. The severity of myelosuppression may be increased if topotecan is administered in combination with cisplatin. The use of a granulocyte CSF may be indicated in severe neutropenia.

Common adverse reactions are mild to moderate nausea and vomiting, stomatitis, anorexia, abdominal pain, diarrhea, constipation, dyspnea, fever, and fatigue. Headache is the most commonly reported CNS toxicity. Most patients will experience at least some alopecia, with about 30% having total alopecia.[17,19,35-37,52]

CHEMOTHERAPY ADMINISTRATION CONSIDERATIONS

Because of the caustic properties of many chemotherapeutic agents and their potential for severe complications (Table 13-1), much consideration needs to be given to the venous access. Small peripheral veins with low blood flow cause higher concentration of drugs than larger veins with rapid flow. Even though the vessels in the antecubital fossa are large and venipuncture is easily accomplished, it should be avoided. Because it is such a common site of venipuncture for blood draws, if there is an extravasation, the local damage is severe.

The recommended peripheral administration site is the proximal forearm over muscle bulk. The dorsum of the hand is discouraged because of the scant amount of tissue surrounding the area, so there is less tissue for solution absorption. The guiding principle for selecting a site is to choose an area that offers the best protection to tendons and nerves and results in the least loss of function if an extravasation occurs.

The safest way to determine vein integrity is always to use a newly established venipuncture. Only a site that provides a good blood return should be used. A site in which there was difficulty threading the catheter should not be used. If a venipuncture is unsuccessful, a second attempt should be made in the opposite arm. If it is necessary to use the same arm, a different vein at a site proximal to the first venipuncture is used. The choice of catheter and site depend on the expertise and dexterity of the nurse and the condition of the veins in each patient.

Chemotherapy administration using the sidearm method with a free-flowing IV is preferred over a straight push. This method provides the greatest margin of safety and allows frequent checks on vein integrity.

Central venous access decreases the chance of phlebitis, and the increased blood flow results in an increased and more rapid dilution of the drug. Central lines contribute their own set of

Text continued on p. 273

Table 13-1   Common and Life-Threatening Side Effects of Chemotherapeutic Agents

Drug (Chemical Name, Trade Name, Class)	Nadir	Hematologic	Gastrointestinal	Dermatologic	Other Systems	Vesicant/ Irritant	Special Considerations
Asparaginase Elspar Miscellaneous	7-10 days	Anemia, leukopenia, prolonged clotting factors	Mild nausea/vomiting	Allergic/anaphylactic reactions	Renal failure, hepatotoxicity, hemorrhagic pancreatitis, fatal hyperthermia, coma		■ Intradermal skin testing recommended before first dose ■ Chance of anaphylactic reaction increases with each dose ■ Reactions more common in adults than in children
Bleomycin Blenoxane Antitumor antibiotic	10 days	0 → mild myelosuppression	Mild nausea/vomiting	Rashes, hyper-pigmentation, nail changes, alopecia 47%, photosensitivity	Fever/chills, pneumonitis, pulmonary fibrosis		■ Baseline chest radiograph ■ Pulmonary toxicity higher in patients >70 yr ■ Test dose before first 2 doses ■ Lifetime cumulative dose limit 400 units or 220 U/m^2
Carboplatin Paraplatin Alkylating	14-21 days	Severe myelosuppression	30%-60% moderate to severe nausea/ vomiting, mild anorexia, taste changes	Alopecia 50%	Anaphylaxis, cardiac failure, embolism, cerebrovascular accident	I	■ Steel needles only; reacts with aluminum ■ Premedicate with antiemetics ■ Instruct patient to avoid aspirin
Carmustine BCNU Alkylating	4-6 wk	Delayed cumulative myelosuppression	60%-90% severe nausea/vomiting, stomatitis	Intense pain at injection site	Nephrotoxicity, hepatotoxicity, pulmonary fibrosis	I	■ Premedicate with antiemetics ■ Intense pain at infusion site: slow infusion; place ice above site ■ Stains skin brown on contact
Cisplatin Platinol Alkylating	18-23 days	Myelosuppression dose dependent	>90% severe nausea/vomiting, taste changes		Ototoxicity, cumulative peripheral neuropathy, renal toxicity	V/I	■ Vesicant if >20 ml of 0.5 mg/ml extravasated ■ Vigorous hydration before and after treatment ■ Reacts with aluminum; only use stainless steel needles ■ KCl and magnesium should be added to IV fluids
Cyclophosphamide Cytoxan Alkylating	8-14 days	Dose-dependent myelosuppression, thrombocytopenia with high dosages	60%-90% nausea/ vomiting	Alopecia 50%	Hemorrhagic cystitis, pulmonary fibrosis, cardio-toxicity with high dosages, hyper-sensitivity reactions	I	■ Vigorous hydration before and after treatment ■ Patient should void frequently ■ Cardiotoxicity may occur when combined with doxorubicin ■ Rapid infusions increase nausea/vomiting

Continued

Data from References 1, 3, 9, 17, 19, 23, 25, 35-39, 41, 42, 45, and 47-55.
IV, Intravenous; *NSAIDs,* nonsteroidal antiinflammatory drugs.

Table 13-1   Common and Life-Threatening Side Effects of Chemotherapeutic Agents—cont'd

Drug (Chemical Name, Trade Name, Class)	Nadir	Hematologic	Gastrointestinal	Dermatologic	Other Systems	Vesicant/ Irritant	Special Considerations
Cytarabine Ara-C Antimetabolite	7-9 days, second nadir 15-24 days	Dose-limiting myelosuppression	30%-60% severe nausea/vomiting, anorexia, diarrhea, stomatitis	Alopecia, rashes, hand-foot syndrome	Tumor lysis syndrome, conjunctivitis		▪ Corticosteroid eyedrops prevent conjunctivitis ▪ Rapid infusions increase nausea/vomiting ▪ Incompatible with 5-fluorouracil and heparin
Dacarbazine DTIC-DOME Alkylating	7-14 days	Myelosuppression	90% nausea/vomiting, metallic taste	Photosensitivity, pruritus, erythema, pain at infusion site	Flulike syndrome	V/I	▪ Incompatible in same tubing with heparin ▪ Diluting drug, slowing infusion and ice above site may help pain
Dactinomycin Cosmegen Antitumor antibiotic	10 days	Severe myelosuppression	>90% nausea/ vomiting, severe anorexia, diarrhea	Alopecia 47%, radiation recall, erythema	Hepatotoxicity, anaphylaxis	V	▪ Contraindicated in patients with exposure to chickenpox or herpes zoster
Daunorubicin HCl Cerubidine Antitumor antibiotic	10-14 days	Myelosuppression	Nausea/vomiting mild to moderate, diarrhea, mucositis	Alopecia 90%, photosensitivity, flare reaction, radiation recall	Cardiotoxicity	V	▪ Do not mix with heparin or dexamethasone in the same line ▪ Cumulative lifetime dose is 500-600 mg/m^2 ▪ Chronic cardiotoxicity presents as congestive heart failure ▪ Acute cardiotoxicity presents as superventricular arrhythmias
Daunorubicin citrate liposome DaunoXome Liposomal anthracycline	May be same as above	Myelosuppression, stomatitis	Nausea/vomiting (rare)	Alopecia (rare), hand-foot syndrome	Allergic reactions, tachycardia, palpitations, chest pain	I	▪ Do not filter ▪ Do not mix with saline, bacteriostatic agents or any other solution
Denileukin diftitox ONTAK Miscellaneous		None to very mild myelosuppression	Nausea/vomiting	Rash	Acute hypersensitivity reactions, flulike syndrome, hypoalbuminemia, vascular leak syndrome		▪ Do not prepare or administer in a glass container ▪ Do not filter ▪ Premedicate ▪ Have crash cart available ▪ Monitor weight, edema, blood pressure and serum albumin between doses
Docetaxel Taxotere Miscellaneous	7 days	Myelosuppression	Mild to moderate nausea/vomiting, stomatitis, diarrhea	Alopecia 80%	Weakness, fluid retention, severe hypersensitivity reactions		▪ Premedicate with corticosteroids ▪ Contraindicated in patients with a known allergy to polysorbate 80

Drug	Nadir (days)	Myelosuppression	Nausea/Vomiting	Alopecia/Skin	Cardiotoxicity/Other	Vesicant	Special considerations
Doxorubicin HCl / Adriamycin / Antitumor antibiotic	10-14 days	Myelosuppression; severity dose related	Severe nausea/vomiting dose related	Alopecia 90%-100%, flare reaction, radiation recall	Cardiotoxicity	V severe	■ Baseline cardiac assessment ■ Must have careful cardiac monitoring ■ Cumulative lifetime dose 550 mg/m² ■ Red-colored urine for 1-2 days ■ Do not mix in same line with heparin or 5-fluorouracil
Doxorubicin hydrochloride liposome / Doxil / Liposomal anthracycline	May be same as above	Myelosuppression, stomatitis	Nausea/vomiting (rare)	Alopecia (rare), hand-foot syndrome	Allergic reactions, tachycardia, palpitations, chest pain	—	■ *Do not filter* ■ Does not discolor urine ■ *Do not shake* ■ Do not mix with saline, bacteriostatic agents, or any other solution
Etoposide / Vepesid / Plant alkaloid	7-14 days	Myelosuppression	Mild to moderate nausea/vomiting, anorexia, diarrhea, metallic aftertaste	Alopecia 66%, radiation	Anaphylactic reactions	—	■ Severe hypotension occurs if infused too rapidly ■ Baseline blood pressure for all doses ■ First dose: baseline blood pressure and monitor every 15 min ■ Anaphylactic reactions more common with first dose ■ Crash cart available
Floxuridine / FUDR / Antimetabolite		Mild myelosuppression	Nausea/vomiting, anorexia, abdominal pain, stomatitis, diarrhea	Alopecia, dermatitis, hyperpigmentation, photosensitivity			■ Administered intra-arterially for liver tumors ■ Use sunscreen, hat, long sleeves when outside
Fludarabine / Fludara / Antimetabolite	Day 13, range 3-25 days	Severe myelosuppression	Nausea/vomiting, anorexia, diarrhea, gastrointestinal bleeding	Rash	Confusion, coma, death with higher dosages, fever, chills, fatigue, cardiotoxicity, pulmonary toxicity, tumor lysis syndrome		■ Do not give concurrently with pentostatin, 5-fluorouracil or methotrexate ■ Tumor lysis syndrome presents as flank pain and hematuria

Continued

Table 13-1 Common and Life-Threatening Side Effects of Chemotherapeutic Agents—cont'd

Drug (Chemical Name, Trade Name, Class)	Nadir	Hematologic	Gastrointestinal	Dermatologic	Other Systems	Vesicant/ Irritant	Special Considerations
5-Fluorouracil 5-FU Antimetabolite	7-14 days	Myelosuppression	Nausea/vomiting (dose related), stomatitis, diarrhea, anorexia	Alopecia, photosensitivity, hyperpigmentation, hand-foot syndrome			• Avoid prolonged sun exposure • Use sunscreen SPF ≥15 • Protect drug from light • Premedicate with antiemetic • Diligent oral hygiene
Gemcitabine HCl Gemzar Antimetabolite		Myelosuppression	Nausea/vomiting, diarrhea, stomatitis, constipation	Rashes, alopecia 15%	Fever, flulike symptoms		• Dyspnea and bronchospasm may occur in patients with previous lung conditions
Idarubicin HCl Idamycin Antitumor antibiotic	10-14 days	Severe myelosuppression	Severe nausea/ vomiting, diarrhea, cramps, mucositis	Alopecia, rashes, hand-foot syndrome, radiation recall, flare reaction	Dose-limiting cardiotoxicity (severe to fatal)	V	• Baseline cardiac function and assess throughout treatments • Incompatible with heparin • Red-colored urine
Ifosfamide Ifex Alkylating	10-14 days	Myelosuppression	Nausea/vomiting 50%	Alopecia 83%	Somnolence, hemorrhagic cystitis, confusion, coma, seizures	I	• Vigorous pretreatment hydration • Uroprotector (Mesna) recommended • Patient should void frequently
Irinotecan HCl Camptosar Topoisomerase I inhibitor	14-21 days	Severe myelosuppression	Severe diarrhea: acute or late onset; nausea/vomiting, anorexia, flatulence, abdominal enlargement, constipation	Alopecia	Severe sweating, flushing, insomnia, dizziness, headache, back pain, muscle weakness, orthostatic hypotension	I	• Strict intake and output • Frequent checks of electrolyte balances • Warn patient, no laxatives • Contact irritant; wear gloves to administer
Mechlorethamine HCl (nitrogen mustard) Mustargen Alkylating	6-14 days	Myelosuppression	Immediate, severe nausea/vomiting, anorexia, diarrhea, metallic taste	Alopecia (thinning)	Delayed menses	V severe	• Very unstable; infuse over 3 minutes and within 15 min of preparation • Avoid skin contact • Premedicate with antiemetics
Methotrexate Folex Antimetabolite	5-14 days	Myelosuppression	Stomatitis, esophagitis (dose related may be severe), nausea/vomiting, anorexia, gastrointestinal ulceration and bleeding	Photosensitivity, alopecia, rashes	Pneumonitis, sudden death, hepatotoxicity		• Incompatible with 5-fluorouracil, asparaginase, and vincristine • Warn patient against use of aspirin, NSAIDs, folic acid preparations, vaccines, and alcohol • Use sunscreen • Leucovorin must be given on time

Drug	Nadir	Myelosuppression	GI effects	Skin/other	Other toxicities	Route	Nursing considerations
Mitomycin Mutamycin Antitumor antibiotic	4-8 wk	Myelosuppression (delayed and cumulative)	Mild nausea/vomiting <30 min, after treatment, anorexia, diarrhea	Alopecia, purple bands on nails, pain at IV site	Interstitial pneumonitis	V	▪ May cause respiratory distress if given with vinca alkaloids
Mitoxantrone Novantrone Antitumor antibiotic	10-14 days	Myelosuppression	Nausea/vomiting, mucositis, diarrhea, abdominal pain	Alopecia, rash	Dyspnea, headache, seizures, cardiotoxicity	IV	▪ Vesicant potential increases with dose concentration ▪ Incompatible with heparin ▪ Blue-green urine ▪ Bluish discoloration of sclera ▪ Hydrate before and after treatment
Paclitaxel Taxol Vinca alkaloid	14 days	Dose-related myelosuppression	Nausea/vomiting, mucositis, diarrhea	Flushing, rashes, alopecia 80%	Peripheral neuropathy, hypersensitivity reactions, tachycardia, dyspnea, hypotension, arrhythmias	V	▪ If given with cisplatin, paclitaxel must be given first ▪ Prepare in glass container only ▪ Must use polyethylene lined tubing and 0.2-micron filter ▪ Premedicate ▪ Baseline electrocardiogram ▪ Depression and nervousness are common
Pentostatin Nipent Antimetabolite	15 days	Severe myelosuppression	Nausea/vomiting, stomatitis, abdominal pain, diarrhea	Rashes	Pulmonary toxicity, infections, hypersensitivity reactions, coma, cardiotoxicity fatigue, headache	I	
Streptozocin Zanosar Alkylating	1-2 wk	Mild myelosuppression	Severe nausea/vomiting	Pain at IV site	Renal toxicity (severe and often fatal), hepatotoxicity	I	▪ Baseline renal function studies before treatment ▪ Slowing infusion, dilution of drug and ice above IV site may help infusion pain
Thiotepa Thioplex Alkylating	7-10 days	Myelosuppression	Nausea/vomiting (dose dependent)	Alopecia, pain at IV site	Allergic reactions	I	▪ Advise patients not to use aspirin products ▪ Dilute drug further, slow infusion or place ice above IV site for pain at IV site
Topotecan HCl Hycamtin Topoisomerase I inhibitor	11-15 days	Myelosuppression	Nausea/vomiting, stomatitis, anorexia, abdominal pain, diarrhea, constipation	Alopecia 30%	Dyspnea, fever, fatigue, headache	I	▪ Severe myelosuppression if given in combination with cisplatin

Continued

Table 13-1 Common and Life-Threatening Side Effects of Chemotherapeutic Agents—cont'd

Drug (Chemical Name, Trade Name, Class)	Nadir	Hematologic	Gastrointestinal	Dermatologic	Other Systems	Vesicant/ Irritant	Special Considerations
Vinblastine Velban Vinca alkaloid	5-10 days	Myelosuppression	Mild nausea/vomiting, constipation	Alopecia	Neurotoxicity Jaw pain Loss of deep tendon reflexes Peripheral neuropathy	V severe	▪ Prophylactic stool softener ▪ Watch for foot drop and difficulty with buttons ▪ Recommended 7 days between doses ▪ Bronchospasm with dyspnea if receiving mitomycin
Vincristine Oncovin Vinca alkaloid	10-14 days	Mild myelosuppression	Mild nausea/vomiting, constipation	Alopecia	Neurotoxicity, jaw pain, loss of deep tendon reflexes, peripheral neuropathy	V severe	▪ Prophylactic stool softener ▪ Watch for foot drop, difficulty walking, fastening buttons ▪ Maximum dose at one administration is 2 mg ▪ Doses should be 7 days apart
Vinorelbine Navelbine Vinca alkaloid	7-10 days	Myelosuppression	Nausea/vomiting, stomatitis, anorexia, diarrhea	Alopecia	Fatigue, neuro-toxicity, jaw pain, loss of deep tendon reflexes, peripheral neuropathy	V severe	▪ Bone marrow suppression may be increased if given with cisplatin ▪ Contact irritant; wear gloves for administration ▪ Bronchospasm and dyspnea may occur if given with mitomycin

potential difficulties, primarily infection and large vein thrombosis.

Use of electronic pumps for chemotherapy administration provides a margin of safety with infusion times; however, the nurse is responsible for monitoring the flow rate and patency of the site. If an electronic pump is used, it should be a nonpressure device.

Continuous monitoring of the site is imperative. Blood return is checked frequently with drip infusions and every 1 to 2 ml when pushing a vesicant or irritant drug. If the patient complains of burning or stinging at the site, the infusion should be discontinued even if the site is unremarkable and a blood return is evident. *The presence of a blood return cannot be totally relied upon because the catheter may have nicked the posterior vein wall causing a slow leakage.*[1,5-7,10]

Biohazard safety

Safety for the patient, nurse, and ancillary staff should not be overlooked. The standard is never to expose the patient, the nurse, or the environment unnecessarily to potentially hazardous substances. Special care in preparing and administering chemotherapeutic agents eliminates accidental exposure from spills and sprays. Unpowdered latex gloves of 0.007- to 0.009-mm thickness should always be worn when handling chemotherapeutic agents. Some experts recommend double-gloving during chemotherapy preparation and changing the gloves every 30 to 60 minutes. The use of gowns and masks is controversial because they may have a negative psychologic effect on the patient; however, the nurse must comply with standard precautions and OSHA (Occupational Safety and Health Administration) guidelines. If there is the possibility of a splash, eye protection should be worn. In the case of an accidental spray of chemotherapeutic agent into the eye, the eye must be flushed with copious amounts of water. Depending on the agent and the degree of eye irritation, steroid drops may be administered.

A vertical laminar flow hood, class II biologic safety cabinet, is imperative for the preparation of chemotherapeutic agents to prevent the release of aerosol spray in the air and potential exposure to toxic substances. Bottles and bags should be spiked and tubing primed in the chemotherapy preparation area before adding the antineoplastic agent. This provides an added safety margin for the nurse when connecting the infusion to the patient. After the infusion has been completed, the tubing should be flushed with saline to eliminate the potential for an accidental spill while disconnecting the tubing. If a chemotherapeutic agent comes in contact with the skin, the area must be thoroughly cleansed with mild soap and large amounts of water.

Inadvertent spills should be cleaned up immediately. Most institutions have a chemotherapy spill kit that contains a sawdustlike substance or an absorbent, plastic-backed sheet to soak up the solution. Spills are cleaned starting from the outside edges and working toward the center. Traffic in the spill area needs to be limited to prevent spread of the contamination. Broken glass is gathered with a disposable scoop. The involved area should be washed with copious amounts of soap and water at least three times. Protective clothing, including a low-permeability gown or cover-up and safety glasses, face shield, or goggles, are to be worn while cleaning a spill of chemotherapeutic agents and disposed of properly.

All contaminated material, such as gloves, tubing, and filters, should be discarded in a double-thick, leak-proof, and sealable plastic bag and labeled as a biohazard. Sharp instruments, including needles, syringes, and ampules, should be placed in a leak-proof, puncture-resistant container and disposed of in accordance with federal, EPA (Environmental Protection Agency), and OSHA regulations. State regulations may vary and have other specific requirements that must be followed.

Many chemotherapy drugs are excreted in the urine and stool. Some studies have shown drug levels in the saliva. The nurse needs to exercise caution when handling sputum, emesis, or excreta from patients receiving chemotherapy. Gloves should always be worn when cleaning an incontinent patient or when emptying a Foley catheter or bedpan. The primary caregiver needs to be aware of and use standard precautions when caring for the patient. Hands should always be washed before applying and after removing gloves.[1,5,9,10,37]

ALTERNATIVE THERAPIES

Alternative therapies are nonconventional therapies not taught in medical school; they are not available in hospitals and are considered outside traditional medicine. These therapies continue to flourish, reflecting the trend toward holistic, self-care medicine. Cancer patients spend more than $5 billion a year on alternative therapies, and most do not inform their physicians. Most of these patients are young adults with above-average income and education.

Practitioners of these therapies exploit the patient's fear and promise painless, nontoxic treatments with good results. A common thread is the theory that all cancers have one cause, hence one cure. Currently, more than 90 alternative therapies are available.

The most popular are metabolic and nutritional therapies, of which the macrobiotic diet is the best known. This natural, preservative-free diet using limited protein may appear healthy, but it could lead to nutritional deficiencies. Food preparation is time-consuming and some foods are expensive and difficult to find.

Other therapies use vitamins and minerals, high colonics, and mind-body control techniques such as imagery, music, and aromatherapy for relaxation. Herbal remedies are popular, but herbal supplements are not standardized and some can be dangerous. Therapeutic touch, acupuncture, acupressure, and chiropractic techniques are common but remain controversial.

Cancer patients are susceptible to claims for miracle cures. When they ask questions about alternative therapies, it is best to be nonjudgmental and to provide factual information so that the patient can make an informed choice.[1,5,56,57]

ONCOLOGY IN THE NEW CENTURY

Cancer prevention and continued new research will be the key issues of this new century. Current literature suggests that 75% of all cancers could be eliminated by changes in lifestyle (e.g., not smoking). Studies show that some cancers are caused or promoted by viruses, others by contact with chemical agents such as tar or hydrocarbons and physical agents such as radiation, asbestos, and ultraviolet light. Other possible carcinogens, such as estrogen therapy, remain controversial.

Age, sex, geographic location, occupation, heredity, diet, stress, and precancerous lesions all affect an individual's chances of getting cancer.

The new century will bring improved selection, dosing, and scheduling of combination antineoplastics, genetic engineering, DNA testing for cancer predisposition, and cancer vaccines. Not only will there be new antineoplastics and drugs to minimize or prevent side effects, but there will be new ways to improve tumor response and cell kill. Hyperthermia, which increases the core temperature of the tumor, will enhance cell kill when combined with chemotherapy. Photodynamic therapy using Photofrin, a light-sensitive drug administered intravenously, enables chemotherapeutic agents to be retained by the cancer cells. Laser light is used to activate the compound and produce cell death. The development of multidrug-resistant modulators such as Valspodar for preventing or delaying the common problem of drug resistance will be a major advance in cancer care.[1,5,58-60]

REFERENCES

1. Itano JK, Taoka KN: *Core curriculum for oncology nursing,* ed 3, Philadelphia, 1998, WB Saunders.
2. Black JM, Matassarin-Jacobs E: *Medical-surgical nursing: clinical management for continuity of care,* ed 5, Philadelphia, 1997, WB Saunders.
3. Lehne RA: *Pharmacology for nursing care,* ed 3, Philadelphia, 1998, WB Saunders.
4. Krozier E, Wilkerson B: *Fundamentals of nursing concepts, process and practice,* ed 5, Menlo Park, Calif, 1998, Addison, Wesley, Longman.
5. McCorkle R, et al: *Cancer Nursing,* ed 2, Philadelphia, 1996, WB Saunders.
6. Smeltzer SC, Bare BG: *Brunner and Suddareth's textbook of medical-surgical nursing,* ed 8, Philadelphia, 1996, Lippincott-Raven.
7. Intravenous Nurses Society: Infusion nursing standards of practice, *JIN* (suppl) 23(6S), 2000.
8. Tucker SM, et al: *Patient care standards: collaborative practice planning guides,* ed 6, St Louis, 1996, Mosby.
9. Berkery R, Cleri LB, Skarin AT: *Oncology pocket guide to chemotherapy,* ed 3, St Louis, 1997, Mosby.
10. Phillips LD: *Manual of I.V. therapeutics,* ed 2, Philadelphia, 1997, FA Davis.
11. Ezzone S, Baker C, Rosselet R, Terepka E: Music as an adjunct to antiemetic therapy, *Oncol Nurs Forum* 25(9):1551, 1998.
12. Anzemet, package insert, 1997, Hoechst Marion Rouse Inc.
13. Zofran, package insert, 1999, GlaxoWellcome Inc.
14. Hawkins R: Amifostine, *Clin J Oncol Nurs* 3(3):128, 1999.
15. Heinemann L, et al: *Clinical management of chemotherapy-induced nausea and vomiting: focus on oral 5-HT3-receptor antagonists,* Springfield, NJ, 1999, Scientific Therapeutics Information.
16. Doherty KM: Closing the gap in prophylactic antimetic therapy: patient factors in calculating the emetogenic potential of chemotherapy, *Clin J Oncol Nurs* 3(3):113, 1999.
17. Doyle RM, et al: *Nursing 99 drug handbook,* Springhouse, Penn, 1999, Springhouse Corp.
18. Neupogen, package insert, 1998 Amgen, Inc.
19. Skidmore RL: *Mosby's drug guide for nurses,* ed 2, St Louis, 1999, Mosby.
20. Frankel C: *Antibody therapies: nursing management considerations,* 1998 Annual Congress–Symposia Highlights, Yardley, Penn, 1998, Medical Association Communications and the Oncology Nursing Society.
21. Neumega, package insert, 1998, Genetics Institute, Inc.
22. Rust DM, Wood LS, Battiato LA: Oprelvekin: an alternative treatment for thrombocytopenia, *Clin J Oncol Nurs* 3(2):57, 1999.
23. Ellerby R, Ault S, Kubli B: *Quick reference handbook of oncology drugs,* Philadelphia, 1996, WB Saunders.
24. Procrit, package insert, 1999, Ortho Biotech Inc.
25. Aikin JL: Docetaxel, *Clin J Oncol Nurs* 2:83, 1999.
26. Abraham JL: *Promoting symptom control in palliative care: seminars in oncology nursing,* Philadelphia, 1998, WB Saunders.
27. Wickham RS, et al: Taste changes experienced by patients receiving chemotherapy, *Oncol Nurs Forum* 26(4):697, 1999.
28. Engelking C: Cancer treatment-related diarrhea: challenges and barriers to clinical practice, *Oncol Nurs Updates* 5(2):1, 1998:
29. O'Rourke ME, Lee C: From research to clinical practice: chemotherapy-associated fatigue, *Clin J Oncol Nurs* 2(4):152, 1998.
30. Rieger PT: Assessing the phenomenon of cancer-related fatigue is an important nursing consideration, *Fatigue Forum Newslett* 3(1): 82, 1999.
31. Vincent L: Clinical assessment of fatigue: where are the essentials? *Fatigue Forum Newslett Oncol Educ Serv* 3(1):1, 1999.
32. Camp-Sorrell D: Surviving the cancer, surviving the treatment: acute cardiac and pulmonary toxicity, *Oncol Nurs Forum* 26(6): 983, 1999.
33. Zinecard, package insert, 1998, Pharmacia & Upjohn.
34. Almadrones L, Armstrong T, Thigpen J: *Assessment and management of chemotherapy-induced neurotoxicities,* 1998 annual congress–Symposia Highlights, Yardley, Penn, 1998, Medical Association Communications and the Oncology Nursing Society.
35. Micromedex, USP DI Editorial Group: *Oncology drug information,* ed 3, Versailles, Ky, 1999-2000, World Color Book Services.
36. *Drug facts and comparisons.* St Louis, 2000, Facts and Comparisons.
37. Editors from the American Society of Health-System Pharmacists, Inc: *American Hospital Formulary Service drug information,* Bethesda, Md, 1999, American Society of Health-System Pharmacists, Inc.
38. Frankel C: *Strategies for the nursing management of gemcitabine for the treatment of pancreatic cancer,* 1998 Annual Congress–Symposia Highlights, Yardley, Penn, 1998, Medical Association Communications and the Oncology Nursing Society.
39. Gemzar, package insert, 1999, Eli Lily & Co.
40. Engulfing C, Berg D, Bushels J: *Treating colorectal cancer,* 1998 Annual Congress–Symposia Highlights, Yardley, Penn, 1998, Medical Association Communications and the Oncology Nursing Society.
41. Taxol, package insert, 1998, Mead Johnson Oncology Products.
42. Boyle DA, Goldspiel BR: A review of paclitaxel [Taxol] administration, stability, and compatibility issues, *Clin J Oncol Nurs* 2(4):141, 1998.
43. Clark JM, et al: *The role of cytoprotection in maximizing therapies, minimizing toxicities,* New York, 1998, Medical Educational Technologies.
44. Mesnex, package insert, 1998, Mead Johnson Oncology Products.
45. Ifex, package insert, 1998, Mead Johnson Oncology Products.
46. Ethyol, package insert, 1999, U.S. Bioscience Inc.
47. Steingass SK: *Liposomal anthracyclines: Doxil and DaunoXome administration guidelines and nursing management,* 1998 Annual Congress–Symposia Highlights, Yardley, Penn, 1998, Medical Association Communications and the Oncology Nursing Society.

48. Doxil, package insert, 1997, SEQUUS Pharmaceuticals, Inc.

49. Taxotere, package insert, 1998, Rhone-Poulenc Rorer Pharmaceuticals Inc.

50. Liebman MC: Docetaxel, *Clin J Oncol Nurs* 2:83, 1999.

51. ONTAK, package insert, 1999, San Diego, Calif, Ligand Pharmaceuticals Inc.

52. Door A, et al: *Clinical management of ovarian cancer: role of topoisomerase-I inhibitors,* Springfield, NJ, 1999, Scientific Therapeutics Information.

53. Perez-Solar R: *1998 camptothecin analogues: a new therapeutic option for the treatment of small-cell lung cancer,* 1998 annual congress–symposia highlights, Yardley, Penn, 1998, Medical Association Communications and the Oncology Nursing Society.

54. Camptosar, package insert, 1999, Pharmacia & Upjohn Co.

55. Hycamtin, package insert, 1998, SmithKline Beecham Pharmaceuticals.

56. Costco J, Decker G, Hawthorne L: *Shark cartilage to soy protein: healing or hurting patients,* 1998 annual congress–symposia highlights, Yardley, Penn, 1998, Medical Association Communications and the Oncology Nursing Society.

57. Montbriand MJ: Past and present herbs used to treat cancer: medicine, magic or poison? *Oncol Nurs Forum* 26(1):49, 1999.

58. Loescher LJ: DNA testing for cancer predisposition, *Oncol Nurs Forum* 25(8):1317, 1998.

59. Berg D, et al: Overcoming multidrug resistance: Valspodar as a paradigm for nursing care, *Oncol Nurs Forum* 26(4):711, 1999.

60. Camp-Sorrell D: 1999 newsbriefs: vaccine therapy, *Clin J Oncol Nurs* 3(2):56, 1999.

Chapter

14

Pain Management

Barbara St. Marie, MA, CNP

Pain Management

Patient advocacy is at the forefront of pain management, whether it involves acute pain, chronic pain, or cancer pain. Nurses in any setting are obligated to stand up for the patient's right to appropriate pain management. In order to do this, nurses must be armed with the knowledge of what is appropriate—of what constitutes undertreatment and overtreatment. When technologies are used, one must be able to assess their appropriateness and whether they fit into the patient's lifestyle, frame of mind, and support system. The Joint Commission on Accreditation of Healthcare Organization now requires that hospitals provide pain management across the continuum of care. This means that the pain management plan is outlined from admission to discharge and that patients are part of that planning process when possible. Nurses need to

ensure that patients and their families are well educated regarding what is available for pain management intervention and what to expect from each intervention, including side effects and complications.

Categories of pain

People are now more aware of pain and the significant problems associated with it than in any time in history. "Pain is a more terrible lord of mankind than even death itself."[1] Therefore it is important that nurses and other health care professionals have up-to-date knowledge of pain as well as know how to define it and how to intervene. The International Association for the Study of Pain has established three different categories of pain: acute, chronic, and cancer.[2]

Acute pain. Acute pain is caused by such occurrences as traumatic injury, a surgical procedure, or a medical disorder. With acute pain, the patient may show a clinical picture of tachycardia, hypertension, tachypnea, shallow respirations, agitation or restlessness, facial grimace, or splinting. The incidence of acute pain is astounding. Each year, more than 100 million people have acute pain, 30 million of whom are disabled for 12 days, with a loss of 360 million days of work worth $1 billion.[3] The International Association for the Study of Pain has now published a textbook titled *Epidemiology of Pain*, which provides an in-depth look at pain and how it affects our society.[4] The challenges of acute pain become greater when individuals also suffer from chronic pain or have a history of chemical dependency.

Chronic pain. Chronic pain is persistent, often lasting more than 6 months. However, some practitioners believe that chronic pain may exist before this 6-month period. An individual who has chronic pain may show the same clinical picture as the person suffering from acute pain, or their body may condition all signs of pain with normal heart rate, normal blood pressure, and no facial grimace. It is estimated that back pain alone disables approximately 11.7 million Americans; 2.6 million are temporarily disabled, and 2.6 million are permanently disabled.[4]

Cancer pain. Millions of cancer patients throughout the world experience pain they rate from moderate to severe. Approximately 30% to 40% of cancer patients in the intermediate stages of cancer and 55% to 90% of terminal cancer patients have pain; 60% of patients reporting pain express it as moderate or great severity.[4] Some may achieve pain relief, but only at the expense of losing consciousness before death because of massive doses of narcotics. This supports the need to do a better job of controlling pain.

Barriers to effective pain control

Many health care professionals have inadequate knowledge and skills regarding the pharmacology of pain medications, physiology of pain, and pain control techniques. This lack remains despite efforts to set standards of practice and to educate physicians and nurses. The Agency for Health Care Policy and Research developed and distributed pain management guidelines in the early and mid 1990s, yet pain control for acute pain conditions continues to be inadequate. Attitudes of health care professionals serve as a barrier to effective pain control. Some professionals believe that pain is normal or innocuous, whereas others fear addiction.[5,6] The daily media is filled with information about drug abuse and addiction that feeds the fears of physicians, nurses, and the public about potential drug addiction. Even popular television shows, when they portray pain management in an acute pain situation, fail to show the newer modalities and manners of assessment. Laws and regulations impose penalties designed to prohibit the use of narcotics except in severely limited circumstances. These concerns and prohibitions can inhibit the use of certain drugs even when recent studies clearly show they can provide more effective pain control without addiction and that patients can maintain awareness of their environment.

State cancer pain initiatives, which began in Wisconsin, are organized efforts to overcome the lack of knowledge and prohibitions of law by educating physicians and nurses and lobbying legislators and regulatory authorities. Many of those participating in these initiatives are volunteers who have been close to someone who needlessly suffered cancer pain. The cancer patient's quality of life is threatened by the caregiver's fear of professional penalties for the misuse of narcotics and the lack of understanding of a cancer patient's often increased needs for systemic narcotics.

The provision for physician-assisted suicide, part of the Oregon Death with Dignity Act passed by referendum in October 1997, adds another dimension to pain management. This act allows physicians to write prescriptions for lethal overdoses. Over the first year of this act, researchers from the Oregon Health Division in Portland compared people who took lethal medications prescribed under the act (group 1) with those who died of natural causes from similar illnesses (group 2). The data were collected by physician interviews, physician reports, and death certificates. The data were not the result of interviews with patients' families. There were 23 patients in group 1 and 43 patients in group 2. In group 1, one patient expressed concern about inadequate control of pain. In group 2, 15 patients expressed concern about inadequate control of pain. The fact that inadequate pain control was a concern is a challenge to health care providers. It demonstrates the need to educate patients in ways of controlling intractable pain and to establish systems in hospitals and home care agencies to rapidly meet the need for adequate pain control.

A landmark study published in the *Annals of Internal Medicine* showed that pain is greatly undertreated. This study revealed that physicians underprescribe analgesic agents, nurses administer fewer analgesics than prescribed, patients request fewer analgesic medications than they need, and the as-needed regimen of administering intramuscular (IM) narcotic agents

ensures that the patient will experience pain.[7] Pain warns the individual that something is wrong, but once it serves that purpose, it should be relieved. Pain is harmful to the body if left untreated. There are significant endocrine responses to pain—increased heart rate and vasoconstriction and decreased gastrointestinal (GI) motility. Pain also causes muscle splinting, which can diminish pulmonary function and lead to atelectasis or pneumonia. These findings make it even more evident that health care professionals need to take pain control seriously to reduce postoperative complications, reduce the length of the hospital stay, and improve the quality of patients' lives.[6]

DISCIPLINES INVOLVED

The discipline of pain management is rapidly taking form. Physicians from anesthesiology, neurology, and oncology specialties have chosen to be involved with pain management. Anesthesiology offers a pain fellowship that includes the practice of acute, chronic, and cancer pain management as an adjunct to the practice of traditional pain control in the operating room. The technique of preemptive analgesia was initially introduced by anesthesiologists to prevent pain from being transmitted through the nerves by anesthetizing the skin and deeper tissues before the insult of the scalpel in surgery. The anesthetizing of skin can be through deep infiltration in the involved tissue or by epidural or intrathecal local anesthetics and opioids. The theory behind preemptive analgesia is that it reduces the use of postoperative opioids and improves pain control. Further investigation is needed to study the various methods of preemptive analgesia and its affect on postoperative analgesia, length of hospital stay, and reduction of complications.[8] The oncologist deals with cancer pain while focusing on curing patients of their cancer. The neurologist concentrates on the management of pain that has a neurologic component, which is usually chronic, nonmalignant pain. Headache management is advancing as new drugs are released. Research on pain in the chemically dependent population provides possibilities for controlling pain in this challenging population. The new and rapidly developing discipline of pain management could quickly become obsolete if the supportive foundation of these disciplines were to falter. To prevent this, societies and associations have been organized to advance the art of pain management, provide support for nurses and physicians with educational programs, and promote clinical networking.

The need for improving pain management systems for acute, chronic, and cancer pain is apparent and should be recognized by all health care entities.[9] The American Society of Pain Management Nurses, founded in 1991, recognizes this need and responds by educating nurses and supporting nursing research in pain management. The society's goals are to develop a core curriculum, establish the role of the nurse in pain management, and eventually offer certification. As more information becomes available about pain pathways, different opiate receptor sites, new medications, and new routes of analgesia administration, nurses are invited to help implement advances in pain management. These advances include patient-controlled analgesia, intraspinal narcotics, local anesthetics administered topically and spinally, nonsteroidal antiinflammatory drugs (NSAIDs), and anticonvulsant agents. Continuing education regarding advances in pain management warrants high priority.

Knowledge gained through infection control and advances in intravenous (IV) technology have provided the IV nurse with a background that can make it easy to gain proficiency in pain management. Pain management includes such procedures as piggybacking narcotic infusions and supplying patient-controlled doses of narcotic into maintenance lines. It also involves the delivery of narcotics and local anesthetics into the epidural and intrathecal spaces. Infusion pumps are becoming "smarter," and one must understand computer technology to program these sophisticated pumps correctly.

IV nurses can be valuable members of the health care team concerned with pain management. They have knowledge and expertise that can help resolve the problems that occur with pain management. For example, IV nurses know what constitutes an inappropriate dosage of narcotics. They are familiar with the ways that the equipment used to deliver pain-relief medications can fail. Finally, they are aware of the complications and adverse reactions that can occur when a patient is subjected to the procedures and medications the IV nurse provides. Special challenges arise when patients receive these therapies in a variety of settings, such as homes, hospitals, and outpatient clinics. As people become more aware of new technology for providing pain relief, they will demand it in every setting. The IV nurse is positioned to provide pain relief with present technologic skills supplemented by additional training.

PHYSIOLOGY OF PAIN

Matching clinical indicators with the appropriate pain intervention requires knowledge of the biochemical response to pain, the pain pathway, and opiate receptor sites. Also, correctly interpreting what the patient is communicating about pain requires a predisposition to hear and believe what the patient says.[10]

When the skin is cut, a chemical called a *prostaglandin* is released. Prostaglandin is thought to be the precursor to the pain impulse, the substance that allows the impulse to be carried through the afferent or peripheral nerve fibers into the spinal cord. In the spinal cord, the nerve endings release a neurotransmitter called *substance P*.[11] Substance P allows the pain impulse to be carried through the dorsal horn and ascend to the brain, which interprets the signal as pain at the site of the cut. Fig. 14-1 is a simplified cross section of the spinal cord; the heavy black line traces the pain path. Substance P is released at the presynaptic junction and carries the pain impulse forward to the laminae. At the laminae there is a synapse, or firing, which impels the pain impulse through each lamina to the postsynaptic junction.

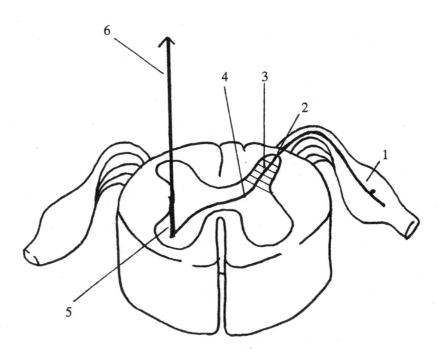

1. Dorsal Root Ganglion
2. Presynaptic Junction
3. Laminae
4. Postsynaptic Junction
5. Contralateral Spinothalamic Tract
6. Brain (Conscious Level)

FIG. 14-1 *Cross section of the spinal cord.*

Substance P continues to be released, and the pain impulse is transmitted through the spinothalamic tract to the brain—in particular, the thalamus. The pathway continues as the impulse travels to the cerebral cortex, where the pain becomes conscious, and down the descending pathway, where a withdrawal reflex makes the individual pull away from the painful stimuli.[2]

Many other factors affect the pain response. These factors include past experiences of pain; anxiety and anticipatory pain; emotional, physical, or sexual abuse; history of chemical dependency; and the patient's support structures. Because studies of these factors are lacking, we must rely on our own perceptions of what the patient is experiencing. This allows myth and misconception, rather than fact, to guide our treatment of patients in pain. However, experts in pain management have defined the patient's self-report as the gold standard for measuring acute pain, and this practice guides health care providers who take pain management seriously.

Endogenous opiates

The body has its own protection, called *endogenous opiates,* against pain.[12] These substances keep us pain free through normal daily living. Endogenous opiates include the endorphins and the enkephalins. Endorphins, which are located in the brain, are mimicked by the systemic administration of narcotics. Enkephalins, which are located in the spinal cord, are mimicked by the intraspinal administration of narcotics.

Activities that promote the release of endogenous opiates are physical exercise, deep relaxation, sexual activity, crying, and laughter. Situations that decrease the release of endogenous opiates are stress, chronic pain, chemical dependency, and depression.

Opiate receptors

Understanding opiate receptors helps us understand how narcotics work to break the painful impulses. Opiate receptors are parts of cells that link with particular opiates to create analgesia and various side effects. There are five known opiate receptor sites. Researchers have learned the most about three—mu, kappa, and sigma. Each t opiate receptor has particular characteristics. Table 14-1 lists the receptors, their opiates, the effects of the opiates, and their antagonists.[2]

The most effective opiate receptor for producing superior analgesia is the mu receptor. The kappa receptor is weaker and less likely to produce physical dependency. The sigma receptor is very weak; when linked with narcotics, it tends to produce agitation and respiratory stimulation. Little is known about the delta and epsilon receptors. All five opiate receptors are located near the thalamus in the brain and in the dorsal horn of the spinal cord.[13] Naloxone can reverse any combination of opioids to their respective receptor sites. It has been discovered that there are subsets of the mu receptor, mu-1 and mu-2. Mu-1 is responsible for analgesic effects and mu-2 for side effects. Efforts are now being made to find narcotics that can combine only with mu-1.

Antagonist and agonist-antagonist

The advantage of administering narcotics for pain management is that their effects can always be reversed. Early intervention allows narcotic side effects to be reversed before the situation becomes an emergency. Two types of medication can reverse a mu-receptor narcotic. A commonly used pure antagonist is naloxone hydrochloride (Narcan). This drug competitively inhibits narcotics at the opiate receptor sites and thus reverses their side effects. However, some reports have indicated that the reversal of the kappa agonist may not be predictable.

An agonist-antagonist can also reverse a mu-receptor narcotic.[14] Agonist-antagonist narcotics combine at the kappa receptor site, thus producing lower-quality analgesia than would a mu agonist. A commonly used agonist-antagonist that combines with the kappa opiate receptor site is nalbuphine hydrochloride (Nubain). Working with agonist-antagonist medications requires understanding when this kappa agonist is administered in relation to a mu agonist. When given alone, nalbuphine hydrochloride produces mild analgesia. However, if it is given while a mu agonist is in the patient's system, it acts to reverse the mu agonist's analgesia and side effects. For example, a cancer patient who is accustomed to taking oral morphine solution (300 mg/day) is admitted to the hospital for pain control. An order is written to administer 10 mg nalbuphine hydrochloride intravenously every 3 to 4 hours as needed for pain to supplement the oral morphine. The nalbuphine hydrochloride may be ordered because it has fewer side effects, but in this situation, it will reverse the effects of the oral morphine, thereby producing severe pain and, most likely, symptoms of withdrawal.

Pain nerve fibers

Specialized nerve endings in the skin and viscera send messages of noxious stimuli, such as mechanical, chemical, or thermal, to

Table 14-1	Opiate Receptors and the Effects of Opiates		
OPIATE RECEPTOR	**AGONIST**	**ANTAGONIST**	**EFFECT OF AGONIST**
Mu	Morphine Meperidine Fentanyl Sufentanil Alfentanil	Naloxone (Narcan) Pentazocine (Talwin) Nalbuphine (Nubain)	Analgesia; decreased respirations; decreased heart rate; physical dependence; euphoria
Kappa	Pentazocine Nalbuphine Butorphanol (Stadol) Buprenorphine (Buprenex)	Naloxone (?)	Analgesia; sedation; decreased respirations; miosis
Sigma	Pentazocine Ketamine	Naloxone	Dysphoria; hypertonia; tachycardia; tachypnea

From St. Marie B: Narcotic infusions: a changing scene, *JIN* 14:334, 1991.

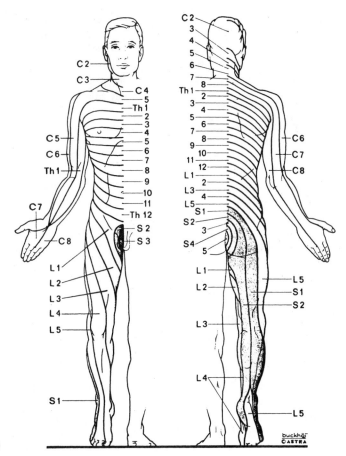

FIG. 14-2 *Dermatome chart.* (Courtesy Astra Pharmaceuticals.)

the brain. These specialized nerve endings, or receptors, send impulses along specific fiber types, all of which are peripheral nerves. These fiber types, identified as *A, B,* and *C,* differ in their rate of impulse conduction and their diameter. The myelinated A-fibers are the largest and most rapid conductors. Lightly myelinated B-fibers are smaller and somewhat slower conductors. Unmyelinated C-fibers have the smallest diameter and are the slowest conductors. A-fibers tend to conduct intense pain but are more receptive to local anesthetics and NSAIDs. B-fibers conduct both sympathetic and parasympathetic impulses. C-fibers tend to conduct dull pain and are most responsive to narcotics by any route.[2]

Dermatomes constitute the segmental distribution of the spinal nerve sensations and are labeled according to their exit point on the spinal cord. Dermatome charts (Fig. 14-2) are useful for tracking the nerves innervating the area of pain. With a nerve block or the intraspinal route of analgesia, medications can be delivered directly to those nerves that are the origin of an individual's pain.[2]

The IV nurse, with a knowledge of pharmacology, can intervene for those with poorly managed pain by evaluating the patient's narcotic regimen. Antagonism between the mu and kappa agonists is easily identified. If a kappa agonist is being used for analgesia and is providing inadequate analgesia, the IV nurse may recommend a mu agonist for superior analgesia.

Understanding the function of the A-delta fibers and C-fibers in pain conduction can help the IV nurse identify whether the intervention being used for the type of pain the patient describes is appropriate.

By understanding the dermatomal distribution of pain when working with epidural infusions of narcotics and local anesthetics, the IV nurse can work with the anesthesiologist to determine the appropriate dermatomal distribution of narcotic and local anesthetic to the painful area. For example, the volume of infusion of lipid-soluble narcotic may need to be increased to widen the spread of analgesia (see Fig. 14-2).

PARENTERAL NARCOTICS

The quality of pain management depends on the knowledge and expertise of health care professionals. In the ideal health care setting, the professionals are knowledgeable in conventional methods of pain control and recent advances, and they are willing to practice quality, up-to-date pain management for their patients.

Parenteral narcotic administration is available to patients in a variety of forms, for example, continuous infusions of narcotics, intermittent doses of narcotics, and combinations of these. Selection of the type of parenteral narcotics depends on the type of pain indicated by the patient and the availability of the nursing staff for administering it appropriately.

Continuous infusion

A patient may receive a continuous infusion of narcotics when pain management is desired at a steady state.[15] For example, if the patient states that the pain is rather constant, a continuous infusion of narcotics may be indicated. Before the continuous infusion is given, it is best to administer small doses of narcotic frequently until the proper blood level is achieved to control pain. The continuous infusion is then begun. Continuous infusions of narcotics are appropriately used in trauma, postsurgical, and terminal care settings. The routes of continuous infusion include the intravenous, subcutaneous, and intraspinal (epidural or intrathecal) routes.

Intermittent doses

Patients may receive intermittent doses of narcotics when they state that the pain is episodic. In these cases, it may be more desirable to treat pain only when experienced, with fast-acting narcotics that are effective for short periods. For example, if the patient has a kidney stone that produces only intermittent yet severe pain, an intermittent dose of narcotic can be effective. Frequent intermittent doses of narcotics can be administered through the oral, sublingual, buccal, rectal, IM, IV, subcutaneous, or intraspinal routes. Administering narcotics less frequently in larger doses can create periods of oversedation interrupted by periods of inadequate pain relief (Fig. 14-3). It is more desirable to use small doses of narcotic frequently than large doses infrequently. Although the frequent administration of narcotic is time-consuming for the nurse, it is the safest method for administering narcotics. To solve this dilemma, the nurse should consider administering small, frequent doses of narcotics through a patient-controlled analgesia (PCA) delivery system.[16]

Combination

A patient may receive a combination of continuous narcotic infusion and intermittent doses of narcotics when it is desirable to produce a steady state of analgesia[17] during painful procedures, increased activity levels, or painful episodes that result from surgery or trauma to organs or tissues.

Routes of administration

Narcotics can be administered in combination through the IV, subcutaneous, or intraspinal routes. A continuous infusion of narcotics, with the patient capability to bolus additional doses, is beneficial for cancer pain management. With some infusion pumps, the patient can push the bolus button to administer the dose of narcotic needed. After 12 to 24 hours, the nurse can determine how much the patient has used and adjust the hourly rate accordingly. The appropriate assessment of the patient's pain is especially important in determining whether the pain is intermittent, constant, or related to activity.[18]

Intravenous administration. Narcotics administered intravenously may be delivered through central or peripheral venous access. Because these routes direct narcotics to bind

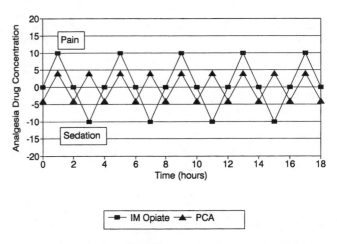

FIG. 14-3 *Comparison of analgesic levels between intramuscular and patient-controlled analgesia narcotics.*

primarily at the opiate receptor sites located in the brain, central nervous system effects such as sedation or respiratory depression may easily occur in a narcotic-naive patient. The physician may order narcotics for intermittent injections to be administered by the nurse, for constant infusion, or for PCA. The mechanisms of delivering these narcotics need to be given careful consideration in all settings.

Intermittent injections of narcotics administered by the nurse allow small doses of narcotics to be given frequently and require that the nurse be available to the patient for these frequent administrations. Although this may be feasible for nurses attending to patients in critical care settings and postanesthesia care units (PACU), it is not feasible for nurses who work on postsurgical, oncology, or medical-surgical floors, where the patient/nurse ratio is larger.

A constant infusion is a convenient method for administration and provides the patient with a steady state of analgesia. The problem with this system is that accumulation may occur, causing the patient to feel oversedated and to later develop respiratory depression. To ascertain the appropriate hourly dose, consideration needs to be given to the patient's age, size, disease process, concurrent diseases, and narcotic tolerance.

PCA allows patients to deliver their own narcotics for pain control. PCA involves small doses of a narcotic administered frequently, with the patient's goal being to provide a steady state of analgesia, thus avoiding the peaks and valleys of analgesia, sedation, and pain.[19] PCA delivery does not, however, prevent the accumulation of a narcotic and its subsequent side effects. Therefore patients need to be assessed regularly for respiratory effects and mental status changes. A successful PCA program needs to be safe for the patient while providing adequate pain relief. PCA protocol involves the following: (1) defining the type of patient who can use PCA devices and preparing a list of teaching tools, (2) selecting the appropriate equipment, (3) selecting the medications and concentrations used, (4) establishing consistency of use and dosage, (5) defining who can handle the side effects, and (6) providing an appropriate avenue of communication between the patient and nurse to determine the quality of pain relief experienced by the patient. The types of patients who are candidates for PCA are listed in Box 14-1.

Choosing the proper equipment for PCA administration is imperative (Box 14-2).[20]

Specific patient populations require different guidelines for setting the PCA dose and frequency. Most narcotics are metabolized in the liver or kidney, so any impairment in these systems may cause accumulation. Precautions such as lowering the drug dose and increasing the time between PCA doses decrease the likelihood of narcotic accumulation. Frequent nursing assessment of the patient's mental status can detect early signs of accumulation so that doses can be adjusted accordingly.

In the elderly population, higher peak effects of a narcotic and longer duration of pain relief may be observed after the administration of narcotic.[21] Cognitive impairment creates barriers to pain management because pain assessment may not be accurate. Pain control for the elderly population must be individualized, making the "routine procedure" of pain management obsolete.[22]

PCA is being increasingly used in the substance-abuse population once the cause of pain has been determined (e.g., postoperative pain). The dosage limits must be increased to achieve analgesia because of the patient's tolerance to opioids.[23] The delivery system for PCA must allow lock-out intervals and dosage limits to be set, and it must be tamper resistant. By using nonopioid therapies such as transcutaneous electrical nerve stimulation, NSAIDs, or epidural local anesthetics, the amount of narcotics given can be significantly reduced. The nurse must monitor the patient for substance abuse of other narcotics or sedatives during PCA to prevent the inadvertent potentiation of the narcotic, resulting in overdose. Thorough discussion with the patient may determine this potential, and a toxicology screen can exclude or confirm any suspicions of inaccuracies in the patient's report.

The cooperation of nursing personnel is necessary for a successful PCA program. Infusion devices are sometimes difficult to program, lock out, and troubleshoot. When patients sense a nurse's frustration in trying to program the infusion device, their faith in the pain management program can waiver. IV nurses provide a valuable service by selecting the appropriate pain-control delivery systems for their facility (see Box 14-2).

The importance of the questions listed in Box 14-2 varies with each setting. By answering these questions, the nurse can select an infusion device that is appropriate for the facility. Nurses should receive in-service training about the infusion device before implementation and should be tested regularly for competency in operating the device.

The Intravenous Nurses Society *Infusion Nursing Standards of Practice*[24] emphasizes the nurse's vital role in educating the patient. The patient should become familiar with the PCA infusion pump before surgery because the stress of surgery along with amnesic medications received perioperatively may cause the patient to forget any teaching that occurred in the preinduction area, in the PACU, or on the surgical floor postoperatively. Patient education should include discussion of the following:

- How to use patient-controlled analgesia
- When to push the bolus button
- When to communicate with the nurse (e.g., pain not controlled with PCA, feeling of sedation)
- Fear of administering too much medication
- Fear of addiction to narcotics with PCA therapy
- Expected outcomes for the patient (e.g., pain rating of 1 or 2, early ambulation)

Efforts in establishing a PCA program are worthwhile. Patients who use PCA are more comfortable. They have control over their own pain management and can keep their narcotic blood level within therapeutic range, allowing them to effectively ambulate and breathe deeply. As Lehman has stated, "PCA is not only suitable to establish and maintain adequate postoperative pain relief but can also yield important information about pain behavior and the patient's pain measurement."[25] An expansion of the idea of patient-controlled analgesia is parent-controlled analgesia, family-controlled analgesia, or nurse-controlled analgesia. Before an institution decides to initiate these forms of analgesia, careful consideration should be given to the quality of education given to the person who will push the button for bolus dosing.

To summarize, there are definite advantages to administering IV narcotics to achieve pain control. Most nurses are familiar with the IV route, there is a rapid onset of action, and it is therefore easier to titrate increasing narcotic requirements with

Box 14-3   Necessary Items for Accessing Subcutaneous Tissue

Small-gauge scalp-vein needle, cannula, or subcutaneous access needles
Povidone-iodine swab
Adhesive bandage
Transparent dressing

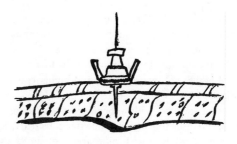

FIG. 14-4 *Subcutaneous access for narcotic administration.* (Courtesy MiniMed Technologies.)

Table 14-2   Conversion Chart

	Equianalgesic Dose (mg)	
Analgesic	PO	IM or SC
Morphine sulfate	30.0	10.0
Hydromorphone hydrochloride	7.5	1.5
Levorphanol tartrate	4.0	2.0
Methadone hydrochloride	20.0	10.0

From Agency for Health Care Policy and Research: *Clinical practice guidelines: acute pain management: operative or medical procedures and trauma*, Rockville, Md, 1992, US Department of Health and Human Services.

escalating pain. The disadvantages are that vascular access is sometimes difficult to maintain, the accumulation of IV narcotics may not be predictable, and side effects such as somnolence can interfere with the patient's quality of life. Further studies are needed on outcome measures of PCA because there are conflicting studies as to whether PCA reduces postoperative complications, length of hospital stay, and nursing time.[26,27]

Subcutaneous administration. A nurse who readily accepts the role of patient advocate needs to allow patients to choose which narcotic administration route is amenable to them. Regardless of the cause of pain, patients can be made aware of the advantages and disadvantages of their options.

Patients who are intolerant of or unable to take oral or rectal pain medications or patients in whom vascular access is not reliable or desired may want to consider the subcutaneous route of narcotic administration. This route is less invasive and less costly than other parenteral narcotic routes. Studies have shown that continuous infusions of subcutaneous narcotics have all of the advantages of IV narcotic administration, without the need for vascular access. Subcutaneous and IV narcotic infusions produce similar blood levels and provide comparable analgesia and side effects.[28,29] However, the American Pain Society Guidelines, fourth edition, state that IV and IM dosing of narcotics are not equal as was originally written in equianalgesic charts.[25] This needs to be considered in conversion for subcutaneous dosing of narcotics as well.

The technique for accessing the subcutaneous tissue is a simple procedure. The ease of use makes subcutaneous narcotic infusions desirable for home infusion personnel (Box 14-3).

To begin a subcutaneous narcotic infusion, the nurse preps the skin with a povidone-iodine swab over the desired access site. Commonly used subcutaneous sites are the subclavicular area, anterior chest wall, and abdomen.[30] A small-gauge scalp-vein needle is inserted at an angle under the skin. An adhesive bandage is applied over the plastic wings of the needle for stability, and the site is covered with a transparent dressing. A Teflon catheter inserted into the subcutaneous tissue is shown in Fig. 14-4.

Narcotics used for subcutaneous infusions include morphine sulfate, hydromorphone hydrochloride, levorphanol tartrate, and methadone hydrochloride. Morphine sulfate and hydromorphone hydrochloride are most often used, and no difference has been found between these two narcotics in regard to pain control or side effects.[25,28] Hydromorphone has a high analgesic potency per milliliter—five to six times higher than that of morphine. This property minimizes the volume of infusion and is useful in opioid-tolerant patients who require higher hourly

dosages for adequate pain relief. The effective elimination half-life of hydromorphone is 2.6 hours. Morphine has a slightly longer effective elimination half-life of 3.1 hours.[29] It has been speculated that higher lipid solubility creates a depot effect and that higher water solubility (such as that of morphine) decreases absorption from the subcutaneous compartment into the systemic circulation, resulting in decreased bioavailability. Neither hypothesis has been substantiated through research.[29]

If the patient has a history of oral narcotic use, a conversion chart (Table 14-2) can be used to facilitate the initiation of a subcutaneous narcotic infusion.

The following steps can be taken to convert an oral narcotic to the subcutaneous route:

1. Calculate the previous 24-hour oral dose of narcotic.
2. Convert the oral dose to the subcutaneous dose (see Table 14-2).
3. Divide this number by 24 to obtain the hourly subcutaneous infusion.
4. Program the pump.

Individual absorption characteristics must be factored in to any route conversions.

In their study, Moulin and Kreeft showed that although plasma concentrations of narcotic subcutaneous and IV infusions are similar at 24 hours, at 48 hours the plasma concentration of a subcutaneous infusion drops to 78% of an IV infusion.[29] Therefore adjustments may need to be made during the second day.

Subcutaneous infusions or boluses of narcotics are limited to the absorption of the narcotic at the subcutaneous site. Absorption from injections of a subcutaneous or IM narcotic follows comparable time frames.[30] The subcutaneous tissue can tolerate narcotic infusions with less irritation if the infusion rate is slower than 2 ml/hr. The preparation of narcotic concentrations is therefore important to the success of subcutaneous infusions for pain control. Local toxicity from chemical irritation of the narcotic is uncommon but is more likely to occur with the extremes of higher volume infusions and higher concentrations of narcotic.

Problems associated with subcutaneous infusions are skin irritation at the insertion site and subcutaneous scarring.[30] Skin irritation can be resolved with more frequent site changes and less-concentrated narcotics. Subcutaneous scarring interferes with the absorption of the narcotic, resulting in unpredictable analgesia. Reducing narcotic volume and rotating the site more often prevents scarring.

IV nurses, with their experience in monitoring vascular access sites and performing vascular site rotations, are in a good position to support the patient receiving subcutaneous infusions. The IV nurse can identify chemical irritation of subcutaneous tissue, make recommendations to change the site and concentrate the narcotic infusion, rotate the site, secure the subcutaneous needle, and change the dressing.

Transdermal analgesia is an exciting new technology that merits discussion here. Duragesic (Janssen) patches come in various doses of fentanyl citrate gel, such as 25, 50, 75, and 100 µg/hr. Applied to the skin, this patch allows fentanyl to diffuse into the subcutaneous tissue through a rate-controlling membrane. A depot of fentanyl is deposited in the upper skin layers and is carried into the systemic circulation. The patch is applied to the torso area. Before a transdermal patch is placed, the skin surface needs to be dry and the body hair clipped, not shaved. No soap, oil, or lotions can be used on the skin surface where the patch is to be placed. Areas of abrasion on the skin surface need to be avoided. On the first patch application, the initial concentrations of fentanyl require 12 to 15 hours to peak, and each patch lasts 3 days. Because of the delayed initial peak, fast-acting narcotics are needed to provide relief for breakthrough pain until adequate plasma concentrations have been reached. With subsequent patches, a more stable plasma level can be maintained.

Nursing care

Monitoring. Monitoring patients receiving parenteral narcotic medications requires that the nurse document consistently on a flow sheet. The nurse should have knowledge of the pharmacologic implications of the medications along with baseline information about the patient, such as pulse, respirations, blood pressure, known drug allergies, and history of narcotic use, before narcotics are given.[23] Flow sheets are useful in the hospital or home setting and should enable the nurse to monitor the patient for therapeutic response, record untoward side effects, and document nursing interventions. The flow sheet should be part of the medical record. Two samples of flow sheets that can be used in the hospital or home setting are found in Appendix A. State and federal regulations require that controlled substances be discarded appropriately and documented.

Monitoring for respiratory depression is routine to most nurses who administer narcotics. Respiratory depression is usually preceded by signs of changes in mental status, such as confusion or sedation. If the nurse monitors the patient's mental status regularly, such as every hour, respiratory depression can be identified early. Early identification allows the narcotic dose to be reduced or stopped or IV naloxone to be given before the respiratory depression sets in.[31] Respiratory rates should be counted for a full minute. If they drop below a predefined limit, such as 8 or 10 respirations/min, or become shallow with poor quality and the patient is difficult to arouse, the narcotic is stopped and reversal of the narcotic is necessary. Reversal of narcotic overdose can be accomplished with pure antagonist or agonist-antagonist narcotics (if the primary narcotic combines with the mu receptor). IV naloxone can be administered frequently in small increments, such as 0.1 or 0.2 mg every 1 to 2 minutes, or with a full ampule (0.4 mg). An abrupt reversal of all analgesia, because of the sudden onset of severe pain, may produce hypertension, tachycardia, rapid respirations, decreased GI motility, and hypercoagulability. By titrating naloxone hydrochloride slowly, the nurse can reverse the side effects without reversing the analgesia. When reversal takes place, the patient should still be monitored for return of decreased mental status and respiratory depression; because the duration of some narcotics can be longer than the duration of naloxone, naloxone may need to be repeated. A low-dose infusion of naloxone might even be considered.

The apnea monitor is a plethysmographic device that detects movements of the thorax, which it records as a ventilation rate. It varies in reliability from one patient to another and occasionally can emit loud false alarms that disrupt normal sleep in monitored patients. In many people, normal sleep is characterized by intermittent periodic breathing and short periods of apnea. Patients may develop progressive respiratory depression characterized by rapid, shallow breathing, and this is not detected by plethysmographic apnea monitors. Significant respiratory depression with infusions of opiates is consistently accompanied by progressive somnolence and obtundation. Therefore the best monitoring involves hourly nursing checks, with observation of ventilatory patterns and assessment of mental status. During nighttime sleep, patients need only be touched to see that they arouse easily, and the ventilatory rate can be counted without disturbing sleep. Sleep deprivation related to apnea monitor false alarms may have adverse medical consequences. The use of apnea monitors on cancer patients who are tolerant to the side effects of narcotics may be objected to by the patient as bothersome and may even be considered punitive.

Complications. Nursing management of complications related to the parenteral administration of narcotics requires knowledge and prompt intervention to remedy the situation. Complications include inadequate pain relief and respiratory depression.

Inadequate pain relief. Nurses often do not know how to respond when patients do not receive adequate pain control from their medications. This frustration may reflect a disbelief that the patient has pain or a desire to withhold narcotics because for fear of addiction.[32] These conditions often occur after a pain-control measure sedates the patient to allow sleep, but when awake, the patient complains of pain. The nurse needs to realize that patients in pain often do sleep and that sleep is not a good indicator of a pain-free state. It can be reassuring to the nurse whose patient does not have adequate pain control to realize that there is no perfect method of pain control. Breakthrough pain may occur with any pain control method, but constant attempts to control pain should continue. In general, treating breakthrough pain with small, repetitive doses of IV narcotic is a safe and effective practice that should be used routinely until the medication can be adjusted or the technique of pain management altered. Certain PCA infusion pumps allow the nurse to give small, repetitive doses of IV narcotics to patients without using up the doses patients can give themselves; or the nurse may choose to bypass the PCA pump to administer IV push narcotic boluses directly. Regardless of the means of administration, one should continually monitor the patient and keep track of the pain medication used (amount, type, time, and patient response).

Respiratory depression.
Respiratory depression is a serious complication resulting from overnarcotizing the patient. It may occur with any route of narcotic administration. The important thing to remember is that narcotics that bind with the mu receptor can always be reversed with an antagonist.[33] Respiratory depression is uniformly associated with somnolence or confusion. Therefore, if nurses assess mental status and respirations frequently (e.g., every hour), they can identify and treat the occasional individual who has ventilation depression. It is important to assess mental status with respiratory rate because some people slow their breathing rate or breathe irregularly during normal sleep or at times of rest during the day. If these patients are awake, alert, and appropriate, it is doubtful that they have clinically significant respiratory depression. However, confusion or somnolence is cause for alarm, even if breathing is not slowed.

Side effects.
Side effects occur with all routes of narcotic administration and include excessive somnolence or confusion, nausea and vomiting, urinary retention, pruritus, and constipation.

Excessive somnolence or confusion may indicate that significant levels of the narcotic are present in the brain, a cause for concern. Excessive somnolence may herald impending respiratory depression. The narcotic infusion should be stopped, the respiration rate counted for 1 full minute while observing the quality of respirations, and the physician notified. The administration of naloxone may be necessary if the mental status is markedly abnormal or if there is poor-quality respiratory status.

Nausea and vomiting may result from a number of causes unrelated to the use of narcotics, including postsurgical ileus, certain nonnarcotic medications, and the effects of general anesthetics. Nausea is often associated with narcotics by any route.[34] Narcotic-related nausea tends to occur when patients are ambulatory rather than recumbent and may be the result of narcotic-enhanced labyrinthine sensitivity to motion.[35] Many antiemetics can alleviate nausea, or the narcotic can be counteracted by an antagonist such as nalbuphine or naloxone.

Urinary retention is not a common side effect of systemically administered narcotics. However, when it does occur, and if there is no mechanical urinary obstruction, it can be treated with medications that contract the bladder, such as bethanechol chloride. A single bladder catheterization may also reverse the retention problem, but it may expose the patient to the risk of urinary tract infection.

Pruritus is a side effect that may be related to a sensitivity or allergy to the drug or its vehicle. Administering an antihistamine is often effective, or the narcotic effects can be reversed with an antagonist. Use of another narcotic should be considered.

Narcotics can slow bowel function, resulting in constipation. Bowel sounds need to be monitored, elimination patterns tracked, and stool softeners given when necessary. Managing pain in terminal cancer patients needs to be done simultaneously with managing or preventing constipation. In these patients, poorly managed pain, immobility, poor diet, and dehydration, as well as narcotics, can reduce GI motility. Elimination patterns must be monitored to facilitate a bowel movement at least every 3 days. A stool softener combined with a peristaltic agent is most likely necessary. If bowel evacuation is delayed for longer than 3 days, the physician should be notified immediately and a more aggressive bowel program defined.

Special considerations

Nonnarcotic adjuvant medications can be useful in pain control, either by themselves or in combination with narcotics. These drugs include NSAIDs, tricyclic antidepressants, topical local anesthetic agents, and anticonvulsants. These medications need to be considered when evaluating patients with acute, chronic, or cancer pain.

NSAIDs, which can be given orally, intramuscularly, or rectally, inhibit the synthesis of prostaglandin by inhibiting cyclooxygenase. Because of this prostaglandin-inhibiting activity, studies have shown that the adjuvant use of NSAIDs reduces the amount of narcotics necessary to control pain.[36] Careful consideration should be given to the patient before administering NSAIDs. The patient's medical history and physical condition should be evaluated, and current medications need to be identified. For instance, if a patient has a history of renal disease or has an elevated creatinine level, the use of NSAIDs may be contraindicated. If the patient has a coagulopathy or is taking anticoagulants, the use of NSAIDs needs to be evaluated carefully. Because certain NSAIDs can be irritating to the stomach, patients with a history of peptic ulcer disease need to be evaluated carefully for this method of pain control because NSAIDs inhibit the production of the very prostaglandins that protect the stomach lining from gastric acids.

Researchers recently learned that there are two types of cyclooxygenase. Cyclooxygenase type 1 produces prostaglandins that are beneficial to renal and gastric function. Cyclooxygenase type 2 produces prostaglandins related to the inflammatory process. Cyclooxygenase 2 inhibitors (COX-2 inhibitors) selectively inhibit cyclooxygenase type 2. When this happens, inflammation is reduced. COX-2 inhibitors introduced in December 1998, provide the benefit of analgesia by blocking cyclooxygenase type 2, thus keeping cyclooxygenase type 1 working to benefit the kidneys and stomach lining. It has yet to be determined whether COX-2 inhibitors can be used to manage acute pain. Two brands of COX-2 inhibitors are rofecoxib (Vioxx) and celecoxib (Celebrex). Patients allergic to aspirin need to be questioned carefully to see whether it is a true allergic reaction. Cross allergies to some NSAIDs occur.[25]

Tricyclic antidepressants are important medications for deafferentation or neuropathic pain caused by surgical trauma, radiation therapy, chemotherapy, or malignant nerve infiltration. They are beneficial in pain control because they contribute to an increase in serotonin in the descending pain pathway, resulting in a release of enkephalin in the spinal cord and a decrease in pain. Because of this function, tricyclic antidepressants are physiologically responsible for terminating nerve-transmitting activity. Side effects include hypotension, sedation, and dry mouth. Contraindications are coronary disease in patients with ventricular arrhythmias.

Anticonvulsants are used to relieve brief, lancinating pain arising from the peripheral nerve. They can be used to treat conditions such as trigeminal neuralgia and postherpetic neuralgia. Gabapentin has been a popular anticonvulsant because it has a low side effect profile, has no metabolite, and does not interfere with other medications. However, the gabapentin dose must be reduced in patients with renal insufficiency.

Clonidine has been approved by the U.S. Food and Drug Administration for the treatment of pain. This is available for epidural administration in a 100 mg/ml concentration. Hypotension and bradycardia are possible side effects, but these are uncommon at low dosages.

Pain management in the home setting or long-term care facility involves the transfer of knowledge to the staff. Transfer of care needs to be well defined in protocol. Documentation of pain level and compliance with the pain treatment plan is important. Nurses in home health care and long-term care need to be familiar with the use of narcotics, NSAIDs, and tricyclic antidepressants for their terminal cancer patients suffering from intractable pain. They need to be able to communicate effectively to determine the patient's goals for pain management. The patient needs to be educated regarding the various methods and routes of pain control; only by being educated can the patient be involved in the decision-making process.[19] Given the lack of available resources in the home setting, it is particularly important that home health care nurses be able to recognize side effects and complications and know how to intervene immediately.

EPIDURAL NARCOTICS

The epidural route can be used for acute, chronic, and cancer pain management. There are various approaches to the administration of narcotics by the epidural route, and each has its own clinical indication. These approaches include a single bolus injection of narcotic or local anesthetic, a continuous infusion of narcotic with or without local anesthetic, and a continuous infusion of narcotic with a patient-activated bolus. Preservatives can cause nerve damage and need to be avoided in narcotics or local anesthetics used in the epidural or intrathecal spaces.[37,38]

Nurses are better prepared to work with patients receiving epidural or intrathecal analgesic agents if they know the lipid- and water-solubility properties of the drugs with which they are working. Lipid- and water-solubility factors determine the length of time an intraspinal narcotic provides analgesia, the degree of rostral spread (distribution of the narcotic) in the cerebrospinal fluid, and the amount of vascular uptake.[39] When fat-soluble or lipophilic medications are administered in the epidural space, they quickly diffuse through the dura and arach-

noid mater and bind at the spinal cord, where analgesia is achieved. Because these medications bind at the spinal cord, there is limited rostral spread and the analgesia that is achieved is segmental rather than generalized. Because of the lipid-solubility factors of certain narcotics, catheters may need to be placed close to the appropriate dermatome for successful analgesia. This allows lipid-soluble medications to be delivered to specific dermatome levels of the nerves that innervate the lesion or incision. An infusion using a lipid-soluble narcotic and local anesthetic can achieve a wider segmental spread of analgesia with higher rates of infusion. The amount of narcotic administered and the amount of local anesthetic need to be calculated to prevent toxicity from either medication. Conversely, when water-soluble or hydrophilic medications are administered in the epidural space, diffusion across the dura and arachnoid mater is slower. These medications do not bind as quickly along the spinal cord, thereby allowing more time for the drug to diffuse rostrally through the spinal fluid.[36] The analgesia created has a broader segment. The rostral spread of a water-soluble narcotic may produce a delayed respiratory depression when it reaches the respiratory center or medulla.[40] Fentanyl citrate, sufentanil citrate, and hydromorphone hydrochloride are commonly used lipid-soluble narcotics, and morphine sulfate is a commonly used water-soluble narcotic.

Local anesthetic agents are often used with epidural narcotics and are instrumental in controlling pain and reducing postoperative complications. Thus they may reduce the length of a hospital stay.[41] Knowledge of the autonomic nervous system is necessary to understand the advantages of adding local anesthetic agents to an epidural narcotic infusion. The autonomic nervous system consists of two systems: the sympathetic and the parasympathetic. Table 14-3 presents a summary of the physiologic responses of each system. With the administration of local anesthetics, the sympathetic system is blocked, thereby reducing postoperative complications such as paralytic ileus,[42] pulmonary complications, and thrombophlebitis.[41] By combining local anesthetics with narcotics in epidural infusions, the amount of narcotics required to control the pain is also reduced.

Contraindications for the epidural or intrathecal routes for analgesic administration include patients with head injuries (increased intracranial pressure), in whom mental status is difficult to monitor, and those with coagulopathies, infections, and tumor infiltration. Patients who have had back surgery need to be evaluated further by an anesthesiologist before the intraspinal space is accessed.

Table 14-3	**Physiologic Responses of the Autonomic Nervous System**
PARASYMPATHETIC SYSTEM	**SYMPATHETIC SYSTEM**
Decreased heart rate	Increased heart rate
Decreased respirations	Increased respirations
Decreased blood pressure	Increased blood pressure
Increased gastrointestinal function	Decreased gastrointestinal function
Vasodilation and enhanced vascular return and flow	Vasoconstriction and decreased vascular return and flow

Mechanisms of delivery

Single shot. A single injection of epidural narcotic such as fentanyl or morphine may be used for procedures that produce a short course of postoperative pain.[41] A single injection of epidural morphine may be appropriate for patients having a cesarean section or vaginal hysterectomy, as well as for some orthopedic surgeries.[43] The advantages of this type of analgesia are that the duration is approximately 12 hours, the analgesia onset is 10 to 15 minutes, and no other type of analgesia may be necessary while the narcotic is in the epidural space. The disadvantage is that respiratory depression may occur in the first 10 minutes from the vascular uptake of the morphine sulfate in the epidural veins or may be delayed 6 to 8 hours because of the rostral spread of the morphine.[39,40] Therefore narcotic-naive patients need to be monitored for excessive somnolence and respiratory depression for the duration of the medication, from 12 to 24 hours. Another disadvantage is that if the patient has had a previous, unidentified injection of intraspinal narcotic, the inadvertent administration of additional narcotic by another route may overnarcotize the patient, causing respiratory depression. It is also impossible to predict when the medication will wear off. When breakthrough pain occurs, a narcotic is more safely administered in small, frequent doses rather than by large, infrequent doses. The breakthrough pain may also be handled with an NSAID if the patient passes the aforementioned screening for their use (refer to Special Considerations section). For patients receiving same-day surgical procedures, epidural fentanyl provides short-term, postoperative analgesia and normally is eliminated before they go home, creating no danger to narcotic-naive patients who may not be monitored closely at home for delayed respiratory depression.[44]

Continuous infusion. Epidural narcotic infusions can be administered short or long term. Indications for a short-term epidural narcotic infusion include patients with pain from surgery, trauma, and acute medical disorders creating severe pain.[41,45] It may also be indicated for a cancer patient with an acute exacerbation of pain in whom systemic narcotics cloud the sensorium or the systemic administration of analgesic agents is not effective in controlling pain, despite rapid elevations of dosages.

Continuous infusion with local anesthetic agents. Epidural local anesthetic agents break the pain pathway at the sympathetic chain ganglion outside the spinal cord. By using local anesthetics, narcotic levels are reduced, vascular graft blood flow is improved, the incidence of deep vein thrombosis in the lower extremities is reduced, and there is a decreased incidence of paralytic ileus.[41] Patients who are predisposed to postoperative complications may be considered for the administration of epidural narcotic with local anesthetic for their postoperative recovery period.

Patient-controlled epidural analgesia. Epidural narcotics are safely administered by patient control in the postoperative setting using a lipid-soluble narcotic. This allows the patient to administer medications beyond their low infusion rate to accommodate pain from ambulation, incentive spirometry, and coughing. The onset of analgesia is within 2 minutes, and the analgesia level is superior to that obtained with the IV administration of narcotics.[41]

Cancer patients with chronic, intractable pain may be a candidate for epidural narcotic. Allowing for limited PCA in addition to a continuous infusion is helpful in controlling these patients' pain. These patients are tolerant to the side effects of narcotic because of their history of pain control using a systemic narcotic, therefore the epidural narcotic used may be lipophilic or hydrophilic, with few side effects. With hydrophilic narcotics, the onset of analgesia is within 15 to 30 minutes.

External catheters. A temporary or permanent epidural catheter may be used externally. A temporary catheter may be appropriate for epidural therapy if it is used for a short period, such as for trauma pain, postoperative pain management for adults and children,[46] or cancer pain using a trial epidural catheter system. When an epidural catheter is placed, the location of the insertion site and the distance the catheter is advanced cephalad should be documented. The catheter should be labeled "for epidural use only" to avoid the injection of potentially neurolytic substances. A temporary catheter is commonly used for as few as 3 days up to 1 week. Manufacturers do not guarantee a temporary catheter's integrity for long-term use. The long-term use of temporary epidural catheters has been associated with catheter-related problems such as catheter dislodgment and migration.[47,48] The advantage of the temporary epidural catheter is its ease and speed of insertion. Its disadvantage (even for temporary, short-term use) is that it cannot be easily secured, and thus falls out readily or begins leaking around the insertion site. Manufacturers have not yet perfected temporary epidural catheter systems and should be challenged to do so.[49]

Permanent epidural catheters are used for long-term therapy for patients with intractable cancer pain[50-52] and for patients with nonmalignant pain, if deemed appropriate. A permanent epidural catheter threads between the spinous processes and is tunnelled subcutaneously until it exits around the rib, where it can be intermittently accessed or connected to an external catheter. The advantage of the permanent, exteriorized epidural catheter is the length of dwell time. Permanent epidural catheters have been left in place and functional for more than a year. The disadvantage of the permanent epidural catheter is the chance of infection. Although the incidence of infection is low, the epidural catheter is external, thus creating some risk of infection.

Internal catheters. The epidural portal system (Fig. 14-5) has the same clinical indications as the external epidural catheter. There are two main advantages of having an epidural catheter connected subcutaneously to an implanted port. First, the catheter is not so easily dislodged because the device is under the skin. Second, there are no external components to trail bacteria into the epidural space. The disadvantage of the epidural portal system for patients who have continuous infusions is that the metal needle may be irritating to the skin or become dislodged. Securing the epidural port appropriately may alleviate this concern.[52] Labeling should be clear to ensure epidural use only.

Implantable infusion pump technology (Fig. 14-6) is available as a specialty of anesthesiology and neurosurgery.[53,54] One type of implantable infusion pump may be programmed from outside the body by using a laptop computer with a telemetry device that can be placed over the implanted pump. Another type of implanted infusion pump provides a set rate of narcotic infusion. When the concentration of the narcotic is changed inside the pump, the dosage the patient receives is changed and the rate stays the same. These exciting products hold much promise for a number of applications, including long-term pain relief.

The advantages of an implantable pump are the following:

1. The risk of infection is low.
2. The catheter can be placed epidurally or intrathecally.
3. Because the pump reservoir holds 10 to 20 ml of fluid,

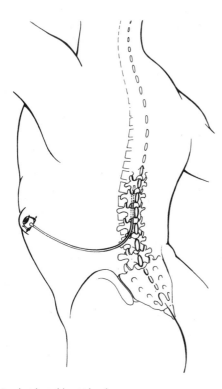

FIG. 14-5 *Implantable epidural access system.* (Courtesy Sims Deltec.)

refills are required only every 1 to 3 months, depending on the concentration and dose of the medication.

4. Infusion rates can be changed either by a computer or by changing the concentration of the medication.

The disadvantages are as follows:

1. The initial cost of the equipment and implantation is high (the longer the pump is used, the more cost-effective it becomes).
2. The complexity of the technology requires health care professionals who can adapt well to computer technology and internal pump access.
3. Each fill necessitates a needlestick, which some patients may find uncomfortable without the site being anesthetized with subcutaneous lidocaine.
4. No one knows exactly what problems long-term epidural or intrathecal infusions can cause within the spinal canal because the technology has only been available for a few years.
5. Because the life of the pump may be shorter than the patient's life expectancy, it may have to be surgically replaced. More research is needed to document outcomes over long periods, and case studies continue to be reported in the literature.[55]

Nursing care

Monitoring. A flow sheet is used to monitor the patient's response when using epidural technology for pain control. This allows the nurse to track the patient's analgesia and side effects and enhances the continuity of care. Items on the flow sheet may include the patient's mental status, respiratory status, numbness in the lower extremities, signs of infection, bowel function, and bladder function; the integrity of the epidural system; the narcotic dose; and the patient's pain rating.[48,49,55] Flow sheets can be used in any care setting.

Monitoring mental status when narcotics are being used is a

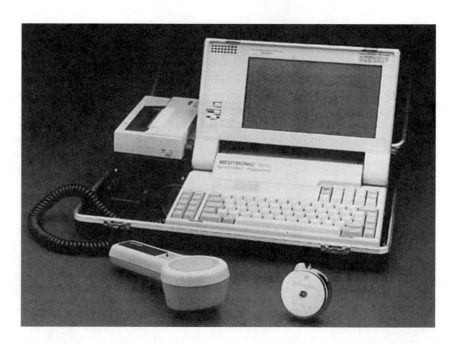

FIG. 14-6 *Implantable, programmable pump.*
(Courtesy Medtronic, Inc.)

priority. Alteration of mental status is the first indicator that the patient is receiving too much narcotic. Using a level-of-consciousness scale may be helpful (Table 14-4).

Evaluation of the respiratory status is also necessary (i.e., counting respirations for 1 minute and noting the quality of the respirations). The respiratory rate and mental status should be checked hourly, and the frequency of mental status checks is the same as when IV narcotics are being infused.[56]

Patient education is important when local anesthetics are infused. The patient should know that when they ambulate for the first time, they must assess how strong their legs are and whether they can walk. Monitoring for numbness in the lower extremities when local anesthetics are used protects the patient from an accidental fall. Numbness in the pelvic area does not impede ambulation, but if the local anesthetic used in the epidural infusion is not reduced or eliminated, the numbness gradually goes to the knees and significantly impedes ambulation. This can be prevented by good communication between the nurse and an educated patient.

Infection rarely occurs with short-term epidural infusions, but infections have been documented during long-term infusions of narcotics. Localized infections may occur at the exit site of the catheter, whether the catheter is permanent or temporary. When this occurs, the catheter should be removed, the tip of the catheter cultured, and the patient placed on antibiotic therapy. Subarachnoid infection appears as a temperature elevation (unless the patient is immunosuppressed), along with severe pain in the back where the catheter was inserted, or pain in the neck with an inability to flex the neck forward without severe pain. This requires immediate intervention by a physician.

Constipation is a problem associated with narcotics administered by any route. With epidural infusion of narcotics, constipation is less likely because of the tremendous reduction of narcotic that is used. However, bowel sounds and bowel status should be part of the nursing assessment.

Integrity of the epidural system always needs close attention. Research is continuing on the development of epidural systems that do not leak or fall apart, but until these problems are remedied, the nursing assessment needs to include catheter integrity.[49] Signs and symptoms of catheter malfunction include leaking at the distal end of the catheter and leaking at the insertion site.

Narcotic-tolerant patients receiving epidural infusions at home for intractable cancer pain should be monitored daily by the home infusion nurse, either by phone or a home visit, until the patient is stabilized. Monitoring includes mental status

evaluation, level of pain relief, side effects, and skin condition around the epidural system.

Site care. Temporary epidural catheters should be handled carefully during site care because they are easily dislodged. Proper dressing change technique is presented in Box 14-4. The dressing change frequency in the hospital or home care setting should follow the Intravenous Nurses Society *Infusion Nursing Standards of Practice.*[24]

Permanent external epidural catheters require dressing changes. The frequency of dressing changes is according to *Infusion Nursing Standards of Practice,*[24] and the technique is the same as with a temporary epidural catheter. Permanent epidural catheters have a Dacron cuff that acts as a protective barrier against bacterial migration along the catheter tract. The Dacron cuff also secures the catheter placement, so securing the catheter during dressing changes is not as great a concern.

Epidural portal systems allow the patient to have the epidural system implanted under the skin. The port requires needle access for the narcotic infusion or narcotic intermittent injection. Skin preparation for needle access includes the use of nonalcohol, antimicrobial solutions applied in a circular motion at the insertion site, working outward. The solution is allowed to air dry, and the port is accessed using sterile technique. The epidural portal system requires access with a noncoring needle. A 90-degree, shaped, noncoring needle may be used for longer narcotic infusions. The manufacturer requires that these needles be changed weekly. Minimizing irritation of the needle in the port or preventing displacement of the needle can be accomplished by securing the needle adequately.

Site preparation for accessing implantable epidural or intrathecal infusion pumps requires sterile technique using the same preparations as for an epidural portal system.

Successful epidural pain management in the home setting is totally dependent on the care provided by home infusion nurses. Home infusion nurses must be able to perform all of the nursing functions mentioned and to evaluate the patient's response to intervention. Appendix B shows an example of standing orders for permanent epidural catheter management in the home setting. Because pain management incorporates all of the complexities of a patient and the support systems, the home infusion nurse is challenged to assess the whole individual in addition to the technology.[57]

Table 14-4   Consciousness Scale for Monitoring Mental Status

Level	Patient Response
I	Alert
II	Sleepy
III	Lethargic
IV	Responds only to maximal stimulation; response to painful stimulus still present
V	Coma

Box 14-4   Dressing Change Technique

1. Wash hands.
2. Secure the temporary catheter close to the exit site with a piece of tape.
3. Remove the old dressing carefully and slowly. Discard appropriately.
4. Apply antimicrobial solution without alcohol in a circular motion, starting at the exit site and working outward.
5. Allow the solution to air dry.
6. Apply the desired dressing, gauze, or transparent, making sure that the catheter is well secured and cannot dislodge accidentally.
7. Document the dressing change, reporting the inspection of the exit site and how the patient tolerated the change.

Complications. The nursing management of complications and side effects is important to the safety and efficacy of epidural pain administration.[58] Complications include inadequate pain relief, respiratory depression, infection, and epidural catheter migration.[59] The role of the IV nurse is to educate patients and troubleshoot complications of epidural narcotics, taking appropriate measures to remedy these complications.

Inadequate pain relief. Patients receiving epidural analgesia must receive effective pain control, whether for acute, chronic, or cancer pain. Therefore the nurse should treat inadequate pain control seriously. Pain control is no longer viewed as a luxury. Pain can harm the patient by creating a sympathetic response, which delays a postoperative patient's recovery and prevents the terminal cancer patient from having quality of life during their time remaining.

Inadequate pain relief for patients with acute pain may occur for three reasons: (1) epidural catheter migration, (2) insufficient dosages of narcotics and local anesthetics, or (3) an undetermined surgical complication. Inadequate pain relief for cancer patients with intractable pain may occur for three reasons: (1) epidural catheter migration, (2) insufficient dosages of narcotics and local anesthetics, or (3) advancing disease process.

Respiratory depression. Respiratory depression related to epidural narcotics occurs when the narcotics affect the brain (similar to parenteral narcotics). It is managed in the same manner as respiratory depression from IV narcotics.[48,49]

Infection. Infections caused by using epidural catheters are rare, but precautions should be instituted to keep the catheter insertion process and exit site sterile. For a patient who is not immunosuppressed, an infection in the epidural space causes temperature elevation, pain in the back where the catheter is placed, drainage at the exit site, and inadequate pain relief. If these symptoms are present, they should be reported to an anesthesiologist and consideration given to removing the catheter immediately. If the infection develops elsewhere, the patient should also be evaluated for removal of the epidural catheter. For cancer pain management, infection may be evident in the epidural space without temperature elevation in immunosuppressed patients; therefore other signs and symptoms need to be monitored. Infection may exist with symptoms of pain in the back at the catheter site, drainage at the exit site, or inadequate pain control. This can be confirmed by an epidurogram, which is an x-ray examination of the epidural space following injection of radiopaque dye through the catheter.

Catheter migration. Epidural catheter migration may occur in two different ways. The catheter may migrate through the dura mater into the intrathecal space, creating an overdose of narcotic, or the catheter may migrate into an epidural vein or subcutaneous space, creating inadequate pain relief. Catheter migration with permanent epidural catheter systems is almost unheard of, but catheter migration of a temporary epidural catheter, although not common, has occurred. Catheter migration must be evaluated if pain is suddenly uncontrolled. Aspirating the epidural catheter to check for blood return is not a reliable means of evaluating catheter displacement into an epidural vein because epidural veins are pliable and collapse easily with aspiration.[60] A more reliable method of checking catheter placement is by injecting the epidural catheter with a local anesthetic and epinephrine hydrochloride. The patient is monitored for temperature sensation changes around the dermatome area and for tachycardia. If tachycardia is present, the epidural catheter is venous, and no further medication should be injected until the anesthesiologist evaluates the catheter. If there is a temperature sensation change, it can be assumed that the epidural catheter is functional. Policies and procedures should be available and proper training with approval from the State Board of Nursing should be obtained before a nurse injects a local anesthetic into the epidural space.

Evaluating epidural catheter migration into the intrathecal space is easier. Cerebrospinal fluid, 10 ml, is easily aspirated when the catheter is in the intrathecal space. The anesthesiologist should be notified and the patient evaluated for decreased mental status and respiratory depression.

Side effects. Side effects of epidural narcotics are excessive somnolence and confusion, nausea and vomiting, urinary retention, and pruritus.[48,49] The use of an antagonist or agonist-antagonist is helpful in handling the side effects of epidural narcotics. If the respiratory rate is low and mental status is changed, and pruritus, urinary retention, or nausea occurs, a pure antagonist such as naloxone hydrochloride or an agonist-antagonist such as nalbuphine hydrochloride can be used at dosages low enough to reverse the side effects without reversing the analgesia. However, some physicians prefer to treat side effects by other means.

The goal in managing the side effects of epidural narcotics is to provide early intervention. The IV therapy department can work collaboratively with the anesthesiology department to establish protocols so that side effects can be managed by the nurse at the bedside. The IV nurse, as an educator, can reinforce the use of this protocol to the staff nurse.

Excessive somnolence or confusion occurs when too much narcotic is being administered. Somnolence improves by decreasing the epidural narcotic infusion and by administering naloxone hydrochloride in a small dose, such as 0.1 or 0.2 mg IV push. By titrating naloxone hydrochloride to effect, there is a reverse in somnolence without reversing the analgesia.

Nausea and vomiting can be controlled with antiemetics, such as prochlorperazine, droperidol, or a scopolamine patch.[61] An antagonist such as IV naloxone 0.2 mg, which can be titrated to effect, or an agonist-antagonist such as nalbuphine hydrochloride 5 to 10 mg subcutaneously, can reverse the narcotic enough to reverse the side effects without reversing the analgesia.

Urinary retention may occur 10 to 20 hours after the first injection of intraspinal narcotic. Bethanechol chloride or antagonist drugs can be given for relief. Intraspinal narcotics may prevent the bladder from emptying and therefore cause it to overdistend. This may require catheterization if medical intervention proves inadequate. For postoperative patients, some physicians prefer to maintain the Foley catheter until the epidural catheter is ready to be discontinued.[62]

Pruritus from intraspinal narcotics is not caused by histamine release but by the opiate interacting with the opiate receptor sites in the dorsal horn.[63] It is best treated with an antagonist rather than with diphenhydramine.[64] After an epidural injection, 8.5% of all patients experience pruritus; after an intrathecal injection, 46% experience pruritus. Table 14-5 compares side effects with various routes of analgesic agents.

Table 14-5 Comparison of Side Effects of Different Administration Routes*

Side Effect of Analgesic	IV and SC Opiates	Intraspinal Opiates	Intraspinal Local Anesthetics
Respiratory depression	Yes	Yes	No
Nausea	Yes	Yes	No†
Constipation	Yes	No	No
Sedation	Yes	Less frequent	No
Urinary retention	Less frequent	Yes	No
Pruritus	Less frequent	Yes	No
Postural hypotension	Less frequent	No	Yes
Numbness	No	No	Yes

From St. Marie B: Narcotic infusions: a changing scene, *JIN* 14:334, 1991.
*There are few absolutes in the patient's response while administering narcotic infusions. The reports in this table are based on trends in clinical practice.
†If the hypotension occurs from local anesthetics, nausea may follow.

Special considerations

Adjuvant medications, such as NSAIDs, tricyclic antidepressants, topical local anesthetic agents, and anticonvulsant medications, can be used with epidural analgesia and with narcotics administered by other routes.

INTRATHECAL NARCOTICS

Intrathecal narcotic infusions can be considered for cancer patients who have a life expectancy of more than a few months; who do not receive adequate pain relief with systemic narcotics, tricyclic antidepressants, or NSAIDs; and who have pain located below the midcervical dermatomes. Intrathecal narcotic infusions require an implanted infusion pump, not an external pump, because of the risk of infection. Patients have been reported to receive pain relief for 6 months or longer, which merits consideration of this therapy for cancer patients whose effects from systemic narcotics interfere with their quality of life.[65]

An implantable infusion pump (see Fig. 14-6) is indicated for long-term intrathecal infusions, using the same types of implantable pumps used in epidural infusions.[13] There are differences between the epidural space and the intrathecal space that affect clinical practice. The epidural space contains a vascular system, creating leukocytic activity that decreases the likelihood of an epidural infection. The intrathecal space affords a greater risk for infection and may also cause a spinal headache from a cerebrospinal fluid leak. An intrathecal injection of morphine requires approximately 10 to 12 times less medication than that needed in the epidural space. For example, if 5 mg of morphine is injected into the epidural space to produce analgesia, an equivalent dose of morphine injected into the intrathecal space is 0.2 to 0.5 mg. Guidelines for monitoring, site care, and managing complications and side effects are the same as those for epidural infusions. Providing support in the home setting requires knowledge of computer technology to access the implantable pump program through telemetry and refilling the pump.

Intrathecal narcotics given as a single injection are commonly used for postoperative pain management, especially when using preservative-free morphine sulfate. Analgesia from an injection of intrathecal morphine has a rapid onset and may last 18 to 24 hours. This is commonly used for cesarean surgeries, vaginal hysterectomies, and some orthopedic surgeries. The advantages of this delivery method are the following: (1) there is no external catheter creating a risk of dislodgment or infection, (2) prolonged analgesia is offered, and (3) the catheter is relatively simple to access. The disadvantages are as follows: (1) high levels of pain may be experienced as the narcotic wears off, leaving the patient with inadequate pain control; (2) respiratory depression may occur[66]; and (3) the risk of infection is greater than that with epidural delivery because the cerebrospinal fluid is a good medium for bacterial growth. Spinal headache may occur, especially in young women. A spinal headache is caused by needle puncture through the dura that does not seal off and results in cerebrospinal fluid continuing to leak epidurally. The patient could experience a spinal headache for 3 days after the intrathecal injection. Diagnosis of the cause of the headache is confirmed if the patient's headache gets worse when sitting up and improves when lying down. The pain may be located at the back of the head, at the top of the head, or across the forehead. The most effective remedy for spinal headache is a blood patch. This is performed by drawing approximately 10 ml of blood from the patient's arm and injecting the blood epidurally near the level of the original insertion site of the intrathecal needle. This blood gels over the dural puncture, preventing cerebrospinal fluid from leaking out of the dural hole, and displaces the lost fluid from the space, stopping the headache. Patients are instructed to rest and not to exert themselves for 24 hours after placement of the blood patch.

EQUIPMENT USED FOR NARCOTIC INFUSIONS

Having knowledge of various types of infusion devices and supportive equipment allows IV nurses to participate in the decision-making process of their respective hospital, home care organization, outpatient clinic, or long-term facility.

The clinical use of filters with epidural infusions is variable. Bioassay research has confirmed that the stability of medication in cassettes is not a problem.[67] Therefore 5-micron filters are not necessary, but bacterial studies are not documented. The Intravenous Nurses Society *Infusion Nursing Standards of Practice*[24] supports using a 0.22-micron filter without surfactant for epidural infusions. This should be considered for home and hospital care.

Medication containers for epidural infusions may include a regular IV bag containing preservative-free medication or a container that is compatible with an infusion pump. In either case, the containers need to be well marked for epidural use only so that they are not mistaken for an IV medication or vice versa.

Because one purpose of epidural analgesia is to achieve early ambulation, ambulatory infusion pumps should be considered. A variety of ambulatory infusion pumps are available, and careful consideration needs to be given to the selection of a pump. The important features of an infusion pump for administering narcotics have been presented (see Box 14-2). The technology is advancing, challenging the IV nurse to continue to evaluate new infusion pumps in the marketplace.

NURSING AND PAIN MANAGEMENT

Pain management is an aspect of patient care in which patient advocacy is exceedingly important. Nurses who work at the patient's bedside hear what the patient tells them and know when their patients are experiencing pain. Nurses need to be organized in their approach to pain and can use the nursing process to assist in this organization. Nurses can communicate effectively with other members of the health care team and also need to teach patients how to manage their pain effectively.

It is the responsibility of each nurse caring for a patient to ensure quality pain management. Nurses in various health care settings need to be cognizant of this fact. Interdisciplinary approaches have been implemented successfully throughout the United States. Health care professionals from various disciplines, such as anesthesiology, neurology, nursing, oncology, and physical therapy, have developed pain management strategies, and these team members share the responsibilities of care.

Teams of nurses responsible for pain management have been formed in some hospitals, hospices, and home health agencies. The nursing responsibilities of these teams range from actually administering the pain medications to educating nurses about proper dosing and delivery. A pain team may also identify and solve problems associated with pain management.

A pain management medical director is usually a physician who specializes in pain management. The medical director serves as a resource to those involved in pain management and also acts as liaison and educator of other physicians. The medical director needs to understand and respect the nursing role in pain management, thereby enhancing the care that nurses give to patients in pain.

Assessment of pain

Pain assessment requires an extensive knowledge of pain, its causes, and its management. An in-depth study of pain assessment is beyond the limitations of this treatise but is essential to conducting clinical pain assessments that can guide initial pain therapy. A number of resources are available.[5,68-72] The nurse must be sure to document the assessment of pain, the intervention used, and the reassessment of pain to determine the effectiveness of the pain management intervention.

Assessing the patient's pain is necessary for effective control. The clinician involved in pain control can use either a brief or a comprehensive assessment.

A brief assessment of pain is performed when the patient is in absolute distress and delaying pain management would have harmful effects. A brief assessment includes the patient's description and rating of the pain, its timing, and location; any associated symptoms; what lessens the pain or makes it worse; what medications are being used; and the identification of any behavioral component. The brief assessment is beneficial for postoperative pain, trauma pain, and acute medical disorders, including acute exacerbations of cancer pain. The goal of a brief

---

Box 14-5   Components of a Comprehensive Assessment of Chronic Pain

- Overview of pain history
- Sites of pain
- Quality and quantity descriptors, timing
- Exacerbating and relieving factors
- Social evaluation
- Psychologic evaluation

---

assessment is to determine what pathways the pain is taking and to intervene with medications that affect those pathways directly.

A comprehensive assessment of pain is used to formulate a long-term plan for pain management. This approach is useful for cancer pain and for chronic pain from nonmalignant disorders (Box 14-5).

Appendix C presents an example of a pain assessment form. When the variables of the pain have been determined and systemic narcotics have been administered, it is essential to evaluate the effectiveness of the intervention by asking the following questions:

1. Is pain adequately controlled with systemic narcotics, NSAIDs, and tricyclic antidepressants, where applicable?
2. Are the side effects of the systemic narcotics severe enough to affect the quality of the patient's remaining life adversely?

If the answer to either question is yes, the patient should be evaluated for epidural or intrathecal narcotic administration. While attempting to control the patient's pain, the nurse should continue to assess variables to evaluate the effectiveness of these pain interventions. These variables include vital signs, urinary and bowel function, integument, mental status, pain rating (using a pain flow sheet), and coping capability of the patient and family. "The single most reliable indicator of the existence and intensity of acute pain and any resultant affective discomfort or distress—is the patient's self-report."[73] By looking at the whole picture, the nurse can identify and anticipate problems.

Nursing diagnosis

Nursing diagnosis "is a clinical judgment about individual . . . responses to actual and potential health problems."[74] The nursing diagnoses listed in Box 14-6, among others, can be used to assist in the development of a care plan.

Care plan. When a particular problem or problems with pain management have been identified, the nursing process continues with planning. Nursing diagnosis is critical to the development of nursing care plans, providing a basis for selecting nursing interventions to achieve desired outcomes for which nursing is accountable. Nursing care plans help communicate the plan of care to the nurse's peers. In developing the care plan, the nurse needs to be informed of patients' goals for pain management. For example, cancer patients with intractable pain may express a desire to achieve pain relief but to remain alert and oriented so that they can continue to interact with their loved ones. Care plans should not only consider the patient's

Box 14-6   Nursing Diagnoses for Pain Management

Anxiety: characterized by sympathetic stimulation, trembling, voice quivering, facial tension, diaphoresis

Fatigue: characterized by emotional irritability and decreased performance

Knowledge deficit: inaccurate follow-through of instruction

Activity intolerance: related to exertional discomfort

Sleep pattern disturbance: characterized by irritability, restlessness, disorientation, lethargy, slight hand tremor, ptosis of eyelid, and mild, fleeting nystagmus

Altered thought processes: characterized by cognitive dissonance, inaccurate interpretation of environment, memory deficit

wishes, but also communicate and accommodate them. The nursing care plan also helps provide continuity of care, which is so important to a patient in pain. The nursing care plan can be used for postoperative pain, pain caused by acute medical disorders, trauma pain, and acute and chronic cancer pain.

Implementation. When the plan has been determined, implementing the plan in the hospital requires 24-hour cooperation among all nurses. In the home setting, implementation initially includes daily assessment of the patient by telephone or visit; after the patient is stabilized, daily contact may not be necessary.

The importance of continuity of care for patients in pain cannot be stressed enough. If one or two nurses caring for the patient are not knowledgeable about the level of care given, the patient is left feeling isolated, helpless, and in pain. A variety of methods can be used to communicate knowledge and care:

- Educational in-service training with speakers, videos, audio tapes, and self-guided learning packets
- Staff meetings at which pain management is a regularly discussed topic
- Verbal "reporting off" on each shift (taking the time to emphasize nursing care given for pain control)
- Written documentation in the nursing progress notes for each shift and documentation on a flow sheet that is left conveniently at the bedside
- Preceptors or nursing instructors who may "buddy" with nurses to facilitate the focus on pain management and serve as models
- Home care case conferences and verbal reports between involved team members.

Implementation also includes teaching the patient. Patients with all types of pain benefit from teaching about pain management; education helps put them at ease regarding the pain management interventions that may be used on their behalf. Box 14-7 lists a few important concepts that can be applied to any pain control intervention for postoperative, trauma, chronic nonmalignant pain disorders, and cancer pain.

Important concepts for patient instruction regarding PCA have been discussed (see Parenteral Narcotics: Intravenous Administration). Concepts important for instruction in intraspinal narcotics (epidural and intrathecal) are described in Box 14-8.

Box 14-7   Important Concepts in Pain Control

1. Pain rating—explain that patient will be asked to rate pain on a pain scale (define your pain scale). The usual pain scale is 0 to 10, where 0 equals no pain and 10 equals excruciating pain.
2. Tell the patient to let you know when the pain becomes worse.
3. Explain that side effects may occur and say what they are. Explain the importance of notifying the nurse immediately if side effects are experienced so that they can be treated.
4. Ask the patient to notify the nurse immediately if the medication does not relieve the pain.
5. The patient may be concerned about addiction to narcotics during the postoperative recovery. This fear should be addressed directly. For postoperative pain, the nurse should stress that people do not become addicted if they are taking narcotics directly for short-term pain relief. For patients who have a long recovery and probably need narcotic pain relief during the painful recovery period, clarify the two different types of addiction: physical dependence and psychologic dependence. Explain that physical dependence can occur when the body is accustomed to receiving narcotics and that if use of the narcotic is abruptly terminated, the patient may go through withdrawal. This is the easiest type of addiction to handle because the patient is weaned off the narcotic over a short period and withdrawal is prevented.[26] However, psychologic dependence occurs when the patient craves the narcotic and uses it for reasons other than pain control. Psychologic dependence from postoperative pain management is rare. This type of addiction is difficult to treat in the usual health care setting, and the patient may need to be referred to a chemical dependency setting. Once patients are educated about these differences, their fears are relieved.

Box 14-8   Patient Teaching Concepts for Intraspinal Narcotics

1. The infusion pump is preset to deliver medication near the nerve root.
2. If epidural local anesthetic is used, explain to patients that they may experience numbness, but should not be alarmed. They should report numbness to the nurse, so that adjustments can be made.
3. Physical dependence on an epidural infusion for acute pain has not been documented or noted in clinical practice. The infusion can be stopped abruptly and patients do not go through withdrawal.
4. Patients may ask whether epidural narcotics can take away all their pain. An appropriate response is that this technique helps keep their pain at a minimum with less narcotic and fewer side effects. If they *do* have pain, the nurse should be told, and they can be supplemented with additional medication and the epidural dosages adjusted.

Evaluation

Patient. The patient's response to any pain intervention may be evaluated through nurse-patient communication, vital sign monitoring, and observation of pupil size and mental status. If the side effects of narcotics become severe while the patient is still having increased pain, a nonnarcotic approach should be evaluated (e.g., NSAIDs). For example, if a patient has received 12 mg of IV morphine sulfate over 30 minutes and cannot keep his or her eyes open but still complains of pain, an injection of ketorolac tromethamine may be helpful to control the pain without producing more sedation.

Monitoring the outcome of all patients receiving treatment for pain validates the need for advanced pain management interventions to patients, physicians, nurses, and insurance carriers.[75] Any problems in pain intervention can be readily identified and communicated to authorities designated to make recommendations. Improving the quality of pain management means having pain intervention accessible to patients in a timely manner and ensuring that the intervention has the desired effect. The goals of effective pain management are presented in Box 14-9.

Clinical indications for quality improvement.

Organizational trends in pain management can be improved through a process of continuous quality improvement. Predetermined clinical indicators related to pain management can be identified, such as respiratory depression, breakthrough pain, and somnolence, and these can be monitored quarterly. Other measurements can be determined by using patient satisfaction surveys and monitoring costs and charges for pain management interventions. It is through these measures that health care professionals can link cause and effect to intervention and outcome.

In recent years, new therapies have been developed that have increased the effectiveness of pain management. There is reason to hope that patients with intractable cancer, surgical, and trauma pain can benefit even more in the future from advances in pain control.

It is clear that there are valuable benefits to having a well-organized system in place for delivering pain management services. Good communication among physicians and nurses can empower nurses to provide effective analgesia to their patients, and it is well documented that effective pain management reduces complications, thereby decreasing length of hospital stay. A good system also ensures that up-to-date approaches to pain management are used efficiently.

There have been many discoveries in the field of pain management—pain pathways, opiate receptor sites, NSAIDs, and new ways to use old methods—so many that pain management is evolving into a specialty of its own. These discoveries should help improve patient outcomes, but it takes motivated personnel to keep up with the latest information. IV nurses should seize the opportunity presented by these advancements and accumulate the knowledge needed to facilitate pain control for their patients. Reading journals that focus on pain management, one might be surprised by what can be done to improve patient outcomes. Now is the time for IV nurses and nurses in other disciplines to open their minds to improved methods of achieving analgesia.

REFERENCES

1. Schweitzer A: *On the edge of the primeval forest,* New York, 1931, Macmillan.
2. Bonica J: *The management of pain,* ed 2, vol 1, Philadelphia, 1990, Lea & Febiger.
3. Bamberger A, Tanelian DK, Klein K: Pain management for the postoperative patient, *Tex Med* 90:54, 1994.
4. Crombie I, et al: *Epidemiology of pain,* London, 1999, IASP Press.
5. Ahmedzai S: Current strategies for pain control, *Ann Oncol* 3(suppl 8):S21, 1997.
6. Nimmo WS, Duthie DJ: Pain relief after surgery, *Anaesth Intensive Care* 15:68, 1987.
7. Marks RM, Sacher EJ: Undertreatment of medical inpatients with narcotic analgesic, *Ann Intern Med* 78(2):173, 1973.
8. Grass J: Preemptive analgesia, *Probl Anesth* 10(1):107, 1998.
9. McCaffery M, Beebe A: *Pain: clinical manual for nursing practice,* St Louis, 1989, Mosby.
10. Mettler FA: Pain I: what is it? *J Med Soc NJ* 61(1):10, 1964.
11. Sjostrom S, et al: Cerebrospinal fluid concentrations of substance P and (met) Enkephalin-Arg6-Phe7 during surgery and patient-controlled analgesia, *Anesth Analg* 67:976, 1988.
12. Hughes J: Isolation of an endogenous compound from the brain with pharmacological properties similar to morphine, *Brain Res* 88:295, 1975.
13. Atweh SF, Kuhar MJ: Autoradiographic localization of opiate receptors in rat brain: I, spinal cord and lower medulla, *Brain Res* 124:53, 1977.
14. Scott DB: *Techniques of regional anaesthesia,* Norwalk, Conn, 1989, Appleton and Lange.
15. Hauer M, et al: Intravenous patient-controlled analgesia in critically ill postoperative-trauma patients: research-based practice recommendations, *Dimens Crit Care Nurs* 14:144, 1995.
16. Hadaway LC: Evaluation and use of advanced I.V. technology: part 2 patient-controlled analgesia, *JIN* 12:184, 1989.
17. Hansen LA, Noyes MA, Lehman ME: Evaluation of patient-controlled analgesia (PCA) versus PCA plus continuous infusion in postoperative cancer patients, *J Pain Symptom Manage* 6:4, 1991.
18. Allcock N: Factors affecting the assessment of postoperative pain: literature review, *J Adv Nurs* 24:1144, 1996.
19. White PF: Use of patient-controlled analgesia for management of acute pain, *JAMA* 259:243, 1988.
20. St. Marie B: Narcotic infusions: a changing scene, *JIN* 14:334, 1991.
21. American Geriatrics Society Panel on Chronic Pain in Older Persons: Clinical practice guideline: the management of chronic pain in the older person, *JAGS* 46:635, 1998.
22. Egbert AM: Postoperative pain management in the frail elderly, *Clin Geriatr Med* 12:583, 1996.
23. Agency for Health Care Policy and Research: *Clinical practice guidelines: acute pain management: operative or medical procedures and trauma,* Rockville, Md, 1992, US Department of Health and Human Services.
24. Intravenous Nurses Society: Infusion nursing standards of practice, *JIN* (suppl) 23(6S), 2000.

Box 14-9 Goals of Providing Quality Pain Management

- Provide better analgesia with less sedation
- Improve pulmonary function
- Decrease the stress response evident in people with pain
- Produce earlier ambulation
- Shorten intensive care unit stay
- Facilitate earlier hospital discharge

25. Lehman K, Ribbert N, Horricks-Haermeyer G: Postoperative patient-controlled analgesia with alfentanil: analgesic efficacy and minimum effective concentrations, *J Pain Symptom Manage* 5:249, 1990.

26. American Pain Society: *Principles of analgesic use in the treatment of acute pain and cancer pain,* ed 4, Glenview, Ill, 1999, American Pain Society.

27. Jackson D: A study of pain management: patient-controlled analgesia versus intramuscular analgesia, *JIN* 12:42, 1989.

28. Bruera E, et al: Use of the subcutaneous route for the administration of narcotics in patients with cancer pain, *Cancer* 62:407, 1988.

29. Moulin E, Kreeft J, Murray-Parson N, Bouquillon AI: Comparison of continuous subcutaneous and intravenous hydromorphone infusions for management of cancer pain, *Lancet* 337:465, 1991.

30. Coyle N, Mauskop A, Moggard J, Foley KM: Continuous subcutaneous infusions of opiates in cancer patients with pain, *Oncol Nurs Forum* 13:53, 1986.

31. Carey SJ, et al: Improving pain management in an acute care setting: The Crawford Long Hospital of Emory University experience, *Ortho Nurs* 16:29, 1997.

32. Borrmeo AR, Windle PE: Benchmarking for unrelieved pain in a postanesthesia care unit, *Best Practice Benchmarking Healthcare* 2:20, 1997.

33. Gueneron JP, et al: Effect of naloxone infusion on analgesia and respiratory depression after epidural fentanyl, *Anesth Analg* 67:35, 1988.

34. Barber D: The physiology and pharmacology of pain: a review of opioids, *J Perianesthesia Nurs* 12:95, 1997.

35. Ferris FD, et al: Transdermal scopolamine use in the control of narcotic-induced nausea, *J Pain Symptom Manage* 6(6):389, 1991.

36. Gillis JC, Brogden RN: Ketoralac: a reappraisal of its pharmacodynamic and pharmacokinetic properties and therapeutic use in pain management, *Drugs* 53(1):139, 1997.

37. Warfield CA, Dohlman LE: Intraspinal narcotics for pain control, *Hosp Pract* 12(9):148B, 1984.

38. DuPen SL: *Epidural morphine sulfate: preservatives or not?* Seattle, 1987, Swedish Hospital Medical Center (Reprint).

39. Hicks RJ, et al: The radionuclide assessment of a system for a low intrathecal infusion of drugs, *Clin Nucl Med* 14:275, 1989.

40. Yaksh TL: Spinal opiate analgesia: characteristics and principles of action, *Pain* 11:293, 1981.

41. DeLeon-Casasola OA, Lema MJ: Postoperative epidural opioid analgesia: what are the choices? *Anesth Analg* 83:867, 1996.

42. Wattwil M, et al: Epidural analgesia with bupivacaine reduces postoperative paralytic ileus after hysterectomy, *Anesth Analg* 68:353, 1989.

43. Loper KA, Ready LB: Epidural morphine after anterior cruciate ligament repair: a comparison with patient-controlled intravenous morphine, *Anesth Analg* 68:350, 1989.

44. Hansdottir V, et al: The CSF and plasma pharmacokinetics of sufentanil after intrathecal administration, *Anesthesiology* 74:264, 1991.

45. Ready LB: Spinal opioids in the management of acute and postoperative pain, *J Pain Symptom Manage* 5:138, 1990.

46. Gladd NL: Pediatric postoperative pain management, *Anesth Analg* 28(suppl), 1998.

47. Wulf H, Maier C, Streipling E: Pharmacokinetics and protein binding of Bupivacaine in postoperative epidural analgesia, *Acta Anaesthesiol Scand* 32:530, 1988.

48. Strathern D: Epidural analgesia: educating patients and nurses, *Nursing Standard* 10(25):33, 1996.

49. Naber L, Jones G, Halm M: Epidural analgesia for effective pain control, *Crit Care Nurse* 69, Oct 1994.

50. Waldman SD: The role of spinal opioids in the management of cancer pain, *J Pain Symptom Manage* 5:163, 1990.

51. DuPen SL, et al: A new permanent exteriorized epidural catheter for narcotic self-administration to control cancer pain, *Cancer* 59:986, 1987.

52. Waldman SD, Feldstein G, Allen M: Troubleshooting intraspinal narcotic delivery systems, *Am J Nurs* 87(1):63, 1987.

53. Caballero GA, Ausmen RK, Hemo J: Epidural morphine by continuous infusion with an external pump for pain management in oncology patients, *Am Surgeon* 52:8, 1986.

54. Yaksh TL, Onofrio BM: Retrospective consideration of the doses of morphine given intrathecally by chronic infusion in 163 patients by 19 physicians, *Pain* 31:211, 1987.

55. Paice JA: New delivery systems in pain management, *Nurs Clin North Am* 22:715, 1987.

56. Harmer M, Davies KA: The effect of education, assessment and a standardized prescription on postoperative pain management, *Anesthesia* 53:424, 1998.

57. St. Marie B, Henrickson K: Intraspinal narcotic infusions for terminal cancer pain, *JIN* 11:161, 1988.

58. Chrubasik J, Magra F: Postoperative epidural opiate pharmacokinetics, *Anesth Analg* 74:S44, 1992.

59. Krames ES, et al: Continuous infusion of spinally administered narcotics for the relief of pain due to malignant disorders, *Cancer* 56:696, 1985.

60. Makie K, Lam AM: The epinephrine-containing test dose during beta-blockade, *Anesthesiology* 71:A1146, 1989.

61. Loper KA, Ready LD, Horman BH: Prophylactic transdermal scopolamine patches reduce nausea in postoperative patients receiving epidural morphine, *Anesth Analg* 68:144, 1989.

62. Carpenter RL: Optimizing postoperative pain management, *Am Fam Physician* 56:835, 1997.

63. Ackerman WE, Guneja MM, Kaczorowski DM: A comparison of the incidence of pruritus following epidural opioid administration in the parturient, *Can J Anaesth* 36:388, 1989.

64. Davies GG, From R: A blinded study using nalbuphine for prevention of pruritus induced by epidural fentanyl, *Anesthesiology* 69:763, 1988.

65. Penn RD, Paice JA: Chronic intrathecal morphine for intractable pain, *J Neurosurg* 67:182, 1987.

66. Etches RC, Sandler AN, Daley MD: Respiratory depression and spinal opioids, *Can J Anaesth* 36:165, 1989.

67. Allen LV, Stiles MI, Yu-Hsing TU: Stability of fentanyl citrate in 0.9% sodium chloride solutions prefilled in ambulatory infusion reservoirs, *Am J Hosp Pharm* 1572, 1990.

68. Turk D, Melzack R: *Handbook of pain assessment,* New York, 1992 The Guilford Press.

69. Kerns RD, Turk DC, Rudy TE: The West Haven-Yale Multidimensional Pain Inventory (WHYMPI), *Pain* 23:345, 1985.

70. Fishman B, et al: The memorial pain assessment card: a valid instrument for the evaluation of cancer pain, *Cancer* 60:1151, 1987.

71. Melzack R: The McGill pain questionnaire: major properties and scoring methods, *Pain* 1:277, 1975.

72. Dau RL, Clerland CS: Development of the Wisconsin brief pain questionnaire to assess pain in cancer and other diseases, *Pain* 17:197, 1983.

73. Agency for Health Care Policy and Research: *Clinical practice guidelines. acute pain management: operative or medical procedures and trauma,* Rockville, Md, 1992, US Department of Health and Human Services.

74. North American Nursing Diagnosis Association: *Nursing diagnosis: definitions and classification, 1999-2000,* Philadelphia, 1999.

75. American Pain Society Quality of Care Committee: *Quality improvement guidelines for the treatment of acute pain and cancer pain,* Glenview, Ill, 1995, American Pain Society.

NORTH MEMORIAL
MEDICAL CENTER
3300 North Oakdale,
Robbinsdale, MN 55422
(612) 520-5200

CONTROLLED SUBSTANCE

INFUSION

FLOW SHEET

DRUG: **CONCENTRATION:**

DATE/TIME DISPENSED: **BY:**

RECEIVED BY: RN **VOLUME:**

Date										
Time										
RES VOL										
CONC. mg/ml (Epidural: Set screen at 0)										
Rate										
Bolus Dose										
Dose Min/Dose Hr										
Dose Given										
Clinician Bolus										
Given 0600-1400-2200 mg or ml										
Other Analgesics (Yes/No)										
LOC *										
Pain Rating **										
Epidural: Qh LOC and Resp. Rate (✓)										
Epidural: Numbness (+/-)										
Epidural: Orthostatic Changes (Yes/No)										
Pruritus (+/-)										
Nausea (+/-)										
Dressing/Connection Check (✓)										
Nurse's Initials										

INITIALS	SIGNATURE	INITIALS	SIGNATURE	INITIALS	SIGNATURE

LEVEL OF CONSCIOUSNESS KEY (LOC) *

1. Alert, engages in conversation; purposefully travels with eyes, if mute.
2. Lethargic, drowsy, sedate - focuses on personal interchange - but unable to maintain focus.
3. Responds only to maximal stimulation (shaking). Response only a grunt or moan - not a clear sentence.
4. Coma - unable to respond at all.

PAIN RATING (INTENSITY) **

5	Overwhelming
4	Severe
3	Distressing
2	Moderate
1	Mild
0	No Pain

Mix expiration = 7 days
Hang expiration = 72 hrs

Mix date/time_____ Exp_____
Hang date/time_____ Exp_____

Cassette changed or DC'd by_____

Amount Wasted = RES VOL_____

Witness to Wasting of Drug_____

F431 11/92   **Original White = Chart, Yellow = Pharmacy, Pink = Pharmacy**   N21411.dop/bb

APPENDIX 14-A-1

Courtesy of North Memorial Medical Center, Robbinsville, MN.

USE IN ACCORDANCE WITH PROCEDURE AND PROTOCOL

<u>CIRCLE</u> **PAIN TREATMENT MODALITY:**

1. PO
2. SUBLINGUAL
3. PATIENT CONTROLLED ANALGESIA
4. CONTINUOUS IV OPIOID INFUSION
5. TEMPORARY EPIDURAL INTERMITTENT INJECTION
6. PERMANENT EPIDURAL INTERMITTENT INJECTION

7. IM
8. RECTAL
9. CONTINUOUS SUBCUTANEOUS OPIOID INFUSION
10. INTERMITTENT IV OPIOID INJECTION
11. TEMPORARY EPIDURAL CONTINUOUS INFUSION
12. PERMANENT EPIDURAL CONTINUOUS INFUSION

PAIN SCALE:
0 = none
1 = mild
2
3 = moderate
4
5 = severe

SEDATION SCALE:
3 = Awake and responding
2 = Sleeping, but responds to normal voice
1 = Sleeping, but responds to loud voice or movement
0 = Sedated, doesn't respond

DATE	TIME	MED	BAG OR SYRINGE #	ROUTE #	BOLUS	CONT. RATE or basal	DOSE	PCA DELAY (min)	8 hr total	BP	P/RR	SEDATION SCALE	PAIN	SKIN ANESTHESIA N=Normal T=Tingling Nb=Numbness A=Absent	SITE	CHECK	Tubing filter &/or SQ needle change	COMMENTS	INITIALS

NURSE INITIALS & SIGNATURE:

ADDRESSOGRAPH:

SWEDISH HOSPITAL MEDICAL CENTER

PAIN MANAGEMENT
NU-1153 Rev. 1/91 FC/SHMC SN-5885

APPENDIX 14-A-2

Courtesy of Swedish Hospital Medical Center, Seattle, WA.

DATE	TIME	PHYSICIAN'S ORDERS	NOTED BY

PERMANENT EPIDURAL CATHETERS STANDING ORDERS

MD: Please indicate selections with an "X" and fill in all blanks.

Intermittent Injections:
1. Opioid: _____ every _____ hours
   Dilute with _____ ml preservative-free normal saline

Continuous Infusion per Micro Abbott Pump:
1. Opioid: _____
2. Local anesthetic agent and percentage: _____
   Other additive: _____
3. Start infusion at _____ ml/hour
4. ( ) Discontinue intermittent epidural injections previously ordered.

Patient Controlled Epidural Analgesia (PCEA) per Bard pump:
1. PCEA syringe medication same as continuous infusion drug   3. Delay interval _____ minutes
2. PCEA dose _____ ml   4. Basal "OFF"

For inadequate pain relief: (Pain Scale 0 = None, 1 = Mild, 3 = Moderate, 5 = Severe)

   <u>**Intermittent Injections**</u>
     Opioid _____ every _____ hours
     Dilute with _____ ml preservative-free normal saline
     Breakthrough pain relief – Opioid: _____

   <u>**Continuous infusion per Micro Abbott pump**</u>
     If pain level 3: increase rate to _____ ml/hr.
     If pain level 4: increase rate to _____ ml/hr.
     If pain level 5: increase rate to _____ ml/hr.

   <u>**PCEA per Bard pump**</u> (Pain level ≥ 3)
     Increase PCA dose to _____ ml.   Decrease delay interval to _____ minutes

   Call Pain Service STAT (Ext. 2323) (or attending MD) if patient's pain level increases or sustains at a 3 - 5 level.

IV Therapy:
1. IV fluid solution _____ at _____ ml/hr
2. For initiation of local anesthetic agent, patient must have IV access x 48 hrs

Treatment of side effects:
1. For nausea/vomiting:
      ( ) Prochlorperazine (Compazine) 5 - 10 mg IV q 6 hrs prn
      ( ) Lorazepam (Ativan) 0.5 - 1.0 mg IV q 4 hrs prn
      ( ) Metoclopramide (Reglan) 5 - 10 mg IV q 4 hrs prn
      ( ) Other _____
2. Call Pain Service and/or attending MD for the following:
      Sedation level 1 (responds to loud voice or noise) or 0 (no response)   dysphoria
      RR < 8/min   urinary retention
      If BP < _____ or > _____
      Significant increase or sudden onset of numbness or motor weakness
3. If sedation level ≤ 1 **and** RR < 8/min:
      Decrease continuous infusion by 50%.
      Stat oximetry
      Naloxone (Narcan) 0.1 mg IV **slow** push q 5 min x 4; reassess sedation & RR before each dose to determine need for continued dosing. Call Pain Service or attending M.D.
4. If urinary retention: straight cath x 1.
5. Bowel care by nurses

Monitoring:
1. P, RR, BP, sedation, pain, and skin anesthesia (only with local anesthetic agents) q 1 hr x 2, then q 4 hr
2. Postural BP (only with local anesthetic agents) q 8 hr until stable
3. Urinary output q 8 hr – monitor for retention
4. Contact Infusion Therapy instructors at Ext. 6023

☐ _____ _____ , M.D.
     PHONE

☐ Stuart DuPen, M.D.   991-5751   _____
☐ Anna Williams, R.N.   998-6495   _____

A DRUG EQUIVALENT MAY BE DISPENSED UNLESS CHECKED ☐

SIGNATURE IS REQUIRED FOLLOWING ENTRY OF EACH ORDER

SWEDISH MEDICAL CENTER
747 Summit Avenue   Seattle, WA 98104-2196

NU-1756   Rev. 9/93   FC/SMC

PHYSICIAN'S ORDERS
APPENDIX 14-B

Courtesy of Swedish Hospital Medical Center, Seattle, WA.

PAIN ASSESSMENT FORM

1. Intensity:

NURSE: _____
PATIENT: _____
DATE: _____

PAIN SCALE

```
        0   1   2   3   4   5   6   7   8   9   10
No     |___|___|___|___|___|___|___|___|___|___|
Pain
```

Worst Pain Imaginable

Pain Rating _____ mm

2. Where is your pain located?   (I = Internal)
   Patient or Nurse mark drawing.   (E = External)

3. How and when did your pain begin?
   Does something trigger your pain?
   _____
   _____

4. How long have you had the pain?
   Is it continuous or intermittent?
   Describe any patterns or changes.
   _____
   _____
   _____

5. Describe in your own words what your pain feels like: _____
   _____
   _____
   _____

6. What makes the pain better? _____
   _____

7. What makes the pain worse? _____
   _____

8. What has helped in the past? _____
   _____

9. What has not helped in the past? _____
   _____

10. What other symptoms accompany your pain? _____
    _____

11. How does your pain affect your: _____
    Sleep? _____
    Appetite? _____
    Physical activity? _____
    Concentration? _____
    Emotions? _____
    Social relationships? _____

12. What do you think is causing your pain now?
    _____

13. Current Analgesic Regimen? _____
    _____

14. Plan/comments _____
    _____
    _____

JPI-DR-019-4A

APPENDIX 14-C

Chapter

15

Infusion Therapy Equipment: Types of Infusion Therapy Equipment

Roxanne Perucca, MSN, CRNI*

FLUID CONTAINERS
Glass containers
Plastic containers
Semirigid containers
Other fluid containers
Venting rigid containers
Light sensitivity
Use-activated containers
ADMINISTRATION SETS
Primary administration sets
Secondary administration sets
Vented and nonvented sets
Metered-volume chamber sets
Drop factors
Primary Y sets
Internal diameter of tubing
In-line rate-control clamps
Add-on manual flow control devices
Resealable Y injection ports
Back-check valves
Connections
Pressure bags
Nitroglycerin administration sets
Fat emulsion–specific sets
Blood administration sets
Add-on devices
INFUSION FILTERS
Purpose
Characteristics
Configuration
Blood filters

INFUSION CATHETERS AND CANNULAS
Peripheral catheters/cannulas
Central infusion catheters
Types of central line devices
Alternative access devices
DRESSINGS
Gauze
Transparent dressings
Securement devices
Antimicrobial barrier materials
INFUSION DEVICES
Mechanical infusion devices
Electronic infusion devices
Mechanisms of delivery
INFUSION PUMPS
Characteristics
Types
Cost considerations in infusion pump technology
Infusion pumps in various settings

The equipment used in health care is changing rapidly to meet the demands of consumers. In the health care market, the consumers are the health care providers and patients. The patient is rarely involved in the decision-making process of equipment acquisition, so the patient's role is more that of a recipient than an actively participating consumer. Because of this unique situation, the nurse makes product decisions for the patient, thereby reinforcing the traditional role of the nurse as the patient advocate. The nurse's role in equipment selection is to ensure the safe, effective delivery of health care to the patient.

*The author and editors wish to acknowledge the contributions made by Brenda Jensen, as author of this chapter in the first edition of *Intravenous Nursing: Clinical Principles and Practice*.

The nurse must be aware of the almost unlimited amount of information available from the health care industry. Because of their desire to anticipate needs, representatives of the health care industry are aware of medical research in the early stages. Research and clinical validation of products can reveal a great deal of information about product capabilities and limitations. These factors make the manufacturer a rich source of information that cumulatively can aid in product selection. The nurse should look at all brands of a specific product to separate salesmanship from product performance before determining the product's acceptability.

Financial accountability is a necessity in health care. The financial profile of specific populations should guide reimbursement expectations. This information is necessary for the formulation of plans to evaluate and procure equipment in a cost-effective manner. Medical manufacturers pride themselves on the extensive research and clinical activity used to design and develop medical products. Many companies have departments of medical professionals who are involved in the evolution of medical products, and reimbursement potential is always a consideration. Research and development departments are an invaluable source of information for the nurse. Not only do manufacturers research the products they develop, but most also submit products for third-party research to validate their findings. A part of product acquisition is the sharing of research information with users, nurses, and physicians. The product's capabilities and supporting data are available to anyone who is interested and are often cataloged in the institution's purchasing department.

Manufacturers are subject to the laws of supply and demand. If the supply is ample and the demand steady, the cost is usually reasonable. If the demand is high and the supplies are scarce, the cost can be high. Professional networking can help identify substandard products and consequently decrease demand.

In summary, the relationship among industry, health care providers, and patients is one of mutual dependence. The role of each exists because of the presence of the other two. The public holds industry, medical institutions, and professionals accountable for the safe and effective delivery of health care. Medical products and equipment are the collaborative responsibility of industry and medical professionals.

FLUID CONTAINERS
Glass containers

The first intravenous (IV) infusion container to be mass produced was made of glass. Glass was and is easy to sterilize, and graduations on glass can be easily and accurately read. However, after 50 years of use, glass remains the container of choice only for infusates that cannot adapt to plastic bags because of incompatibilities with the chemicals or properties of plastic.

Nitroglycerin adheres to the plastic container, reducing the amount of drug available for infusion. Administration is therefore difficult to measure accurately. Drug dosages are titrated to patient condition.

Closed-system glass bottles are sealed with a thick, hard, rubber disk. The center is designated with a target area, which can be easily perforated with the administration-tubing spike.

The hard rubber disk is covered with an easily removable vacuum seal. Once the seal is removed, the bottle should be used immediately to ensure sterility. The seal must be removed before it is spiked with an administration set and cannot be reapplied or resealed. In a sterile admixture program, infusates can be mixed and a second sterile cover applied for delivery to the patient care area.

Because they are noncollapsible, glass bottles must also be vented. For the solution to empty from the bottle, air must replace the solution, which can occur through a venting straw or with vented tubing. If the bottle is made with a venting straw, it runs the length of the bottle to allow air to be pulled in as the solution infuses. The potential for contamination of the solution is increased with the use of a venting straw because no barrier exists between the external sources of contamination and the interior of the bottle.

Most glass bottles are made without venting straws, and vented administration sets are used to relieve the vacuum in the bottle. The tubing spike has a regular channel for the flow of fluid and a very small side channel to introduce air into the bottle. The infusion set may be made specifically as a vented set, or may be considered a universal infusion set with a capped air channel, requiring the nurse to uncap the air inlet channel when it is used with a glass fluid container (Fig. 15-1).

Plastic containers

The first real commitment to large-scale conversion to plastic IV fluid containers came with the need to transport soldiers from the battlefield or field triage areas with treatment already initiated. The same pressure for plastic came from improved emergency care in regular hospitals. As emergency personnel and treatments evolved and many more treatments were initiated outside the hospital, the need for the safety of plastic became critical for the patient and for the health care provider.

The introduction of polyvinyl chloride (PVC) plastic fluid containers has met many compatibility requirements. The health care industry predominantly uses plastic bags as primary fluid containers. However, many concerns have been raised recently regarding the leaching of Di-2-ethylhexyl-phthalate (DHEP) into the blood exposing the patient to carcinogens. DHEP is known as a *plasticizer*, a substance that imparts certain qualities to plastics. DHEP is added to plastic to make it pliable, but it is not chemically bonded to the vinyl and can leach out.[1] The issue is being widely discussed, and several federal panels have been mandated to evaluate the data on plasticizers.

Infusates that remain a concern with regard to compatibility to plastic are insulin, nitroglycerin, fat emulsions, lorazepam, and others.[2] Research on the combination of these drugs, plastic bags, and administration sets is ongoing and remains controversial.

Besides compatibility, another concern is accuracy—of the graduations marked on plastic containers and of volume readings taken by health care workers. A study reported by Coles and Fanning in 1987 found that measurements in Viaflex plastic bags were within plus or minus 10% for increments 1 through 9. However, the first and last graduations were as much as 40% inaccurate.[3]

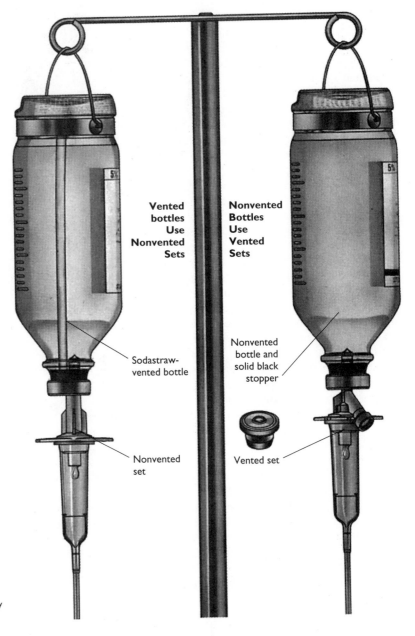

Vented bottles Use Nonvented Sets

Nonvented Bottles Use Vented Sets

Sodastraw-vented bottle

Nonvented bottle and solid black stopper

Nonvented set

Vented set

FIG. 15-1 *Vented and nonvented bottle tubing.* (Courtesy Baxter Healthcare Corporation.)

Plastic fluid containers should be inspected carefully before they are used. All fluid ports should be examined to ensure that they are sealed and intact. The container can be perforated during use. Attention should be taken to avoid tearing the side of the container when it is spiked. The tear may result in fluid contamination and leakage of the infusate.

Plastic fluid containers collapse when they empty, eliminating the need for a venting device either in the bag or on the solution administration set. Because air is not introduced into the bag, very little air can be accidentally infused.

Because it is relatively light and unbreakable, the plastic container is safer and more practical to store, stack, and move from one place to another. Most plastic containers are not sensitive to fluctuations in temperature or changes in environment. Because plastic can withstand freezing and thawing, many drugs are provided in prefrozen minibags.

With the trend toward ambulatory and home care infusion, the plastic fluid container has added a significant degree of safety and convenience. The expanding outpatient delivery of infusion therapy is possible because of the development of plastic fluid containers.

Semirigid containers

Semirigid containers were developed to capture the best qualities of both glass and plastic containers. Although they do not share the popularity of the plastic bag, they also do not share its shortcomings. The semirigid container holds its shape independent of its contents and is made of rigid plastic. The rigid plastic does not contain plasticizers, reducing drug compatibility issues. The semirigid container is as safe as glass for most drugs that are incompatible with plastic.

The container does not collapse during infusion, so graduations are easily read and reliable. The semirigid container does not perforate during spiking and is difficult to puncture accidentally during admixing.

The semirigid container is lightweight and unbreakable, making storage, stacking, and transportation safe. However, the container is more bulky and less flexible. It is easy to use in ambulatory and home care infusion services, but it does not adapt well to being worn inside pouches or concealed in ambulatory packs.

Besides being too rigid for ambulatory uses, semirigid containers must be vented to add air to the infusion system. As is the case with glass, venting straws or vented tubing must be used for the fluid to flow correctly. The continuous addition of air to the system contraindicates the use of a semirigid container for many ambulatory situations. Semirigid containers can be cracked if handled roughly or subjected to environmental temperature extremes. This type of container is not well suited to being frozen.

Other fluid containers

Syringes can be correctly identified as primary infusion containers. The syringe, when used in conjunction with a syringe-loaded electronic infusion pump, acts as a primary container for either intermittent or continuous use. If the syringe contents are withdrawn or aspirated by the pumping mechanism, the tubing must be vented to allow air to displace the fluid being extracted. If the pump mechanism only compresses the syringe, any tubing may be used with the syringe.

A syringe is easily and accurately readable for volume given or volume remaining. The syringe is unbreakable, easy to store and transport, and impossible to perforate accidentally. The syringe, in comparison with other fluid containers, is inexpensive and available worldwide. The syringe can be prefilled and prefrozen with an almost unlimited number of fluids and drugs.

The limiting feature of the syringe is the volume it holds. Syringes are seldom seen with volume capabilities of greater than 50 to 60 ml because syringes of this size are awkward to handle. This is not a limiting feature in neonatal and pediatric applications. In these areas, syringes can be the primary container for all types of infusions, such as crystalloids, blood products, fat emulsions, medications, and parenteral nutrition. In adults, the syringe is most often used for intermittent medications. Continuous infusion via the syringe may be used for small volumes required by such therapies as pain control and nontitrated concentrated medications.

Infusion pump–specific containers also fall in the category of fluid containers. Most of these are reservoirs made specifically for use with a single, unique infusion device. They are not interchangeable. Efforts to use most of these fluid containers in devices other than the one for which they were produced may lead to serious and harmful effects. Some are dedicated not only to a specific infusion system but also to a specific therapy, such as chemotherapy or pain control.

The container systems used for specific devices have unique limitations, depending on pump functions and therapies delivered. Limitations include lack of testing for a wider variety of uses and problems arising with commonly used drugs in uncommon concentrations or infusion modes.

Venting rigid containers

Whether rigid, inflexible containers or collapsible bags are used, the nurse must understand the differences in systems and how to promote the exchange of air and fluid. Air must be introduced into the fluid container if the container does not collapse as the infusate empties. The most acceptable method of introducing air into the system is to use vented tubing designed to allow air to enter the bottle or rigid container.

The venting mechanism provided by the manufacturer is intended to allow air to enter without allowing fluid to leak from the venting device. Although this might appear simple, it requires an understanding of droplet formation and the physical make-up of the venting outlet. In the absence of a vented administration set, filter needles are available to provide a filtered air source. It is not acceptable to vent a bottle or rigid container with a needle through the rubber disk; this method creates a risk of solution contamination and an open entry for infection. This is also an unsafe use of a needle. When a needle is used inappropriately in this way, fluid often leaks from the bottle.

When noncollapsible containers are used, air must be introduced into the bottle to allow the fluid to flow correctly. Risk is associated with air being introduced into the fluid administration system, but there are many built-in safeguards to counter that risk. These safeguards are addressed throughout this chapter.

Light sensitivity

Certain drugs, such as nitroprusside, are degraded when the agents have prolonged exposure to light during infusion. With regard to plastic versus glass, there is apparently no distinct advantage of one material over another. Efforts have been made to provide a container material that would protect light-sensitive drugs, but such development is not economically practical. A simple solution is to protect the infusate container from light by placing a dark material over the bag.

Use-activated containers

Several types of complex fluid containers are available. Use-activated containers are compartmentalized and have premeasured ingredients that form an admixture when mixed. These containers are very helpful for high-use infusions with a relatively short shelf life after admixture. Although they are more expensive than the individually supplied products, use-activated containers offer considerable savings of personnel time for admixture. These containers play a significant time-saving role in emergency care and are easy to use in acute situations, such as in ambulances, field use, or transport. Ambulatory and home care settings can also benefit from use-activated containers.

To activate the container, the nurse deliberately ruptures the container's seal or diaphragm by compressing opposing parts or applying pressure to rupture the internal reservoir. The primary disadvantage of the system occurs when this step is not completed appropriately. It is not always apparent when the admixture has not occurred, leaving the primary fluid infusing without the medication. A more severe concern is the belated rupture of the medication reservoir with a potentially harmful concentration of drug being administered.

ADMINISTRATION SETS

Primary administration sets

A primary set is typically the main tubing used to carry the infusing fluid from the container to the patient. It can be a single entity, or it can have many attachments and features. Primary sets can be gravity tubing, infusion pump tubing, or even microbore–syringe-pump tubing if the main fluid is being infused with the syringe pump.

The primary set can be selected with varying drop size and length, depending on the intended use, the patient's condition, and the rate of infusion. The spike should be designed with a finger guard to help spike the fluid container with ease and prevent contamination. Tubing length depends on the patient's needs and whether other equipment is used. Tubing should be long enough to allow patient activity and for appropriate placement of the IV fluid container and an infusion device. Standard primary sets can range from 60 to 110 inches in length.

Any tubing or set attached to a primary set is considered an add-on device and is generally discouraged. If used with a primary set, add-on devices should have a specific purpose, and their use should be strictly limited. Each add-on device is a potential source of contamination, misuse, and accidental disconnection. Examples of add-on devices are filters, extension sets, stopcocks, and multiflow adapters.

Primary administration sets should have Luer connectors to prevent accidental disconnection. The use of needles to access administration set ports should be avoided; needleless or needle-protective systems should be used. Fig. 15-2 depicts a primary administration.

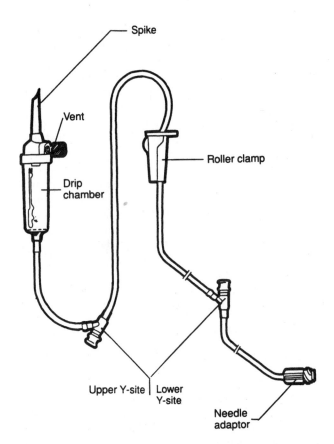

FIG. 15-2 *Primary administration set.* (Courtesy MiniMed Technologies.)

Secondary administration sets

A secondary set is usually defined as tubing that attaches to the primary administration set for a specific purpose, which is generally to administer medication. The set may be used for intermittent or continuous infusion, which must be compatible with the primary fluid.

Secondary sets are usually between 18 and 70 inches long, but the most commonly used length is 30 to 36 inches. Secondary sets can be macrodrop or microdrop, depending on the volume and rate of the secondary fluid and the patient's condition. The drip chamber should have a finger guard at the spike for ease of use and to prevent touch contamination.

Secondary administration sets can be attached to the primary set by using one of several types of needleless systems. One system uses a blunt, hard-plastic cannula to penetrate a soft latex cap that locks in place with Luer connectors. Another device is a recessed needle in a rigid cap that penetrates the traditional injection port on the primary set and locks securely. Other needleless systems feature back-check valves, which prevent the retrograde of blood or the medication being administered. Using a secondary administration set and a needleless system greatly reduces the risk of accidental disconnection or needle injury and promotes safety.

Vented and nonvented sets

Vented sets allow air to enter the infusion container to displace the infusing fluid. These sets are necessary for containers that do not collapse when emptying (glass or semirigid plastic). A vented set is designed with a small air inlet on the spike portion of the tubing. The fit into the container may be tighter than a nonvented spike, requiring more effort to spike the container. This characteristic is not considered a problem, but the nurse should be aware of it to ensure that the spike is fully inserted into the bottle, preventing accidental dislodgment or impeded flow. Vented sets are available in gravity-infusion administration sets and infusion pump sets.

Some manufacturers prefer to offer a universal set that can be vented or nonvented, depending on need. In these sets, a removable cap exists for the air inlet vent. To create a vented set, the capping device is simply removed.

Collapsible plastic containers can physically accommodate a vented spike. If a bag is vented, the infusing fluid is displaced by air entering the bag. Therefore air is introduced into the infusing system, creating unnecessary risk for the patient.

Nonvented tubing is designed for collapsible plastic containers. No air is admitted into the system; the infusing fluid creates a small vacuum that allows the bag to collapse as it empties. This is an important characteristic when a sterile, closed infusion system is the goal. Nonvented tubing cannot be used with glass or rigid plastic.

Many administration sets are marketed for use with a specific system or with limited-fluid containers. It is crucial that all users know these limitations. The universal adaptability of administration sets is more common in add-on devices than in primary sets. The best and safest connections are achieved when fluid containers of the same manufacturer are used.

Metered-volume chamber sets

A metered set contains a small-volume chamber between the primary fluid container and the administration set. The metered chamber may or may not be attached to the administration set. It can easily be obtained as a stand-alone item, which enables its use with various administration sets. It is available with a large variety of preattached tubing. Many pump manufacturers also provide pump sets that have a metered chamber or can adapt to one.

The metered chamber is calibrated in much smaller increments than are other infusion sets. Some may be calibrated precisely, down to 2 ml, but most are very accurate at 5 ml. They are semirigid and may have a ball float at the bottom of the chamber to prevent air from entering the infusion line when the chamber empties.

Metered-chamber sets are designed to limit the amount of fluid available to the patient and are often used to administer intermittent infusions. The chamber is usually 100 or 150 ml. Some neonatal chambers may be only 10 to 50 ml.

The use of a controlled-volume chamber is crucial for critical care drugs, titrated drugs, and fluids infusing into severely volume-restricted patients. Some pediatric and most neonatal units require metered-volume chamber administration sets on all patients receiving IV infusions. Many use a 1- or 2-hour fill limit of fluid for infusion. This limit prevents adverse consequences in the event of uncontrolled IV infusions, rates set too high, or tampering mishaps. Metered-volume chamber administration sets are equally important in adults receiving critical care drugs such as aminophylline or lidocaine. Metered sets are contraindicated when non-PVC tubing must be used to infuse a specific fluid, such as fat emulsions or nitroglycerin.

Another application of the metered chamber is the intermittent infusion of medication. The chamber is filled to a prescribed level to achieve a correct dilution, and the medication is added through an injection port at the top of the chamber. This method is useful when the medication is available in a syringe, the medication is admixed immediately before infusion, or the patient's volume is restricted. The primary infusing fluid then becomes the diluent. The drawback to this method is that the medication administration rate varies greatly from the primary infusion rate. There is also a problem when the medication is not compatible with the primary fluid. Fig. 15-3 depicts a metered-volume set.

Drop factors

The *drop factor* is the number of drops delivered that equal 1 ml. The drop factor is a specific measurement that is perfected to deliver exact amounts over long periods. Each administration set has a predetermined drop factor and can be relied on to deliver fluid accurately, plus or minus 10% (the industry standard). The user calculates flow rates based on the number of drops allowed to fall each minute.

Drop factors are manufacturer specific. Each administration set manufacturer has very rigid standards set for its products and their unique drop size, and there is very little variance among the thousands of sets of like kind. Drop sizes vary from 10 to 60 drops/ml. Drop factors are usually divided into two categories: *macrodrop* and *microdrop*.

Macrodrop is also called *regular drop size.* The 10-, 12-, 15-,

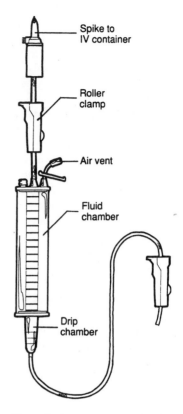

FIG. 15-3 *Metered-volume set.* (Courtesy MiniMed Technologies.)

Labels: Spike to IV container; Roller clamp; Air vent; Fluid chamber; Drip chamber

and 20-drop/ml sets are macrodrop sets. This common set can be used in any application, although its accuracy decreases as the rate per hour decreases.

Microdrop tubing is the most suitable for infusion rates of less than 100 ml/hr. Microdrop tubing is usually termed *pediatric,* although it is used as often or even more often in adults in whom high rates are not necessary. Microdrop sizes are usually 50 to 60 drops/ml.

Microdrop tubing, by restricting the flow even with the control clamp wide open, allows an added safety feature against runaway IV lines or free flow. Both phenomena can still occur, but they are slowed considerably with microdrop tubing. This characteristic makes microdrop tubing especially safe for pediatric, geriatric, or volume-restricted patients.

Electronic infusion pumps sometimes offer administration sets with macrodrop or microdrop options, which should be a consideration if the administration sets are routinely taken from the infusion pumps for use as gravity administration sets. The size of the drop does not factor into the delivery of fluid by an electronic infusion device. These devices measure by fluid displacement or mechanical movement and do not measure drop size or count drops. Any consideration for drop size on infusion pump tubing would be relevant only for use outside the infusion device or as free-flow protection if the infusion pump does not offer that safeguard.

Primary Y sets

Primary Y sets are used for rapid infusion or dual administration, usually in critical care, trauma, or surgery patients and can be found in gravity as well as in infusion pump configurations. Each leg of the Y set is capable of being the primary set. The Y set has two separate spikes, with a separate drip chamber and a short length of tubing with individual clamps. The joining occurs usually 12 to 20 inches below the spikes. At this junction, another drip chamber may be present. The fluids mix fully at this point. Primary Y tubing cannot be used to infuse incompatible fluids.

Because they are meant to infuse large amounts in acute situations, primary Y sets are commonly made with very large-bore tubing and clamps that lack the fine-tuning capabilities of general-use tubing. These sets are not intended for general use and pose a risk if used for general-purpose infusion. The risk of accidental bolus or a runaway IV line is very high because of the design of the tubing.

The primary Y set is ideal, however, for the infusion of blood and some blood products. The infusion leg opposite the portion infusing the unit of blood is commonly used to administer the 0.9% sodium chloride given before and after a unit of blood product is infused. The large inner lumen allows the more-viscous blood solution to infuse with ease and decreases trauma to infusing blood cells. Blood can be infused very rapidly with a primary Y set.

A word of caution about the primary Y set: if it is used with a noncollapsible fluid container or glass bottle, the air vent will not only fill the bottle, but the air will continue to flow with the infusing fluid from the other side into the patient. Primary Y sets are not provided as vented sets, so this caution applies to bottles with venting straws or a venting apparatus added to the bottle. Any air emboli associated with tubing of this inner lumen size would be significant.

Internal diameter of tubing

Internal lumen sizes of fluid administration tubing are manufacturer specific. Industry standards refer to a range of inner lumen sizes, and each manufacturer is allowed to market products that are compatible but not uniform. Tubing can be categorized into types based on lumen size, but uniformity among manufacturers cannot be assumed. Usually, minuscule differences are acceptable and do not affect performance in situations not calling for such precision. In other instances, these differences can be critical. If performance problems are suspected, the manufacturer of the products should always be consulted to confirm or rule out tubing conflicts. (A tubing conflict means that one piece of tubing interferes with the performance of another.)

Macrobore tubing is commonly used on blood administration sets or primary Y sets for use in trauma or operating room situations. Macrobore means that the tubing inner lumen is larger than standard tubing to facilitate high flow rates. How much larger depends on the manufacturer. Anesthesia sets and some specialty sets are designed specifically with macrobore tubing.

The large inner lumen makes macrobore tubing stiffer and makes it more difficult to accommodate a controlling mechanism such as a roller clamp. The clamp is less reliable for long-term infusion control. Macrobore tubing should never be used in electronic infusion pumps that accommodate generic tubing.

Microbore tubing has a smaller-than-standard inner lumen. Because small tubing is very flimsy, microbore tubing often has a smaller inner lumen but a thicker wall, making it resistant to kinking. Many microbore sets are termed *kink resistant* or *noncompliant* (meaning the tubing does not bend or stretch). Again, because tubing is manufacturer specific, the qualities of each microbore set should be investigated, not assumed.

Because microbore sets have a narrowed inner lumen, flow is somewhat restricted. Microbore sets can be used as a safeguard against runaway or bolus infusions and offer a very low priming volume, making them suitable for pediatrics, neonatal units, and volume-restricted adult care areas such as cardiology or renal units. Microbore tubing is often the tubing of choice for syringe pumps, epidural infusion pumps, or ambulatory infusion devices that are designed to deliver small quantities over a long period, such as low-dose chemotherapy or pain-control medications.

Standard-lumen tubing makes up most sets, and almost all infusions can be accomplished with standard-bore administration sets. All standard-bore sets have a common inner lumen size with very little variation from manufacturer to manufacturer. Again, the standard-bore sets are within a common range but should never be assumed to be exactly the same.

In-line rate-control clamps

Roller clamps. Roller clamps are found on all standard administration sets and are in-line, which means that they are attached during the manufacturing of the set. The roller clamp allows the tubing to be incrementally occluded by pinching the tubing as the roller clamp is tightened. Most roller clamps are easily regulated with one hand. The clamp is designed to hold its place on the tubing, keeping the infusion rate constant between adjustments. The primary purpose of the roller clamp is to control flow rates of infusion. Standard roller clamps on standard-bore tubing can be as accurate as plus or minus 10%.

The accuracy of standard roller clamps is directly dependent on the number of variables involved in each administration. Patient movement, ambulation, patient transfer, and the height of the fluid container are just a few of the things that can affect the accuracy of an adjusted roller clamp. Safe rate control with roller clamps requires vigilant observation at frequent intervals by the caregiver to confirm the infusion rates.

Roller clamps should be positioned on the upper third of the tubing near the fluid container. This placement is convenient for the nurse and, more importantly, is out of the way of the patient, thus preventing accidental manipulation. The clamp should be repositioned on the tubing at periodic intervals because the tubing develops "memory," making it difficult to regulate. This memory can work in two ways. In the event of "cold creep," the tubing tries to retain its round shape, pushing the clamp open. The other form of memory creates a pinched section of tubing that does not reopen when the clamp is removed. Both of these problems can be avoided by using a set for only the designated number of hours and moving the clamp to an unused portion of tubing when the rate is readjusted.

Some standard sets have a more advanced roller clamp, called a *stationary clamp,* which is positioned on the tubing as an insert. A portion of the PVC tubing is replaced with a small segment of softer silicone tubing. Cold creep and memory do not affect the silicone tubing; therefore the rate is more easily maintained. This tubing is somewhat more expensive and remains accurate at plus or minus 10%.

Slide and pinch clamps. Slide and pinch clamps are provided on some sets but are not regulating clamps. Both are simple, one-handed clamps whose sole purpose is to provide on-off control. Infusions should never be regulated with slide or pinch clamps because these clamps are not accompanied by accuracy claims. Both of these clamps are capable of creating a serious crimp or crease in the tubing that can be hazardous.

Screw clamps. Screw clamps function by turning a screw device to incrementally apply pressure to a point on the tubing, thereby pinching it off. They are easy to adjust with one hand and should be positioned on the upper third of the tubing. Unlike the roller clamp, the screw clamp cannot migrate back, making cold creep impossible. The screw clamp can be moved easily, however, even if it is accidentally bumped. Manufacturers of screw clamps do not make claims of substantially greater accuracy than for traditional roller clamps, but most users believe them to be more reliable.

Add-on manual flow control devices

Add-on manual flow control devices are readily available in many types and shapes. Recent years have brought new developments in sophisticated flow regulators. These devices are added to a gravity infusion line at the distal end of the administration set, proximal to the patient. They are used to regulate the flow of fluid instead of using the clamp on the administration set.

These flow regulators generally provide a more consistent flow rate than do preattached roller clamps. They are accurate within plus or minus 10%, which is the same for the clamp on standard tubing. In actual practice, however, some of these clamps have been shown to provide added safety, a benefit that is not easily quantified. With most add-on controlling devices, significant added protection exists against crimped tubing, cold creep, and drifting of the roller clamp. The add-on controlling devices are not likely to be accidentally reset when bumped or jostled because of patient activity. In addition, they provide added protection from accidental free flow.

In recent years, some manufacturers have claimed the ability to compensate for the changes in head height. Head height is the vertical distance between the solution container and the IV site. Changes in patient position or the height of the fluid container in relation to the patient can either increase or decrease fluid flow. This feature could be an important asset in the care of ambulatory patients.

An issue that has arisen with some models of add-on regulators is the accuracy of predetermined settings. On these devices, the nurse sets the dial or indicator to a given number, and the set supposedly delivers at that rate. In actuality, many variables in the patient care setting can alter that rate, such as change in patient position, sharp changes in room temperature, or even decreased volume in the fluid container. The nurse cannot rely on the numbered setting to indicate the actual flow being delivered. Although the numbered dial may have some advan-

tages of add-on control devices, the number on the indicator may not be what is actually being delivered. Great harm can occur when the caregiver assumes that the delivery rate is the same as the value on the dial indicator and the drop rate is not counted for confirmation.

Whether to use add-on controlling devices must be determined by close examination of real versus perceived need. The proficiency of the nursing staff, the level of illness being treated, the type of patient population, and the care environment need to be considered. Add-on regulators add significantly to the cost per IV line in any setting, and they must be changed with the routine tubing changes.

An add-on-controlling device is not a substitute for an infusion pump. If patient acuity and drug therapy indicate that an electronic infusion pump is necessary to safely deliver care, an add-on regulator cannot possibly provide any degree of that safety. However, if gravity administration is indicated, some add-on devices may provide an extra measure of safety.

Resealable Y injection ports

Most primary IV infusion administration sets are made with one to three injection Y ports located in strategic places along the line. Resealable ports, or injection ports, provide a significant advantage in the administration of multiple infusions. Injection ports are made of dense latex or a nonlatex rubber and are secured to a portion of the infusion line where a hard, molded Y exits the main infusion line. These rubber caps are tightly secured with a heat-shrunk band to prevent any movement or break in the sterility of the infusion line.

The port is able to reseal after it is penetrated with a needle or, if it is part of a needleless system, a dull plastic spike. This characteristic makes it possible for the nurse to administer other medications through the existing primary infusion line after confirming compatibility. The port should be able to accommodate numerous punctures, although a definitive number does not exist. The port can usually be safely used through the limited life of the infusion line. Caution should be taken if an extraordinary number of punctures are made. If the port is compromised by excessive penetrations, air emboli may occur and bacteria may enter the infusion line.

Coring occurs when a large needle or numerous small needles remove a piece of the rubber from the port during needle penetration. The chance of coring increases with large-gauge needles and some vulnerable rubber materials. Coring may occur after only one puncture or after repeated punctures. The nurse should suspect coring if little resistance is felt when inserting the needle or spike into the port. When this happens, the tubing should be changed immediately.

The injection port that is found on the upper third of the infusion line nearest the fluid container is used for piggyback administration. It is common practice for the piggyback infusion to be attached at this level to administer infusions concurrently or sequentially with the main IV fluid. The administration set attached is referred to as the *secondary set.*

The injection port that is found nearest the patient is used for IV push medications. This port is often 6 to 12 inches from the distal end of the tubing; because of its close proximity to the patient, it should never be used for the attachment of a secondary set. One or more other injection ports may be located at various points on the primary administration set.

Back-check valves

Back-check valves, or one-way valves, are an integral part of many administration sets. These valves allow the fluid to flow in one direction only. Back-check valves work much like a float. When the fluid is passing through the disk, a small float device holds the passage open. If the flow is reversed, the float device closes off the passageway. Another one-way valve appears similar to a flap valve in the fluid path. When fluid is passing correctly, the flap flows open. When the flow is reversed, the flap is forced shut, stopping the flow. Back-check valves have no other purpose than to direct the flow of fluid.

The most common use of back-check valves is to administer piggyback medications. The piggyback medication is attached to the injection port on the upper third of the primary administration set. The back-check valve is between this junction and the primary fluid container. This configuration prevents the secondary piggyback from flowing into the primary infusion container if there is resistance in the infusion system at the patient end. As long as the piggyback solution hangs higher than the primary container, the primary fluid does not flow into the secondary container.

This same premise applies for back-check valves used in patient-controlled analgesia (PCA) pump sets. To ensure that the pain medication is flowing from the pump to the patient, the PCA tubing incorporates a back-check valve where the PCA tubing attaches to the primary set. The valve is on the leg of the Y that infuses the primary fluid. This configuration prevents the pain medication from flowing upstream into the primary infusion should the IV access device become occluded.

In all cases, the back-check valve prevents the retrograde flow of fluid. This measure is necessary in many dual-infusion systems and also inhibits the backflow of blood into the tubing.

Back-check valves are standard additions to many infusion systems (Fig. 15-4).

Connections

Manufacturers of IV tubing connections strive to make them universal, which means that male and female fittings for standard devices should make a correct fit when connected. This standard exists for reasons of safety and efficiency.

Two basic types of standard connections exist: slip and Luer. Slip connections provide fittings that simply slide into each other and provide a tight connection when twisted. These connections are not absolute in preventing accidental disconnects. Luer connections screw together two compatible ends. Deliberate twisting motions are required to disconnect a Luer connector, making accidental disconnection almost impossible. Most major medical manufacturers offer tubing and add-on devices with Luer connections. Luer connections are an industry standard and do not add to the cost of the device or tubing.

Pressure bags

A pressure bag for the infusion of gravity-drip fluids should be reserved for trauma, anesthesiology, surgery, and critical care needs. Pressure bags maintain consistent pressure on the infusing fluid to hasten the pace of the infusion. Because this pressure is difficult to regulate and maintain safely, pressure bags are not routinely used. Infusion pumps are the method of choice when rapid infusion is necessary.

The most routine use of pressure bags is the maintenance of pressurized arterial lines. The pressure bag maintains consistent pressure on the infusing heparin infusate or 0.9% sodium chloride, which infuses through a restricted access that maintains flow at a very minimal amount (usually 3 ml/hr). The pressure does not allow any backflow of blood, maintaining patency of the arterial catheter.

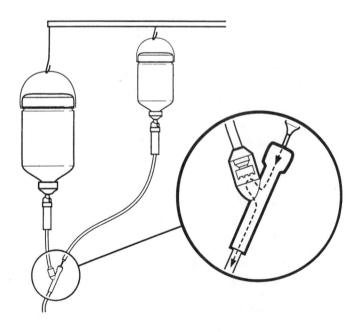

FIG. 15-4 *Back-check valve or one-way valve.* (Courtesy MiniMed Technologies.)

Nitroglycerin administration sets

Continuous IV nitroglycerin infusions are common in critical care nursing. Nitroglycerin tubing is available in certain infusion pump sets and gravity administration sets. Because of the critical nature of the drug, nitroglycerin should never be infused by gravity.

Nitroglycerin is somewhat of a challenge because it is incompatible with standard PVC tubing. Studies have shown that nitroglycerin adheres to the plastic in the tubing and fluid bag.[2] The percentage of drug lost to bag adherence depends on the exact nature of the plastic, which varies by manufacturer, the length and type of tubing, and the length of exposure to the plastic.

This phenomenon of nitroglycerin adhering to PVC tubing prevents the prescribing physician and the nurse administering the infusion from knowing exactly what percentage of nitroglycerin is being delivered. In the clinical setting, the drug is titrated, so the concentration delivered depends on the patient's symptoms, making the actual concentration less critical. Not knowing the actual concentration could be problematic if certain interventions are initiated based on the assumption that a predetermined limit of drug infusion has been reached. The saturation point must be reached with each tubing change, potentially creating fluctuations in the drug concentrations delivered. Many clinicians are uncomfortable dealing with such an unknown factor in conjunction with such a critical drug.

Nitroglycerin sets can be made with non-PVC material, or the inner lumen can be coated with polyethylene or similarly compatible material. Used with glass containers, both of these alternatives offer a system that does not create an adhering surface for nitroglycerin. Minimal drug loss occurs, making the infusing concentration constant. These nitroglycerin-specific sets are more expensive than standard PVC sets. The use of specialty sets remains controversial and much debated. Safe care can be accomplished with or without nitroglycerin-specific administration sets, as long as the potential risks are understood.

Fat emulsion–specific sets

The infusion of fat emulsions has been a topic of discussion in recent years. The essence of the controversy was that the plasticizer DHEP was found to leach from the plastic container and tubing into the fat emulsion. The final disposition of the DHEP into the human recipient is the focus of the controversy; of special concern are neonates and children.

Fat emulsions are provided in glass containers only. Some researchers believe that the length of time the lipids are in contact with the plastic tubing does not constitute a risk. Regardless, fat emulsions in glass containers necessitate a vented administration set.

Blood administration sets

Blood-specific administration sets are designed to accommodate the viscous properties of blood, allow rapid transfusion (if needed), and provide a dual line for the infusion of 0.9% sodium chloride before and after the blood product is infused.

Blood-specific sets can be gravity or pump specific and should be used only for their stated purpose. The large-bore tubing and flow regulation clamp in these sets are not intended for routine infusion of crystalloids or medications.

Blood sets usually contain a large-screen filter to remove coarse fibrin and byproducts of stored blood. This filter is usually 170 to 220 microns in size. Add-on filters of smaller pore size, including microaggregate and leukocyte-depletion filters, may be added and are discussed later in this chapter.

Some blood sets incorporate an in-line hand pump to push blood along when rapid infusion is needed. The hand pump should be used with caution. Adverse effects of inappropriate use of a hand pump include damaged vasculature, loss of the IV site, and severe infiltration. Other potential problems can be damage to the infusing red blood cells, pulmonary emboli, and speed shock.

Blood should be given only through blood-specific sets (Fig. 15-5). Most electronic infusion devices offer blood-specific sets that are able to safely infuse blood without damaging blood cells. Infusion pump manufacturers who do not offer these sets should be consulted before blood is infused through one of their devices. Most blood is infused by gravity through sets specially designed for the safe infusion of blood.

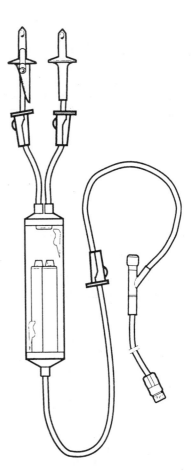

FIG. 15-5 *Sample blood tubing.* (Courtesy MiniMed Technologies.)

Add-on devices

The health care market offers an unlimited number of devices that can be attached to any infusion tubing. Devices are available for attachment to the proximal and the distal connections and to access ports between them. The routine use of add-on devices is discouraged. Limiting their use reduces the incidence of contamination and accidental disconnection, minimizes the manipulation of the sterile closed system, and reduces the costs associated with their use.

Add-on devices are numerous because they serve many functions. They are used to add length, filtering capability, or increased overall function to the infusion system. Increased function is realized with stopcocks, manifolds, multiflow devices, or specialized flow regulators. Although their use is discouraged, they are sometimes necessary to accomplish a specific purpose. Health care workers should constantly justify the use of add-on devices to ensure they are not used habitually or routinely.

Stopcocks. A stopcock is a manually manipulated device used to direct the flow of fluid. The stopcock is generally a three-way or four-way device. For example, the stopcock has an inlet from the main infusion line and a second portal to direct the fluid to the patient. Turning the stopcock to the third portal allows fluid to flow from a second container and from the primary container. The fourth portal is an off port, so the first three can be used in any combination of two or three.

Because of its versatility, this device is very useful in critical care, anesthesia, and trauma settings. As useful as it is in these settings, however, the general use of stopcocks is strongly discouraged. Misuse of stopcocks has become a major factor contributing to their unavailability in many health care settings.

The issue of contamination of stopcocks has been addressed in multiple arenas. When the stopcock portals are uncapped, they are vulnerable to touch contamination. The stopcock itself is small and must be handled in such a way that sterility is not compromised. Often, syringes are attached for IV push administration, and the portal is poorly protected after use. Many stopcocks are made without Luer connections, making accidental disconnection a major issue. If the stopcock is accidentally turned, the infusion may be interrupted or administered incorrectly. The potential for error with stopcocks makes their use worthy of caution.

Extension sets. Extension sets are used to add length or clamping capability or to restrict flow. To add length, extension sets can be 20, 30, or 60 inches long. Many specialty sets may be just about any length imaginable. Sets that are made to add clamping capability are usually much shorter, even as short as 2 to 3 inches. It might be advisable to restrict flow with an extension set if a standard set is used for a volume-restricted patient and an infusion pump is not available to protect against fluid overload. An extension set of microbore tubing would add a measure of safety in this case.

Extension sets should not be added routinely or for convenience; there must be a clearly defined purpose. The potential for contamination exists with any add-on device, especially if excessive length allows tubing to lay on the floor or become entangled. To ensure patient safety, only extension sets with Luer connectors should be used.

Multiflow adapters and Y connectors. Multiflow adapters and Y connectors allow two or three infusions to be joined into one infusion. These devices are usually designed to connect directly as opposed to requiring a needle. Multiflow adapters and Y connectors should have Luer connections. Some have color-coded hubs or clamps attached. The versatility of the these devices is enhanced by adding pinch or slide clamps on each leg of the device.

The caps provided with many multiflow adaptors and Y connectors are air vented for easy priming. It is important to remember to prime all infusion legs of the device before their use to prevent small air emboli. Because these caps allow movement of air, they cannot be left in place after the system is primed. The system is not closed because contamination can occur through the cap at this point. If an infusion line is not attached to each leg of the multiflow adapter, a sterile injection cap must be attached. If the cap provided with the multiflow adapter or Y connector provides a sterile, airtight seal, it will need to be removed to accommodate priming; the end should then be recapped with a sterile cap. If the multiflow adapter or Y connector does not have capped ends, it is unlikely the device can be used without being contaminated during set-up.

Catheter connection devices. T ports have become common add-on devices. The T port is usually 4 to 6 inches long and is made of standard or microbore tubing with a hard, plastic, T-shaped connector on one end. One side of the T attaches to the IV device, and the other is a resealable port. The long leg of the T attaches to standard administration tubing and often has a simple slide or pinch clamp attached.

The T connector has a clamp that allows safe disconnection of the administration tubing without fear of backflow of blood or air emboli. If the IV device is locked for intermittent use, many patients and practitioners feel more comfortable with the T connector clamped.

If the T connector is used on children, care should also be taken to ensure that the slide or pinch clamp is not removable. Some manufacturers make the slide clamp optional and easy to remove. This feature poses a risk to small children, who find the clamps an irresistible item for small fingers and mouths.

J loops and U connectors have the same intended use as T connectors. Both are rigid and hold their shape when attached to the IV site. Their predetermined shape creates a disadvantage at times because the distal end can be in only a specific area depending on the site, even if the point of connection is in an awkward spot. Their rigid shape does not help prevent catheter movement when the connection is manipulated.

Fig. 15-6 depicts several types of add-on devices.

Injection ports/caps. Injection ports, or caps, are small, hard-molded devices with resealable rubber caps that are used to cap an IV catheter or female opening on an administration set or an add-on device. This description implies that the device is designed to accommodate needle punctures or, if designed for needleless systems, will reseal after puncture by a specially designed, blunt-tipped spike. Some hard-plastic caps solidly occlude an opening and are not included in this discussion because they serve no purpose except to provide an impenetrable cap. All of these devices should have Luer connections.

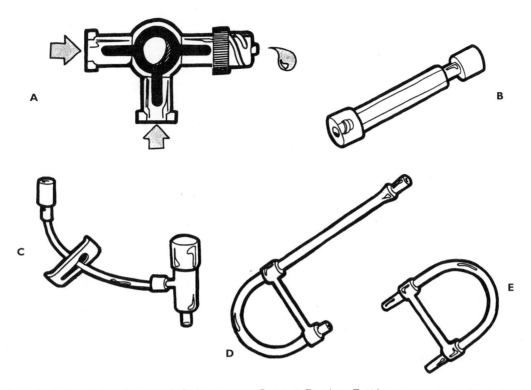

FIG. 15-6 *Add-on devices.* **A,** *Stopcock.* **B,** *Injection cap.* **C,** T *port.* **D,** J *loop.* **E,** U *loop.* (Courtesy MiniMed Technologies.)

Although injection ports are small, simple devices, they are worthy of close consideration. One important aspect is their length; injection ports are available in lengths of less than ½ inch to 2 inches. There are benefits of a shorter cap. Its smaller bulk helps during dressing, its lower weight helps during securing, and it creates less dead space during priming, which is an important consideration in neonatal use. Inversely, a short injection port may allow needles to penetrate the hub of the infusion catheter, potentially puncturing or compromising the catheter or tubing. The use of the needleless design eliminates the need for needles completely in this context.

Coring is a hazard that occurs when large-bore needles or frequent needle punctures remove a plug of rubber from the port, compromising the intact seal. Because coring is difficult to predict, injection caps should be changed routinely in accordance with Intravenous Nurses Society *Infusion Nursing Standards of Practice* and institutional protocol. If an injection port is penetrated multiple times daily, it is recommended to change it more frequently than scheduled. Again, the hazard of coring is greatly diminished and possibly eliminated when a needleless system is used.

Another hazard of injection ports that is often overlooked occurs when blood is withdrawn from the infusion device with the through-the-cap technique. In this technique, the injection cap is left in place and blood is aspirated with a needle or blunt spike through the cap. Adequate flushing after the infusion often fails to remove blood cells from under the rubber, and the residual blood provides a medium for bacterial growth. Profuse

flushing is required while the needle or spike is withdrawn, or a new injection cap must be applied.

INFUSION FILTERS
Purpose

Infusion Nursing Standards of Practice states that a 0.2-micron filter containing a membrane that is both bacteria/particulate retentive and air eliminating should be used for non–lipid-containing solutions that require filtration.[4]

Indications for filters include infusions administered via the peripheral and central venous systems or intraspinal and intraosseous routes. Blood filters are advocated for the routine infusion of blood and blood components. Arterial routes are not filtered, although the introduction of particulate matter or contaminates into the arterial system has great potential for causing injury. Arterial routes are most often used for monitoring rather than for infusion. An infusion filter on an arterial system negates the clinician's ability to accurately perform hemodynamic monitoring.

Filters are contraindicated for use with certain medications, which are retained on the filter material. Blanket statements cannot be made because filter materials vary greatly. Most adjunct filter tubing is made from PVC, however, and drugs mentioned previously with an incompatibility to the plasticizer in PVC are also contraindicated for use with filters. Filters should also be avoided when administering very small volumes of drugs because unknown retention by the filter might seriously decrease the volume of medication received by the patient.

Characteristics

Filters are characterized numerically to differentiate filter pore size. The universal scale of measurement is the micron. Common filters are 5.0-, 1.2-, 0.45-, and 0.2-micron retentive filters for use with common IV fluids and medications. Larger filters must be used to filter blood products because they capture large particulate matter and allow red blood cells to pass. Blood filters are discussed separately in this section.

The micron number attached to the filter tells the user that to a degree of certainty, the filter will retain 98% of a given micron size or larger. For example, a 1.2-micron filter will retain 98% of all the particles in the infusate that are greater than 1.2 microns.

Modern infusion filters have many functions. Their design and construction must allow them to maintain high flow rates while automatically venting air; to retain bacteria, fungi, particulate matter, and endotoxins; to tolerate pressures generated by infusion pumps; and to act in a nonbinding fashion with drugs. Particulate matter may include undissolved drug particles, glass, and other debris from the manufacturing process. The presence of these particles is acceptable in a sterile infusate to a certain tolerance set by the U.S. Food and Drug Administration. Although these particles do not pose an infectious risk, they have been implicated as being at least partially responsible for adverse systemic effects related to obstructing blood flow in the microvasculature of the lungs, spleen, renal medulla, and liver, which could lead to pulmonary embolism.[5]

Another function of the infusion filter is protection from air emboli. The hydrophobic characteristic that provides this effect blocks the passage of air and successfully vents the excess air out of the system. All filters currently on the market are air eliminating, which means that air passes through the infusion line and is vented out of the system by the filter. Adding a surfactant to the filter surface prevents filters from becoming air locked. This occurs when an air bubble is trapped in the filter, preventing the flow of solution. The air-venting feature is important in gravity flow situations and when using infusion pumps. Because modern filters are not position dependent, the air-elimination feature works well in almost all positions.

Filters should have high flow capabilities and incorporate hydrophilic and hydrophobic membranes. Hydrophilic filters are easily wetted and pull the fluid forward, overcoming flow resistance. Most reputable filters can accommodate extremely high flow rates, as much as several liters per hour. The better filters allow high flow rates despite medications being added or being given IV push.

Pressure tolerance is sometimes a misunderstood feature of an IV filter. Filters used in conjunction with a pressure bag or IV pumps may pose a certain risk if the filter membrane ruptures as a result of excessive pressure. Rupture can also occur if an IV push medication is administered upstream or above the filter. If undue pressure causes the filter membrane to rupture, the patient could receive a concentrated infusion of particulate and infectious matter. To prevent this situation from happening, the filter is made with pounds per square inch (psi) tolerance in the housing. The housing of the filter is designed to rupture, leaving the filter membrane intact and protecting the downstream flow of fluid. When this rupture occurs, the integrity of the infusion system is broken, and the infusate flows from the filter, necessitating a change in tubing.

Most users associate filter breakage with a malfunctioning filter. However, filter breakage is a patient-protection mechanism intended to warn the user to examine the activity that precipitated the breakage. If the situation calls for extremely high pressure to be used, such as in trauma cases, the filter should not be used. If the filter breaks during routine use, the event precipitating the breakage should be examined carefully. Pressure powerful enough to break the filter could also damage the vasculature or rupture softer infusion catheters.

The various designs of filter membranes are the products of much research and medical consumer feedback. The goal of all filters is to economically provide high-flow sterilizing (0.2-micron) filtration. The *surface area* of a filter refers to the type of filter configuration and the amount of surface area promoting flow capabilities. Filters with increased surface areas are able to achieve higher flow rates.

The depth filter consists of multiple layers of material through which fluid must pass. Because the pore size of the different layers is not uniform, the filter captures various-sized particles at different layers. The flow rates provided by the depth filter are usually very good. However, these filters clog when large amounts of particulate are retained. A depth filter is not easily discernible from other filters on examination. It usually appears to be a disk with fluid passing through from the top or the side to the bottom. Depth filters prime easily and can eliminate air.

The membrane filter differs from a depth filter in that the layer of screening material is of uniform pore size. Its advantage is more efficient retention of uniform particle size. Its disadvantage is that when particles are retained on one plane, the filter clogs more easily, restricting flow rates. The membrane filter is not visually differentiated from the depth filter in most cases.

The screen filter, one of the original concepts in filtering devices, is now rarely used. The screen filter has a very limited surface area that easily coats with particles, thereby obstructing flow. The screen filter is often difficult to prime, depending on the hydrophilic properties of the screen material.

Hollow-fiber filters are designed in the fashion of dialysis filters, providing a very high surface area to achieve very high flow. The hollow-fiber filter housing is cylindrical and consists of many very fine tubes, each of which is porous and allows the passage of fluid through sterilizing membranes. The number of tubes makes high flow rates possible and minimizes clogging over long periods. The hollow-fiber filter achieves good air elimination and primes easily.

Configuration

An in-line filter is an infusion filter that is preattached to the primary infusion administration set. It is a 0.2-micron filter and is not removable. In-line filters also provide total filtration and give consistency and uniformity of care. Because not all infusates can be filtered, administration sets that do not contain a filter must also be available, which increases inventory and cost.

Add-on filters can be any micron size, but the 0.2-micron filter is recommended for routine IV infusions. It is critical that the filter provide Luer connections. Add-on filters allow flexibility in use, product choice, and features desired. Add-on filters can be added to the proximal or distal end of the administration set, depending on the intended benefit of the filter. If the filter is added to the proximal end, it is between the fluid container and the tubing spike. Placing the filter at this end ensures sterility and particulate removal from the infusate container. It also prevents a dry fluid container with the possibility of air being infused through the line to the patient. The filter attached to the distal end of the administration set filters the contents of the container, as well as any contaminants introduced from add-on devices, secondary administrations, or interruptions to the primary system, including touch contamination. Adding the filter at the distal position also safely negates any air particles.

Filter sets commonly include an injection port after the filter, situated between the filter and the patient. This design allows the nurse to give small-volume IV push medications, avoiding the filter.

Blood filters

The routine use of blood filters is institution specific. *Infusion Nursing Standards of Practice* states that blood filters are used to remove particulate matter during blood administration.[4] The American Association of Blood Banks states that blood must be transfused through a sterile, pyrogen-free transfusion set that has a filter capable of retaining particles that are potentially harmful to the recipient.[6]

Routine IV fluid and blood filters are not interchangeable. The size of a red blood cell is several hundred times the size of the microorganisms being filtered from routine IV fluids. Available blood filters are 20, 40, 80, and 170 microns.

The filter found in-line in some blood administration sets is 170 to 220 microns. A filter of this great pore size removes only coagulated products, microclots, and debris resulting from collection and storage. The 170-micron filters are a safety net because the particles retained are potentially lethal to the patient. They are visible in the mesh filter after transfusion. Without the large-screen filter, debris and microclots can be a potential source for emboli in pulmonary or cerebral circulation.

The 20-, 40-, and 80-micron filters are regarded as microaggregate filters. The 20-micron filter does an excellent job of removing most debris from the transfusion product. Because of the natural presence of a certain amount of debris in all blood products, the 20-micron filter can slow the administration of blood to an undesirable rate. The 40-micron filter allows blood to transfuse easily in the specified time, but the filtration is less refined. The 80-micron filter is the filter of choice in many institutions because of its safe level of filtration and high flow rate potential. All three are considered adequate.

Leukocyte-depletion filters are designed to remove leukocytes and leukocyte-mediated viruses, which greatly increases the safety of transfusions to patients who have received multiple transfusions. They have been shown to improve patient response to blood products in persons requiring frequent, repeated transfusions and to prevent febrile reactions in patients who have experienced transfusion reactions. Leukocyte-depletion filters are classified according to efficiency level, not micron size, and can remove up to 99.9% of leukocytes from the blood transfusions and platelets.

INFUSION CATHETERS AND CANNULAS

The first devices used to access the vascular system were hollow feather quills. They were followed by catheters, which are hollow tubes inserted into a body passage. The next generation of products was called *cannulas,* because a cannula has an obturator or something inside the tube that is later removed. Most peripheral access devices, which are routinely used, are actually cannulas. The terms *catheter* and *cannula* have become interchangeable. Industry usually refers to most of the venous infusion devices manufactured as catheters. Some clinicians refer to a winged infusion set as a *butterfly.*

Peripheral catheters/cannulas

A peripheral catheter, or cannula, is one that begins and terminates in an extremity (arm, hand, leg, foot, or head). The external jugular access is considered a peripheral access if the catheter does not extend into the subclavian vein. Peripheral catheters may be any length and include midline catheters or those that extend 8 to 12 inches from the antecubital insertion site. Intraosseous access is not considered a peripheral route.

Catheter configurations. An incredible evolution of infusion devices has occurred in the past 20 years. Once performed as a procedure by physicians in the hospital setting, IV cannulation is now commonly performed in the home care setting and in 90% of all hospitalized patients.

One of the most basic and time-tested devices is the winged infusion set, which is available with a steel needle or as an over-the-needle catheter with wings. The winged infusion set, or butterfly, as it is commonly called, has flexible plastic wings or flaps protruding from either side of the needle hub (Fig. 15-7). The hub is usually plastic and is color-coded for gauge identification. Attached to the hub is a short length of PVC tubing ranging from 3 to 12 inches in length. Syringes or IV administration sets attach easily to the connector at the end of the tubing. Winged infusion sets with safety sheaths are also available to prevent accidental needlestick injuries.

The winged infusion set is biocompatible. Low rates of inflammation or phlebitis have been documented with its use. Because they are easy to use and cause little trauma to the vein and blood cells, winged infusion sets are often used to obtain blood for laboratory specimens. Users believe that the winged infusion set is easier to insert than other devices because there are no parts to manipulate.

The major drawback of the traditional winged steel-needle set is its rigidity and the inability of the needle to soften next to the vein wall. The steel tip easily punctures the vasculature after placement, and the risk for an infiltration increases proportionately to the time the needle is in place. The winged steel-needle

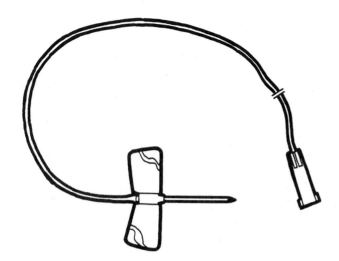

FIG. 15-7 Winged steel-needle (butterfly or scalp vein). (Courtesy MiniMed Technologies.)

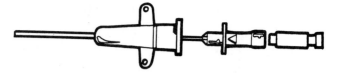

FIG. 15-8 Over-the-needle catheter. (Courtesy MiniMed Technologies.)

infusion set is recommended for infusions lasting fewer than 24 hours. Because of the short interval of use, steel needles are associated with minimal phlebitis.

The most widely used infusion device is the over-the-needle catheter (Fig. 15-8). This device is a soft catheter usually made of plastic or plasticlike material with a rigid, color-coded plastic hub. A hollow metal stylet (needle) is preinserted into the catheter and protrudes through the distal tip of the catheter to allow puncture of the vessel to guide the catheter as the venipuncture is performed. When the vein is punctured, the flashback appears in a closed chamber behind the catheter hub. The catheter is then threaded off the stylet into the vein, and the stylet is completely removed, leaving the softer, plastic catheter in place. Several safety-enhancing over-the-needle catheter designs are available with retracting stylets to protect the health care worker from accidental needlestick injury. In some of these designs, the catheter has preattached PVC tubing that is similar to the scalp-vein or butterfly needle, and a stylet that is attached to a wire, enabling its complete withdrawal from the tubing. This design reduces risk of blood contamination and needlestick injury.

The through-the-needle catheter with a nonremovable needle for peripheral infusion is rarely used today. The steel needle makes the venipuncture, then the softer plastic catheter slides through the needle and into the vein. The sharp needle is pulled back out of the skin after the vein is cannulated and is left attached to the apparatus. A protective device covers the needle to prevent catheter shearing or patient trauma.

Newer versions of through-the-needle catheters are designed for central and peripheral placement. (The distinction is the proximal tip location of the catheter.) Most of these catheters use a through-the-needle design, but the needles are of steel or plastic that splits or peels away, leaving only a soft catheter exiting the skin. The breakaway needle introduced a new generation of access devices.

Catheter material.
Generically speaking, almost all peripheral catheter materials are a variation of plastic. Some are

simple plastic and have very limited use. Some are new extrapolations of plastic that are very close to being a new category.

Polytetrafluoroethylene (Teflon) is a plastic-coated material that is less thrombogenic and less inflammatory than simple PVC or polyurethane, both of which are bioreactive and thrombogenic. When coated with polytetrafluoroethylene, however, they become much more compatible with the vasculature.

Vialon is a nonhemolytic, hemocompatible polymer that is free of plasticizers. This material is very slick when wet and softens after insertion, minimizing vein trauma and clot induction. Each year, new and improved polymers for catheter materials are introduced, not all of which are discussed here.

Catheter sizes.
The gauges and lengths of catheters are as varied as their uses. Steel is the most limited material. A small steel needle for infusion may be ⅜ to 1½ inches long and 27 to 13 gauge.

Plastic catheters have a greater flexibility of length. Typically, the length ranges from ⅝ to 2 inches, but it can be as long as 12 inches. The catheter sizes range from 27 to 12 gauge, with the most common adult sizes being 22, 20, and 18 gauge.

Catheters inserted and advanced 3 to 10 inches are commonly called *midline catheters*. Their use has increased in recent years. Gauge sizes range from 16 to 24. Some are available in dual-lumen configurations. Midline catheter insertions are increasing. The insertion technique for a midline catheter is more technical and complex than that of short, peripheral catheters. Midlines are inserted and managed like long-term peripherally inserted central catheters. Peripheral catheters that are designed to terminate in the superior vena cava are discussed appropriately as central catheters.

Catheter design.
The thin-walled catheter is constructed of plastic, and its thinner wall provides higher flow rates because of its larger internal lumen. Thin-walled catheters are smoother on insertion because they have a more tapered fit to the inner stylet. The thin-walled construction also causes the catheter to become less able to hold its shape once it is inserted and warmed to body temperature. This soft, "flimsy" catheter is easier on the intima of the vein but collapses with negative pressure. Catheters manufactured from soft polymers are more difficult to use when aspirating blood and less desirable for use as arterial catheters.

Plastic catheters were originally manufactured using a thick-walled construction design. Users of these catheters claim to be more confident in the insertion process because they feel the vein "give" or "pop" with successful cannulation. A thick-walled catheter may be sturdier in such applications as arterial and jugular puncture. If the arterial line is used to monitor blood pressure, some clinicians believe that the readings have improved accuracy because of the less flexible or noncompliant quality of the thick-walled catheter.

The stylet inside the plastic catheter must be held stationary and in a bevel-up position during insertion to prevent vein trauma and to receive early flashback. Ideally, the nurse must control the stylet assembly or the catheter must be notched. The notch locks the catheter and stylet in a preset, clinically correct position with the bevel up. This feature is increasingly popular and is now standard on many products.

The flashback chamber is a small space at the hub of the stylet. When the stylet punctures the vein during catheter insertion, the increased pressure in the vein is immediately relieved into the catheter stylet with a flow of blood in the flashback chamber. Catheters have a closed flashback chamber that allows air to escape and blood to enter.

Some flashback chambers are remarkable feats of engineering, allowing blood to travel a micropathway like a maze or an endlessly convoluted path. This capability allows the nurse to see that the blood return is continuing as the catheter is advanced and secured. The safest catheters use a flashback chamber that allows the rapid return of blood but prohibits any blood spillage, even with abnormally high flashback pressures. A well-designed flashback chamber minimizes the amount of blood needed to make the flashback apparent.

Adding wings to the design of IV catheters and scalp-vein needles was intended to improve insertion technique and catheter maintenance. The wings are usually flexible plastic protrusions from the hub of the device that conform to curves in skin contour. Many nurses think that a winged catheter allows more flexibility during the securing of the device, without requiring the placement of tape directly over the skin puncture.

Winged catheters also provide more control when the catheter is manipulated. The nurse's fingers never touch the catheter hub during insertion, decreasing the potential of contamination. The preference of wings is user dependent. Wings are offered with a variety of products, including catheters with preattached tubing. Catheters without wings are also very popular, widely used, and accepted.

Short peripheral catheter hubs incorporate international color-coding standards. Universal color-coding standards allow visual recognition of the catheter gauge size. This standard has not been applied to the gauge sizes of midline or central infusion catheters. An inherent danger exists in color-coding of IV catheters, medical products, and other devices because color-coding implies that products can be identified without reading the label. For ease of sorting, supplying, or reaching for a product, color codes are useful. After the product is in hand, the label must be read. Color-coding should never substitute for reading the package label.

X-rays do not penetrate radiopaque materials, making a radiopaque device visible on an x-ray film. Infusion catheters are made radiopaque by adding barium sulfate to the catheter material or a barium sulfate stripe to the catheter. Although the radiopacity is provided to help identify a catheter embolus, the incidence of catheter severance is rare. The radiopaque striping is also so small that it may be difficult to see in many cases. Nonetheless, industry has taken steps to provide high-quality peripheral catheters that are radiopaque.

Dual-lumen peripheral IV catheters may also be used and are available in a range of catheter gauges with corresponding lumen sizes. These catheters have a larger total lumen size, necessitating cannulation of a larger vessel to accommodate both lumens. They have two infusion channels, making it possible to infuse two fluids. Because two infusions may be delivered simultaneously, it is necessary to have as much hemodilution as possible to protect the vessel. Some investigators recommend the antecubital fossa as the site of choice, although this vessel is not the only one that is able to accommodate a dual-lumen catheter. Simultaneous infusions of fluids or medications known to be incompatible are controversial because of the proximity of the outlets and the limited hemodilution achievable in peripheral vessels.

Catheters designed for safety. Although the goal of all manufacturers is to design products that perform well and make treatments less troublesome for the patient, increased emphasis is on safety in the work environment. The caregiver also needs to be protected from harm in the administration of routine and emergent care. Medical manufacturers are providing an array of products that safeguard personnel.

The latest designs for infusion devices are moving away from the traditional stylet into newer technology that eliminates exposure of health care workers to blood and body fluids and prevents accidental needlestick injuries. One safety product design is a self-sheathing stylet that is recessed into a rigid chamber at the hub of the catheter when insertion is complete. Another design puts the stylet at the end of a flexible wire, making accidental needle sticks unlikely. A newly designed scalp-vein set allows the steel needle to recess into the hub and wing assembly.

Central infusion catheters

A central infusion catheter is commonly called a *central line,* the line being the device threaded into the central vasculature. The central line has evolved from being used for emergent access or long-term access to one that is commonplace in all aspects of health care. Central lines are commonly seen at home, in non–acute care facilities, and in the entire range of hospital units.

Medical manufacturers, in conjunction with health care professionals and patients, have worked together to make many central lines safe and functional for many uses and in many settings. Home health nurses and some patients independently manage the delivery of complex infusion regimens via central access at home, greatly enhancing the continuum of care from the hospital to ambulatory care to home. Although many central lines are used for emergent or trauma care, they are increasingly inserted to provide long-term, chronic infusion access.

Although central lines are becoming commonplace and are easily managed, their insertion and use necessitate current knowledge of national standards of care, and clinical competency must be validated. Before they are used, all central catheters should have tip location confirmed by x-ray. It is imperative that the managing physician, nurse, and patient/family member have a thorough knowledge of the benefits and limitations of available infusion devices and that they make the final selection together. The overall goal of device selection should focus on inserting the infusion device which best meets the patient's long-term needs.

Percutaneously inserted devices. A central line that is inserted by direct skin puncture into the vein is a *percutaneous device,* which means that a steel needle (which may be a through-the-needle or over-the-needle device) punctures the skin and is advanced until the vein is entered. The vessel is then cannulated with the central venous catheter. A catheter inserted by this method is usually not considered a long-term device because it is not tunneled under the skin. A percutaneously inserted catheter may consist of polyurethane, a stiffer material, which makes the catheter easy to advance, allowing catheter insertion outside the operating room. Examples of a percutaneously inserted catheter include single-, dual-, triple-, and quadruple-lumen subclavian and jugular catheters.

Another percutaneously inserted device is the peripherally inserted central catheter. This is a long-term catheter that has the advantage of being tunneled. Most of these catheters are designed to stay in place for weeks to months because of their biocompatible composition.

Tunneled catheters. *Tunneling* is the technique for placing silicone, cuffed catheters. This technique allows long dwell times and permits self-care. Proper placement of silicone catheters is crucial to their usefulness and to patient acceptance. The catheter ideally exits low on the patient's chest so that the patient can easily participate in self-care and to hide the catheter under clothing. Types of tunneled catheters include Hickman, Broviac, Raaf, and Groshong catheters. They may have single or multiple (up to four) lumens.

A very small incision called the *entrance site* is made at a point near the subclavian vein. From this point to a predetermined point lower on the chest where the catheter will exit, a small, pencil-like device called a *tunneler* is passed. The catheter is drawn through the subcutaneous layer while the tunneler is removed. The tunnel may be 2 to 12 inches long for placement on the chest. If the catheter has a nontraditional entrance and exit site, the tunnel may be even longer. For example, a catheter with a femoral entry site could exit midsternum.

Placement is determined by the terminal end location of the catheter in the central circulation. Catheters, which may be trimmed at the terminal end, are placed in the previously described manner. Catheters unable to be trimmed because of their unique design at the terminal end (e.g., valve-tip or staggered lumen ends) must be inserted in reverse. The catheter is placed in the central vessel, and the hub ends (minus the large connectors) are threaded (with the tunneling device) through the skin from the entrance site to the exit site. Any trimming to make the catheter shorter occurs at the hub end before the Luer connectors are attached. A schematic of tunneling technique is presented in Fig. 15-9.

Catheter characteristics and properties. When evaluating which infusion devices to use, some qualities are essential, others are optional. In determining which catheter is best suited to a particular situation, the physician and nurse should define the infusion requirements with the patient and together select the product that best meets the patient's needs. Approaching product selection in this manner improves patient satisfaction, achieves outcomes, and results in quality, cost-effective infusion care.

Radiopacity. All infusion devices should be radiopaque. For central catheters, radiopacity helps determine catheter tip placement and location of catheter emboli in event of catheter shearing or breakage. Although catheter embolism is rare, it does occur; being able to locate the catheter determines the treatment. The degree of radiopacity varies between manufacturers.

Thrombogenicity. Thrombogenicity is the rate of thrombus occurrence. All catheters are thrombogenic; they differ only in degree. New catheter materials are thoroughly researched to determine their thrombogenicity. Thrombogenicity is evaluated by simulating normal body conditions under time-elapsed measurement. The amount and type of thrombogenic matter that accumulates on the catheter surface determines thrombogenicity.

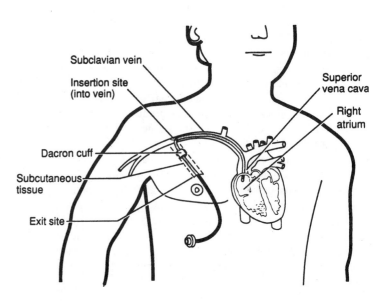

FIG. 15-9 *Schematic of tunneling technique.* (Courtesy MiniMed Technologies.)

Biocompatibility. Biocompatibility, or bioinertness, is a beneficial characteristic that has become a goal of most catheter material research. When a material is bioinert, the body does not perceive it as a foreign substance; therefore inflammation and irritation do not occur. Silicone is the most bioinert material currently used in catheter construction.

Central catheter cuffs. A cuff is a strip of material about 1 cm wide and less than 18 cm deep that encircles a catheter. The cuff can be made of various materials, such as nylon or Dacron, although the texture of the cuff before insertion is roughened like Velcro. Approximately 14 days after catheter insertion, the cuff, positioned in the subcutaneous tunnel, becomes firmly attached by the growth of a connective-tissue seal. The tissue seal around the cuff stabilizes the catheter and reduces the risk of a catheter-related infection by inhibiting the migration of microorganisms along the catheter track. Because the cuff is firmly adhered to the tissue, the catheter is designed to pull loose from the cuff when sharp tension is applied. This feature prevents tissue tearing if the catheter is accidentally pulled. After the catheter is removed, the cuff can be left behind or surgically removed using local anesthesia.

The silver-impregnated collagen matrix cuff has been shown to reduce the incidence of catheter colonization or catheter-related infections with central venous catheters that have been inserted for less than 2 weeks.[7] The cuff can be used on short- or long-term catheters made of either plastic or silicone.

Chemical bonding. Several different types of chemically bonded catheters are available. Initially, the bonding product of choice was heparin. Manufacturers introduced heparin-bonded catheters for two reasons. With heparin bonding, less expensive plastic can be used, making the catheter much more biocompatible at a reduced cost. Second, the heparin bond reduces the thrombogenicity of the product. The distinct disadvantage of the heparin-bonded catheter is that it is unsuitable for use in patients who have heparin antibodies, heparin sensitivity, or coagulation disorders of unknown cause.

A newer bonding concept is antiseptic bonding. A recent study of patients with polyurethane catheters bonded with silver sulfadiazine and chlorhexidine showed that they demonstrated nearly a fivefold lower likelihood of catheter-related bloodstream infections than patients in a control group with noncoated polyurethane catheters. Highly sensitive assays found no evidence of the bonding material in the bloodstream.[8]

Another bonding concept uses surfactant and antibiotics. In a trial study, catheters coated with penicillin and cephalosporin had an almost sevenfold reduction in the incidence of infection. However, there is some concern about the widespread use of antibiotic-bonded catheters and the potential development of resistant microorganisms.[7]

Safety-tipped catheters. A concern from use of all central catheters is the potential damage to the inner lining of the vessel or the myocardium from the chronic rubbing of the catheter tip. Because of this, few central vascular catheters are placed in the right atrium; the superior vena cava is considered the position of choice. The safety tip on some catheters is designed to decrease the rubbing caused by the rush of blood with each beat of the heart. The tip is a very soft material, usually silicone, which enhances the safety of the catheter.

Suturability. A standard feature on most central catheters is a cuff or wing for suturing. The cuff or wing may be stationary, making placement more difficult in some cases. In some catheters, the cuff or wing is attached to the catheter after placement, allowing more flexibility in catheter positioning. If the cuff or wing is not preattached, care must be taken not to damage the catheter or cause it to kink during application and suturing. Catheters that do not provide a suture wing may be predisposed to catheter damage and skin stress because the catheter must be sutured directly onto the skin. The suture wing does not affect the overall performance of the catheter but makes it easier to use and more comfortable for the patient. Many catheter suture wings do not require suturing; they are attached to a catheter-locking device that adheres to the skin. The suture wing holes are placed on the pegs of the catheter-locking device to firmly secure the catheter.

Clampability. The type of material used to construct the catheter determines whether it can be clamped. Silicone is easily damaged and can be clamped only with soft, smooth, toothless clamps. Even plastic catheters can be damaged when clamped too aggressively. Catheters with preattached clamps have an area distal to the skin exit site that is made of PVC tubing to allow safe clamping. Several makers of silicone and polyurethane central lines attach these extensions to ensure product safety and to satisfy the need for clamping. The clamps are nonregulating, and suitable only for on-off control.

Repairability. Most plastic central infusion catheters are not repairable. Silicone does not tolerate high pressures and ruptures easily during pressure injections. Because of its elasticity, it can be pressure-fitted over a repair coupling to make the catheter whole again. The main criterion for successful catheter repair is to leave enough external catheter to allow repair. Usually, tears or ruptures can be trimmed and a new connecting hub applied. This characteristic of silicone is one of many benefits of using this catheter in home or extended care settings.

Introducers. The use of an introducer, or dilator, or the incorporation of a guidewire can be a tremendous benefit in percutaneous central catheter insertion. An introducer is used to cannulate a vessel and allow nontraumatic cannulation. Introducers can be left in place or removed. Introducers left in place must be specifically designed for use after insertion. Using an insertion guidewire and introducer is more complex than are traditional through-the-needle or over-the-needle insertions. The risks associated with introducers are greater, but the types of catheters that require introducers and guidewires have advantages that well outweigh the risks.

In some instances, the introducer is deliberately left in place and may incorporate an added infusion port. This feature is most common with the insertion of a Swan-Ganz catheter. With these introducers, the opening that permits insertion of the catheter may have a rubber disk through which the catheter is inserted. This rubber seal holds tight around the catheter, preventing the introduction of air or bacteria. In the absence of a sealing disk, air and bacteria are prevented from entering the port only by the snug fit of the catheter inside the introducer.

An added infusion port appears as a side "pigtail" and exits at the internal tip of the catheter. This side port provides an extra infusion lumen, but it is not necessary for the function of the introducer. The side port does not have a separate lumen but allows flow around the catheter inside the introducer.

The introducer must not be thought of as a central line. The introducer by design is shorter and stiffer than a typical central line and its intended purpose it not that of an infusion device. When the catheter is removed from the introducer, the introducer should also be removed. The act of removing the catheter may dislodge the introducer. After the rubber seal has been held in an open position embracing the catheter, it may not seal satisfactorily after the catheter is removed. Its short length and more rigid material may be harmful to the vasculature at the point at which the infusate enters the bloodstream. Because not all introducers have the rubber seal, the open port must be capped. Although in some cases a cap can be obtained to fit the open end of the introducer, it is not a universal cap because that port is quite large. Having an injection cap specific to the introducer, yet compatible with other infusion catheters, creates additional risk to the patient.

Types of central line devices

Implanted ports. Implanted ports are different from the long-term catheters mentioned earlier because they are implanted under the surface of the skin, alleviating the need for daily care. (Many manufacturers incorporate the word *port* in their brands names. Use of the word here does not imply any particular brand.) When an implanted device is used, it must be accessed with a noncoring needle. Implanted ports may be single or dual lumen; a dual port has two separate ports, and a single catheter has two lumens. The description of implanted catheters here does not include intraosseous accesses, although their use is very similar. The intraosseous access port terminates in the bone marrow, whereas those addressed in this section are central venous catheters. Implanted ports are best suited for long-term intermittent needs. If the implanted port must be used daily for extended periods, it may not be the access device of choice.

The implantation procedure is surgical and requires a knowledgeable physician. An implantable port can also be inserted by an interventional radiologist. The incision is made on the chest in a site below the clavicle. At the incision, the subclavian or internal jugular vein is cannulated with a silicone catheter via a splittable introducer. The catheter is trimmed and attached to the reservoir, or if it is preattached to the reservoir, it is trimmed before it is inserted through the introducer. The reservoir is sutured in place in a small pocket located superficially above the breast tissue. The incision is sutured or suture-taped, leaving no external apparatus.

The implanted port has a strong, well-made reservoir that is attached to a soft silicone or polyurethane catheter. The catheter is trimmed so that it does not extend into the right atrium, and the terminal end may have staggered lumen openings or may be valve tipped.

Ports are made of plastic, titanium, steel, silicone rubber, and various combinations. Steel is not used as often any more because it interferes with electromagnetic imaging procedures and is quite heavy compared with the other materials. Titanium has the advantages of steel without the interference problems

and is very lightweight. Silicone is rarely used alone but is used in conjunction with hard rubber or plastic. Plastic comes in many types and properties; when coated with high-quality silicone material, it can be a satisfactory port material. Apart from the decreasing use of steel, the market has shown no major preference for one port material over another.

Reservoirs for implanted ports come in many sizes. Most reservoirs are less than 1 inch in height and have a quarter-size diameter. Ports must be easily palpable to be accessed and are available in different sizes for children and adults. Smaller ports are called *low-profile ports,* are no more than ½ inch high and ½ inch wide, and they have a very low priming volume. If they are placed in the arm, a port designed specifically for that area should be used. The location of the port may be stabilized by suturing the holes on the portal base or through the latex or plastic base to the muscle fascia. The reservoir itself should be designed to allow thorough and complete flushing, with no dead space or corners that would allow for build-up of sludge, a blood product residue that impairs use of the catheter. The outlet to the catheter should be located at the base of the port and should be of lumen size that correlates to the catheter. Fig. 15-10 depicts a cross section of an implanted port.

The septum that accommodates the injection needle is critical to the success of the device. The septum is denser and thicker in an implanted reservoir than in routine injection caps because it not only allows the needle to enter, but is also the only means of stabilizing the needle. The septum must hold the needle tightly upright to prevent damage to the septum, which would render the device unusable, and to prevent tearing or coring of the skin.

The septum is the point of injection and must be palpable through the skin. Some implanted ports recess the septum for ease in identification, whereas others have a domed configuration. Experience has not shown remarkable superiority of one design over another. The tissue over the septum commonly becomes calloused or scarred, with a loss of sensitivity resulting from the chronic presence of the device and the needlesticks

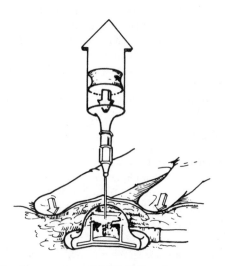

FIG. 15-10 *Cross section of implanted port.* (Courtesy Bard Access Systems.)

associated with its use. Experience has shown that ports with softly molded angles cause minimal skin breakdown.

The septum must be protected because it is the key to the implanted port. If traditional needles are used to penetrate the septum, coring and leakage occur after a few punctures, rendering the device useless. Noncoring needles are used exclusively to prevent this complication.

A noncoring needle has the penetration effect of a knife, so when the needle is removed, the septum closes cleanly behind it. The bevel opens on the side of the needle instead of on the end. These needles are very effective and allow the port to be accessed more than 1000 times. Use of smaller-gauge noncoring needles adds to the longevity of the septum. Fig. 15-11 compares the construction of coring and noncoring needles.

The silicone catheter attaches to the implanted port at the base. It may be preattached or attached during the insertion procedure. The fluid path must make a 90-degree angle at this point. When the implanted device is evaluated, the outlet of the port into the catheter must be thoroughly examined. Some manufacturers have silicone catheters that are designed to accommodate high flow rates and blood infusions, but the outlet coupling is far smaller than the catheter itself and impairs flow. Implanted catheters with this design often have occlusion and low-flow problems.

Silicone tunneled catheters.
The most traditional silicone catheter is the tunneled catheter; the most popular and widely used is the Hickman. Tunneled catheters are between 20 and 30 inches long and have an internal lumen diameter of 22 to 17 gauge. The thickness of the silicone varies by manufacturer. A thin silicone wall may be more supple in the vasculature but is prone to rupture and easily pinches off if it is placed near the clavicle and rib cross point. A thicker-walled catheter is less likely to rupture or pinch. However, if it is structured so that the thickness of the wall narrows the lumen, the catheter is sluggish, clots easily, and resists high flow rates. Quality silicone catheters have a tougher, thinner wall that does not impede flow or increase risk of rupture.

The insertion of a tunneled catheter is a surgical procedure and requires a knowledgeable physician or an interventional radiologist. The incision is made on the chest in a site below the clavicle. Tunneled catheters have a small cuff of slightly abrasive material located on the catheter at a point that would normally be in the subcutaneous tissue. This cuff is usually no more than 1 cm wide and acts to initiate the formation of a scar band, which has a twofold purpose. The scar band eliminates the need

for the catheter to be sutured in place. If sutures are placed during insertion, they may be removed 5 to 7 days after insertion. Some physicians prefer to leave the suture in place as long as they are free from redness, tenderness, or drainage. The scar is well developed after 7 to 14 days, and the catheter is usually secure by this time, making accidental dislodgment less likely.

The second vital role of the cuff is to terminate epithelialization of the tunnel. The bioinert properties of silicone allow the skin at the exit site to attempt to fully heal, uninterrupted by the presence of the catheter. The epithelium begins to repair, and because it cannot cover the catheter, it follows the catheter up the tunnel. The cuff and scar band stops the epithelialization at that point, making an intact tunnel to the cuff. This well-healed and protected tunnel prevents bacterial migration up the catheter beyond the cuff, and most bacteria are held harmless in contact with the epithelialized surface of the tunnel.

Silicone catheters can be dual, single, or triple lumen. Careful consideration of patient need before placement is important because the silicone catheter can stay in place for an indefinite period. Additional lumens may be convenient during the initial phase of treatment but are an added care responsibility over a long period. If the life span of the catheter is many months to years, an unused lumen may represent an unnecessary risk and patient cost.

The Broviac catheter is a smaller-lumen tunneled catheter. Tunneled catheters made for children are designed with the cuff located with regard to smaller anatomy. Large-lumen catheters are available for children if desired.

When the catheter has multiple lumens, the exterior design of the catheter should be round to ensure that no leakage occurs when the catheter enters the vein wall. Irregular shapes are difficult for the vasculature to seal around and to use with an introducer, necessitating a cut-down procedure to cannulate the vein.

The inner tip of the silicone catheter has traditionally been a blunt cut, which allows the inserting physician to trim the catheter to the appropriate length before insertion. The Groshong catheter has a closed end with a slit valve located on the side near the tip and should not be trimmed at the terminal end. Some versions of the valve tip have two slit valves, one above the other, to ensure catheter function if one valve fails. With infusion, the valve flows open, and with aspiration, the valve opening flows inward. With no pressure exerted in either direction, the valve lies closed, preventing blood flow into the catheter or airflow into the system (Fig. 15-12). The catheter hub can be open to air without an adverse affect if the valve is functioning properly. Because blood does not normally flux into the catheter, patency is easily maintained without heparin. A weekly saline flush is recommended.

Many variations exist in the design of silicone catheters. Listing all of them is not possible, and distinguishing one from another is difficult. However, a basic understanding of structure and function is necessary for working with these catheters.

Plastic catheters.
Plastic is the most widely used material for catheter construction. Many kinds of plastic are used, each with its own indications and associated problems. The cross mixing of types of plastics makes it difficult to rate them or to make general statements about their performance.

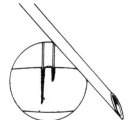
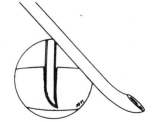

FIG. 15-11 *Comparison of coring versus noncoring needle.* (Courtesy Bard Access Systems.)

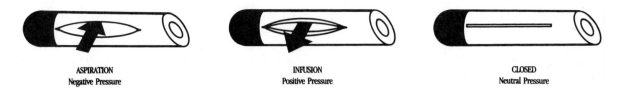

ASPIRATION
Negative Pressure

INFUSION
Positive Pressure

CLOSED
Neutral Pressure

FIG. 15-12   *Valve-tipped catheter. The three-way Groshong valve opens inward for aspiration, opens outward for infusion, and remains closed when not in use.* (Courtesy Bard Access Systems.)

PVC is a familiar type of plastic, but it is not the plastic of choice for internal dwelling catheters. PVC is relatively rigid and has been criticized for possible vascular erosion resulting from trauma of the inner vessel wall from constant rubbing. PVC catheters are radiographic and are easy to insert, but they are not tolerated well by body tissue. PVC can be coated to improve biocompatibility.

Polyurethane is more commonly used in catheters because it is less thrombogenic and softens considerably when it is warmed in the bloodstream. Increased pliability equates to increased patient safety. Polyurethane is marginally radiopaque; many manufacturers have embedded radiopaque beads or striping to make it more visible.

Polyethylene is a polymer used in central catheter structure. This material is available in heparin-coated and non–heparin-coated design. Polyethylene has been implicated in a higher incidence and size of radiologic thrombi than have silicone elastomer catheters.[9]

Alternative access devices

Swan-Ganz catheters. The Swan-Ganz catheter is a hemodynamic monitoring catheter. Its lumens are function specific, and the catheter is primarily used in critical care nursing. The lumens of a Swan-Ganz catheter are for the attachment of data-monitoring devices to determine core temperature, cardiac output, and hemodynamic analysis. The catheter itself is longer than 3 feet and is used in fully monitored intensive care units and specialty care areas.

Dialysis/pheresis catheters. Dialysis catheters are rarely considered for the routine use of infusions; they are strictly reserved for dialysis, primarily because of the many problems associated with occlusion and the increased risk of a catheter-related infection. However, pheresis catheters may be used for the purpose of plasmapheresis and for the routine administration of medications.

Dialysis and pheresis catheters are available in plastic for short-term needs and in silicone materials for long-term needs. Short-term dialysis catheters are primarily used to provide temporary dialysis access.

Dialysis and pheresis catheters have a much larger lumen (usually 13 to 16 gauge) and are shorter and less flexible than those of regular central lines. They have traditionally been more rigid than other lines to allow high blood volumes and rates. The high flow rates for dialysis and pheresis are necessary to provide blood volume for aspiration and infusion. A catheter that becomes soft and collapses with large-flow dynamics is unacceptable for dialysis or pheresis.

Plastic dialysis and pheresis catheters are problematic in that they are difficult to secure and maintain because of their rigidity. Their large size makes them more painful to the patient during movement. The site bleeds easily, making it difficult to keep the dressing clean, dry, and intact. Plastic dialysis and pheresis catheters do not have long-term dwell times.

The newer silicone dialysis and pheresis catheters are softer and more comfortable to the patient. Because they are not as obtrusive as previously designed silicone catheters, they are easier to secure and maintain, and bleeding at the site is more easily controlled. These catheters may have a cuff to encourage epithelialization of the entrance wound. The connecting hubs are color-coded to facilitate the identification of lumens. These silicone products may stay in place for months.

Shunts. Shunts can be placed for many reasons. Only the artificial venous shunt is discussed here as a vascular access device. Modern shunts are made of Gor-Tex or silicone material. A shunt bridges two vessels: an artery and a vein. The shunt is usually placed in the forearm between the radial artery and the brachial or cephalic vein. It is accessed with a large-bore dialysis needle and is used for routine hemodialysis.

Newer shunts are able to withstand many needlesticks and are used routinely in some places for infusion purposes other than dialysis. Only knowledgeable persons should access a shunt. If it is inadvertently damaged, surgical replacement is necessary.

Arterial catheters. Catheters that are introduced into the arterial circulation can be used for two purposes: monitoring or organ-specific infusions. When the purpose is monitoring, the arterial catheter provides an access for blood sampling (including blood gases) and blood pressure monitoring, usually at the radial artery located at the wrist.

The catheter must be able to sustain its shape and be long enough to cannulate the artery, which is normally deeper than a peripheral vein. Some of the newer catheter materials are designed to be softer and more pliable after insertion, making them less desirable for arterial cannulation. When properly placed, the arterial catheter may have to bend as it descends to the artery. If the catheter kinks at the bend or collapses on itself with negative pressure, it does not function well as an arterial catheter. As mentioned earlier, many anesthesiologists prefer to use thick-walled catheters as arterial catheters because of their sturdy design. Most peripheral catheters can be used as arterial catheters, and some have superior performance for monitoring and for blood sampling (for arterial blood gases and general laboratory testing). Arterial catheters are routinely used to monitor blood pressure when they are attached to the appropriate nondistensible tubing and transducer set-up.

Peripherally placed arterial catheters are not used for the infusion of fluids. Medication infused into an artery, even in benign volumes and concentrations, can cause tissue damage because of the close proximity to the capillary bed or terminal point of circulation. Hemodilution is not sufficient to prevent tissue saturation of the drug and resulting cellular hypoxia.

Arterial catheters placed for infusion are organ specific, with the most common being the hepatic artery catheter. These therapies are for specialized infusions, such as regionalized chemotherapy to a particular diseased organ. Some are attached to an implanted pump or reservoir that is accessible with a special needle.

Intraspinal catheters. *Intraspinal* means located within the spinal space. Technically speaking, this area can include the epidural and the intrathecal spaces. The intraspinal route has been accessed for many years for many forms of medical treatment, injections, diagnostic tests, and infusions. Advancements in anesthesia have made the intraspinal space more accessible, medically functional, and respected as a route for fluid and medication administration.

The catheters used for intraspinal infusion are 22 to 26 gauge and are approximately 10 to 30 inches long. They are made of biocompatible formulas of polyurethane or silicone-like polymers. They can extend several inches into the epidural space, especially if the catheter is intended to be in place long term. Intraspinal catheters can exit directly from the spinal puncture site or can be threaded subcutaneously to a remote site.

Once successful spinal puncture has been performed, the catheters are threaded through an introducer apparatus. If the catheter is intended for a one-time infusion, it is lightly secured until the procedure is over. The rigid needle is not left in place for any length of time. If the catheter is to be left in place for extended periods, it is threaded farther into the epidural space and taped securely.

Another device that introduces infusate into the spinal fluid is the Ommaya reservoir (Fig. 15-13). This is a very specific therapy reservoir that attaches to a catheter and terminates in the cerebral ventricular space. The medication most often infused is concentrated morphine sulfate without preservative. This drug bathes the neurons of the brain and spine directly to achieve maximum pain control. This is also called *intraventricular therapy.*

Needles. A needle is a sterile steel or aluminum tube through which fluids flow. It can be as small as a coarse hair or large enough to drink through. When used to infuse, the needle must be inserted into a fluid space, fluid path, or compartment that can accommodate the introduction of fluids.

Hypodermic needles are those that are inserted beneath the skin. IV access can be gained with a hypodermic needle. If a needle is used to perform venipuncture, the vein is easily perforated by the needle's rigid and sharp construction. Hypodermic needles easily penetrate leathery skin and tough vein walls. The disadvantage of these needles is that after penetrating the wall of the vein, they often penetrate the opposite wall as well.

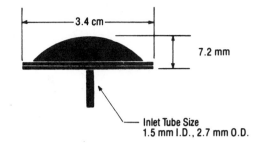

FIG. 15-13 *Ommaya reservoir.* (Courtesy American V. Mueller.)

Venous perforation and infiltration are common with hypodermic needle venipuncture. This method of venipuncture is reserved for blood drawing and delivering one-time IV push medications. If the needle is to remain in the vein more than momentarily, an IV catheter is the device of choice. The scalp-vein set does not fall into the category of hypodermic needles, although both are made of metal. The scalp-vein needle's design greatly increases its dwell time and patient safety.

Subcutaneous needles are inserted into the fatty tissue below the skin, providing the name for this procedure, *subcutaneous infusion* or *hypodermoclysis.* The subcutaneous tissue has minimal pain sensors but good absorption rates, making medications and fluid infused into this compartment effective therapy. Needles used to access this space can be regular hypodermic needles less than 1 inch long. The needle is inserted at a 10- to 20-degree angle, depending on the patient's fatty tissue depth. Specially designed subcutaneous needles that appear to have a flat disk at the hub to enable leaving the needle in place for a period are also available. The needles are ⅜ to ⅞ inch long and are inserted directly into the skin with the disk resting on the skin. These needles are comfortable for the patient and do not dislodge easily.

Intraosseous needles. Intraosseous needles, those inserted into the bone, are categorized with steel needles. The marrow space of the human bone, especially in children, is capable of providing an infusion route for any IV drug or fluid.

Several designs of intraosseous needles are available. The tip end of an intraosseous needle is solidly protected by an obturator, is very sharp, and may have circular screwing threads to help penetrate the bone. The hub end has a large, solid handle that fits into the palm so that pressure can be exerted. Fig. 15-14 depicts intraosseous needle placement.

The needle recommended for a child is 18 gauge, and a 15- to 16-gauge needle is used for adults. The long bones of the leg or iliac crest are usually the point of insertion. Intraosseous administration is thought of as a pediatric procedure, but it can be used in adults. The sternum of adults has been used with mixed opinions.[10] Complications include bone breakage, infiltration, bone infection, and cellulitis. This technology is reserved for problems that cannot be resolved by routine means.

An implanting technique in which the bone is cannulated and a reservoir sits on the bone under the skin to allow an intermittent access to the bone has been developed. This method allows medications such as antibiotics or chemotherapy agents to be administered directly into the bone.

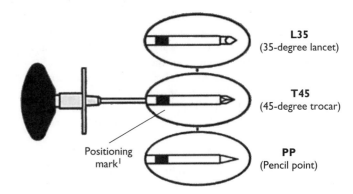

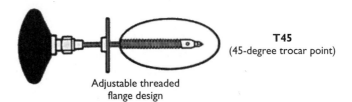

FIG. 15-14 *Intraosseous needle placement.* (Courtesy Cook Critical Care.)

DRESSINGS

Many different types of dressings materials are available, ranging from gauze and tape to adhesive bandages to sterile, specialized, semipermeable membranes. Each type of dressing material has specific recommendations for optimal use. However, much controversy exists as to which dressing material is optimal, whether ointment should be incorporated under a dressing, whether a dressing change necessitates the use of a mask and gloves, and at what interval the dressing should be changed. These questions are access specific and must be answered in the context of the equipment used, the patient, the treatment delivered, and the practice setting.

Gauze

Cotton and cotton blends with synthetics are used to make gauze sponges. Finer-quality sponges have very little lint or are lint free. *Lint free* means that small flecks of cotton do not adhere to tissue. Lint adhering to soft tissue or granulating areas hinders wound healing.

Gauze, which has a higher cotton or all-cotton content, may be more absorbent than synthetic blended gauze. If the intent of the dressing is to cushion or pad an area, blended gauze is an excellent choice because it is very soft. If the intent is to absorb, all-cotton gauze may be superior.

Appealing aspects of gauze are its absorptive quality and clean appearance. A gauze dressing is less costly than other dressings, easily applied, and readily available in most health care environments. Disadvantages are few but significant. A gauze dressing prevents visual inspection of the IV site. Once the dressing is lifted to observe the condition of the catheter and the insertion site, a new dressing must be applied.

Transparent dressings

Transparent dressings are also called *semipermeable membrane dressings.* They are designed to allow moisture to pass through the dressing away from the skin surface. The rate of moisture release varies greatly among products. Even with the best semipermeable membranes, the adhering ability of the dressing is severely tested by wound drainage and perspiration.

Semipermeable dressings are occlusive. Moisture, and therefore microorganisms, cannot permeate the dressing, a characteristic that makes it an effective shield against contamination. They are able to adhere satisfactorily most of the time, minimizing the tape necessary to secure the dressing and the IV device.

Transparent dressings are provided in individually wrapped sterile packaging. Each brand has a specific application method. Because transparent dressings remain in place for longer periods, the user must be vigilant to protect against contamination with handling and application. If the dressing is poorly designed or the application technique is complex, there is a greater chance that the dressing will be contaminated. Therefore, there is a greater chance for colonization because of the extended time the dressing stays in place.

Securement devices

There are a variety of securement devices available that will serve as a venipuncture device dressing or as a supplement to dressing materials. The securement dressings come in a variety of sizes to cover peripheral venipuncture devices as well as central line catheters. Some of the securement devices include a mechanism that allows the venipuncture device to be snapped in place. This prevents movement of the catheter, thus helping prevent mechanical phlebitis. These products, like the transparent dressings, come in individually wrapped sterile packaging and have a specific application method depending on the brand. This may lead to waste and improper use of these products. Care should be taken to ensure proper application and the area should be monitored on a regular basis per institutional protocol.

Antimicrobial barrier materials

An antimicrobial patch is applied under a dressing or used alone. This patch releases chlorhexidine gluconate incrementally over several days. Chlorhexidine reduces gram-positive and gram-negative colonization significantly.[7] Patches are smaller than a regular dressing and have a precut radial slit to allow the catheter to exit at the center. Patches are also absorptive, nontoxic, and nonirritating.

The indications for routine use of these patches are institution specific, but they are especially useful in patients with high infection risks. Children with short-gut syndrome, immunosuppressed patients, or patients with recurring line failures may benefit from the use of these patches on any invasive line, such as chest tubes, orthopedic pins, or drains.

Infusion Devices

Many options are available for the infusion of parenteral fluids other than by gravity. To simplify this discussion, infusion devices have been categorized based on certain similarities. Specific pumps are not evaluated in this discussion, and the merits and drawbacks of these devices are discussed generally rather than specifically.

The proliferation of infusion devices is directly related to massive cost-cutting efforts in the health care industry. Research and development laboratories continue to redesign cost-effective devices that allow nontraditional caregivers to provide safe infusion therapy in many alternative care settings.

An infusion device controls the rate or monitors the flow of fluid or medication. Some of these devices are very basic, whereas others are very sophisticated. Two kinds of infusion devices exist: mechanical and electronic. Mechanical devices have no outside power source; they operate on the physical principle of matter retaining its own shape, such as a balloon or spring. Electronic devices are powered by internal batteries or alternating current.

Mechanical infusion devices

Mechanical infusion devices are simple and compact, although not necessarily cost-effective. Two types of mechanical devices exist: the balloon and the simple spring.

Elastomeric balloons. Elastomeric balloons are made of a soft rubberized material. They are inflated to a predetermined volume of infusate, which is infused over a specified time. They deliver the infusate over the time determined by the balloon and tubing. The balloon is safely encapsulated inside a rigid, transparent container. The container shape is manufacturer specific; some are round, cylindrical, or shaped liked a disk. There is a tamper-proof port for injecting the medication into the balloon, which prevents accidental opening and contamination. There is an outlet port with preattached tubing or a

hub to which kink-resistant tubing can be attached. The tubing must have a low priming volume and Luer connections.

These balloon devices are used primarily to deliver antibiotics. Other therapies can be delivered, but intermittent, small-volume parenteral therapies are ideal. Volume-replacement therapy requires larger volumes of solutions. The typical volumes for this device are 50 to 100 ml; however, elastomeric balloons are available in sizes up to 250 ml. Elastomeric balloon devices are not reusable.

The balloons are capable of delivering their preset volume in intervals ranging from 30 minutes to several days. The rate of infusion is not dependent on any characteristic of the balloon. The role of the balloon is to exert constant pressure. The balloon deflates at a rate determined by the diameter of the restricting outlet located in the preattached tubing or in the neck of the container, where the tubing exits from the balloon. The restricting outlet is a very simple and ingenious method of ensuring safe rate control. The outlet is much like a glass capillary with a microscopic tunnel. The size of the tunnel controls the passage of fluid. There are no parts to malfunction and no dials to set in error. Examples of elastomeric balloons are shown in Fig. 15-15.

The elastomeric balloons have been tested extensively for drug compatibility and stability. Most drugs are compatible with this method, and many can be premixed, frozen or refrigerated for long periods, thawed, and safely infused.

The PCA elastomeric balloon functions in the same manner, but the controlling mechanism is unique. A restricting orifice exists in the neck of the rigid container. The patient-control option is a push-button regulator on the tubing leading to the patient. The push-button holds a dose of prescribed analgesia, which the patient administers to himself or herself when the need arises. The restricting orifice refills the tiny reservoir under the push-button at a rate safe enough to prevent an overdose of analgesia.

There are only a few factors to consider when evaluating elastomeric balloon devices, but they are significant. The devices are so simple that not many aspects create controversy; their simplicity is their best attribute.

There is a 0.2-micron in-line filter in the kink-resistant tubing. Particulate matter is retained at this point, keeping the orifice free from occlusion. The elastomeric balloon is considered an ambulatory home infusion device because, given the large number of small-volume parenteral infusions administered in hospitals, it is more economical to use traditional methods for inpatients.

Spring-coil piston syringes. The volume of a spring-coil piston syringe ranges from 30 to 60 ml. The syringe piston is equipped with a spring, which powers the plunger in the absence of manual pressure. The device is not sensitive to change or interference, such as increased resistance from infiltration. Like the balloon device mentioned earlier, the spring-coil piston syringe has limited applications and can be used only once.

The syringe piston is filled by withdrawing the piston and overextending the spring. As the spring attempts to regain its shape, it forces the piston back down, expelling the contents. The orifice at the outlet of the syringe has a restricting tube that allows the syringe to empty at a preset rate. Spring syringes are more bulky than elastomeric balloons, and care must be taken not to interfere with the piston as it collapses. Volume is

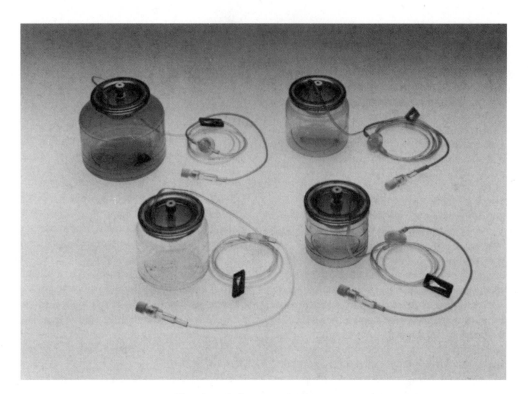

FIG. 15-15 *Elastomeric balloon construction.* (Courtesy McGraw, Inc.)

restricted to the size of the syringe, which limits medications that can be administered.

The syringe has no incompatibilities associated with its use, which makes it ideal for the infusion of problematic drugs. Its volumes are easy to read. Syringes can be prefilled and frozen.

Spring-coil container. The spring-coil container is a combination of the spring coil and a collapsible, flattened disk. The overextended spring is in an enclosed space between two disks and seeks to collapse, pulling the top and bottom together and forcing the contents out of the restricting orifice. This shape can accommodate many infusions and volumes. Its round, flat shape makes it easy to carry in a pocket while it is infusing. Unlike spring-syringe devices, spring-coil containers can have multiple uses for the administration of small-volume doses.

Electronic infusion devices

Controllers. Infusion pumps are devices that push with pressure until certain levels are reached. The term *pumps* indicates positive-pressure devices, whereas the term *controllers* indicates infusion-assist devices that do not *create* pressure, but rather rely on gravity for infusion. Pressure is exerted from the head height of the infusion bag, which is usually 2 psi. Some controllers can reach a psi of 5, but this pressure is uncommon. The function of the controller is to monitor the infusion for constant operation, to sound an alarm if flow is interrupted, and to provide even, consistent flow. This level of function is adequate for general populations with uncomplicated problems. Controllers are safe because they usually do not contribute to large infiltrations or vascular trauma. They are very safe for use on neonatal, pediatric, and oncology patients.

Most controllers use drop-sensor technology. In some devices, a drop sensor attaches to the drip chamber of the administration set and counts drops as they fall into the drip chamber. The accuracy of a drop sensor is dependent on uniform drop size. The absence of a drop tells the controller that no flow is occurring. The controller then sounds an alarm to alert the nurse. A controller has many other features, and these are discussed in conjunction with positive-pressure pumps.

Positive-pressure infusion pumps. A pump creates pressure to infuse. This pressure overcomes vascular resistance, such as excessive tubing length, low head height of the infusion container, and tape applied too tightly. The term used to describe the measurement of pressure exerted by an infusion device is *psi*. Ten psi is the average for pumps, although newer pumps are set at psi rates as low as 5. Older pumps may pump at dangerous pressures of 16 to 22 psi. Pressures greater than 10 to 12 psi should be used with extreme caution. Unusual applications for high-psi pumps are discussed later.

Pumps are important for high-volume, high-acuity situations, which include complex therapies. By increasing the infusion resistance for alarms, electronic infusion pumps are being designed to have fewer nuisance alarms. The pump delivers at an accurate rate and has many features to safeguard the patient. Positive-pressure pumps account for most of the infusion devices used in alternative care settings and in the hospitals.

Mechanisms of delivery

Volumetric. *Volumetric* means that the pump calculates the volume delivered by measuring the volume displaced in a reservoir that is part of the disposable administration set. The pump calculates every fill and empty cycle of the reservoir to deliver a given amount of fluid.

The reservoir is manipulated internally by a specific action of the pump. This action may be similar to that of a syringe; the piston withdraws to fill and pushes to pump. Another action is linear peristaltic; peristaltic fingers in the pump move in a wavelike manner, pushing the fluid out of the chamber. The most accurate mechanism is a series of microreservoirs that fill and empty in sequence and are measurable in hundredths of a milliliter.

The key to accuracy for volumetric devices is that the reservoir is able to fill and deliver a volume in increments of one to several milliliters. If the delivery increment is very small, the degree of accuracy increases. The pump counts to the nearest milliliter the amount of fluid that is emptied out of the reservoir and delivered. In the case of pediatric micropumps, the pump counts the amount emptied out of the reservoir to the nearest tenth of a milliliter.

Volumetric pumps and controllers represent some of the finest equipment available in health care today. Although some pump manufacturers believed that they have progressed beyond volumetric pumps, the functional basis of the pumps is unchanged and, for the most part, acceptable.

Drop sensors. The drop sensors mentioned earlier are also applicable to a discussion of drop counters. In a controller, the purpose of the drop sensor is to confirm the presence or absence of flow. In some drop sensors, the device is specially designed to count the number of drops, thus calculating the volume. The drop sensor can be located internally on the controller where the flow passes through a chamber, but it is usually attached to the drip chamber of the administration set.

A problem associated with drop sensors is the change in the microvolume of each drop with solution changes. The variance of drop size equates to errors in flow rate. In addition, the drop chamber must remain completely still to ensure that the counter senses or detects each drop as it falls. This feature can be a problem if the counter detects splashes or fails to catch multiple drops in sudden rate changes.

Syringe pumps. Piston-driven infusion pumps use a syringe. Because of volume limitations, their use is infusion specific. Most syringe pumps are used to administer antibiotics and small-volume parenteral infusions. The use of syringe pump technology for PCA infusions, together with some significant enhancements, has kept syringe pumps in the forefront of infusion therapy. Numerous syringe pumps are specific to anesthesia, oncology, and obstetric applications.

Syringe pump volume is limited to the size of the syringe used in the device. Certain devices accommodate syringes ranging from 5 to 60 ml. The rate is controlled by the drive speed of the piston attached to the syringe plunger. Although infusion rates vary widely, some syringe pumps infuse over 1 hour or less, whereas others are capable of continuous infusion.

Syringe pumps eliminate the concern for drop size or fluid viscosity, but they are unable to detect no-flow situations unless significant backpressure is exerted. They are not equipped with air sensors or various other safety and convenience alarms. The tubing usually consists of a single, uninterrupted length of kink-resistant tubing without Y injection ports. Syringe pump tubing can be the primary set or the secondary set, depending on the intended use.

INFUSION PUMPS
Characteristics

The alarms on infusion devices should never be assumed to be part of the basic device, nor should it be assumed that every device is equally endowed with the alarms necessary to make it safe. For example, not all pumps have free-flow alarms, but those that do not are considered safe by current regulatory standards. A free-flow alarm or prevention device is considered a necessary feature not only by nurses but also by risk managers. However, an abundance of alarms does not ensure a high-performance pump. Each health care environment must establish which alarms are necessary and which are merely "busy," adding nothing to the performance of the device or the care delivered. The nurse should always remember that alarms are for the protection of the patient, not the caregiver.

The features noted in the general discussion of infusion pumps are important to the largest application of the pumps—the hospital bedside. Pumps used in the home may not have the same features as those used in the hospital. However, they are absolutely safe and applicable to the alternative health care setting. For example, the following air-in-line discussion refers to air-in-line alarms that are crucial to patient safety when fluids are pumped. Several home ambulatory devices are positive-pressure pumps and do not incorporate air-in-line alarms because the infusates and containers are vacuum filled and closed, thereby eliminating the risk of air. The type of therapy and the setting must dictate what is necessary and safe. General rules regarding safety cover the predominant applications but are not absolute.

Alarms
Air-in-line. The *air-in-line* alarm is a basic, necessary alarm. The air-detector device is located on the pump where the administration set exits the device. The detector can be designed to detect only visible bubbles or microscopic bubbles, commonly called *champagne bubbles.*

Volumetric pumps are usually equipped with air-in-line detectors. Some pumps, such as rotary peristaltic or syringe pumps, are rarely equipped with air-in-line detectors because of the types of infusions and fluid containers used. The piston delivers a finite amount in a closed system, and the rotary pump stops functioning when the flow is interrupted, making it unlikely the pump would infuse with air in the line.

The importance of the air-in-line alarm is not to create anxiety over small particles of air, but rather to alert the nurse that the integrity of the system may be compromised. Air may be entering the infusion line, or it may not have been properly removed before the infusion commenced. Microscopic bubbles are more frustrating than visible ones because their origin is harder to determine. The presence of microbubbles can also alert the nurse to other problems, such as an incompatibility or gas being released by the solution. Conversely, microbubbles may be meaningless, having come from vigorous movement of the tubing or infusate.

Although air-in-line alarms were designed to protect the patient, it has long been established that many of the air bubbles detected and tediously removed are far too small to have a harmful effect. Because of this, some pumps allow the nurse to simply push the air through the line by advancing the bubble with a microbolus. The pump supposedly quantifies the air bubble and does not advance a bubble that is greater than a certain volume. Another pump uses a waste collection bag for air purged through the pumping mechanism and vents this air into the bag. This self-purging process is automatic.

Air-in-line alarms are a necessity for all positive-pressure pumps and infusion controllers. Although the alarm is sometimes annoying, it serves as a legitimate safety factor in infusion therapy.

Occlusion. *Occlusion* alarms have become standard for infusion pumps and controllers. Controllers are able to indicate upstream (between the pump and the container) or downstream (between the patient and the pump) occlusion by absence of flow. Some infusion devices can be made to perform as positive-pressure pumps or controllers by simply pressing a keypad on the device.

Because of their positive-pressure design, infusion pumps are able to detect when flow is interrupted above the device and when resistance to flow occurs below the device. Many newer pumps are able to differentiate the message in the alarm, alerting the nurse that the occlusion is "upstream" or "downstream."

An upstream alarm is triggered when the fill stroke is unable to complete because of the vacuum created in the upstream line or fill reservoir. The resistance to fill might be from a completely collapsed and empty plastic fluid container or from clamped tubing. The newer pumps detect this problem very early in the fill cycle.

Downstream alarms are older technology but are more refined today. A downstream alarm occurs when the pressure required by the pump to push the solution forward exceeds a certain psi limit. The psi on some pumps is preset by the manufacturer and can usually be adjusted only by biomedical engineering departments. Even then, the range is very limited. On most new infusion devices, pressure can be adjusted at the bedside. The psi can be set to a maximum to infuse in problematic situations, such as positional central lines or long-line catheters, although the maximum is rarely greater than 10 psi. Caution must be used when increasing the psi of an infusion pump. Increasing the flow pressure can result in infiltration, extravasation, and damage to or rupture of the catheter.

The pressure can be set as low as 2 to 5 psi for infusion of vesicants or routine fluids through healthy veins. Occlusion alarms with low psi settings are common because the pumps are sensitive to slight changes in pressure. Nurses often call these low-pressure occlusion alarms *nuisance* alarms because changes as simple as the patient turning from one side to the other can create pressure. For this reason, the average variable-pressure setting is not as low as it could be.

Another variation of the occlusion pressure alarm is the ability of the pumps to register a central venous pressure or to detect infiltration or venous occlusion before it is clinically detectable. These features are discussed more fully in the section on pump enhancements.

Infusion complete. An *infusion-complete* alarm sounds when a preset volume limit has been reached. Infusion-complete alarms are available only on pumps that allow the user to program infusion volume. The infusion pump calculates the volume delivered and sounds an alarm when the programmed volume is reached. Because the alarm can be set to sound before the fluid container is completely infused, it helps prevent pumping the reservoir dry. This feature has replaced many drop sensors because the infusion-complete alarm calls attention to empty or near-empty infusion containers.

Low battery or low power. *Low-battery* alarms give the user warning of the pump's impending inability to function. A low-battery alarm means that the batteries need to be replaced immediately or an external power source connected. Many battery-powered pumps can be recharged while they run on regular electrical current. Others, less ideally, must be recharged while the pump is not being used. Still others have no capacity for external power and require only a battery replacement.

A *low-power* alarm usually indicates a slightly different power problem. The low-power alarm indicates that power received from an alternating current is not adequate to support the pump or is causing the pump to pull from battery power. This alarm alerts the user that insufficient power is endangering the accurate flow or proper operation of the device. This situation could occur in a home when power is interrupted or in a hospital when outlets are not fully supplied during peak demand times or when emergency generators are inadequate.

As a protective measure, when low-battery and low-power alarms are continued over a preset number of minutes, the pumps are usually designed to convert to a "keep vein open" (KVO) rate. The actual time frame is manufacturer specific and can range from a few minutes to several hours depending on the pump. The preset KVO can be 0.1 to 5.0 ml and continues until the battery power is exhausted. The pump may simply cease to function or may sound an alarm one last time. When this occurs, the programmed infusion information and volume counts may be lost.

In almost every infusion device, the safety of the patient is well protected by adequate alarms. The pumps also hold the programmed information and maintain the set rate until lack of power triggers the KVO rate. The devices are designed not to drift or to slowly fluctuate downward. The programs or settings are usually safely maintained until all the power is exhausted.

Nonfunctional. The *nonfunctional* alarm can be expressed in many ways. It may be a series of scrambled letters or numbers on a display screen, a light that is completely alien to any other known alarm, or a sound unlike any other alarm sound. A nonfunctional alarm means the pump has malfunctioned and the problem cannot be resolved. Pumps may go into a nonfunctional status spontaneously or because of improper use or programming.

Regardless of the reason, a pump that indicates malfunction or nonfunction or resists corrective action should be disconnected from the patient immediately. The pump should not be used again unless it is thoroughly checked by a biomedical engineering specialist or the manufacturer.

Not infusing. The *not-infusing* alarm indicates that the pump infusion settings have not been programmed. Most devices require a deliberate act for operation to begin. This feature prevents tampering or changing settings accidentally. The pump must be programmed or changed and then told to start. Without the start command, the pump does not begin infusing, nor does it make the designated changes. Instead, it sounds the not-infusing alarm.

Parameter. *Parameter* alarms are those that tell the user or programmer that not all of the settings have been completed. These alarms are manufacturer specific. They include set rate, set volume to be infused, secondary rate, and secondary volume. These alarms are instrumental in helping the user program the pump correctly and in safeguarding against misuse.

Tubing. *Tubing* alarms are provided to ensure proper use of the device. They prevent the wrong tubing from being used or the correct tubing from being loaded into the pump incorrectly. The tubing alarm can also instruct or remind the user to load the tubing into the pump.

Door. *Door* alarms indicate that the door that secures the tubing is not closed or is closed incorrectly. In most pumps, the door plays an integral part in the correct operation of the pumping mechanism. If the door is not securely in place, the pump can deliver in error. In other cases, the door is part of the free-flow protection mechanism, and incorrect placement of the door jeopardizes this feature.

Free flow. *Free-flow* alarms, although not available on every infusion device, are lifesaving if the administration set can be gravity primed. More simply stated, if the tubing has no restrictive valves or reservoirs that require the motion of the pump to propel the fluid, it can be gravity primed. Many users see this feature as a significant advantage because, if necessary, the tubing can be removed from the pump and used as a gravity administration set. The danger in this process occurs when the set is removed from the pump and the tubing is not immediately clamped or regulated. Free flow is the unobstructed, wide-open flow of an infusate to the patient. This situation has created many fatal and near-fatal situations.

To prevent errors, most pumps have a free-flow alarm that detects the rapid infusion of fluid that results when the pumping or controlling mechanism is partially disengaged. The alarm also sounds if a tubing clamping device is circumvented.

Many newer gravity-primed sets are designed with clamps that lock into place when the tubing is removed from the pump, thereby preventing free flow. The tubing is fully usable as gravity tubing when the user disengages the clamps. Disengaging the clamp requires a deliberate act and cannot occur accidentally.

Additional safety features. The wide range of safety features are usually taken for granted until they are compromised. An excellent example is the actual pump housing. The housing should be sealed to prevent fluid from entering the internal mechanisms of the pump. Although the housing is not important to most users, biomedical engineers have witnessed the amazing efforts of infusion devices to function while mired in dextrose solutions. The seal of the housing includes the face, where the indicators and control knobs are located. To achieve a more effective seal, most devices use touch pad technology with liquid crystal display.

The seal cannot be perfect. There must be a vent somewhere on the housing to allow gas to escape from the pump. Gas is a product of battery storage and pump operation, and although minuscule in volume, gaseous build-up can cause the pump housing to rupture. The vent is usually not readily visible, is extremely small, and must be clear to ventilate the device.

Automatic KVO features are not available on all devices but are considered highly desirable. An automatic KVO feature ensures that instead of a device shutting down when an alarm sounds, such as low battery or infusion complete, the pump goes into a KVO rate. The KVO rate is pump specific but usually ranges from 0.1 to 5.0 ml/hr.

Size is considered a safety feature in the current climate of health care delivery. Smaller pumps pose fewer risks to the caregiver and patient in terms of transport and ambulation. Size can cause significant problems in terms of excess weight, bulk, and cumbersome management.

Size should be considered inversely as well. When pumps are miniaturized, certain features, such as the back-up battery, the air-in-line alarm, or the free-flow features, may be affected. Smaller is not always better or safer. Infusion devices must be evaluated in terms of safety features, availability, and ability to meet the needs of required therapy.

A tamper-proof feature requires that a deliberate series of steps be taken to affect the action of the pump. These steps may not be complex; in fact, they may include nothing more than having to start the pump after it is reprogrammed or started. Tamper-proof features may also include lock-out programs, which require the nurse to enter a sequence of numbers to access the programming capabilities of the pump. For both hospital and alternative care settings, tamper-proof devices are often desirable.

Tamper-proof pumps are beneficial safety features, but they must be tailored to fit the situation. A tamper-proof feature could prove hazardous if it is used in conjunction with life-threatening medications because the time required to override the tamper-proof feature could hinder quick action. All pumps should provide some degree of tamper-proof consideration; especially those used for geriatric and pediatric populations.

Another safety feature is the inability to bypass alarms. Most devices feature an alarm silence button, which is usually self-terminating in less than 5 minutes. This means the alarm can be silenced for only 5 minutes or less. This self-terminating feature prevents the safety features from being overlooked or deliberately ignored. Repeated attempts to fool a safety feature can result in the pump going into a nonfunctional mode, completely refusing to operate.

Electrical safety is a concern with any equipment connected to an alternating current outlet. Electrical cords should be equipped with grounded plugs and a grounded outlet. Many devices even call attention to their power source if it is in any way inadequate. When any device is used, both the caregiver and patient must be protected from electrical hazards.

Accuracy. The industry standard for accuracy of an electronic IV infusion pump is plus or minus 5%. This standard has been fluctuating widely with the introduction of infusion-specific pumps and the wide array of devices designed for alternative care settings. Some have claimed that accuracy is not an issue for the home infusion of a small-volume parenteral infusion. This claim has been answered with concern that the absence of medical support in the home should underscore the need for accuracy in home devices, not diminish it.

Most devices do not have problems, and their error rate is well below 5%. New technology in which micromeasures of solution can be dispensed makes accuracy easier to achieve. In a device that delivers each milliliter in $\frac{1}{100}$ increments, accuracy is minutely measurable.

Pressure capabilities. Pressure terminology includes the terms *fixed* and *variable*. With fixed infusion pressure, the pump is set internally to infuse up to a certain psi but no more. Occlusion-limit alarms sound at that point. Some fixed-pressure pumps can be internally altered by the manufacturer or by biomedical engineering departments. Any fixed-pressure pump that has been altered by increasing the psi should be clearly marked on the outside to inform all users and should be restricted to certain applications, such as hyperbaric units or dialysis.

Variable-pressure pumps allow the user to determine the psi needed to safely deliver therapy. With a simple programming designation, the nurse can adjust a variable-pressure pump, or a lock-out sequence that limits access to a few persons may be used. Variable-pressure devices have a conservative upper limit, usually around 10 psi, and a lower limit that makes the pump function more like a controller, with a two-psi setting. A psi setting of 4 to 8 is common.

Pressures greater than 12 to 14 psi are rarely necessary. However, in some instances, pressures up to 22 psi are appropriate. Greater-than-normal pressures are needed when infusion pumps are used in conjunction with specialized high-volume, high-pressure treatments, such as hemodialysis, plasmapheresis, cardiothoracic surgeries, and arterial occlusion procedures. In each of these cases, which require close medical supervision and specialized nursing personnel, high pressures are used for purposes other than simple fluid infusion.

Another arena for very high pressure is the hyperbaric chamber. Pressures required for the chamber must exceed the greatly exaggerated atmospheric pressure of the therapy. The infusion pump is ideally outside the chamber or room because its pumping function cannot be guaranteed under high pressure. An extension piece allows the pump to reach the patient through a sealed portal. A psi greater than 16 and up to 22 is necessary.

The psi rating on infusion pumps is a safety factor for the patient. Nurses commonly increase the psi limit to decrease alarms, thereby allowing pressure to reach a higher limit before detecting an occlusion or infiltration. This should be done with caution; there is a very fine line between eliminating a nuisance alarm and disabling a safety feature.

Standard programming capabilities

Rate. *Rate* is expressed as the volume of fluid that infuses over a unit of time. For example a 1000-ml volume infusing over 6 hours will be infused at a rate of 2.7 ml/min or 166 ml/hr. With very rare exceptions, infusion pumps deliver in increments of milliliters per hour. Therapy-specific pumps, such as those used to administer anesthesia, can be programmed in milligrams per hour.

For regular infusion pumps, the increment of measure is 1.0 ml, and the most common rate settings are from 1.0 to 999.0 ml/hr. For microinfusion pumps, the increment of measure is 0.1 ml, and the settings range from 0.1 to 99.9 ml/hr.

These numbers represent generalities, and some pumps offer a variation or a combination of these settings.

Many newer pumps are capable of setting rates that satisfy both regular infusion and microinfusion needs. These pumps usually allow volume to be set in 0.1-ml increments up to 99.9 ml, and then in 1-ml increments up to 999.0 ml. Many users are excited to have this option because it eliminates the need for having both a pediatric and an adult pump on hand. The simplification of infusion sets and distribution of pumps are two reasons this combination pump option is widely accepted.

A word of caution, however. The decision to use a combination pump should be weighed heavily against the possible dangers associated with its use. If the pump cannot be programmed to limit the rate in certain situations, the potential for error exists. The danger exists in a health care setting that does not have a designated number of pumps with preset rate limits for use in pediatric applications. When pumps are used for both adults and children, a nurse may program a pump for a child without noticing that the decimal is in the wrong place, thereby setting a rate of 440 ml/hr instead of 44.0 ml/hr.

Better-quality pumps that offer combination rates do not allow the rate to be set above 99.9 without a deliberate act to enter the adult values. Some pumps must be set into one mode or the other which prevent programming until the adult/child designation has been made. Another safety feature prevents the volume to be infused from being programmed above 99.9 ml when the rate includes a decimal.

Volume to be infused. The volume to be infused is usually the amount of infusate hanging in the fluid container. However, it could be a lesser amount if only part of the fluid is to be administered. The pump is designed to sound an alarm when the volume to be infused is reached according to the volume measured by the pump.

Like the rate, the volume to be infused on a regular adult pump is usually between 1.0 and 999.0 ml, measured in 1-ml increments. In a microinfusion pump, the volume to be infused is between 0.1 and 99.9 ml and measured in 0.1-ml increments.

As stated earlier, the potential for error is present with combination pumps that can be regular or microinfusion devices unless the pump has built-in safeguards. These safeguards include a deliberate action to limit the threshold to 99.9 ml.

As stated earlier, unless the pump has built-in safeguards, combination pumps that serve as both regular and microinfusion devices create a potential for error. One safeguard that works well is the inability to set the volume threshold above 99.9 ml without deliberate action confirming the user's intent.

Volume infused. The volume infused is a common measurement provided by the infusion pump, not a programmable capability. This measurement is the amount the pump has supposedly delivered since it was last set to zero. By setting the counter to zero at the start of an infusion, the nurse can determine how much fluid has been infused. By setting the counter to zero at the beginning of each shift, the nurse can determine how much fluid has been infused during the shift. This counter can be extremely valuable to a home health nurse who can only occasionally monitor the infusion during the day or over several days. The volume infused measurement is a standard feature on most devices.

Optional programming capabilities

Tapering or ramping. *Tapering* and *ramping* are terms used to describe the progressive increase or decrease of the infusion rate. Some infusates, specifically those with high dextrose concentrations, such as total parenteral nutrition, are tapered when they are cycled, discontinued, or initiated. Once the pump is programmed to the patient's needs, it begins infusing at a low rate, usually one quarter to one third of the final rate. Then, at 1- or 2-hour intervals, the rate increases to half, then to three quarters of the final rate, until the full rate is achieved. The hourly increment is individualized, as is the rate increase. Many patients accustomed to the cycle of total parenteral nutrition may taper or ramp in a one- or two-step process over 1 to 2 hours. Tapering is also used in reverse for a patient coming off of total parenteral nutrition. Again, patients accustomed to the process can taper or ramp down more quickly.

Tapering and ramping are not new ideas, and pumps that will do this automatically are gaining popularity. The pump can use its own program to mathematically calculate the ramping rate once the duration of infusion and total volume to be infused is given. These preprogrammed ramping schedules are satisfactory for most applications. The pumps are also able to accommodate individualized schedules.

Timed infusion. *Timed infusion* refers to an infusion governed by a 24-hour clock within the device. With timed infusion, the device must have a sufficient internal back-up battery to maintain the clock accurately at all times. Timed infusions are used for ramping and tapering, automatic piggybacking, and intermittent dosing. Timed-infusion features can greatly simplify many infusion regimens both inside and outside the hospital. A smaller ambulatory pump with this feature must be checked frequently to ensure that the internal power source is sufficient to maintain the accuracy of the internal clock.

Other infusion device considerations

Miscellaneous enhancements. Although the following enhancements are described as miscellaneous, they are part of the total infusion device package. If the infusion device has most of the previously mentioned characteristics, the enhancements described in this section complete the potential of the device. By purchasing infusion devices with these enhancements, hospitals and home care agencies ensure the devices are completely suited to their intended use.

Preprogrammed drug compatibility. The preprogrammed drug compatibility feature provides compatibility information on the display screen. When an infusion is initiated, drug dosing and the prescribed concentration are programmed into the device. The pump is then able to alert the user to compatibility problems.

Retrievable historical data. The retrievable historical data feature is available on the display screen of pain-control pumps, chemotherapy pumps, and other common devices. Upon request, the device displays how much fluid has infused in a given period (even over days); gives a record of rate changes; and tallies patient requests for pain medications, intermittent doses delivered, and alarm situations sensed by the pump.

Infiltration or thrombus detection. The infiltration or thrombus detection feature, which accurately detects the needed infusion pressure, is a technical sophistication of variable occlusion pressure capability. The pump displays the infusion pressure on the display screen. When monitoring the pressure, the user is alerted to the increased likelihood of infiltration or inflammation as pressure increases incrementally over time. An increase in pressure alone is not an indication to remove a catheter from the current site. However, the pressure-monitoring capability combined with careful observation can play a part in early detection of problems.

Central venous pressure monitor. The central venous pressure monitor is a sideline enhancement of positive-pressure devices that are able to accurately measure vascular flow resistance. In the same manner that infiltration is detected in the previous description, infusion pumps attached to central catheters measure central venous pressure. The internal pump sensor, which monitors for occlusion, does not differentiate between kinked tubing below the pump and vascular resistance. Ideally, the pressure detected by an uncompromised infusion system is the central venous pressure. The value of this enhancement should be carefully weighed to determine whether care interventions would be initiated based on the readings of the infusion pump.

Positive-pressure fill stroke. The positive-pressure fill stroke feature is important in applications in which no tolerance exists for the intermittent loss of positive pressure or for intermittent negative pressure. This feature is very important in arterial pumping, neonatal infusion, or infusion of sensitively maintained, titrated medications. The fill stroke occurs when the pump momentum is temporarily interrupted while the pump reservoir refills. If, during the refill phase, the pressure in the infusion line is reduced or allowed to "backstroke" even a fraction of a milliliter, blood is drawn into the catheter. If the line is a tiny catheter threaded into an umbilical vessel, the catheter and the infusion are compromised. If the fill stroke stops the consistent forward pressure of medication, blood pressure may fluctuate, cardiac indicators may vary, and hemodynamic status may be compromised.

Modular self-diagnosing capabilities. The self-diagnosing feature has made infusion pumps much easier to maintain and repair. It allows the clinical engineering department to perform certain tests on the infusion device to isolate and communicate mechanical or potential infusion problems. The mechanisms within the device are modular, allowing repairs to a specific compartment without affecting the remaining parts. Personnel from bioengineering departments perform repairs quickly and return devices to service readily. In addition, pumps can be upgraded or enhanced by replacing a specific part. With technology changing so rapidly, infusion pumps are able to keep pace with changing needs.

Printer read-out. The ability to get a printer read-out of pump activity is available from several manufacturers. The printer may be centrally located and electrically connected to the infusion device, or the printer can be moved from pump to pump with information being passed to the printer, much like information is downloaded into a computer. Some pumps have their own printers, which print on self-contained paper much like the narrow strips generated by a cash register.

The printer is able to print all of the pump's activity over a certain time frame. In the case of PCA, this activity might include milligrams and milliliters infused, patient requests, and infusion limits programmed into the pump. Other pumps print out drugs infused, total volumes, alarms experienced, and interruptions in use.

Nurse call systems. Infusion devices are being attached to nurse call systems. With these systems, the patient's bedside call light can be activated if the pump sounds an alarm, or the signal can be relayed to a central pump diagnostic station. The pump diagnosis screen may be at the nurses' station, where the nurse can problem solve without going to the bedside. The screen at the nurses' station is scored, giving each bedside pump a portion of the screen. The section that lights up corresponds to a specific bedside and a specific device. The screen also indicates the type of alarm sounding.

Remote site programming. Remote programming is accomplished by using computer technology, which allows communication with the pump by telephone modem. The pump can literally be hundreds of miles from the base unit or can be down the hall. The base unit may be at the pharmacy or home health agency. The pump's activities can be monitored from the base unit, making it possible for the caregiver to monitor the pump without being present. The base unit has the ability to change the pump's infusion settings once an assessment has been made. This development has proven to be cost-effective and efficient. The goal is to monitor the infusion more frequently and more accurately. This capability does not circumvent nursing assessment, but rather supports it.

Syringe use for secondary infusion. Syringe use for secondary infusion is becoming a practical alternative to small-volume piggybacks or tedious IV push medications. The syringe is attached directly to the pump administration set and is vented, allowing the solution to flow from the syringe without requiring pressure to be exerted on the syringe piston.

This option is available with the primary fluid in the syringe or with the syringe attached to the primary set as a secondary infusion container. Both options offer considerable cost savings if they eliminate the need for syringe pumps in addition to regular pumps. The largest cost savings are realized by using inexpensive syringes in place of more expensive, small-volume plastic bags.

Adjustable occlusion pressures. Another feature allows the user to program the pump at the bedside to sound an alarm at high or low occlusion pressures. Most nurses use this feature as a convenience because its clinical potential is not fully appreciated. Adjusting the pressure upward and silencing a persistent occlusion alarm that needs attention can compromise patient safety.

The real value of being able to adjust occlusion pressure is to ensure patient safety during infusion. The oncology nurse may want to use very low occlusion pressures to prevent vesicant extravasations associated with peripheral chemotherapy. The pediatric nurse may want to use a very low pressure to prevent an infiltration while infusing through a scalp vein but may choose a higher occlusion pressure for a central line infusion on an active, inconsolable 2-year-old. Critical care nurses may use high infusion pressures to administer sensitive medications through a central catheter, but they use lower pressures to infuse the same medications at the same rate through a peripheral site.

Opaque infusions. Opaque infusions have not always been easily administered through pumps because of their opaque nature. Pumps that rely on certain air-in-line detectors are unable to infuse opaque fluids. Opaque infusates are blood, fat emulsions, and some heavily darkened solutions such as iron dextran. The air-in-line detectors were bypassed in these cases in the past, which was an unsafe practice.

Newer pumps easily accommodate opaque fluids. The technology of air detection has moved from optic sensors, which are unable to distinguish between infusates of various clarity, to ultrasonography. Because ultrasound does not rely on clarity of fluids, accurate administration of opaque infusates is accomplished.

Secondary rate settings. Secondary rate settings are achieved in the same manner as secondary infusions by gravity administration. The secondary container is hung at a higher level than is the primary infusion, so the secondary automatically infuses first. The pump settings are designed to program two separate rates and two separate volumes. After the secondary volume is reached, the pump switches to the primary rate and resumes counting the primary volume. The pump is unable to tell which fluid is infusing because it counts volume infused only. Fluid containers must be hung at the correct height to ensure that the pump infuses correctly.

Bar coding. Amazing new microtechnology has made it possible for the pharmacist to generate the prescription for infusion into a bar code label. An appropriately equipped infusion device reads the bar code using an attached scanner and programs the pump at the ordered rate. The nurse can check the settings for accuracy by reviewing the display screen. This technology has significantly reduced human error. The pump can be changed immediately to override the system if unplanned interventions become necessary. This device is ideal in home infusion practice because it eliminates any accidental program changes or tampering.

Types

Ambulatory infusion pumps. Ambulatory infusion pumps are small enough to be easily carried, allowing the patient full ambulation. They were developed with the patient's home in mind. Ambulatory devices allow the patient the freedom to return to work, to school, or to a more normal life pattern. Ambulatory devices are capable of delivering most infusion therapies delivered by larger pumps, including critical care drugs and blood products.

Ambulatory devices range in size and weight; some are small enough to fit into the palm of the hand, whereas others are large enough to necessitate a backpack. Most of these pumps weigh less than 6 pounds. The fluid container is often more cumbersome than the actual pump. Ambulatory pumps have pump-specific tubing made to accommodate only the therapies for which each device is designed. Reducing the number of programming options is one factor that enables the manufacturer to miniaturize the pump.

Ambulatory pumps have the advantage of being small, but they have limitations that prevent the small size from being incorporated into the hospital setting. The main inhibiting factor is the power supply. Ambulatory pumps use a battery system that necessitates frequent recharging and battery replacement. The lack of a significant power source built into the pump may limit the in-hospital use of these pumps. Most hospital uses are so rigorous that the ambulatory pump's battery is quickly depleted. Ambulatory devices usually infuse at lower rates or intermittently, requiring significantly less power. Hospitals using battery-powered infusion pumps report significant battery replacement costs.

Ambulatory pumps have many features that have improved the quality of life for persons who require infusions outside the hospital. Because one pump cannot perform all of the infusion therapies, pumps have been designed to address a wide range of therapies. Currently, a pump exists that can be synchronized with the patient's biorhythms, giving medications when needed instead of on a schedule. Another pump is able to deliver several different dose sizes at several different intervals to replicate the secretion of hormones. Several medications may be given sequentially by an internal clock, freeing the patient or caregiver from all interventions except reloading of the device. These pumps retain memory of programs, use informational display screens, and have safety alarms that alert the user of potential problems.

Patient-controlled analgesia pumps.
The concept of PCA is not new, but the technology to provide this type of pain control is advancing rapidly. PCA pumps are available as ambulatory, semiportable, or full-sized devices. The smallest pumps use microprocessors to achieve miniaturization. The pumps can be programmed in milliliters or milligrams. The programming options are somewhat standardized, although accessory features vary with each pump.

The PCA pumps most widely used are volumetric and syringe-type. Volumetric pumps move the medication through the pump by a fill-and-empty cycle of very small increments. The syringe pump forces down on the syringe piston, administering the syringe volume at a preset rate.

The distinguishing feature of a PCA device is the ability of the pump to deliver doses on demand, which occurs when the patient or caregiver pushes a button on a cord similar to a nurse call light. The pump responds by delivering or denying the dose, recording the request, and perhaps making a small sound to assure the patient that the request was received. Whether the dose is delivered is determined by preset limits set on the pump.

Infusion options of a PCA pump can be categorized into three types: basal, continuous, and demand. All three afford some type of pain control with varying degrees of patient interaction. The nurse and physician must understand the terminology of the therapy offered so that PCA pumps can be used to the maximum potential.

The continuous mode of therapy is designed for the patient who needs maximum pain relief without the option of demand dosing. Continuous pain infusions usually do not fluctuate from hour to hour and should completely relieve pain or achieve a constant affect. This mode is used for epidural narcotic infusions, neonatal infusions, pain-control administration to persons unable to use the demand feature, or any application requiring a constant rate.

The basal mode differs from the continuous mode in that a basal rate can be accompanied by intermittent doses requested by the patient. The basal dose is designed to achieve pain relief with minimal medication, but not necessarily to achieve a pain-free state, allowing the patient to be alert and active without sedation.

The demand dose is delivered by intermittent infusion when a button attached to the pump is pushed. The demand dose can be used alone or supplemented by the basal rate. Demand doses are limited by a physician-designated maximum amount. Demand doses are prescribed with the amount per dose, the interval between doses, and the total hourly limit of medication.

The PCA pump must be programmed with a lock-out interval to prevent overmedication. A lock-out interval on a PCA device ensures that over a set period the patient can receive only a prescribed dose of medication.

PCA pumps are also capable of dispensing a bolus dose. Practitioners sometimes call the initial bolus dose a *loading dose.* After an initial bolus dose or after a short lapse in medication, the patient may benefit from a one-time dose of medication that is significantly higher than a demand dose to achieve immediate pain relief. After the bolus dose is delivered, the basal or demand doses provide the sustained effect of pain control. The bolus dose is not calculated into the hourly limit of medication and cannot be accidentally delivered.

PCA devices may offer a lock-out feature designed for patient safety. Lock out differs from tamper resistance in that tamper-proof pumps require the nurse to repeat a series of simple steps known to any user to change pump settings. *Lock out* means that a key or a combination of numbers must be used to gain access to the pump controls. Because PCA pumps normally house a container of narcotic medication, the lock-out capability prevents tampering with the narcotic and the pump settings. In the hospital setting, the PCA device is commonly locked to the IV pole for added security. Narcotic accountability is more defined with the PCA device because the drug is in one reservoir, and all deliveries are automated and recorded on the pump memory.

PCA pumps are built with extensive memory capability, which includes the pump programming, any interventions by the patient or the nurse, and the times of the interventions. The memory is critical for the pump's effective use in pain management. The frequency of patient requests, the tolerated time intervals, and the numbers of bolus injections are a few of the assessments needed to monitor pain tolerance or change in pain intensity. The programming and memory can be viewed on a display screen.

Ambulatory PCA pumps may have the same limitations of use as regular ambulatory devices. They are not built to withstand the rigors of hospital environments unless a small specialty group uses them. The number of different staff, patient transfers, pump distribution factors, pump accountability, and potential interactions make ambulatory PCA devices more prone to breakdown and malfunction in a hospital environment.

Multichannel and dual-channel pumps.
The changing hospital environment dictates infusion pump needs,

and rising acuity has resulted in the development of multichannel and dual-channel infusion pumps. These pumps may consist of two devices with an attached housing or of several infusion channels within a single device. The best effect is achieved when multiple infusion channels can be regulated independently of each other in a device that stays within the size and shape configurations of a single pump. Depending on the design, this goal can be achieved with two or more incoming solution lines, each regulated independently and leaving the pump in a single infusing line to the patient. Another design allows each incoming independent line to remain independent.

Many dual-channel and multichannel pumps are available. Some require little adaptation because they appear to be two single-channel devices fused side by side. Others have two pump mechanisms with common control and programming panels. These types of dual-channel pumps use one administration set for each channel, and if one channel is idle, no tubing is used. Multichannel pumps requiring manifold-type sets that provide all channels, whether used or not, save significant dollars if all the channels are in use. If one or more channels are idle, the sets are no longer cost-effective. Each channel must be programmed independently, or the pump is not really dual channel or multichannel.

Intermittent, automatic IV piggyback capability does not fit the description of dual channel unless the IV piggyback is regulated by an internal clock that turns the infusion off and on following a schedule. This feature makes a dual-channel pump invaluable. If the IV piggyback feature is based on head height to deliver a single dose, it does not have dual-channel capability.

Multichannel pumps have three or four channels. Programming a multichannel pump can be complex, and the potential for confusion rises sharply. The need for a three- or four-channel pump should be clearly defined before this complex technology is routinely used. These pumps offer an exciting capacity for infusion, but they are not routinely used in general care.

Cost considerations in infusion pump technology

The continued theme of defining the patient's need applies to infusion pump technology more than to any other type of IV equipment. If the need is a consistent low-acuity patient situation and the pump is a convenience item, a great investment in the latest technology will probably never pay off. On the other hand, older technology with few capabilities may create a significant risk to certain patient populations. The acuity and technology needs are by no means confined to the hospital setting.

Responsible care involves assessing and delivering affordable care. Infusion devices too sophisticated for the intended purpose confuse and complicate care unnecessarily. A safe rule of thumb is to use the least difficult equipment and the least amount of supplies necessary to safely and effectively provide the care needed.

The financial investment in infusion devices is significant. Infusion devices are expensive, and the disposable tubing costs far outweigh the price of the devices in just a few months. The

entire picture should be analyzed, including any changes that will be made when a new system is implemented. These costs should be calculated over the entire length of a contract because costs are often inflated during the start-up period.

Institutions can use one of several financial options when considering reusable equipment such as infusion pumps. When equipment is rented, the title to the property stays with the original owner (the agency from which the institution is getting the equipment). In a rental agreement, the upkeep and repair are the responsibility of the owner. There is also more flexibility in obtaining additional devices or upgrading to newer technology with the same device. Rental agreements usually cover disposable supplies as well.

Leasing equipment is similar to renting. In a lease, it is possible to own the devices at the end of the agreement or to terminate the lease with intent to buy. In many lease agreements, repair and upkeep are the responsibility of the user institution, and disposable supplies are part of the agreement. Lease options are almost unlimited. In a lease agreement, the receiving institution has temporary ownership.

Purchase options result in transfer of ownership, equipment warrantees, repair contracts, and institutional upkeep. The cost of disposable supplies is usually less when purchasing the pumps, which sometimes results in the total cost over several years being much less than with rent or lease agreements. The manufacturer has made the profit initially, theoretically making the long-term investment less costly to the buyer. Technology bought with a purchase agreement is static unless the purchase contract stipulates periodic updating of equipment.

Infusion pumps in various settings

Acute care. The acute care setting can be a traditional hospital setting, a short-term treatment center, or a surgery center. The diversity of need is great in the hospital, requiring infusion devices to withstand the rigors of the environment. The number of different users that come in contact with a pump in a hospital include the nurse, the physician, and the persons involved in transporting, cleaning, and storing the device.

Infusion devices in a hospital must meet the infusion requirements of the patient moving through the system, from the intensive care unit, to surgery, to general care. The device must be user friendly, allowing the constantly changing staff and multiple disciplines to work with it easily.

Infusion devices that have specific functions may not be cost-effective for hospitals. Tubing and additional accessory items, education, biomedical engineering related to parts and service, and many other related costs make lack of equipment standardization expensive. Potential user error is a nonquantifiable cost that could outweigh all other considerations.

Alternative care. Alternative care settings represent many different types of health care. Active treatment is offered in many settings once reserved for diagnosis or long-term care. Chemotherapy, blood products, and antibiotics are now commonly given in long-term care facilities, physician's clinics, or outpatient treatment centers. These therapies are given safely when adequate medical support is present and the equipment selected is intended for such a setting. An infusion-specific pump is most likely to have programming features that prompt the user to input information necessary to infuse a specific treatment correctly.

Home care. The fastest growing environment for the delivery of health care is the home. Specialized treatment regimens and equipment variations needed to serve patients receiving home health care has generated an evolution in the infusion equipment market.

Equipment used at home must offer the best safety features because the caregiver in most situations is the patient. Priming, setup, and troubleshooting should be easy, uncomplicated, and directed by the pump. Certain settings of particular treatments may even be locked out, with the patient able to only start and stop the infusion. Such strategies are popular in pain control or ramping of parenteral nutrition.

Home care infusion devices are designed to allow the patient maximum portability and freedom with minimum interference and inconvenience. Small, quiet, lightweight infusion pumps, with pouches to enclose the infusion container, are available for almost all therapies.

As with alternative care settings, the use of infusion pumps in home care is often challenged. Knowing the patient's reimbursement status simplifies selection of the appropriate infusion device. If an infusion device is necessary for safe administration of IV medications or fluids in the home, lack of payment should not prevent the use of the equipment. The physician and the payer should collaborate with the health care provider to ensure the safe treatment of the patient in the home.

REFERENCES

1. Kaplan LK: Vinyl debate heats up, *Infusion (Newsline)* 5(8):6, 10, 1999.
2. Trissel LA: *Handbook on injectable drugs,* ed 11, Bethesda, Md, 2000, American Society of Health-System Pharmacists.
3. Coles D, Fanning J: Accuracy of Viaflex container graduation marks, *NITA* 14:422, 1987.
4. Intravenous Nurses Society: Infusion nursing standards of practice, *JIN* (suppl) 23(6S), 2000.
5. Kaplan LK: Filtration: an overview, *Infusion* 3(1):29, 1996.
6. Menitore J, editor: *Standards for blood banks and transfusion services,* ed 19, Bethesda, Md, 1999, American Association of Blood Banks.
7. Maki DG: Infections due to infusion therapy. In Bennett JV, Brachman PS, editors: *Hospital infections,* ed 4, Philadelphia, 1998, Lippincott-Raven.
8. Maki DG, et al: Prevention of central venous catheter-related bloodstream infection by use of an antiseptic-impregnated catheter, *Ann Intern Med* 128(4):257, 1997.
9. Smith JP: Thrombotic complications in intravenous access, *JIN* 21(2):96, 1998.
10. West VL: Alternative routes of administration, *JIN* 21(4):221, 1998.

Intravenous Therapy Equipment: Preparation, Maintenance, and Problem Solving

Krisha S. Scharnweber, BSN, CRNI*

Intravenous (IV) therapy devices and equipment are well represented in the medical marketplace. They can be classified into three types: durable medical goods, reusable products, and disposable products. The aspects of product care vary greatly between the three types. This chapter deals with product preparation before use, handling of products after use, and care and maintenance required between uses.

Durable medical goods are defined as equipment that is used for long periods, is cleaned between uses, and may be considered property or capital equipment. Examples of durable medical equipment are IV poles, infusion pumps, wheelchairs, and walkers.

Reusable products are those that are used for limited periods and are cleaned and disinfected between use. A reusable item must be specifically designated as reusable. Few items are reused in IV therapy because IV devices are usually sterile, one-time-use products.

Disposable products can be used only once. They are discarded after being used one time with a single patient. Most IV products are disposable, including solution containers, administration sets, IV catheters, and dressing supplies.

This chapter underscores the need for users to be aware of all aspects of devices and products used to administer IV treatments. The caregiver's duty to protect patients from harm resulting from misused or malfunctioning equipment has many ramifications. Equipment must be checked for electrical hazards and mechanical malfunctions, and any equipment known to be malfunctioning must be removed from use until it is repaired. Equipment must be used according to manufacturer specifications, and only for the purposes intended. All personnel operating equipment must be properly trained in its safe and effective use. The care provider must also protect patients from infectious hazards resulting from inadequately cleaned equipment, reuse of disposable products, or procedures performed with poor aseptic technique.

The safety of the nurse and other caregivers is of great importance in the development, use, and maintenance of infusion products and equipment. For decades, top priorities for manufacturers have included the protection of patients and health care workers and ease of use. The addition of finger guards to administration sets at the top of the drip chamber to make spiking containers easier and safer is an example of a small change that represents the safety consciousness of the industry.

Employee protection is the responsibility of the health care facility and each worker. This does not mean that the facility has to purchase every device that enhances safety; it does mean that product purchases must be made with patient and employee safety in mind. Employees and patients have the right to be protected from electrical hazards by proper grounding of electronic devices and by routine safety checks. Mechanical hazards can be avoided by proper inspection of equipment and thorough, up-to-date education regarding the use and upkeep of equipment. For any device brought into an institution, in-service training should be held for the users and for those responsible for the upkeep and maintenance of the equipment.

Prevention of chemical hazards requires that employees be well informed regarding the use and risks associated with haz-

*The author and editors wish to acknowledge the contributions made by Brenda L. Jensen and Dawn G. Frederick, as coauthors of this chapter in the first edition of *Intravenous Nursing: Clinical Principles and Practice*.

ardous chemicals. Proper disposal receptacles for hazardous wastes must be provided, and employees must have access to the accessory supplies needed to use hazardous materials properly, such as gloves, gowns/aprons, and protective eye wear.

IV therapy has always posed a high level of infectious risk to nurses, but protecting against infectious hazards has a new urgency since the rapid spread of human immunodeficiency virus and associated diseases. However, a thorough understanding of the risk factors and the products and procedures used can reduce the risk. Infectious risks can be minimized further with the introduction of devices developed specifically for infusion safety, but education plays a far greater role.

Protecting employees in the workplace starts with education. Education begins with a thorough employee orientation and continues with new product in-services and continuous education. Employees should be provided with written information regarding equipment instructions, procedures, and handling of nonroutine or emergency situations. In-service instruction should be provided when new equipment is introduced, and periodically thereafter as long as it remains in use. Attendance at educational programs or completion of competencies should be validated in the employee record.

The intended outcome of these extensive efforts is the safe use of medical devices and equipment and, ultimately, the protection of the public. Prevention of infectious risk to employees and the patients is a constant and deliberate focus.

PREPARING EQUIPMENT FOR USE
Ensuring sterility and fitness for use

The nurse is responsible for confirming that equipment is cleaned and checked for safety before it is used. Although others perform these functions, the nurse must ensure the usability of equipment. All infusion equipment must be inspected for product integrity before, during, and after use. If the product's integrity is compromised, that product is not to be used. If inspection reveals any defects during or after use, appropriate intervention is initiated and the defective product retained and reported.[1]

Materials management and sterile processing departments are responsible for the flow of equipment and supplies from the manufacturer to the user. These two departments share the tasks of ensuring product supply and confirming that products and equipment arrive ready for use at the patient care area. Ensuring usability in the home setting is the responsibility of the health care provider, regardless of who delivers the products.

Other departments, such as biomedical engineering and infection control, have a continuing role in product monitoring and testing. The infection control department usually gets involved in monitoring products after an adverse situation has been identified (e.g., contaminated antimicrobial prep solution). The biomedical engineering department is directed to maintain a log of electrical safety checks for all equipment and to confirm usability and the accuracy of calibrations at regular intervals, as determined by hospital policy or the manufacturer's recommendation. Any devices with a history of problems are evaluated more frequently.

The increased use of home infusion therapy, with its complexity and inherent risks, make at-home use of infusion pumps an area of expanding public health importance.[2] Equipment rental companies may validate safety and performance, and infection control resources may be regional rather than office specific.

Ensuring proper use of equipment

Before products are purchased, their intended use should be clearly defined. Products cannot be used for purposes other than that specified by the manufacturer. Manufacturers are not liable for problems resulting from misuse of their products. The U.S. Food and Drug Administration (FDA) warns against misuse of products and approves only those products whose documentation clearly states the intended purpose, complete with support studies and data.

Proper product use requires education of all users. This education should occur when the product is introduced and as often as necessary during sustained use of the product to ensure continued safe practice. Validation of education is mandated by the Joint Commission on Accreditation of Healthcare Organizations (JCAHO). This validation should appear in the employee record or a central education database. Employees responsible for safe product handling and cleaning also require education.

Quality improvement criteria should be developed to measure progress toward meeting equipment education goals. Quality improvement requires intense planning and effort and is meant to be an ongoing initiative.[3] The criteria may include educational in-service attendance on device use and care or time spent viewing an educational program about the product. They may involve spontaneous checks for procedural compliance during use of the product. Variance reports or problem-reporting mechanisms also demonstrate educational need.

Every institution should implement and maintain a device education model. A model will define a series of progressive steps necessary to successfully educate personnel who will use the devices. The model should address the most basic understanding of a device function. The model then becomes a checklist that can be used to evaluate devices before they are purchased.

Ensuring proper cost allocation and reimbursement

Being accountable for product use means being mindful of costs and reimbursement. Without payment, the health care system is unable to function. To safeguard the financial integrity of the institution, health care providers are held accountable for the items being charged, and reimbursement is being scrutinized as never before.

Nurses involved in product selection and education are also responsible for ensuring that users understand how to appropriately charge for materials and for confirming patient use of durable equipment. Moving equipment from one patient to another without using an accountability system may put the patient at risk. Tracking and accountability are instrumental in ensuring not only that equipment is appropriately charged, but also that it is cleaned and, if necessary, that a safety check is performed between uses.

Correct charging for products and equipment facilitates the reimbursement process. Meticulous care in charging eliminates suspect charges, which further delay reimbursement. Product cost and charging are seldom included as a part of nursing curriculum; however, it is part of the whole picture that sustains the financial cycle. When products and equipment are introduced into any health care setting, correct patient charging should be taught and validated.

CONTROL OF EQUIPMENT

Storage

Medical equipment can be seriously affected by temperature extremes or damaged from excessive dryness or humidity. Although these factors are difficult to control in a warehouse, they are important to consider. Generally, disposable products are able to tolerate environmental fluctuations, but they should never be exposed to moisture or allowed to freeze. If stored in areas that are subject to extreme temperature changes, mechanical equipment should be flagged to alert the biomedical engineering department to possible function variations.

Electronic equipment stored away from nursing care areas should be plugged into continuous electric current to prevent depletion of internal batteries, especially under very cold storage situations. Equipment powered only by batteries can be rendered useless by cold, leaving them unusable until returned to room temperature. Equipment powered by commercial, 9-volt, or "AA" batteries should be stored without the batteries in place, because batteries corrode and can leak into the internal mechanisms of equipment.

Cleanliness is critical for storage of medical products. The storage area should be free of dust, lint, rodents, and insects. Mechanical equipment should be covered and protected, and products should be stored to prevent damage from stacking or crowding.

Equipment and supplies that are stored off site, requiring movement and transport, are especially vulnerable to damage. Persons responsible for moving equipment should be educated about the nature of the products entrusted to their care as well as the hazards of damage. If equipment must be transported to the patient care area, proper function and safety should be verified on delivery. In home health care, the verification may be performed by the nurse or by a driver trained in equipment set-up.

Allocation

Allocation of equipment should be delegated to a central resource. In most cases, allocation is a materials management or distribution function that is largely taken for granted. In hospitals, where equipment is kept in the nursing areas and moved from patient to patient as needed, critical elements for equipment upkeep and accountability, such as knowing the equipment's location and how it is being used, are often unattended.

Centralized management of equipment is often a specialized function of the materials management department, as is charging a daily fee for equipment use. Ideally, it is not the function of the professional nurse. This process is best performed by persons dedicated to the goal of equipment accountability. Just as nurses' knowledge and skills are advancing, so too are the job requirements of biomedical technicians, as the medical equipment of today becomes the "front end" of tomorrow's medical information and processing systems.[4]

There must be physical accountability of equipment at all times, even if the equipment is not returned to a central pool at the end of each use. Tracking equipment is an important record-keeping obligation. If a recall were to occur, a system must be in place to locate the equipment. Logs must be kept to keep track of safety and calibration checks and to validate that equipment is cleaned between uses. Any equipment leaving the system must be fully checked by the biomedical engineering department before it is returned to use. Any interruption in accountability necessitates that the equipment's function and safety be confirmed.

On discontinuation of therapy, the nurse is responsible for notifying the central equipment pool or, in the case of home health care, the billing office. This action ensures that the patient is not charged needlessly and that the equipment can be retrieved, cleaned, and reallocated as soon as it is needed. The nurse must ensure that the persons responsible for cleaning the equipment are aware of its availability.

Disinfection of durable medical equipment

Sterilization and *disinfection* are not synonymous. *Disinfection* describes a process that eliminates all microorganisms except bacterial spores from an inanimate object. *Sterilization* is the complete elimination or destruction of all forms of microbial life.[5]

Items intended for use in a sterile procedure must be sterilized. Mechanical equipment is not sterilized because it cannot be subjected to a sterilization process to remove all microorganisms. Devices or objects that are in constant use or are considered reusable parts of a system are also unable to be sterilized. Items such as IV poles, electric cords, sinks, floors, and walls cannot be sterilized. Items that can be sterilized include drapes, certain instruments, implanted products, catheters, and needles.

Products coming from the manufacturer in sterile packaging do not need to be sterilized before use. In IV therapy, sterilization is used for reusable items. Because most IV products are provided in sterile packages for immediate use, there are few reusable items that require sterilization.

Methods used to sterilize products are not legislated or directed by any single source or authority. Processes most used in health care settings are determined by the written policy of each institution and manufacturer's recommendations. Sterilization chemicals are registered with the Environmental Protection Agency, which monitors the claims made by manufacturers but does not recommend products used for sterilization or disinfection.

The FDA, however, does make recommendations regarding the reuse and sterilization of products. They do not specifically direct the process by stating what method is most suitable for a specific product. Rather, the FDA suggests the best method of sterilizing types of material; the institution then decides which materials fit that category.

Recommendations made by the Centers for Disease Control and Prevention are also in the form of general guidelines; they do not deal with performance of specific products. JCAHO recommends that all sterilization and disinfection procedures should be written and that policies should be provided to govern all aspects of disinfection and sterilization.

A primary agent for sterilization is ethylene oxide, which is a gas that easily permeates all surfaces of items. This gas must be used with caution to prevent employee exposure during sterilization and aeration. Strict guidelines for the use of ethylene oxide sterilization are available from such organizations as the Association of periOperative Registered Nurses.

Another method of sterilization effective against pathogens is pressurized steam. It is important to fully educate employees in the process of steam sterilization. Equipment that is poorly maintained or improperly used will not sterilize properly and may injure the operator.

Disinfection is more applicable to IV therapy equipment than is sterilization. Disinfection requirements, which should be established by an institution's policies and procedures, are applicable to durable medical equipment, which includes IV poles, infusion pumps, teaching models, and nondisposable arm boards. The agent used to disinfect durable equipment should effectively prevent cross-contamination,[6,7] which is defined as the movement of pathogens from one source to another.

IV equipment is usually disinfected by being wiped down or immersed in a germicidal solution. Chemicals used for either of these processes should always be considered dangerous. Once a product is disinfected, it should be allowed to thoroughly dry, and fumes should be avoided. Manufacturers of some chemical disinfection products suggest that the product be aerated for a certain time before reusing.

Several chemicals are acceptable for use in disinfection. Alcohol, which is bactericidal rather than bacteriostatic, is also tuberculocidal, fungicidal, and virucidal, but it does not destroy spores. It is used extensively in hospitals, but never as a sterilizing agent. Chlorine is inexpensive, fast acting, and widely used, but it is associated with noxious vapors and corrosive properties. Chlorine compounds are difficult to control because they are relatively unstable and are easily inactivated by organic matter. Other acceptable products are formaldehyde, glutaraldehyde, iodophors, and phenolics.

Policies regarding the use of chemical disinfectants should include guidelines that protect employees from exposure and harm. Gloves should be worn to protect the hands. The work area should be adequately ventilated. The product being disinfected should be allowed to aerate and dry before it is reused, wrapped, or packaged. Although proper aeration is seemingly a minor point, nurses have reported ill effects from fumes emitted by disinfected products in closed areas, even from face masks removed from sterile packs.

Durable equipment should be disinfected between each patient use. This means that an infusion pump cannot be moved from one patient to another without validating that it has been thoroughly disinfected. In the absence of a centralized equipment pool, knowledgeable personnel on the nursing unit are responsible for such validation; the task should be assigned to a specific person to ensure its completion.

Disinfection should also be performed intermittently during patient use, weekly in the hospital or monthly in the home. The institution should set the precise interval, and this task should also be delegated to a specific department or person.

The responsibility for ensuring that equipment is disinfected rests with the professional nurse. Although the actual task can be assigned, the nurse should not use any durable medical product without confirming that the product does not represent a risk of infection. Items should be tagged or repackaged to clearly indicate fitness for use. Properly identifying sterile products is often not a high priority, but it is necessary to complete the disinfection process, which is a critical aspect of health care delivery.

BIOMEDICAL CONSIDERATIONS
Routine maintenance

No single authority exists to set standards for equipment validation by biomedical engineering departments. Guidelines are set by manufacturers for periodic checks of equipment function using standardized tests. JCAHO requires that periodic safety and function tests be performed on all electronic equipment. However, this requirement does not include checking for accuracy. Several other agencies give input into what constitutes acceptable levels of equipment monitoring by biomedical departments.

Institutional policy has priority over other guidelines and standards regarding equipment safety checks and the frequency with which they are performed. When new equipment is introduced to an institution, all aspects of its performance should be checked. After the initial inspection, further performance checks may not be necessary unless a situation arises that indicates a need for testing.

The biomedical department might perform diagnostic tests on any equipment that is considered to have been under undue stress as a result of prolonged use (e.g., an ambulatory pump that is used continuously for many months on the same patient).

The age and service history of a product should be considered when scheduling maintenance checks. Older devices may have impeccable service histories but should be watched with care because all devices have a predictable life span. However, many infusion pumps from past generations still infuse with the accuracy and reliability of new devices. Older equipment, or equipment that malfunctions often, should be logged and tracked to validate poor performance and extra expense resulting from repairs, supplies, and personnel time.

In the case of rented infusion equipment, some agencies prefer to monitor performance between each patient use. Because infusion equipment supplied for home care may be located far from the provider or support systems, equipment malfunction or failure is inconvenient, at best, and can be dangerous. To minimize these situations, care of equipment is a full-time effort that requires many more hours and tests than are mandated by regulatory agencies.

All tests and uses of equipment are clearly logged and kept as permanent records, as mandated by JCAHO; this regimen should also be a part of institutional policy. The maintenance of equipment is a focus of risk management in hospital and home care alike for the safety of the public, the institution, and the employee.

The nurse facilitates problem solving by clearly noting suspected and actual occurrences of malfunction, including questionable product performance. Without clear observation and communication, equipment malfunction may continue undetected. If equipment users and services do not work closely together, the assumptions each make about the other can lead to serious compromises in safety.[8]

When equipment is found to be functioning in error or is suspected of operating outside normal parameters, its use should be discontinued immediately. The exact problem should be documented, and a detailed description should be attached to the device. If the problem is poorly stated, it may not be found in routine examination. For example, if an infusion pump is not delivering at the prescribed rate, a nonspecific complaint of malfunction to the biomedical engineering department will result in diagnostic tests that do not include long-term infusion-accuracy tests. The scope of routine diagnostic procedures may have to be expanded to isolate a problem that has already been identified by the nurse but that was not clearly stated.

It is also helpful if the nurse can describe the situation that precipitated the problem. User errors can result from unfamiliarity with the operational controls of a device or from fundamental misconceptions about functions and capabilities. Knowing what precipitated the error can greatly facilitate its correction.

If user error is confirmed, it is the responsibility of the nurse and the institution to prevent further error from occurring. Corrective action can include product education to confirm that all users are knowledgeable in problem solving and in recognizing situations that might cause the problem to recur.

The nurse should keep records of product problems. Some institutions keep records in a centralized location, such as the IV therapy, biomedical engineering, purchasing, materials management, or nursing education departments. Isolated incidents rarely receive attention until a central party notices that the complaints and problems represent a trend. Problems with devices should always be considered for inclusion in the medical device reporting program discussed later in this chapter.

Recognition of malfunction

Statistically, the equipment provided for use in health care is very safe. No allowances are made for critical-error acceptability, and the health care industry has tried to design equipment that errs on the side of the patient. This means that if a certain aspect of performance malfunctions, it should decrease danger to the patient rather than increase it. For example, if a microinfusion device for pain medication fails, it should cease to infuse rather than overinfuse. The patient would experience discomfort and inconvenience but not oversedation or death.

By law, situations that cause permanent injury and death as a result of infusion devices must be reported to the FDA and the manufacturer. The exact cause need not be confirmed at the time of the incident, but the occurrence must be reported within 10 working days.[9]

Malfunction indicators are built into devices to protect the patient and caregiver. Alarms on infusion devices should never be circumvented. Some devices are still made that allow alarms to be silenced, a feature that invites certain hazards. All alarms have a specific purpose, and using equipment properly is the correct way to silence alarms.

Some device problems are not detected by alarms but are discovered by alert caregivers. At times, caregivers confirm that the equipment is functioning without double checking its performance. An example of this type of performance problem is an infusion device set to infuse at a given rate. The nurse monitors the patient, notes that the pump is infusing, reads the amount infused, and charts the data provided by the pump on the amount infused. Eventually, an observant nurse notices that the solution should have totally infused hours earlier if the pump had actually delivered the amount calculated. In this case, the device is not operating according to its programming, but no alarm has sounded. The infusion device must be used as an adjunct to providing safe care, not as a substitution for careful nursing. From legal, professional, and clinical perspectives, competency is vital to IV specialists, nurses, nursing staff, non-RN staff, and family members. It is paramount to patients who depend on the health care team to deliver the best care possible.[10]

Equipment malfunction should always be suspected in situations with negative outcomes. Complications, unexpected deterioration of the patient, or development of a patient crisis should always cue the caregiver to check the equipment. If a device or product is even remotely involved in a negative patient outcome, the device should be removed, not altered in any way, and taken to the biomedical engineering department; a full written report should be made. If the equipment appears to be functioning appropriately but cannot be ruled out as a potential problem, it should be removed as soon as safely possible and checked completely.

The nurse must never allow equipment to substitute for nursing judgment or assessment. If the equipment indicates that the patient is doing well but nursing assessment does not confirm it, the nurse's professional skills should supersede the equipment.[1] It is not necessary to calculate drop factors for infusion pumps, but monitoring the pump's performance is mandatory. If the patient is using a patient-controlled anesthesia device, is pain controlled? If not, is the device functioning? If the patient is somnolent, is the pump delivering medication as programmed? These questions should be answered before changing the infusion settings to attain improved patient response.

User-induced malfunctions fall into four categories. These problems are the most dangerous, most challenging to identify, and most difficult to correct. The first type of malfunction is created when the user bypasses a normal function of the device, such as the air-in-line alarm. New pumps make such bypassing more difficult, but if the feature is circumvented, the patient is subject to the uninhibited infusion of air. Another example is bypassing the patient lock-out feature on a patient-controlled anesthesia device because the nurse finds it cumbersome. This can result in tampering by the patient, family, or staff members and possible oversedation of the patient.

The second category of user-induced malfunctions is using disposables not approved for use with a specific device. This problem happens with application or implementation of dedicated and generic tubing. Infusion devices are tested in controlled situations, and accuracy data are based only on use with specific tubing. When tubing is adapted by the user to function in nonapproved situations, the result can be overinfusion or underinfusion.

Another problem in the second category is use of different brands of gravity tubing in pumps designed to use generic gravity administration sets. These pumps are calibrated for use with only one brand of gravity infusion set at a time. Alternating between brands causes great fluctuations in performance. Not all tubing is alike, internally or externally, and tubing cannot be used interchangeably without seriously affecting the performance of the device. This is also true of secondary tubing added to pump infusion sets. The infusion device manufacturer must approve of tubing used in conjunction with pump sets, or performance claims may be null and void. Manufacturers condone the mixing of sets if the device is capable of maintaining adequate performance with various sets. However, if the manufacturer is noncommittal, alternative sets should be avoided.

Ignorance or disregard of equipment operation is the third category of user-induced malfunction. All health care providers agree that proper use of equipment depends on understanding normal operation, yet some nurses assume that all equipment and related supplies operate alike. Some caregivers may not be properly educated in device operation. These caregivers are unfamiliar with the equipment, which may represent a potential problem. Competency-based learning programs can prevent many errors generated by ignorance.

The fourth category of user-induced problems is the misuse of equipment—using it for purposes other than those intended by the manufacturer. Health care journals are full of documented cases of death or injury resulting from unapproved equipment use. A dangerous example is the use of infusion pumps and administration sets with Y injection sites attached to epidural drips. The pump may be capable of performing the function correctly, but numerous safety violations are associated with this application. The infusion pump can easily be mistaken for an IV infusion, and the presence of the Y injection sites on the tubing increases the likelihood of accidental infusion.

All of these user-induced problems can be prevented with education, but they continue to plague health care. The health care industry as well as health care professionals must make a concerted effort to address these issues through quality improvement programs designed to identify and correct potential errors.

PRODUCT DEFECT REPORTING
Role of the federal government

Under the administrative jurisdiction of the U.S. Department of Health and Human Services, the FDA has monitored health care since 1938. In 1976, the Medical Devices Amendment was enacted to ensure that medical devices are safe and effective for their intended purpose. This is accomplished through the coordinating efforts of the *United States Pharmacopeia.* To advance the goal of product safety, the FDA Medical Products Reporting Program (MedWatch) was developed and put into action. This program is a national effort to encourage product reporting by all health care workers without fear of confrontation. The purpose of the reporting program is to objectively catalog problems in an effort to safeguard the public from inappropriate or hazardous medical devices.

The Safe Medical Devices Act of 1990 (P. L. 101-629) and its final ruling of 1996 mandate the reporting of serious injury, illness, or death related to the use of medical devices. Highlights of the final ruling include the statement that facilities using medical devices must submit a medical device report to the manufacturer within 10 working days after becoming aware of a reportable death or serious injury, or illness. If the event involves a device-related death or if the identity of the manufacturer is not known, the report must be sent to the FDA. Device users also must submit a semiannual summary of reports to the FDA.[11] The law defines the penalties for not reporting and actions to be taken by the FDA. The FDA notifies the manufacturer that a report has been filed and ensures follow-up by the manufacturer. If the follow-up is deemed inadequate by the FDA, further action is necessary. The FDA fully investigates all device-related deaths that are reported.

The role of the government with regard to medical devices appears to be one of collaboration. Medical manufacturers are allowed to study and report device issues to the FDA, many times without government intervention or FDA confirmation of test results. The approval process is considered rigorous.

Role of nongovernmental agencies

Another organization that monitors and independently tests medical devices and products is the Emergency Care Research Institute (ECRI), located in Plymouth Meeting, Pennsylvania. ECRI is a nonprofit, tax-exempt institute that has gained worldwide recognition for nonbiased evaluation and data collection regarding medical products. ECRI publishes volumes of material annually to help health care agencies develop cost-effective and practical approaches for the acquisition of technology. ECRI has an impeccable reputation for representing products in a fair and analytical manner; their endorsement is highly prized by medical manufacturers. ECRI provides many excellent publications to help medical professionals and patients evaluate and select medical products.

The Health Industry Manufacturers Association (HIMA), located in Washington, D.C., is also a powerful force in medical device monitoring. This association's members include the manufacturers of more than 90% of the health care devices on the market today. Addressing the common concerns of quality, education, marketing, and legislation, HIMA acts as a self-monitoring association to safeguard the public and ensure consistent quality. A major emphasis of this organization is educating the government about how impending legislation will affect health care.

Professional nursing organizations are also influential public safety advocates. Nursing organizations such as the Intravenous Nurses Society, the Association of periOperative Registered Nurses, and the Association for Professionals in Infection Control and Epidemiology strive to educate their members about the hazards or potential problems of medical devices. These organizations offer feedback to manufacturers to initiate needed changes.

Role of the nurse

Nurses can provide a high volume of input to product-defect recognition and reporting. The nursing profession is usually represented in all health care settings and is in a position to observe and document the proper functioning or malfunctioning of medical devices and products. However, problems with products may be identified, but not reported, by nurses.

By being informed about available equipment and technology, the nurse can be a credible source of information. Reading professional nursing journals is an important form of continuing education, especially in today's environment of ever-shrinking budgets for in-service education and staff development.[12] An informed nurse is able to understand new concepts and is quick to recognize potential problems. Nurses must take the initiative to be self-educated in this regard, learning how and why a product works instead of simply acknowledging its presence.

The FDA's MedWatch provides a way for nurses to report adverse events and product problems. Although anyone can use this program, it is specifically designed for ease of use by nurses or other health care professionals. Many nurses are reluctant to report product problems because they are not confident in their ability to recognize situations that are appropriate for reporting.

MedWatch encourages reporting of any device suspected of malfunctioning or of being undependable. Examples include catheters that break easily, tubing that consistently comes apart with tension, labels that do not include enough information or create confusion, packaging that causes problems when opened, instructions that are incomplete, and user errors that occur at a higher-than-acceptable rate. Products that can be reported include pumps, gloves, transducers, catheters, testing kits, implanted devices, connectors, tubing, and dressings. Death or injury does not have to occur for a report to be initiated; simple observations, if based on intelligent assessment, are all that is necessary.

When reporting a problem, one must be aware of the whole picture regarding the device. Is it cleaned on the nursing unit or in a specialized department? Was the infusion pump delivered to the patient by a rental equipment company or by the home health agency? Professional networking is not necessary before reporting a device, but it can add useful insight into the total scope of the product's uses and reputation. The specialty practice of IV nursing lends itself to this type of collegial communication.

Any device suspected of causing injury or death should be impounded immediately and reported to the FDA within 10 working days. The device should not be cleaned, safety checked, or manipulated in any way. In the case of an infusion pump, the programming data and history display should be verified by two persons not related to the incident before the pump is turned off. If the pump is battery powered, the battery should not be removed. Legal counsel should be consulted for further action regarding the device.

When to report a problem

Medical devices suspected of malfunction should be reported as soon as the product defect can be defined and user error can be ruled out. Manufacturers cannot be held accountable for problems that can be attributed to the user. Corrective action includes education and competency-based skills testing to verify the ability of the user.

User problems are a common explanation for many device faults. Although many problems arise from caregivers being inadequately prepared to use products, this excuse is acceptable only to a certain point. If the staff must be taught an excessive number of times and they continue to experience problems, perhaps the problem lies with the device and not the users. The device may be functional and may operate flawlessly, but if the staff cannot use the product efficiently and safely in a reasonable amount of time, then the product may be the source of the problem. The product may be too difficult, complex, or time-consuming. A product that continues to be difficult to use 6 months after acquisition poses user-error risks; this is a reportable product defect.

A recurring problem, even when it can be explained, should raise a red flag. Problems may appear to be isolated incidents to the users who experience them, but a centralized reporting mechanism can analyze all of the reports to spot trends and identify potentially serious situations. Most institutions have a committee for material standardization and review. A progressive committee of this type invites product comments by all disciplines to ensure quality and to prevent risk.

Any product-related injury or death of a patient or employee should be immediately reported to the FDA. Suspicion alone is enough to warrant reporting because careful investigation must begin immediately and the role of the device must be clarified. The Role of the Federal Government section presented earlier in this chapter gives more details regarding reporting death or injury.

Active communication with the manufacturer should always be a first step when problems are suspected. The manufacturer must report problems to the FDA and is obligated to investigate all communications that describe problems. Most companies have toll-free numbers for consumer questions and complaints.

The nurse should be realistic about the expected response from the manufacturer. The company is not obligated to release information about other reported negative occurrences regarding the product in question. The company will record the complaint or comment and investigate. It is in their own best interest to address and resolve issues before professional publications or nurse networking reveals product safety issues.

If the product problem is significant and urgent, manufacturers should be notified so that corrective action can be taken immediately. When identifying problems with disposable products, the nurse should keep defective samples. Both the FDA and the manufacturer can use the samples to discover the source of the problem, and defective samples can help protect the organization if litigation occurs. The labels on packaging, including the lot number and any other identifying numbers or markings, should be provided to the manufacturer and kept in the institution's records. All details of the negative occurrence should be documented immediately. Institutional risk management departments should also be apprised of any negative product occurrences. Simple problems, such as misleading labels on packaging or unclear instructions, can be resolved with the manufacturer alone, and the results of the requested change can be almost immediate.

How to report a problem

MedWatch, the FDA Medical Products Reporting Program, supplies reporting forms to anyone who needs them. Institutions may stock these forms in nursing administration, clinical engineering, materials management, or purchasing offices. These one-page forms are simple, straightforward, and concise (Fig. 16-1). They can be reproduced without permission, but original forms are postage free and can be mailed without an envelope. If assistance is needed in filling out the form, an 800 number is available. The report can also be made online, faxed, or given orally.

The report form asks for the name of the product and a brief description, including gauge numbers, lot numbers, and any identifying characteristics. If known, the manufacturer's name and address, as well as the product's serial number, manufacturer's product number, and expiration date should be included.

Reporter information includes the name, facility, and address of the person initiating the problem report. The report can be held in strict confidence with no public disclosure. In this case, the reporter's name and address are still important because the investigator may want to contact the reporter to confirm that the report was received, request additional information, or offer information regarding the intended course of action.

The reporter's second option is to disclose the problem report to the manufacturer only. This option allows the maker to respond to problems and to investigate along with the reporter. In most cases, the manufacturer seeks to reassure the user that the complaint has been received and will be investigated. A problem cannot be corrected unless the manufacturer or distributor is fully informed, and the reporter of the problem is the most accurate source of information.

The third identification option is to make the reporter's name available to the manufacturer and to anyone who requests a copy of the report from the FDA. This openness may be intimidating to persons who worry about being confronted. However, the availability of the reporting person lends credibility to the report and makes the free flow of information much easier. Problem identification is often difficult because of the wide variety of possible contributing factors. The availability of the reporter makes quantifying and qualifying problems much easier. Reporter identification is strictly voluntary, and reports that limit the identity of the author are given as much attention as those that do not.

The report form asks for a detailed description of the problem as seen by the reporter. Facts are necessary, but suspected flaws or perceived problems can also be included. Sometimes, reports reflect nothing more than a concern that a problem *might* occur. No facts exist in these cases; the report serves only to predict or to warn. User-related issues are acceptable problems to report, as are specific product function concerns.

It is acceptable to copy the report to the manufacturer; this action will speed the process of response. Ideally, the maker of a product should be informed of suspected product defects as soon as they occur, which may be some time before the problem is perceived to be widespread enough to warrant a report to the FDA. Nurses should openly communicate with manufacturers to solicit help in education and problem solving. This interaction could resolve many issues early in the process. Typically, a nurse who is a caregiver assumes that nursing administration communicates with vendors. The irony is that the administrative nurse is rarely the product user or the caregiver and therefore has limited hands-on perspective of the problem. Manufacturers respond to the bedside nurse and consider input from the actual caregiver to be of significant value. Problem reports submitted by primary care nurses are very important contributions; they are always welcome by the FDA and the health care industry alike.

All health care institutions have internal reporting mechanisms as well in the form of variance or incident reports. These are reporting tools for quality improvement and risk management programs; they provide written, ongoing communication regarding real and potential risks in the work environment. Any situation requiring manufacturer or FDA communication should also be processed through quality improvement or risk management programs.

Biomedical engineering departments should be notified first in cases of suspected equipment problems. This department can provide insight into potential risks. The biomedical engineering department may have to impound the device, even if temporarily, to service and test the product before an accurate report can be made. This department is trained to evaluate and anticipate potential and real problems. If the equipment is rented or leased, the owner or distributor should be notified by the biomedical engineering department.

When a nurse articulates a problem, the report must be written in a professional manner to be considered a credible resource. This means that the report must be free of bias or prejudicial comments. Stating that a product is not as good as that of a competitor is not a problem. The report must provide facts, including dates and times. The report should not stress blame or fault because these will become evident when the defect is properly identified. The reporter must be interested in corrective action and patient safety more than in assigning fault.

Risk management

Notifying the risk management department does not always imply that action is needed. The risk management department

MED**W**ATCH

THE FDA MEDICAL PRODUCTS REPORTING PROGRAM

For **VOLUNTARY** reporting
by health professionals of adverse
events and product problems

Page ____ of ____

Form Approved: OMB No. 0910-0291 Expires: 8/31/00
See OMB statement on reverse

FDA Use Only

Triage unit
sequence #

PLEASE TYPE OR USE BLACK INK

A. Patient information

1. Patient identifier	2. Age at time of event: or _____ Date of birth:	3. Sex ☐ female ☐ male	4. Weight ____ lbs or ____ kgs
In confidence			

B. Adverse event or product problem

1. ☐ **Adverse event**   and/or   ☐ **Product problem** (e.g., defects/malfunctions)

2. **Outcomes attributed to adverse event**
(check all that apply)

☐ death _____ (mo/day/yr)
☐ life-threatening
☐ hospitalization – initial or prolonged

☐ disability
☐ congenital anomaly
☐ required intervention to prevent permanent impairment/damage
☐ other: _____

3. Date of event (mo/day/yr)	4. Date of this report (mo/day/yr)

5. **Describe event or problem**

6. **Relevant tests/laboratory data, including dates**

7. **Other relevant history, including preexisting medical conditions** (e.g., allergies, race, pregnancy, smoking and alcohol use, hepatic/renal dysfunction, etc.)

C. Suspect medication(s)

1. **Name** (give labeled strength & mfr/labeler, if known)

#1

#2

2. **Dose, frequency & route used** #1 #2	3. **Therapy dates** (if unknown, give duration) from/to (or best estimate) #1 #2

4. **Diagnosis for use** (indication)

#1

#2

6. **Lot #** (if known) #1 #2	7. **Exp. date** (if known) #1 #2

9. **NDC #** (for product problems only)
– –

5. **Event abated after use stopped or dose reduced**

#1 ☐ yes ☐ no ☐ doesn't apply

#2 ☐ yes ☐ no ☐ doesn't apply

8. **Event reappeared after reintroduction**

#1 ☐ yes ☐ no ☐ doesn't apply

#2 ☐ yes ☐ no ☐ doesn't apply

10. **Concomitant medical products** and therapy dates (exclude treatment of event)

D. Suspect medical device

1. **Brand name**

2. **Type of device**

3. **Manufacturer name & address**

4. **Operator of device**
☐ health professional
☐ lay user/patient
☐ other: _____

5. **Expiration date** (mo/day/yr)

6.
model # _____
catalog # _____
serial # _____
lot # _____
other #

7. **If implanted, give date** (mo/day/yr)

8. **If explanted, give date** (mo/day/yr)

9. **Device available for evaluation?**   (Do not send to FDA)
☐ yes   ☐ no   ☐ returned to manufacturer on _____ (mo/day/yr)

10. **Concomitant medical products** and therapy dates (exclude treatment of event)

E. Reporter (see confidentiality section on back)

1. **Name & address**   phone #

2. Health professional? ☐ yes ☐ no	3. Occupation	4. Also reported to ☐ manufacturer ☐ user facility ☐ distributor

5. **If you do NOT want your identity disclosed to the manufacturer, place an " X " in this box.** ☐

Mail to: MED**W**ATCH   **or FAX to:**
5600 Fishers Lane   1-800-FDA-0178
Rockville, MD 20852-9787

FDA Form 3500

Submission of a report does not constitute an admission that medical personnel or the product caused or contributed to the event.

FIG. 16-1 *Voluntary reporting form for MedWatch, the FDA Medical Products Reporting Program.*

often collects and categorizes information just to have it available if a problem does occur. Allowing this department to collect information and be aware of potential problems allows the institution to better protect itself and the safety of the public.

Legal counsel is notified at the discretion of the risk management department. Usually, legal counsel advises the institution's personnel and perhaps corresponds with manufacturers regarding situations or events. This action gives more authority to a product complaint issue. Legal counsel is always involved immediately in the case of injury or death.

The risk management department should always be consulted if equipment is to be returned to use after a suspected problem of major impact. The risk management department is able to advise users if problems with the product have been resolved sufficiently to support its return to use.

Summary

The caregiver must be knowledgeable about the equipment used and must be motivated to initiate change when indicated. The governing institution or agency can provide the access or avenue to action, but it is the responsibility of the person providing patient care to initiate the process. The nurse is a patient advocate who strives for the patient's total well-being, a goal that should include not only the care provided but also awareness of the equipment used and corrective action to take, should it be necessary.

References

1. Intravenous Nurses Society: Infusion nursing standards of practice, *JIN* (suppl) 23(6S), 2000.
2. Brown SL, et al: Infusion pump adverse events: experience from medical device reports, *JIN* 20(1):41, 1997.
3. Messner K: Barriers to implementing a quality improvement program, *Nurs Manage* 29 (1):33, 1998.
4. Zambuto RP: Current health care trends and their impact on clinical engineering, *Biomed Instrum Technol* 31:228, 1997.
5. Rutala WA: APIC guideline for selection and use of disinfectants, *Am J Infect Control* 18(2):100, 1990.
6. Joint Commission on Accreditation of Healthcare Organizations: *Comprehensive accreditation manual for hospitals,* Oakbrook Terrace, Ill, 1999-2000, JCAHO.
7. Joint Commission on Accreditation of Healthcare Organizations: *Comprehensive accreditation manual for home care,* Oakbrook Terrace, Ill, 1999-2000, JCAHO.
8. Stockmaster MO: There's no such thing as "safe equipment," *Biomed Instrum Technol* 34 (9):301, 1996.
9. US Department of Health and Human Services: Safe Medical Devices Act. Medical Device Reporting for User Facilities. Public Law 101-629. Washington, DC: DHHS, April 1996.
10. Dugger B: Intravenous nursing competency: why is it important? *JIN* 20(6):287, 1997.
11. Cuthrell P: Managing equipment failures: nursing practice requirements for meeting the challenges of the safe medical devices act, *JIN* 19(5):264, 1996.
12. McConnell EA: Medical device use by nurses: a review of published nursing literature, *Biomed Instrum Technol* 32(5):471, 1998.

Product Selection and Evaluation

Mary C. Alexander, BS, CRNI

Product selection and evaluation of intravenous (IV) therapy equipment are critical to effective IV nursing practice. With the vast number of products on the market, a methodical approach to product selection and evaluation will help the IV nurse specialist and health care administrator identify cost-effective, appropriate IV products for safe, high-quality patient care delivery.

Important steps in the process of selecting a product include recognizing and documenting the need for equipment, scanning the market, and identifying essential features of the device. Once the product has been selected, each member of the product evaluation committee plays a specific role in the comprehensive evaluation process. Verbal and written communication of the process must be conveyed to the users of the equipment to ensure proper evaluation. Finally, the financial aspects of purchasing or leasing new products must be considered. Product pricing must not be the primary factor in product selection because poor-quality products may lead to increased use, patient trauma, or liability issues. Cost analysis and justification will enable efficient and appropriate decisions to be made in choosing a new product or in demonstrating the need to continue using an existing product.

This chapter discusses the related processes of product selection and evaluation. The chapter is intended to help the IV nurse specialist make educated and informed selections of IV products, ensuring safe delivery of IV therapy without compromising quality patient care.

THE ROLE OF NURSES IN PRODUCT SELECTION AND EVALUATION

As the most likely end-users of IV products, nurses possess the expertise, knowledge, and experience to participate in product evaluation. The nurse's awareness of the cost-effectiveness of current products and new technology is critical to the evaluation process.[1] Because the nurse provides direct patient care, he or she is cognizant of the benefits and complications associated with infusion products.

The nurse's education and experience should be considered before a product is replaced or a new product is introduced. The health care professional's educational background and clinical orientation will determine his or her understanding of the scientific principles of the product's application. Depending on the facility's policies and procedures, the practitioner's professional status may determine who uses the equipment. For instance, a licensed practical nurse may not be permitted to regulate IV infusions via an infusion pump but may operate an infusion controller. If the facility's nursing population is largely made up of licensed practical nurses, the most appropriate choice for that institution would be to purchase controllers.

The practitioner must know how to operate the equipment to ensure that safe IV therapy is delivered to the patient and operator error is minimized. Reading the product literature, familiarizing oneself with the product, and observing precautions are necessary measures to guarantee safe, efficient operation. Health care professionals must be educated in the use and operation of the product. References should be available and supervision provided if the nurse requires additional assistance.

Educational programs should include the reasons for the product evaluation because staff cooperation and understanding can greatly enhance the effectiveness of the evaluation. During the evaluation, the nurse should be aware of the importance of reporting a product defect or malfunction. Documenting the problem, using another product, returning to the formerly used product until the problem is corrected, and contacting the company representative are appropriate responses to a defect or malfunction. By taking an active role in the evaluation, the practitioner develops a sense of accomplishment as his or her suggestions and recommendations are applied to clinical practice.[2]

PRODUCT SELECTION PROCESS
Identifying the need for a product change

To begin the product selection process, the facility must determine a need for changing equipment or purchasing a new product. Patient care requirements drive this process. The rationale for change should fall into one of the following categories: cost considerations, safety considerations, or product effectiveness.

Because cost containment and fiscal constraints are critical issues, product prices must be carefully compared. Lower prices may not be equated with cost-efficiency. Therefore purchasing a less costly item may not be cost-effective if poor product performance leads to increased product use. If custom-made products are desired, the associated high cost may preclude their use in the facility.

Some products require associated equipment. The tubing of an infusion control device may require a dedicated set, whereas extension tubing and latex injection ports may be necessary to complete a catheter insertion component. In the case of IV start kits, buying each item individually may be less expensive than purchasing an assembled kit. When calculating the cost of a device, the extra expense of the added equipment must be included to reflect the true cost of the product.

Operating costs must be taken into account in addition to acquisition costs. One product may cost less than another, but if priming the device or training the patient is very time-consuming, any cost advantage may be outweighed by the additional labor involved.[3]

In addition to the price of the product, the manufacturer's product support capabilities need to be considered. Manufacturers' proposals and competitive bidding should be compared to ensure an appropriate and cost-effective arrangement for the institution.

Safety must be considered when initiating the product selection process. As stated in *Infusion Nursing Standards of Practice,* "the infusion nurse . . . should interact with other members of the health care team to provide safe, quality infusion therapy."[4] Technologic advancement has resulted in product innovation, evident in the more-concentrated and potent forms of medications being administered. Therefore, when products are selected and evaluated, specific product safety features should be considered. For instance, infusion control devices should have features that reduce the risk of accidental free flow and alarms that detect air, malfunctions, or occlusions. A lock-out mechanism may be necessary to make the device tamper proof. When evaluating administration devices, needlestick protection features should be assessed. Safety components that capture or resheath needles or those that make it difficult to accidentally or intentionally defeat a safety mechanism need to be considered. Inserting catheters with protected-needle features can reduce the risk of accidental needlesticks to the patient and the practitioner. Safer products, although sometimes more expensive, may actually save money by reducing the institution's exposure to liability claims.

The consistency of the product's effectiveness also needs to be assessed. A review of maintenance records and product features will help determine how consistently the product produces the desired results. Technologic advances and the product's ease and range of use should be examined.

Technologic changes have resulted in improved quality and technique. Infusion control devices have become more sophisticated to accommodate the administration of potent medications and therefore are more valuable in acute care settings. Conversely, some infusion control devices have been designed simply enough that the patient can be taught to use them; these devices have become assets in home care settings. Another change has been the development of new catheter materials that make insertion less painful for the patient.

Improved technique can be demonstrated by the use of transparent semipermeable membrane dressings. If these dressings, instead of gauze dressings, are applied on an IV insertion site, the area can be seen and inspected without removal of the dressing.

The ease of product use should be investigated. The practitioner's education and experience may affect the success of a product's introduction. If an institution has a high staff turnover rate, less complicated equipment may facilitate orientation and decrease errors. For home care patients, the complexity of a product may be an issue because the patient and caregiver will need to be taught how to use it competently and be prepared for troubleshooting when necessary.

A product's range of use depends on several factors, including the needs of the patient, the anticipated uses for the product, the patient population using the product, and the clinical settings in which the product will be used.

Patient needs must be considered when assessing new products. Particular patient populations have varying needs. For example, home care patients whose homes are not equipped with electricity will require battery-powered infusion devices to administer their therapy. The size and weight of ambulatory pumps are concerns for patients who wish to maintain their normal activities.

Anticipated product uses must be defined. For instance, when evaluating infusion control devices, the types of solutions and medications to be administered should be considered. Specific features may be required to infuse such therapies as narcotics, chemotherapy, and total parenteral nutrition. IV catheters, whether being used for short- or long-term therapy, vary in terms of product design and materials. Many types of peripheral, central, and peripherally inserted central catheters are available.

The patient population using the product is another consideration. An infusion pump used in the hospital may be a more sophisticated device than one used in the home. For instance, in the acute care setting, medications may need to be titrated to a tenth of a milliliter. Patients requiring the administration of epidural anesthesia, vasoconstrictors, or chemotherapy may need specific equipment to closely monitor drug delivery. In the case of the home care patient requiring cyclic total parenteral nutrition during the night, the infusion device would need a specialized titrating feature. Also, patients with implantable ports usually require infusion devices to deliver their treatments. Therefore the nurse should be aware of the patient's clinical conditions that warrant specific products to deliver the appropriate treatments.

The clinical setting in which the product will be used should be considered. If an infusion pump is used primarily in an intensive care unit, the size of the device (i.e., can several pumps be attached safely to one IV pole?) and its ability to titrate medications may be major considerations. The size of a pump would also be a concern for a home care patient who wishes to maintain normal activities; a compact, portable device would be preferred. In the case of the patient receiving long-term antibiotic therapy at home, a peripherally inserted central catheter instead of a short peripheral catheter may be the appropriate method for medication delivery. The peripherally inserted central catheter may remain in place indefinitely, whereas a peripheral catheter has to be changed every 72 hours, or sooner if complications such as phlebitis or infiltration occur. Scheduled follow-up visits by the home care nurse could be planned to change dressings and evaluate the condition of the peripherally inserted central catheter, as opposed to frequent calls to replace the peripheral catheter.

Timing a product change

Incident reports may indicate the need for product change. Evolving patterns that demonstrate product errors or defects can threaten safe IV delivery and patient outcomes, warranting a product change.

It is important to review the patient care areas that will be affected by a product change to ensure that the product selected is representative of the institution's needs. The facility should then determine whether the proposed product is a necessity or a luxury. For example, an infusion control device should have alarms that detect air, occlusion, and malfunction, but a feature for titration may not be necessary if that mode is seldom used.

Researching for product selection

Once the need for a product has been established, the next step is to document that need, draft a proposal of intention, and research the market. Reviewing current literature, attending trade shows, and interviewing facilities currently using the product are effective ways to obtain product information.

Conducting a literature review provides material about current products. Marketing brochures and articles on IV therapy in nursing and pharmacy journals provide useful information on IV equipment. Scientific, health, and cost-outcomes research that objectively identifies the qualities of patients who will benefit from various types of infusion technology should be requested from manufacturers.[5] Information from the Emergency Care Research Institute may be beneficial. This independent organization evaluates medical equipment,

publishes journals featuring comparative evaluations and ratings of products, and reports hazards and problems of medical devices.

Attending trade shows is another way to obtain product information. At these exhibits, many products can be viewed in one place. Trade shows offer the opportunity to see and use devices and to speak with company representatives. Manufacturing representatives demonstrate their products, enabling cursory evaluations. This helps narrow the field of available products early in the selection process by eliminating equipment inappropriate for the facility.

In addition, interviewing other facilities regarding their experiences with products can provide useful information about equipment, including advantages and disadvantages. Researching available products helps the health care professional make an educated choice.

Identifying necessary product features

Before a product is changed or a new product selected, written criteria should be developed that include the product's necessary features. To ensure that all aspects of a product are considered, the most important as well as the least important features should be included in the criteria.[2] Input from all departments using the product should be considered when developing the guidelines because each practitioner's perspective is valuable. This material will be used to narrow the field for the final hands-on evaluation. In addition, this information will be incorporated into a preliminary evaluation form for product selection. Table 17-1 identifies characteristics worth assessing in four products: catheters, transparent semipermeable membrane dressings, administration sets, and needleless systems.

Preliminary evaluation form for product selection

Once product guidelines are established, a product evaluation form is created. The evaluation form may be designed by the IV team, the product evaluation committee, or a task force that is specifically addressing a particular product. This evaluation form is helpful in preliminary product selection. The form encourages objective ratings and product comparisons. This process also encourages price bidding and may result in lower costs.

As many products as possible should be evaluated during this initial phase, which helps narrow the field for the actual hands-on evaluations. It is not feasible to evaluate all the devices on the market; the cost of doing so, in time and money, is prohibitive.

To facilitate product selection, the entries on the form should coincide with the product guidelines. Spaces for the product name, manufacturer, person evaluating the product, dates of evaluation, and comments should be included. Fig. 17-1 illustrates the information to be included on a preliminary product evaluation form, and Table 17-2 and Box 17-1 provide guidelines for its use.

Table 17-1	**Product Guidelines**

FEATURES	CONSIDERATIONS
CATHETERS	
Packaging	Is the package easy to open? Is sterility easily maintained after the package is opened? Can the package be easily stored or discarded?
Handling	Is the catheter easy to hold? Do features make it awkward to handle?
Length	What lengths are available?
Gauge	What gauge sizes are available?
Lumens	Is it available with multiple lumens?
Radiopacity	Is it radiopaque?
Ease of insertion	Does the needle penetrate the skin easily or with resistance? Does the needle appear dull?
Catheter advancement	Does the catheter advance easily? Is sterility maintained while it is advanced?
Catheter flexibility	Is the catheter too flexible or too rigid?
Blood return	Is blood return quickly visible? Are features available to prevent blood contamination?
Needleless feature	Does the needleless feature capture or resheath the stylet after insertion? Is user activation necessary? Can it be determined whether the safety feature is activated? Can the safety feature be deactivated? Does the safety feature remain protective through disposal?
Catheter stabilization	Can the catheter be easily secured to prevent movement? Can a dressing be applied that does not interfere with assessment of the insertion site?
TRANSPARENT SEMIPERMEABLE MEMBRANE DRESSINGS	
Ease of application	Is the dressing easy to apply? Is sterility maintained when applying? Is a one- or two-handed method needed for application?
Adhesive quality	Does the dressing adhere adequately to the skin? Is it difficult to remove?
Water resistance	Is it water resistant?
Air permeability	Is it air permeable?
ADMINISTRATION SETS	
Injection ports	How many injection ports are available?
Clamps	How many clamps are available? What types of clamps are on the tubing?
Drop size	What drop sizes are available?
Filters	Is an in-line filter available on the tubing? Can a filter be added to the tubing?
Length	What lengths are available?
Luer-Lok design	Is a Luer-Lok feature available?
Types of infusates	Can all types of infusates infuse through the tubing or are other types of sets required?
Compatibility with existing equipment	Can the tubing be used with existing products or devices?
NEEDLELESS SYSTEMS	
Packaging	Is the packaging easy to open? Is sterility maintained after opening? Will storage and disposal be a problem?
Number of components	How many components are necessary to complete the system?
Ease of use	Is the system easy to handle? Are there features that make it awkward to handle?
Compatibility with existing equipment	Can it be used with existing equipment?
Injection port	Is it self-sealing? How many repeated insertions can be made into it?
Types of infusates	Can all types of infusates be delivered via this system?
Injury prevention	Does it automatically guard itself? Is it rendered useless after a single use?
Safety feature	Is the safety feature difficult to accidentally defeat? Is it difficult to intentionally defeat? Does it remain in effect after disposal?
Patient comfort	Is patient comfort compromised; that is, are more insertion attempts necessary or is needle penetration painful? Is it difficult to tape or secure the device to the patient?
Infection control	Does the device increase the risk of infection? Does it prevent changing of needles, which may be necessary to maintain sterile technique? To obtain access, does the system have to be opened to the air?

PRELIMINARY PRODUCT EVALUATION REVIEW FORM

Product _____   Evaluation Date _____

Evaluator _____

RATING: 4 = highly satisfactory; 3 = more than satisfactory;
2 = satisfactory; 1 = less than satisfactory;
0 = not acceptable

Guidelines	Manufacturer				
Alarms					
Battery life					
Rate range					
Accuracy					
PSI					
Size of machine					
Titration					
Types of infusates					
Easy to read					
Directions on machine					
Free-flow protection					
Tamper proof					
Piggyback mode					
Associated equipment needs					
Total					

Comments:

FIG. 17-1   *Example of a preliminary product evaluation form.*

Table 17-2   **Infusion Pump Evaluation Guidelines***

FEATURES	CONSIDERATIONS
Alarms	What alarms are included: air, occlusion, door open, malfunction, low battery, infusion complete?
Battery life	How long will the pump operate on battery power?
Rate range	What is the rate range? Are tenths-of-milliliter increments available?
Accuracy	What is the percentage of margin of error?
psi	What is the maximum psi exerted?
Size of machine	Can the pump fit easily on an IV pole? Can several fit safely on one IV pole? Is the size of the ambulatory pump conducive to the patient's normal daily activities?
Titration	Can the pump titrate solutions?
Types of infusates	Can all types of infusates, including opaque total parenteral nutrition solutions, be infused?
Easy to read	Are commands and buttons easy to read? Are panel lights available to illuminate in a dark room?
Directions on machine	Are there permanent directions on the pump for quick reference? Are they easy to understand?
Free-flow protection	Are there safeguards against free flow of infusates?
Tamper-proof characteristics	Is there a lock-out mechanism to prevent unauthorized tampering?
Piggyback mode	Is this mode available?
Associated equipment needs	Does the pump need dedicated infusion sets?

IV, Intravenous; *psi,* pounds per square inch.
*Use these guidelines when completing the corresponding preliminary product evaluation form.

Box 17-1   Completing the Evaluation Form
(see also Fig. 17-1)

1. Identify the type of product to be evaluated (e.g., peripheral catheter or infusion device).
2. Complete the evaluation date and evaluator's name.
3. Insert product name and model number.
4. Rate each product feature according to a given scale.
5. Add the ratings for each product to determine the total score.
6. Add comments as necessary.

Compile ratings from the evaluation forms: Once a total rating is determined for each product, the committee can narrow the field to a few products for the final hands-on evaluation. The products with the highest scores are chosen to be evaluated. The "Comments" section must be taken into consideration because negative comments may override a high score.

CONDUCTING A PRODUCT EVALUATION
Product evaluation committee

A product evaluation committee facilitates product selection and evaluation with decision making. This group should be broad based and multidisciplinary; it should include representatives from departments affected directly or indirectly by the use of the product. This committee participates in the preliminary selection process (Box 17-2) and ongoing product evaluations, and acts as an end reviewer for product decisions. The product evaluation committee considers the product's merits and assesses its range of use within the facility before deciding to either support or deny support for the purchase.[2,3,6-8] The committee should include representatives from the IV therapy, nursing, medical, infection control, pharmacy, materials management, purchasing, and biomedical engineering departments. Each person will have specific concerns relative to his or her discipline. In some situations, one committee member may represent more than one discipline. For instance, in a small home care company, the pharmacist may also be the purchasing agent and the materials management director. Subcommittees or task force groups may be convened to evaluate a specific infusion product.

IV therapy department representatives are integral members of the evaluation committee. Their clinical expertise is beneficial to the process, and they can identify favorable and unfavorable features of a product. In addition, they review products for appropriate and safe clinical use. Because IV nurses are likely the clinicians most involved with the hands-on evaluation, one of them could be the committee chairperson who leads the process. They should be used as resources by others during the evaluation process, and their comments are valuable at the point of final product selection. If IV nurses are not available in an institution, the Intravenous Nurses Society or other professional networks may provide useful product information or clinical insight.

The committee should include members of the nursing department. Depending on the product to be tested, the staff nurses may participate in the hands-on evaluation of the devices. The evaluators must be aware of the importance of completing the evaluation forms and conveying any comments about the product to the designated person on the committee.

Box 17-2   Product Selection Process

1. Identify and document the need to purchase or change to a new product. Is the product being considered to improve cost-effectiveness, safety, or efficiency?
2. Research competing products by conducting a literature review, attending trade shows, and interviewing facilities using the product.
3. Develop product guidelines by including the most and least important features desired.
4. Complete the preliminary product evaluation form by rating the product using the corresponding guidelines.
5. Narrow the field for hands-on evaluations; compile the results from the evaluation forms and select the product.

Suggestions from physicians are beneficial because they may identify advantages and disadvantages of the product from a different perspective. Physicians may be involved in the hands-on evaluation. For example, the interventional radiologist and the neonatologist may be asked to evaluate a new brand of peripherally inserted central catheters for pediatric patients.

Pharmacists should be represented on the evaluation committee. Their knowledge of medication administration and infusion capabilities, including guidelines to safeguard the patient, can be valuable. They can advise the committee on the appropriate distribution of products, particularly infusion control devices, within the facility.

Input regarding the efficacy and safety of a product from the infection control department may be important to the evaluation. For instance, when evaluating needleless systems, infection control professionals may assist IV nurses in monitoring sharps injuries or nosocomial infection rates related to a specific product. The infection control department may also be helpful when interpreting data from a manufacturer's clinical trials and scientific studies.

A representative from the biomedical engineering department (also referred to as the *medical* or *clinical engineering department*) should be included on the committee. Representatives from this department perform accuracy and pressure tests and disassemble devices to evaluate the quality of design and workmanship. They also provide information on a product's approximate repair and replacement time and cost. Engineering professionals can warn of any design flaws, possible power inadequacies, or incompatibilities with equipment already in use. They may have information on future upgrade capability and vendor histories.[7]

Materials management representatives on the committee provide valuable information regarding a product's storage requirements. The overall size of product packaging determines the amount that can be put on the IV nurses' carts and in department storage units. The materials management department is responsible for storing products in easily accessible, sterile places. They address issues that may limit product distribution and raise awareness of similar products in stock that may be confused with the product in question.

Input from the purchasing department is imperative. This department manages information on product prices, shipping costs, and buying groups and contract negotiations that encourage competitive bidding. Their goal is to purchase products at low cost without sacrificing quality. With many facilities facing increasing economic pressures, the price of a product may dictate purchasing decisions. Elaborating on patient safety issues may demonstrate the need to buy a more costly product. In addition, the purchasing department performs cost comparisons. For example, the cost of an infusion pump may be low, but the price of the dedicated tubing required for its operation may be higher than regular tubing. If a custom-designed product is desired, comparisons with other products need to be performed. This department also has insight into equipment and product reimbursement issues.

Other departments, including radiology, anesthesiology, and the emergency and operating rooms, may be affected by a product change as well. Inquiries should be made to determine the impact the change may have on different units, and representatives of these departments may wish to be on the committee.

With all committee members working as a team, an informed product choice can be made. Each representative contributes valuable information (Box 17-3). The product evaluation committee's goal is to choose safe, cost-efficient products that are appropriate for the patient and facility; product selections should never compromise quality patient care.

Evaluation process

Once the preliminary selection process has been completed, the final evaluation procedure can begin (Box 17-4). The IV team or the product evaluation committee rates products using established guidelines. Literature reviews, product demonstrations, and manufacturer recommendations help complete the preliminary selection process. When the field is narrowed, the products chosen should be those that are appropriate for the institution based on established criteria. Once all the products have been rated, the committee determines the number to be evaluated by the staff. Usually, no more than two or three products are selected for hands-on evaluation.

Once the committee establishes the number of products to be evaluated, the group delineates the actual evaluation process. The committee then considers such factors as the length of time for the evaluation, the number of products to be evaluated, the location of the evaluation, and the staff involved with the hands-on process.

The length of time for the evaluation varies depending on the product. Weeks or months may be needed to complete an effective evaluation. When evaluating electronic infusion devices, it is important to allow sufficient time. Educating the staff in the correct use of the product could take 1 or 2 weeks; therefore 2 to 4 weeks per product may be necessary for all evaluators to have the opportunity to evaluate the products. Some evaluators may like a product because it is new, and others will dislike it for the same reason. The length of the evaluation should be sufficient to diminish the novelty effect. When a product is used many times each day, staff will make the transition more quickly than with a product that is used once a day or once a week.

The number of items that will be rated must also be determined. For example, when catheters are tested, the committee will determine how many catheters must be inserted to allow a thorough evaluation. Another way to rate products may be to have a predetermined time frame, such as 3 to 4 weeks. A sufficiently long trial period helps overcome the learning curve required by some products.

The committee must establish the location of the evaluation. In a large institution, the committee may select several units to participate in the study, whereas in a small hospital, the evaluation may be conducted throughout the hospital. One of the advantages of selecting certain units within a facility is that by limiting the number of staff involved, the facility can reduce the number of in-service hours dedicated to training. Another advantage is the ability to select hospital units that use the product often and represent diverse patient populations. Units in which central and peripheral catheters are used, multiple types of IV medications are administered, and blood components are transfused can improve the evaluation process because of the varied delivery methods. Data are generated quickly if the selected department uses the product often. There are also disadvantages to limiting the evaluation to a small number of departments. When a patient is transferred to a unit that is not evaluating the product, the likelihood of incorrect use and errors in operation increases because the staff may not be familiar with the device. When the entire facility is not represented in the evaluation, it may be difficult for staff in nonparticipating units to obtain comprehensive product information.

Guidelines for evaluations must also be established in home care and alternative settings. Select nurses may test the product or all staff members may participate, depending on the size of the organization.

The next step is communicating the evaluation procedure to those involved. An explanation of the importance of the process is essential. When the evaluators understand the purpose of the evaluation, they are more likely to cooperate with the process.

User education

The next step in preparing for the hands-on evaluation is the education of all evaluators. In-service sessions should be scheduled with the product manufacturer's representative once the product's availability, evaluation start date, and completion date are established. IV nurses and all other evaluators need to know how to use the product correctly, so time should be allowed for

---

Box 17-3   Product Selection Committee*

IV therapy	Biomedical engineering
Nursing	Pharmacy
Medical (physicians)	Materials management
Infection control	Purchasing

*Other departments may include radiology, anesthesiology, emergency, operating room, and so on, as appropriate.

Box 17-4   Final Evaluation Process

1. Determine the length of time for the evaluation.
2. Identify the location for the evaluation (i.e., several departments or facilitywide testing).
3. Convey to the evaluators the importance of completing the product evaluation forms.
4. Schedule in-service sessions for proper product operation as near to the evaluation start date as possible.
5. Compile evaluation results and make the final decision for product selection.
6. Communicate throughout the facility which product was chosen.
7. Continuously evaluate new products, as well as the ones in use, to ensure that the appropriate product is being used in patient care.

hands-on practice. To lessen the chance of forgotten details about product operation, the in-service sessions should be conducted as near to the evaluation start date as possible. Written instructions, operating manuals, and videos should be available as resource materials.

Evaluation form

The evaluation form is essential to product evaluation. Data can be obtained in various ways. One method is to have the evaluators rank product performance on a scale ranging from 0 to 5, from "highly satisfactory" to "not acceptable," or from "strongly agree" to "strongly disagree." Another way is to ask closed-ended or open-ended questions. Closed-ended questions require only "yes" and "no" answers and may ask evaluators to compare products. Conversely, open-ended questions allow the evaluators to respond with subjective comments. An effective evaluation combines both types of questions on the evaluation form. Closed-ended questions take less time to answer, but additional information can be obtained from responses to the open-ended questions.[2]

The evaluation form can be generic or specific to the product. Either type should be clear and concise. Fig. 17-2 is an example of a generic evaluation form that can be used for any

---

GENERAL PRODUCT EVALUATION
REVIEW FORM

Department conducting evaluation _____

Evaluation period to last _____ Days from _____ to _____

	Existing Product	Proposed Product
Description		
Manufacturer		
Model		

Your comments are important to help conduct a thorough product evaluation; please complete this questionnaire and forward to your supervisor.

		YES	NO
1.	Have you been in-serviced on the proper use of the product?	____	____
2.	Does the product open from its packaging with ease?	____	____
3.	If the product is sterile, does it permit sterile transfer from packaging to use site?	____	____
4.	Does this product contain all the components necessary for the procedure to be performed?	____	____
	If no, which additional items are required?		

_____

| 5. | Does this product contain unnecessary components (resulting in excessive costs) for the procedure to be performed? | ____ | ____ |

If yes, which ones? _____

6. Which characteristics of this product are inferior to those of the existing product? _____

_____

Which characteristics of this product are superior to those of the existing product? _____

_____

| 7. | Do you recommend this product for use in the hospital? | ____ | ____ |

_____   _____   _____
(Name)   (Date)   (Ext.)

Comments:

FIG. 17-2 *Example of a generic product evaluation form.*

PRODUCT EVALUATION FORM FOR INFUSION DEVICES

Product _____   Evaluation date _____

Manufacturer _____   Evaluator _____

Complete this form by rating each statement and adding any comments. Return to the Product Evaluation Committee representative.

RATING: 4 = highly satisfactory; 3 = more than satisfactory; 2 = satisfactory;
1 = less than satisfactory; 0 = not acceptable

1. The alarms were easy to identify and troubleshoot.   _____

2. The pump was accurate and reliable.   _____

3. The pump could be easily positioned at the bedside or on an IV pole. The weight of the machine did not hinder patient ambulation or transport.   _____

4. The command panel was easy to read.   _____

5. The pump was easy to prime and load.   _____

6. The pump was easy to operate.   _____

7. The directions on the pump were easy to understand.   _____

8. The lock-out mechanism provided additional patient safety.   _____

9. The featured safeguards prevent accidental free-flow of infusates.   _____

10. The in-service education for operation was adequate.   _____

11. Approximately how many times did you use the pump?   _____

Comments:

FIG. 17-3 *Example of a product evaluation form for infusion devices.*

product. If a particular product requires a detailed evaluation, the committee should solicit specific information. Fig. 17-3 is an evaluation form specific to infusion pumps.

Evaluators must understand the importance of returning their completed forms after they have taken sufficient time to evaluate the device. The frequency of responses should be determined: the evaluators may respond each time they use a product or after using the product for a specified period. A designated area may be assigned where the forms can be placed, or a specific person may have the responsibility of collecting them. Oral comments, both positive and negative, need to be documented to ensure that all information received about a product is compiled for comparison. Evaluators must report equipment problems and complaints. An evaluation may be terminated before the completion date if extensive difficulties are encountered.

Manufacturer support

Manufacturer support is an important component of product evaluation. The manufacturer's availability and responsiveness when problems occur during the evaluation should be assessed.

During the trial, the accessibility and receptiveness of the company representative should be observed. Brochures and teaching materials should be available as references. The quality of the representative's in-service training to the staff needs to be

noted. In addition, the manufacturer's follow-up efforts when responding to requests from staff or resolving product difficulties should be observed. When serious problems occur, it is important to note the representative's response as well as that of the company's management. These characteristics indicate the company's quality of service.

Cost considerations

Infusion Nursing Standards of Practice states that the nurse should be actively involved in and accountable for establishing and maintaining the budgetary process that encompasses staffing, education, and products used in IV nursing.[4] Responsible financial decisions regarding new products can be made when the IV nurse specialist takes an active role in product selection.

The cost of the product needs to be justified, and consideration must be given to associated equipment needs. The cost of custom-made items needs to be assessed because they may prove to be exceedingly high. With custom-made products, the prototype should be retained until the actual item is obtained. If problems arise, a comparison of the item with the prototype is warranted. Written evaluations may substantiate product quality.

When the committee narrows the field to a few products, a cost analysis should be conducted. The costs of the different products, including associated equipment requirements, must be compared. In addition to the price of the product, labor costs need to be included. Nurses' time can be calculated relative to the frequency of product use and the time necessary to educate a patient or caregiver on the product's use.[2] In a home care agency, reducing the time nurses spend training patients may justify using a more expensive product. In a facility where nursing and pharmacy costs are fixed and staffing is not expected to be reduced, the advantage of shorter training times may not be sufficient to warrant a product change.[3]

To encourage competitive bidding, hospital negotiators should carefully compare manufacturers' proposals. The evaluation's cost also needs to be considered; the evaluation price can be reduced by having the manufacturer provide the products, as opposed to the institution's purchasing them.

At this stage of the evaluation, the purchasing department takes a more active role. New equipment can be obtained in many ways: the institution may purchase, rent, or lease the products. Renting or leasing may be more advantageous than purchasing because when the lease agreement expires, an updated version of the product may be obtained. Purchase options may include volume discounts, selected option programs, and maintenance contracts.

Group purchasing arrangements may be available to reduce costs. Depending on the product, bidding may be structured in such a way that allows several manufacturers to bid on an individual item rather than a group of products. With the rapid development of new technology, it may be advantageous to limit the duration of a contract, thus allowing the facility to replace outdated equipment more quickly.

Product selection

When the product trials are completed, a final selection can be made. The product evaluation committee or specific task force tallies the results of the completed evaluation forms and compiles the evaluators' comments. The committee compares product advantages and disadvantages. At this point, if the products are comparable, an enhanced feature may be the determining factor in the final decision. Whether the institution plans to standardize the product throughout the facility may influence the selection; some products may not be suited to universal use. The manufacturer may offer a product mix to satisfy the facility's varied needs.

Final product selection involves several factors, including product performance, cost, overall evaluation results, and the manufacturer's performance. Product performance must be acceptable and meet the committee's criteria. From a financial standpoint, the least expensive product may not be a high-quality or efficient device; therefore cost should not be the only consideration. To justify purchasing an expensive or superior product, features that reduce user time or eliminate complications may be favorable. For example, needle safety devices decrease the risk of needlestick injuries and the associated complications. Comments from the overall evaluation may illuminate product or service problems. Finally, the company representative's responsiveness must be assessed with regard to the effectiveness of the in-service training, the frequency of follow-up calls, and the response to problems.

Communication of product selection

Once the product evaluation committee selects the final product, it must be communicated throughout the institution. Memoranda should be distributed to all units stating which product will be used and when implementation will begin. Policies and procedures will need to be developed for use of the product. IV nurse specialists should be involved in establishing the new product's procedures and guidelines for use. Nursing procedure committees, staff education departments, and nursing management may also participate in this process.

The new product may be introduced immediately or gradually, depending on the size of the institution. Smaller institutions may immediately implement the product throughout the facility, whereas large hospitals may find it more effective to educate the staff unit by unit.

In-service sessions must be scheduled, with duration dependent on the complexity and sophistication of the product and staff members' skills and training. Because the sessions may be time-consuming, staffing levels may have to be increased during the evaluation and implementation processes. Around-the-clock in-service sessions with the manufacturer may be necessary for one product, whereas viewing of a video may be sufficient instruction for another. For example, operation of an electronic infusion device will probably require in-depth instruction, whereas application of a transparent semipermeable membrane dressing may be demonstrated adequately on a video.

POSTEVALUATION EDUCATION

Once a product has been selected, postevaluation education and problem solving are necessary. Written procedures, training manuals, or posters describing proper operation should be available. Resource materials and personnel should be readily accessible to the staff using the product. IV nurse specialists' knowledge and clinical expertise make them excellent resources. Staff members should be allowed sufficient time to learn how to operate the product and should be supported until they are comfortable doing so. If staff members appear to have difficulty using the product, additional in-service programs conducted by the company representative may be needed to ensure proper use of the device.

When a product malfunctions or a defect in the device is identified, the serial and lot numbers of the item should be documented. This information helps the vendor locate a problem that may have developed during the manufacturing process. Incident reports should be filed. Accumulated information on the product's performance may demonstrate a need for immediate intervention by the manufacturer. According to the Safe Medical Devices Act of 1990, product defects and failures causing serious injury, illness, or death must be reported to the Food and Drug Administration (see Chapter 16).

To ensure quality IV care, product evaluation must be ongoing. Practitioners may like the product initially, but over time, they may cease using it. Reasons for this failure need to be identified. Additional in-service education may be needed, the device may be faulty, or there may be an inadequate supply to meet the facility's needs. Institutions should participate in ongoing evaluations of products in use and those new to the market. This continuous assessment guarantees that the most appropriate device is used for patient care.

SUMMARY

The IV nurse specialist plays an important role in the product selection and evaluation processes. Educated product selection choices enable safe, efficient delivery of IV therapy to the patient. A methodic approach facilitates this process. Written evaluations help demonstrate objective rationales for selecting particular products. The process may show that a product can improve technique or patient safety and be cost-efficient, or it may conclude that the product in use is appropriate for the patient and the institution. Ongoing evaluation of products in use is important in the delivery of high-quality patient care. The IV nurse specialist's participation with his or her colleagues from other departments enhances commitment to the specialty and to the facility and provides personal satisfaction. Assuming an active role in product selection and evaluation contributes to the IV nurse specialist's sense of professional accomplishment as his or her suggestions and recommendations are applied to clinical practice.

REFERENCES

1. Intravenous Nurses Society: Position paper: the registered nurse's role in product purchase, *JIN* 20(2):69, 1997.
2. DiGirolamo D: Professional product evaluation, *JIN* 18(2):79, 1995.
3. Schleis TG, Tice AD: Selecting infusion devices for use in ambulatory care, *Am J Health Syst Pharm* 53(8):868, 1996.
4. Intravenous Nurses Society: Infusion nursing standards of practice, *JIN* (suppl) 23(6S), 2000.
5. McConnell EA: Infusion devices require educated users, *Nurs Manage* 29(11):55, 1998.
6. Hinson EK, Blough LD: Skilled IV therapy clinicians' product evaluation of open-ended versus closed-ended valve PICC lines, *JIN* 19(4):198, 1996.
7. Hostutler JJ: A better way to select medical equipment, *Nurs Manage* 27(9):32M, 1996.
8. Valenti WM, Herwaldt LA: Product evaluation, *Infect Control Hosp Epidemiol* 18(10):722, 1997.

Chapter
18

Patient Assessment

Rose Anne Waldman Lonsway, BSN, MA, CRNI

ASSESSMENT TECHNIQUES
PATIENT HISTORY
   Current status
   Medications
   Intake and output
CLINICAL ASSESSMENT
   Body weight
   Intake and output
   Urine volume and concentration
   Vital signs
   Hemodynamic monitoring
   Tissue turgor
   Thirst
   Appearance of the skin
   Edema
   Tearing and salivation
   Behavioral and sensory changes
LABORATORY DATA
SUMMARY

Knowledge and recognition of potential problems associated with a fluid or electrolyte imbalance are critical to patient care. This chapter describes basic patient assessment as it relates to fluid volume and electrolyte dynamics. Patient history, clinical assessment, and correct interpretation of laboratory data are valuable components of this process.

ASSESSMENT TECHNIQUES

The physical assessment of a patient is one of the most important functions that a nurse performs. The results of the initial assessment develop the baseline for the patient's care and treatment. Ongoing assessment charts the patient's response to treatment and provides data to measure outcomes. The nurse uses many skills during the assessment and builds a relational database by synthesizing bits of information into a total picture of the patient.

The skills used in assessment include inspection, auscultation, palpation, and percussion, as well as observation, inquiry, and listening. These skills are used in combination, system by system, as the assessment progresses. This chapter focuses on those aspects of physical assessment related to alterations in fluid and electrolyte balance.

PATIENT HISTORY

To understand how the body responds to its internal environment, a description of the patient's fluid and electrolyte status must be obtained from the patient. It is difficult to determine the absolute amount of total body water and the relationship between that amount and other mechanisms within the body. The more accurate the history obtained from the patient, the more sensitive the monitoring process will be for specific alterations.

Information obtained from the patient should include medical and family history. For example, although the patient may not exhibit signs or symptoms of diabetes, there may be a familial history of diabetes. As the course of the patient's treatment unfolds, latent diabetes may manifest itself. When this information is obtained from a comprehensive patient history, the nurse can be watchful for signs and symptoms indicating the beginning of diabetic changes in the patient's electrolyte status.

The patient's medical history indicates whether there is risk for or a history of fluid and electrolyte alterations and how the alteration and course of treatment were tolerated. Although the information may not currently be clinically significant, it may be applied to future treatment.

Current status

When reviewing body systems in conjunction with a physical assessment, the nurse should listen carefully to the patient's description of the chief complaint. If the patient has suffered an injury, the type and degree of injury should be ascertained because injury may affect the patient's fluid and electrolyte balance (Table 18-1).

---

*The author and editors wish to acknowledge the contributions made by Maxine Acevedo, co-author of this chapter in the first edition of *Intravenous Nursing: Clinical Principles and Practice.*

Table 18-1   Fluid and Electrolyte Imbalances Associated with Selected Diseases or Conditions

DISEASE OR CONDITION	POTENTIAL IMBALANCE
Crushing injuries	Potassium excess
	Plasma to interstitial fluid shift
Head injury	Sodium deficit
SIADH	Sodium deficit
Congestive heart failure	Fluid volume excess
Acute pancreatitis	Calcium deficit
	Magnesium deficit
	Hypovolemia
Selected tumors	Calcium excess
Diabetes	Metabolic acidosis
	Fluid volume deficit
Emphysema	Respiratory acidosis
Diuretic therapy	Potassium excess
	Potassium deficit
Prolonged immobilization	Calcium excess
Cirrhosis (hepatic)	Fluid volume excess
	Sodium deficit

SIADH, Syndrome of inappropriate antidiuretic hormone secretion.

Patients should be questioned to determine whether they suffer from any illness that may affect fluid and electrolyte balance. For example, in congestive heart failure, the patient is at risk for fluid volume excess. Metabolic aberrations, such as diabetes mellitus, can put the patient at risk for metabolic acidosis and fluid volume deficits. Episodes of acute pancreatitis can result in calcium deficits. Conditions such as emphysema cause a respiratory acidosis that results from the patient's inability to exchange carbon dioxide. Some tumors interfere with the use or uptake of calcium, leading to calcium excess.

Many fluid and electrolyte imbalances are insidious and require careful history taking and monitoring to prevent further problems. Prolonged immobilization of a patient may cause calcium excess caused by loss of calcium from the bone into the extracellular fluid. A patient who drinks excessive amounts of plain water may wash out electrolytes, causing potassium or sodium deficits or metabolic alkalosis if the condition is not corrected.

Medications

A thorough medication history should be obtained because any medications or therapeutic regimens, such as steroids or total parenteral nutrition, can disrupt fluid or electrolyte balance. For example, potassium-depleting diuretics may cause this problem. Conversely, potassium-sparing diuretics may cause potassium excess, the opposite of problems anticipated with diuretics. Overuse of laxatives may result in potassium deficits.

Intake and output

The nurse must ascertain whether the patient has experienced a large loss of body fluids from vomiting, diarrhea, or lack of intake. An assessment of dietary alterations or medically imposed dietary restrictions should be made. Questions are asked of the patient to try to elicit any discrepancies in intake and output. Is the patient producing copious amounts of urine, or is the patient drinking large amounts of plain water? Has the patient experienced any draining wounds or high-output fistulas that would cause a discrepancy between intake and output? The answers to these questions must be examined carefully when the history is analyzed and must be kept in mind as the clinical assessment is begun.

CLINICAL ASSESSMENT

The clinical assessment of a patient includes the initial intake assessment as well as ongoing assessment to monitor a patient's progress and response to therapy. A systems approach is recommended to assess for fluid and electrolyte balances related to infusion therapy.

Body weight

An accurate body weight is one of the initial clinical assessment parameters. Changes in body weight accurately reflect fluid loss or gain. An accurate determination of change in weight provides important information and is sometimes easier to obtain than an accurate intake and output record. Rapid changes in the patient's body weight can reflect problems with the fluid balance status. One way to approximate the amount of fluid gain or loss is to compare the equivalent between kilograms and liters of fluid. One kilogram, or 2.2 pounds of body weight, is thought to be approximately equivalent to the gain or loss of 1 L of fluid. Expressed in pounds, a gain or loss of 1 pound is equivalent to 500 ml of fluid.

This gain or loss is usually rapid. It is usually compared with what is called the *dry weight* of an individual. Even under conditions of starvation, a person will lose no more than one third to one half of a pound of dry weight a day. When monitoring for rapid weight gain or loss (and therefore fluid gain or loss), it is important to assess weight daily. Fluid gains or losses are categorized as mild, moderate, or severe, as described in Table 18-2.

The phenomenon of third spacing may complicate the fluid balance picture. Third spacing occurs when a patient has a fluid volume deficit of the extracellular space. Body weight is basically unchanged, however, because the fluid loss is from the extracellular space to other body compartments.

To ensure that accurate weights are obtained, the patient should be weighed at the same time every day, preferably in the morning before breakfast and after voiding. The same scale should be used for each weighing, and the patient should wear the same or similar-weight clothing. It is also important to ensure that the scale is accurate. This requires verifying the scale reading at regular intervals as recommended by the manufacturer.

Intake and output

Intake and output is a clinical measurement that is used daily; unfortunately, the accuracy of this measurement may not always be dependable. Intake and output can be recorded as a result of nursing judgment and may be initiated by nursing order; a physician's order is not necessary. The intake and output should approximate one another, maintaining a balance between all sources in and all sources out in any 24-hour period.

Table 18-2	Rapid Fluid Gain or Loss in the Adult	
CATEGORY	FLUID VOLUME EXCESS (%)	FLUID VOLUME DEFICIT (%)
Mild	2	2
Moderate	5	5
Severe	≥8	≥8

Box 18-1   Questions Used to Assess Intake and Output

- How much is the patient drinking? If the patient is allowed oral fluids, is at least 1500 ml of fluid per day ingested?
- How much is the patient urinating?
- What does the urine look like? Is it dilute without odor, or is it very concentrated and highly odoriferous?
- What is the texture of the skin? Is it dry? Is it loose? Is it overly moist or firm?
- Does the patient have a fever?
- Is the patient perspiring excessively?
- Is the patient experiencing excessive drainage anywhere, including nasogastric tubes, fistulas, or any portal from which the patient could lose fluids? It is important to include those amounts in the daily intake and output record.

Box 18-1 provides a series of questions the nurse can ask to develop a complete picture of intake and output.

There are many ways to ensure accurate recording of intake and output. First, the importance of the patient's record should be stressed to the clinical staff and to the patient and family so that all may assist in recording intake and output. If the patient is undergoing parenteral fluid replacement, it is important to remember that IV fluid containers may be overfilled by up to 10%. This means that a liter container may actually contain 1100 ml of fluid rather than the 1000 ml printed on the container. When possible, intake and output amounts should be measured rather than guessed. In addition, *all* input, such as ice chips (a 200-ml glass of ice chips could equal approximately 100 ml of water) must be recorded.

Output is often referred to as either *sensible* or *insensible* loss. Sensible loss is measurable output, whereas insensible loss is difficult to measure, such as perspiration. Water loss by perspiration should be estimated with labels such as excessive, moderate, or mild. The amount of insensible loss in an adult is 500 to 1000 ml/day.[1] Estimates of fluid from incontinence of stool or urine, wound exudate, and irrigating solutions for bladder or wounds are important parts of intake and output records. Insensible loss increases if respirations increase.[2] For a patient who is in a delicate state of fluid balance or imbalance, it is important to review 8-hour intake and output totals in addition to the 24-hour totals.

Urine volume and concentration

During clinical assessment, a nurse needs to synthesize several pieces of information to understand and evaluate urine volume and concentration. Naturally, an accurate intake and output record is extremely important.

Normal urine output averages about 1 ml/kg body weight per hour, or approximately 1500 ml in a 24-hour period in a healthy adult. The urine output can be as small as 1000 ml or as great as 2000 ml in 24 hours, which is an average of approximately 40 to 80 ml/hr in a healthy adult. Children have lesser amounts of urine volume, based on their age and weight (see Chapter 30). When the body is under stress, urine output may be less than normal because of increased secretion of aldosterone and antidiuretic hormone. In periods of stress, this may lead to an average output of 30 to 50 ml/hr.

Low or high urine volumes may indicate a fluid imbalance. Urine osmolality and specific gravity give further information on this issue. Urine osmolality is the measure of the number of particles per unit of water. The average normal value is 200 to 1200 mOsm/kg H_2O.[3]

Urine osmolality depends on the amount of antidiuretic hormone that is in the bloodstream and the rate that solutes are excreted through the kidneys. It more accurately reflects changes in urine content and the ability of the kidneys to concentrate urine than does specific gravity. Urine osmolality depends on the state of hydration; measuring serum and urine osmolality at the same time yields a more accurate reflection of renal concentrating ability than does urine-specific gravity.[1]

Urine-specific gravity, which ranges from 1.016 to 1.022,[3] measures the amount of solutes in the urine, gives a picture of the patient's state of hydration, and reflects the kidneys' ability to regulate fluid balance. Urine-specific gravity increases with any condition that causes hypoperfusion in the kidneys. Hypoperfusion may lead to oliguria, shock, or severe dehydration. The urine-specific gravity decreases when the renal tubules are no longer able to reabsorb water and concentrate urine. This phenomenon would occur, for example, during the early stages of pyelonephritis.

It is also wise to look at urine pH, which may range from 4.6 to 8.0, with an average of 6.0. Urine pH increases in metabolic and respiratory alkalosis and decreases in the presence of uric acid stones or metabolic and respiratory acidosis.

It is important to understand and discriminate between the differences in water diuresis and solute diuresis. A low urinary specific gravity, a low urinary osmolality, and a normal or elevated serum sodium level can indicate either a lack of antidiuretic hormone or the inability of the renal tubules to respond properly. These findings indicate water diuresis.

Solute diuresis occurs when tubular absorption of a solute is impaired. Symptoms of solute diuresis are high urinary specific gravity, high urinary osmolality, and normal or low serum sodium. Solute diuresis may occur in patients with diabetes mellitus or those who have had bladder obstructions corrected.

Water diuresis and solute diuresis usually occur in conjunction with polyuria. The interplay and responsiveness to feedback systems between filtration, reabsorption, and secretion determine the volume and composition of urine released from the body. Diluting and concentrating mechanisms of the nephrons maintain fluid volume in the presence of normal renal blood flow. Dilution results when the kidneys reabsorb solute but not the accompanying water. Concentration of urine is the result of reabsorption of water without solute.

Based on this information, it is apparent that the amount of solute and the amount of waste product in the urine can influence volume. In other words, urine volume would be increased in conditions that cause high levels of solute in the urine. The amount of circulating volume in the extracellular space also affects urine volume. Hypovolemia can result in decreased urinary output. Hypervolemia can cause increased urinary output in the presence of normal renal function.

The color of urine normally ranges from pale yellow to deep amber, depending on the degree of urine concentration. Some color changes can occur because of medications or foods ingested.

Vital signs

The measurement of vital signs provides important information regarding the patient's fluid and electrolyte status.

Blood pressure. Changes in blood pressure may be associated with fluid volume status. Postural hypotension may indicate a fluid volume deficit. Electrolyte alterations may cause fluctuations in blood pressure as well. For example, magnesium deficits or excess extracellular fluid volume may cause hypertension. Potassium alterations may cause hypotension. Accurate baseline blood pressure measurements and blood pressure monitoring assist in early recognition and monitoring of fluid and electrolyte status. It is critical that the equipment used to measure blood pressure be calibrated for accuracy regularly and that the cuff of the sphygmomanometer is the proper size for the patient's arm circumference.

Respirations. Respirations should be assessed for their depth, rate, and effectiveness. Respiration is affected by various alterations. Potassium alterations may cause weakness or possible paralysis of respiratory muscles. Fluid volume excess affects respirations because of the increased effort required to move air in and out of the lungs. Respiration is also altered, as a compensatory mechanism, in the presence of acid-base balance deficiencies. Moist rales in the absence of cardiopulmonary disease indicate fluid volume excess.[1]

Pulse. The quality, amplitude, rhythm, and rate of the pulse yields information about cardiac status and how the patient is tolerating excesses or deficits of extracellular fluid. Major pulse points should be examined regularly to determine circulatory status and vascular integrity. Areas to assess include the carotid, brachial, radial, ulnar, femoral, popliteal, posterior tibial, and dorsalis pedis arteries. Tachycardia, pulsus alternans, and irregular rhythms may indicate left ventricular failure. A rapid, weak, thready pulse may signal hyponatremia. Hyponatremia accompanied by fluid volume excess may result in a rapid pulse rate with a full quality.

Temperature. Body temperature may increase or decrease in response to fluid and electrolyte imbalances. The skin and core body temperature should be noted when the fluid and electrolyte status is assessed. Changes in skin temperature are discussed later in this chapter.

Core body temperature may be decreased in the presence of fluid deficit, or it may become elevated in response to electrolyte imbalances. For example, hypernatremia may cause an elevation of body temperature.

Temperature elevations increase the fluid requirements of the body. A temperature between 101° and 103° F increases the 24-hour fluid requirement by at least 500 ml. A temperature above 103° F increases it by a minimum of 1000 ml. Because of increased fluid requirements with fever or temperature elevation, additional fluid and electrolyte imbalances may occur if extra fluid requirements are not met.

Hemodynamic monitoring

Fluid volume alterations may be detected through various hemodynamic monitoring techniques. Central venous pressure (CVP) gives information on the status of intravascular volume. The CVP may be measured with a water manometer or with an electronic transducer. Normal CVP values are 8 to 10 cm H_2O.

The CVP measurement reflects right atrial pressure or the filling of the right side of the heart, known as *preload;* this measurement can be used to guide volume replacement. When fluid challenges are performed, the response of right atrial pressure provides important information regarding the patient's fluid and cardiovascular status.

The CVP can be estimated during the physical examination. With a patient in a supine position, the jugular veins are visually examined for distension. The jugular vein should be distended in this position because it is then at the same level as the right atrium. The patient can then be slowly raised to a sitting position. As the patient rises to the sitting position, the upper portion of the jugular vein will collapse, and a bulge may be seen where blood vessel distension is still occurring within the vessel.

The distance between the bulge, or point of distension, and the right atrium is then a measure of CVP. When a person is fully upright, the sternal notch is approximately 5 cm above the right atrium. Measurable distension of the jugular vein above the sternal notch in centimeters is added to the 5 cm: the resulting value is the CVP. If the jugular veins are not visible above the clavicle, it is assumed that the CVP is less than 5 cm H_2O. CVP adequately reflects right atrial pressure only in a person with a normal cardiac status. When myocardial dysfunction exists, especially in the presence of right-sided heart failure, the jugular venous pressure is elevated regardless of the patient's extracellular volume.

Various pressures within the cardiac and pulmonary systems can be measured by use of a Swan-Ganz catheter. Single pressure measurements may be useful, but an advantage of IV pressure monitoring is the ability to evaluate pressures over time. The CVP or the pulmonary artery catheter can provide a means to monitor a patient's response to therapy for the correction of volume depletion and help determine volume status.[4]

Tissue turgor

Assessing tissue turgor helps the nurse evaluate the amount of fluid available to the tissues. Tissue turgor is tested by grasping the skin between the fingers in a pinching action and then releasing the tissue and observing the "tented" skin. If a person is in fluid volume deficit, the skin remains in the pinched or tented position for an extended period of time—usually longer than 3 seconds.

Tissue turgor describes the elasticity available to the skin, which depends in part on the presence of interstitial fluid. Tissue turgor is an age-related phenomenon; the geriatric patient commonly has poor skin turgor because the skin loses elasticity with age. Turgor may also be tested over the sternum, the forehead, or the inner aspect of the thighs. Using the skin over the sternum gives the best indication of skin turgor.

The tongue can also give information on fluid balance. A person with normal hydration status has one longitudinal furrow. In a dehydrated patient, additional furrows are present, and the tongue may actually appear smaller. Tongue turgor is generally not affected by age, as is skin turgor.

Thirst

The sensation of thirst is a normal function of the body that encourages the system to ingest sufficient amounts of water for metabolism. If a person has suffered water losses, the thirst mechanism encourages the intake of more water. If the thirst mechanism fails for some reason, a patient may be at risk for developing hypernatremia as a result of decreased circulating fluid.

The thirst mechanism is affected by a rise in plasma osmolarity or a decrease in fluid volume. Cells of the thirst center respond to the movement of water from the cells to the extracellular fluid by shrinking, thus causing the urge to consume fluid.[5] Psychogenic alterations can also encourage the patient to drink copious amounts of water, thereby leading to water intoxication and placing the patient in danger of fluid volume overload. People expressing a sense of thirst may often complain of a dry mouth; however, a dry mouth may also result from excessive mouth breathing. Oral dryness resulting from mouth breathing can be differentiated from dryness resulting from fluid volume deficit by an examination of the membrane inside the cheek and gum. When this area is dry, the dry mouth results from fluid volume deficit.

Appearance of the skin

Assessing the skin may provide clues to the patient's fluid status because skin changes are related to the amount of fluid in the interstitium. For example, in extracellular fluid volume deficits, the skin and mucous membranes are dry. Skin appears cold and clammy and possibly cyanotic if the patient is progressing to shock. Conversely, in intracellular fluid volume deficit, the skin may be warm and flushed. The skin may feel cool and clammy in acute pancreatitis, whereas in respiratory acidosis, it may appear warm and flushed.

Edema

Edema is the retention of excessive fluid in the interstitial space. Edema may be classified as *pitting* or *dependent*. Systemic symptoms seen in edema are weight gain, high blood pressure, and dyspnea. Inspection of hand veins is a means for evaluating plasma volume. When the hand is elevated, the veins will empty in 3 to 5 seconds; when it is lowered, they will fill in the same amount of time. Filling that takes longer than 3 to 5 seconds may indicate compromised circulation.[4] Hand veins that remain engorged when held higher than the heart for 10 seconds signify overhydration and excessive blood volume.[4]

Pitting edema is generally not seen until there is a weight gain of 10 to 15 pounds related to retention of excess fluid.[4] Pitting edema is identified by pressing the tissue with the fingers; if an indentation remains, pitting edema is present. It is best to test the ankles or feet of an ambulatory person or the sacral area of a bedridden person. A more accurate means of determining edema is by daily measurement with a measuring tape. Pitting is classified from a +1 to a +4, with +4 being the most severe.

Dependent edema is generally related to gravity. Fluid accumulates in any portion of the body that is dependent. If a person is ambulatory, dependent edema may be seen mostly in the feet and ankles, or possibly in the buttocks if the patient has been sitting for a long period. The sacral area of the patient confined to bed rest should be evaluated for dependent edema.

Some edema is refractory, meaning that it persists after appropriate therapy, such as diuretics or salt-restricted diets, has been implemented. Persons with refractory edema may have persistent weight gain and are usually hypertensive. Edema usually results from an increase in the total body sodium content. Circulatory overload may cause edema and is generally associated with either heart failure or renal failure caused by sodium and water retention.

Edema may be associated with overly aggressive infusion of hypertonic IV solutions. The cause of this edema is generally thought to be a rise in plasma hydrostatic pressure, which forces fluid into the interstitial spaces. Edema may occur when plasma protein is low, resulting in decreased plasma oncotic pressure. A decrease in plasma protein occurs in kidney disease, when there is a loss of protein, cirrhosis, serous drainage, or hemorrhage. Edema may also be associated with interference in venous return or obstruction of the lymphatic system.

It is important to remember that edema may manifest itself in various ways, not just in dependent areas of the body. The patient's history may reveal such symptoms as swollen feet, the feeling of tightness in the lower legs, or puffiness of the face or fingers. Rings may fit too tightly. A patient may complain of a rapid weight gain. If the lungs or heart are involved, a patient may speak of dyspnea on exertion or at night. Obtaining daily weights can be beneficial in identifying and monitoring the edematous state and its treatment.

Tearing and salivation

Tearing and salivation are most useful in assessing fluid balance in an infant or child. A child suffering from a fluid volume deficit of moderate proportions will not produce tears or salivate.

Behavioral and sensory changes

Behavioral changes may occur in relation to fluid and electrolyte imbalance. A patient suffering from a fluid deficit may be apprehensive and restless. Coma may occur in severe cases. Fluid volume excess may cause hyperirritability, disorientation, and mental disturbances. Metabolic acidosis may cause apathy, disorientation, delirium, or stupor. Metabolic alkalosis may cause belligerence, irritability, disorientation, or lethargy. Potassium deficit may cause changes in speech, lethargy, apathy, irritability,

Table 18-3 Selected Laboratory Values

LABORATORY TEST	PARAMETER	LABORATORY TEST	PARAMETER
BLOOD CHEMISTRY/ ELECTROLYTES	**NORMAL VALUES**	Calcium (ionized)	4.6-5.3 mg/dl
		Magnesium	1.6-2.6 mg/dl
Blood urea nitrogen (BUN)	6-20 mg/dl	Chloride	98-107 mEq/L
Serum creatinine	Male: 0.6-1.1 mg/dl	Carbon dioxide	22-28 mEq/L
	Female: 0.7-1.3 mg/dl	Phosphorus	2.3-4.1 mg/dl
Creatinine clearance	Male: 94-140 ml/min	Zinc	70-120 µg/dl
	Female: 72-110 ml/min	Lithium	Therapeutic: 0.5-1.4 mEq/L
Hematocrit	Male: 39%-49%	Serum proteins	Total: 6.4-8.3 g/dl
	Female: 35%-45%	Albumin	3.5-5.2 g/dl
Hemoglobin	Male: 13.2-17.3 g/dl	Lactic acid	Venous: 8.1-15.3 mg/dl
	Female: 11.7-15.5 g/dl		Arterial: <11.3 mg/dl
Red blood cells	Male: 4.5-5.9×10^{12}/L	Serum salicylates	Therapeutic range:
	Female: 4.1-5.1×10^{12}/L		Anagesia <100 µg/ml
Mean corpuscular volume (MCV)	80-96 fL		Antiinflammatory 150-300 µg/ml
Mean corpuscular hemoglobin (MCH)	27.5-33.2 pg		Toxic range >500 µg/ml
Mean corpuscular hemoglobin concentration (MCHC)	33.4%-35.5%	Anion gap	10-20 mEq/L
		Aspartate aminotransferase (AST) (SGOT)	8-20 units/L
COMPLETE BLOOD COUNT		Alanine aminotransferase (ALT) (SGPT)	Male: 10-40 units/L
Total leukocytes	4.5-11.0×10^{3}/µl		Female: 7-35 units/L
Segmented neutrophils	1.8-7.8×10^{9}/L	Alkaline phosphatase	4.5-13 units/L
Lymphocytes	1.0-4.8×10^{9}/L	**SERUM BILIRUBIN**	
Monocytes	0.0-0.8×10^{9}/L	Total	0.3-1.2 mg/dl
Eosinophils	0.0-0.45×10^{9}/L	Direct (conjugated)	<0.2 mg/dl
Basophils	0.0-0.2×10^{9}/L	Indirect (unconjugated)	<1.1 mg/dl
Platelets	150-400×10^{9}/L	Lactate dehydrogenase (LDH)	100-190 units/L
Reticulocytes	25-75×10^{9}/L	**URINE CHEMISTRY/ ELECTROLYTES**	
Prothrombin time	10-15 sec		
	Standard therapeutic: 2.0-3.0 INR	Sodium	75-200 mEq/day (varies with Na$^+$ intake)
	High-dose therapeutic: 3.0-4.5 INR	Potassium	40-80 mEq/day (varies with dietary intake)
Iron	Male: 65-175 µg/dl	Chloride	140-250 mEq/day
	Female: 50-170 µg/dl	Calcium	100-240 mg/day (varies with dietary intake)
Ferritin	Male: 20-250 ng/ml	Osmolality	300-900 mOsm/kg H$_2$O
	Female: 10-120 ng/ml		(usually about 1.0-3.0 times
Total iron-binding capacity (TIBC)	250-425 µg/dl		greater than serum osmolality)
Transferrin	215-380 mg/dl	Specific gravity (SG)	Random samples have an SG of 1.016-1.022
Partial thromboplastin time	Activated: <35 sec		
Fibrinogen	200-400 mg/dl	pH	4.6-8.0
Serum osmolality	275-295 mOsm/kg	**ARTERIAL BLOOD GASES**	
Serum amylase	27-131 units/L	pH	7.35-7.45
Serum glucose	74-106 mg/dl	Pao$_2$	83-108 mm Hg
SERUM ELECTROLYTES*		Paco$_2$	32-48 mm Hg
Sodium	136-145 mEq/L	Bicarbonate	19.8-24.8 mEq/L
Potassium	3.5-5.0 mEq/L	Base excess	−2 to +3
Calcium (total)	8.6-10.0 mg/dl		

Adapted from Burtis CA, Ashwood ER: *Tietz textbook of clinical chemistry,* ed 3, Philadelphia, 1999, WB Saunders; Henry JB: *Clinical diagnosis and management by laboratory methods,* ed 19, Philadelphia, 1996, WB Saunders; and Cavanaugh BM: *Nurse's manual of laboratory and diagnostic tests,* ed 3, Philadelphia, 1999, FA Davis.
*Measurement of electrolytes may be of limited value because of recent administration of diuretics or lack of knowledge of dietary intake.

and mental confusion. Calcium excess may cause lethargy, exhaustion, mental confusion, a loss of interest in surroundings, and irritability. Magnesium deficiency may cause hallucinations, illusions, extreme confusion, or aggressive behavior. As seen by these examples, it is important to have a baseline understanding of a patient's normal behavior and reaction to surroundings so that subtle changes in behavior can be recognized.

LABORATORY DATA

Obtaining and evaluating a patient's laboratory data are important adjuncts to the physical and clinical assessment. Laboratory data most useful in evaluating fluid and electrolyte status are the blood urea nitrogen, serum creatinine, hematocrit, hemoglobin, serum osmolality, serum electrolyte values (sodium, potassium, chloride, calcium, magnesium, phosphate, and bicarbonate), and arterial blood gases (pH, Pa_{O_2}, Pa_{CO_2}, bicarbonate, and base excess). Table 18-3[1,3,5] provides normal values for these and other tests that are useful in evaluating patients with problems related to IV therapy. (These values may vary among facilities. "Normal" values must be referenced with the laboratory performing the tests.)

SUMMARY

Although not primarily responsible for a complete physical assessment, it is imperative that the infusion nurse demonstrate competency in assessing fluid volume and electrolyte imbalances. By using the systems approach for clinical assessment and obtaining information from the patient's medical history, one can more accurately determine a patient's current fluid and electrolyte status. Accurate and timely assessment allows astute observation of subtle changes in the patient's condition. Rapid recognition of these nuances leads to improved outcomes for patients experiencing fluid and electrolyte alterations.

REFERENCES

1. Metheny NM: *Fluid and electrolyte balance: nursing considerations,* ed 3, Philadelphia, 1996, JB Lippincott.
2. Corrigan A, Pelletier G, Alexander M: *Core curriculum for intravenous nursing,* ed 2, Philadelphia, 2000, Lippincott.
3. Chernecky C, Berger BJ: *Laboratory tests and diagnostic procedures,* ed 2, Philadelphia, 1997, WB Saunders.
4. Ignatavicius DD, Workman L, Mishler M: *Medical-surgical nursing across the continuum,* ed 3, Philadelphia, 1999, WB Saunders.
5. LeFever Kee J, Paulanka BJ: *Handbook of fluid, electrolyte and acid-base imbalances,* Albany, 2000, Delmar.

Intravenous Therapy Calculations

Gloria Pelletier, CRNI

A physician is responsible for prescribing patient medications, but the nurse must ensure that the medication order is accurate and will be safe for the patient. This chapter primarily focuses on a variety of calculations that will ensure that the ordered medication can be administered correctly.

The responsibility for preparing intravenous (IV) medications often rests with the nurse. This is especially true in institutions that have limited pharmacy coverage and in others that function without the benefit of a comprehensive pharmacy IV admixture program.

Even when a health care institution has a comprehensive IV admixture program, it is important for the nurse to remember that the person administering the drug must verify that it is the correct drug for the correct patient and that it is administered at the correct dose, rate, route, and time.

Many nurses tend to have difficulty with calculations. With our increasing reliance on technology and the increasing complexity and specialization of our health care system, nurses have come to depend on calculations performed by machines or by other health care workers. Therefore it is not surprising if some nurses find calculations intimidating.

This chapter is intended to facilitate the various calculations associated with IV administration of medication. It is hoped that this review can help the reader recall knowledge previously acquired.

MEASUREMENTS: METRIC SYSTEM

The metric system is universally accepted by the medical profession. It provides the most accurate means for calculating drug dosages. The effects of a drug administered directly into the vascular system may be immediate, so accuracy is very important. The precise measurements attainable by using the metric system make it preferable to apothecaries and household measuring systems.

Abbreviations

The units of the metric system are based on measurements of weight, volume, and length (Table 19-1). For IV drug calculations, the four most commonly used weights, ranging from largest to smallest, are the kilogram (kg), gram (g), milligram (mg), and microgram (µg). The liter (L) and milliliter (ml) are units of volume. To reduce confusion, liter is usually abbreviated as the upper case letter, because the lower case letter (l) could be mistaken for the number one. Milliliter and cubic centimeter (cc) are identical measurements (1 ml = 1 cc), but milliliter is preferred. Although units of length such as millimeter (mm) and centimeter (cm) are also used in health care, they are seldom required for IV dose calculations.

Conversions

The metric system uses decimals to calculate fractional amounts. Any metric unit can be converted to the next smaller unit by moving the decimal point one place to the right. Conversely, any unit can be converted to the next larger unit by moving the decimal point one place to the left.

When working with the metric measures that are common in health care and listed in Table 19-1, it is important to remember that they do not differ by magnitudes of 10, but rather by magnitudes of 1000. Therefore one of these units can be converted to the next smaller unit by moving the decimal point three places to the right.

Example 1: A kilogram is larger than a gram, so the decimal point should be moved three places to the right.

$$1 \text{ kilogram} = 1.000. \text{ grams}$$

$$1 \text{ milligram} = 1.000. \text{ micrograms}$$

$$1 \text{ liter} = 1.000. \text{ milliliters}$$

Conversely, a unit from Table 19-1 can be converted to the next larger unit by moving the decimal point three places to the left.

Table 19-1	**Metric System Abbreviations**	
WEIGHT	**VOLUME**	**LENGTH**
Kilogram = kg	Liter = L	Centimeter = cm
Gram = g	Milliliter = ml	Millimeter = mm
Milligram = mg	Cubic	
Microgram = μg	centimeter = cc	

Table 19-2	**Metric Conversion Factors**			
WEIGHT				
kilogram	×	1000	=	1000 grams
1 gram	×	1000	=	1000 milligrams
1 milligram	×	1000	=	1000 micrograms
1 microgram	÷	1000	=	0.001 milligram
1 milligram	÷	1000	=	0.001 gram
1 gram	÷	1000	=	0.001 kilogram
VOLUME				
1 liter	×	1000	=	1000 milliliters
1 milliliter	÷	1000	=	0.001 liter

Example 2: A gram is smaller than a kilogram, so the decimal point should be moved three places to the left.*

$$1 \text{ gram} = 0.001. \text{ kilograms}$$

$$1 \text{ microgram} = 0.001. \text{ milligrams}$$

$$1 \text{ milliliter} = 0.001. \text{ liters}$$

An alternative method for converting a larger unit to the next smaller unit is to multiply by 1000. To convert a smaller unit to a larger unit, divide by 1000 (Table 19-2).

CALCULATIONS
Drug dosage determinations

In determining dosages, most nurses are familiar with either the ratio-proportion or formula method. Each method is reviewed here, but it is not necessary to learn both. Readers should use their preferred method.

Ratio-proportion method. To use this method effectively, it must be remembered that a ratio is a comparison between two related items, and a proportion is the equality of two ratios.

When setting up a proportion, start with what you know about the drug from the label; the strength of the drug on hand (H) and volume of the drug on hand (V). Place this information in the form of a ratio (H:V) on the left of the equal sign (=). The ratio for the dose desired is the relationship of the dose ordered (D) and the amount to give (G), and this is placed on the right of the equal sign (=):

$$H:V = D:G$$

---

*A zero should always be placed to the left of the decimal point when the number is less than 1. This is a precautionary measure to prevent dosage calculation errors.

Thus the strength on hand (H) is related (:) to the volume (V) as (=) the dose ordered (D) is related (:) to the amount to give (G).

For an answer to be correct, the product of the means must equal the product of the extremes. The extremes are always the two outside numbers, as in the following example. The means are the two inside numbers.

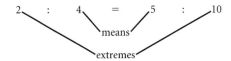

Multiply the extremes together ($2 \times 10 = 20$). Multiply the means together ($4 \times 5 = 20$). Thus the product of the means equals the product of the extremes.

When one of the numbers in the proportion is unknown, it is identified with an X. Using the same example as above, the 10 is replaced with an *X*:

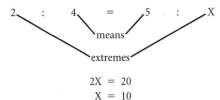

$$2X = 20$$
$$X = 10$$

To prove the answer is correct, replace the X with 10 and repeat the proofing process. If the product of the means equals the product of the extremes, the answer is correct.

Never assume the initial answer is correct without completing the second equation for proof. When administering drugs into the vascular system, it is imperative that the correct dose be administered.

Formula method. The terminology applied to the ratio-proportion method remains the same for the formula method; the equation, however, is changed to the following:

$$\text{Amount to give (G)} = \frac{\text{Dose ordered (D)}}{\text{Strength on hand (H)}} \times \text{Volume (V)}$$

In the ratio-proportion method, the example was presented as follows:

$$2:4 = 5:X$$

In the formula method, this example is expressed by the following formula:

$$X = \frac{5}{2} \times 4 = \frac{20}{2} = 20 \div 2 = 10$$

The answer remains as 10.

Example 1: A vial contains clindamycin phosphate, 600 mg/4 ml. What volume must be given to administer 300 mg?

Ratio-Proportion Method

$$H \text{ (mg)}:V \text{ (ml)} = D \text{ (mg)}:G \text{ (ml)}$$
$$600:4 = 300:X$$
$$600X = 1200$$
$$X = 2 \text{ ml of clindamycin phosphate}$$

Proof:

$$600:4 = 300:2$$
$$600 \times 2 = 4 \times 300$$
$$1200 = 1200$$

The product of the means equals the product of the extremes.

Formula Method

$$G = \frac{D}{H} \times V$$

$$\text{Amount to give} = \frac{\text{Dose ordered}}{\text{Dose on hand}} \times \text{Volume}$$

$$X = \frac{300 \text{ mg}}{600 \text{ mg}} \times 4 \text{ ml} = \frac{1200}{600} = 1200 \div 600$$

$$= 2 \text{ ml of clindamycin phosphate}$$

Example 2: A 10-ml vial contains calcium gluconate, 0.45 mEq/ml. What volume must be given to administer 2.25 mEq?

Ratio-Proportion Method

$$H \text{ (mEq)}:V \text{ (ml)} = D \text{ (mEq)}:G \text{ (ml)}$$
$$0.45:1 = 2.25:X$$
$$0.45X = 2.25$$
$$X = 5 \text{ ml of calcium gluconate}$$

Proof:

$$0.45:1 = 2.25:5$$
$$0.45 \times 5 = 1 \times 2.25$$
$$2.25 = 2.25$$

The product of the means equals the product of the extremes.

Formula Method

$$G = \frac{D}{H} \times V$$

$$\text{Amount to give} = \frac{\text{Dose ordered}}{\text{Dose on hand}} \times \text{Volume}$$

$$X = \frac{2.25 \text{ mEq}}{0.45 \text{ mEq}} \times 1 \text{ ml} = \frac{2.25}{0.45} \times 1 = 2.25 \div 0.45$$

$$= 5 \text{ ml of calcium gluconate}$$

Example 3: A vial contains cefuroxime sodium, 1.5 g/ml. What volume must be given to administer 750 mg? The dose on hand and dose ordered are not identical units of measure. Through use of the metric conversion factors (Table 19-2), grams can be converted to milligrams:

$$1.5 \text{ g} \times 1000 = 1500 \text{ mg}$$

Ratio-Proportion Method

$$H \text{ (mg)}:V \text{ (ml)} = D \text{ (mg)}:G \text{ (ml)}$$
$$1500:1 = 750:X$$
$$1500X = 750$$
$$X = 0.5 \text{ ml of cefuroxime sodium}$$

Proof:

$$1500:1 = 750:0.5$$
$$1500 \times 0.05 = 1 \times 750$$
$$750 = 750$$

The product of the means equals the product of the extremes.

Formula Method

$$G = \frac{D}{H} \times V$$

$$\text{Amount to give} = \frac{\text{Dose ordered}}{\text{Dose on hand}} \times \text{Volume}$$

$$X = \frac{750}{1500} \times 1 = \frac{750}{1500} = 750 \div 1500$$

$$= 0.5 \text{ ml of cefuroxime sodium}$$

Percent solutions. MOST solutions administered intravenously are in the form of a percent solution. These solutions are administered routinely with little consideration of their composition until the nurse is required to calculate and prepare a solution that is not routinely available.

It should be understood that a percent solution is a measure of parts per hundred. This means that 1 g of a drug in 100 ml of solution is a 1% solution. A 100-ml solution containing 10 g of a drug is a 10% solution. To make 1000 ml of a 10% solution, 100 g of a drug is necessary. This can be determined through either the ratio-proportion or formula method.

Ratio-Proportion Method

$$g:ml = g:ml$$
$$10:100 = X:1000$$
$$100X = 10,000$$
$$X = 100 \text{ g of drug required for a 10\% solution}$$

Proof:

$$10:100 = 100:1000$$
$$10 \times 1000 = 100 \times 100$$
$$10,000 = 10,000$$

The product of the means equals the product of the extremes.

Formula Method

$$X = \frac{10}{100} \times 1000 = \frac{10,000}{100} = 10,000 \div 100$$
$$= 100 \text{ g of drug required for a 10\% solution}$$

In the Drug Dosage Determinations section, the examples demonstrated how to determine the amount of drug to give. When applying these methods to percent calculations, the amount of drug to be added to the solution must be determined.

Example 1: The time is 2:00 AM and the pharmacy is not open. A flexible container of 1000-ml solution of 10% dextrose and 5% amino acids is inadvertently punctured. Available supplies are 50% dextrose in water, 7% amino acids, sterile water for injection, and a 1000-ml empty evacuated container. Prepare the 1000-ml solution of 10% dextrose and 5% amino acids.

Step 1: Determine the amount of 7% amino acids needed.

Ratio-Proportion Method

$$\% : ml = \% : ml$$
$$7 : 1000 = 5 : X$$
$$7X = 5000$$
$$X = 714 \text{ ml of 7% amino acids needed}$$

The proof of this solution is simple and has been adequately demonstrated. Remember, however, that the nurse should never administer drugs without completing the proof.

Formula Method

$$X = \frac{5}{7} \times 1000 = \frac{5000}{7} = 5000 \div 7$$
$$= 714 \text{ ml of 7% amino acids needed}$$

Step 2: Determine the amount of 50% dextrose in water needed.

Ratio-Proportion Method

$$\% : ml = \% : ml$$
$$50 : 1000 = 10 : X$$
$$50X = 10,000$$
$$X = 200 \text{ ml of 50% dextrose in water needed}$$

Formula Method

$$X = \frac{10}{50} \times 1,000 = \frac{10,000}{50} = 10,000 \div 50$$
$$= 200 \text{ ml of 50% dextrose in water needed}$$

Step 3: Using the results of the first two steps, determine the amount of water needed.

714 ml of 7% amino acids
+ 200 ml of 50% dextrose in water
914 ml

A total volume of 1000 ml is needed.

1000 ml
− 914 ml
86 ml of water for injection is needed

The combination of these three solutions in the empty evacuated container provides the 1000 ml of 10% dextrose and 5% amino acids solution.

An alternative and perhaps more difficult way to solve this problem is by using grams. As previously indicated, grams and percentages are interchangeable. The following computations test this hypothesis.

Step 1: A 7% amino acid solution contains 7 g/100 ml.

$$g : ml = g : ml$$
$$7 : 100 = X : 1000$$
$$100X = 7000$$
$$X = 70 \text{ g in 1000 ml}$$

Needed: 5% amino acid solution

$$g : ml = g : ml$$
$$5 : 100 = X : 1000$$
$$100X = 5000$$
$$X = 50 \text{ g in 1000 ml}$$

It has been determined that there are 70 g in 1000 ml of 7% amino acids, and that 50 g are needed.

$$g : ml = g : ml$$
$$70 : 1,000 = 50 : X$$
$$70X = 50,000$$
$$X = 714 \text{ ml of 7% amino acids needed}$$

Step 2: 50% dextrose in water contains 50 g/100 ml.

$$g : ml = g : ml$$
$$50 : 100 = X : 1000$$
$$100X = 50,000$$
$$X = 500 \text{ g in 1000 ml}$$

Needed: 10% dextrose in water

$$g : ml = g : ml$$
$$10 : 100 = X : 1000$$
$$100X = 10,000$$
$$X = 100 \text{ g in 1000 ml}$$

It is now known that there are 500 g in 1000 ml of 50% dextrose in water and that 100 g are needed.

$$g : ml = g : ml$$
$$500 : 1,000 = 100 : X$$
$$500X = 100,000$$
$$X = 200 \text{ ml in 1000 ml}$$

714 ml of 7% amino acids
+ 200 ml of 50% dextrose in water
914 ml, which is identical to the previous,
less complicated calculation

Example 2: A 10-ml vial contains 10% calcium chloride. What volume must be given to administer 700 mg? (Recall that a 10% solution contains 10 g of drug in 100 ml and that grams and percentages are interchangeable.)

Ratio-Proportion Method

$$g : ml = g : ml$$
$$10 : 100 = X : 10$$
$$100X = 100$$
$$X = 1 \text{ g of calcium chloride in 10 ml}$$

Formula Method

$$X = \frac{10 \text{ g}}{100 \text{ ml}} \times 10 \text{ ml} = \frac{100}{100}$$
$$= 1 \text{ g of calcium chloride in 10 ml}$$

Grams and milligrams are not identical units of measure, so convert the gram to milligrams (Table 19-2).

$$1 \text{ g} \times 1000 = 1000 \text{ mg}$$

Ratio-Proportion Method

$$mg:ml = mg:ml$$
$$1000:10 = 700:X$$
$$1000X = 7000$$
$$X = 7 \text{ ml of 10\% calcium chloride,}$$
which is equal to 700 mg

Formula Method

$$X = \frac{700 \text{ mg}}{1000 \text{ mg}} \times 10 \text{ ml} = \frac{7000}{1000} = 7000 \div 1000$$
$$= 7 \text{ ml of calcium chloride}$$

Example 3: A 30-ml vial contains 23.4% sodium chloride. What volume must be added to 500 ml of 10% dextrose in water to make a 10% dextrose in 0.225% sodium chloride solution?

Ratio-Proportion Method

$$\%:ml = \%:ml$$
$$23.4:500 = 0.225:X$$
$$23.4X = 112.5$$
$$X = 4.8 \text{ ml (rounded to nearest}$$
0.1 ml of 23.4% sodium chloride)

Formula Method

$$X = \frac{0.225\%}{23.4\%} \times 500 \text{ ml} = \frac{112.5}{23.4} = 112.5 \div 23.4 = 4.8 \text{ ml}$$
(rounded to nearest 0.1 ml of 23.4% sodium chloride)

Units. A unit may be defined as a measurement of a specific drug. The number of units in a specific drug is based on the strength of that drug. A unit is not interchangeable with any other measurement, but dosages can be calculated through use of the methods discussed earlier.

An abbreviation for unit is U. Accuracy is crucial when administering a drug based on unit strength, and it is imperative that the ordered dose not be exceeded. The abbreviation of U may erroneously be interpreted as a zero, so it is recommended that the term *unit* always be written out.

Insulin was formerly available as 40 and 80 units/ml. To standardize the concentration and reduce the potential for dosage error, production of these preparations is on the decline.

The following examples of insulin calculations refer to 100 units/ml, which is the concentration most commonly used. Some institutions have eliminated use of the 100-unit syringe for the administration of 100 units/ml insulin. They believe that the availability of 100 units/ml insulin reduces the absolute need for an insulin syringe. An identical level of accuracy can be obtained with the 1-ml tuberculin (TB) syringe. The number of insulin units required is always equal to an equivalent number of hundredths of a milliliter. Although the syringe adopted by the institution should prevail, profound attention and caution by the nurse are required when the 1-ml TB syringe is used to administer 100 units/ml insulin. On one side of the syringe is the 1-ml scale. The calibration is broken down to tenths and hundredths of a milliliter. Next to the 1-ml scale is a section not identified but recognized as a minim scale. There is absolutely no reason to use minims in drug calculations. Personnel using the TB syringe must use extreme caution so that the minim scale is not used when preparing drugs.

Profound attention is mandatory. *Do not* relate tenths of milliliters with units. For example, when drawing up 8 units of insulin, there is a tendency to draw up 0.8 ml, which equals 80 units rather than 8 units.

Example 1: How much 100 units/ml insulin is needed to administer 40 units? (When using a 100-unit syringe, draw insulin up to the 40-unit calibration mark.)

When using a TB syringe, either of the following methods can help in preparing the correct dose.

Ratio-Proportion Method

$$units:ml = units:ml$$
$$100:1 = 40:X$$
$$100X = 40$$
$$X = 0.4 \text{ ml of 100 units/ml needed to give 40 units}$$

Formula Method

$$X = \frac{40 \text{ units}}{100 \text{ units}} \times 1 \text{ ml} = \frac{40}{100} = 40 \div 100$$
$$= 0.4 \text{ ml of 100 units/ml needed to give 40 units}$$

Example 2: A heparin solution contains 25,000 units in 500 ml of 5% dextrose in water. The administration rate is 16 ml/hr. What is the hourly heparin dose?

Ratio-Proportion Method

$$units:ml = units:ml$$
$$25,000:500 = X:16$$
$$500X = 400,000$$
$$X = 800 \text{ units/hr}$$

Formula Method

$$X = \frac{16 \text{ ml}}{500 \text{ ml}} \times 25,000 \text{ units} = \frac{400,000}{500}$$
$$= 400,000 \div 500 = 800 \text{ units/hr}$$

Example 3: A vial of penicillin G potassium contains 200,000 units/ml. What volume must be added to a solution to administer 4,000,000 units?

Ratio-Proportion Method

$$units:ml = units:ml$$
$$200,000:1 = 4,000,000:X$$
$$200,000X = 4,000,000$$
$$X = 20 \text{ ml of drug are needed}$$

Formula Method

$$X = \frac{4,000,000 \text{ units}}{200,000 \text{ units}} \times 1 \text{ ml} = \frac{4,000,000}{200,000} = 4,000,000 \div 200,000$$
$$= 20 \text{ ml of drug are needed}$$

Milliequivalents. A milliequivalent (mEq) is not interchangeable with any other measurement, but dosages can be calculated by the methods discussed earlier.

Example 1: A vial of calcium gluconate contains 0.45 mEq of calcium/ml. How much must be added to a solution for a dose of 9 mEq?

Ratio-Proportion Method

$$mEq:ml = mEq:ml$$
$$0.45:1 = 9:X$$
$$0.45X = 9$$
$$X = 20 \text{ ml of drug are needed}$$

Formula Method

$$X = \frac{9 \text{ mEq}}{0.45 \text{ mEq}} \times 1 \text{ ml} = \frac{9}{0.45} = 9 \div 0.45$$
$$= 20 \text{ ml of drug are needed}$$

Example 2: A 500-ml solution contains 40 mEq of potassium acetate. The rate ordered is 50 ml/hr. How much potassium is being administered hourly?

Ratio-Proportion Method

$$mEq:ml = mEq:ml$$
$$40:500 = X:50$$
$$500X = 2000$$
$$X = 4 \text{ mEq/hr}$$

Formula Method

$$X = \frac{50 \text{ ml}}{500 \text{ ml}} \times 40 \text{ mEq} = \frac{2000}{500} = 2000 \div 500$$
$$= 4 \text{ mEq/hr}$$

Example 3: A 50-ml vial of sodium bicarbonate contains 44.6 mEq. What volume must be given to administer 25 mEq?

Ratio-Proportion Method

$$mEq:ml = mEq:ml$$
$$44.6:50 = 25:X$$
$$44.6X = 1250$$
$$X = 28 \text{ ml need to be given}$$

Formula Method

$$X = \frac{25 \text{ mEq}}{44.6 \text{ mEq}} \times 50 \text{ ml} = \frac{1250}{44.6} = 1250 \div 44.6$$
$$= 28 \text{ ml need to be given}$$

Body surface area. Use of the body surface area (BSA) is one of the most accurate methods for calculating adult drug dosages. This method is often used to determine dosages for antineoplastic agents.

To determine the BSA, the height and weight of the patient must be known and a nomogram chart must be available. The West nomogram (Fig. 19-1), most applicable for determining the BSA in children, is also appropriate for adults. This nomogram is one of several available for this purpose.

Example 1: What is the BSA for a patient who weighs 130 pounds and is 68 inches tall?

PROCEDURE *for Nomogram*

1. Find the patient's height in the column labeled height
2. Find the patient's weight in the column labeled weight.
3. Using a ruler or straight edge, draw a straight line between these two values.
4. In the BSA column, note where the line intersects. This value represents the BSA in square meters (m²).

Drawing a line between 68 inches and 130 pounds on the West nomogram indicates that the BSA is 1.7 m².

Example 2: Applying the 1.7 m² answer just obtained, what dose should be prepared for a patient who requires doxorubicin hydrochloride (Adriamycin) 70 mg/m²?

$$70 \text{ mg} \times 1.7 \text{ m}^2 = 119 \text{ mg of doxorubicin hydrochloride}$$

Body weight. There are many drugs whose dose is calculated according to the weight of a person in kilograms. Using kilograms instead of pounds provides a more precise calculation of dosage. The need for accuracy when preparing drugs in the form of units was discussed. Drugs based on kilograms of body weight require the same respect. An error in dosage calculations can result in irreversible consequences.

The universal conversion formula between kilograms and pounds is as follows:

$$1 \text{ kilogram (kg)} = 2.2 \text{ pounds (lb)}$$

Divide pounds by 2.2 to convert body weight in pounds to kilograms. For example,

$$88 \text{ lb} \div 2.2 = 40 \text{ kg}$$

To prove the answer, multiply the kilograms by the 2.2 figure. The answer is in pounds:

$$40 \text{ kg} \times 2.2 = 88 \text{ lb}$$

When deciding whether to multiply or divide to determine the kilogram weight, remember to look for a smaller number to work with so that the number of kilograms is always smaller than the pound weight. Note that a gain or loss in body weight may necessitate dosage adjustments when additional doses are ordered.

Example 1: An aminophylline dose of 6 mg/kg has been ordered for a patient who weighs 198 pounds. How much aminophylline should be administered?

Step 1: Convert pounds to kilograms.

$$198 \text{ lb} \div 2.2 = 90 \text{ kg}$$

Proof:

$$90 \text{ kg} \times 2.2 = 198 \text{ lb}$$

Step 2: Determine the ordered dose to be administered.

Ratio-Proportion Method

$$mg : kg = mg : kg$$
$$6 : 1 = X : 90$$
$$1X = 540$$
$$X = 540 \text{ mg of aminophylline}$$

Formula Method

$$X = \frac{6 \text{ mg}}{1 \text{ mg}} \times 90 \text{ kg} = \frac{540}{1} = 540 \text{ mg of aminophylline}$$

Example 2: An acyclovir sodium (Zovirax) dose of 15 mg/kg in three divided doses has been ordered for a 132-pound patient. How much acyclovir should be administered with each dose?

Step 1: Convert pounds to kilograms.

$$132 \text{ lb} \div 2.2 = 60 \text{ kg}$$

Proof:

$$60 \text{ kg} \times 2.2 = 132 \text{ lb}$$

Step 2: Determine the total dose ordered.

Ratio-Proportion Method

$$mg : kg = mg : kg$$
$$15 : 1 = X : 60$$
$$1X = 900$$
$$X = 900 \text{ mg of acyclovir}$$

Formula Method

$$X = \frac{15 \text{ mg}}{1 \text{ mg}} \times 60 \text{ kg} = \frac{900}{1} = 900 \text{ mg of acyclovir}$$

Step 3: Determine the amount in each dose to be administered.

$$900 \text{ mg} \div 3 = 300 \text{ mg}$$

Acyclovir sodium (Zovirax) 300 mg should be administered times three doses for a total dose of 900 mg.

Example 3: An infusion of lidocaine hydrochloride (Xylocaine), 1 g in 500 ml of 5% dextrose in water at a rate of 20 µg/kg/min, has been ordered. The patient weighs 154 pounds. Determine the rate in ml/min.

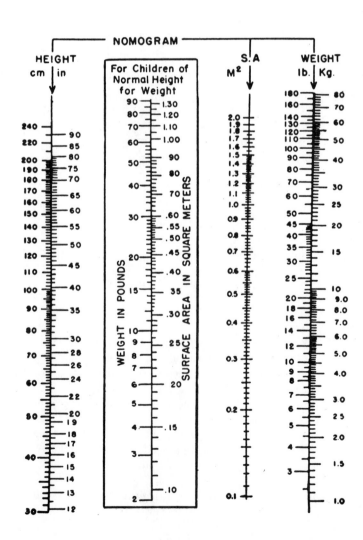

FIG. 19-1 *The West nomogram for body surface area (BSA).* (From Behrman RE, Vaughan VC: *Nelson textbook of pediatrics,* ed 14, Philadelphia, 1992, WB Saunders.)

Step 1: Convert pounds to kilograms.

$$154 \text{ lb} \div 2.2 = 70 \text{ kg}$$

Step 2: Determine the ordered dose/min.

$$20 \text{ mg} \times 70 \text{ kg} = 1400 \text{ mg/min}$$

Step 3: Determine the number of micrograms in solution.

$$1 \text{ g} \times 1000 = 1000 \text{ mg}$$
$$1 \text{ mg} \times 1000 = 1,000,000 \text{ μg}$$

Step 4: Determine the ml/min dose.

Ratio-Proportion Method

$$\text{μg} : \text{ml} = \text{μg} : \text{ml}$$
$$1,000,000 : 500 = 1,400 : \text{X}$$
$$1,000,000 \text{X} = 700,000$$
$$\text{X} = 0.7 \text{ ml/min can deliver } 20 \text{ μg/kg/min}$$

Formula Method

$$\frac{1400 \text{ μg}}{1,000,000 \text{ μg}} \times 500 \text{ ml} = \frac{700,000}{1,000,000}$$
$$= 700,000 \div 1,000,000 = 0.7 \text{ ml/min can deliver } 20 \text{ μg/min}$$

Pediatric dosage formulas

The formulas reviewed here are not considered to be absolutely accurate for dosage determination. Dosing for the child and, in particular, the neonate necessitates the evaluation of other factors, such as clinical and laboratory values. The BSA and body weight formulas are commonly used. The remaining formulas in this section are of limited value; they are provided as a reference for the reader.

The therapeutic range for neonates and children may be small and a calculation error could prove fatal. Be careful when rounding off dose calculations using the following guidelines:

Body surface area. As discussed earlier, the use of BSA is one of the most accurate methods for calculating drug dosage. There are two ways to determine a pediatric BSA:

1. If the child is considered to be of normal height and weight, refer to the section on the right of the West nomogram (see Fig. 19-1). The figure opposite the weight in pounds represents the BSA in square meters.
2. Use the actual height and weight of the child. Determine the BSA from the nomogram procedure given earlier. The BSA method is used when a dose in square meters is ordered.

WEIGHT
Less than 1 mg: round to two decimal places.
1 to 10 mg: round to one decimal place.
More than 10 mg: round to a whole number.
VOLUME
Less than 1 ml: round to two decimal places.
More than 1 ml: round to one decimal place.

As an alternative, a pediatric dose based on an accepted adult BSA of 1.73 m² and the recommended adult dose can be determined. The formula is as follows:

$$\frac{\text{BSA of child (m}^2\text{)} \times \text{recommended adult dose}}{\text{BSA of adult (1.73 m}^2\text{)}} = \text{pediatric dose}$$

Example 1: A child weighs 22.7 kg and is 50 inches tall. What is the BSA? Drawing a line between 22.7 kg and 50 inches on the West nomogram indicates that the BSA is 0.9 m².

Example 2: A child of normal height weighs 10 kg. What is the BSA?

1. Convert 10 kg to pounds: $10 \text{ kg} \times 2.2 = 22 \text{ lb}$.
2. In accordance with the section on the right of the West nomogram (see Fig. 19-1), the BSA is 0.465 m².

Example 3: What is the dose for a child with a BSA of 0.7 m² if the recommended adult dose is 750 mg?

$$\frac{\text{BSA of child (m}^2\text{)} \times \text{recommended adult dose}}{\text{BSA of adult (1.73 m}^2\text{)}} = \text{pediatric dose}$$

$$\frac{0.7 \text{ m}^2 \times 750 \text{ mg}}{1.73 \text{ m}^2} = \frac{525}{1.73} = 525 \div 1.73 = 303 \text{ mg (rounded to nearest mg)}$$

Body weight. Calculations based on body weight or BSA are the most common methods used for pediatric drug dosing. Body weight calculations appear simple, because all that is required is to convert the weight in pounds to kilograms and then multiply by the ordered dose per kilogram. Because it is one of the most commonly used methods, there is an increased potential for error because many people use calculators or mental recall to obtain the answer. It is very important, especially with pediatric dosing, to verify the answers on paper.

Remember that 1 kg = 2.2 lb. Divide by 2.2 to convert body weight in pounds to kilograms.
For example,

$$22 \text{ lb} \div 2.2 = 10 \text{ kg}$$

To prove your answer, multiply the kilograms by the 2.2 figure. The answer is in pounds.

Example 1: A physician has ordered 10 mg/kg of phenytoin (Dilantin) to be administered at a rate of 0.5 mg/kg/min. The child weighs 35 pounds. Determine the total dose ordered, dose per minute, and administration time.

Step 1: Convert pounds to kilograms.

$$35 \text{ lb} \div 2.2 = 15.9 \text{ kg}$$

Step 2: Determine the total dose.

$$10 \text{ mg} \times 15.9 \text{ kg} = 159 \text{ mg}$$

Step 3: Determine the dose per minute.

Ratio-Proportion Method

$$mg/kg = mg/kg$$
$$0.5:1 = X:15.9$$
$$1X = 7.95$$
$$X = 7.95 \text{ mg/min}$$

Step 4: Determine the administration time.

$$mg/min = mg/min$$
$$7.95:1 = 159:X$$
$$7.95X = 159$$
$$X = 20 \text{ minutes}$$

Formula Method
(Steps 1 and 2 remain the same.)

Step 3: Determine the dose per minute.

$$\frac{\text{Dose ordered}}{\text{per kg}} \times \text{total kg} = \text{dose/min}$$

$$\frac{0.5}{1} \times 15.9 = 7.95 \text{ mg/min}$$

Step 4: Determine the administration time.

$$\frac{\text{Min}}{\text{Dose/min}} \times \text{Total dose} = \text{Administration time}$$

$$\frac{1}{7.95} \times 159 = \frac{159}{7.95} = 159 \div 7.95 = 20 \text{ minutes}$$

Example 2: Tobramycin sulfate (Nebcin) 4 mg/kg has been ordered in two divided doses for a neonate who weighs 2.86 pounds. How much should be given with each dose?

Step 1: Convert pounds to kilograms.

$$2.86 \text{ lb} \div 2.2 = 1.3 \text{ kg}$$

Step 2: Determine the total dose.

$$4 \text{ mg} \times 1.3 \text{ kg} = 5.2 \text{ mg}$$

Step 3: Determine the amount to be given with each dose.

$$5.2 \text{ mg} \div 2 \text{ doses} = 2.6 \text{ mg/dose}$$

The ratio-proportion or formula method can also be used.

Ratio-Proportion Method

$$mg:dose = mg:dose$$
$$5.2:2 = X:1$$
$$2X = 5.2$$
$$X = 2.6 \text{ mg/dose}$$

Formula Method

$$mg/dose = \frac{\text{Dose ordered}}{\text{Number of doses}} \times \text{Each dose}$$

$$X = \frac{5.2}{2} \times 1 = \frac{5.2}{2} = 5.2 \div 2 = 2.6 \text{ mg/dose}$$

Bastedo's rule. Bastedo's rule determines the child's dose based on the child's age + 3 divided by 30, and on the average adult dose.

$$\frac{\text{Age (years)} + 3}{30} \times \text{Average adult dose} = \text{Child's dose}$$

Clark's rule. Clark's rule determines the child's dose based on the child's weight in relation to the average adult body weight and dose.

$$\frac{\text{Weight (lb)}}{\text{Average adult weight (150 lb)}} \times \text{Average adult dose} = \text{Child's dose}$$

Cowling's rule. Cowling's rule determines the child's dose based on the child's age and the average adult dose, divided by 24.

$$\frac{\text{Age (years) on next birthday}}{24} \times \text{Average adult dose} = \text{Child's dose}$$

Dilling's rule. Dilling's rule determines the child's dose based on the child's age and average adult dose, divided by 20.

$$\frac{\text{Age (years)}}{20} \times \text{Average adult dose} = \text{Child's dose}$$

Fried's rule. Fried's rule determines the infant's dose based on the infant's age in relation to the average adult body weight and dose. This rule is effective only for infants younger than 1 year old.

$$\frac{\text{Age (in months)}}{\text{Averge adult weight (150 lb)}} \times \text{Average adult dose} = \text{Infant's dose}$$

Young's rule. Young's rule determines the child's dose based on the child's age and average adult dose, divided by the child's age + 12.

$$\frac{\text{Age (in years)}}{(\text{Age [in years]} + 12)} \times \text{Average adult dose} = \text{Child's dose}$$

ADMINISTRATION OF INTRAVENOUS SOLUTIONS
Flow rate determination

To administer an IV solution accurately, the flow rate must be regulated carefully. Flow rates may be expressed in the form of an infusion over a period of hours, milliliters per hour or minute, or number of drops per minute. The responsibility for administering the solution rests on the nurse, who should evaluate the available sets and select the one most appropriate for administering the solution. Criteria for set selection include its ability to deliver the required flow rate.

Because it is impossible to deliver a part or fraction of a drop, drop rates (per minute) should be rounded to the nearest whole number. The milliliters per hour rate also needs to be rounded to a whole number when solutions are to be administered by gravity. (Electronic infusion devices are available that permit the administration of solutions in fractions of milliliters.)

Milliliters per hour. Several formulas provide the information necessary for the delivery of a precise flow rate.

Three-step method. The three-step method is a comprehensive flow rate calculation because it determines the rate in milliliters per hour and milliliters per minute, as well as the number of drops per minute for solution administration.

Example: A physician has ordered 3000 ml of solution to be administered over 24 hours.

Step 1: Determine the flow rate per hour.

Formula Method

Total volume ÷ Administration time = milliliters per hour

3000 ml ÷ 24 hours = 125 ml/hr

Step 2: Determine the rate per minute.

Formula Method

Milliliters per hour ÷ minutes per hour (60) = milliliters per minute

125 ml ÷ 60 min = 2.08 ml/min

Step 3: The administration set drop factor is 15 drops (gtt)/ml. Determine the number of drops per minute.

Formula Method

Milliliters per minute × Drop factor = Drops per minute

2.08 ml × 15 gtt = 31.2 gtt/min (rounded to 31 gtt/min)

An infusion at this rate administers the 3000 ml over 24 hours.

Ratio-proportion method.
The example used to illustrate three-step method can be used with the ratio-proportion method to determine whether the answers are identical. Again, a physician has ordered 3000 ml of solution to be administered over 24 hours.

Step 1: Determine the rate per hour.

Ratio-Proportion Method

$$ml:hr = ml:hr$$
$$3000:24 = X:1$$
$$24X = 3000$$
$$X = 125 \text{ ml/hr}$$

(The drops per minute calculation is identical to the three-step method, so we will skip it here.)

Step 2: Determine the rate per minute. Hours and minutes are not interchangeable, so convert the hour to minutes (60).

$$ml:min = ml:min$$
$$125:60 = X:1$$
$$60X = 125$$
$$X = 2.08 \text{ ml/min}$$

Step 3: The administration set drop factor is 15 gtt/min. Determine the number of drops per minute.

$$gtt:ml = gtt:ml$$
$$15:1 = X:2.08$$
$$1X = 31.2 \text{ gtt/min (rounded to 31 gtt/min)}$$

The two methods produce the same result.

Formula method.
For the benefit of those who prefer the formula method, the same example is presented. It was given that a physician ordered 3000 ml of solution to be administered over 24 hours.

Step 1: Determine the rate per hour.

$$\frac{3000 \text{ ml}}{24 \text{ hr}} = X \text{ ml/hr}$$

$$\frac{3000}{24} = 3000 \div 24 = 125 \text{ ml/hr}$$

Step 2: Determine the rate per minute. Hours and minutes are not interchangeable, so convert the hour to minutes (60).

$$\frac{125 \text{ ml}}{60 \text{ min}} = X \text{ ml/min}$$

$$\frac{125}{60} = 125 \div 60 = 2.08 \text{ ml/min}$$

Step 3: The administration set drop factor is 15 gtt/min. Determine the number of drops per minute.

$$\frac{15 \text{ gtt}}{1 \text{ ml}} \times 2.08 \text{ ml/min} = \frac{31.2}{1} = 31.2 \text{ gtt/min (rounded to 31 gtt/min)}$$

This method also produces the same result.

Milliliters per minute.
The ratio-proportion and formula methods may also be used to calculate a rate per minute in milliliters.

Example: A 10-ml vial (800 mg) of quinidine gluconate has been added to 40 ml of 5% dextrose in water. A rate of 16 mg/min is ordered. What is the milliliter per minute rate? The total volume of the solution is 50 ml (10 ml of drug + 40 ml of solution).

Ratio-Proportion Method

$$mg:ml = mg:ml$$
$$800:50 = 16:X$$
$$800X = 800 \text{ ml}$$
$$X = 1 \text{ ml/min can deliver 16 mg/min}$$

Formula Method

$$\text{Amount to give (G)} = \frac{\text{Dose ordered (D)}}{\text{Strength on hand (H)}} \times \text{volume (V)}$$

$$X = \frac{16 \text{ mg}}{800 \text{ mg}} \times 50 \text{ ml} = 800/800 = 1 \text{ ml/min can deliver 16 mg/min}$$

Drops per minute.
To regulate a solution accurately by the gravity method, the number of drops per minute for the infusion is required. Several methods can be used to determine the infusion rate. (Some electronic infusion devices require that the drops per minute be programmed. Others require programming in milliliters per hour.)

The drip chamber inlet determines how many drops per minute the set can deliver. The larger the inlet, the fewer drops required to equal 1 ml. The smaller the inlet, the more drops required to equal 1 ml. The drop factor is usually determined by the set brand and can be found on the outer packaging. We will review the following administration-set drop factors:

$$10 \text{ gtt} = 1 \text{ ml}$$
$$15 \text{ gtt} = 1 \text{ ml}$$
$$20 \text{ gtt} = 1 \text{ ml}$$
$$60 \text{ gtt} = 1 \text{ ml}$$

Excluding the 60 gtt/ml factor, all of these sets are known as *macrodrop* sets. The 60 gtt/ml set is known as a *microdrop* set; it is often indicated for use in pediatrics and for adult infusions of solutions at rates lower than 60 ml/hr.

Method 1: This is the longest method presented because it requires that the ml/min be known before the gtt/min can be determined.

Step 1: Determine the milliliters per minute.

$$\text{ml/hr} \div 60 \text{ min/hr} = \text{ml/min}$$

Step 2: Determine the drops per minute.

$$\text{ml/min} \times \text{drop factor} = \text{gtt/min}$$

Examples: The flow rate is 90 ml/hr. What is the rate in drops per minute?

$$90 \text{ ml/hr} \div 60 \text{ min/hr} = 1.5 \text{ ml/min}$$

$$1.5 \text{ ml/min} \times 10 \text{ (drop factor)} = 15 \text{ gtt/min}$$
$$1.5 \text{ ml/min} \times 15 \text{ (drop factor)} = 23 \text{ gtt/min}$$
$$1.5 \text{ ml/min} \times 20 \text{ (drop factor)} = 30 \text{ gtt/min}$$
$$1.5 \text{ ml/min} \times 60 \text{ (drop factor)} = 90 \text{ gtt/min}$$

Method 2:

$$\frac{\text{Drop factor}}{\text{Time}} \times \text{Volume} = \text{Flow rate}$$

The drop factor is determined by the brand or type of set to be used. The time is always 60 because there are 60 minutes in 1 hour. The volume is the amount to be infused in 1 hour. The flow rate is the infusion rate in drops per minute.

Examples:

$$\frac{10 \text{ gtt/ml set}}{60 \text{ min/hr}} \times 125 \text{ ml/hr} = \frac{1250}{60} = 1250 \div 60 = 21 \text{ gtt/min}$$

$$\frac{15 \text{ gtt/ml set}}{60 \text{ min/hr}} \times 125 \text{ ml/hr} = \frac{1875}{60} = 1875 \div 60 = 31 \text{ gtt/min}$$

$$\frac{20 \text{ gtt/ml set}}{60 \text{ min/hr}} \times 125 \text{ ml/hr} = \frac{2500}{60} = 2500 \div 60 = 42 \text{ gtt/min}$$

$$\frac{60 \text{ gtt/ml set}}{60 \text{ min/hr}} \times 125 \text{ ml/hr} = \frac{7500}{60} = 7500 \div 60 = 125 \text{ gtt/min}$$

A macrodrop set is recommended for infusions over 60 ml per hour.

Method 3: This is a simple way to determine drops per minute. The milliliter per hour rate is simply divided by a specific number associated with the drop factor.

As an example, a drop factor of 15 gtt/ml means that 1 ml contains 15 drops. Mentally, associate the "15" with minutes rather than drops. There are 60 minutes in 1 hour. Divide 60 minutes by 15 "minutes" and the answer is 4. Once the milliliters per hour are known, divide this rate by 4 to obtain the drops per minute.

In Table 19-3, it is necessary to remember only the specific number related to the brand of administration set.

Examples: The flow rate is 120 ml/hr. What is the rate in gtt/min?

The drop factor is 10 gtt/ml; the specific number is 6.

$$120 \div 6 = 20 \text{ gtt/min}$$

The drop factor is 15 gtt/ml; the specific number is 4.

$$120 \div 4 = 30 \text{ gtt/min}$$

The drop factor is 20 gtt/ml; the specific number is 3.

$$120 \div 3 = 40 \text{ gtt/min}$$

The drop factor is 60 gtt/ml; the specific number is 1.

$$120 \div 1 = 120 \text{ gtt/min}$$

The drop factor can also determine the milliliters per minute a solution is infusing.

Examples: A solution is being infused at a rate of 21 gtt/min. What is the ml/min rate?

The drop factor is 10 gtt/ml.

$$\frac{21}{10} = 21 \div 10 = 2.1 \text{ ml/min}$$

The drop factor is 15 gtt/ml.

$$\frac{21}{15} = 21 \div 15 = 1.4 \text{ ml/min}$$

The drop factor is 20 gtt/ml.

$$\frac{21}{20} = 21 \div 20 = 1.05 \text{ ml/min}$$

The drop factor is 60 gtt/ml.

$$\frac{21}{60} = 21 \div 60 = 0.35 \text{ ml/min}$$

Total volume based on milliliters per hour. For accurate documentation, the ability to calculate the total

Table 19-3   Drop Factor Conversions

DROP FACTOR	SPECIFIC NUMBER
10 gtt/ml	6
15 gtt/ml	4
20 gtt/ml	3
60 gtt/ml	1

amount of solution a patient has received is required. This total may also need to be determined as part of the patient assessment process.

Example 1: A 1000-ml solution container has been infusing at a rate of 50 ml/hr. At the start of the shift, 150 ml have been infused. What amount of solution should be documented as IV input for an 8-hour shift?

Formula Method

Milliliters per hour × Hours infused = Amount of fluid infused

50 ml × 8 hours = 400 ml infused on the 8-hour shift

Example 2: A 500-ml solution was ordered to be infused at a rate of 40 ml/hr. The rate was increased to 75 ml/hr after 3 hours. Two hours later, it was decreased to 60 ml/hr for 3 hours. What volume did the patient receive during the 8-hour period?

ml/hr × Hours = Fluid infused

$$40 \text{ ml/hr} \times 3 \text{ hours} = 120 \text{ ml infused}$$
$$75 \text{ ml/hr} \times 2 \text{ hours} = 150 \text{ ml infused}$$
$$60 \text{ ml/hr} \times 3 \text{ hours} = \underline{180 \text{ ml infused}}$$
$$450 \text{ ml infused during the 8-hour period}$$

Length of administration and flow rate

The hours for administration are based on milliliters per hour. On occasion, it may be necessary to determine the hours required for an infusion. The calculation can be completed through the use of simple arithmetic.

Formula Method

Volume to be infused (ml) ÷ ml/hr = Number of hours

Example: A physician orders that a patient receive 1000 ml of solution at a rate of 80 ml/hr and then be discharged. Seven hours later, the patient requests an approximate discharge time. How much longer must the patient receive the infusion?

80 ml/hr × 7 hr = 560 ml infused

$$\begin{array}{ll} 1000 \text{ ml} & \text{total solution to be infused} \\ - \ 560 \text{ ml} & \text{infused} \\ \hline 440 \text{ ml} & \text{remains to be infused} \end{array}$$

Volume to be infused ÷ ml/hr = Number of hours
440 ml ÷ 80 ml/hr = 5.5 hours to infusion completion

The ratio-proportion or formula methods are also appropriate for calculating this example.

Previously discussed were formulas for converting milliliters per hour to drops per minute. The conversion of drops per minute to milliliters per hour can also be determined.

Formula Method

$$\frac{\text{Drops/min}}{\text{Drop factor}} \times 60 \text{ min/hr} = \text{ml/hr rate}$$

Example: An administration set with a drop factor of 15 gtt/ml is infusing a solution at a rate of 25 gtt/min. What is the hourly rate?

$$\frac{\text{gtt/min}}{\text{Drop factor}} \times 60 \text{ min/hr} = \text{ml/hr rate}$$

$$\frac{25}{15} \times 60 = 1500 \div 15 = 100 \text{ ml/hr rate}$$

Solution container overfill

The infusion of a medication through an administration set is known as *drip administration*. The infusion may take place over a period of minutes or hours. The infusion of a small volume (usually 100 ml or less) over a short period or at specific intervals is known as *intermittent infusion*. The infusion of a large volume (usually over 100 ml) over a period of hours is known as *continuous infusion*.

When an infusion is not completed within the calculated time frame, blame is usually placed on factors such as the administration set, roller clamp, or container head pressure. The most important factor, which is usually overlooked, is container overfill.

The exact amount of solution in a manufacturer's container is unknown. When a solution is ordered at a specific rate, it must be assumed that the total volume, including additives, is as listed either on the manufacturer's or institution's admixture label. The most accurate solution container volumes are those compounded by the institution using an empty container. The volume listed on the admixture label, although perhaps not absolute, is the most accurate listing.

Containers of IV solutions compounded by manufacturers may be overfilled. Table 19-4 presents information regarding the volume of IV solution containers. In the table, *target* indicates the proposed amount to be put into a specific solution container. *Acceptable range* represents the minimum and maximum amounts of solution permitted for a specific container. Some of these containers, such as the 150-ml glass container, may contain a 33% overfill.

Table 19-4   Intravenous Solution Container Volumes

Label	Target (ml)	Acceptable Range (ml)
5-ml syringe	5.5	5.3-5.8
10-ml syringe	10.8	10.3-11.3
20-ml syringe	21.6	20.5-22.5
150-ml glass	175	150-200
250-ml glass	275	250-300
500-ml glass	535	500-570
1000-ml glass	1035	1000-1070
250-ml plastic	280	250-310
500-ml plastic	545	500-565
1000-ml plastic	1065	1000-1090

Because the exact amount of solution in a container is not precise, institution policy should indicate the preferred method for calculating the infusion rate. In policy development, consideration should be given to the following:

- Whether it is the intent of the physician that the patient receives fluids at the rate ordered
- Whether the physician is aware of solution container overfills
- The importance, if any, of infusions being completed over a specific number of hours
- Drug classifications and requirements for a consistent infusion rate

If policy determines that the ordered rate be divided by the stated container volume, the infusion time for each container should be fairly constant.

For example, a 1000-ml plastic container of 5% dextrose in water to which 1 g of aminophylline has been added could actually contain 1130 ml (see Table 19-4):

$$
\begin{array}{ll}
1090\ \text{ml} & \text{5\% dextrose in water} \\
\underline{40\ \text{ml}} & \underline{\text{aminophylline (1 g)}} \\
1130\ \text{ml} & \text{total}
\end{array}
$$

The ordered infusion rate is 75 ml/hr.

Depending on institution policy, if the infusion is administered at a rate exactly as ordered, it may take up to 15 hours for completion:

$$1130\ \text{ml} \div 75\ \text{ml/hr} = 15\ \text{hr of infusion time}$$

If the infusion rate is to be based on a 1000-ml container, on the other hand, rate adjustments may be necessary. This method requires the nurse to determine the amount of solution remaining to be infused at some point after the infusion has been started but before it is complete. Based on the container calibrations, the volume remaining is divided by the hours of infusion time remaining and the rate is adjusted:

$$
\begin{array}{ll}
1130\ \text{ml} & \text{total infusion over 13 hours} \\
\underline{-\ 150\ \text{ml}} & \underline{\text{75 ml/hr} \times 2\ \text{hours}} \\
980\ \text{ml} & \text{remains to be infused 2 hours after initiation}
\end{array}
$$

$$980\ \text{ml} \div 11\ \text{hours} = 89\ \text{ml/hr}$$

Increasing the rate from 75 ml/hr to 89 ml/hr at the start of the third hour should result in complete infusion over 13 hours.

SUMMARY

The author recommends that the reader select a preferred method (ratio-proportion versus formula) for specific calculations. The consistent use of a particular method results in ease of use, saved time, and increased accuracy of dose determinations.

Caution should be observed when calculators are used—calculators are fallible. Mistakes can be attributed to low battery power and human error. The slightest calculation error could be detrimental to a patient. Nurses should not rely solely on the results obtained from these devices. Calculations should be completed on paper and then, if necessary, a calculator used as a proofing tool.

As stated at the beginning of this chapter, the information presented here should help the reader recall knowledge previously acquired. Applying this knowledge diligently and regularly will ensure that doses are calculated accurately.

BIBLIOGRAPHY

Aurigemma A, Bohny B: *Dosage calculation: method and workbook,* ed 3, New York, 1987, National League for Nursing.

Hunt ML: *Training manual for intravenous admixture personnel,* ed 5, Round Lake, Ill, 1995, Baxter Healthcare Corporation.

Kressin K: *Understanding mathematics: from counting to calculus,* Colorado Springs, 1997, K Sq, Squared Publishing, Inc.

Lacy C, et al: *Drug information handbook,* ed 7, Hudson, Ohio, 1999, Lexi-Comp Inc.

McEvoy G: *AHFS drug information 99,* Bethesda, Md, 1999, American Society of Health-System Pharmacists.

Medici GA: *Drug dosage calculations,* ed 2, Norwalk, Conn, 1988, Appleton and Lange.

Norville MAF: *Drug dosages and solutions: a workbook,* Norwalk, Conn, 1988, Appleton and Lange.

Phillips LD: *Manual of I.V. therapeutics,* ed 2, Philadelphia, 1997, FA Davis.

Wilson BA, Shannon MT: *A unified approach to dosage calculation,* Norwalk, Conn, 1991, Appleton and Lange.

Chapter 20

Obtaining Vascular Access

Roxanne Perucca, MSN, CRNI

PREPARATION OF PATIENT AND EQUIPMENT
   Verification of prescribed therapy
   Compatibility check
   Equipment check
   Initiating the intravenous set-up
   Patient identification and orientation
VASCULAR ASSESSMENT
   Patient preparation
PERIPHERAL INTRAVENOUS ADMINISTRATION
   Site selection
   Site preparation
   Cannula selection
   Cannula placement
   Midline catheter insertion
   Cannula securement/dressing
ARTERIAL ADMINISTRATION
   Site selection
   Site preparation
   Cannula selection
   Cannula placement and securement
CENTRAL VASCULAR ADMINISTRATION
   Site selection
   Site preparation
   Catheter selection
   Catheter placement
   Implantable port access
   Blood sampling
   Cannula securement
   Postinsertion verification
NURSING DIAGNOSES
PATIENT OUTCOMES

When nurses first began to administer infusion therapy, the sole requisite was the ability to perform a venipuncture skillfully. Today, with the technologic development of vascular access devices, the use of multiple delivery systems, and the administration of highly specialized treatment modalities, the nurse must be knowledgeable and clinically competent to ensure the safe delivery of infusion therapy. The nurse must be committed to the delivery of safe, cost-effective, quality infusion care.

Before infusion therapy can be initiated, consideration must be given to the nursing process. A holistic approach is used to assess the patient's health care status, develop and implement nursing interventions, and evaluate patient outcomes. A nursing history is obtained to help describe the whole patient. The nursing history provides patients with an opportunity to express their concerns and fears related to infusion therapy and to be active participants in their care. The following questions may be asked during a nursing history interview:

1. Has the patient had previous experience with intravenous (IV) placement?
2. What was the patient's outcome?
3. What are the ramifications for the present infusion interventions?
4. What are the patient's perceptions and expectations of the prescribed therapy?

The nursing history interview provides the nurse with an opportunity to assess the patient. Assessment data are collected to provide a database from which all health care team members can formulate conclusions about the patient's problems.[1] The assessment of a patient includes subjective and objective information. Subjective data are contained in the patient's clinical record, including the patient's medical history and progress notes.

Examples of information that might be documented in the patient's history include previous surgeries of an upper extremity that would contraindicate future catheter placement, previous complications associated with vascular access placement, or history of IV drug abuse. The progress notes might provide information about the patient's coping mechanisms regarding IV treatment, the family support system, or the patient's compliance regarding health care.

Objective information consists of the nurse's observations and the overall status of the patient. Laboratory data, such as an abnormal red or white blood cell count, decreased platelet count, or altered coagulation factors, require nursing consideration and judgment. The condition of the skin, the availability of the veins, and the patient's comfort level are evaluated. Nursing observations of torn, thin, or bruised skin require that special consideration be given to catheter insertion techniques and the application of dressings. A hypotensive, diaphoretic patient with labored respirations requires nursing interventions and decisions regarding the type and size of the infusion device to be inserted. Nursing judgments are required before the placement of an IV catheter. The patient who is confused, combative, or physically restrained requires decisions ensuring safety. The nurse must decide how the IV catheter can be protected to prevent the patient from pulling it out, and how to protect the patient from harm if an infiltration occurs.

The decisions made and interventions taken are determined by the information acquired in the patient assessment. Nursing judgments are based on a synthesis of knowledge, experience, and observation. The needs and problems of the patient are identified and prioritized into nursing diagnoses. Commonly encountered nursing diagnoses in the administration of infusion therapy include the potential for infection, anxiety, impairment of skin integrity, and potential for fluid and electrolyte imbalance. A nursing care plan is developed and implemented to organize and provide goal-directed nursing care. In many organizations, clinical pathways are used to organize and provide goals for patient care. Establishing good, sound, clinical pathways ensures that care is goal directed, cost-effective, and high quality. The goals of a nursing care plan or clinical pathway are developed in consultation with the patient and must be documented and communicated to the patient and other members of the health care team. The infusion nurse must plan and provide the necessary specialized interventions. An ongoing evaluation process delineates the patient outcomes achieved.

Expected patient outcomes result from the use of the nursing process and from the delivery of infusion care according to established policies and procedures. Policies and procedures describe acceptable nursing interventions and actions to promote the delivery of safe, high-quality infusion care. The development and implementation of infusion policies and procedures should be based on established professional standards of practice. The Intravenous Nurses Society has established professional standards in the publication *Infusion Nursing Standards of Practice.*[2]

PREPARATION OF PATIENT AND EQUIPMENT
Verification of prescribed therapy

The initiation of IV therapy requires an order by the physician or other authorized individual, which must be written in the patient's medical record. The order must be complete and consist of the name of the solution or medication to be used; the dosage; the volume to be infused; and the rate, frequency, and route of administration. The nurse must assess and ensure that the order is appropriate for the patient. If the order is incomplete, illegible, unclear, or inappropriate, the physician should be contacted for clarification.

Compatibility check

After the order has been verified, the nurse assesses the order and its implications for the patient. Particular attention is given to identifying allergies to medications, iodine, latex, and tape. The patient's status is evaluated, and the outcome goal is reviewed.

When multiple solutions or medications are to be infused, consideration must be given to compatibility. More than one infusion site may be required if the medications to be infused are incompatible. A pharmacist or pharmaceutical compatibility reference guide should be consulted to determine compatibilities.

If the compatibility of the solution or medications is not known, the IV system must be flushed with a compatible solution. The IV administration set or device can be flushed by using a syringe filled with 0.9% sodium chloride or by establishing a 0.9% sodium chloride or 5% dextrose and water administration system that is used before and after the administration of incompatible medications. Some facilities have established flushing policies that take into consideration the number of medications to be administered per day. For example, if two or fewer medications are administered per day, the sodium chloride syringe method can be used to flush the IV line. If more than two medications are to be administered per day, a separate administration system to flush the IV line must be established.

Equipment check

After the orders have been verified and the type of infusion system has been determined, the nurse gathers the equipment. The fluid container is examined to verify that the type and volume of parenteral fluid match the order, taking note of any medications that are to be added. The container is checked for leaks, and the expiration date is verified. The fluid is observed for clarity and particulate matter. If there are any doubts regarding the suitability of the parenteral fluid, it must be returned to the dispensing department.

Initiating the intravenous set-up

The procedure in Box 20-1 may be used to prepare a fluid container and an IV administration tubing set for use.

If the IV device is to be inserted for intermittent therapy, a 2-ml syringe of 0.9% sodium chloride and an injection cap must be collected. The remaining venipuncture equipment is gathered. Start kits are advantageous because they can contain all the necessary insertion equipment except the cannula. When equip-

---

PROCEDURE *for Preparing a Fluid Container and Administration Tubing Set*   **Box 20-1**

1. Verify physician's order.
2. Gather administration set, electronic infusion device if needed, and labels.
3. Wash hands.
4. Remove container outer wrap and discard, if applicable.
5. Examine container and fluid, checking for particulate matter, cloudiness, and leaks.
6. Close roller clamp on tubing.
7. Remove protective cap from fluid container.
8. Remove protective cap from spike of administration tubing. Caution must be taken to avoid touch contamination of the spike. If it is accidentally contaminated, new tubing must be obtained.
9. Insert administration set spike into container.
10. Hang container on IV pole.
11. Squeeze chamber to at least $\frac{1}{3}$ to $\frac{1}{2}$ full.
12. Open clamp slightly and allow tubing to fill slowly.
13. Invert medication ports and tap to clear air. If an electronic infusion device is used, purge air from tubing according to manufacturer's recommendations.
14. Close roller clamp.
15. Write date and time initiated on a time strip, and tape it to fluid container.

ment is gathered separately, an item may be forgotten and therefore unavailable when needed. Many start kits are available that provide any combination of the following venipuncture equipment: 70% isopropyl alcohol, antimicrobial solution, sterile gauze, transparent dressing, tape, tourniquet, and label. The institution's policies and procedures for IV cannula insertion determine the required venipuncture equipment for use.

Patient identification and orientation

Before the infusion device is inserted, the patient's identity must be confirmed. The patient should be asked to state his or her name. The nurse should orally repeat the patient's name to ensure accuracy and correct patient identification. The nurse should then check the patient's identification band to confirm the patient's identity. The patient's given name should be verified with the medical record and the physician's order sheet.

After the patient has been properly identified, the nurse identifies himself or herself to the patient. The nurse then assesses the patient's psychologic preparedness while explaining the following: the purpose of therapy, possible duration of therapy, method of administration, insertion procedure, expected side effects, care and maintenance of the device, and any limitations or restrictions on mobility.

It is essential for the nurse to establish trust. The patient should be approached in a calm and reassuring manner. Encouraging the patient to ask questions provides information that helps alleviate fear and anxiety. When answering a patient's questions, the nurse must be honest and forthright. The nurse should always convey self-assurance and appear confident.

Occasionally, despite appropriate patient teaching and reassurance, the patient remains uncooperative. These situations require careful nursing assessment and judgment. The patient has the right to refuse treatment. When the patient refuses to cooperate with the ordered medical intervention, the rationale for therapy should be explained again and the patient's physician notified. Possible alternative routes of medication administration should be assessed with the physician and the patient. The nurse's actions and the physician's orders are recorded in the patient's medical record.

VASCULAR ASSESSMENT
Patient preparation

After the patient has been properly identified, the nurse must provide privacy by pulling the curtain around the patient's bed, asking visitors to step outside the room, and closing the door to the patient's room. In addition, adequate lighting of the environment is essential for performing accurate venous assessment and cannula insertion. If the lighting in the patient's room is inadequate, the patient may be transported to a treatment room that has adequate lighting.

To prepare a patient before inserting any vascular access IV device, the nurse should explain the rationale for the procedure, and the type of catheter, placement procedure, common complications, and expected outcome. The patient is encouraged to ask questions. The nurse can reduce the patient's anxiety by encouraging him or her to be an active participant in the placement process; active participation communicates that the patient's concerns are important and that the nurse is interested in the whole person and not just in performing the technical procedure. The patient should also be encouraged to report any discomfort experienced during or after the insertion procedure.

The nurse should also ensure that the patient is comfortable. The patient should be able to extend and stabilize his or her arm on a firm, flat surface. Sometimes, it is helpful to place a pillow or roll a blanket or towel under the extended arm. Attention must also be given to the comfort of the nurse. The height of the bed can be adjusted, if necessary, to prevent unnecessary bending.

In alternative care settings, particularly the home, the nurse may have to adapt to poor lighting, not having an adjustable bed, and lack of privacy. Creative thinking and forethought will often allow the nurse to change a given situation to provide patient comfort, privacy, and safety. For example, if a patient lives in a one-room apartment with another individual, the caregiver may want to take a walk or run an errand while care is being given. The patient is provided privacy and the caregiver has the opportunity to complete an errand.

A large flashlight can provide better visibility when lighting is poor. Because most beds in the home are not adjustable, the nurse may sit at the bedside in a chair to perform the venipuncture. Regardless of the circumstances, the nurse should be creative and manipulate the environment as needed to provide quality infusion care.

After ensuring privacy and comfort, the nurse's hands must be washed before the vascular assessment is performed. Before the venous access of the patient is evaluated, the nurse needs to consider the following questions regarding the prescribed therapy: What is the anticipated duration of the prescribed therapy? What clinical procedures are to be performed? What extremity or location does the patient prefer? and Which arm is dominant? Prior consideration of these factors often determines the success of the infusion, which ultimately results in preserving the patient's veins. To determine which arm should be selected, the nurse performs an overall assessment of the patient's upper extremities. Any injury or absence of sensation to the arm restricts the use of the extremity for venipuncture.

An extremity with an arteriovenous (AV) fistula or graft should not be used for routine peripheral cannula insertion. An AV fistula or graft is inserted usually for dialysis only and requires special consideration for cannula placement. The cannulation of grafts and AV fistulas should be established within institutional policies and procedures.

The nurse should avoid placing a cannula into the affected extremity of a patient who has undergone a cerebrovascular accident because of the extremity's decreased or absent neurologic sensation. If the infusion device infiltrates or develops phlebitis, the patient might be unable to detect these problems. Often, because of decreased mobility, the affected extremity has limited venous access potential.

According to *Infusion Nursing Standards of Practice,* a physician's order is required for cannula placement in the arm of a patient who has undergone a mastectomy or axillary node removal.[2] Before these veins are accessed, the nurse should evaluate the patient for the presence of lymphedema and ascertain when the surgical procedure was performed. If the physician gives permission for cannulation, the patient's arm must be monitored closely for any increase in swelling or indications of infection.

Applying a tourniquet promotes venous distension. The tourniquet should be applied snugly enough to impede the venous, but not the arterial, flow. To prevent the spread of nosocomial or community-acquired infection, tourniquets are for single-patient use. The tourniquet is applied 5 to 6 inches above the intended insertion site to promote the dilation of the veins. A blood pressure cuff may also be used to distend veins. The cuff should be inflated and the pressure released to just below the diastolic pressure. When a patient has extremely fragile veins, the tourniquet must be applied very loosely. Sometimes, nurses elect not to apply a tourniquet if a patient bruises easily.

After the tourniquet has been applied, the veins must be given time to fill. Another method for promoting venous distension is lowering the extremity below the level of the heart and having the patient open and close his or her fist. Lightly tapping the vein promotes venous distension; however, caution must be taken when using this method. If a vein is tapped too hard, pain may occur and cause vasoconstriction, or the vein may rupture, creating a hematoma. When these methods fail to promote venous distension, warm, moist compresses may be applied to the extremity for 10 to 15 minutes before insertion. The compresses increase blood flow to the area, which promotes venous filling.

With an edematous patient or an individual who has extremely limited venous access, the nurse may be able to locate a vein by its anatomic location. For example, the cephalic vein is located on the lateral wrist extending along the radial forearm and the lateral aspect of the antecubital fossa and biceps; the nurse, by assessment and palpation, may be able to find it. Several commercial products may also help identify the location of veins.

Veins that are tender, phlebitic, sclerotic, or located in a previously infiltrated area are unacceptable for venipuncture. If damaged veins are used for venipuncture, greater injury to the skin tissue and vascular system will occur. Also, if previous phlebitic or infiltrated areas are used for cannulation, accurate site assessments cannot be performed.

Cannulation of the lower extremities in adults should be avoided because of the increased risk of phlebitis.[3] The cannulation of lower extremity veins is acceptable in children until they are of walking age. If a cannula is inserted in the lower extremity of an adult patient, it should be changed as soon as a central line or an appropriate site in an upper extremity can be established. Institutional policy should define the authorization and approval process for cannulation of a lower extremity.[2]

Palpation of the vein is an important assessment tool used to evaluate the condition of a vessel. By always using the same finger to palpate veins, one develops the sensitivity required for accurate assessment. Usually, the index finger and the third forefinger of the nondominant hand have the most sensitivity for palpating veins. A hard, cordlike feeling can identify a sclerosed vein. Successful venipuncture requires a healthy vein that feels soft and bouncy as one palpates over and across the vessel. Valves can be detected by a hard lump or knotlike feeling. Resilient veins, which are easily depressed, are required for venipuncture. Palpation helps determine whether the vein is located in the superficial fascia or deep tissues. Stroking the vessel downward and observing the venous refill is helpful in determining the condition of the vein. Performing venipuncture in areas where valves are palpated or where two veins bifurcate should be avoided. The insertion site should be proximal to a valve or a bifurcation (Fig. 20-1).

Palpation also helps differentiate arteries and veins. The selected vein must not pulsate; aberrant arteries pulsate and are located superficially in an unusual location. Often, aberrant arteries occur bilaterally on the hand or wrist, usually on a thin, emaciated person. An aberrant artery should not be used for peripheral cannula insertion.

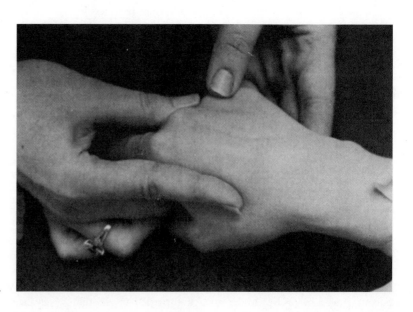

FIG. 20-1 *Vein assessment.*

PERIPHERAL INTRAVENOUS ADMINISTRATION

Site selection

The most distal site on the extremity should be selected for peripheral cannula insertion. Peripheral infusion therapy can be maintained longer by starting at the lowest point on the arm and working upward with future cannula insertions. Sites located below previous insertion sites, as well as phlebitic, infiltrated, or bruised areas, should be avoided. Areas of flexion, such as the wrist or antecubital fossa, are also not recommended. The antecubital veins should be preserved for as long as possible and are not used for routine IV therapy. A short peripheral cannula inserted into an antecubital fossa vein is at greater risk for the occurrence of mechanical phlebitis and infiltration. The metacarpal, cephalic, basilic, and median veins are recommended for venipuncture because of their size and location.

The antecubital fossa is the recommended site for the insertion of a midline catheter. A midline catheter is introduced one fingerbreadth below the bend of the arm or two to three fingerbreadths above the bend of the arm with the tip terminating in the upper arm.

Site preparation

Health care personnel must wash their hands before and immediately after all clinical procedures. Washing with soap and water is adequate for inserting a peripheral cannula. However, if long-term IV catheters are being inserted, antiseptic handwashing solutions should be used.

Standard precautions must be used for cannula placement. Gloves are worn to prevent contact with blood and to provide protection for the patient and the health care worker. When splashing of blood is likely to occur (e.g., with the use of a breakaway needle), protective eyewear must be used.

If the patient is unusually dirty, the selected extremity should be washed with soap and water before the insertion site is prepared. If hair removal is necessary, it should be clipped with scissors. Shaving can be harmful to the skin because it can cause microabrasions, which can harbor bacteria. Depilatories are not recommended because of allergic reactions, which can cause skin eruptions. Surgical clippers with disposable clipper heads are acceptable for removing excess hair. To prevent cross-contamination, the clipper heads should be changed after each patient use.

Acceptable antimicrobial solutions to prepare the skin include 1% to 2% tincture of iodine, iodophors (povidone-iodine), alcohol, or chlorhexidine.[3] Antimicrobial preparations that combine 70% ethyl alcohol and 10% povidone-iodine are available. The combination antimicrobial preparations are applied in one step and dry in 45 seconds. Unacceptable antimicrobial solutions are aqueous benzalkonium-like solutions and hexachlorophene.[2]

Preparation for peripheral IV insertion begins with the application of alcohol to remove fatty acids from the skin. Alcohol should be applied with friction, working from the insertion site outward. The prepared area should be 2 to 3 inches in diameter. After the alcohol is allowed to air dry, the povidone-iodine is applied in a circular motion, working outward from the insertion site (Fig. 20-2). For the antimicrobial solution to be effective, it should be allowed to air dry for a minimum of 30 seconds. Fanning, blowing, or blotting the prepared area are contraindicated.

If a patient is allergic to iodine, the site should be cleansed with alcohol. The alcohol should be applied with friction for a minimum of 30 seconds; the area should be cleansed until the final applicator is visually clean. Applicators are intended for single-patient, one-time use only.

The routine use of 1% lidocaine hydrochloride (Xylocaine) for cannula insertion is a controversial practice and is not recommended. Some clinicians believe that lidocaine use before catheter insertion increases patient comfort and decreases anxiety. However, its use increases the risks for a potential allergic reaction, anaphylaxis, for example, possible inadvertent injec-

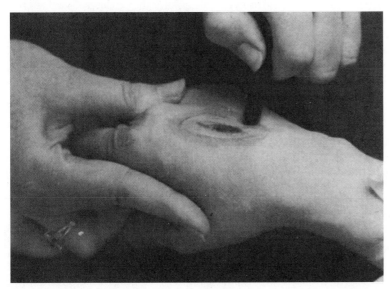

FIG. 20-2 *Prepping solution is applied in a circular motion, working outward from the insertion site.*

tion of the drug into the vascular system, and obliteration of the vein.[2] One alternative to lidocaine is intradermal injection of 0.9% sodium chloride to the side of the vein before the cannula is inserted; this method produces an anesthetic effect but does not increase patient risk, except for the potential for infections.

Another alternative is the application of a transdermal analgesic cream to produce anesthesia. A disadvantage to using an analgesic transdermal cream is that it must be applied 60 minutes before the venipuncture procedure. Vasoconstriction and venospasm have also been reported with the use of transdermal analgesic cream.[4] Transdermal cream is contraindicated in patients who have a known allergy or sensitivity to local anesthetics of the amide type.

Local dermal anesthesia can also be obtained by using iontophoresis. This method uses a drug electrode, which is applied to the area of the skin to be anesthetized. Then, using a small, battery-powered electronic unit, the drug molecule (lidocaine HCl 2% and epinephrine 1:100,000 topical solution) is actively pushed into the skin by a low-level direct current. The area of skin under the electrode is anesthetized within 7 to 10 minutes and has a penetration depth of 10 mm.[5]

Cannula selection

The overall goal of infusion therapy is a positive patient outcome. Selecting the vascular access device that best meets the patient's needs is the means of achieving this goal. The increased availability of different cannula designs and configurations adds complexity to the selection process. The duration and composition of the infusion, clinical condition and age of the patient, and size and condition of the vein are some of the factors to consider when selecting the best device for the patient.

Cannulas or over-the-needle catheter-type devices are the most commonly used peripheral IV devices. Dual-lumen peripheral cannula devices are available for multiple infusions. The plastic cannula was first introduced in 1945.[6] As the dwell time of cannulas has lengthened, the prevalence of sepsis and phlebitis has increased. Catheter composition has evolved from polyvinyl chloride and polytetrafluoroethylene (Teflon) to various polyurethane materials, and there is still controversy over the advantages and disadvantages of the available cannula materials. Ongoing research in polymer technology seeks to develop a catheter material that further decreases thrombogenicity. To promote patient safety, IV cannulas are radiopaque. Safety-enhancing designs of over-the-needle catheters and valved cannulas prevent accidental needlesticks, exposure to blood and body fluids, and promotes the safety of health care workers.

The smallest gauge and the shortest length of cannula that will accommodate the prescribed therapy should be selected (Table 20-1). A small-gauge cannula results in fewer traumas to the vessel, promotes proper hemodilution of the infusate, and allows adequate blood flow around the catheter wall. All of these factors promote increased cannula dwell time.

Stainless steel winged needles are intended for short-term duration, usually 1 to 4 hours. Winged stainless steel needles are often used to administer a single dose of medication. A winged set with a flexible catheter is also available for intermittent or

Table 20-1	Recommendations for Cannula Selection
CANNULA SIZE	CLINICAL APPLICATIONS
14, 16, 18 gauge	Trauma, surgery, blood transfusion
20 gauge	Continuous or intermittent infusions, blood transfusion
22 gauge	Intermittent general infusions, children, and elderly patients
24 gauge	Fragile veins for intermittent or continuous infusions

general infusion therapy. The device is available with a Y adapter or with an injection cap.

A midline catheter is indicated for patients who require frequent restarts of their peripheral IV cannulas, depending on the type of therapy they are receiving. The midline catheter is also indicated for patients who are to receive 2 to 4 weeks of infusion therapy.[7] Consideration should to be given to the composition of the infusate to be administered. Midline catheters may be appropriate for the infusion of IV fluids, electrolytes, and isoosmotic or near-isoosmotic medications that are appropriate for infusion into a peripheral vein.[7] Midline catheters should be inserted by persons who have clinical expertise in IV insertion or should be supervised by someone who is skilled in such insertion.

If venous access will be needed for weeks or months, multiple venipunctures can be prevented by inserting a peripherally inserted central catheter (PICC). Nurses who have advanced IV therapy skills and specialized education pertaining to PICCs may insert these catheters.

Initiating the cannula on the distal area of the upper extremity can preserve veins. Subsequent cannulation should be performed proximal to previously cannulated sites. The condition of the patient influences cannula selection. In emergency situations, larger catheter access is necessary to accommodate the rapid infusion of fluids. Cannulas inserted in emergency situations should be restarted as soon as the patient has stabilized but within 24 hours of the emergency. These cannulas are restarted because one cannot ensure that the site was adequately prepared or that aseptic technique was maintained during insertion.

The diameter of the vein and the ordered therapy to be delivered determine the size of the cannula inserted. A smaller-gauge catheter allows greater blood flow around the catheter, which promotes less irritation to the vessel wall. Small veins should not be used for vesicants or irritants. If a large-gauge cannula is required, a larger vein should be selected.

Increased osmolality of the solution increases venous irritation. Hyperosmotic solutions of greater than 320 mOsm must be administered through veins with large blood volume to dilute the IV solution and to reduce vein wall irritation. Examples of hyperosmotic solutions are 5% dextrose in Ringer's lactate solution (527 mOsm), and 5% dextrose in 0.45% sodium chloride (405 mOsm).[8]

Fluids with a greater viscosity, such as packed red cells, require a larger cannula. An 18- or 20-gauge catheter has a larger

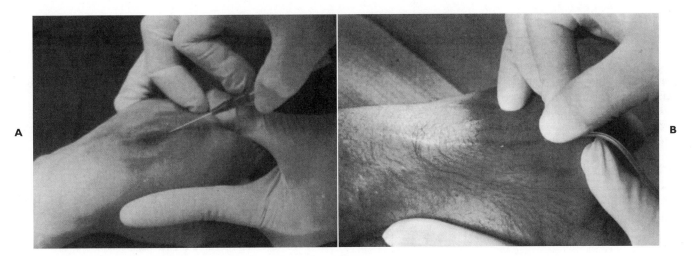

FIG. 20-3   A, *The cannula is held at a 10- to 30-degree angle as it enters the skin.* **B,** *After the skin has been penetrated, the angle of the needle is decreased as the cannula is advanced into the vein.*

inner lumen, which permits the flow of viscous components. A smaller-gauge cannula may be used in children.

Cannula placement

Before the venipuncture is performed, the cannula bevel is inspected for product integrity. The patient is informed of the venipuncture. Skin stabilization is an important element of successful venipuncture. Veins are stabilized by applying traction to the side of the insertion site with the nondominant hand to prevent the vein from rolling. Traction may be applied to the forearm by the palm of the nondominant hand, which is holding the whole forearm while the index finger and the thumb pull the skin away from the insertion site. For patients with poor muscle tone, it may be helpful to apply three-way traction. This method requires that a second person apply traction, pulling the skin upward, while the inserter applies traction downward.

With the bevel up, the cannula is held at a 10- to 30-degree angle as it penetrates the skin (Fig. 20-3). The angle used to enter the skin varies slightly with cannulas from different manufacturers. The depth of the vein in the subcutaneous tissue also determines the angle used to enter the skin. A vein located superficially requires a smaller cannula angle. However, a vein located deeper in the subcutaneous tissue requires a greater cannula angle. A direct or an indirect approach into the vein can accomplish venipuncture. Using the direct method, the cannula enters the skin directly into the vein. An advantage of the direct method is that the vein is entered immediately. The disadvantage of this method is that with small, fragile veins, direct insertion can cause the vein to bruise more easily or can pierce the opposite side of the vein wall. With the indirect method, the cannula is inserted through the skin, the vein is relocated, and the cannula is then advanced into the vein. An advantage of this method is that a small tunnel space exists between the area of entry through the skin and the vein. This method approaches the vein more easily with a gentle entry into the vessel. When

small, fragile veins are cannulated by the indirect method, bruising is less likely to occur.

After the skin has been penetrated, the angle of the needle is decreased to prevent puncturing the posterior wall of the vein. The flashback chamber is checked for a blood return. With small-gauge catheters or hypotensive patients, a slow or minimal blood return may be obtained. If a blood return is obtained, the cannula should be advanced an additional $\frac{1}{16}$ inch before the stylet is withdrawn. The cannula is advanced gently into the vein. The catheter can be threaded into the vein by use of a one-handed or a two-handed technique. With the one-handed technique, the same hand that performs the venipuncture also withdraws the stylet while advancing the catheter into the vein. This technique allows skin traction to be maintained while the catheter is advanced. It is also an advantage with the uncooperative patient because the skin traction and the hold on the patient are maintained. In the two-handed technique, one hand performs the venipuncture and the opposite hand grasps the catheter hub while the hand performing the venipuncture withdraws the stylet and advances the catheter with the dominant hand. This method requires the release of skin traction while the stylet is pulled back.

Once the cannula is totally advanced into the vein, the tourniquet is removed. If any bruising occurs while the venipuncture is performed, the tourniquet is removed immediately to prevent a hematoma from forming. A stylet must not be reinserted into a catheter; doing so can puncture or sever the catheter wall, possibly resulting in catheter fragmentation and catheter embolism. Sometimes, the stylet is removed from the cannula and the solution in a syringe or administration set is used to advance the catheter into the vein. If any difficulty is encountered advancing the cannula or if it cannot be advanced in its entirety, the insertion should be discontinued and a new attempt at cannulation should be made.

If a venipuncture is unsuccessful, a new catheter must be used with each attempt. Once a catheter has been used, it is contaminated. As the cannula enters the skin, it acquires any microorganisms that are on the skin. Also, once a cannula has been used to puncture the skin, catheter tip fraying is likely to occur. No more than two attempts at cannulation are recommended. If a nurse has made two unsuccessful insertion attempts, the nurse with the most advanced IV skills should evaluate the patient's venous access. Further insertion attempts should be made only if the venous access is deemed adequate. Multiple unsuccessful attempts limit future vascular access and cause unnecessary trauma to the patient. When the patient has limited venous access and the veins cannot be cannulated successfully, the patient's physician should be notified; another type of vascular access device needs to be established or alternative routes for medication administration evaluated. Cannula stabilization and care are discussed in detail in Chapter 21.

Box 20-2 contains a suggested procedure for the insertion of a peripheral IV cannula.

Midline catheter insertion

Only nurses who have validated competency and clinical proficiency in the insertion of short peripheral cannulas should insert midline catheters. There is some controversy regarding the necessity of obtaining informed consent signed by the patient or significant other for this procedure. Some agencies require a physician's order because of the increased dwell time of the catheter; other agencies do not require a physician's order because the catheter is not entering the central venous system. Each institution should have a written policy regarding the necessity of obtaining documentation of informed consent before the insertion of a midline device.

Although the actual procedure varies slightly with different midline devices, Box 20-3 contains a sample procedure for the insertion of a midline catheter.

PROCEDURE for Peripheral Intravenous Line Insertion   **Box 20-2**

1. Gather equipment.
2. Wash hands using antiseptic soap.
3. Ascertain the presence of allergies.
4. Explain procedure and rationale for therapy to patient.
5. Set up equipment.
6. Apply tourniquet.
7. Assess veins, keeping in mind the rationale for therapy and the duration of therapy.
8. Apply alcohol with friction in circular motion for a minimum of 30 seconds. Allow to air dry.
9. If antimicrobial preparation is used, apply in circular motion. Allow to air dry for a minimum of 30 seconds.
10. Don gloves.
11. Perform venipuncture while stabilizing skin with the nondominant hand.
12. Enter skin at a 10- to 30-degree angle. Decrease angle when skin has been penetrated. When blood is obtained in flashback chamber, advance catheter 1/16 inch, then slightly pull stylet back, advancing catheter gently into vessel.
13. Remove tourniquet.
14. Remove stylet and connect IV administration set. Begin infusing fluids slowly. Observe insertion site for any signs of swelling. If catheter is inserted for intermittent therapy, attach injection cap or needleless device and flush slowly with 2 ml of 0.9% sodium chloride solution.
15. Stabilize cannula with chevron taping, if necessary.
16. Apply dressing.
17. Write date, time, gauge, and length of catheter and name of nurse inserting catheter on the dressing label.
18. Document insertion in medical record.

PROCEDURE for Midline Catheter Insertion   **Box 20-3**

1. Gather supplies and equipment.
2. Explain the procedure and rationale for the therapy to the patient.
3. Assist the patient to a comfortable supine position.
4. Fully extend the patient's arm, which should be supported by a towel roll.
5. Abduct the arm at a 45-degree angle.
6. Prepare the work area.
7. Position protective covering under the patient's arm.
8. Place tourniquet on the mid-upper arm for final vein assessment.
9. Clip hair 8 to 10 inches from around the antecubital fossa.
10. Don sterile gloves.
11. Flush catheter with 0.9% sodium chloride solution.
12. Cleanse insertion area three times with alcohol swab sticks, starting at the insertion site; apply in a circular motion, working outward to an area 4 to 5 inches in diameter.
13. Repeat cleansing with povidone-iodine swab sticks. Allow to air dry.
14. Remove and discard gloves.
15. Apply tourniquet.
16. Don second pair of sterile gloves.
17. Drape arm with a fenestrated drape or sterile towels, leaving an opening for the venipuncture. The venipuncture site should be two to three fingerbreadths above the bend of the arm or one fingerbreadth below the bend of the arm.
18. Perform venipuncture using the technique recommended by the manufacturer.
19. Slowly continue to advance the catheter to the desired initial length. Intermittently flush with 0.9% sodium chloride alternating with aspiration for a blood return. *Caution:* If resistance is met during advancement, stop immediately. Techniques that can be used if resistance is met include changing the angle of the arm, rotating the wrist, or having the patient open and close his or her fist. Catheter may be slightly withdrawn, until blood return is aspirated, and slowly advanced while continuing to flush with 0.9% sodium chloride. If resistance continues to be met, catheter insertion must be discontinued.
20. Remove tourniquet.
21. Attach IV administration set or injection cap. Begin infusion slowly while observing upper arm for swelling. If catheter is to be used for intermittent therapy, slowly flush with 0.9% sodium chloride solution, followed by heparinized saline solution.
22. If available, secure catheter with catheter stabilization device. Cover with sterile occlusive dressing.

Cannula securement/dressing

Peripheral cannulas may be secured using various taping methods. Some midline catheters may be stabilized with catheter-securement devices. Minimizing cannula movement helps prevent mechanical irritation to the lining of the vein. Transparent and gauze dressings are commonly used dressing materials. Transparent dressings are popular because they allow direct observation of the insertion site. If gauze dressings are used, all the edges must be taped to occlude air flow.

ARTERIAL ADMINISTRATION
Site selection

The placement of an arterial cannula may be indicated for drawing samples for arterial blood gas determinations, obtaining continuous and accurate arterial pressure readings, and assessing the cardiovascular effects of vasoactive drugs. The vessel should be assessed for the presence of a pulse. The radial and brachial arteries are recommended insertion sites because these locations promote ease of insertion and reduce the risk of infection. Occasionally, the femoral artery may be used. In the radial and brachial areas, it is much easier to keep an occlusive dressing intact than in the femoral area. When the radial or brachial artery is used, the Allen test should be performed to assess the collateral circulation to the hand (see Chapter 23).

Site preparation

Arterial site preparation follows the same procedure for site preparation as for a peripheral site, except that it is a sterile procedure. Arterial cannula insertion necessitates the application of a mask, sterile gloves, and a face shield when splashing of blood could occur.

Cannula selection

Indwelling continuous arterial access requires the use of a radiopaque catheter in the smallest gauge and shortest length possible. Stainless steel needles may be used for intermittent arterial blood sampling. Cannulas are available that are specially made for arterial cannulation.

Cannula placement and securement

See Chapter 23 for a basic step-by-step procedure for arterial insertion. Arterial catheters may be secured by sterile tape or sutures and covered by a sterile air-occlusive dressing.

CENTRAL VASCULAR ADMINISTRATION
Site selection

Peripherally inserted central catheters. When the therapy is anticipated to be a few weeks' to several months' duration, the placement of a PICC may be indicated. The administration of long-term antibiotic therapy, total parenteral nutrition, pain control, and vesicant or irritant medications are some of the clinical situations warranting PICC insertion. Long-term antibiotic therapy is usually defined as lasting from 2 or 3 weeks to several months. If the duration of the catheter exceeds 1 year, consideration should be given to placement of an alternative long-term central venous catheter.[9]

One of the risks associated with inserting central lines is the inadvertent puncturing of the lung because of the anatomic proximity of the lung to the subclavian vein. When the pleural space is inadvertently punctured, a pneumothorax occurs. Because the needle used for PICC insertion cannulates the antecubital vein, the risk of a pneumothorax is eliminated.

The basilic and cephalic antecubital fossa veins are the preferred sites for PICC placement. The basilic vein is the largest and usually the best vein. The cephalic vein is smaller, and the curvature is greater where it anastomoses with the subclavian vein. Because of the risk of additional injury to the vessel and surrounding tissue, previously damaged, sclerotic veins should not be used for PICC insertion; an increase in the occurrence of complications, such as phlebitis and infection, could result. An extremity affected by a mastectomy or axillary node removal, an AV graft, or a fistula is also not recommended for PICC placement.

Short-term percutaneously inserted central venous catheters. A short-term percutaneous central venous catheter (CVC) is inserted in patients who require vascular access for a few days to several weeks. These catheters are considered short term because no tunneling of the device is involved. For this reason, these catheters may be associated with an increased risk of complications. Occasionally, with proper maintenance and meticulous site care, these catheters may remain in place longer than several weeks.

A percutaneously inserted catheter enters through the skin directly into the vein. The subclavian and internal jugular veins are the most common locations for placement of a CVC. The preferred vein for most CVCs is the subclavian vein. At jugular insertion sites, an intact sterile dressing is difficult to maintain, and the patient's mobility and comfort are altered. Subclavian insertion is contraindicated in patients who have superior vena cava syndrome, subclavian stenosis, tumor blockage, bilateral neck dissection, upper torso trauma, or a history of central placement problems. In these patients, the femoral vein may be used. The femoral veins are primarily used for short-term vascular access. At femoral insertion sites, an occlusive sterile dressing is difficult to maintain, and the catheter inhibits the patient's mobility and may be associated with an increased risk of infection.

Site preparation

Central site preparation is a sterile procedure. The insertion of a PICC requires the use of a mask, sterile gloves, a gown, a surgical scrub, and sterile drapes. Protective eyewear should be worn if a breakaway needle is used. Sterile towels and drapes are used to create a sterile field.

Long-term venous access devices, such as tunneled devices and implantable ports, are usually inserted in specialized surgical areas. Short-term percutaneously inserted CVCs may be inserted at the patient's bedside, and nurses may be required to prepare the site before these devices are placed. The method of site preparation for the insertion of a CVC follows the same principals as those detailed earlier for preparing a peripheral site, except that it is a sterile procedure. The same antimicrobial solutions recommended for preparing a peripheral site (alcohol, 1% to 2% tincture of iodine, 10% povidone-iodine, and chlorhexidine as single agents or in combination) are also recommended for CVC site preparation. The intended insertion site, if unusually dirty, is cleansed with soap and water, and any excess hair at the intended insertion site is removed with surgical clippers. Sterile surgical preparation consists of cleansing in a circular motion with alcohol from the intended insertion site, working outward. The actual size of the prepared area varies depending on the specific CVC to be inserted, but usually an area of 8 to 10 inches is prepared before placing a CVC. Starting at the intended insertion site and working outward, cleansing is repeated with povidone-iodine. Some facilities use a povidone-iodine scrub, which is removed with a sterile towel, and then apply povidone-iodine paint. Regardless of the actual preparatory method used, the povidone-iodine solution is allowed to air dry and is not removed. The prepared area is draped with sterile towels, creating a wide sterile field.

Catheter selection

Some of the types of central venous access devices available are single-lumen and multilumen PICCs, tunneled catheters, and implantable ports. Central vascular access devices are available in many catheter materials that are designed for short- and long-term therapy. Catheters used for long-term therapy, such as PICCs, tunneled catheters, and implantable ports, are usually made from a soft material such as silicone. Short-term catheters are usually made of polyurethane and may have multiple lumens. Multiple-lumen catheters allow the simultaneous administration of incompatible medications and fluids. Catheters with multiple lumens may be associated with increased catheter-related infection and sepsis because the IV system has increased manipulation, which increases the risk for contamination.

Central vascular access devices are inserted either percutaneously or surgically. PICCs and various short-term subclavian and jugular multilumen catheters are inserted percutaneously, and tunneled catheters and implantable ports are inserted surgically. Factors to consider when a vascular access device is chosen include the patient's diagnosis, the length of therapy, the maintenance requirements of the device, and the patient's preferences.

A PICC is a long, radiopaque, flexible catheter that is introduced into an antecubital vein with the distal tip terminating in the superior vena cava. Tip placement should be confirmed by radiology. If the tip of a PICC terminates in the proximal axillary or subclavian vein, the catheter is considered midclavicular. Consideration should be given to the properties of the infusate administered through a midclavicular catheter. Midclavicular catheters are appropriate for the infusion of IV fluids, electrolytes, and isomotic or near-isomotic medications. Hypertonic solutions should not be administrated through a midclavicular catheter.

The physician's order for PICC placement must be verified and documented in the medical record. The patient or legal guardian must sign an informed consent. Before consent is obtained, the physician or nurse should explain to the patient the rationale for inserting a PICC, the insertion procedure, potential complications, and maintenance requirements of the catheter.

Short-term percutaneously inserted CVCs are available in many lengths and gauges. Smaller-gauge, shorter catheters are used in children and neonates. CVCs are available in lengths of 15, 20, and 30 cm. An average-size adult requires a 20-cm catheter for the tip to be properly located in the superior vena cava. Larger adults or left-sided insertions may require a 30-cm catheter for the tip to be in the superior vena cava.

Some short-term CVCs are large-bore dual lumen catheters designed for pheresis, hemodialysis, or rapid infusion of IV solutions. Dialysis catheters are often inserted temporarily to maintain dialysis/pheresis capability until permanent access has matured. The preferred insertion site is the right internal jugular. Dialysis/pheresis catheters are also available as tunneled cuffed catheters.

A tunneled catheter is a long-term catheter that exits through the skin. Tunneled catheters have a Dacron cuff, around which fibrous tissue grows. The cuff and tunnel anchor the catheter and impede the migration of microorganisms through the subcutaneous tract. Inserting a tunneled catheter is considered a surgical procedure. A very small incision is made at the point of entry near the subclavian vein. Next, a subcutaneous tunnel from the subclavian vein is formed between the sternum and the nipple. The lower point is called the *exit site*.

After the catheter has been tunneled under the skin, it is inserted into the vein percutaneously or by cutdown. Usually, the catheter is inserted percutaneously by using a breakaway introducer. Placement is determined by the specific design of the tunneled catheter. Catheters that can be trimmed at the terminal end are inserted in the manner just described. If the terminal end is closed and not able to be trimmed, it is inserted in reverse. The catheter is inserted in the superior vena cava, and the hub end (the hub connectors are absent) is tunneled subcutaneously through the skin from the entrance site to the exit site. The closed-end tunneled catheter is trimmed at the hub end before the connectors are attached.

An implantable port is a system for IV, intraarterial, epidural, or intraperitoneal delivery of drugs and fluids. It permits repeated access for the administration of medications by bolus injection or infusion, administration of blood products and total parenteral nutrition, and withdrawal of blood specimens. The system consists of a stainless steel or plastic chamber with a silicone septum in the center. A silicone catheter locks onto the portal chamber. The catheter system is surgically implanted into the subcutaneous tissues and sutured, and the catheter is threaded into the superior vena cava, right atrium, or the appropriate cavity. A surgeon performs the procedure in the operating room with the patient under local or general anesthesia. The implantable port can be accessed only with a noncoring needle, which has a specially designed bevel that prevents coring or placing a hole in the rubber diaphragm when the needle is inserted.

The nurse should explain the advantages and disadvantages of the various types of venous access devices. The nurse, patient,

PROCEDURE *for Insertion of a Peripherally Inserted Central Catheter*   Box 20-4

1. Explain procedure to patient.
2. Assist patient to dorsal recumbent position.
3. Ascertain patient's allergies.
4. Scrub hands using antiseptic soap for 60 seconds.
5. Don mask.
6. Prepare work area.
7. Position protective covering under patient's arm.
8. Place tourniquet on mid-upper arm.
9. Measure arm with sterile tape. For peripherally inserted central catheter (PICC) placement in the superior vena cava, measure two to three fingerbreadths above the bend of the arm or one fingerbreadth below the antecubital fossa, up the arm to the shoulder and across the shoulder. Continue to the sternal notch and down to the third intercostal space.
10. Select vein and release tourniquet.
11. Clip hair 8 to 10 inches around antecubital fossa.
12. Don nonpowdered sterile gloves.
13. Flush catheter with 0.9% sodium chloride solution.
14. Cleanse with alcohol, starting at insertion site and cleansing outward in a circular motion in an area 8 to 10 inches in diameter. Repeat three to five times.
15. Repeat cleansing with povidone-iodine.
16. Remove and discard gloves.
17. Apply tourniquet snugly.
18. Don second pair of sterile gloves.
19. Drape arm with sterile towels or sterile sheet drape, creating a large sterile field.
20. Inject subcutaneously 0.5 ml or less of 1% lidocaine to anesthetize the insertion site. (Omitted if a local dermal anesthetic agent has been used.)
21. Perform venipuncture while applying reverse traction with the other hand to stabilize the vein.
22. After venipuncture is obtained, pull back stylet and slowly advance introducer (Fig. 20-4, *A*).
23. Remove stylet (Fig. 20-4, *B*).
24. Slowly advance catheter to prevent damage to the vein (Fig. 20-4, *C*). Intermittently, aspirate for a blood return and alternately flush catheter with 0.9% sodium chloride solution.
25. Release tourniquet.
26. Continue to advance catheter slowly over 5 to 10 minutes.
27. When catheter is advanced midway, have the patient turn his or her head toward the insertion site with the chin placed downward on the clavicle.
28. Remove the introducer (Fig. 20-4, *D*).
29. Slowly advance the remaining catheter to the measured length that was determined before insertion.
30. Gently remove guidewire from catheter.
31. Prime and attach extension tubing and injection cap.
32. Flush with 0.5 ml of 0.9% sodium chloride solution.
33. Aspirate with 0.9% sodium chloride to check for blood return.
34. Assess blood for type of flow, color, consistency, and pulsation.
35. Flush vigorously with remaining sodium chloride, followed by heparinized saline.
36. Secure catheter with Steri-Strips, catheter stabilization device, or suture.
37. Cover with 4 × 4 gauze and a sterile wrap for 24 hours.
38. Obtain chest radiograph for catheter tip placement. Tip should be in the superior vena cava.
39. Document in medical record.
40. After 24 hours, assess insertion site and upper forearm by changing the sterile dressing. Intermittent warm moist packs may be applied to the upper forearm to prevent phlebitis.

and physician should decide which vascular access device is in the best interest of the patient. Information regarding other vascular access, the insertion procedure, potential complications, and the care and maintenance of each catheter is provided to enable the patient to make an informed decision.

Catheter placement

Peripherally inserted central catheters. Only nurses who have advanced IV therapy skills and have validated clinical competency in the insertion of short peripheral infusion devices should insert PICCs. The insertion procedure varies slightly depending on the PICC product used. PICC cannulas come in several designs. The catheter may be inserted through a breakaway needle or cannula with or without a guidewire. With the breakaway needle design, the catheter is passed through a splittable needle. After the catheter is placed, the needle is split and peeled from around the catheter. With the cannula design, an over-the-needle plastic cannula is used as the introducer for the catheter. The over-the-needle design is also available with a valved safety introducer. The needle is removed, leaving the cannula in place, and the catheter is threaded through the plastic cannula.

Some catheter designs have a guidewire, which adds firmness

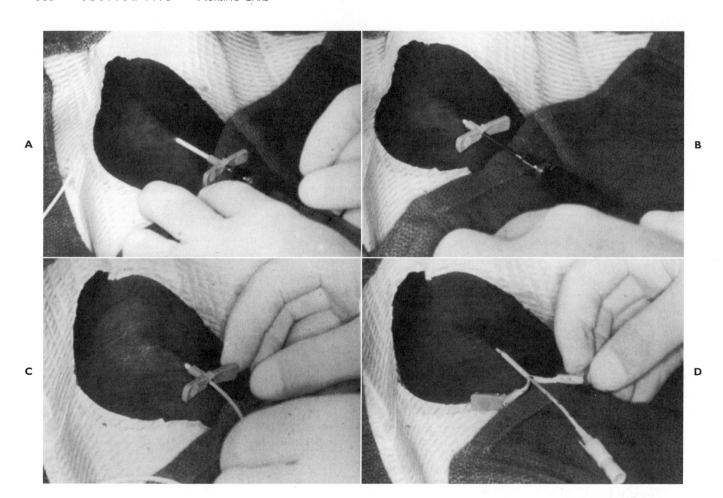

FIG. 20-4 **A,** *After venipuncture has been obtained, aspirate with a syringe to verify blood return.* **B,** *Remove the stylet.* **C,** *Slowly advance the catheter to prevent trauma to the vein intima.* **D,** *Remove the breakaway introducer before advancing the remaining catheter.*

to the silicone catheter, enhances the advancement of the catheter, and increases the visibility of the catheter on the radiograph. Guidewires are seldom used with the smaller-gauge PICC catheters or in children, who have smaller vein diameters. The guidewire design requires that venous access be established with a needle. A guidewire is then threaded through the needle, the needle is removed, and the catheter is threaded over the guidewire. This technique is commonly referred to as the *Seldinger method.* A microintroducer is also available to facilitate placement in smaller, more difficult veins. In patients with limited venous access, PICCs may be inserted using ultrasound technology.

Although the procedure varies with different manufacturer's products, the procedure in Box 20-4 is suggested for the insertion of a PICC.

Short-term percutaneously inserted central venous catheters. A physician must perform the insertion of a short-term percutaneously inserted CVC. Nurses may assist physicians with the placement of these catheters. Often, nurses are responsible for gathering the supplies, positioning the patient, preparing the skin before catheter insertion, and flushing

the catheter before and after insertion. Before insertion, signed consent should be obtained from the patient or legal guardian.

The procedure varies depending on the physician performing the insertion and the type of CVC used. Box 20-5 contains a suggested procedure using the Seldinger technique, which is the most commonly used technique.

Implantable port access

Because an implantable port is placed totally under the skin and out of view, the nurse must be familiar with the patient's specific type of port. Numerous portal devices are available. Palpation of the portal device helps determine the type of port and the length of needle to use for accessing. If the port is located in deeper subcutaneous tissue, a longer needle must be used. Many types of noncoring needles are available in different gauges and lengths. A bent or 90-degree, curved, noncoring needle is used for continuous infusion. A straight, noncoring needle may be used for aspirating blood, heparinizing, or injecting a bolus. Patency is always determined by obtaining a blood return before any medication is infused or injected. IV and intraarterial ports

PROCEDURE *for Insertion of a Central Venous Catheter Using the Seldinger Technique* — Box 20-5

1. Explain the technique to the patient.
2. Position patient in the Trendelenburg or supine position, with a rolled towel between the shoulders.
3. Ascertain patient's allergies.
4. Wash hands using antiseptic soap for 60 seconds.
5. Don mask.
6. Prepare work area.
7. Clip hair around intended insertion site area.
8. Position protective covering underneath patient's shoulder and neck.
9. Apply sterile gloves (to prepare site [if established in organizational policy] or to assist physician).
10. Cleanse with alcohol, starting at insertion site and working outward in circular motion to an area 8 to 10 inches in diameter (actual prepared area may vary in size according to physician's discretion).
11. Apply povidone-iodine detergent scrub for 2 minutes.
12. Pat dry with sterile towel.
13. Apply povidone-iodine for 2 minutes. Allow to air dry.
14. Drape insertion site with sterile towels, creating a wide sterile field. (*Note:* the physician performs the remaining procedure.)
15. Apply second pair of sterile gloves to assist the physician.
16. Anesthetize the insertion site with 1% lidocaine.
17. Perform venipuncture into jugular, subclavian, or femoral vein.
18. Remove syringe from needle.
19. Insert spring guidewire through the needle.
20. Remove needle. Sometimes, vein dilator is used.
21. Thread catheter over the guidewire.
22. Suture catheter into place if necessary.
23. Flush catheter with 0.9% sodium chloride; aspirate for blood return, flush with remaining sodium chloride solution, then flush with heparin.
24. Attach injection caps or needleless device as needed.
25. Apply sterile occlusive dressing over insertion site.
26. Obtain chest radiograph to verify tip placement and to rule out pneumothorax before initiating therapy. The correct catheter tip placement should be in the superior vena cava. If the femoral vein was used for insertion, the correct tip location is the inferior vena cava.
27. Document patient tolerance during insertion and monitoring in the medical record.

PROCEDURE *for Accessing an Implantable Port* — Box 20-6

1. Gather supplies and equipment.
2. Explain procedure to patient.
3. Wash hands thoroughly for 1 minute with antiseptic soap.
4. Palpate site to locate septum.
5. Don mask and sterile gloves.
6. Cleanse with three swab sticks of alcohol, starting with the center of the septum and moving outward in a circular motion. Cover an area that is 4 inches in diameter.
7. Repeat cleansing with povidone-iodine solution. Allow to air dry.
8. Remove and discard gloves.
9. Don second pair of sterile gloves.
10. Locate port by palpation.
11. Immobilize port with index finger and forefinger.
12. Insert needle perpendicular to the septum. Push firmly through the skin and septum until the needle tip contacts the back of the port.
13. Aspirate for blood return to establish patency.
14. Flush with 10 ml of 0.9% sodium chloride solution if medication is going to be administered. Use heparinized saline if the port is not going to be used. To prevent reflux, maintain positive injection pressure while simultaneously withdrawing the needle and syringe from the port.
15. If port is to remain accessed, anchor noncoring needle using sterile tape and sterile 2×2 gauze pad and support needle. To prevent portal erosion and needle dislodgment, secure needle to eliminate any to-and-fro movement.
16. Cover needle and gauze with sterile occlusive dressing.
17. Label dressing with date, time, needle gauge, and length.
18. Document procedure in the medical record.

must always be flushed with heparinized saline between uses. If an IV port is not in use, it may be flushed every 4 weeks. An intraarterial port that remains unaccessed must be flushed every week.

A procedure for accessing an implantable port is described in Box 20-6.

Blood sampling

1. After aspirating to establish patency, withdraw 5 ml of blood and discard.
2. Attach sterile syringe and withdraw blood volume.
3. Flush vigorously with 10 to 20 ml of 0.9% sodium chloride solution, followed by heparinized saline if port is being used intermittently.

Cannula securement

Sterile tape, a catheter securement device, or sutures may secure PICCs and short-term percutaneously inserted CVCs. Several catheters are available with wings, which snap and lock to a securement device that adheres to the patient's skin. After the catheter is secured, it is covered with a sterile transparent dressing. Some providers cover the insertion site with a 2×2 gauze and a transparent dressing. IV tubing junctions must be secured, preferably with Luer-Lok connections, clasping devices, or tape. Accidental tubing separations can cause air embolism, hemorrhage, and contamination of the infusion system.

Postinsertion verification

The insertion of infusion devices requires verification that the placement is correct. The presence of a blood return does not always provide absolute verification. If the tip of the IV catheter punctures the posterior wall of the vein, leaving the greater part of the cannula in the vessel, a blood return may be obtained, but at the same time, the fluid could be infiltrating into the tissue. It is important to assess the insertion site for swelling, hardness, coolness, and any patient discomfort. Comparing the infusion site with the same area on the opposite extremity helps determine whether any swelling is present. To ascertain whether an infiltration has occurred, a tourniquet can be applied proximally to the insertion site. When a tourniquet is applied, the venous flow is restricted. However, if the infusion continues regardless of the applied venous obstruction, infiltration of the fluid is confirmed. If there are any questions regarding the patency of the device, the site should be discontinued immediately and a new cannula restarted.

Arterial placement can be verified by observing the pulsation of blood into the tubing or a syringe without applying any traction on the syringe. Central venous placement is verified by obtaining a blood return and by radiologic confirmation. If any questions remain regarding CVC placement, fluoroscopic and radiologic examination can confirm catheter placement.

NURSING DIAGNOSES

With the recent technologic advancements in vascular access devices and infusion equipment and the evolution of nursing research, infusion therapy has developed into a highly specialized practice. The nurse must be able to readily identify and define patient care problems and plan and provide the necessary specialized interventions. The identified problems are referred to as *potential nursing diagnoses*. Commonly encountered problems related to infusion administration are fluid volume excess or deficit; altered nutrition: less than body requirements; impairment of skin integrity; potential for injury in relation to infection; knowledge deficit; anxiety; and noncompliance.

Fluid volume deficit or excess can be prevented by performing an ongoing assessment of the patient and the prescribed therapy and by frequently monitoring the infusion. Determining intake and output, monitoring weight, and assessing the integrity of the patient's skin can be used to verify that the patient's daily nutritional requirements are being met. The potential for infection and impairment of skin integrity result whenever an infusion device is inserted. Careful site preparation, skillful insertion technique, and meticulous assessment of the insertion site during site care all reduce the occurrence of infections from IV cannulas. A knowledge deficit exists for most patients receiving IV therapy. One of the most important aspects of care is the education of the patient and the family. Teaching begins before the cannula is placed and continues through the duration of therapy until the cannula is discontinued. By providing teaching, patient and family anxiety will be reduced and compliance will be increased.

PATIENT OUTCOMES

The nurse continuously evaluates patient outcomes to determine whether the nursing interventions are appropriate. Expected outcome statements for the patient receiving infusion therapy include the following: maintaining adequate intake of fluid and electrolytes as evidenced by the relief of symptoms of dehydration, exhibiting decreased peripheral edema, identifying factors that increase the potential for injury, verbalizing fears and anxiety related to health care needs, and describing the rationale and procedure for treatment.

Although infusion therapy has seen great technologic advancements, from steel needles to a variety of long-dwelling catheters, from the acute care setting to the home, from continuous to intermittent administration, it is paramount that the nurse provide quality patient care. To ensure the delivery of quality infusion care, potential patient problems must be identified rapidly. Nursing care must be goal directed, and appropriate nursing interventions must be provided. The delivery of infusion therapy is practiced according to policies and procedures that are based on established professional standards of practice. Patient outcomes are evaluated, and appropriate interventions are implemented and communicated to all members of the health care team.

REFERENCES

1. Perry AG, Potter PA: *Clinical nursing skills and techniques,* ed 4, St Louis, 1998, Mosby.
2. Intravenous Nurses Society: Infusion nursing standards of practice, *JIN* (suppl) 23(6S), 2000.
3. US Department of Health and Human Services, Public Health Service, Centers for Disease Control and Prevention: Guideline for prevention of intravascular device-related infections, *Am J Infect Control* 24(4):262, 1996.
4. Bahruth AJ: Peripherally inserted central catheter insertion problems associated with topical anesthesia, *JIN* 19(1);32, 1996.
5. Iomed Clinical Systems: *Iontoaine* (product literature), Salt Lake City, 1996, Iomed, Inc.
6. Millam D: The history of intravenous therapy, *JIN* 19(1):5, 1996.
7. Intravenous Nurses Society: Position paper: midline and midclavicular catheters, *JIN* 20(4):175, 1997.
8. Klotz RS: The effects of intravenous solutions on fluid and electrolyte balance, *JIN* 21(1):20, 1998.
9. Intravenous Nurses Society: Position paper: peripherally inserted central catheters, *JIN* 20(4):172, 1997.

Infusion Monitoring and Catheter Care

Roxanne Perucca, MSN, CRNI

The administration of intravenous (IV) therapy subjects the patient to numerous risks, such as local or systemic complications. Local complications, such as phlebitis, infiltration, and needle or cannula occlusion, occur more often than systemic complications. However, systemic complications, such as septicemia, circulatory overload, and embolism, can be life-threatening. For this reason, patient monitoring and catheter care are critical components of IV administration; early detection can prevent many of these complications. Monitoring provides information regarding the patient's response to therapy, confirms the accurate delivery of fluid and medications, and detects imminent complications. Catheter care is essential in preventing, detecting, and decreasing the occurrence of complications.

The nurse is responsible for observing and assessing the patient's response and providing appropriate nursing interventions. For example, after beginning the infusion of a newly ordered antibiotic, if a nurse observes that the patient is extremely anxious, is short of breath, and has hives on the face and chest, the nurse should intervene immediately. Interventions for this situation include stopping the remaining antibiotic infusion, notifying the patient's physician, and assessing the patient's vital signs. The patient's response to the administration of IV fluids or medications must be documented in the medical record and communicated to the other members of the health care team.

MONITORING PERIPHERAL SITES

The following aspects of the IV administration system should be monitored: fluid container, administration tubing and flow rate, electronic infusion device, IV site dressing, vascular access device, and insertion site. The frequency for monitoring a periph-

eral IV site is determined by the prescribed therapy, the condition and age of the patient, and the practice setting. IV sites in acute care settings are often monitored at 1- to 2-hour intervals. The pediatric, geriatric, or critically ill patient requires more frequent site assessments. A thorough assessment of the insertion site should be performed when the dressing is changed. The patient receiving care in the home should be taught how to assess his or her infusion device and insertion site several times daily. If administering any medications, the patient should be taught to assess the insertion site before the catheter is flushed or any medication is administered. The home care nurse must provide frequent follow up and supervision.

A systematic and organized assessment of the IV administration system begins with the fluid container and progresses down the tubing to the vascular access device and insertion site. The type of fluids and medications added are verified against the physician's or other licensed authority's order, as is the information printed on the fluid container label. The container must be labeled with the date and time that it was hung. Several types of flow strips are manufactured that can be used to identify the time the container was hung and have interval markings indicating the fluid level at specified times. Sometimes, a tape strip is placed on the container that indicates the time when the container was hung and the fluid level. No matter how the hang time of the container is labeled, the label should not be placed over important information printed on the fluid container, such as the name of the fluid or the "medication added" label. The fluid container should not be labeled by writing with a pen or a felt tip marker on the plastic surface because the ink can penetrate the plastic and leak into the infusate.

The next monitoring criterion to note is the amount of fluid remaining in the container. The nurse determines how much fluid should remain in the fluid container based on the prescribed flow rate and the indicated time. The appearance of the fluid remaining in the container is noted: the fluid should be clear—free from cloudiness and particulate matter.

The correct type of tubing should be hanging with the fluid container and the electronic infusion device. Infusates contained in glass bottles require vented IV tubing. Most electronic infusion devices require that a specific manufacturer's tubing be used. If an infusion is being administered by gravity at a very slow infusion rate, microdrop tubing should be used.

Armboards may be used when an insertion site is located near an area of flexion. Care must be taken when an extremity is placed on an armboard to ensure that it remains in a functional position. Contractures, unnecessary discomfort, skin tears, and neural injuries to the extremity can occur if an armboard is applied incorrectly. Tape or gauze may secure the armboard. If tape is used, it should be back-strapped (tape placed back-to-back) to avoid placing tape directly on the patient's skin. Tape should never encircle an extremity because such practice impairs circulation. If gauze is used to secure an armboard, a window should be left to allow easy observation of the insertion site.

The viscosity of fluids affects the flow rate. Fluids that are thick, including blood, lipid emulsions, or colloidal solutions (e.g., albumin, dextran), can alter flow rates. It may be necessary to administer viscous fluids through a larger-gauge cannula. The temperature of an infusate also affects the flow rate. Refrigerated fluid should be removed and allowed to reach room temperature before infusing. Cool fluids can induce venous spasm, which further slows the flow rate. Infusates cannot be submerged in warm water to hasten warming.

The administration tubing can alter the flow rate if it is crimped or dangling below the bed, a filter is occluded, or the air vent is occluded (with vented administration sets). When the administration tubing is assessed, it is usually helpful to start the evaluation at the drip chamber and work down the length of the tubing, assessing tubing and piggyback junctions, then continuing down to the cannula-tubing junction site. If the filter or an air vent becomes occluded, a new administration set must be used.

If the position of an IV cannula changes, the flow rate can be altered. The cannula tip may become occluded if it lies against the vessel wall or next to a bifurcation in the vein. This condition can sometimes be corrected by pulling the cannula back 1/8 inch or less. When the cannula is pulled back, care must be taken to avoid withdrawing it from the vessel, or an infiltration will occur. In addition, the IV cannula can become occluded if venous pressure increases. An increase in venous pressure occurs when a blood pressure reading is taken on an extremity that has an IV site or when a wrist restraint is placed on or above the IV cannula. Blood pressure readings should be taken on an extremity that does not have a vascular access device. Wrist restraints must be applied loosely and should never be placed directly over an IV cannula.

The flow rate changes if an undetected infiltration, phlebitis, or thrombus is present. As the infiltration progresses, the infusion rate decreases, and the electronic infusion device might sound an alarm. If the electronic infusion device infuses fluid using positive pressure, it may not detect an infiltration, in which case it continues to infuse the fluid into the subcutaneous tissues. The insertion site must be assessed when any alteration in the flow rate occurs or when the electronic control device sounds an alarm.

The monitoring of the IV infusion system continues with assessment of the electronic infusion device. The electronic infusion device is evaluated to determine whether it is infusing at the prescribed flow rate. When a gravity administration set is being used, the drops of fluid per minute are counted to determine the flow rate. The flow rate is altered if the fluid container is placed higher or lower than the optimal height, which is 30 to 36 inches above the patient. Raising the height of the container increases the flow rate. The flow rate can also be altered by any change in the patient's position. If the venipuncture site is located on an extremity near a point of flexion,

bending of the patient's arm or wrist will alter the flow rate. Sporadic flow rates should be avoided because they result in an inaccurate delivery of fluids and medications.

Many electronic infusion devices are available, and health care professionals must be familiar with the IV equipment being used for each patient. The nurse oversees the overall mechanical operation and troubleshooting when an alarm sounds. Equipment should be monitored to ensure that the prescribed therapy is delivered with minimal deviation. To ensure accurate flow rates, the fluid container should be labeled with the date and time it was hung. Some electronic infusion devices decrease the flow rate when the programmed amount of fluid has been administered. Other electronic control devices decrease the flow rate if the battery is low. When the electronic infusion device is assessed, it is helpful to read the display panel to note the amount of fluid infused and compare this reading with the volume remaining in the container to ensure that the machine is operating properly.

If the cannula-tubing junction site has already been assessed, the nurse can proceed to the IV site dressing. The dressing is monitored to ensure that it remains dry, closed, and intact. An intact dressing is one in which all edges of the dressing are sealed to the skin. If the dressing is damp or its integrity compromised, it must be changed immediately. IV dressing changes are discussed in detail later in this chapter (see Catheter Care).

The monitoring of the IV system proceeds to the assessment of the insertion site. To thoroughly assess the IV device, the nurse must know the type and length of the IV device. Many types of vascular access devices, both peripheral and central, are available in various gauges and lengths. Peripheral IV cannulas may be as short as 0.7 mm or as long as 65 cm when the tip of the catheter is located centrally. The length of the IV device determines the area of the patient's arm that requires assessment. If the catheter length is 65 cm, the area of the patient's arm to be assessed begins at the insertion site and follows the catheter tract up the arm, around the shoulder, and down to the third intercostal space. For this reason, the length of the vascular access device should be documented on the insertion-site dressing and in the medical record.

The IV site must be assessed for pain and tenderness. If a patient experiences pain or discomfort from a peripheral cannula, the site should be discontinued and a new cannula should be inserted because pain can be a precursor to phlebitis. Another cause of discomfort is infusing fluids that are cool. The tunica media, or the middle layer of the vein, contains nerve fibers. When cool fluids are administered, the veins constrict, and venospasm can occur. Therefore refrigerated infusates should be allowed to reach room temperature before they are infused. Fluids can be warmed to room temperature by removing them from the refrigerator 1 hour before they are to be administered. If the infusate cannot be warmed in this way, such as when blood is administered, the infusion should be started slowly and the fluid allowed time to warm before the infusion rate is increased. Application of warm moist packs to the vein promotes vasodilation, relieves venospasm, increases blood flow, and relieves pain.

The peripheral IV site must be assessed for any signs of swelling at or above the venipuncture site. If the tip of the IV catheter punctures the posterior wall of the vein, leaving the greater part of the cannula in the vessel, a blood return may be obtained, but the fluid could be leaking into the tissues. The size of the arm with the inserted IV device should be compared with that of the opposite extremity. If the arm with the IV device is larger or if swelling is observed above the insertion site, the cannula must be removed.

Blanching is a white, shiny appearance at or above the insertion site. It is an indicator of an infiltration or a fluid leak into the tissue. If any fluid leakage is noted at or above the insertion site, the IV site should be changed. Leaking at or above the insertion site compromises the integrity of the skin tissue. Any IV site from which fluid leaks should be evaluated for signs of cellulitis, which manifests as edema, redness, pain, and irritation that is usually accompanied by weeping skin. *Cellulitis* is an inflammatory response within the subcutaneous tissue that can be caused by the infiltration or extravasation of irritating medications, the lack of aseptic technique during site preparation, or the use of contaminated equipment or fluid. Any indications of cellulitis should be reported promptly to the patient's physician.

Redness at the insertion site indicates phlebitis, which is an inflammation of the vein. An IV site should be discontinued when the first signs of erythema (redness) are observed. Some of the other clinical indicators of phlebitis are swelling, induration, tenderness, and palpation of a venous cord. The degree of phlebitis should be measured according to a uniform phlebitis scale, which provides a consistent standard for measuring the degree of phlebitis. A recommended phlebitis scale is available in *Infusion Nursing Standards of Practice.*[1] The accepted phlebitis rate is 5% or less in any given patient population.[1] The degree of phlebitis should be documented in the patient's medical record. The presence of phlebitis may require the application of warm, moist compresses or a medical intervention, such as changing medications, doses, dilution, method of delivery, or vascular access devices.

Septic (suppurative) thrombophlebitis can occur when purulent drainage is present at the insertion site. The occurrence of septic thrombophlebitis is related to the presence of an intravascular abscess, which discharges myriad microorganisms into the bloodstream.[2] A swab culture of the drainage is obtained, blood cultures are drawn, and the hub and catheter tip are cultured. Removing the cannula does not make the infection disappear. In fact, if any of the infecting organisms are present in the circulatory system, bacteremia can result. The first signs of a catheter-related infection may appear while the catheter is in use or 2 to 10 days after the cannula is removed.

MONITORING CENTRAL SITES

All of the previously mentioned IV monitoring criteria apply to the assessment of central sites as well. The monitoring of a central site starts with the fluid container and progresses down the tubing to the vascular access device. Monitoring criteria for central IV sites depend on the type of vascular access device used. The nurse must be knowledgeable about the various types of vascular access devices that are available. When a central vascular access device is assessed, the nurse must differentiate a tunneled catheter from an implantable one. The various types of vascular access devices, regardless of where or how they are inserted (subclavian, jugular, tunneled, implanted, or peripheral), have similar monitoring guidelines.

The insertion site, catheter tract, and adjacent skin must be evaluated for swelling and induration. Swelling around the neck or clavicles is an indicator of superior vena cava syndrome. Obtaining a blood return does not guarantee catheter integrity; the integrity of the catheter and any leakage of parenteral fluid can be confirmed by fluoroscopy. If catheter integrity is compromised, the physician should be notified and medical intervention should be undertaken immediately.

The insertion site, the catheter tunnel and exit site, the portal pocket, and the catheter tract are assessed for pain and tenderness. To thoroughly evaluate the catheter tract, the nurse must know the length of the inserted catheter and the location of the catheter tract. The insertion site, the entire length of the catheter tract or tunnel, the sutures, and the portal pocket are assessed for erythema, which is an indicator of inflammation. The size of the erythematous area should be documented in the medical record and communicated to the other members of the health care team for continued assessment. An inflamed portal pocket of an implantable device is usually left unaccessed until the redness and inflammation are resolved. Any painful, reddened, or inflamed insertion site, catheter tract, or portal pocket should be monitored closely. The assessment should be reported to the physician, and medical intervention may be necessary.

The catheter insertion site should be assessed for drainage. If drainage is present, the amount, color, and consistency should be noted. A swab culture of the drainage (according to organizational policy) should be sent to the laboratory, and the physician should be notified immediately. A description of the drainage and nursing actions implemented should be documented in the patient's medical record. A catheter insertion site that has purulent drainage, is inflamed, and is possibly infected, needs to be monitored closely. The catheter usually is discontinued, and systemic antibiotics are prescribed for the patient. If fever is present, semiquantitative blood cultures should be performed to determine the causative organisms and the source of the infection. The definitive method to determine catheter sepsis is to perform a culture of the catheter tip. The most commonly used method to perform a culture of the catheter tip is the semiquantitative culture. A disadvantage of using this method is that the catheter must be discontinued. The growth of 15 or more colony-forming units is regarded as positive culture and indicates significant growth or colonization.[2]

Quantitative cultures may be obtained to facilitate the diagnosis of a catheter-related infection without discontinuing the intravascular device. To obtain a quantitative culture, blood cultures are drawn percutaneously and compared with blood drawn from the suspected intravascular device. The concordant microbial growth between catheter-drawn and percutaneously drawn blood cultures is 4:1 or greater (catheter-drawn/percutaneously drawn).[2]

Allowing an infected catheter to remain in place can result in hematogenous seeding of the organism throughout the bloodstream. Hematogenous seeding can result in a catheter-related infection if another source or site of infection seeds microorganisms on the intravascular catheter. Examples of hematogenous seeding include urinary tract infections, wound infections, and osteomyelitis. It is often difficult to identify the single source of infection responsible for the catheter-related infection with absolute certainty.

Many factors affect catheter seeding, such as the patient's clinical status, the type of catheter inserted (i.e., number of lumens, catheter size), location of insertion site, dwell time, and the degree, type, and duration of the causative pathogen. If a fever is present with positive blood cultures, the intravascular catheter must be removed immediately.

MONITORING OTHER SPECIALTY SITES

The condition and age of the patient, the prescribed therapy, and the practice setting determine the frequency of monitoring of subcutaneous, epidural, intrathecal, ventricular reservoir, and intraosseous sites. Flow rate is one of the evaluation parameters for all of these infusion devices.

The catheter insertion site of subcutaneous, epidural, intrathecal, ventricular reservoir, and intraosseous infusions should be monitored and assessed for pain, tenderness, inflammation, and swelling. If swelling occurs, catheter placement should be assessed. Aspiration and the absence of spinal fluid determine epidural catheter placement. Any external catheter should be measured regularly to assess for catheter migration.

Aspiration and the presence of spinal fluid ascertain intrathecal and ventricular reservoir placement. Before any fluid or medication is injected into the reservoir, placement is confirmed by slightly depressing the dome several times. If patent, there will be a free flow of cerebrospinal fluid from the ventricle into the dome. The site above and around the dome should be monitored for tenderness and erythema.

Once an intraosseous needle has been inserted, it must be securely anchored to prevent migration out of the bone marrow. To prevent dislodgment, a plastic site-protector may be placed over the insertion site. Intraosseous needle placement is determined by the aspiration of bone marrow. If the infusion slows,

the marrow may have clotted in the needle. Flushing the intraosseous needle with 0.9% sodium chloride may restore patency. If flushing does not improve a sluggish infusion, the needle may have extravasated into the surrounding tissue. Hourly measurements of leg circumference should be made, particularly if the dwell time is expected to last more than a short time.[3] (See Chapter 14 for further details on the care and maintenance of epidural and intrathecal catheters; see Chapter 30 for details on intraosseous infusions.)

CATHETER CARE
Peripheral

Peripheral catheter care should be performed after an IV catheter is inserted, or on a routine basis with catheter site rotation, and when the dressing is soiled or no longer intact. The guidelines for peripheral site care are established in *Infusion Nursing Standards of Practice*.[1] First, the skin-cannula junction should be cleansed with an acceptable antiseptic solution (tincture of iodine 2%, 10% povidone-iodine, alcohol, or chlorhexidine).

During catheter care, the cannula should be stabilized so that movement of the cannula is minimized. Stabilization of the cannula reduces the risk of phlebitis, infiltration, infection, and cannula migration. Various chevron-taping methods may be used to stabilize the cannula. When chevron tape is used to anchor a cannula, the sterility of the tape must be maintained. Care should be taken to avoid tearing the tape and sticking it to contaminated overbed tables and side rails before insertion. Any microorganisms present on an inanimate object will be transmitted on the tape. When the contaminated tape is placed on the skin-cannula junction site, it may be a potential source of infection. Anchor tape should be applied only to the wings-cannula hub so that the insertion site remains visible and assessment and monitoring of the skin-cannula junction site are not interrupted (Fig. 21-1). Tape should never be placed over the insertion site.

Many types of dressing materials for IV catheters are available. Some of the desired qualities for IV dressings are ease of

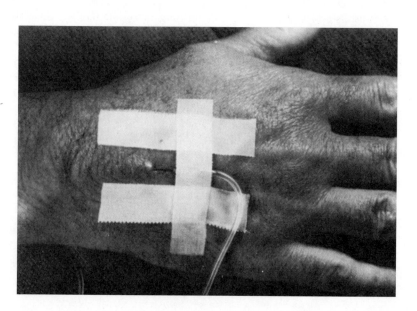

FIG. 21-1 *Apply chevron tape to the wings and cannula hub only to allow assessment and monitoring of the insertion site.*

application, viewing capacity, proper adhesion, appropriate size, moisture-proof characteristics, permeability, durability, patient comfort, ability to immobilize the catheter, ease of removal, and cost-effectiveness. A sterile dressing is applied over the cannula-catheter insertion site to prevent the introduction of microorganisms into the intravascular system.

Infusion Nursing Standards of Practice recommends that a sterile gauze or a transparent semipermeable membrane dressing be aseptically applied over the insertion site.[1] The most commonly used dressing materials are gauze or a transparent semipermeable membrane. Because it is nonocclusive, a Band-Aid dressing is not recommended. If gauze is used, the entire surface and all edges must be secured with tape to ensure that the dressing is closed and intact.

The transparent semipermeable membrane is the most commonly used cannula-site dressing. It is a water-resistant sterile dressing, permeable to air, that enables continual visual inspection and observation of the insertion site, adheres well, and reliably secures the cannula. After the dressing has been aseptically applied on a peripheral IV cannula, a label should be attached to the dressing identifying the date and time, the gauge and length of the cannula, and the name of the nurse who inserted the cannula. If tubing is being attached to the peripheral cannula, the tubing should be looped and the loop taped to the patient's skin. This measure helps stabilize the cannula and keeps the tubing out of the patient's way. Several tubing devices and microextension sets are available that attach to the tubing and the cannula, forming a loop. A transparent semipermeable dressing is not routinely changed on short peripheral cannulas unless it becomes soiled, becomes damp, or is no longer intact. The dressing should be changed at the time the catheter site is rotated.

Although the tip of a midline catheter is not in a central vein, the dressing is changed using sterile technique. Most agencies administer catheter care for midline catheters by following the same policies and procedures as those used for central vascular access devices. Central IV, subclavian, jugular, peripherally inserted central catheters (PICCs), and implanted ports require sterile dressing changes. Prepackaged dressing kits ensure the availability of all the required supplies and promote continuity in the delivery of care. A sterile dressing change requires the use of a mask and sterile gloves.

Central

The benefit of applying ointment at the central catheter insertion site remains unestablished.[4] Clinical trials regarding the use of ointment have not been conclusive and do not firmly establish decreased infection rates with its use. Polyantibiotic ointments, which are not fungicidal, may significantly increase the colonization rate of *Candida* species.[5]

For central catheters, a transparent, semipermeable polyurethane is the most commonly used dressing material.[4] Sometimes, dressing materials are combined and gauze is applied under a transparent dressing. *Infusion Nursing Standards of Practice* states that when a transparent semipermeable membrane is placed over gauze, it is considered a gauze dressing and must be changed when the administration set is changed.[1]

Much controversy exists over the colonization of bacteria and the best type of dressing material to be used with vascular access devices.[6,7] Regardless of the type of dressing material applied, dressings should be kept dry, sterile, and intact. After the dressing is applied, it should be labeled with the date and time of the dressing change and the name of the nurse who changed the dressing.

Jugular cannulation dressings are difficult to maintain in a manner that is intact and occlusive to air. The jugular area of catheter insertion and movement of the neck create a challenge in applying a dressing that is comfortable to the patient and that remains occlusive. If the jugular insertion site is located near a tracheostomy, moisture repellency is a requirement. With diaphoretic patients, adhesion can be enhanced by applying a skin sealant around the outer perimeter before and after applying the dressing. Numerous skin protectants are available in sterile, single-application packages. If the upper layer of the skin is broken or denuded, the application of a skin sealant is contraindicated because of the alcohol content in these preparations. The application of tincture of benzoin is not recommended because of its drying effect on the skin, which can cause skin irritation.

The optimal time frequency for changing central line dressings has not been established.[8] *Infusion Nursing Standards of Practice* recommends that gauze dressings on central cannula sites be routinely changed every 48 hours and that semipermeable transparent dressings be changed at least every 3 to 7 days, sooner if the integrity of the dressing is compromised.[1]

Transparent dressings are preferred because they promote stabilization of the catheter and allow observation of the insertion site. If the catheter is secured with sterile wound-closure strips or a catheter securement device, they should be replaced with each dressing change. The dressing should be changed immediately when it becomes damp or soiled or if the integrity is compromised. Some patients receiving home care (if they are not immunocompromised) have family members or caregivers change their PICC dressings using clean technique. Dressing changes are required if the dressing is damp, soiled, or no longer intact. More frequent dressing changes are necessary if visual inspection of the insertion site is required.

Box 21-1 contains an example of a procedure incorporating the recommendations of the *Infusion Nursing Standards of Practice* for administering site care and changing the dressing on a central venous catheter.

When not in use, unaccessed implanted ports do not require any site care except flushing with a heparinized saline solution every 28 days to maintain patency. Because accessing an implanted port is a sterile procedure, sterile gloves and a mask should be used. When the port is accessed, the noncoring needle should be changed at least every 7 days.[1] A sterile occlusive dressing should be placed over the noncoring needle to anchor it and stabilize the needle. The noncoring needle is often anchored with gauze and a transparent membrane dressing is applied over the needle, which allows the insertion site to be observed. This method of applying a dressing permits detection of any edema caused by infiltration of a dislodged noncoring needle. The dressing must be changed if it becomes damp or soiled or is no longer intact.

PROCEDURE for Site Care and Dressing Change on a Central Venous Catheter — Box 21-1

1. Wash hands with antimicrobial soap.
2. Ascertain allergies of patient.
3. Instruct patient to keep head turned away from insertion site.
4. Apply mask.
5. Apply nonsterile gloves.
6. Remove old dressing.
7. Assess insertion site for signs of inflammation, tenderness, or drainage.
8. Remove nonsterile gloves and apply sterile gloves.
9. Cleanse site with alcohol, beginning at insertion site and applying outward in a circular pattern. Repeat with second swab stick. Cleanse catheter and sutures with third swab stick.
10. Repeat with iodophor solution (Fig. 21-2).
11. Allow to air dry.
12. Apply either a transparent or sterile gauze dressing and tape over the entire gauze dressing, securing all edges.
13. Write date, time, and signature of nurse on label and attach to dressing (Fig. 21-3).
14. Document the dressing change and site assessment in medical record.

Injection caps and needleless systems

Peripheral IV cannulas and central IV catheters are often used for intermittent infusions and injections. Latex injection caps are placed on catheters and cannulas that are used intermittently. All injection caps should have a Luer-Lok design to decrease the risk of an air embolus. A latex injection cap attached to a peripheral cannula should be changed when a new cannula is inserted or if the integrity of the cap becomes compromised. The integrity of the injection cap depends on the number of needle punctures, the gauge of the needle inserted, and the composition of the latex. The integrity of the injection cap should be confirmed before and immediately after each use. If the integrity of the cap is compromised, it should be changed immediately. The optimal period for changing a latex injection cap on a peripherally inserted central or midline catheter is unknown. However, the latex injection caps on all central catheters should be changed at least every 7 days.[1] Ideally, the injection cap change should coincide with the dressing change and flushing of the catheter.

The needleless system is the preferred method for accessing infusion devices. Various needleless systems are available. Blunt-ended plastic insertion devices and reflux valves eliminate latex injection caps that require standard needle access. The integrity of the valve system is verified before use. Valved and needleless systems should be used according to the manufacturer's guidelines. Most needleless devices require minimal change in administration techniques or methods.

Although needleless and needle-safe devices have reduced needlestick injuries to health care workers, they raise concerns regarding patient safety. Several studies have reported an increased potential for bloodstream infections associated with the improper use of needleless devices.[9-11]

The greatest risk for bloodstream infections from safety devices appears to be when the caps are improperly cleaned or when total parenteral nutrition or lipids are administered through central catheters.[12]

Current guidelines from the Centers for Disease Control and Prevention do not provide recommendations for the use, maintenance, or frequency for changing needleless infusion devices.[8] Additional research exploring the risks of infection associated with needleless devices is needed before clinical standards of practice can be developed.

Flushes

After an IV cannula is used at routine intervals, the patency of the cannula can be maintained by flushing with a heparinized saline solution. A Groshong catheter, which has a two-way slit valve next to a rounded, closed tip, is routinely flushed with 5 ml of 0.9% sodium chloride solution. To maintain catheter patency, the lowest possible concentration of heparin should be used. The strength of heparin used varies from 10 to 1000 units/ml, depending on the patient's condition. The volume of the heparinized saline flush should be equal to twice the internal volume capacity of the catheter and the add-on device.[2] Information on the internal volume of a catheter can be obtained from the manufacturer. Many institutions flush intermittent peripheral cannulas with 0.9% sodium chloride solution only. Most studies that have compared the use of saline versus heparin recommend the saline for use with peripheral venous access devices.[13,14]

When a vascular access device is flushed, positive pressure must be maintained on the lumen of the cannula to prevent a reflux of blood into the cannula lumen. Positive pressure is maintained by keeping a forward motion on the syringe plunger as the needle is removed from the injection port. If resistance is met during flushing, no further attempts to flush should be made. Pressure should not be exerted on the catheter in an attempt to restore patency; applying pressure to an occluded catheter can dislodge the clot into the vascular system or can rupture the catheter. The amount and the frequency of the flush should be such that the patient's clotting factors are not altered. If a patient has decreased coagulation factors, a more dilute heparinized saline may be indicated. Devices are available that will maintain positive pressure as the stylet is removed.

The catheter should be heparinized as soon as a medication is infused or when blood samples have been withdrawn. When blood samples have been withdrawn, the catheter should be flushed with 0.9% sodium chloride to remove the residual red blood cells before flushing the catheter with the heparinized saline solution. The cannula should also be flushed when continuous fluids are discontinued and when the cannula is left in place for intermittent therapy. If a catheter is capped and no medication is being administered intravenously, the catheter must be flushed to maintain patency. The frequency of flushing vascular access devices varies from institution to institution. IV catheters may be flushed with a heparinized saline solution every 12 to 24 hours. Implantable venous ports are usually routinely flushed with a heparinized saline solution every 28

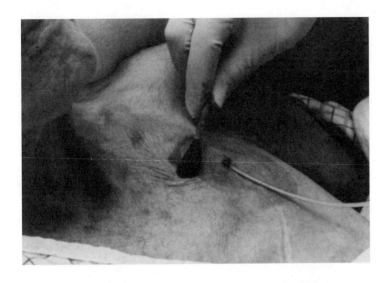

FIG. 21-2 *Cleanse with iodophor solution, beginning at the insertion site and applying outward in a circular pattern.*

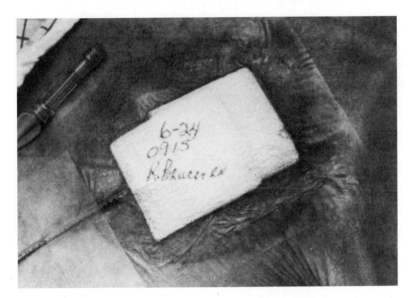

FIG. 21-3 *After the dressing is changed, label with date, time, and signature of the nurse.*

days to maintain catheter patency. Because of the closed-valve feature of Groshong catheters, they may be flushed weekly with 0.9% sodium chloride solution. To decrease some of the confusion regarding the amount, frequency, and concentration of routine flushes, many institutions have established standardized flushing protocols for the various vascular access devices.

BLOOD WITHDRAWAL

Central venous catheters are often placed in patients who have limited peripheral access and are therefore commonly used for withdrawing blood specimens. Some institutions require a physician's order permitting these devices to be used for this purpose. Serious consideration must be given when blood specimens for prothrombin time or partial prothrombin time determinations are to be drawn from a heparinized catheter. Erroneous laboratory values have been reported on blood specimens obtained from central catheters. For example, altered

aminoglycoside serum concentration results have been reported when blood is withdrawn from central venous silastic catheters. In addition, errors in measuring potassium levels have been identified when laboratory specimens have been withdrawn from newly inserted central catheters. These erroneous laboratory values were secondarily attributed to the sensitivity of certain analyzers to the presence of benzalkonium salts on newly inserted central catheters.[15] If laboratory values for blood withdrawn from a central vascular access device are significantly altered in a previously stable patient, the laboratory test should be repeated before any treatment is implemented.

When multiple-lumen catheters are used to withdraw blood specimens, the proximal lumen is the preferred site from which the specimen should be obtained. Before the blood is withdrawn, the nurse must wash his or her hands and don gloves. All infusions being administered through the catheter must be stopped before the blood sample is obtained. Some organizations flush the catheter with 5 to 10 ml of 0.9% sodium chloride to confirm catheter patency and to remove any drug within the catheter lumen before drawing the blood for discard. Approximately 5 to 10 ml of blood is commonly withdrawn and discarded. Smaller waste volumes are used for neonates and children. An alternative waste method is to flush the catheter with 0.9% sodium chloride and then aspirate or flush back and forth multiple times to clear the catheter before withdrawing the laboratory sample. Occasionally, when central catheters are used to withdraw blood specimens, the blood may be difficult to aspirate. If this occurs, it is sometimes helpful to ask the patient to sit, lie down, turn from side to side, or cough. After the blood has been withdrawn, the catheter should be flushed with 10 to 20 ml of 0.9% sodium chloride solution to remove any residual red blood cells. The catheter may then be flushed with a heparinized saline solution as established in the flushing protocol.

Many patients are discharged from the hospital with IV catheters. Patients and caregivers are taught to manage the catheters and are provided with professional support from a home care nurse. The frequency of visits to determine compliance depends on the patient's condition and age, caregiver support, and therapy being administered. Compliance visits by the home care nurse should reinforce the need for the patient or caregiver to use aseptic technique while changing dressings and administering medications. The nurse should encourage the patient or caregiver to report immediately any abnormal findings, such as elevated temperature, inflamed insertion or exit site, unusual catheter discomfort, or equipment or catheter malfunction.

NURSING DIAGNOSES

When nurses are knowledgeable about the array of vascular access devices, monitoring criteria associated with each device, and catheter care requirements, quality patient care is given and the risks to the patient are minimized. Nurses must be able to quickly identify the wide variety of IV devices and to plan and make appropriate nursing interventions to prevent complications. The identification of problems is referred to as *potential nursing diagnoses*. Appropriate nursing diagnoses associated with intravascular devices include alteration in comfort (including acute pain), impairment of skin integrity related to a potential for infection, knowledge deficit in relation to vascular access devices, anxiety, and noncompliance.

Alteration in comfort, including acute pain, can occur with the insertion of any intravascular device. Patients should be encouraged to promptly report any unusual discomfort related to their infusion device. Whenever an IV catheter is in place, the integrity of the skin is impaired and a potential for infection exists. Many patients who require central IV catheters are immunocompromised and at increased risk for acquiring a nosocomial or community-acquired infection. Many patients are discharged from the hospital with an infusion device intended for long-term use. Whenever a patient has an IV catheter, a knowledge deficit may exist regarding the purpose and the function of the device. Patients and caregivers are often anxious about the management of the intravascular device. After discharge from the hospital, some patients may be noncompliant in administering their medications or maintaining their catheter.

PATIENT OUTCOMES

The desired outcome for all patients receiving infusion therapy is to complete treatment with minimal or no complications. When nurses deliver infusion care according to established policies and procedures that are based on professional nursing standards of practice, the risks associated with an intravascular device are significantly decreased.

When the patient's pain is acknowledged, desired patient outcomes regarding an alteration in comfort are achieved. If the intravascular device is a peripheral cannula, the device should be discontinued and a new one started. Application of warm, moist packs may be required if the pain is associated with phlebitis. If the pain experienced is from a central venous catheter, the insertion site should be monitored often, and meticulous catheter care should be administered.

If phlebitis occurs with a peripheral or central venous cannula, close monitoring and possible treatment with warm, moist compresses may be required. It is important that patients express their fears and anxiety related to health needs. Compliance is increased when the patient's ability and willingness to learn has been properly assessed. Consideration must be given to the home environment, the availability of the caregiver, and the family's previous IV experience and expectations. Much anxiety can be alleviated when the patient and caregiver are instructed on the purpose and management of the IV device. When patients and caregivers are taught the importance of good handwashing, administering medications on time, and assessing the insertion site accurately, they will be more compliant in the care and maintenance of their infusion device. After such instruction, the patient and caregiver should be able to identify factors that decrease the occurrence of potential complications.

REFERENCES

1. Intravenous Nurses Society: Infusion nursing standards of practice, *JIN* (suppl) 23(6S), 2000.
2. Maki DG: Infections due to infusion therapy. In Bennett JV, Brachman PS, editors: *Hospital infections*, ed 4, Philadelphia, 1998, Lippincott-Raven.
3. West VL: Alternate routes of administration, *JIN* 21(4):221, 1998.
4. Collins E, et al: Care of central venous catheters for total parenteral nutrition, *Nutr Clin Pract* 11(3):109, 1996.
5. Clemence MA, Walker D, Farr B: Central venous catheter practices: results of a survey, *Am J Infect Control* 23(1):5, 1995.
6. Treston-Aurand J, et al: Impact of dressing materials on central venous catheter infection rate, *JIN* 20(4):201, 1997.
7. Lau CE: Transparent and gauze dressings and their effect on infection rates of central venous catheters: a review of past and current literature, *JIN* 19(5):240, 1996.
8. US Department of Health and Human Services, Public Health Service Centers for Disease Control and Prevention: Guideline for prevention of intravascular device-related infections, *Am J Infect Control* 24(4):262, 1996
9. Danzig LE, et al: Bloodstream infections associated with a needleless intravenous infusion system in patients receiving home infusion therapy, *JAMA* 273:1862, 1995.
10. Arduino MJ, et al: Microbiologic evaluation of needleless and needle-access devices, *Am J Infect Control* 26:377, 1997.

11. Hanchett M, Kung LY: Do needleless intravenous systems increase the risk of infection? *JIN* 22(3):117, 1999.

12. Orenstein, R: The benefits and limitations of needle protectors and needleless intravenous systems, *JIN* 22(3):122, 1999.

13. Goode CJ, et al: A meta-analysis of effects of heparin flush, and saline flush: quality and cost implications, *Nurs Res* 40(6):324, 1991.

14. Kamitomo V, Olson K: Using normal saline to lock peripheral intravenous catheters in ambulatory cancer patients, *JIN* 19(2):75, 1996.

15. Johnston JB, Messina M: Erroneous laboratory values obtained from central catheters, *JIN* 14(1):13, 1991.

Changing and Discontinuing Infusion Therapy

Roxanne Perucca, MSN, CRNI

The delivery of safe, quality infusion care requires changing fluid containers and administration sets, rotating peripheral intravenous (IV) cannulas, changing dressings, and performing site assessments. Careful maintenance of the infusion system, performance of appropriate nursing interventions, and close monitoring minimize risks to the patient and improve expected patient outcomes. The nurse administering infusion therapy must be knowledgeable about the risks involved and must be able to implement measures to prevent their occurrence.

CHANGING THERAPY

A physician's order is necessary to change the fluids or medications being administered. The physician's order should be clearly written. The nurse uses the nursing process to evaluate the rationale for changing the therapy and intervenes appropriately. Before changing or administering IV fluid or medication, the nurse should assess the appropriateness of the prescribed order by evaluating the patient's age and condition and the dosage, route, and rate of the IV fluid or medication to be administered. The nurse must be knowledgeable about the indications, actions, dosage, side effects, and adverse reactions associated with each fluid and medication administered.

The nurse is accountable for administering medications and fluids safely and for making appropriate nursing interventions. For example, if the nurse questions the prescribed dosage or determines that the patient's condition does not warrant the prescribed medication or fluid, the order should not be carried out until it is clarified. If there are any questions regarding the prescribed therapy, the physician should be contacted to clarify the plan of care and to verify the medication order.

The nurse closely monitors the infusion system and the patient's response to the fluid or medication being administered. The type and degree of change in the patient's status determine how promptly the nurse must intervene. It may be necessary to discontinue therapy before notifying the physician. For example, if a patient develops hives, hypotension, diaphoresis, or respiratory distress, the nurse must intervene immediately by stopping the medication. These signs and symptoms are indicators of an anaphylactic reaction, and appropriate therapy must be initiated immediately to reverse the complications of the reaction.

Fluid containers

IV fluid containers may be changed to add a sequential container, to avoid exceeding "hang time" restrictions, or in response to a change in the prescribed therapy. Before a new IV fluid container is used, the fluid in the container should be inspected for clarity and the presence of particulate matter. The infusate container should be inspected for cracks, leaks, or punctures, and the expiration date should be verified. If the appearance of the fluid is questionable or if the integrity of the container is compromised, the container should be returned to the pharmacy or dispensing department and should be clearly labeled with the reason for the return. If the expiration date has passed or will pass during the infusion, the container should be returned to the originating department or disposed of according to institutional policy.

After a medication has been added to the fluid container or when an administration set has been attached, the fluid container must be used or discarded within 24 hours. Once the fluid container has been accessed, the potential for bacterial growth is increased; therefore IV fluid containers must not hang longer than 24 hours.[1] The fluid container should be labeled with the date and time that it was initiated.

Administration sets

Changing the primary administration set should coincide with the hanging of a new IV fluid container or with the changing of the peripheral IV cannula. Each entry into the IV delivery system increases the risk of inadvertent contamination. *Infusion Nursing Standards of Practice* has established that continuous peripheral and central primary sets and secondary administration sets should be changed every 72 hours. However, failure to maintain an ongoing phlebitis rate of 5% or less, or any increased rate of catheter-related bacteremia, requires a return to 48-hour administration set change.[2]

Administration tubing for total parenteral nutrition and

primary intermittent sets should be changed every 24 hours.[2] Primary intermittent sets deliver medication through latex injection caps or needleless system devices. Intermittent devices have a greater risk of touch contamination than continuous devices because of the interruption involved in initiating and discontinuing infusates.

Guidelines from the Centers for Disease Control and Prevention (CDC) recommend that administration sets that include intermittent tubing not be changed any more frequently than every 72 hours. Tubing used to administer blood, blood products, or lipid emulsions should be changed within 24 hours. Total parenteral nutrition requires the administration set to be changed every 24 hours because of the greater potential for bacterial and fungal contamination.[3]

The administration set should be labeled with the date and time that it was initiated and should be documented according to institutional policy. The tubing should be labeled to communicate to subsequent shifts, home care nurses, or caregivers when it must be changed.

The administration set, dome, and pressure tubing used for hemodynamic and arterial pressure monitoring should be changed every 96 hours.[3] If the integrity of the system has been compromised and contamination has occurred, the system must be changed immediately. The tubing change is performed using aseptic technique. Greater detail about the hemodynamic and arterial pressure monitoring system can be found in Chapter 23.

Box 22-1 details a procedure that can be used to add a fluid container to an existing administration set. The initiation of a fluid container with a new administration set is described in Chapter 20.

Dressings

The IV insertion-site dressing should be changed simultaneously with the administration set change. Each break into the IV system increases the risk of contamination and infection. The procedure to perform peripheral cannula care and to change a central line dressing is detailed in Chapter 21. Peripheral cannula care is performed using aseptic technique. If the catheter is a peripherally inserted central catheter (PICC), the dressing should be changed using sterile technique. Changing the IV insertion-site dressing allows observation and evaluation of the skin-cannula junction. Transparent semipermeable dressings on short peripheral cannulas are changed at the time of site rotation or if the dressing becomes damp or soiled or becomes no longer intact. If a transparent dressing is placed over gauze on a peripheral or central catheter insertion site, it is considered a gauze dressing and should be changed every 48 hours.[2]

The ideal frequency to change transparent central line dressings has not been established. Regardless of the established dressing change policy, dressing changes are required if the dressing is damp, soiled, or becomes no longer intact. If visual inspection of the insertion site is required, more frequent dressing changes may be necessary.

Vascular access devices

When infusion therapy is changed, the nurse must assess whether the current IV device and equipment can be used with the new therapy. For instance, if the patient has been receiving peripheral parenteral nutrition and the order is changed to total parenteral nutrition, a central venous access device will need to be inserted. When the glucose concentration of a solution exceeds 10%, the solution becomes very irritating to small peripheral veins. Solutions whose glucose concentration exceeds 10% or whose protein concentration exceeds 5% must be administered through a central venous access device.

Peripheral cannulas

Infusion Nursing Standards of Practice recommends that short peripheral cannulas be removed every 72 hours and immediately upon suspected contamination, complication, or when therapy has been discontinued. However, failure to maintain an ongoing phlebitis rate of 5% or less with a 72-hour site rotation policy requires that practice return to a 48-hour site rotation interval.[2]

When a peripheral rotation policy is strictly followed, venous access may be prolonged, and the complications of phlebitis and infiltration are reduced. For routine peripheral site rotation, the extremities should be alternated whenever possible. Using the opposite extremity allows previous insertion sites time to rest and phlebitic or infiltrated areas time to resolve. If a subsequent insertion site is restarted in the same extremity, it must be located proximal to the previously cannulated site. Inserting a cannula proximal to a previously infiltrated or phlebitic site prevents further damage to the tissues.

Some institutions have policies that allow cannula dwell time to be extended in patients who have limited venous access. In these situations, an order must be obtained from the physician to continue the present site, and the physician's order must be documented in the patient's medical record. Peripheral venous sites that are extended beyond the 72-hour catheter dwell time must be monitored very closely and discontinued at the first

---

PROCEDURE *for Adding a Fluid*   **Box 22-1**
Container to an Existing
Administration Set

1. Close the flow control clamp or shut off the electronic flow device.
2. Remove the protective cap from the new container.
3. Remove the old fluid container from the intravenous pole.
4. Remove the spike from the old container and insert it into the new container. Be careful to avoid touch contamination of the administration set spike or the fluid port.
5. Hang the new container.
6. Regulate the flow clamp or turn on the electronic flow device.
7. Label the new container with the date and time it was initiated.
8. Discard the old container according to institutional policy.
9. Document in medical record the type and volume of fluid, the date and time initiated, the rate of flow, and the amount infused.

indication of tenderness, infiltration, or phlebitis. Documentation by the nurse should include the location and appearance of the insertion site; site care, if administered; and any nursing actions taken to resolve problems associated with the cannula.

Cannulas that have been placed in emergency situations should be replaced as soon as possible because aseptic technique or skin preparation may have been compromised. Peripheral cannulas must be removed immediately if phlebitis, infiltration, or cannula occlusion occurs. If the peripheral cannula appears to be infected, the cannula and insertion site should be cultured when the cannula is removed. Culturing will identify microorganisms that are the source of the infection and will determine the medical interventions that follow.

The CDC guidelines do not have any recommendations regarding the routine frequency change of a midline catheter.[3]

Central catheters

The optimal time interval for the routine changing of central venous catheters has not been established. The guidelines from the CDC recommend that percutaneously inserted nontunneled catheters not be routinely changed by rotating insertion sites or by guidewire-assisted catheter exchange. The guidelines recommend that PICCs be exchanged every 6 weeks. However, no recommendations exist regarding the frequency for changing PICCs when the duration of therapy is expected to exceed 6 weeks.[3]

PICCs must be removed when an infection or inflammatory process is evident. Because of their small diameter and the insertion procedure used, veins in the upper extremities may develop mechanical phlebitis within 24 hours after catheter insertion. Mazzola reported that the mean time for the development of postinsertion phlebitis for PICCs was 4.8 days.[4] Depending on the patient's condition, conservative treatment with the application of warm, moist compresses and elevation may resolve the phlebitis, or catheter removal may be required.[5]

A catheter tip is considered *malpositioned* if it does not maintain a direct course with the tip ending in the superior vena cava. The most common malpositioned locations are the internal jugular and axillary veins. Malpositioning can be caused by curling, knotting, misdirection, or spontaneous migration after insertion.[6] Nurses may successfully reposition a malpositioned PICC tip by using a noninvasive technique such as rapid flushing of the catheter with 0.9% sodium chloride, positive-pressure infusion pumps, or catheter exchange using a guidewire (dependent on institutional policy). If these interventions are unsuccessful, a physician's order is obtained to have the catheter tip repositioned in radiology using fluoroscopy.

Catheter tip placement should be confirmed intermittently by radiography. Occasionally, the tip of a PICC migrates outside of the superior vena cava or the subclavian vein. If this situation occurs, the catheter can no longer be considered a central line. The catheter must be removed if the prescribed therapy requires central access, such as the administration of total parenteral nutrition. A catheter that has been partially withdrawn from the vein cannot be readvanced because the external portion of the withdrawn catheter is no longer sterile

and introduces microorganisms into the vascular system if it is reintroduced.

Long-term catheters, such as tunneled catheters and implantable ports, are often left in place for several years. If complications occur (e.g., fever or sepsis), the catheter must be considered a possible source of the infection. Blood cultures should be drawn through the device and compared with peripherally obtained blood cultures. A long-term catheter should be removed if the source of infection cannot be identified. The feasibility of treating a catheter-related infection while allowing the catheter to remain in place must be evaluated repeatedly through the course of antibiotic therapy.[7]

It is important to explain to the patient the rationale for the medication being administered, the purpose for changing the IV access device, and the reason for changing the dressing over the insertion site. A patient's anxiety and apprehension are decreased when he or she understands the reason for changing the therapy. For example, if a patient receiving IV therapy at home understands the importance of maintaining a dry and intact central venous catheter dressing to decrease the risk of infection, compliance will be increased.

Any change in the IV therapy fluid or medication, the administration set, the cannula, or the insertion-site dressing should be documented in the patient's medical record. The date and time of the change and the nurse's name should be charted. When a cannula or a dressing is changed, the condition of the site and the reason for changing the site should be documented. With peripheral cannula changes, the type, gauge, and length of the cannula and the location of the insertion site must be documented. When patient education is provided on the care of an IV catheter, the communication should be documented.

DISCONTINUING THERAPY

The physician's order to discontinue IV therapy must be clearly written. The nurse uses the nursing process of assessment, planning, and implementation to evaluate the rationale for discontinuing the therapy. IV access may be discontinued because the patient no longer requires it or because the patient decides not to continue treatment. Because of the risk of complications carried by central venous catheters, they are usually removed when they are no longer indicated. A catheter should be removed immediately if its integrity is compromised; for example, a hole or tear in the catheter wall greatly increases the risk of infection if the catheter is left in place. If a catheter is removed because it is defective, it should be saved and the problem reported to risk management, the manufacturer, and the U.S. Food and Drug Administration.

Before an IV cannula is removed, the procedure should be explained to the patient. The patient should be encouraged to ask questions regarding the process; answering a patient's questions decreases anxiety and alleviates apprehension.

At any time during the therapy, the patient or the legally authorized representative has the right to request that the treatment be discontinued. Any intervention that results in the discontinuation of therapy should be communicated to the physician and documented.

1. Verify physician's order.
2. Wash hands with antiseptic soap.
3. Explain cannula removal to the patient.
4. Close the flow clamp if administration set is attached.
5. Assess the cannula insertion site for evidence of local complication.
6. Don gloves.
7. Remove the tape and dressing, and stabilize the cannula with one hand. Do not use scissors to remove the tape.
8. Cover the site with sterile gauze as the cannula is withdrawn; use a slow steady movement and keep the hub parallel to the skin.
9. With the extremity elevated, gently apply pressure with sterile dry gauze to the insertion site until the bleeding stops.
10. Assess cannula integrity and length.
11. Tape a sterile dressing over the insertion site.
12. Remove gloves. Wash hands.
13. Document the type, gauge, and length of the cannula removed; the assessment of the insertion site; and the date and time the cannula was removed.

Peripheral cannulas

Peripheral cannulas should be removed (Box 22-2) immediately if contamination is suspected, the patient experiences discomfort, or phlebitis or infiltration is detected. The delayed withdrawal of an infiltrated or phlebitic IV catheter extends the duration and the severity of the tissue damage. If the insertion site is tender or reddened with a palpable cord after the cannula is removed, warm, moist compresses may be applied for 20 minutes several times a day to alleviate the discomfort associated with phlebitis. If a vesicant medication has been administered and extravasated, the treatment protocol should be initiated before the cannula is removed. The severity of the tissue damage is decreased if the extravasation protocol is implemented immediately.

After the cannula has been removed, the insertion site requires ongoing observation and assessment because postinfusion phlebitis can occur after the cannula has been removed. Usually, postinfusion phlebitis is evident within 48 hours after cannula removal. Some investigators have reported that more than 40% of catheter-associated phlebitis occurs more than 24 hours after the cannula has been discontinued.[8] Depending on the severity of the phlebitis, nursing interventions may include applying intermittent, warm, moist compresses to the phlebitic area. In cases of severe phlebitis, medical intervention may be necessary. The treatment of severe phlebitis may include the administration of systemic antibiotics or lysis of the phlebitic vein.

Arterial catheters

Infusion Nursing Standards of Practice recommends that peripheral arterial catheters be removed every 96 hours.[2] If the arterial catheter becomes contaminated, occluded, infiltrated, or infected or if circulatory impairment develops, the catheter should be discontinued immediately. Arterial catheter removal is detailed in Chapter 23.

Central catheters

Before a central venous access device is removed, the nurse must determine whether the intervention is a medical act. In many health care settings, subclavian, jugular, and peripherally inserted central catheters are removed by a registered nurse in accordance with the institution's policies and procedures. The removal of central catheters requires that precautions be taken to minimize the risk of an air embolism. Two such precautions are positioning the patient to a dorsal recumbent position with the head of the bed in a flat position and having the patient perform the Valsalva maneuver while the catheter is being withdrawn. The Valsalva maneuver raises intrathoracic pressure, which impedes air from entering the vein. A patient may be instructed to perform the Valsalva maneuver by bearing down against a closed glottis after taking a deep breath.[9]

Precautions should also be taken to prevent an air embolism when a PICC is removed. The patient's arm should be abducted, and if resistance is encountered as the catheter is withdrawn, the nurse should not remove the catheter. A PICC may resist removal because of venous spasm, vasoconstriction, phlebitis, valve inflammation, or thrombophlebitis or when a fibrin sheath is present.[10] The application of warm, moist compresses may alleviate venous spasm and vasoconstriction, resulting in easier removal of the catheter. Any catheter that is not withdrawn with smooth, gentle pressure should be left in place and covered with a sterile dressing, and the physician should be notified. A catheter embolism can occur if too much withdrawal pressure is applied to a resistant catheter.

A physician must remove a tunneled catheter. This procedure may require the dissection of the Dacron cuff from the subcutaneous tissue. After a tunneled catheter is removed, the exit site should be covered with a sterile, dry dressing. The nurse is then responsible for observing the exit site and making appropriate interventions, such as notifying the physician if signs of infection occur or if the site does not heal appropriately.

Implanted ports may be surgically removed when infusion therapy is no longer necessary. After removal of an implantable port, the insertion site must be assessed for signs of inflammation. Tunneled catheters and implantable ports are often removed as an outpatient procedure; in these cases, the patient must be instructed to monitor their temperature and the incision site for signs of tenderness, redness, and drainage. If any signs of inflammation are observed or if the patient has a fever, the physician should be contacted.

If a catheter has purulent drainage at the insertion site or is considered a source of infection, it should be cultured as it is removed. This measure will identify any microorganisms that are present on the catheter surface.

The procedure in Box 22-3 may be used to remove a central catheter.

PROCEDURE *for Central Catheter Removal*   Box 22-3

1. Wash hands with antiseptic soap.
2. Assist patient to dorsal recumbent position. *Note:* The head of the bed must be in a flat position.
3. Close the flow clamp if administration set is attached.
4. Don gloves.
5. Remove the tape and dressing.
6. Assess the insertion site.
7. Clip and remove sutures, if present.
8. Instruct the patient to perform the Valsalva maneuver.
9. Remove the catheter with gentle pulling motion (Fig. 22-1).
10. Instruct patient to breathe normally.
11. Apply gentle pressure at the insertion site with sterile, dry gauze until bleeding stops.
12. Cleanse with an antiseptic solution and apply a small amount of antimicrobial ointment at the insertion site.
13. Apply sterile, air-occlusive dressing over the insertion site to prevent a delayed air embolism (Fig. 22-2).
14. Assess the length and integrity of the discontinued catheter and visually inspect the tip for smoothness.
15. Document the date, time, site assessment, patient response, and nursing interventions in the patient's medical record.

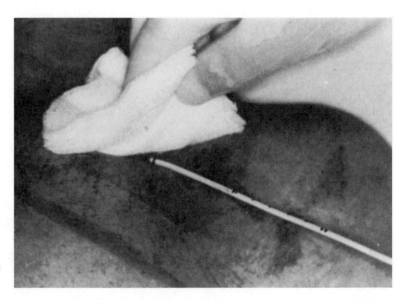

FIG. 22-1 *Remove catheter with a gentle pulling motion. Apply pressure at the insertion site with sterile gauze until bleeding stops.*

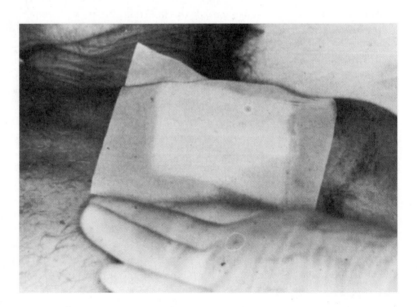

FIG. 22-2 *Apply a sterile, air-occlusive dressing over the insertion site to prevent a delayed air embolism.*

After the catheter has been removed, monitoring of the patient's condition must continue. The patient should remain flat and supine for a short time after central catheter removal; this position helps maintain a positive intrathoracic pressure and allows the tissue tract time to seal. The condition of the insertion site and surrounding tissues should continue to be assessed and documented. The insertion-site dressing should be changed, and the site should be assessed every 24 hours after central line removal until the site has epithelialized. Large-bore catheters or devices that have a longer dwell time require a longer period for the insertion site to close.

NURSING DIAGNOSES

Maintaining and monitoring the infusion system are nursing responsibilities. Commonly encountered nursing diagnoses related to changing and discontinuing IV therapy are knowledge deficit in relation to infusion devices, potential for injury related to infection, impairment of skin integrity, and noncompliance.

Many patients who have IV devices have a knowledge deficit. It is important for patients to understand that if their peripheral cannula site is tender or painful while their antibiotic is infusing, they should report it to the nurse. Failure of patients to be honest when they are asked about the comfort of their IV site results in increased phlebitis and inflammation.

Today, many patients are sent home with long-term central venous catheters. Some of these catheters are inserted during the patient's hospitalization, and the patient and caregiver are instructed regarding catheter care and management before the patient is discharged. Usually, the catheter is inserted as an outpatient procedure; the patient is discharged immediately with a long-term central venous catheter. Patients must be instructed on the potential for injury and infection related to the maintenance of an IV catheter. The signs of inflammation (redness, tenderness, drainage, and temperature elevation) should be explained to the patient or caregiver. If the patient observes inflammatory indicators, it is essential that he or she immediately notify the physician or home care nurse. When patients or caregivers do not understand the risks involved, they may become noncompliant in reporting discomfort.

Impairment in skin integrity results in an increased risk of local or systemic complications. The nurse delivering IV care must understand the importance of changing the administration set and fluid container according to established professional standards of practice. The nurse must understand the risks involved to the patient when aseptic technique is not used while a peripheral cannula is restarted.

PATIENT OUTCOMES

The delivery of quality infusion care requires that the nurse continually evaluate patient outcomes. The evaluation of patient outcomes determines whether the nursing interventions used are appropriate. Desired patient outcomes related to changing and discontinuing treatment are completing therapy with minimal or no complications, identifying factors that decrease the potential for injury, and verbalizing the rationale for treatment.

Rotating cannula sites, changing central line dressings and administration sets, and assessing insertion sites allow many patients to complete their course of IV therapy with minimal or no local complications. When patients receiving IV therapy in the home understand the risk factors related to their therapy, they are more compliant in the administration of their catheter care. Compliance is increased when patients understand the rationale for monitoring their insertion site for signs of inflammation.

Nurses must be knowledgeable about the risks involved in IV therapy. Today, many patients are immunocompromised, have extended hospitalizations, and are critically ill; these patients are at risk for developing local and systemic complications. To prevent complications, the nurse must be committed to the principles and rationale involved in changing and discontinuing IV devices and equipment. When the nurse adheres to professional standards of practice, safe, quality infusion care will be delivered.

REFERENCES

1. Maki DG: Infections due to infusion therapy. In Bennett JV, Brachman PS, editors: *Hospital infections*, ed 4, Philadelphia, 1998, Lippincott-Raven.
2. Intravenous Nurses Society: Infusion nursing standards of practice, *JIN* (suppl) 23(6S), 2000.
3. U.S. Department of Health and Human Service, Public Health Service, Centers for Disease Control and Prevention: Guideline for prevention of intravascular device-related infections, *Am J Infect Control* 24(4):262, 1996.
4. Mazzola JR, Schott-Baer DS, Addy L: Clinical factors associated with the development of phlebitis after insertion of a peripherally inserted central catheter, *JIN* 22(1):36, 1999.
5. Duerksen DR, Papineau N, Siemens J, Yaffe C: Peripherally inserted central catheters for parenteral nutrition: a comparison with centrally inserted catheters, *J Parenenter Enteral Nutr* 23(2): 85, 1999.
6. Banks N: Positive outcome after looped peripherally inserted central catheter malposition, *JIN* 22(1):14, 1999.
7. Jones GR: A practical guide to evaluation and treatment of infections in patients with central venous catheter, *JIN* 21(5S):134, 1998.
8. Hershey CO, et al: Natural history of intravenous catheter-associated phlebitis, *Arch Intern Med* 144(7):1373, 1984.
9. Thielen JB, Nyquist J: Subclavian catheter removal: nursing implications to prevent air emboli, *JIN* 14(2):114, 1991.
10. Marx M: The management of the difficult peripherally inserted central venous catheter line removal, *JIN* 18(5):246, 1995.

Chapter

23

Hemodynamic Monitoring

Barbara A. Ciano, RN, MSN*

Hemodynamics is "the forces involved in the circulation of the blood."[1] The effectiveness of the heart to contract and circulate blood depends on the strength of the heart muscle itself and the pressures surrounding it. These pressures within the surrounding major vessels, heart valves, and lungs are generated by the blood volume with contraction (systole) and relaxation (diastole) of the heart. Hemodynamic monitoring catheters and equipment translate the pressures into graphs and numbers.

Arterial, venous, and balloon flotation or pulmonary artery catheters have been developed to allow measurement of these pressures. Bedside monitoring of these pressure values, *or readings,* aids the physician in preoperative and postoperative evaluation of cardiac function, fluid volume delivery, and intravenous (IV) medication administration for optimal cardiac function.

Nurses are responsible for maintaining many of these invasive monitoring catheters while caring for patients in a critical care setting. To ensure proper care of the patient, the nurse should have a basic understanding of the pressures within the circulatory system, be familiar with the similarities among catheter systems, recognize normal and abnormal pressure patterns, and respond with appropriate nursing actions.

GENERAL HEMODYNAMIC MONITORING

Arterial and venous pressure waveforms reflect atrial and ventricular contraction (systole) and relaxation (diastole). The closing of the heart valves may sometimes be seen. The contraction of the heart chamber is an upward (positive) stroke on the pressure tracing, and the relaxation is the downward (negative) stroke. Valvular closure, when seen, is also an upstroke, reflecting the increased pressure in the monitored chamber of the heart. Central venous, arterial, and pulmonary artery monitor tracings are represented by a, v, and c waveforms, which refer to atrial, ventricular, and valvular-closure pressures in all of the monitoring systems.

Intraarterial blood pressure, central venous pressure (CVP), pulmonary artery pressure, and pulmonary wedge pressure (PWP) are the basic pressure waveforms monitored in the critical care setting. Pulmonary artery catheters also have the ability to determine cardiac output and mixed venous oxygenation, and may have a port for pacing wires.[2]

These types of monitoring require the same basic equipment. A fluid system, a transducer, and a monitor translate the pressures in the vascular system into digital values and visible waveforms, which appear on the bedside monitor. Most critical care units have a central monitor system that is capable of displaying the information and storing it for later printout.

The fluid system needed to translate the patient pressures to the transducer is pressurized by a pressure bag at 300 mm Hg. The IV solutions used may be heparinized 0.9% sodium chloride in a concentration of 1 to 4 units of heparin per milliliter of solution. Patients with clotting disorders or low platelet counts may be given only saline (0.9% sodium chloride) flush solutions.

The bag used to pressurize the flush solution may have a pressure gauge attached for proper inflation via a bulb or handle that automatically reaches proper pressure when it is fully cranked and locked. Either method gives a continuous infusion at 3 to 5 ml/hr when the bag is inflated to 300 mm Hg. The system can also be flushed intermittently via a fast-flush device. Fig. 23-1 depicts the various components of a disposable single-pressure transducer system.

The tubing for this system is stiff and noncompliant and contains stopcocks for calibration to zero and for blood sampling. The length of tubing is kept to a minimum to prevent distortion of the signal; it is generally 3 to 4 feet long.

The fluid system is connected to the transducer, which senses changes in flow, temperature, concentration, pressure, light intensity, and other physiologic variables. Disposable and reusable transducers are available. External, disposable, strain gauge, and pressure transducers are the most widely used. Each system

*The author and editors wish to acknowledge the contributions made by Terri A. Miller, as author of this chapter in the first edition of *Intravenous Nursing: Clinical Principles and Practice.*

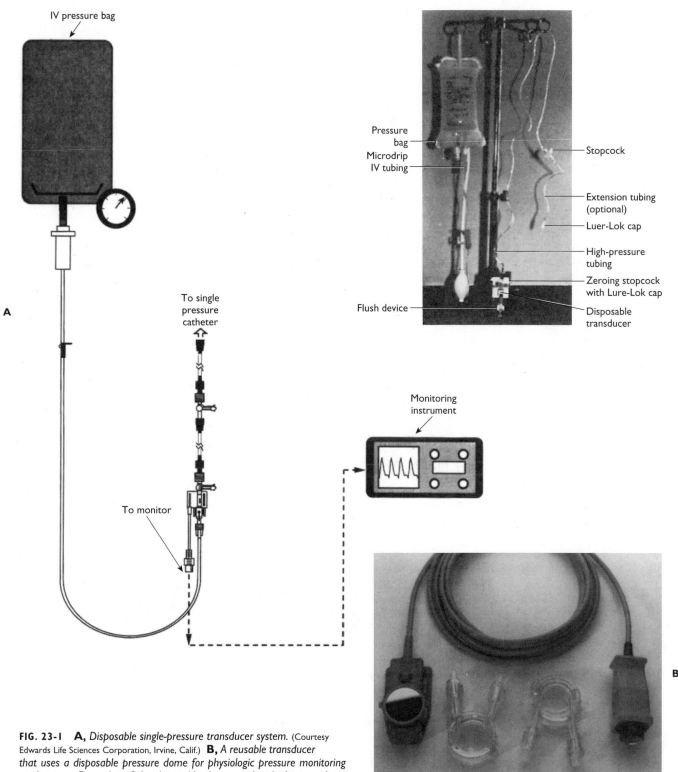

FIG. 23-1   **A,** *Disposable single-pressure transducer system.* (Courtesy Edwards Life Sciences Corporation, Irvine, Calif.) **B,** *A reusable transducer that uses a disposable pressure dome for physiologic pressure monitoring applications. Examples of the disposable dome used with the transducer are also shown.* (Courtesy Hewlett-Packard Company, Andover, Mass.)

has a diaphragm that transfers the pressure it senses to a bedside monitoring system.

Placing the transducer level with the patient's right atrium negates the effect of atmospheric pressure. This plane is known as the *phlebostatic axis* and is located at the fourth intercostal space, at the midaxillary line.[2-6] Marking the phlebostatic axis position on the patient's chest ensures the accuracy of each reading. Figs. 23-2 and 23-3 demonstrate the process of leveling a transducer to the phlebostatic axis.

The patient is placed in a supine position when the transducer is set to zero to facilitate the accuracy of the reading. If the transducer is below the level of the heart, a falsely high pressure can be recorded. When placed too high, the transducer reflects a falsely low reading.[5] Setting the monitor at zero on the scale will cancel the effect of atmospheric pressure and allow the pressures within the circulatory system to be recorded.

If the patient's head is kept elevated (e.g., because of cerebral injury), the phlebostatic axis should be marked on the patient's chest with an indelible marker, and the degree of elevation should be noted. Some institutions lock the bed in this position to ensure that it is kept elevated to the ordered degree and to ensure the accuracy of hemodynamic readings.

A cable attached to the transducer carries the signals to the bedside monitor, which is an amplifying device for these pressure readings. Basic monitor functions include digital read-outs, an oscilloscope to display waveforms, indicators for the various pressures being obtained, alarm systems with high and low adjustments, waveform size (gain) control, and controls for setting the machine to zero and for calibration. Simultaneous monitoring of various pressures is possible with newer monitoring systems.

Inserting a hemodynamic catheter is a sterile procedure. Equipment for insertion may be gathered from unit supplies, or prepackaged insertion kits may be used. Supplies needed include sterile gowns, gloves, masks, hats, drapes, towels, gauze, dressing, local anesthetic, suture equipment, flush solution, and a catheter. A stocked cart containing additional supplies in case of defect or contamination may be taken to the patient's bedside.

Preparation

Placement of a hemodynamic catheter requires obtaining informed consent from the patient, or from the family if the patient cannot consent. Ample time should be provided for the patient and family to ask questions; lessening patient apprehension can facilitate insertion. The patient should be told that the nurse will assist with the procedure, answer questions, and explain the steps as the procedure progresses. After consent is obtained, the system should be prepared (Box 23-1). Then the patient should be prepared to provide a sterile entry area. The insertion site should be scrubbed and prepared with povidone-iodine, alcohol, or both, and allowed to dry before venipuncture.[7] The catheter may be inserted into the antecubital area or directly into the central system by the subclavian, internal or external jugular, or femoral vein.

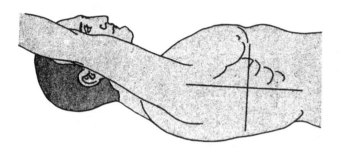

FIG. 23-2 *Transducer leveling from different positions.* (From Boggs RL, Wooldridge-King M: *AACN procedure manual for critical care*, ed 3, Philadelphia, 1993, WB Saunders.)

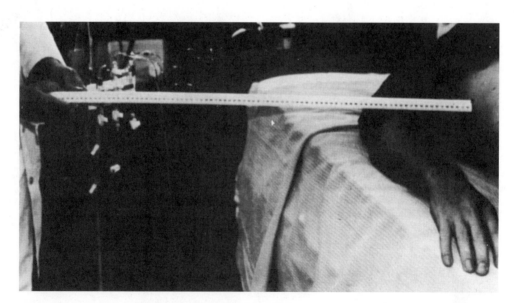

FIG. 23-3 *Leveling transducer to phlebostatic axis.* (From Boggs RL, Wooldridge-King M: *AACN procedure manual for critical care*, ed 3, Philadelphia, 1993, WB Saunders.)

A sterile field is prepared either during preparation of the equipment and fluid system or while the patient is being prepared. In some institutions, the physician prepares the patient while the nurse prepares the equipment and field. In other institutions, two nurses may prepare the patient and sterile field and are available to help with the insertion.

When a pulmonary artery catheter is placed, the balloon is checked for leakage before the catheter is inserted. If a multilumen catheter is used, the ports are preflushed with a heparinized solution. A 0.9% sodium chloride solution may be used for patients with known heparin allergy or when heparin use is contraindicated. Other items placed on the sterile field include a local anesthetic, suture equipment, sponges, and dressing equipment. A separate table may be used for sterile gowns, drapes, and towels. The nurse preparing the field dons a gown and gloves and may help the physician don gown and gloves, if necessary.

Insertion

The patient is placed in the Trendelenburg position unless it is contraindicated. This position engorges the jugular and subclavian vessels to ease insertion. The antecubital or femoral insertion does not require the Trendelenburg position. The assisting nurse passes equipment to the physician, observes the monitor for cardiac and waveform changes, inflates the balloon if a pulmonary artery catheter is inserted, reassures the patient, and places the sterile dressing over the insertion site. Transparent or traditional gauze dressings may be used to cover the catheter after it is inserted. Dressings are changed at established intervals according to organizational policy and procedure, when the dressing becomes damp, loosened, or soiled; or when inspection of the site is necessary.[7,8] Some institutions use a second nurse to attach the transducer tubing to the catheter. The nurse calibrates the bedside monitor, observes the patient's cardiac status, and records all waveform pressures as noted by the physician. This second nurse may obtain additional equipment, if needed, and may provide additional reassurance to the patient during the procedure.

Most monitors are able to run continuously, which is a convenient feature if only one nurse is assisting. These monitors store the digital pressure readings and waveforms so that they can be placed in the chart when the catheter insertion is completed. The type of catheter placed and its location, the person inserting it, and how the patient tolerated the procedure are recorded in the narrative section of the patient's chart.

Complications occurring with subclavian or jugular vein placement include hematoma, pneumothorax, and hemothorax. Arterial puncture or laceration and nerve damage can occur with both venous and arterial insertions.[2-5] A chest radiograph is taken to verify proper location of the catheter tip after any central line insertion. The radiograph is also used to assess for lung complications if the catheter placement is in the jugular or subclavian vein (see Chapter 24 for treatment of insertion complications).

Initiating therapy

Patient care after hemodynamic line placement focuses on patient safety and interpretation of hemodynamic values. Many patients may need restraints to prevent catheter or line dislodgement. If restraints are needed, institutional policies regarding their use should be followed.

In most institutions, blood samples for laboratory testing can be drawn by registered nurses and physicians. When heparin is used to maintain line patency, the results of coagulation studies may be altered. Care must be taken to maintain the monitoring system integrity because contamination and accidental blood

---

PROCEDURE *for System Preparation before Hemodynamic Catheter Insertion*   **Box 23-1**

1. Turn on the monitor. Allow it to warm up according to manufacturer's recommendation.
2. Prepare and label the flush solution, spike the bag with microdrop tubing, and prime the tubing.
3. Carefully remove the transducer tubing from the package. Tighten all connections and replace the open stopcock caps with dead-end caps.
4. If using a disposable dome, a drop of sterile 0.9% sodium chloride may be placed atop the transducer to facilitate transmission before the dome is attached.
5. Attach the transducer system to the monitor.
6. Attach the flush solution and tubing to the stopcock at the transducer.
7. Use the fast-flush device on the transducer tubing to prime it. Inspect tubing for air bubbles and prime again as needed.
8. Place the pressure bag over the flush solution. Wait to inflate the pressure bag until the monitor has been set to zero to avoid contamination or electrical hazard from leakage of fluid. This measure also will decrease pressure on the transducer tubing created by the system being closed to itself, and will lessen the chance of diaphragm rupture.
9. Align the transducer to the phlebostatic axis by using a carpenter's level. Mark the spot on the patient's chest with a waterproof marker.
10. If the patient cannot be supine, note the degree of elevation used for leveling the transducer on the flow sheet or other designated area.
11. Inflate the pressure bag. The system can now be calibrated, and a pressure monitoring range selected.
12. Follow the manufacturer's directions for calibrating and setting the monitor to zero. This may be accomplished by pushing a button and holding it in until the monitor has been set to zero and calibrated, or the monitor will perform its functions automatically after the desired function is selected.

loss may result if the line is disconnected. Blood loss from an arterial line can be rapid. A transparent dressing permits observation of the arterial insertion site. High and low alarm limits should always be set to assess significant changes and to detect accidental line disconnection.

The recording of pressure readings varies according to the severity of the patient's illness and institutional guidelines. Readings every 15 to 30 minutes are commonly required for unstable patients, whereas readings obtained every 2 hours may be routine after the patient is stabilized. Wedge pressures from a pulmonary artery catheter are not obtained as frequently in an effort to prevent vessel trauma and balloon rupture. The pulmonary artery diastolic pressure may be recorded instead of repeated inflation of the balloon. The care provided and pressure readings may be documented on a flow sheet. Clinically significant changes should always be recorded in the narrative section of the patient's chart.

Discontinuing therapy

The physician writes an order to remove the catheter when hemodynamic monitoring is no longer needed. The central catheter placed for hemodynamic monitoring is removed using the method noted in Chapter 22. The pulmonary artery catheter balloon must be deflated before it is removed to prevent damage to the cardiac valves. Pressure is applied at the insertion site for 5 to 10 minutes after the device is removed. Pressure should be held longer when arterial lines or other lines are removed from patients with coagulation abnormalities. These patients should be assessed after 10 to 15 minutes. A sterile dressing should be placed on the site after bleeding ceases.

After arterial and or central lines are removed, the condition of the insertion sites should be documented in the narrative section of the patient's chart. Early recognition of signs of infection, phlebitis, or hematoma facilitates early intervention. Documentation includes when and how the line was removed, the type of dressing applied, and how the patient tolerated the procedure.

TYPES OF HEMODYNAMIC MONITORING
Intraarterial monitoring

As the heart contracts, pressure from the blood volume is exerted against the arterial walls. The amount of blood in the left ventricle, the elasticity, and the integrity of the arterial system determine the amount of pressure needed for contraction.[2] Intraarterial monitoring is used to obtain direct measurements of the systolic and diastolic pressures occurring during the cardiac cycle.

The arterial line waveform has three separate components that reflect the cardiac cycle (Fig. 23-4). The upstroke, or positive deflection, occurs at the peak of systole and ranges from 90 to 140 mm Hg. The dicrotic notch occurs with aortic valve closure and reflects the beginning of diastole. The lowest point of the waveform is end-diastole and ranges from 60 to 90 mm Hg.

Most bedside monitors provide mean arterial pressure (MAP) in addition to systolic and diastolic values. MAP, which is an indicator of organ perfusion, is determined by the following equation:

$$MAP = Systole + 2 (Diastole)/3$$

Factors affecting MAP include the cardiac output and the elasticity of the vessels (systemic vascular resistance). MAP is reflected on the monitor screen by a number that is a weighted average of the systolic and diastolic readings, or it can be measured alone by use of an aneroid sphygmomanometer gauge. A normal MAP ranges from 70 to 105 mm Hg. Catheter size and location can cause pressure readings to vary, but the MAP is not affected by these characteristics.

Intraarterial monitoring is used with patients who require frequent blood gas samplings, patients receiving vasoactive drugs, critically ill patients undergoing other invasive monitoring, and patients who have undergone or will undergo surgical procedures.

Arterial catheter placement is determined by the collateral circulation and the size of the artery to be cannulated. The Allen test (Fig. 23-5) or a modified version of it is used to determine

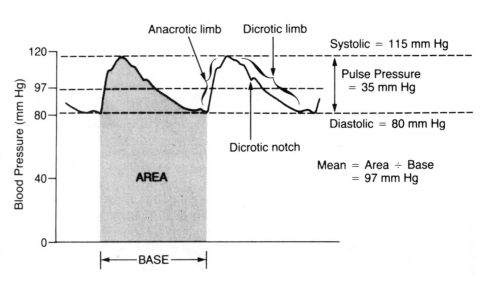

FIG. 23-4 *Normal arterial waveform.*
(From Darovic GO: *Hemodynamic monitoring,* Philadelphia, 1987, WB Saunders.)

adequate collateral circulation. Both arteries on the limb being used for insertion are occluded simultaneously. The limb is raised slightly above the torso while the hand is clenched several times. The pressure on each artery is released separately, and the hand is observed for return of color, which indicates adequate collateral circulation. Slowed return of color is a negative test result, and another site should be selected.[2]

Catheters are usually placed in the radial, brachial, or femoral arteries; the dorsalis pedis, axillary, temporal, and umbilical arteries are lesser-used sights. The catheter is placed either by direct arterial puncture or by cut-down if the vessel cannot be cannulated. Catheter changes are recommended every 3 to 5 days.

Preparation and insertion.
The system and patient are prepared as previously described. A short length of pressure tubing is added to the sterile tray. This tubing has a stopcock near the proximal end, which will be attached to the catheter after it is inserted. The tubing may be preflushed with a syringe or is flushed just before arterial insertion by connecting the distal end to the transducer tubing. After the pressure tubing is attached to the transducer tubing, it may be held by the assisting nurse or covered with a sterile towel and clamped on the field.

After the catheter is inserted, the system is set to zero and calibrated, the stopcock is opened to the patient, and readings are obtained. The nurse assists the physician either by being scrubbed and handing equipment to the physician or by attaching the monitoring tubing and recording pressure readings. The catheter is usually sutured in place, and a sterile dressing is applied. A pressure dressing is recommended if bleeding from the site occurs.

Types of catheters used for arterial monitoring include an over-the-needle catheter and an over-needle catheter with a guidewire. Some catheters are designed solely for arterial use, or a venous access catheter may be used. The length of the catheter depends on which artery is used, the size of the patient, and the preference of the inserter. Catheters made out of material such as silicone are soft and may affect pressure readings (i.e., the radial artery waveform may appear rounded or dampened as a result of kinking or an occlusion of the catheter).

Nursing considerations.
Nursing care of the patient with an arterial line includes assessing the catheter, system, and pressure waveform. The site should be observed for redness, tenderness, swelling, or drainage. The involved extremity should be inspected for color, size, warmth, and sensation distal to the insertion site. The dressing should be changed as previously described and when the catheter is changed. Nursing care is documented on the appropriate form according to institution policy.

The system should be checked for loose connections, proper pressure on the flush solution, dead-end caps on the stopcocks, and proper labeling of the tubing, including any changes. The system should be maintained as a closed system and changed every 96 hours.[7] The monitor should be set for the proper range (300 mm Hg), and alarms should be turned on. The high and low alarm limits need to be set according to the patient's blood pressure. Usually, these limits are 10 to 20 mm Hg above or below the patient's pressure, or as indicated by the physician order when vasoactive medications are administered.

Changes in the waveform may signify a change in the patient's condition or a change within the system. The physical status of the patient should be assessed, and if no changes are noted, the system should be evaluated.

A poorly defined or dampened waveform is softer, rounder, and less clearly defined on the monitor (Fig. 23-6). A dampened waveform can be caused by air or blood in the tubing, inadequate pressure on the flush solution bag, inaccurate calibration, or a positional catheter. Blood or air can be removed by aspiration followed by fast-flushing through a stopcock. The blood or air should always be aspirated before the fast-flush device is used to ensure that a clot or air embolus is not introduced into the patient.

The pressure on the flush solution bag should remain at 300 mm Hg. The system should be recalibrated and set to zero with each shift change, change of the line and solution, or whenever the waveform changes character. The phlebostatic axis should be verified before the system is recalibrated and set to zero.

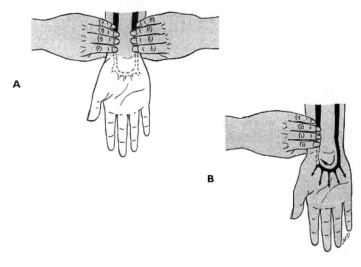

FIG. 23-5 *In the Allen test, the hand is raised and clenched several times. The radial and ulnar arteries are compressed, and then the hand is lowered. **A,** When the hand is opened and arteries are still occluded, the client's hand is pale. **B,** When either the ulnar or the radial artery is released, the entire hand should become pink as a result of collateral circulation.* (From Black JM, Matassarin-Jacobs E, editors: *Luckmann and Sorensen's medical surgical nursing: a psychophysiologic approach,* ed 4, Philadelphia, 1993, WB Saunders.)

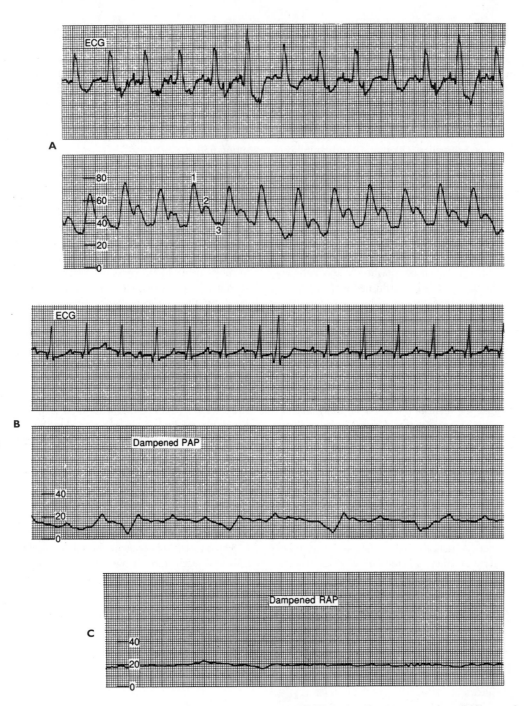

FIG. 23-6 *Effects of dampening on pulmonary artery pressure (PAP) and right atrium pressure (RAP) waveforms.* **A,** *Normal PAP waveform. 1, PA systole; 2, dicrotic notch; 3, PA diastole.* **B,** *Dampened PAP waveform.* **C,** *Dampening of RAP waveform. Dampening of the waveform may result from clots at catheter tip, catheter against vessel or heart wall, air in lines, partially closed stopcock, deflated pressure bag, or patient hypotension.* (From Boggs RL, Wooldridge-King M: AACN *procedure manual for critical care,* ed 3, Philadelphia, 1993, WB Saunders.)

Observing the blood pressure and reporting changes is a major responsibility of nurses caring for patients with arterial lines. If a significant drop or elevation is noted and the system is intact, a cuff blood pressure should also be obtained. Catheter size and location can cause variations between cuff and arterial pressures between 5 and 20 mm Hg. Hospital protocol may pro-vide guidelines for assessing the arterial line blood pressure's correlation with cuff pressure.

If the patient is taking medication that affects blood pressure, specific orders for notification of the physician are written. The nurse should always assess the patient's physical status when interpreting arterial monitoring changes.

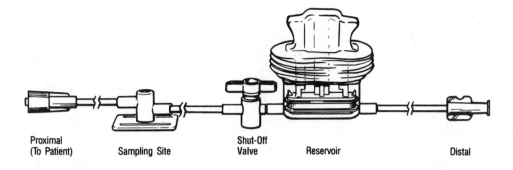

Proximal
(To Patient)   Sampling Site   Shut-Off Valve   Reservoir   Distal

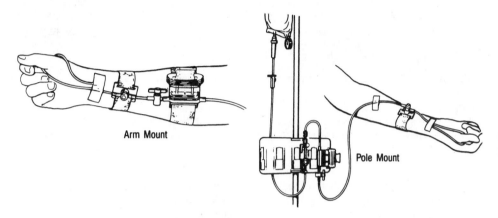

Arm Mount   Pole Mount

FIG. 23-7   *VAMP system for needleless blood withdrawal from hemodynamic lines.* (Courtesy Edwards Life Sciences Corporation, Irvine, Calif.)

PROCEDURE *for Obtaining Arterial Blood Samples by the Syringe Method*   **Box 23-2**

1. Obtain necessary supplies, including syringes in the appropriate volume for specimen collection, clean gloves, 4 × 4-inch gauze pads, new stopcock caps.
2. Remove the cap from the stopcock closest to the insertion site, and attach a sterile syringe to the portal.
3. Turn the stopcock off to the solution, and aspirate 3 to 5 ml of blood into the syringe.
4. Turn the stopcock off to the syringe, remove it, and replace with a second syringe. This syringe may contain heparin if it is needed for the test being performed.
5. Turn the stopcock off to the solution and aspirate the amount of blood needed.
6. Turn the stopcock off to the syringe and remove it. Use the fast-flush device to clear the line of blood distal to the stopcock.
7. Turn the stopcock off to the patient, and flush the portal free of blood. Turn the stopcock off to the portal, and recap with a new, sterile cap.
8. Document the amount of blood withdrawn, the type of laboratory test for which it was drawn, and the return of the initial waveform after flushing the portal free of blood.
9. Recalibrate if needed.

Blood samples can be obtained from an arterial line. The system may have a reservoir to withdraw blood (Fig. 23-7), or the syringe method with aspiration may be used (Box 23-2). Gloves should be worn when blood is obtained from an arterial line.

As previously stated, care and observation of the line can be documented on a flow sheet designed for that purpose. Abnormal findings or a change of site should be recorded in the narrative section of the patient's chart.

Complications. Complications occurring with arterial line placement include bleeding, infection, arterial spasm, pain, nerve damage, circulatory decrease in the ipsilateral side, throm-

bus formation, and air embolism. If complications occur, catheter removal is indicated in most cases. Infection is usually treated with systemic antibiotics. Fasciotomy or arterial repair (or both) may be indicated if thrombus formation and occlusion, severe swelling with circulatory decrease, or excessive, uncontrolled bleeding occur.[2-6,9-14]

Discontinuing therapy. A minimum of 5 minutes of direct pressure should be applied to an upper extremity artery after the line is removed. Femoral catheters or those in patients with abnormal coagulation study results should have pressure applied to the insertion site for at least 15 minutes after the catheter is removed. In patients receiving coagulation therapy,

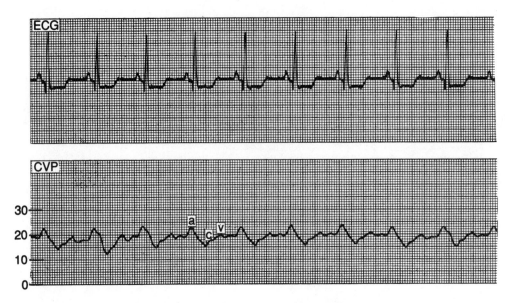

FIG. 23-8 *Central venous pressure waveform with a, c, and v waves present. The a wave usually is seen just after the P wave of the electrocardiogram (ECG). The c wave appears at the time of the RST junction on the ECG. The v wave is seen in the TP interval.* (From Boggs RL, Wooldridge-King M: *AACN procedure manual for critical care,* ed 3, Philadelphia, 1993, WB Saunders.)

the therapy may be discontinued for 1 or 2 hours before the line is removed. All bleeding should cease before a pressure dressing is applied. Physicians commonly order bed rest for 6 to 8 hours after removal of a femoral line.[2-6,9-14] The site should be checked at each assessment and redressed if bleeding occurs. The nurse should always check under the affected limb for bleeding. Patients should notify the nurse at once if they feel wet, warm, or sticky sensations under the dressing or affected extremity.

Central venous pressure monitoring

CVP is a measure of right-sided heart function, or the pressure of blood in the right atrium or vena cava. The waveform for a CVP tracing reflects the contraction of the atria and the concurrent effect of the ventricles and surrounding major vessels. It consists of a, c, and v ascending (positive) waves and x and y descending (negative) waves (Fig. 23-8). Because systolic atrial pressure (a) and diastolic (v) pressure are almost the same, the reading is taken as an average or mean of the two.

Normal values may vary, depending on the method used for measurement and on the patient's underlying condition. CVP values are affected by circulating volume, cardiac contractility, and vascular tone. Water manometer pressures range between 4 and 12 cm H_2O. If a transducer and monitor are used, the pressures are between 0 and 8 mm Hg. Physician orders direct the frequency of CVP readings and interventions for abnormal values.

The approach for placing a CVP line varies. Some lines are inserted by the antecubital route, whereas others are inserted via the subclavian or jugular routes. The tip of any device placed for CVP readings should lie in the distal superior vena cava to prevent right atrial irritation, arrhythmia, and erosion of the catheter through the atrium. Because no valves exist between the right atrium and the superior vena cava, a tip in this location provides accurate values from the right side of the heart.

Pressure monitoring setups for CVP readings are identical to those previously noted. The monitor is set to the desired scale before reading the CVP.

CVP readings can also be obtained by use of a water manometer. This method is most commonly used outside the critical care setting when other hemodynamic tracings are not needed. Water manometers use a fluid column and continuous-drip IV solution instead of a pressure line to keep the system patent. Infusion is performed with a three-way stopcock (Fig. 23-9).

When readings are needed, the stopcock is turned off to the solution and on to a fluid chamber. The pressure in the right atrium is reflected in this fluid. When the pressures equalize, the reading is taken from the markings on the fluid chamber.

The distal port of a multilumen catheter is used to measure CVP. The proximal port of a pulmonary artery catheter is used. Infusions through the other ports on both types of catheters may need to be turned off during readings to obtain an accurate pressure. However, if infusates cannot be temporarily stopped, this inability is documented to maintain consistency between persons performing the measurement.

Nursing considerations. Routine care of hemodynamic catheters has previously been described. Dressing, administration, setup of the line, and changes should all be performed and charted according to the Intravenous Nurses Society's *Infusion Nursing Standards of Practice.*

CVP readings indicate changes in the preload (filling pressure in the right ventricle) of the heart. Abnormal readings may result from inadequate or increased preload, decreased contractility, or increased afterload (pressure the left ventricle contracts against). If the waveform is low or dampened, line integrity should be assessed. Abnormal CVP readings are seen in patients with tricuspid stenosis and regurgitation, cardiac tamponade, constrictive pericarditis, pulmonary hypertension, chronic left ventricular failure, and volume overload or depletion.

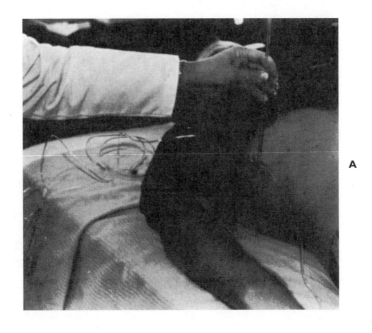

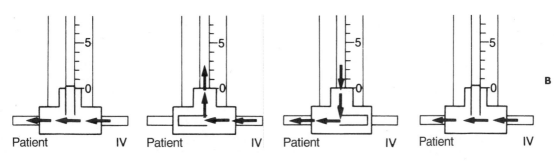

Fluid flow = ⬅ ⬅ ⬅

FIG. 23-9   A, *Water manometer placed at phlebostatic axis on patient.* (From Boggs RL, Wooldridge-King M: *AACN procedure manual for critical care,* ed 3, Philadelphia, 1993, WB Saunders.) **B,** *Proper stopcock positioning sequence in a venous pressure manometer.* (From Darovic GO: *Hemodynamic monitoring,* Philadelphia, 1987, WB Saunders.)

Complications. Complications occurring with CVP lines are the same as those previously noted. If the antecubital approach is used, the patient may experience mechanical phlebitis after the insertion. Application of warm moist heat is used to treat the phlebitis.[15] If the phlebitis is not resolved in 24 to 36 hours, the catheter is removed.

Pulmonary artery catheter monitoring

Pulmonary artery catheter (or balloon floatation) pressures reflect left ventricular function. The catheter passes through the right side of the heart into the pulmonary vessels. When the balloon of the catheter is inflated, it wedges in a pulmonary artery (Fig. 23-10). Wedge pressures reflect left ventricular end-diastolic pressure in patients with normally functioning mitral valves. Pulmonary artery pressure can be assessed preoperatively or postoperatively to give the physician more extensive knowledge of the patients' cardiac and circulatory status. Pulmonary artery catheters are also placed in trauma patients and

patients with acute respiratory and cardiac impairment. Pulmonary artery catheters are used only in critical care settings.

Pulmonary artery catheters are multiluminal and can be used to measure CVP, pulmonary artery pressure, PWP, cardiac output, and mixed venous oxygen saturation; they can also be used for temporary pacing of the heart. The number of lumens within the catheter dictates how many functions the catheter is able to perform (Fig. 23-11).

Normal pulmonary artery pressure ranges from 20 to 30 mm Hg systolic/8 to 12 mm Hg diastolic. Pulmonary artery pressure reflects pulmonary blood volume and vascular resistance. Systolic pressure represents right ventricular contraction, and diastolic pressure represents resistance to blood flow within the small arterioles and pulmonary capillaries. If there are no obstructions to blood flow, the diastolic pressure reflects the PWP. Normal PWP readings range from 4 to 12 mm Hg.[2-6]

The cardiac output reflects how well the heart is pumping; specifically, cardiac output equals the amount of blood the left ventricle ejects in 1 minute. A specialized computer measures

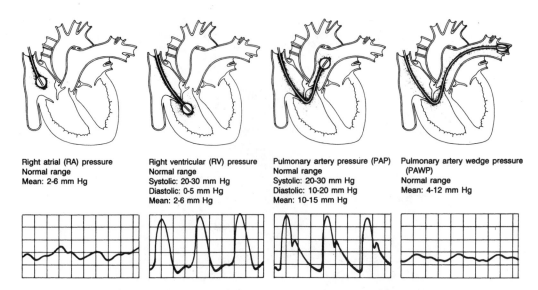

Right atrial (RA) pressure
Normal range
Mean: 2-6 mm Hg

Right ventricular (RV) pressure
Normal range
Systolic: 20-30 mm Hg
Diastolic: 0-5 mm Hg
Mean: 2-6 mm Hg

Pulmonary artery pressure (PAP)
Normal range
Systolic: 20-30 mm Hg
Diastolic: 10-20 mm Hg
Mean: 10-15 mm Hg

Pulmonary artery wedge pressure
(PAWP)
Normal range
Mean: 4-12 mm Hg

FIG. 23-10 *Flow-directed balloon-tipped catheter as it passes through the right side of the heart, wedging in a distal pulmonary artery with corresponding pressure waveforms and normal values.* (From Alspach JG: AACN core curriculum for critical care nursing, ed 4, Philadelphia, 1991, WB Saunders.)

the cardiac output by determining the length of time it takes a predetermined amount of solution to reach the temperature thermistor at the tip of the catheter. The normal cardiac output ranges from 4 to 8 L/min.[2-6]

The vessels of choice for placement of a pulmonary artery catheter are the subclavian and jugular veins; the femoral and antecubital veins are less commonly used. As the catheter is passed through the heart, pressure readings in the right atrium, right ventricle, and pulmonary artery and the PWP are noted. The waveform on the monitor changes with the passage of the catheter through the heart and reflects the specific location of the tip. Characteristic waveform variations and pressure measurements facilitate passage at the patient's bedside without the need for fluoroscopy (see Fig. 23-10).

Commonly observed waveforms when pulmonary artery catheters with bedside monitoring are used include the pulmonary artery and PWP. The pulmonary artery waveform has an abrupt upstroke (systole) with a gradual downstroke followed by a dicrotic notch (pulmonic valve closure, designated *c*). The PWP has a and v waves owing to atrial contraction and ventricular systole (Fig. 23-12).

Preparation and insertion.
Along with the routine setup previously described, preparation for inserting a pulmonary artery catheter includes checking the integrity of the balloon. The balloon is inflated and placed in a cup of sterile water or saline to observe for leaks. Care must be taken not to rupture the balloon by overinflation. The balloon port is labeled with the inflation amount (0.8 to 1.5 ml). The nurse who prepares the sterile field and scrubs with the physician is responsible for checking the balloon, preflushing the other ports, and attaching the sterile sheath to the catheter.

After the catheter is placed, a routine dressing for central lines is applied. Documentation should include the insertion site location, length of the catheter inserted to obtain PWP, initial readings, and patient's tolerance of the procedure. Subsequent pressure readings can be documented on a flow sheet.

Nursing considerations.
The frequency and type of readings obtained depend on the severity of the patient's condition and the physician's orders. Various medications to help improve or ease preload and afterload may be ordered based on pulmonary artery, PWP, or cardiac output readings. The nurse must be sure that each reading is performed accurately to assess trends that indicate need for therapy.

Changes in pressures can be seen in patients with conditions that increase the pulmonary blood flow, including pulmonary hypertension and embolus, mitral stenosis and left ventricular failure, and exacerbation of pulmonary disease (chronic obstructive pulmonary disease). Cardiac tamponade, constrictive pericarditis, or volume overload may also result in elevated pressures. Decreased pressures may indicate hypovolemia or a reduction in afterload, as occurs with vasodilator administration.

Complications.
Insertion complications with a pulmonary artery catheter include those noted for any central line insertion, and arrhythmias as the catheter floats through the right side of the heart. The irritation to the endocardium is the mechanical cause of these arrhythmias. Pulmonary infarction and balloon rupture can also occur.

After the catheter is inserted, the nurse should observe for waveform changes that indicate problems within the system. These changes, which include dampening or poor waveform and respiratory variations from ventilation, may indicate catheter fling, catheter migration into the wedge position, or balloon rupture. If the patient's physical status has not changed, the waveform change may result from system problems.

A dampened wave is less defined and more rounded than a normal wave. The upstroke may be slowed and the dicrotic notch absent (see Fig. 23-6). The pressure bag should be checked

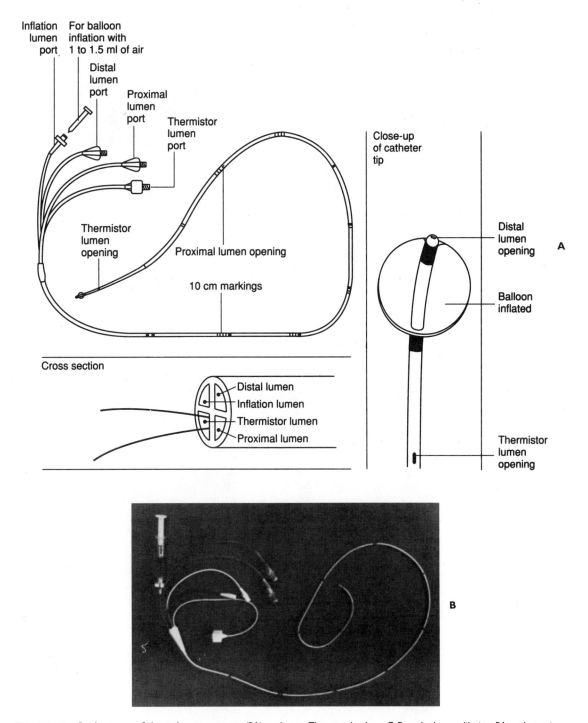

FIG. 23-11   A, *Anatomy of the pulmonary artery (PA) catheter. The standard no. 7 French thermodilution PA catheter is 110 cm in length and contains four lumens.* **B,** *PA catheter with atrial and ventricular pacing lumens.* (From Boggs RL, Wooldridge-King M: *AACN procedure manual for critical care,* ed 3, Philadelphia, 1993, WB Saunders.)

for proper inflation, all connections should be tightened, and any air or blood in line should be removed and the system recalibrated and reset to zero.

If the wave has developed an artifact or is exaggerated, the catheter may have developed "fling" or "whip" as a result of movement at the insertion site as the patient moves. Fling may result from the location of the catheter in the pulmonary artery.

The nurse should be sure the patient is lying flat or at the recorded angle of elevation and is still when values are recorded. The physician may need to pull the line back to compensate for the internal location or may need to reposition it entirely if the catheter has coiled in the ventricle.

When the catheter is inserted in a patient with a ventilator or if the patient is receiving mechanical ventilation after the

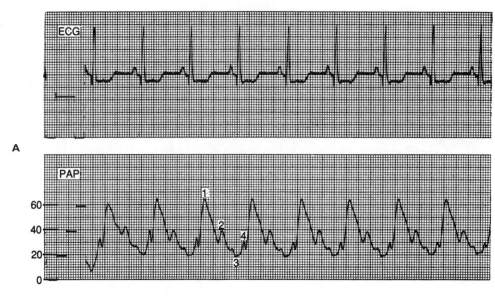

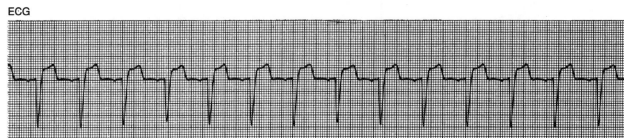

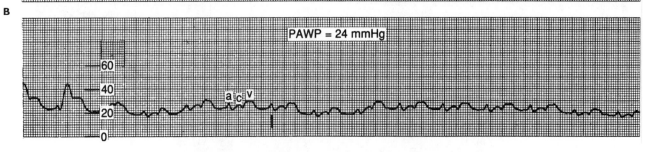

FIG. 23-12 **A,** *Pulmonary artery (PA) waveform and components: 1, PA systole; 2, dicrotic notch; 3, PA end-diastole; 4, anacrotic notch of PA valve opening.* **B,** *Normal PA wedge pressure waveform and components. Note delay in a, c, and v waves as a result of the time it takes for the mechanical events to show a pressure change. This waveform is from a spontaneously breathing patient. The arrow indicates end-expiration, where the height of a wave pressure is measured.* (From Boggs RL, Wooldridge-King M: AACN procedure manual for critical care, ed 3, Philadelphia, 1993, WB Saunders.)

insertion, pulmonary artery pressures may increase as a result of positive thoracic pressure. Readings (PA and PWP) should be taken at the end of the respiratory cycle (end-exhalation). Patients are not routinely taken off ventilators to obtain readings because doing so may jeopardize the patient's respiratory status.

When the catheter migrates into a smaller branch of the pulmonary artery, it may occlude the artery without balloon inflation. This migration results in a "wedge" waveform on the monitor. If the system is intact and the balloon is deflated, migration is suspected. If the initial length of catheter inserted has been documented, the dressing should be removed and the amount of catheter lying outside the patient checked against the length recorded at insertion. If the catheter is farther inside the vein, migration has occurred. Before the physician is called to reposition the catheter, the nurse may attempt to dislodge the wedged catheter. Having the patient cough, suctioning an intubated patient, or turning the patient on either side may cause migration back to a pulmonary artery pattern. If such attempts are unsuccessful, the catheter will need to be pulled back until a pulmonary artery pattern appears on the screen. The balloon is then inflated, and a PWP is obtained. The physician may need to resuture the catheter, or it can be more securely taped.

Balloon rupture can occur if the balloon is overinflated or is frequently inflated. The amount of air needed to obtain PWP

(0.8 to 1.5 ml) should be noted with the initial insertion, and no more than this should be used each time. Using the full balloon capacity may not be necessary to obtain a wedge. After the reading is obtained, the syringe is removed from the port for deflation. If blood is noted in the balloon port or if a wedge pattern cannot be obtained after the system has been thoroughly checked, rupture is suspected. The port should be locked off and taped over to prevent it from being used. The catheter may be replaced, or the pulmonary artery diastolic reading may be used in place of a wedge reading.

Any complications should be documented in the narrative section of the patient's chart. Routine pressure readings and care may be noted on a flow sheet. Documentation of removal of the catheter includes the deflation of the balloon, the position of the patient (Trendelenburg), the amount of time pressure is applied to the site, the type of dressing applied, and how the patient tolerated the procedure.

NURSING DIAGNOSIS

The nursing diagnosis for patients with hemodynamic lines may include reduction of anxiety, recognition and treatment of any insertion complications, potential for bleeding, infection, monitoring problems, and potential problems during or after catheter removal.[14]

The expected patient outcomes will be a less anxious patient and family, complication-free insertion, and absence of or prompt recognition and treatment of any bleeding, infection, mechanical problems, or problems occurring with removal.[14]

OTHER TYPES OF MONITORING

Some catheters enhance cardiac perfusion and measure left atrial pressures, cerebral pressures, and other vital organ pressures. These catheters are considered hemodynamic devices more advanced than those routinely used by all critical care units. Many critical care references describe these types of hemodynamic monitoring devices in detail.[2-6]

SUMMARY

Hemodynamic monitoring reflects advanced nursing practice that requires basic critical care assessment skills and an understanding of basic cardiovascular physiology. Nurses in a critical care setting are familiar with the different types of hemodynamic monitoring catheters. The ability to interpret the waveform and its values in conjunction with physical assessment of the patient enables prompt interventions. When basic knowledge and appropriate infection control techniques with regard to IV therapy are also used, quality patient care is ensured.

REFERENCES

1. *Taber's cyclopedic medical dictionary,* ed 18, Philadelphia, 1997, FA Davis.
2. Daily EK, Schroeder JS: *Techniques in bedside hemodynamic monitoring,* ed 4, St Louis, 1990, Mosby.
3. DeAngelis R: Diagnostic studies. In Alspach J, editor: *Core curriculum for critical care nursing,* ed 5, Philadelphia, 1998, WB Saunders.
4. Kadota LT: Hemodynamic monitoring. In Clochesy JM, Breu C, Cardin S, editors: *Critical care nursing,* Philadelphia, 1993, WB Saunders.
5. Lough M: Introduction to hemodynamic monitoring, *Nurs Clin North Am* 22(1):89, 1987.
6. Yang SS, Bentivoglio LG, Maranhao V: *From cardiac catheterization data to hemodynamic parameters,* ed 3, Philadelphia, 1988, FA Davis.
7. Centers for Disease Control and Prevention: Guideline for prevention of intravascular device-related infections, *Am J Infect Control* 24:262, 1996.
8. Intravenous Nurses Society: Infusion nursing standards of practice, *JIN* (suppl) 23(6S), 2000.
9. Rountree WD: Removal of pulmonary artery catheters by registered nurses: a study in safety and complications, *Focus Crit Care* 18(4):313, 1991.
10. Masters S: Complications of pulmonary artery catheters, *Crit Care Nurse* 9(9):82, 1989.
11. Biga CD, Bethel SA: Hemodynamic monitoring in postanesthesia care units, *Crit Care Nurs Clin North Am* 3(1):83, 1991.
12. Covey M, McLane C, Smith N: Infection related to intravascular pressure monitoring: effects of flush and tubing changes, *Am J Infect Control* 16(5):206, 1988.
13. Crow S, Conrad SA, Chaney-Rowell C: Microbial contamination of arterial infusions used for hemodynamic monitoring: a randomized trial of contamination with sampling through conventional stopcocks versus a novel closed system, *Infect Control Hosp Epidemiol* 10(12):557, 1989.
14. Hazinski M: Hemodynamic monitoring. In Johanson BC, Dungca CU, Hoffmeister D, editors: *Standards for critical care,* ed 2, St Louis, 1985, Mosby.
15. *I.V. therapy made incredibly easy,* Springhouse, Pa, 1998, Springhouse Corp.

Intravenous Complications

Maxine B. Perdue, BSN, MHA, MBA, CRNI, CNAA

LOCAL VERSUS SYSTEMIC COMPLICATIONS
    Local complications
    Systemic complications
COMPLICATIONS ASSOCIATED WITH CENTRAL VENOUS CATHETERS
    Insertion-related complications
    Complications associated with indwelling central venous catheters
NURSING CONSIDERATIONS

Up to 80% to 90% of all hospitalized patients in the United States receive some form of intravenous (IV) therapy. An increasing number of patients receive some form of IV therapy in alternative care settings, such as physician's offices, ambulatory clinics, and homes. Although most IV therapy is administered without problems, complications do occur and range from minor to very serious. Some of the more serious complications can result in death if immediate medical intervention is not provided.

The potential for complications is always present in the patient receiving IV therapy. Complications increase hospital stays, length of therapy, and nursing responsibilities and can put the patient at risk for other medical problems. Furthermore, the patient experiences additional discomfort, and overall expenses are increased.

Fortunately, most of these complications are preventable. A thorough knowledge and understanding of the risks involved with IV therapy and measures to prevent their occurrence can eliminate many of the hazards associated with this treatment. Patient education in recognizing the signs and symptoms of complications and frequent monitoring by the nurse result in early detection and treatment. These measures may prevent further complications and promote prompt healing.

LOCAL VERSUS SYSTEMIC COMPLICATIONS

Complications associated with IV therapy are classified according to their location. *Local complications* are usually seen at or near the insertion site or occur as a result of mechanical failure. These complications are more common than systemic complications and are not usually serious. Immediate recognition of associated signs and symptoms coupled with nursing intervention can prevent more serious complications from occurring.

Systemic complications are those occurring within the vascular system, usually remote from the IV site. Although these complications are uncommon, they are usually very serious and can be life-threatening without appropriate medical interven-

tion. Some local complications can lead to more serious systemic complications. For example, thrombophlebitis can develop into a pulmonary embolism if the thrombus becomes detached and floats free in the vascular system. Systemic complications are more difficult to treat than local complications; preventing systemic complications is far easier than treating them.

Local complications

Local complications result from mechanical problems associated with the infusion system or result from trauma to the intima of the vein (Box 24-1). Mechanical problems can result in depriving the patient of urgently needed fluids or medications if vein access is lost. Trauma to the endothelial lining of the vein can lead to extensive edema, depriving the patient of needed fluids and medications, and to necrosis of surrounding tissue; thrombophlebitis, with the subsequent danger of embolism; and sepsis, if an infection at the site is not detected early or goes untreated. Individuals performing IV procedures must use techniques to prevent trauma to the vein intima and must monitor the system often to detect mechanical difficulties and signs of potential complications. The frequency of monitoring should be stated in established policies and procedures, and compliance should be monitored under the institution's clinical performance improvement program.

Mechanical complications. *Mechanical complications* relate to a failure of the IV system to adequately deliver therapy at the prescribed rate. They are usually resolved by correction of the identified problem. If a mechanical problem is suspected, six major areas should be evaluated (Box 24-2).

Tourniquet. Clinicians have been known to fail to release the tourniquet once catheter placement is complete. Fluid does not flow, or blood may back up the tubing. Potential circulatory problems can occur if the tourniquet is not released.

Intravenous site. The IV site should be checked for swelling at, above, and below the insertion of the cannula. By observing for potential problems associated with the site, one can immediately rule out site-related problems.

Cannula. Proper placement of the cannula should be verified. A cannula tip that lies against a bifurcation, valve, or a cannula that is kinked or bent, can slow or stop the infusion. Pulling back slightly on the cannula can often eliminate this problem. Bent cannulas should be discontinued and replaced to prevent possible cannula breakage and subsequent catheter emboli. Taping the cannula to prevent in-and-out motion can help prevent bending or kinking.

Placement of a cannula in a flexion area can also affect the

Box 24-1   Local Complications of Intravenous Therapy

Mechanical failure
Infiltration
Extravasation
Phlebitis
Postinfusion phlebitis
Thrombosis
Thrombophlebitis
Ecchymosis or hematoma
Site infection
Venous or arterial spasm

Box 24-2   Steps in the Evaluation of Mechanical Complications

Check for tourniquet.
Check the site.
Check the cannula.
Check the solution container.
Check the tubing.
Check the involved extremity.

infusion rate. If not obvious, one can easily check for a positional rate by having the patient flex and extend the extremity. If the flow rate slows or increases, the cannula is *positional*. If venous status is limited and the cannula cannot be changed, the application of an armboard should be considered. Armboards must be used according to agency policy and procedure and in compliance with Joint Commission on Accreditation of Healthcare Organizations (JCAHO) regulations.[1] Sites in flexion areas should be avoided, if possible, because they can lead to further complications.

Occasionally, a cannula may leak at the point where it attaches to the hub, or the cannula may be obstructed as a result of the manufacturing process. If either of these situations occurs, the cannula should be removed. The package and the cannula should be placed in a puncture-resistant container that meets the standards of the Occupational Safety and Health Administration (OSHA)[2] and saved by the designated department (usually Risk Management) in event of litigation related to use of the cannula. The lot number should be noted and the manufacturer should be made aware of the occurrence. Other cannulas from the same lot should be monitored for defects. If serious patient injury results from use of the cannula, the incident should be reported to the U.S. Food and Drug Administration, as noted in Chapter 16.

Partially or completely obstructed cannulas, regardless of cause, should be removed. They should not be flushed because a clot may be dislodged; the resulting embolus could cause a more serious complication.

Solution container.
The solution container should be assessed. An empty container or a lack of adequate gravity flow can lead to an inaccurate flow rate or no flow rate at all. This problem is easily corrected by hanging another bag or by adjusting the height of the IV pole.

The solution container should be checked for a patent air vent. IV solution bags do not need to be vented; however, nonvented bottles require a vented adapter or vented tubing. A vacuum cannot be created within a bottle, and solution will not flow from a bottle unless it is replaced with air. Using a needle to vent a bottle is inappropriate because it opens the system for the entry of bacteria.

Another concern is the bag entry port; if it is obstructed, solution cannot pass. The outlet port seal must be completely penetrated by the administration spike for solutions to flow freely.

Refrigerated solutions should be removed from the refrigerator and allowed to reach room temperature before they are administered. The administration of cold solutions can produce venospasms with vasoconstriction and subsequent slowing of the infusion rate.

Tubing.
Tubing that is pinched, crimped, or kinked prevents the delivery of an accurate flow rate. Tubing may need to be taped to prevent this problem. Filters can become blocked by particulates and can slow the infusion rate, particularly with the administration of certain medications, such as tetracycline. The filter should be changed when this problem occurs.

Patient.
The involved extremity should be checked for constrictive clothing, identification bracelet, jewelry, and restraints. Anything placed above an IV site that constricts the arm may act as a tourniquet and slow or stop the infusion.

Ecchymosis and hematoma.
Ecchymosis is a term used to denote the infiltration of blood into the tissues, whereas *hematoma* usually refers to uncontrolled bleeding at a venipuncture site, usually creating a hard, painful lump. Fig. 24-1 illustrates ecchymosis with hematoma formation. Ecchymosis and hematomas are commonly associated with venipunctures that are performed by unskilled professionals or on patients who have a tendency to bruise easily. Patients receiving anticoagulants and long-term steroid therapy are particularly susceptible to bleeding from vein trauma. Ecchymosis and hematomas often occur when multiple entries are made into a vein, or when attempts are made into hard-to-see veins or those that cannot be palpated.

The presence of ecchymosis and hematomas limits veins for future use and damages tissues. If a hematoma is severe, it may limit the use of an extremity.

Patient assessment.
The IV site and surrounding area should be observed for swelling during cannulation. Ecchymosis may not be noted immediately because of tissue turgor and the amount of blood escaping into the tissues. Ecchymosis occurs first, and if bleeding is allowed to continue a hematoma is formed. If sufficient bleeding is present, it is visible at the moment the cannula pierces the vein as blood escapes into the tissues. Discoloration may be immediate or slow, depending on the amount of subcutaneous tissue between the vein and the skin exterior.

Nursing interventions.
If ecchymosis occurs during venipuncture, the cannula should be removed and light pressure should be applied. If heavy pressure is applied, fragile veins within the area may rupture and increase bleeding. These areas usually feel sore, are unsightly, and take 1 to 2 weeks to disappear.

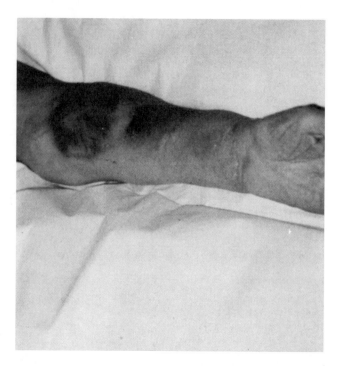

FIG. 24-1 *Ecchymosis with hematoma. The infiltration of blood into the tissues with uncontrolled bleeding can create a hematoma.* (Courtesy of Johnson and Johnson Medical, Inc., Vascular Access, Arlington, Tx.)

If a hematoma is noted during a venipuncture attempt, the cannula is removed immediately, direct pressure is applied to the area, catheter integrity is assessed, and the extremity is elevated until the bleeding has stopped. A dry, sterile dressing is applied to the site and the area is monitored for signs of breakthrough bleeding. Ice may be applied to the area to prevent further enlargement of the hematoma. The extremity is monitored for circulatory, neurologic, and motor function.

Preventive measures. Ecchymosis cannot always be prevented. The best prevention for hematomas is to ensure that venipunctures are performed by highly skilled professionals. Inexperienced individuals should never perform venipunctures on patients with very fragile veins or veins that are not visible or easily palpable.

Hematomas can also result from excessive pressure being applied to a venipuncture site when a cannula is removed. Direct pressure with a dry, sterile dressing should be applied when cannulas are removed. Elevating the extremity while continuing to apply pressure for 1 or 2 minutes helps stop bleeding and prevents hematoma formation. Because alcohol pads inhibit clotting, they should not be used.

Occluded cannula. Peripheral and central venous cannulas can become occluded if monitoring or proper maintenance and care are not carried out. Cannulas can become occluded with blood when solution containers run dry and when flush solutions are not administered appropriately. The administration of incompatible solutions or medications can also lead to precipitate formation within the catheter with subsequent occlusion.

Patient assessment. Usually, the first sign of a partially occluded cannula is the inability to maintain an accurate flow rate. The infusion slows, and readjusting the infusion rate has no effect. When the occlusion intensifies, the infusion stops. Resistance is met when attempts are made to flush an occluded cannula. Prescribed therapy cannot be administered if the cath-

eter is occluded; in addition, a danger exists of thrombophlebitis or pulmonary embolism.

Nursing intervention. Cannulas should never be flushed to remove an occlusion. Clearing a cannula occlusion by force releases the occluding substance directly into the vascular system, creating a potential for an embolus. A peripheral cannula should be removed, the cannula should be examined for integrity, and a dry, sterile dressing should be applied to the site. If therapy is to be continued, a new cannula should be placed in another vein. Interventions for occluded central venous catheters are discussed under Complications Associated with Central Venous Catheters.

Preventive measures. Solution containers should be changed when less than 100 ml of solution remains. The use of time tape to designate the time the solution will reach certain levels is very helpful in determining when a container will empty.

Solutions and medications should be evaluated for compatibilities before they are mixed and administered. The pharmacist should be consulted with questions about compatibilities to prevent the potential for crystallization from the mixing of incompatible solutions.

Policies and procedures should be established for the flushing of cannulas used as intermittent devices. The American Society of Health-System Pharmacists (ASHP) recommends using 0.9% sodium chloride to maintain patency of peripheral indwelling cannulas.[3]

Manufacturers' guidelines should be used when flushing catheters. If heparin is the flush solution of choice, the lowest possible concentration of heparin should be used. The amount and the frequency of the flush should not alter the patient's clotting factors. When medications are administered that are incompatible with heparin, the cannula is flushed with 0.9% sodium chloride before and after the administration of the medication.

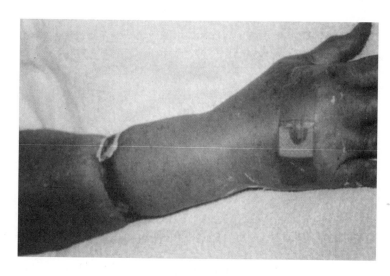

FIG. 24-2 *Infiltration: the inadvertent administration of a nonvesicant solution or medication into surrounding tissues.* (Courtesy of Johnson and Johnson Medical, Inc., Vascular Access, Arlington, Tx.)

All cannulas used as intermittent devices are flushed as follows:

- After each administration of a medication
- After the administration of blood or blood products
- After withdrawal of blood
- When converting a continuous infusion to an intermittent device
- Every 8 to 12 hours when the cannula is not in use

The volume of flushing solution needed to maintain patency is equal to the volume capacity of the cannula times two, plus the volume of the injection cap and extension set (if an extension set is used). When ports or other devices that do not provide a valve or pressure to prevent the reflux of blood into the cannula lumen and the formation of an occlusion are used, positive pressure within the cannula lumen must be maintained during and after the administration of a flush solution. One way of maintaining positive pressure is to exert a continual push on the syringe plunger while withdrawing the syringe during the administration of the last 0.2 ml of flush solution. Withdrawing the syringe while continuing to push on the plunger replaces the space occupied by the needle during flush, thereby preventing reflux of blood within the cannula tip. Some injection ports on tubings and saline/heparin lock systems (extension set with injection port) have a valve that actually prevents blood reflux, and the syringe is not withdrawn until all the flush solution has been given.

Infection at the venipuncture site.
An infection can occur at the venipuncture site in the absence of phlebitis. It is usually a local infection at the cannula-skin entry point.

Patient assessment. The IV site should be assessed frequently for signs of local infection while in use and during dressing and site changes. The site should be monitored after it has been discontinued for the possibility of local inflammation at the site. The cannula-skin entry site should be observed for swelling and inflammation, and the surrounding tissue should be observed for discoloration and purulent drainage. An infection at the site may be apparent before or after the cannula has been removed.

Nursing interventions. If the cannula is in place, it should be removed and cultured to determine whether it is the source of the infection. Any drainage from around the site should be cultured, and the skin should be cleansed with alcohol before the cannula is removed for culture. A sterile dressing should be applied, and the physician should be notified; usually, an antibiotic ointment with sterile dressing changes is ordered. Systemic antibiotic therapy may be necessary, and occasionally surgical intervention is warranted. The site should be monitored until the infection has resolved.

Preventive measures. Usually, the causes of an infection at the site are related to a break in aseptic technique either during catheter insertion, care, or removal. Contaminated equipment or supplies, improper handwashing technique, or the patient's picking at the site can predispose the site to an infection.

Aseptic technique must be maintained during cannula insertion, IV therapy, and catheter removal. An infection at the site provides an excellent opportunity for bacteria to enter the venous system unless it is recognized early and appropriate interventions are carried out.

Infiltration.
Infiltration is the inadvertent administration of a nonvesicant solution or medication into surrounding tissues. It is usually recognized by increasing edema at or near the venipuncture site (Fig. 24-2).

The first symptom recognized by many patients is the feeling of skin tightness at the venipuncture site that makes flexing or extending the involved extremity difficult. If a large amount of fluid is trapped in the subcutaneous tissue, the skin may appear taut or stretched. As more fluid gathers in the tissues, blanching and coolness of the skin may occur, the infusion may slow or stop, and the patient may experience tenderness or discomfort at the site. Discomfort experienced by the patient is determined by the type of solution or medication being infused. Isotonic solutions generally do not produce much discomfort when an infiltration occurs. Solutions with an acidic or alkaline pH or those that are slightly more hypertonic are more irritating and usually cause discomfort.

Unless obvious, an infiltration may go undetected because of dependent edema or the administration of fluid at a very slow rate. The IV site must be monitored frequently to prevent this problem.

Patient assessment. A complete assessment of the patient, the IV site, the involved extremity, and the infusion system may be necessary to determine the presence of an infiltration. The site around the tip of the cannula and the extremity should be inspected for swelling, blanching, stretched skin, firm tissues, and coolness. It may be helpful to compare the site with the same area on the opposite extremity. If both extremities appear edematous, the patient's medical status should be evaluated. Patients with hemodynamic problems, such as congestive heart failure, toxic conditions, compromised kidney function, hypothermia, and vascular insufficiency, are particularly prone to vascular edema. The immobilized patient or the patient with muscular weakness or paralysis of an extremity may experience edema of the extremity that is totally unrelated to a problem at the IV site.

If an assessment of the involved extremity and the patient's medical status are inconclusive, pressure should be applied to the vein with a finger or tourniquet about 2 inches above the insertion site (it must be above the tip of the cannula). If the cannula is in the vein, this pressure will slow or stop the infusion rate. If the infusion continues despite the venous obstruction, an infiltration has occurred.

Checking for a blood return, or backflow of blood, is not a reliable method for determining the absence of an infiltration. A blood return may not be present when small veins are used because they may not permit blood flow around the cannula; one may think the infusion has infiltrated when it has not. In addition, veins that have had previous punctures or that are very fragile may seep fluid at a site above or below the vein cannula entry point; a blood return may be present, yet an infiltration is occurring. The movement of a cannula, such as in-and-out motions, can also cause the skin and the vein entry site to enlarge, allowing fluid to seep at the vein entry site, causing an infiltration.

Nursing interventions. To prevent or minimize infiltration-associated problems (Box 24-3), it is imperative that the cannula be discontinued once an infiltration has been identified. The type of solution being infused should also be considered. If the solution is isotonic and has a normal pH, the patient may not feel much discomfort unless a large amount of fluid has infiltrated. In these cases, warm compresses, such as warm, moist towels or chemical packs, may help alleviate the discomfort and help absorb the infiltration by increasing circulation to the affected area. Sloughing can occur from the application of warm compresses to an area infiltrated with certain medications, such as potassium chloride. In these instances, the application of cold compresses is preferred.[4] Established policies and procedures should dictate the use of compresses. The involved extremity should be elevated to improve circulation and to help absorb infiltrated fluid.

If weeping of the tissues occurs because of an extensive infiltration or loose thin tissue, as is often present in the elderly, it may be necessary to apply a sterile dressing to the affected area. It is usually better to leave these areas open because the dressing necessitates the use of gauze and possibly tape, which can increase tissue damage. If a dressing is used, it should be applied loosely. Extreme care should be given to prevent infection. The physician should be notified and measures should be

---

Box 24-3   Effects of an Infiltration

Deprives the patient of the prescribed rate of medications and solutions essential for successful therapy
Limits mobility of an extremity
Limits availability of veins for therapy
Causes tissue damage
Causes unnecessary patient discomfort

---

carried out as ordered. If an infusion is needed, a cannula is placed in the opposite extremity or in a site above and away from the previous site.

Preventive measures. Not all infiltrations can be prevented, but adherence to certain measures can minimize their severity. Flexion areas should be avoided if possible. The cannula should be taped securely, and the site should be protected from excessive movement or pressure by use of an armboard and restraints. Restraints must be applied with extreme caution and within the guidelines established by JCAHO.[1] Restraints should be well padded and applied in a manner that will not cause nerve damage, constrict circulation, or cause pressure areas. They should be removed at frequent intervals and range-of-motion exercises performed. Inadequate or improper use of armboards or restraints can cause very serious complications; policies and procedures should be established to guide their use.

Patient education can be a key factor in the prevention and early recognition of the signs and symptoms of an infiltration. Patient knowledge about the care of the IV site and system can prevent activities that may cause an infiltration, such as manipulating the cannula, pulling on the tubing, picking at the dressing, and using the extremity excessively. A patient who knows what to look for can alert the nurse to the early signs of an infiltration, and immediate care can be rendered, thereby preventing the possibility of more-serious complications.

Extravasation. *Extravasation* is the inadvertent administration of a vesicant solution or medication into the surrounding tissues. A vesicant solution is a solution or medication that causes the formation of blisters, with subsequent sloughing of tissues occurring from tissue necrosis (Fig. 24-3).

Patient assessment. It is essential that an extravasation be noted early, before extensive fluid is allowed to infiltrate the interstitial tissues. A complete assessment of the patient, the IV site, the involved extremity, and the infusion system should be performed at regular intervals. The flow rate should never be increased to determine the infiltration of a vesicant, nor should a blood return be used as a reliable method to determine an infiltration. Fluid can seep into the tissues from a previous puncture site or around the vein insertion site and increase the potential for tissue necrosis (refer to Infiltration for the assessment process).

Initial indications that tissue sloughing may occur include pain or burning at the site with progression to erythema and edema. Tissue sloughing is usually apparent within 1 to 4 weeks because of tissue necrosis. Necrosis can involve a small or a large area, including underlying connective tissues, muscles, tendons, and bone, necessitating surgical intervention.

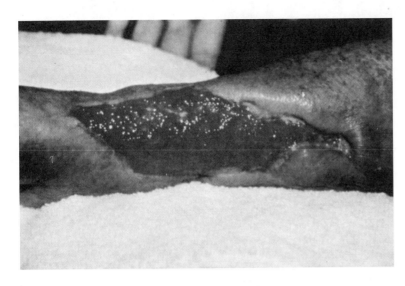

FIG. 24-3 *Tissue sloughing associated with extravasation, the inadvertent administration of a vesicant solution or medication into surrounding tissues.* (Courtesy of Johnson and Johnson Medical, Inc., Vascular Access, Arlington, Tx.)

The severity of damage is directly related to the type, concentration, and volume of fluid infiltrated into the interstitial tissues. The most harmful of the vesicant medications are the antineoplastic agents. Other medications acting as vesicants with the potential for causing tissue necrosis include dopamine hydrochloride (Dopastat, Intropin), norepinephrine (levarterenol bitartrate, Levophed), potassium chloride at high dosages, amphotericin B (Fungizone), calcium, and sodium bicarbonate in high concentrations.

Nursing interventions. When an extravasation is suspected, the infusate is discontinued immediately. Treatment protocols established in written policies and procedures are initiated, and a new site is established, preferably in the opposite extremity or in a site above and away from the extravasated site.

Agency policies vary as to the treatment of the tissues in which an extravasation has occurred. Usually, the cannula is left in place until after any residual medication and blood are aspirated, and an antidote particular to the vesicant is instilled into the tissues. (See Chapter 13 for protocols related to the management of extravasation associated with the administration of chemotherapeutic agents.) After the cannula is removed, a dry, sterile dressing is applied to the site, and either cold or warm compresses are applied. Cold compresses are usually used for the alkalating and antibiotic vesicants, whereas warm compresses are applied to an extravasation of the vinca alkaloids.[4] The extremity is elevated and observed regularly for erythema, induration, and necrosis. The physician is notified, and tissue damage is evaluated for the possibility of surgical intervention.

Preventive measures. Every effort should be made to prevent an extravasation (Box 24-4). Knowledge of the vesicant potential of infusions and medications and identification of associated risk factors are essential to the safe administration of these infusates. The nurse must know if the patient has a history of multiple venipunctures, where they were located, and how long ago the sites were used. Vesicants have been known to seep into the tissues at the vein-entry site of a previous infusion.

The patient should be educated in the care of the infusion, including the recognition of potential problems, what to do if a problem occurs, and the dangers associated with extravasation. A well-educated patient can be a vital asset in preventing an extravasation and in minimizing the effects of an existing extravasation.

Phlebitis. *Phlebitis,* which is the inflammation of the intima of the vein, is a commonly reported complication of IV therapy. Inflammation occurs as a result of irritation to the endothelial cells of the vein intima creating a rough cell wall where platelets readily adhere. Phlebitis is characterized by pain and tenderness along the course of the vein, erythema, and inflammatory swelling with a feeling of warmth at the site. Note the erythema along the vein line in Fig. 24-4.

The following factors substantially increase the risk for infusion-related phlebitis:

- Cannula material, length, and gauge
- Unskilled insertion of the cannula
- Incorrect anatomic site of cannulation
- Prolonged duration of cannulation
- Infrequent dressing changes
- Incompatibility, type, and pH of medications or solutions
- Host factors, such as age and presence of disease

Phlebitis is classified according to its causative factors and can be chemical, mechanical, or bacterial. Phlebitis should be rated according to a uniform scale. The scale recommended by the *Infusion Nursing Standards of Practice* is given in Table 24-1.[5]

Chemical phlebitis. Chemical phlebitis is associated with a response of the vein intima to chemicals producing inflammation. An inflammatory response can be created by the administration of solutions or medications or as a result of certain cannula materials used for access (Box 24-5).

Normal blood pH is 7.35 to 7.45 and is slightly alkaline. The normal pH for solutions is 7.0, which is neutral. The pH for alkaline, or basic, solutions ranges from 7 to 14; that for acid solutions ranges from 7 to 0. The *United States Pharmacopoeia's* specifications for the pH of dextrose solutions range from 3.5 to 6.5.[4] Acidity is necessary to prevent caramelization of the dextrose during sterilization and to maintain the stability of the solution during storage. Some manufacturers also include an additive in the solution to increase the pH. This additive may

Box 24-4   Measures to Reduce Potential for Extravasation

1. Only qualified registered nurses who have been trained in venipuncture and drug administration skills and who have knowledge of drugs with vesicant potential should be allowed to administer vesicants. Their training should include how and over what interval these drugs are administered, early signs of extravasation, preventive measures, and associated treatment protocols.

2. The intravenous site and the surrounding area should be checked for patency before, during, and after the administration of a vesicant. Infusion of 5 to 10 ml of saline before the administration of a vesicant can help determine vein patency.

3. The organization's policies should specify the role of the nurse during the administration of vesicants. Some agency policies state that a nurse must be in constant attendance during the infusion of a vesicant, whereas others state that the patient and the site should be monitored at specified intervals during the infusion. Others require that two licensed nurses verify vein patency before the administration of a vesicant. The degree to which the patient and site are observed may depend on the location of the patient at the time the vesicant is administered.

4. When a vesicant is administered directly into a vein with a syringe, the plunger of the syringe is pulled back every 3 to 4 ml to note blood return. Although a good blood return does not guarantee that an extravasation has not occurred, any change in blood return could indicate the need to investigate the possibility of an extravasation.

5. A vesicant should be administered through a side port of a free-flowing infusion because the vesicant is usually concentrated and the severity of tissue damage is related to the amount and concentration of the vesicant. A free-flowing infusion indicates a patent line.

6. Cannulas should be properly taped to prevent an in-and-out motion, which can enlarge the vein entry site and create an opportunity for the vesicant to seep into interstitial tissues, resulting in an extravasation.

7. Vesicants should not be administered in areas of flexion.

8. The digits, hands, and wrists should be avoided as intravenous sites for vesicant administration because of the close network of tendons and nerves that would be destroyed if an extravasation occurs.

9. Gravity and heat (which maximize vasodilation) should be used to distend small fragile veins, especially those that have been used repeatedly for the administration of chemotherapeutic agents. Venipuncture should be performed without a tourniquet or with a loosely tied tourniquet to decrease the potential for an extravasation in these patients.

10. Sites should be protected from excessive movement by using armboards and restraints when indicated. The use of restraints should be established in written policies and procedures and in compliance with JCAHO standards.[1]

11. If a cannula has been in place longer than 24 hours, consideration should be given to changing the site, preferably to the opposite extremity, before a vesicant is administered.

12. The use of high-pressure infusion pumps must be avoided when administering vesicant medications.

13. Consideration should be given to the placement of a central venous catheter. Some institutions administer vesicants only through central venous catheters, even when good peripheral veins are available. The use of a central venous catheter should not provide false assurance that an extravasation cannot occur; extravasation has been documented from catheter rupture, catheter leakage, backtracking of an infusate along a fibrin sheath, separation of the port, and dislodgment of the port needle.

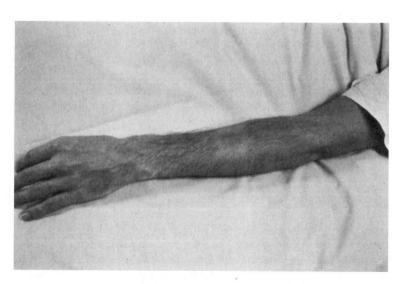

FIG. 24-4 *Phlebitis: inflammation of the vein characterized by pain and tenderness along the course of the vein.* (Courtesy of Johnson and Johnson Medical, Inc., Vascular Access, Arlington, Tx.)

Table 24-1   Assessing the Severity of Phlebitis

0	No clinical symptoms
1	Erythema at access site with or without pain
2	Pain at access site with erythema and/or edema
3	Pain at access site with erythema, streak formation, and/or palpable venous cord ±1 inch in length
4	Pain at access site with erythema, streak formation, palpable venous cord >1 inch in length, and/or purulent drainage

From Intravenous Nurses Society: Infusion nursing standards of practice, *JIN* (suppl) 23(65), 2000.

Box 24-5   Factors Contributing to Chemical Phlebitis

Irritating medications or solutions
Medications improperly mixed or diluted
Medications or solutions administered at a rapid rate
Particulate matter
Cannula structure or material
Extended cannula dwell time

alter the solution's compatibility status when other medications are added.

Solutions or medications with a high pH or osmolality predispose the vein intima to irritation. The more acidic an IV solution, the greater the risk of phlebitis. Glucose-containing admixtures (e.g., amino acids, lipid emulsions used in parenteral nutrition), which are acidic, are far more phlebitogenic than 0.9% sodium chloride. Moreover, additives such as potassium chloride, vancomycin hydrochloride (Vancocin, Vancor), amphotericin B, most beta-lactam antibiotics, benzodiazepines (diazepam and midazolam), and many chemotherapeutic agents can produce severe venous inflammation.

Also, the addition of certain medications can alter the pH of a solution. For instance, adding vitamin C to IV fluids further decreases the pH, whereas the addition of sodium heparin increases the pH, rarely causing phlebitis.

Osmolality refers to the measure of solute concentration and, depending on the solute present, can irritate the vein intima and predispose the patient to phlebitis. Parenteral solutions are classified according to the tonicity of the solution in relation to normal blood plasma. The osmolality of blood plasma is 290 mOsm/L. Solutions that approximate 280 to 300 mOsm/L are considered *isotonic.*[6] Those with an osmolality higher than 300 mOsm/L are considered *hypertonic,* whereas those with an osmolality lower than 280 mOsm/L are *hypotonic.*[6] The tonicity of infused solutions affects not only the patient's physical status but also the vein intima. The vein intima can be traumatized by the administration of hyperosmolar fluids (solutions having an osmolality higher than 300 mOsm/L), especially if they are administered at a rapid rate or through a small vessel. Isotonic solutions may become hyperosmolar when they are mixed with certain medications, such as electrolytes, antibiotics, and nutrients, especially when certain medications are added to solutions less than 100 ml.

Improper mixture or dilution of medications can result in incompatibilities and the possibility of precipitate formation, thus increasing the risk of phlebitis. When medications are mixed without regard to pH or compatibility, the effect of the drug may be altered. Interactions can occur with no apparent change, but rendering one or both of the medications or solutions ineffective or causing a physical change in which crystals are formed and a precipitate is observable.

The infusion rate can be a major factor in the development of phlebitis. A slow rate is thought to cause less venous irritation than a rapid rate. Rapid infusion rates irritate the vessel walls by providing a larger concentration of medications and solutions. Slower rates provide longer absorption times, with hemodilution of smaller amounts of solutions or medications.

Particulate matter within IV solutions or medications may also contribute to the formation of phlebitis. Particulates are formed when medication particles are not fully dissolved during the mixing process. When infused, they irritate the vein intima, causing inflammation. When IV medications are prepared for administration, using a 1- to 5-mm particulate-matter filter eliminates this problem. A 0.2-mm air-eliminating filter may be used to prevent the infusion of particulates formed at the bedside when medications are mixed.[5]

Catheters can predispose the patient to phlebitis. Although several different materials are used in the manufacture of catheters, none is absolutely foolproof for the prevention of phlebitis. Catheters made of silicone elastomer and polyurethane have a smoother microsurface, are thermoplastic and more hydrophilic, become more flexible than polytetrafluoroethylene (Teflon) at body temperature, and induce less venous irritation. In studies performed by Maki and Ringer, peripheral IV catheters made of PEU-Vialon were shown to be much safer for use than those made of polyvinylchloride or polyethylene and were substantially less phlebitogenic than catheters made of FEP-polytetrafluoroethylene. Maki and Ringer also showed that the incidence of phlebitis increased progressively with the increasing period of cannulation. Their studies revealed the risk to be 30% by day 2, and 39% to 40% by day 3.[7]

The basic principles of aseptic technique and measures to prevent chemical phlebitis must be carried out. Many of the problems associated with chemical phlebitis can be eliminated by implementation of the principles in Box 24-6.

The pharmacist should always be consulted for any questions about the mixing of medications or solutions and should be made aware of repeated occurrences of phlebitis associated with certain drugs. Sometimes, the addition of a buffering agent or other additives can help prevent chemical phlebitis. In patient trials in coronary care units, heparin or hydrocortisone significantly reduced the incidence of phlebitis in veins infused with potassium chloride, lidocaine, and antimicrobials.[8]

Mechanical phlebitis. Mechanical phlebitis is associated with the placement of a cannula. Cannulas placed in flexion areas often result in mechanical phlebitis. As the extremity is moved, the cannula irritates the vein intima, causing injury and resultant phlebitis. A large cannula placed in a vein that has a smaller lumen than the cannula also irritates the intima of the vein, causing inflammation and phlebitis. Cannulas that are poorly taped have a tendency to move in and out of the vein,

---

Box 24-6 Principles That Decrease the Potential for Chemical Phlebitis

Use filters.
Use recommended solutions or diluents when mixing medications.
Dilute known irritating medications to the greatest extent possible.
Administer intravenous push medications through a port of a compatible free-flowing infusion.
Administer medications or solutions at the minimal rate recommended.
Rotate peripheral sites at recommended intervals.
Use large veins for the administration of hypertonic or acidic solutions to provide greater hemodilution.
Use the smallest-gauge cannula that will adequately deliver the ordered therapy.

Box 24-7 Factors Contributing to Bacterial Phlebitis

Poor handwashing techniques
Failure to check equipment for compromised integrity
Poor aseptic technique in preparation of the site or system
Poor cannula-insertion techniques
Poorly taped cannula
Extended cannula dwell time
Infrequent site observation with failure to notice early signs of phlebitis

---

allowing the cannula tip to irritate the vein intima and resulting in phlebitis. Extensive, unrestrictive movement of an extremity can also result in unwarranted movement of the cannula within the vein.

The experience of the person inserting an IV cannula clearly influences the risk for phlebitis. In comparative trials, the availability of an IV therapy team of highly experienced nurses who insert IV catheters and provide close surveillance of infusions resulted in a twofold lower rate of infusion-related phlebitis and an even greater reduction in catheter-related sepsis.[7,9]

Bacterial phlebitis. Bacterial phlebitis is an inflammation of the vein intima associated with a bacterial infection. It can be very serious and predispose the patient to the systemic complication of septicemia. Contributing factors include those described in Box 24-7.

Handwashing is the single most important procedure for preventing nosocomial infections.[8,10] The hands should be washed before therapy is initiated and after the procedure has been completed. Standard precautions state that health care providers must wear gloves when performing venipunctures.[11] Even when gloves are provided in the immediate area, the hands should be washed before the gloves are donned; otherwise, contaminants are easily carried into the area and deposited on the gloves.

All equipment and solutions should be checked for expiration date, package integrity, particulate matter, cloudiness, or any signs indicating the presence of contaminants. Bags should be squeezed to reveal punctures, and bottles should be held up to the light and rotated to reveal very fine cracks.

Aseptic technique is essential in the preparation of an insertion site. Appropriate cleansing of the insertion site reduces the potential for infection by minimizing microorganisms on the skin. If the skin is very dirty, it should be washed with soap and water before an antimicrobial solution is applied. Shaving is not recommended because it may cause microabrasions, which can allow microorganisms to enter the vascular system. Antimicrobial solutions that can be used to prepare the skin for venipuncture include 2% tincture of iodine, 10% povidone-iodine, alcohol, and chlorhexidine.[5] The solution should be applied with friction in a circular motion, starting at the intended site for puncture and working outward to prevent contaminants from

being carried from an uncleansed area to a cleansed area. The solution should be allowed to completely air dry; blotting of excess solution should not be allowed.[5]

Aseptic technique should be maintained during the insertion of the cannula. Sterility of the cannula should not be violated by laying the cannula on the skin during insertion or by touching the cannula with the fingers. Only one cannula is used for each venipuncture attempt because cannulas that have penetrated the skin are contaminated. Sterile tape to prevent unwarranted movement of the cannula and a sterile dressing are applied over the cannula site. The cannula is then taped, or a commerically made securement device is used, to prevent in-and-out movement.

Maintenance of the system includes measures to prevent bacteria from entering the system. Routine site care should consist of changing the dressing at established intervals according to the *Infusion Nursing Standards of Practice*.[5] Gauze and transparent dressings should be changed immediately if the integrity of the dressing is compromised. Site care should be routinely given and should consist of cleansing the cannula-skin junction by applying an effective antiseptic solution (e.g., 2% tincture of iodine; 10% povidone-iodine, alcohol, or chlorhexidine) and a sterile dressing. Wearing sterile gloves and a mask should be considered when care is administered to a central venous catheter or to the immunocompromised patient.[5]

Patient assessment. The best treatment for phlebitis, whether chemical, mechanical, or bacterial, is prevention. The site is checked frequently and is changed at the first sign of tenderness, redness, or inflammation. The skin is palpated at the tip of the cannula by use of slight pressure to check for tenderness, and the skin is observed for warmth, edema, and vein induration.

Nursing interventions. If an infection is suspected, the cannula should be removed and cultured using established policies and procedures. The surrounding skin should be cleansed with 70% isopropyl alcohol and allowed to air dry. If purulent drainage is present, a culture of the drainage should be taken before cleansing the skin. The recommended method of culturing is the semiquantitative technique.[5] Consideration should be given to obtaining blood cultures to determine proliferation of cannula-related infections. The cannula should be relocated to the opposite extremity, if possible, or to a vein into which the phlebitic vein does not empty. The application of warm, moist compresses promotes healing and patient comfort.

Postinfusion phlebitis. *Postinfusion phlebitis*, another commonly reported complication of IV therapy, is associated with inflammation of the vein that usually becomes evident within 48 to 96 hours of cannula removal. The following factors contribute to the development of postinfusion phlebitis:

- Poor cannula insertion technique
- Debilitated patient
- Poor vein condition
- Hypertonic or acidic solutions
- Ineffective filtration
- Large-gauge cannula placed in small vessel
- Failure to change tubings, dressings, injection site caps, and cannulas according to *Infusion Nursing Standards of Practice.*[5]

Patient assessment. The patient is assessed for postinfusion phlebitis by monitoring the IV site for signs of inflammation after the IV cannula has been removed. The site is observed for erythema, edema, and drainage. The site is palpated for warmth and for vein induration. The degree of postinfusion phlebitis should be measured according to the uniform scale used to measure phlebitis (Table 24-1).

Nursing interventions. Generally, hot or cold compresses are applied, as described earlier, to the infusion site once a postinfusion phlebitis is detected. Depending on the degree of postinfusion phlebitis, medical intervention may be required.

Preventive measures. Measures to prevent postinfusion phlebitis are the same as those designed to prevent phlebitis and include those outlined in Box 24-8.

Thrombosis. A *thrombosis* is the formation of a blood clot within a blood vessel. It is caused by any injury that breaks the integrity of the endothelial cells of the venous wall and usually occurs at the point at which the cannula touches the intima of the vein. Platelets adhere to the injured wall, and a thrombus is formed. Contributing factors include those listed in Box 24-9.

Patient assessment. When an infusion slows or stops, the causative factors should be assessed. Mechanical and other problems should be ruled out. The possibility of a thrombus should be considered because the formation of a thrombus narrows the lumen of the vein, allowing less fluid to be infused. Usually, a thrombus goes undetected until the infusion stops or the extremity becomes swollen because of circulatory involvement. The area becomes very tender, and redness appears. The degree of circulatory involvement in the involved extremity should be assessed. A thrombosis may impact circulation sufficiently to cause tissue necrosis or result in loss of the involved extremity.

The patient should also be assessed for the possibility of a systemic infection or a pulmonary embolism. Thrombi form an excellent trap for bacteria, whether stationary, carried by the bloodstream from an infectious process located somewhere else in the body, or introduced through a subcutaneous orifice. Although a thrombus is usually well attached, it may in rare circumstances become unattached.

Nursing interventions. If a thrombosis occurs, the infusion should be discontinued immediately and the site should be relocated to the opposite extremity. Cold compresses should be applied to the site initially to decrease the flow of blood and increase platelet adherence to the clot that has already formed. The physician should be notified, and the site should be assessed to determine whether surgical intervention is needed; vein ligation may be necessary if the degree of circulatory impair-

---

Box 24-8   Measures for Preventing Postinfusion Phlebitis

Ensure that venipuncture is performed by a skilled professional.
Use aseptic technique when using or manipulating venous system.
Check compatibility of solutions and medications before mixing and administering.
Use filters when preparing medications and solutions.
Use final filtration when administering medications and solutions.
Add a buffer to known irritating medications and to hypertonic solutions.
Use a cannula that is smaller than the vein to promote hemodilution of infusions.
Use large veins for the administration of hypertonic or acidic solution to promote hemodilution.
Rotate infusion sites as outlined in the *Infusion Nursing Standards of Practice.*[5]
Change solution container every 24 hours.
Change latex injection peripheral ports on intermittent devices at the time of cannula change and when the integrity of the port has been compromised.

Box 24-9   Factors Contributing to the Formation of Thrombosis

Venipuncture by an unskilled professional
Multiple venipuncture attempts
Use of a cannula that is larger than the vein lumen
Poor circulation with venous stasis
Administration of medications incompatible with solutions
Administration of solutions or medications with high pH or tonicity
Ineffective filtration
Use of thrombogenic catheter materials

---

ment is sufficient to cause extensive tissue damage. The site should be monitored until symptoms completely resolve.

Preventive measures. To prevent these injuries, atraumatic venipunctures by skilled professionals are necessary. Cannulation of the lower extremities in adults should be avoided because these veins are very small and allow pooling of blood with subsequent damage to the vein intima and clot formation. The selection of the appropriate venipuncture device is also important; use of the smallest and shortest device possible to deliver the prescribed therapy decreases the potential of injury to the endothelial lining. Veins over flexion areas should be avoided, and cannulas should be anchored securely with tape to avoid in-and-out movements. Consideration should be given to the placement of central venous catheters when venous access is poor.

Thrombophlebitis. *Thrombophlebitis* denotes a twofold injury: the presence of a thrombus and the occurrence of inflammation. Usually, the first symptom noted is inflammation along the vein line that is characterized by erythema. Edema, pain at the site and along the vein line, and a feeling of warmth usually follow. The vein becomes hard and tortuous as it thromboses. Marked erythema, increased edema, marked pain along the vein, and aching of the extremity occur.

Any irritation to the intima of the vein can predispose the vein to inflammation and clot formation as platelets adhere to the traumatized wall of the vein. The incidence and degree of inflammation increase with the duration of the infusion. Other causative factors have been previously discussed under Phlebitis and Thrombosis.

Patient assessment. The IV site and vein line should be observed at frequent intervals for signs and symptoms consistent with thrombophlebitis. The vein should be palpated for induration and tenderness. The patient should be questioned about pain at the site, along the vein line, and in the involved extremity. The patient should also be observed for chills and fever, and laboratory values should be evaluated for an elevated white blood cell count.

If the condition goes untreated, the vein becomes sclerosed and is unavailable for future therapy. Although the inherent danger of an embolism always exists when a thrombus forms, these thrombi are generally well attached to the vein wall and do not migrate. The risk of septicemia or bacterial endocarditis is greater, particularly if the inflammation is the result of sepsis.

The degree of phlebitis should be measured according to the recommended scale (see Table 24-1). Thrombophlebitis is rated a 3 or 4 on this scale because of the presence of a palpable cord.

Nursing interventions. When thrombophlebitis occurs, the infusion should be discontinued immediately and the physician should be notified. If an infection is suspected, the cannula should be cultured using a semiquantitative technique.[5] The skin surrounding the cannula should be cleansed with alcohol and allowed to air dry before the cannula is removed for culture. When a purulent drainage is present, the culture of the drainage should be taken before the skin is cleansed.[5]

If infusion therapy is still necessary, a new cannula with new tubing and solution container should be placed in the opposite extremity, if possible. If using the opposite extremity is impossible, a separate vein that does not form a tributary of the traumatized vein should be used.

Cold compresses should be applied to the site initially to decrease the flow of blood and increase platelet adherence to the clot already formed. Then, warm compresses should be applied. The extremity should be elevated, and the patient should be cautioned that rubbing or massaging the area may cause an embolus. The extremity and the patient are monitored for further complications.

Preventive measures. Thrombophlebitis can lead to serious systemic complications, and measures should be taken to prevent their occurrence. These measures should include those outlined earlier under Phlebitis and Thrombosis.

Venous or arterial spasm. A *spasm* is a sudden, involuntary contraction of a vein or an artery (vasoconstriction) resulting in temporary cessation of blood flow through a vessel. Stimulation by cold infusates or by mechanical or chemical irritation may produce spasms in arteries and veins.

Because arteries supply circulation to large areas of the body, arterial spasms are far more serious than venous spasms. Unlike arteries, many veins supply a particular area, and if one becomes injured, blood is supplied to the area by collateral circulation. In these cases, the supply of blood to the area may be decreased, but not to the extent that it would with injury to an artery.

Patient assessment. It is most important to recognize the signs and symptoms of a spasm. Cramping or pain above an infusion site or a feeling of numbness is usually the first symptom experienced by the patient. Patients experiencing arterial spasms may or may not complain of pain initially; they may not feel pain until tissue damage has occurred. When the patient complains of one of these symptoms, the involved extremity should be observed for localized blanching and the absence of a pulse; these signs would indicate an arterial spasm and a loss of blood flow to the area supplied by the artery.

Nursing interventions. If an arterial spasm occurs, it is usually related to the inadvertent puncture of an artery instead of a vein during venipuncture. If this occurs, the cannula should be removed immediately, pressure should be applied to the site over sufficient time to ensure hemostasis, and a dry, sterile dressing should be applied.

If a venous spasm occurs, discontinuing the infusion is not necessary. The infusion rate should be decreased, and if possible, the medication or solution should be further diluted. If a spasm has occurred as a result of the administration of a cold solution, warm compresses should be applied above the site; the heat provides vasodilation and increases the blood supply, thereby relieving the spasm and the pain.

Some organizational protocols allow the use of 0.25 ml of lidocaine 1% (Xylocaine) to alleviate pain associated with spasms. This medication should be given only with a physician's written order and after an allergy history has been obtained. Established policies and procedures should govern the use of lidocaine for spasms.

Preventive measures. Many spasms can be prevented. Ensuring that venipuncture is performed by skilled, experienced nurses can decrease the possibility of an inadvertent arterial stick. Venous spasms can also be prevented or minimized by infusing medications or solutions known to be irritating at slower rates and by diluting them as much as possible. Blood warmers should be used for rapid transfusions of potent cold agglutinins, exchange transfusions in neonates, and treatment of patients with hypothermia. Fluid warmers may be used to warm IV solutions to prevent or reverse hypothermic conditions. All refrigerated medications and parenteral solutions should be allowed to reach room temperature before they are administered.

Systemic complications

Systemic complications are those occurring in circulation with the possibility of affecting the entire body (Box 24-10). Systemic complications are usually very serious and require immediate interventions.

Septicemia. *Septicemia* is a pathologic state or a pyrogenic reaction that is usually accompanied by systemic illness. It occurs when pathogenic bacteria invade the bloodstream. The incidence of nosocomial bloodstream infections has increased twofold to threefold in the past decade, with central catheter infections accounting for 90% of the catheter-related infections. These infections increase costs by an average of $6000 per patient and have a case-fatality rate of more than 20%.[12]

Box 24-10 **Systemic Complications of Intravenous Therapy**

Septicemia
Pulmonary embolism
Air embolism
Catheter embolism
Pulmonary edema
Speed shock
Allergic reactions

Box 24-11 **Risk Factors Associated with Septicemia**

Patient susceptibility
Advanced age of the patient
Alteration in host defenses
Underlying illness
Presence of other infectious processes
Use of intravenous therapy
Contaminated solution container
Contaminated equipment
Use of three-way stopcocks
Inflexible cannula material or potentially irritating structure
    (larger or multilumen catheters)
Inexperience of professional inserting cannula
Inadequately prepared or maintained insertion sites
Hematogenous seeding
Repeated manipulation of the infusion system
Certain transparent dressings
Use of monitoring devices
Extended duration of cannulation
Lack of handwashing

Patient assessment. Usually, chills, fever, general malaise, and headache are the first symptoms noted when pathogenic bacteria invade the bloodstream. As the fever increases, the pulse rate increases, and extreme weakness occurs. These symptoms may be accompanied by flushed face, backache, nausea and vomiting, and hypotension.

Patients receiving IV therapy should be monitored for these symptoms. If they occur, patients should be evaluated in terms of diagnosis, medications, and any impending conditions that might be present. If no other cause can be found, the diagnosis of septicemia should be considered. If the condition goes undetected or untreated, symptoms become more severe, and cyanosis, increased respirations, or hyperventilation are noted. As the organisms overcome the system, vascular collapse, shock, and death can occur.

Contributing factors. Contributing factors placing the patient at risk for septicemia can be divided into two major categories: those that make the patient susceptible to the infectious process and those that allow microorganisms to enter the system (Box 24-11).

Solution container. The solution container can be a focal point not only for contamination but also for microbial growth. Solutions can become contaminated during the manufacturing process, storage, set-up, or use as a result of manipulation or improper handling. The gram-negative organisms, the *Klebsiella, Serratia,* and *Enterobacter* species, have been associated with contamination during the manufacturing process, whereas *Enterobacter cloacae, Enterobacter agglomerans,* and *Pseudomonas cepacia* have been associated with sepsis from contaminated infusates while in use.[13] In addition, the composition of the infusate may actually promote the growth of microorganisms. *Klebsiella, Enterobacter, Serratia,* and *P. cepacia* show rapid growth within 24 hours in 5% dextrose in water solutions.[14] Blood products also provide an excellent source for *Klebsiella* microorganisms to grow, and total parenteral nutrition solutions support the growth of *Candida* species.

Other characteristics of the solution that can increase the risk of contamination include hypertonicity, acidity, and the presence of particulate matter. Hypertonic solutions containing large amounts of particulates tend to irritate the vascular intima, causing an inflammatory reaction. This situation predisposes the vessel to thrombus formation, which provides a nidus for infection if the area becomes contaminated, either by contiguous infection or by hematogenous seeding.

Contaminated equipment. Equipment may become contaminated at the factory, en route from the factory, during storage, or at the time of use. If the integrity of the package is compromised, it should be discarded and new equipment used.

Stopcocks. Studies have shown that stopcocks used as part of the infusion system have often been the cause of microorganisms entering the IV system.[8] Microorganisms enter the system from (1) the hands of personnel during manipulation of the stopcocks; (2) syringes used to flush or draw blood specimens; (3) residual blood that remains in a port after use, serving as a breeding ground for bacteria; and (4) failure to keep a sterile cap on the stopcock when it is not in use.

Catheter structure and material. The catheter structure and material contribute to the risk of infectious complications associated with the administration of IV therapy. Larger catheters come in contact with a greater skin area, produce a larger hole in the skin and vessel, are more difficult to anchor, and are often used for purposes that require more frequent entries into the system. In nonrandomized trials, multilumen catheters have been associated with a higher risk of infections because of the increased number of entry sites into the vascular system.[9] Stiffer catheters also increase the risk of infection by provoking thrombogenesis and an inflammatory response that may facilitate colonization.

Microorganisms are able to adhere to some catheter materials more readily than to others. In vitro studies show that catheters made of polyvinyl chloride or polyethylene appear to be less resistant to the adherence of microorganisms than Teflon, silicone elastomer, or polyurethane. Some catheter materials also have surface irregularities that may further enhance the microbial adherence of certain species (e.g., CoNS, *Acinetobacter calcoaceticus, Pseudomonas aeruginosa*).[8] Differential adherence of microorganisms to catheters of various compositions may influence the microbiology of infection. Although some catheter materials are less thrombogenic than others, most authorities believe that all catheters become encased in a fibrin sheath within several hours of implantation.[15] Whether this sheath represents an asset or a liability is unclear. Some catheter materials appear to promote the adherence of certain pathogenic strains of microorganisms; in these materials, the fibrin sheath may be relatively protective. Conversely, other catheter materials do not promote microbial adherence; in these materials, the fibrin sheath may represent a nidus for infection.

Experience of practitioner. The technical skill of the person placing the catheter influences the potential for infection. Studies have shown that good insertion techniques actually lower the risks of infection.[8,9,12]

Insertion site. Many authorities believe that the primary route by which microorganisms gain access to the vascular system is by entry along the catheter insertion site, whereas others have demonstrated a rather loose association between skin colonization and subsequent infection by the same organism, with the exception of *Staphylococcus aureus*. Skin organisms gain access to the transcutaneous tract (the space between the catheter and the subcutaneous tissue) at the time the catheter is inserted. IV cannulas can be contaminated during the time of insertion by microorganisms on the hands of personnel.

When serial cultures were performed, two thirds of all persons carried *S. aureus* on their hands. Washing the hands with soap and water while using mechanical friction for a least 10 to 15 seconds is sufficient to remove most transiently acquired bacteria.[12] If not removed, these organisms can be deposited into the bloodstream and can produce bacteremia or fungemia.

Studies have also shown that microbial growth occurs when IV sites are not cleaned appropriately and dressings are not changed. Microorganisms migrate along the tract and enter the bloodstream, producing bacteremia or fungemia. Access to the intravascular portion of the catheter by microbial flora residing in and on the skin depends on several factors, such as insertion technique, catheter composition, microbial adherence to the catheter, and catheter movement in the insertion site.

Hematogenous seeding. Another factor that causes catheter sepsis is *hematogenous seeding* from a distant foci. Current studies suggest that its occurrence is uncommon. Microorganisms are carried from a remote site or from another source of infection, such as a tracheostomy, the urinary tract, or a surgical wound, and actually seed on the intravascular catheter. Most vascular access yeast infections appear to be the result of hematogenous dissemination from another site.[13,14]

Hematogenous seeding can also occur if a catheter is inserted into a patient who has a high-grade bacteremia or candidemia. Factors that affect catheter seeding include the causative pathogen, the degree and duration of bacteremia, the patient's clinical status, and the length of time the catheter has been in place.

Manipulation of the delivery system. Repeated manipulation of the cannula or IV system greatly increases the risk of sepsis. Each time the system is entered, the potential exists for microorganisms to enter the intravascular system. The system may be entered by adding medications to the solution container, injecting medications into the tubing, administering blood products, flushing tubing or cannulas, repositioning catheters, or obtaining blood samples. Because a Swan-Ganz or arterial catheter is manipulated many more times per day than other catheters, it is reasonable to expect the risk of infection to be greater for these devices.[8]

Transparent dressings. In early studies performed by Beam and colleagues,[16] a significant relationship was demonstrated between the application of a polyurethane dressing on central venous catheter sites and the development of infection. These investigators reported a build-up of moisture under these dressings, causing an increase in colonization of the site and the risk of catheter-related infection. Other studies have been controversial and have shown no significant increase in the risk of infection.[8,12] Newer transparent dressings with improved moisture permeability may actually decrease the potential for infection.[17-19]

Pressure monitoring systems. Research has shown that pressure monitoring systems used in conjunction with arterial catheters have been associated with both epidemic and endemic nosocomial intravascular infections.[9] The common pathway for microorganisms to enter the bloodstream, leading to bacteremia, is the fluid column in the tubing between the patient's intravascular catheter and the pressure monitoring apparatus. Microorganisms in a fluid-filled system may move from the pressure monitoring apparatus to the patient or from the patient to the pressure monitoring system. Pressure monitoring systems have also been contaminated by contaminated infusates, nonsterile calibrating devices, ice used to chill syringes, contaminated disinfectant used on the domes, and blind, stagnant columns of fluid between the transducer and infusion system.

Duration of catheterization. Length of exposure is listed by some authorities as the most important risk factor for vascular access infections.[9] Investigators have concluded that an approximate fourfold risk of infection exists for some types of catheters per day of catheterization. Studies have also shown that arterial catheters have an increased incidence of positive catheter cultures after 2 to 4 days.[9] No catheter should be considered as having a low risk of infection, and because the risk is cumulative, no catheter should be left in place any longer than is absolutely necessary.

Catheter hubs. Studies have shown that catheter-related sepsis can have its origin in a highly colonized catheter hub. When the hub becomes colonized, microorganisms are carried into the IV solution to the catheter tip, where they colonize.[12]

Nursing interventions.

Early symptoms of septicemia must be evaluated for possible causes. In the absence of other causes, such as a kidney, respiratory, or wound infection, the solution and delivery system must be considered. Fever in a patient with a central venous catheter should be attributed to the catheter until proven otherwise. Erythema at the insertion site is an unreliable sign of sepsis because catheters under transparent polyurethane dressings may show erythema. However, erythema at the site should be monitored because it could indicate an infectious process that could lead to sepsis. In most of these patients, no other signs of infection are present. Vital signs should be monitored, and if sepsis is suspected, the physician should be notified immediately. If a physician's order is required to perform cultures, the physician should be asked for orders to culture the cannula, the infusate, and the patient's blood.

The cannula should be removed and cultured only after the skin around the cannula has been cleansed with alcohol and allowed to dry. The recommended method of culture is the semiquantitative technique.[5] The infusate should also be cultured. Consideration should be given to obtaining blood cultures to determine the proliferation of an infusate-related infection.

A new infusion site with new tubing and solution container should be initiated as soon as possible. The patient should be monitored for signs of shock, and emergency measures should be carried out, if necessary. The physician usually orders antibiotics, which should be started as quickly as possible after the cultures are drawn.

Some authorities believe that central venous catheters suspected of being infected should not be routinely removed from patients who have limited sites for central venous access or from those who would be put at risk of mechanical complications or bleeding from insertion of a new catheter at a new site. In these patients, quantitative blood cultures are drawn through the catheter and peripherally. Empiric antimicrobial therapy is initiated based on the assessment that a bacteremia is present, and the catheter is removed only if all cultures are positive for infection. Another option is to change the central venous catheter in the same site over a guidewire using aseptic technique. The old catheter is cultured; if it shows heavy colonization, the new catheter that has just been placed is removed because it has been placed into an infected site.[8] The exception to both options is the presence of *Candida* or any other fungus because candidemia cannot be eradicated in a person with a central line. Policies should be established that give specific guidelines on the procedure that should be followed when sepsis from an IV system is suspected.

Preventive measures. The best treatment for septicemia is prevention. Strict adherence to the guidelines listed in Box 24-12 can help prevent septicemia related to the administration of IV therapy.

Numerous studies have shown that catheter-related infections can be greatly reduced by the insertion of peripheral catheters and the administration of care to both peripheral and central venous catheters by a team approach.[8,9] In comparative trials, Maki and Ringer concluded that the availability of a team of nurses who are highly experienced in IV therapy and who insert IV catheters and provide close surveillance of infusions resulted in a twofold lower rate of infusion phlebitis and an even greater reduction in catheter-related sepsis.[7]

Studies have shown that catheter-related infections of central venous catheters can be reduced by using an attachable cuff impregnated with silver ions.[12] Silver ions have a very broad spectrum of antimicrobial activity and are effective against bacteria and fungi that are likely to cause catheter-related infections. The cuff is placed beneath the skin at the insertion site when the catheter is inserted. The cuff inhibits the migration of bacteria along the external surface of the catheter, preventing colonization of the subcutaneous segment and the tip of the catheter. Subcutaneous tissue grows to the cuff, providing a mechanical barrier, and the silver ions provide a chemical barrier against organisms. Studies have shown the use of the cuff to cause a threefold reduction in the incidence of colonization and a fourfold reduction in the incidence of septicemia.[9]

Studies have also shown that catheters molecularly bonded with antimicrobial substances are four times less likely to produce a bacteremia.[8] More recent studies indicate that certain catheters impregnated with silver sulfadiazine and chlorhexidine reduce the incidence of microbial colonization and infection by preventing bacterial adherence to the catheter and decreasing colonization.[20,21]

Pulmonary embolism. A *pulmonary embolism* occurs when a mass of undissolved matter, usually a blood clot, becomes free floating and is carried by venous circulation to the right side of the heart and into the pulmonary artery. The embolus may obstruct the pulmonary artery or its branches that supply the lobes of the lung, thus occluding arterial openings at major bifurcations. If the pulmonary artery is obstructed, the patient will experience cardiac disturbances. If multiple emboli are passed into the pulmonary circulation, the patient will experience pulmonary hypertension and right-sided heart failure.

Patient assessment. The patient receiving IV therapy should be monitored for signs and symptoms of pulmonary embolism. These symptoms include dyspnea, pleuritic pain or discomfort, apprehension, cough, unexplained hemoptysis, sweats, tachypnea, tachycardia, cyanosis, and low-grade fever. If any of these are noted, the chest should be auscultated for a pleural friction rub.

Nursing interventions. If a pulmonary embolism is suspected, the patient should be placed in semi-Fowler's position and the patient's vital signs should be assessed. The physician should be notified. Medical interventions usually include the administration of oxygen to maintain blood gas levels, a lung scan to verify a pulmonary embolism, a prothrombin time determination to have as a baseline clotting time before anticoagulant therapy is initiated, and a bolus of heparin followed by a heparin infusion.

Preventive measures. The best treatment for a pulmonary embolism is prevention. Measures to prevent the formation and the release of pulmonary emboli into the vascular system include those listed in Box 24-13.

Air embolism. An *air embolism* is caused by the entry of a bolus of air into the vascular system. The embolism is propelled into the heart, creating an intracardiac air lock at the pulmonic valve and preventing the ejection of blood from the right side of the heart. The right side of the heart overfills with blood because less blood is ejected from the right ventricle. The force of right ventricular contractions increases in an attempt to eject blood past the air lock. The forceful contractions cause small air bubbles to break loose from the air pocket. These small bubbles are pumped into pulmonary circulation, creating an obstruction to forward blood flow and tissue hypoxia. Pulmonary hypoxia results in vasoconstriction of lung tissue that further increases the workload of the right ventricle and reduces blood flow out of the right side of the heart. This leads to diminished cardiac output, shock, and death.[22]

Patient assessment. When an air embolism occurs, the patient complains of palpitations, chest pain, and shortness of breath and may complain of shoulder or low back pain, depending on the location of the air embolus. The patient appears cyanotic. Assessment reveals hypotension and a weak, rapid

---

BOX 24-12   Guidelines for the Prevention of Septicemia

1. The hands should be washed, rinsed, and dried before initiating an infusion and before handling any part of the intravenous system.
2. All solutions should be checked before administration for clarity, cracks, or leaks and for the presence of a vacuum.
3. The site for cannula placement should be cleansed with an antimicrobial solution applied with friction, working outward from the center to the periphery. To cleanse the site, 2% tincture of iodine, 10% povidone-iodine, alcohol, or chlorhexidine may be used. If both alcohol and a povidone-iodine are used, the alcohol should be applied first, then the povidone-iodine. The povidone-iodine should not be removed with the alcohol, because its action depends on the release of iodine over a period of time. The solution should be allowed to dry completely.
4. Excessive hair over the venipuncture site should be clipped.
5. Cannulas should be secured to prevent an in-and-out movement, which promotes the transport of cutaneous bacteria into the site and the vascular system.
6. Cannula site care should be administered at the time of dressing change and at the intervals stated in the *Infusion Nursing Standards of Practice.* The site should be observed for signs of redness, swelling, or inflammation. The site should be cleansed with an antiseptic solution (e.g., 2% tincture of iodine, 10% povidone-iodine, alcohol, or chlorhexidine). An antimicrobial or antibiotic ointment, as indicated by policy, and a sterile dressing should be applied. Sterile gloves and a mask should be worn during the administration of site care to a central venous catheter.
7. Lines should not be disconnected to allow patients to ambulate or to change gowns.
8. Aseptic technique should be used when initiating therapy or manipulating the line. The cannula should not be touched at any time during insertion. Cannulas inserted in an emergency should be replaced at the earliest opportunity.
9. Peripheral cannulas should be changed according to the *Infusion Nursing Standards of Practice.*
10. Peripheral and central primary and secondary intravenous tubings should be changed according to the *Infusion Nursing Standards of Practice,* and immediately if contamination is suspected or if their integrity has been compromised.
11. Primary intermittent administration sets should be changed according to the *Infusion Nursing Standards of Practice.*
12. Luer-Lok connections should be used when possible, and other connections should be secured with connecting devices to avoid accidental separation.
13. Add-on devices should be used only when absolutely necessary, because the addition of a device allows an opportunity for bacteria to enter the system. If use of an add-on device is necessary, the device should be changed at the same time the administration set is changed.
14. Injection ports should be disinfected with an antimicrobial solution (iodine, 1%-2%, iodophor, isopropyl alcohol, or chlorhexidine) before they are used.
15. Latex injection caps on peripheral lines should be changed when the cannula is changed or whenever the latex injection port is suspected of being compromised. Latex injection caps on central lines should be changed at least every 7 days and when the latex port is suspected of being compromised.
16. Needles should be changed on secondary medication sets before subsequent use. If secondary medication sets are disconnected from the primary line, needles should be changed.
17. Defective equipment or equipment whose package integrity has been broken should never be used.
18. The intravenous site should be observed often and changed at the first signs of inflammation. Policies and procedures should be written specifying the frequency for site checks.
19. Peripheral arterial cannulas should be changed every 96 hours, and pulmonary artery catheters should be changed every fourth or fifth day.
20. Plugged or sluggish cannulas should not be flushed or irrigated. Not only do they represent a nidus for infection, but an embolus can also be released into the vascular system.
21. Intravenous cannulation of the lower extremities should be avoided because of the higher incidence of associated complications.
22. The smallest needle possible should be used when an injection port is used. Needles that are 25 to 20 gauge and do not exceed 1 inch in length are recommended.

---

pulse. On auscultation, a continuous churning sound may be heard over the precordium. The patient may faint or lose consciousness. If signs and symptoms go unrecognized or untreated, shock or cardiac arrest may result.

Nursing interventions. If an air embolism is suspected, the patient should be placed immediately on the left side in Trendelenburg position; this measure keeps the air in the pulmonary outflow tract to a minimum by trapping it in the right heart chambers and great veins proximal to the pulmonic valve. If the air embolism results from an open or leaking infusion line, the line should be changed immediately and replaced with new tubing that is filled with solution. The source of air intake must be corrected immediately, or air will continue to be drawn

into the system. The physician should be notified, and the patient's vital signs should be monitored. Oxygen is usually administered. If hypoxia occurs, arterial blood gases should be monitored and ventilatory support may be necessary.

Preventive measures. Every effort should be made to prevent the formation of an air embolus. Infusion tubings and extensions on catheters should be clamped when tubings are changed. A negative pressure is created within the vein when the extremity receiving the infusion is elevated above the heart, increasing the potential for air to be drawn into the system. Infusions through central venous catheters are at a greater risk of having air drawn into the system; as intrathoracic pressure is decreased below atmospheric pressure, negative pressure occurs

Box 24-13   Measures to Reduce Potential for Pulmonary Emboli

1. Use a filter to remove particulates from solutions or medications being administered.
2. Administer blood and blood components through a filter designed to retain blood clots and other debris.
3. Avoid using the lower extremities for venipuncture in the adult patient.
4. Prevent injuries to the vein intima by ensuring that venipunctures are performed by skilled professionals; using the smallest cannula possible to deliver the prescribed therapy; using large veins to promote hemodilution when irritating solutions or medications are administered; and using proper taping techniques to prevent cannula movement.
5. Use good judgment when intravenous lines are flushed. Positive pressure should never be used to flush an occluded or sluggish line, because a blood clot can be released into the vascular system. Irrigating lines to improve flow rates is dangerous and should not be practiced.
6. Examine solution containers for particulate matter before they are used.
7. Clip excessive hair and cleanse the area to prevent hair from being severed and carried into the vascular system with venipuncture.

within the central vein, causing a sucking effect that can draw air readily into the vein. To prevent this, the patient should lie flat and perform the Valsalva maneuver (forced expiration with the mouth closed) when central lines are inserted or discontinued and when tubings are changed. An air-eliminating filter can remove air before it passes into the vascular system.

Solution containers should be changed before they are completely empty. Leaking infusion tubings should be changed as soon as they are discovered to eliminate the possibility of air being drawn into the vascular system. Luer-Lok connections should be used to prevent the accidental separation of infusion systems, which can also create a negative pressure in the vascular system and pull air into the system. Infusion sets should be purged of all air before an infusion is initiated, and air should be removed from all syringes before medications are administered.

Patient education on the appropriate care and maintenance of a central venous catheter to prevent an air embolism and on recognizing signs and symptoms of an air embolism should be initiated immediately after a central venous catheter is placed.

Catheter embolism. A *catheter embolism* occurs when a piece of catheter is broken in the vein and enters the circulatory system. This event can occur with a through-the-needle catheter; if the catheter is pulled backward and then threaded forward, the needle may pierce or sever the catheter. Catheter embolism can also occur with an over-the-needle catheter if the needle stylet is partially withdrawn and then reinserted into the catheter. In these two instances, the professional inserting the catheter may be aware that the catheter has been severed; however, one does not always have the opportunity to detect an embolism at the time of occurrence because a defective catheter can break or rupture after placement. Silicone catheters may rupture with subsequent catheter breakage and dislodgment if a

medication or a flush solution is administered with positive pressure. Central venous catheters can also rupture as a result of the pinch-off syndrome created by the anatomic structure between the first rib and the clavicle.

Once the catheter is completely severed, or even a small segment is broken, it may be released into circulation. The catheter may block a major vein, causing loss of circulation, or may travel to the heart, causing cardiac irritability and cardiac arrest. A catheter may also rupture without releasing a fragment into circulation, such as could occur with a tunneled catheter; however, the danger of an embolus is always present.

Patient assessment. An immediate sign that a peripheral cannula has broken is cannula and hub separation or a severed cannula on withdrawal. When a central venous catheter has ruptured, the patient may be asymptomatic, and the rupture may not be discovered until the catheter is used. Central venous catheters should be assessed for patency each time they are used. If the nurse suspects that a catheter has been released into the vascular system, the patient should be observed for cyanosis, chest pain, hypotension, increased central venous pressure, tachycardia, fainting, and loss of consciousness. The severity of symptoms is totally dependent on the location of the catheter embolism.

Nursing interventions. Immediate intervention to prevent an embolus from floating in circulation is necessary if a peripheral catheter is severed. A tourniquet is placed on the patient's arm above the venipuncture site, and bed rest is prescribed for the patient to minimize the rapidity with which the cannula travels in the vascular system. The physician is notified immediately, and the patient is monitored for signs of catheter migration. An emergency cart should be readily available in event of a cardiac arrest.

If a central venous catheter embolism is suspected, strict bed rest is prescribed, the physician notified, and the patient monitored for signs of further distress and treated for shock, if necessary.

Radiographic studies are ordered to determine the exact location of the catheter fragment. In most instances, the catheter fragment can be retrieved with a specially designed snare. The procedure involves the IV passage of the snare under fluoroscopic control to remove the catheter fragment. If the fragment cannot be removed successfully, a thoracotomy with operative removal may be required.[23]

Preventive measures. Measures for preventing catheter emboli include those listed in Box 24-14.

Pulmonary edema. *Pulmonary edema* is precipitated by the presence of more fluid volume than the circulatory system can manage. When an excess of fluid volume occurs, there is an increase in venous pressure and the possibility of cardiac dilation. If the condition is allowed to persist, congestive heart failure, shock, and cardiac arrest can result. Pulmonary edema is often precipitated by infusing too much fluid or infusing fluids too fast, which is particularly hazardous to elderly and pediatric patients and patients with renal or cardiac problems.

Patient assessment. The nurse must be alert to the early signs of pulmonary edema. Early signs include restlessness, slow increase in pulse rate, headache, shortness of breath, cough, and possibly flushing. As more fluid continues to build, the patient

---

Box 24-14   Measures for Preventing Catheter Emboli

Inspect cannulas for defects before use.
Never pull through-the-needle catheters back through the needle.
Never withdraw and reinsert over-the-needle catheters once they have been partially or fully threaded.
Do not exert positive pressure when a flush solution or a medication is administered through a silicone catheter.
Consider using syringes of no less than 10 ml when administering medications or flush solutions through silicone catheters.

Box 24-15   Measures for Preventing Pulmonary Edema

Before initiating intravenous therapy, assess patients' previous problems associated with intravenous therapy; a history of cardiac and respiratory problems; and for present status related to their ability to tolerate fluid volume.
Closely monitor patients receiving intravenous therapy for tolerance to the administration of solutions or medications.
Maintain infusion rates as ordered unless such rates would compromise the well being of the patient. Do not increase infusion rates for solutions that are behind schedule.
Slow the infusion rate if signs or symptoms of fluid overload are observed and ask the physician for orders to decrease the infusion rate.
Use volumetric chambers, infusion control devices, or both when administering solutions or medications that require accurate measurement, and when administering solutions or medications to a neonatal, pediatric, or elderly patient whose condition warrants critical management to prevent fluid overload.

---

becomes hypertensive and severely dyspneic, with gurgling respirations, and starts to cough up frothy fluid. The patient should be assessed for venous dilation, which is indicated by engorged neck veins, pitting edema in dependent areas, elevated pulmonary wedge pressure, and moist rales on auscultation. Some patients also experience puffy eyelids as fluids start to collect within the circulatory system.

Nursing interventions. The occurrence of pulmonary edema creates an emergency situation. The infusion should be slowed immediately to a rate that keeps the vein open, and the patient should be placed in a high Fowler's position. The patient's vital signs and fluid balance should be monitored. The physician should be notified, and oxygen should be administered as ordered. Medical intervention may include administering the following: (1) diuretics (intravenously) to produce rapid diuresis; (2) an IV vasodilator, such as sodium nitroprusside, to decrease afterload; (3) morphine sulfate to decrease myocardial workload (by decreasing preload through peripheral venous vasodilation) and afterload (by decreasing arterial blood pressure); and (4) phlebotomy, to relieve the heart's workload and reduce venous pressure.

Preventive measures. Measures for the prevention of pulmonary edema are detailed in Box 24-15.

Speed shock. *Speed shock* is a systemic reaction that occurs when a substance foreign to the body is rapidly introduced into circulation. This phenomenon usually results from the administration of a bolus medication or an infusion containing a medication at a rapid rate. Speed shock should not be confused with pulmonary edema. Pulmonary edema relates to volume, whereas speed shock relates to the rapidity with which a medication is administered; it can occur even when a small volume of medication is given. Rapid injections enter the serum in toxic proportions and flood the heart and the brain with medication.

Patient assessment. When medications are administered, the patient should be observed for dizziness, facial flushing, headache, and medication-specific symptoms. It is vital to note these symptoms early because progression is immediate, with the patient experiencing tightness in the chest, hypotension, irregular pulse, and anaphylactic shock.

Nursing interventions. The infusion should be discontinued immediately with recognition of the first symptom, and an IV line should be maintained for emergency treatment. The

patient should be treated for symptoms of shock, if necessary. The physician should be notified, and the patient should be given additional treatment as needed.

Preventive measures. Speed shock can be prevented. Nurses should know the medication being given and ensure that it is administered at the recommended rate. Gravity flow administration sets should be checked frequently to make sure that they are infusing at the appropriate rate. Solution containers should be time-taped so that the amount that has infused can be readily observed. Electronic flow control devices or volumetric chambers should be used for patients who are at great risk for developing complications and when critical solutions or medications are administered and should also be monitored regularly.

Allergic reactions. An *allergic reaction* is a response to a medication or solution to which the patient is sensitive. Reactions may also occur from the passive transfer of sensitivity to the patient from a blood donor, or the patient may be sensitive to substances normally present in the blood, as is seen in transfusion reactions. Reactions may be immediate or delayed. The most common reactions are those seen as a result of administering antibiotics and blood products. (Reactions to blood and blood products are discussed in Chapter 10.)

Patient assessment. Patients receiving IV therapy should be monitored for symptoms of allergic reactions. The patient may experience chills and fever with or without urticaria, erythema, and itching. Depending on the internal response to the allergen, the patient could experience shortness of breath, with or without wheezing. The patient may also experience angioneurotic edema.

Nursing intervention. The infusion should be stopped immediately, the tubing and solution container changed, and the vein kept open to allow treatment of possible anaphylactic shock. The physician should be notified, and interventions should be carried out as ordered. Antihistamines are usually administered to relieve mild symptoms; epinephrine or steroids are administered for more severe reactions. Sometimes, antihistamines are used prophylactically when an allergic reaction is considered likely.

Preventive measures. Preventive measures include the following:

1. An admission assessment should be performed of the patient's previous drug allergies, sensitivities, or idiosyncrasies. The medical record should be flagged to alert all caregivers of any allergies. In the hospital setting, it is wise to place an allergy alert bracelet on the patient so that all staff members are aware of any allergies. The pharmacy profile should list all allergies so that all medications can be cross-referenced for allergic reactions.

2. Adequate screening of donor and recipient blood can help prevent blood reactions. Policies and procedures should cover drawing blood samples for crossmatching, the crossmatching process, the identification process before blood is administered, and interventions to be carried out if a reaction occurs.

COMPLICATIONS ASSOCIATED WITH CENTRAL VENOUS CATHETERS

As more patients are placed on long-term IV therapies, receive IV therapy within the home, and receive medications or solutions that can produce adverse effects if an infiltration occurs, the use of central venous catheters will continue to rise. The difficulty of maintaining vascular access for the length of extended therapies and the complications associated with using smaller, more fragile blood vessels have required the use of these catheters. In many clinical settings, central venous catheters are being placed early in the treatment process, long before peripheral access is exhausted.

Modern technology has risen to the occasion, and many different types of central catheters have been developed. The availability of these catheters has led to widespread confusion among health care professionals as to which device is best for the therapy prescribed. In addition, each device has its own protocols for insertion, care and maintenance, and removal. Health care providers must establish policies and procedures for the use of each catheter.

Each type of central catheter is unique and has special advantages and disadvantages. The use of these catheters is not without risks or complications. The nurse and the patient must be knowledgeable about and alert to the complications of the catheter being used. Many complications that relate to central catheters have already been discussed under Systemic Complications; however, other complications are specific to central catheters.

Insertion-related complications

Complications associated with the placement of central venous catheters are rare, but they can be very serious. Complications related to the subclavian vein approach include pneumothorax, hemothorax, hydrothorax, extravascular position, chylothorax, and brachial plexus injury, whereas the antecubital cephalic vein approach is associated with hematoma and tendon or nerve

damage. Complications related to both approaches include arrhythmias; perforation of vein, artery, or heart; venous thrombosis; thrombophlebitis; severed catheter; infection; and catheter malposition.

Pneumothorax. A *pneumothorax* is created by the collection of air in the pleural space (the space between the lung and the chest wall). It results from the puncture of the pleural covering of the lung during insertion of a central venous catheter. When this happens, it is usually because of the anatomic proximity of the lung to the subclavian veins. The lung may also be punctured, creating an associated danger of an air embolism from puncture of the vein and of surgical emphysema.

Signs and symptoms depend on the size of the pneumothorax. The patient may experience a sudden onset of chest pain or shortness of breath while the procedure is being performed. On the other hand, the patient may be asymptomatic and the pneumothorax may not be discovered until radiographic confirmation of catheter tip placement is made. On auscultation, a crunching sound is heard with heartbeat; this sound is caused by mediastinal air accumulation. If the pneumothorax is severe, the patient will have marked dyspnea. Other symptoms include tachycardia, persistent cough, and diaphoresis.

If symptoms are noted during catheter insertion, the physician should remove the catheter and insertion needle immediately. The patient's facial color, respirations, and pulse should be monitored. The patient should be observed for signs of pleural shock and effusion. Oxygen is usually administered, and a chest tube may be inserted. If no respiratory distress occurs and the pneumothorax does not create tension within the chest, the pneumothorax may slowly resolve without evacuation of the air. However, if the size of the pneumothorax increases on repeated chest radiographic studies, or if respiratory distress or progressively increasing subcutaneous emphysema occurs, a persistent air leak from the injured lung may be present. The patient should be observed and monitored for these delayed events; if any are present, the physician should be notified, radiographic studies performed, and the patient prepared for chest tubes.

If the pneumothorax is not diagnosed until radiographic confirmation of catheter tip placement is made, the physician should be notified and medical interventions should be carried out as ordered.

Because of the anatomic location of the subclavian veins and the lungs, a pneumothorax cannot always be prevented. However, certain measures may prevent or minimize the effects of a pneumothorax (Box 24-16).

Hemothorax. A *hemothorax* occurs when blood enters the pleural cavity as a result of trauma or transection of a vein during insertion of a central venous catheter. The patient may experience a sudden onset of chest pain with mild to severe dyspnea while the catheter is being inserted, but may be asymptomatic, depending on the amount of blood released into the pleural cavity. Bleeding is often slow and constant into the pleural cavity, which can be particularly alarming if a patient has a clotting problem. Delayed symptoms that may occur as blood accumulates within the chest include tachycardia, hypotension, dusky skin color, diaphoresis, and hemoptysis. Percussion may disclose dullness of the affected side of the chest, and auscultation may detect decreased or absent breath sounds over the affected side.

If symptoms of a hemothorax are noted during catheter insertion, the physician should remove the catheter and the insertion needle, and pressure should be applied to the site. If a tunneled catheter is being inserted, pressure should be applied over the vein entry site. The patient's vital signs should be monitored, and symptoms should be treated. Oxygen is usually administered, and a chest tube may be placed if the hemothorax is associated with a pneumothorax. If symptoms occur after the catheter has been inserted, the physician should be notified and medical interventions carried out as necessary.

The risk of hemothorax may be reduced by following the same guidelines as those for decreasing the risks of a pneumothorax (Box 24-16).

Chylothorax. *Chylothorax* is a condition in which chyle (lymph) enters the pleural cavity as a result of transection of the thoracic duct on the left side, when a catheter is inserted into the subclavian vein. Chyle is the milklike content of the lacteal and lymphatic vessels of the intestines; it consists mainly of absorbed fats and also contains products of digestion. It is carried by the lymphatic vessels to the cisterna chyli and then, by way of the thoracic duct, to the left subclavian vein, where it enters the blood system. Because of the anatomic position of the thoracic duct, the left supraclavicular approach to the subclavian vein is usually avoided.

Symptoms of chylothorax are similar to those of hemothorax. The patient may experience a sudden onset of chest pain with dyspnea as the thoracic duct is transected and lymph fills the pleural cavity. Chylothorax is often noted by the clinician at the time the thoracic duct is transected, because a milklike substance is drawn into the needle or catheter.

The leaking of a cloudy material from around the catheter site suggests the possibility of a chylous fistula. Any cloudy fluid leaking from around the catheter site should be aseptically collected, if possible, and checked for glucose content. A low

glucose content suggests that the liquid is a body fluid, whereas a high glucose content suggests a lymphatic leak. If a lymphatic leak is found, the physician should be notified for removal of the catheter, and the patient's vital signs should be assessed. Oxygen and chest tubes may be necessary, depending on the amount of lymph emptied into the thoracic cavity.

Hydrothorax. *Hydrothorax* occurs when IV fluids are infused directly into the thoracic cavity as a result of transection of the vein and placement of the catheter into the thorax. Signs and symptoms include chest pain with dyspnea, absence of vesicular breath sounds, and a murmur with a flat sound over the location of the fluid.

Medical interventions include removing the catheter, aspirating fluids from the pleural space, and possibly inserting chest tubes. The patient is monitored, and interventions are carried out as necessary. Oxygen may be administered, depending on the severity of the hydrothorax.

A hydrothorax can be prevented or the effects minimized by obtaining radiographic confirmation of catheter tip placement before therapy is initiated. Many institutions now cap central lines as heparin locks or intermittent devices until radiographic confirmation of catheter tip placement is received. This practice prevents fluid from being administered into the thoracic cavity.

Brachial plexus injury. The *brachial plexus* is the network of lower cervical and upper dorsal spinal nerves that supplies the arm, forearm, and hand. Because of the anatomic position of these nerves (Fig. 24-5), they may be injured during the insertion of a central venous catheter. If such an injury occurs, the patient may experience tingling sensations in the fingers, pain shooting down the arm, or paralysis.

The physician is notified, and medication is usually administered for pain. Physical therapy is helpful in the treatment of brachial plexus injuries. Treatment is palliative and does not always resolve the injury. Preventive measures include those listed in Box 24-16.

Inadvertent arterial puncture. Inadvertent puncture of an artery during insertion of a central venous catheter is usually not a serious problem, unless the carotid artery is punctured. If symptoms are noted at the time of insertion and the artery can be located, pressure should be applied to the artery for at least 5 minutes; pressure must be applied longer if a patient has a bleeding or platelet disorder. Pressure cannot be applied to all arteries; the ability to apply pressure to an artery depends on its location.

If symptoms are not recognized immediately, the patient can develop a mediastinal hematoma with signs and symptoms of tracheal compression or respiratory distress. A chest x-ray study should be performed to determine whether a mediastinal hematoma has developed. If a subclavian artery is accidentally catheterized, air or debris may enter the artery and embolize to the brain, creating a central neurologic deficit. Laceration of the subclavian artery can also produce a hemothorax.

Extravascular malposition. An *extravascular malposition* of a central venous catheter exists when the catheter penetrates the vessel and the tip of the catheter lies outside the vascular system. During the process of threading a catheter, the needle or introducer through which the catheter is passed may slip out of the vein. *Hydromediastinum* occurs when the catheter

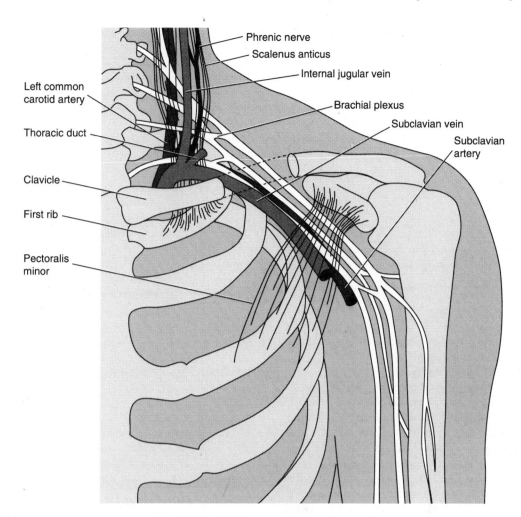

FIG. 24-5 *The brachial plexus in relation to the central vessels.*

tip is placed in the mediastinum and medication is infused into the space where the heart and great vessels are located.

The patient may experience symptoms associated with a pneumothorax if the pleural covering of the lung has been punctured, and of a hemothorax as blood enters the pleural system. If the vein is transected and the catheter tip is placed within the neck or chest area outside the pleural cavity, the patient may not experience any symptoms until the catheter is used. At this time, the patient may experience a hydrothorax as fluid is infused into the chest, or arm or neck swelling as fluid accumulates in the area adjacent to the tip of the catheter.

Radiographic confirmation of catheter tip placement before use can prevent an extravascular malpositioned catheter from being used and from causing more serious complications.

Medical interventions include removing the catheter and treating associated complications. The patient is monitored and vital signs assessed. Oxygen and chest tubes may be necessary if a pneumothorax, hemothorax, or hydrothorax has occurred.

Intravascular malposition. The optimal position for the tip of a central venous catheter is the superior vena cava.[5,15] When a central venous catheter is misplaced, it is usually into the internal jugular vein (rather than the subclavian vein) because of its proximity to the superior vena cava. Misplace-

ments have also been documented in the contralateral innominate, azygos, right and left internal thoracic, superior intercostal, and accessory hemizygous veins. The most common misplacement with the subclavian approach is in the internal jugular vein, and the most common malposition of the cephalic vein is the axillary vein.

Signs and symptoms of catheter malposition are often noted when the catheter is first used. Difficulty with aspiration or infusion through the catheter may be noticed. In addition, the patient may complain of discomfort or pain in the shoulder, neck, or arm. Edema may also be noted in the neck or shoulder area. Infusions through a catheter aberrantly placed in the internal jugular vein have been associated with a benign annoyance called the *ear gurgling* sign, which patients often describe as the sound of a running stream rushing past the ear. The infusion of medications through a catheter located in the internal jugular vein has often produced undesirable neurologic effects resulting from retrograde perfusion into the intracranial venous sinuses and the tributary vein.

A malpositioned catheter is not always removed. Studies have indicated that misplaced central venous catheters can be safely and effectively repositioned without subjecting the patient to the potential morbidity associated with repeated percutaneous cannulation. Most misplaced silicone catheters can be repositioned by rapid flushing of the catheter with 20 ml of 0.9% sodium chloride at 4 to 5 ml/sec. Catheters that loop back into the axillary or peripheral veins in the axilla have a lower rate of successful repositioning. The rapid flushing technique is not successful with double- or triple-lumen catheters or with rigid or semirigid single-lumen catheters because of the inflexibility of the catheters. Obstructed catheters have been known to rupture during rapid flushing; therefore this technique should be performed only when there is no resistance to injection and the patient exhibits no signs of venous occlusion.

It is helpful to reposition the patient when the catheter is repositioned. If the catheter is misplaced into the internal jugular vein, the patient is placed in Fowler's position before the catheter is flushed. If the catheter is in the contralateral vein, the patient is placed in an ipsilateral position with the head of the bed slightly elevated. Finally, for a malpositioned catheter in the axillary vein, the patient is placed in a position contralateral to the insertion, with the head of the bed slightly raised. Catheters with simple looping into the subclavian, innominate, or internal jugular veins can often be repositioned by placing the patient in the aforementioned positions, which allow gravity and blood flow to reposition the catheter overnight.

With experience, malpositioned catheters with the tip in the subclavian, internal jugular, or innominate veins can be replaced in the appropriate vein by guidewire exchange. A catheter malpositioned beyond the superior vena cava into the right atrium or ventricle can be partially withdrawn, provided it is not a nonflexible catheter with memory that is looped in the great vein. Direct fluoroscopic observation is the safest and most reliable method of repositioning a central venous catheter, but radiographic techniques can also be used to reposition catheters.

Certain measures can help reduce the frequency of misplaced central venous catheters. Only well-qualified, highly skilled professionals should place central venous catheters. Measuring the distance from the proposed insertion site to the right atrium can prevent catheter malposition when peripheral central venous catheters are placed. This procedure can easily be performed by measuring the distance from the proposed site on the skin along the presumptive anatomic course of the veins to the right chondrosternal junction, or to one third of the way down the suprasternal notch to the xiphoid process.

Proper positioning of the patient is essential for the appropriate placement of a central venous catheter. For instance, a peripherally placed central catheter inserted through the basilic vein tends to pass along the cephalad wall of the subclavian vein to enter the jugular vein. By turning the patient's head toward the side of insertion to make the angle between the subclavian and the internal jugular vein, this problem can be avoided. Placing a patient in Trendelenburg's position with a rolled towel between the scapulae facilitates the placement of a catheter into the subclavian vein and the threading of it into the superior vena cava by the subclavian approach. However, this position may cause the angle of the clavicle and the first rib to be at its widest on insertion with subsequent catheter pinch-off syndrome.[15,24]

Using soft catheters, such as those made of a silicone elastomer, further enhances the possibility of placing a central cathe-ter into the appropriate vein. The softer catheter materials enhance the blood's ability to carry the catheter tip and allow the catheter to readily follow the contours of the vein.

Radiographic confirmation of tip placement can often prevent complications associated with a malpositioned catheter. However, it may be difficult to determine the correct position of a catheter placed in the left side of the mediastinum because of the proximity of the internal thoracic vein to the superior vena cava when the area is viewed in a frontal chest radiograph. The location can be confirmed by obtaining a lateral chest radiograph and by injecting a contrast medium.

Pericardial tamponade. *Pericardial tamponade* is caused by penetration of the atrium with a centrally placed catheter. Cardiovascular collapse with neck vein distension, a narrow pulse pressure, and hypotension, with or without symptoms of congestive heart failure, suggest that the wall of the atrium has been penetrated. Symptoms are usually delayed because blood or solution must leak into the pericardial space and compress the heart to cause this complication. Symptoms suggestive of this complication require emergency intervention by the physician.

The treatment for pericardial tamponade is aspiration of the pericardial sac from just below the xiphoid process of the sternum. The catheter is removed and replaced only after resuscitative measures are complete.

Preventive measures include ensuring that central vein cannulation is performed by a highly skilled professional and using soft, flexible catheters, such as those made from silicone.

Complications associated with indwelling central venous catheters

Central venous catheters place the patient at risk of complications during insertion, and the patient continues to be at risk while the catheter remains within the vascular system. Central venous catheters must be monitored, and appropriate care must be administered while these catheters are in place. A lack of monitoring or inappropriate care can place patients with these catheters in life-threatening situations.

Dislodgment and twiddler's syndrome. Central venous catheters are usually sutured in place at the time of insertion. However, these catheters can still fall out, be pulled out, or become dislodged. Also, ports can become freely movable and migrate from one area to another, or patients may develop the nervous habit of "twiddling" with their ports, resulting in displacement. The port may actually flip over, preventing access and use.

Although it is fairly obvious when a catheter has been pulled out or when a port moves when accessed, catheter dislodgment may not be so obvious. When an assessment of a central venous catheter is made, the length of the external part of the catheter should be assessed. If the external part appears longer, the catheter tip may no longer be at the position it was on insertion. The exit site and tunnel should be palpated for coiling. In certain catheters, the exposure of a Dacron cuff can also alert the nurse that the catheter has become dislodged. Difficulty with aspiration or infusion through the catheter, leaking of solution from the catheter exit site, edema, a burning sensation, or pain when solution is infused can also indicate a displaced catheter.

Careful observation is sometimes necessary to determine the displacement of a central venous catheter. If displacement is suspected, the physician should be notified. Usually, venographic studies are performed to determine catheter tip placement; depending on radiologic findings, the catheter may or may not be repositioned. If the catheter cannot be repositioned, it should be removed, and a new one with new tubing and solution container should be placed. The catheter should be secured with sutures, and the patient should be taught not to manipulate the catheter.

If a central venous catheter is pulled out, a sterile occlusive pressure dressing, such as Vaseline gauze or Telfa covered with antibiotic ointment, should be applied and the physician should be notified. Usually, the dressing can be removed within 24 to 72 hours. The patient should be prepared for reinsertion of the catheter, if necessary.

Preventive measures for central venous catheter dislodgment include the following:

- Secure the external catheter with sutures, tape, or manufactured securement device and intact dressing.
- Loop and tape the catheter to prevent pulling at the skin exit site.
- Educate the patient in catheter care, physical activities to avoid, and the danger of pulling the catheter out.
- Assess the patient's understanding and compliance with instructions during the entire catheter dwell.

Catheter migration. *Migration* occurs when the tip of an undislodged catheter is displaced from a documented, satisfactory position in the superior vena cava to another position in a neighboring vein.[15] The catheter tip often migrates into the right atrium or into the internal jugular vein after placement. Migrations have also been documented in the axillary veins.

Spontaneous migration of the catheter tip has been reported often. Catheter tip migration may result from forceful flushing of the catheter or from changes in intrathoracic pressure associated with coughing or sneezing. In some instances, migrations have been noted as a result of a disease process. For instance, in patients with congestive heart failure, catheter tip migration has been thought to result from the reduced flow of blood and the dilated vessels associated with the disease. Migrations have also resulted from displacement by invading tissue (tumor) or venous thrombosis.

Although there may not be obvious signs or symptoms of catheter migration, a change in functional capability can be an indication. The inability to flush, infuse, or aspirate can mean the catheter tip is no longer at the desired position. Arrhythmias are very indicative of catheter migration into the right atrium or ventricle. The "ear gurgling" or running stream sound is often heard when a catheter migrates into the internal jugular vein. Palpation of the catheter in the internal jugular can affirm migration to the jugular vein. In addition, complaints of headache or pain, swelling, redness, or discomfort in the shoulder, arm, or neck may indicate catheter migration.

When catheter migration is suspected, the physician should be notified and venographic studies should be performed to verify catheter tip location. The nurse should prepare the patient for either repositioning of the catheter under fluoroscopy or removal and possible reinsertion of another catheter. All infusions should be discontinued.

Catheter migration cannot always be prevented. Confirming that the catheter tip is properly located in the lower portion of the superior vena cava immediately following placement and periodically reassessing tip placement can help prevent or minimize the effects of catheter migration. Preventing trauma to the catheter site, avoiding catheter placement near the site of local disease, and suturing the catheter can help prevent catheter migration.

Catheter occlusion. *Catheter occlusions* are caused by a thrombus formation, drug precipitants, or lipid deposits. They may also be caused by catheter compression, as in catheter pinch-off syndrome (see Catheter Pinch-Off Syndrome). All catheters are subject to fibrin formation at the tip or along the catheter line where the catheter touches the vessel. A catheter occlusion resulting from a thrombus may result from inadequate heparinization, pump malfunction, break in the catheter system, or hypercoagulability of the patient's blood.[15,25,26] Catheters can also become occluded when medications or solutions are incompatible. The most common precipitates are calcium, diazepam, and phenytoin. Patients receiving total nutrient admixtures and lipids piggybacked with parenteral nutrition solutions are at risk for catheter occlusions from lipid accumulation within the catheter.[26]

Signs and symptoms of a partially occluded catheter include the following:

- Discomfort, pain, or edema in the shoulder, neck, arm, or insertion site
- Resistance when a solution, flush, or medication is instilled
- Bubbles in tubing (blood is foamy)
- Leaking of fluid from the insertion site as fluid tracks back along a fibrin trail (fibrin sheath formation)

A catheter is completely occluded when blood cannot be withdrawn from the catheter and complete resistance is met when the catheter is used.

Catheters that are allowed to remain clotted predispose the patient to infection and the possibility of an embolus. When a central venous catheter appears clotted, the nurse must assess the entire line and catheter for patency. The solution container, tubing, and infusion device must be checked for proper operation.

Catheters suspected of being occluded should be assessed for proper placement; the catheter could possibly be pinched between the clavicle and the first rib, or the outlets (particularly on multilumen catheters) could be lying against the wall of the vessel (one-way obstruction). On aspiration, the wall is sucked into the catheter, blocking blood withdrawal; an infusion, however, forces the tip away from the wall and restores patency. Repositioning the patient may restore the ability to aspirate from a port. The patient should change position, sit up, lie down, raise the arm above the head, or cough in an attempt to open the catheter.

To flush a catheter suspected of being occluded, only very light pressure and a 10-ml syringe should be used. If the catheter cannot be flushed without resistance or if flow of an infusion cannot be established, an attempt should be made to aspirate the occlusion using a gentle push-pull technique with 0.9% sodium chloride. If blood cannot be drawn, solution cannot be infused, or aspiration cannot be performed (two-way obstruction), the cause of the occlusion should be determined. Catheters occluded because of precipitant formation are usually removed. Ethanol, hydrochloric acid, and sodium bicarbonate have been used to clear certain precipitates from occluded catheters.[26-28] The organization's policies and procedures should dictate the use of these medications.

If an implanted vascular access device appears occluded, the Huber-point needle should be removed and the device should be reaccessed with a new needle. Often, the needle is pulled out of the septum. The needle should not be pushed back into the portal because this practice could carry microorganisms into the system. Once reaccessed, the system should be reevaluated for patency using 0.9% sodium chloride and a gentle push-pull, as previously stated.

If the occlusion results from a blood clot or a fibrin sheath, the catheter should be declotted using a thrombolytic agent designed specifically for lysis of catheter clots. Urokinase (Abbokinase Open-Cath) was the drug of choice for declotting central venous catheters. The recommended concentration is 5000 IU/ml. The volume administered should be equal to the volume of the catheter. The recent unavailability of Urokinase has promoted the use of alteplase, recombinant (activase, tissue plasminogen activator, tPA). Alteplase, more commonly referred to as *tPA,* is prepared as a 1:1 solution (50 mg/50 ml), and 2 mg/2 ml is instilled into the catheter and allowed to incubate for 2 hours. The dosage may be repeated in 2 hours if catheter patency is not restored. The physician should be notified and the catheter declotted by established policies and procedures. Policies and procedures should specify which catheters may be declotted because not all catheters expand to support the addition of even a small amount of medication when they are occluded.

Central line occlusions and fibrin formation at the catheter tip can often be prevented (Box 24-17).

Catheter pinch-off syndrome.
Catheter pinch-off syndrome results from compression of a central venous catheter between the first rib and the clavicle. Placing the patient in the Trendelenburg position with a rolled towel or sheet between the shoulder blades during catheter insertion may contribute to this condition, particularly if the catheter is inserted medial to the midclavicular line. This position causes the angle of the clavicle and first rib to be at its widest. When the procedure is completed and the patient is returned to an upright position, the weight of the shoulder closes the angle and compresses the catheter.[15]

Catheter pinch-off syndrome is often unrecognized and underreported.[22] It is often identified retrospectively after the catheter fractures from the continuous compression between the first rib and the clavicle.[29] An intermittent positional catheter may indicate catheter pinch-off. Resistance is met when flushing the catheter, infusing solutions, and aspirating blood. The occlusion can usually be relieved immediately by having the patient roll the shoulder backward or raise the arm on the ipsilateral side. The position change opens the angle of the

---

Box 24-17 Recommended Guidelines to Prevent Occlusions of Catheter Tip

1. Comply with established policies and procedures for maintenance of patency.
2. Maintain positive pressure when flushing lines.
3. Use infusion pumps when indicated.
4. Monitor infusion system and catheter often for mechanical difficulties (e.g., empty solution container, kinked tubing, malfunctioning infusion control device).
5. Mix medications with the appropriate diluent and ensure compatibility of medications and solutions.
6. Prevent pulling on catheters and tugging on implanted vascular access devices.
7. Use low-dose oral anticoagulant therapy, especially with patients who have hypercoagulability problems.[15,26]

---

costoclavicular space. This finding is considered a hallmark of catheter pinch-off syndrome.[24]

Clinical findings should be confirmed by a chest radiograph. Proper positioning for the x-ray examination is essential to observing catheter compression. The patient should be positioned upright with the arms straight at his or her sides and not in the standard shoulder raised-and-rolled-forward position. IV contrast and fluoroscopy should be used to evaluate the integrity of the catheter if partial transection is suspected.

Complications of catheter pinch-off syndrome can be serious and include catheter fracture and embolus. Patient complaints of infraclavicular pain or swelling with flushing or infusion are consistent with a partially or completely transected catheter. The patient may be asymptomatic or complain of palpitations or chest pain as the catheter tip embolizes. The catheter should be removed and the embolized segment should be retrieved.

Placing the catheter lateral to the midclavicular line will decrease the risk of catheter pinch-off syndrome.[15,24,30]

Vessel thrombosis (catheter-related thrombosis).
Vessel thrombosis is the formation of a blood clot in a vessel in the neck, chest, or arms in the presence of a central venous catheter. The pathophysiology of a vessel thrombosis has been identified as a triad of thromboses: stasis, vessel wall injury, and hypercoagulability.[15,24] Stasis can result from the effect of intrapulmonary or mediastinal disease. Vessel wall injury can be attributed to the aggregation of platelets on the catheter surface and mechanical irritation of the vessel intima by the catheter tip. Injury to the vessel wall at the site of the catheter's entry can be related to catheter infection or exposure of the vessel wall to total parenteral nutrition solutions and chemotherapeutic agents. Hypercoagulability is often associated with a malignancy; patients with cancer have a tendency for hypercoagulation. Other factors that appear to be associated with thrombosis in tunneled catheters include suboptimal internal catheter tip location and left-sided catheter placement.

Vessel thrombosis should be suspected if the patient complains of chest pain, earache, jaw pain, or edema of the neck, supraclavicular area, or extremities. Associated dangers include pulmonary embolism, cerebral anoxia, laryngeal edema, bronchial obstruction, and death.

The physician should be notified immediately if vessel thrombosis is suspected. Radiographic studies using dye (venography) are usually performed to verify catheter placement. The patient is usually placed on anticoagulant therapy (systemic heparin, warfarin, or both). Depending on the size of the clot and the area of impaired circulation, the clot may have to be lysed; lysis is achieved by imbedding a peripheral catheter into the clot using fluoroscopic guidance and administering a kinase infusion.

Vessel thrombosis can be prevented by using low-dose anticoagulant (warfarin) therapy for patients at high risk of clotting disorders,[15,26] ensuring that central venous catheters are inserted by highly skilled professionals, and placing central venous catheters into the right subclavian vein.

Damaged catheter.
Central venous catheters can easily be damaged if appropriate measures are not used during care and maintenance. Using scissors at or near the catheter during dressing changes can result in the catheter being cut. Catheters are made of a nonresealable material; penetration by a needle creates pinholes with subsequent leaking. Catheters can also rupture when force is exerted, a syringe smaller than 10 ml is used to flush the catheter, or the pinch-off syndrome occurs.

Central venous catheters should be monitored and assessed for pinholes, cuts, leaks, tears, and ruptures at frequent intervals. Assessment should include observation of the dressing, catheter, and area around the catheter. A wet dressing or leaking at the insertion site during an infusion or flushing may indicate catheter damage. Swelling in the chest area may indicate rupture of a catheter and infusion of solution into the chest wall. Tunneled and implanted catheters can usually be palpated to the point at which they enter the subclavian vein; if the rupture is in the tunneled segment of the catheter, swelling may be felt at the point of rupture.

At the very moment an assessment reveals a damaged catheter, a nonserrated clamp should be applied proximal to the damaged part, if possible. The damage should be assessed and the appropriate action taken.

Damaged catheters must be repaired or removed without delay to prevent serious complications. Any opening in the catheter can serve as a portal of entry for bacteria or air into the vascular system. The entrance of bacteria into the system can predispose a debilitated patient to septicemia. Air may also be drawn into the system because of the negative pressure created within the heart, and the patient can suffer an air embolism directly to the heart. Policies and procedures should be established for the repair of a catheter according to the manufacturer's guidelines. If the catheter cannot be repaired, the physician should be notified immediately and the catheter removed.

One of the most serious dangers of an implanted vascular access device is the rupture of the catheter. Implanted vascular access devices are also known for port-catheter separation. Although this phenomenon can cause severe complications if a vesicant is infusing, usually there is less risk of an embolus than there is when the catheter ruptures. If either of these conditions is suspected, the infusion should be discontinued, the patient placed on bed rest, and the physician notified. Radiographic studies should be performed to verify a rupture or a port-

---

Box 24-18   Guidelines for Preventing Damage to Central Venous Catheters

Use clamps on clamping sleeves provided on silicone catheters. If it is necessary to use a clamp at another area on the catheter, use a flat, toothless clamp only.

Avoid using scissors or other sharp objects around the catheter.

Use only small-bore needles (22-25 gauge) with a needle length 1 inch or shorter when accessing latex injection ports on the catheter.

Administer medications without force. Consider using 10-ml syringes when administering medications via a silicone catheter.

Educate the patient regarding the catheter and the problems associated with "twiddling" ports and playing with external catheters.

---

catheter separation, and the patient should be prepared for removal of the port and possible replacement of the catheter. Every effort must be made to prevent damage to central venous catheters (Box 24-18).

Superior vena cava syndrome.
Superior vena cava syndrome is an obstruction of blood flow through the superior vena cava. Extensive vein thrombosis, tumor compression, or enlarged lymph nodes compressing the superior vena cava create obstruction.[15] The cause must be established before it is assumed that the condition results from the central venous catheter.

Signs and symptoms include progressive shortness of breath, dyspnea, cough, sensation of skin tightness, unilateral edema, and cyanosis of the face, neck, shoulder, and arms. Extensive edema of the upper body without edema of the lower body parts, or *short cap edema*, may also be noticed. Edema and cyanosis of the mucous membranes of the mouth, pharynx, larynx, an thorax, and occasionally of the hydropericardium, also occur. The jugular, temporal, and arm veins are engorged and distended. A prominent venous pattern usually is present over the chest as a result of dilated thoracic vessels. If the condition goes unnoticed and untreated, headache may be caused by increased intracranial pressure, visual disturbances, and altered mental status. There is also danger of cerebral anoxia, bronchial obstruction, and death.

The physician must be notified immediately when the first symptoms of superior vena cava syndrome are observed. Diagnosis is confirmed by radiographic studies.

Whether to remove the catheter depends on the severity of symptoms, the ability to initiate an alternate IV route, and the type of catheter in place. Anticoagulant therapy is usually prescribed for the patient, and symptoms are treated. The patient should be placed in a semi-Fowler's position and oxygen should be administered to facilitate breathing. Patients with superior vena cava syndrome become very anxious and fearful because of the feeling of suffocating, so it is important to provide emotional support. The patient's fluid volume status should be monitored to minimize further edema, and cardiovascular and neurologic status should be monitored.

Superior vena cava syndrome is rare but can be very serious. Patient evaluation for tumors or enlarged lymph nodes that compress the superior vena cava is essential before placing a central venous catheter. The benefits versus complications associated with catheter placement must be evaluated when one of these conditions is present. Ensuring that a central venous catheter is inserted by a well-trained, experienced professional can help prevent superior vena cava syndrome. An inexperienced physician can traumatize the endothelial lining of the vein and predispose the vein to clot formation. Anticoagulant therapy, which has proved to be most effective in preventing this syndrome, should be considered, particularly when long-term catheters are used for patients who are at high risk for clotting problems.

Site infection. The insertion and use of a central venous catheter predisposes the patient to the possibility of an infection with subsequent septicemia (septicemia has been discussed under Systemic Complications). However, the patient may experience an infection at the catheter exit site with or without septicemia.

The catheter exit site should be observed for redness, edema, and drainage, and the patient should be questioned about tenderness or pain around the catheter. Laboratory values, such as white blood cell count, should be monitored. If the patient experiences sudden chills with fever, general malaise, headache, nausea and vomiting, hypotension, and cyanosis, he or she should be immediately treated for sepsis.

The physician should be notified immediately of any symptoms related to an infection of the catheter. The physician may have the catheter removed or choose to replace it over a guidewire. Blood cultures are usually drawn peripherally and from the central line. The patient is usually given antibiotic therapy and may be given anticoagulant therapy, because a thrombus within the catheter or at the tip can trap bacteria and predispose the patient to sepsis. If the catheter is removed, consideration should be given to culturing the catheter tip, and care is given until the site is healed. If an implanted vascular access device is in place and has not been accessed, it is not used until the origin of the infection has been determined.

Site infections associated with central venous catheters are preventable. By strictly adhering to the guidelines listed in Box 24-19, the risk of infection is greatly reduced.

Skin erosion. Occasionally, a patient with an implanted vascular access device may experience a skin tear or erosion of the skin over the portal septum. A patient with a tunneled catheter may experience skin erosion over the catheter. Skin erosions are usually seen in patients who, as a consequence of poor nutritional status, are very thin and have experienced a large weight loss. Skin erosions have been seen also as a result of trauma over a tunneled catheter or portal septum. Signs of erosion include visible skin abrasions or tears over a port or catheter with redness or edema.

In response to skin erosion over a port or a catheter, the physician is notified, the catheter is usually removed, and depending on the patient and the therapy being administered, another catheter may be placed.

The possibility of skin erosions over ports or tunneled catheters can be minimized by maintaining a positive nutritional status, avoiding pressure or trauma to the area surrounding the catheter or port, and rotating the site each time the port is accessed.

NURSING CONSIDERATIONS

Nurses must be able to accurately diagnose complications associated with the insertion, use, and removal of venous and arterial devices. By use of the nursing process and the holistic approach, the nurse must implement nursing interventions that provide immediate treatment, promote healing, and prevent further complications. The nurse must constantly evaluate the care rendered in terms of patient outcomes to promote quality improvement in the performance of IV therapies. In forming an accurate diagnosis of complications associated with IV therapy, the nurse should have the requisite knowledge presented in Box 24-20. In addition, the nurse should be able to translate knowledge into practical use when assessing the patient for complications and intervening when necessary.

The clinical diagnosis of complications is related to the nurse's ability to evaluate the patient's signs and symptoms. Using objective, subjective, and cardinal evaluations, the nurse can make an accurate nursing diagnosis. *Objective symptoms* are

---

Box 24-19 Guidelines for Preventing Site Infections Associated with Central Venous Catheters

Maintain aseptic technique during the insertion of a central venous catheter.

Wash hands before gloving to prepare for inserting or manipulating the catheter or changing dressings.

Wear sterile gloves and a mask when performing dressing changes.

Assess all equipment before use for package integrity and sterility.

Change dressings and provide site care according to the *Infusion Nursing Standards of Practice.*[5]

Box 24-20 Necessary Knowledge for the Accurate Diagnosis of Complications Associated with Intravenous Therapy

Anatomy of the vascular system

Disease processes related to therapy and associated complications

Various therapies used, including drug classifications

Recommended dose and volume relative to age, height, and weight, or body surface area

Drug and solution properties, actions, side effects, and adverse reactions

Methods of intravenous administration and use of infusion systems

Interventions necessary for treatment of complications

visible (e.g., edema, erythema, blanching). *Subjective symptoms* have an internal or mental origin; they relate to the patient's perception of what he or she feels (e.g., pain, tingling sensation, feeling of suffocation). *Cardinal symptoms* relate to the physical body (e.g., pulse, temperature, blood pressure). In addition, signs and symptoms occur locally or systemically. Local complications usually appear at the site of the invasion of the body and usually produce visible signs and symptoms. Systemic complications occur within the body and usually affect circulation and other bodily processes.

Other tools often used to evaluate signs and symptoms include differential evaluations, exclusion evaluations, pathologic evaluations, and roentgenographic evaluations. *Differential evaluations* can be extremely helpful, such as comparing one arm against another to determine infiltration. *Exclusion evaluations* are often performed when no other reasonable explanation exists for a complication. For example, a patient with a central venous catheter may suddenly develop an elevated temperature, and no other possible explanation exists for the elevated temperature. Sepsis related to the catheter is considered, and interventions for catheter-induced septicemia are initiated.

Pathologic evaluations are used to verify the presence of pathologic organisms; they are usually performed when drainage from a wound or an elevated temperature occurs, suggesting an infectious process. A good example is the culturing of the catheter site, the catheter, or an infusate when a vascular infection is suspected. A pathologic evaluation is a very good tool because it can verify the disease source. However, it should never be the only tool used because pathologic reports usually take time and complications do not wait to be diagnosed—they often progress very rapidly. *Roentgenographic evaluations* can be used to prevent complications (e.g., obtaining a radiograph to verify placement before using a central venous catheter), or to verify a complication (e.g., verifying a pulmonary embolus). The nurse must be alert to all signs and symptoms and must evaluate each one individually. Early recognition of potential complications can prevent further complications and promote quick healing and restoration of health.

Although observing and evaluating the signs and symptoms of complications is very important, it is far better to prevent complications. The ideal situation is delivering IV therapy that is free of complications, thereby promoting positive patient outcomes. Outcomes should be established that deliver high-quality care, protecting the patient and nurse from risks associated with IV therapy.

Outcome criteria can be written generically to cover an entire aspect of IV nursing care, or to cover only one aspect. An example of a care plan that could apply to all patients receiving peripheral IV therapy is represented in Box 24-21. In comparison, Box 24-22 is a plan of care outlining outcome criteria for a newly implanted vascular access device. Both care plans expect high-quality performance and positive patient outcomes. Goals have been written to define the expected outcomes and the care necessary to achieve the outcome.

Outcome criteria promote the delivery of high-quality IV care by expecting optimal performance. Each model for out-

come criteria promotes delivery of care that prevents complications associated with IV therapy—a goal worth striving for by nurses practicing IV therapy.

In addition to establishing criteria for patient outcomes, nurses should also monitor the actual patient outcomes. Statis-

---

Box 24-21   Outcome Criteria for Peripheral Intravenous Therapy

OUTCOME CRITERIA: THE PATIENT WILL REMAIN FREE OF COMPLICATIONS RELATED TO THE ADMINISTRATION OF IV THERAPY.

1. Goal
The patient will remain free from infection related to IV therapy.

Interventions
IV site will be inspected for signs of infection at least every 4 hours.
IV catheter and tubing will be changed every 72 hours.
IV solution containers will be changed every 24 hours.
IV catheter will be securely taped to prevent movement of catheter in and out of the vein.
IV equipment and solution containers will be inspected for contamination before use.
A final filter will be placed at the distal end of the IV tubing.

2. Goal
The patient will remain free of chemical phlebitis associated with the administration of medications.

Interventions
All medications and solutions will be mixed in the pharmacy under a laminar flow hood. Known irritants will be diluted to the fullest extent possible.
All solutions and medications will be administered at the recommended rate.
The IV site will be checked every 2 hours for redness and inflammation associated with chemical phlebitis.

3. Goal
The patient will remain free of local complications.

Interventions
IV sites over flexion areas will not be used unless absolutely necessary.
Catheters will be taped according to policy and procedure to prevent movement of the catheter.
An armboard will be placed if necessary to limit movement of the extremity, using measures to prevent constriction of circulation and pressure on nerves and skin.

4. Goal
The patient will take part in the care and maintenance of his or her IV system.

Interventions
Patient's level of knowledge for learning will be assessed.
Patient will be taught care of system.
- Performance of routine activities—bathing, movement in bed, and ambulation.
- Emergency measures for pulling out line, loose or wet dressing, kinking of tubing.
- Signs and symptoms of complications.

Developed from policies and procedures at High Point Regional Health System, High Point, North Carolina.
IV, Intravenous.

Box 24-22 Outcome Criteria for a Newly Placed Implanted Vascular Access Device

OUTCOME CRITERIA: THE PATIENT WILL REMAIN FREE OF COMPLICATIONS ASSOCIATED WITH THE IMPLANTATION OF A VASCULAR ACCESS DEVICE.

1. Goal

The patient will remain free from infection associated with placement of implanted vascular access.

Interventions

Site and surrounding area will be checked every 2 hours for swelling, bleeding, and inflammation.

The dressing on the site will be changed daily and as needed using sterile technique.

Dressing changes will be sterile.

The site will be cleansed with alcohol followed by povidone-iodine each time the dressing is changed.

The patient's temperature will be monitored for elevation every 4 hours.

2. Goal

The patient will remain free of infections resulting from use of the device.

Interventions

Solution containers will be checked for possible leaks and contamination.

All equipment will be checked for defects and contamination.

Solution containers will be changed every 24 hours.

Intravenous tubing will be changed every 72 hours.

3. Goal

The patient will experience minimal discomfort at the insertion site.

Interventions

The patient will be assessed often for pain in site area.

Analgesics will be administered as needed.

Relief of pain from analgesics will be evaluated.

Cold compresses will be applied to the site for edema for the first 24 hours after insertion.

Warm compresses will be applied to the site for comfort after the first 24 hours following insertion, unless the site is bleeding.

4. Goal

The patient will be educated regarding care of vascular access device.

Interventions

The patient's ability to learn will be determined.

The patient will develop understanding of how device is used.

The patient will assist in care by taking preventive measures to maintain catheter and dressing.

The patient will be alert to the signs and symptoms of complications.

Developed from policies and procedures at High Point Regional Health System, High Point, North Carolina.

tics should be kept regarding the incidence of complications, interventions, and outcomes. They should be reported to staff, the risk management department, the quality improvement council, and various others involved in the process, and should be used as a tool to recognize areas for improvement.

REFERENCES

1. Joint Commission Accreditation of Health Care Organizations: *CAMH refreshed core: comprehensive accreditation manual for hospitals,* Oakbrook Terrace, Ill, 1999, JCAHO.
2. US Department of Labor, Occupational Safety and Health Administration: *Occupational safe exposure to bloodborne pathogens: final rule,* Washington, DC, OSHA Docket No. H-370, December 6, 1991.
3. American Society of Hospital Pharmacists: ASHP report: ASHP therapeutic position statement on the institutional use of 0.9% sodium chloride injection to maintain patency of peripheral indwelling intermittent infusion devices, *Am Soc Health-Syst Pharm* 51:1572, 1994.
4. Millam DA: Managing complications of I.V. therapy nursing, *Nursing '88* 18(3):34, 1988.
5. Intravenous Nurses Society: Infusion nursing standards of practice, *JIN* (suppl) 23(6S), 2000.
6. Horne MM, Heitz UE, Swearingen Pl: *Pocket guide to fluid, electrolyte, and acid-base balance,* ed 3, St Louis, 1977, Mosby.
7. Maki DG, Ringer M: Risk factors for infusion-related phlebitis with small peripheral catheters, *Am Coll Physicians* 114(10):845, 1991.
8. Pearson ML: Guidelines for prevention of intravascular-device-related infections, *Infect Control Hosp Epidemiol* 17(7):438, 1996.
9. Miller JM, Goetz AM, Squier C, Muder RR: Reduction in nosocomial intravenous device-related bacteremias after institution of an intravenous therapy team, *JIN* 19(2):103, 1996.
10. Association for Professionals in Infection Control and Epidemiology: *Your most powerful defense against infections,* 1998, APIC.
11. West KH, Cohen ML: Standard precautions: a new approach to reducing infection transmission in the hospital setting, *JIN* (suppl) 20(S5):S7, 1997.
12. Crow S: Prevention of intravascular infections ways and means, *JIN* 19(4):175, 1996.
13. Henderson DK: Intravascular device-associated infection: current concepts and controversies, *Infect Surg* 6:365, 1988.
14. Hampton AA. Sherertz RJ: Vascular-access infections in hospitalized patients, *Surg Clin North Am* 68(1):57, 1988.
15. Hadaway LC: Major thrombotic and nonthrombotic complications, *JIN* (suppl) 21(S5):S143, 1998.
16. Beam TR, et al: Preventing central venous catheter-related complications: a roundtable discussion, *Infect Surg* 10:1, 1990.
17. Madeo M, Martin C, Nobbs A: A randomized study comparing IV 3000 (transparent polyurethane dressing) to a dry gauze dressing for peripheral intravenous catheter sites, *JIN* 20(5):253, 1997.
18. Maki DG, Mermel LA: *Transparent polyurethane dressings do not increase the risk of CVC-related BSI: a meta-analysis of prospective randomized trials,* Abstract presented at the annual meeting of the Society for Healthcare Epidemiology of America, St Louis, April 1997.
19. Lau CE: Transparent and gauze dressings and their effect on infection rates of central venous catheters: a review of past and current literature, *JIN* 19(5):240, 1996.
20. Civetta JM: Antiseptic-impregnated non-tunneled central venous catheters: reducing infection risks and associated costs, *Dial Transplantation* 25(11):784, 1996.
21. Maki DG, Stolz SM, Wheeler S, Mermel LA: Prevention of central venous catheter-related bloodstream infection by use of an antiseptic-impregnated catheter: a randomized clinical trial, *Ann Intern Med* 127(4):257, 1997.
22. Phillips LD: *Manual of IV therapeutics,* ed 2, Philadelphia, 1997, FA Davis.
23. Roye GD, Brezeale EE, Brynes JPM, Rue LW: Management of catheter emboli, *South Med J* 89(7):714, 1996.

24. Andris DA, Krzywda EA: Catheter pinch-off syndrome: recognition and management, *JIN* 20(5):233, 1997.

25. O'Farrell L, Griffith JW, Lang CM: Histologic development of the sheath that forms around long-term implanted central venous catheters, *JPEN J Parenter Enteral Nutr* 20(20):156, 1996.

26. Bagnall-Reeb H: Diagnosis of central venous access device occlusions, *JIN* (suppl) 21(5S):S115, 1998.

27. Kepensky DT: Applying current research to influence clinical practice: utilization of midline catheters, *JIN* 21(5):271, 1998.

28. Reed T, Phillips S: Management of central venous catheter occlusions and repair, *JIN* 19(6):28, 1996.

29. Klotz HP, et al: Catheter fracture: a rare complication of totally implantable subclavian venous access devices, *J Surg Oncol* 62:222, 1996.

30. Sansivero GE: Venous anatomy and physiology, *JIN* (suppl) 21(5S):S107, 1998.

Chapter 25

Patient Education

Rebecca Kochheiser Berry, RN, MS, Mary A. Banks, BS, BSN, CRNI

Over the last two decades, the focus of health care has dramatically changed. Factors such as cost containment, emphasis on health and wellness, a renewed commitment to patient satisfaction, and the patient's increased awareness of his or her role as a consumer have created interesting new patient education challenges for the intravenous (IV) nurse. In this current climate, the IV nurse must devise various strategies to provide patients and caregivers with the information and self-care abilities necessary to complete their therapy, prevent complications, and reduce readmissions to the hospital or home care. They must do this while negotiating the current trends in health care, such as decreased length of inpatient hospital stays, payer limitations on the number and frequency of home care visits, and increased reliance by payers and providers on patient self-care. In this environment, patient education must never be considered an optional extra that is "nice to do if you have time." In fact, these very factors make patient education even more significant. They are considered essential components of each nurse's role and are mandated by accrediting bodies such as the Joint Commission on Accreditation of Healthcare Organizations,[1,2] organizations such as the Intravenous Nurses Society,[3] and most state Nursing Practice Acts.

Experience has shown that the benefits of patient education far outweigh the costs incurred—in time and money—teaching patients and families. To effectively meet the educational needs of patients and caregivers, the IV nurse must understand educational principles, be skilled in the educational process, and be knowledgeable about available resources. As a health care provider, the nurse must recognize and accept responsibility for patient education. The legal requirement for nurses to provide patients and their families with education is reflected in most state nursing practice acts. "There are six basic functions covered by most nurse practice acts; the one pertaining to the provision of health guidance and participation in health education establishes the foundation for the professional nurse's involvement in patient education."[4]

The right of a patient to be informed about his condition and care is mandated by law. This information enables the patient to make informed decisions and assume health care responsibilities. Landmark legal cases have supported the right of patients to make informed choices about their care. For example, in *Cantebury v. Spence*[5] and subsequent cases, it was ruled not permissible to withhold information to negate the possibility that the patient will refuse treatment or make a "wrong" decision. Patients rights to information and education are repeatedly emphasized in the American Hospital Association's *A Patient's Bill of Rights*[6] and in the proposed Patients' Bill of Rights Act of 1998.[7] Nurses can help ensure that a patient's consent is truly an informed consent by educating the patient thoroughly and effectively.

Professional organizations also address the nurse's responsibility for patient education. The Intravenous Nurses Society has stated in its *Infusion Nursing Standards of Practice*[3] that "Patients have the right to receive information on all aspects of their care in a manner they can understand, as well as the right to accept or refuse treatment." This standard emphasizes the responsibility of the IV nurse to provide comprehensive patient instruction in a manner that is clear, concise, individualized, and ongoing.

Patients, health care organizations, and society all benefit from effective patient education. Patients benefit by improved outcomes resulting from better compliance with therapy, refined self-care skills, and increased knowledge about their condition and treatments. These positive effects directly translate into increased patient satisfaction with care, decreased anxiety, fewer disruptions in daily functioning, and enhanced self-esteem. They may also result in improved pain control, enhanced patient recovery, and improved physical status.

Health care providers can realize a significant cost savings from effective patient education through more timely hospital discharges, a reduction in the number of nonbillable visits, more appropriate use of services, and reduced need for acute care. They should also experience enhanced patient satisfaction and a reduction in malpractice lawsuits. Nurses, too, may have the opportunity to benefit from patient education. During the educational process, they may develop therapeutic alliances with patients and families; these alliances foster personal and professional satisfaction. A particularly rewarding outcome of this experience is when the nurse sees a patient who is comfortable in his or her knowledge and skills volunteer to teach other patients.

Well-educated health care consumers also provide benefits for society as a whole, including disease prevention, increased control of chronic illness, decreased hospital admissions, reduction in hospital lengths of stay, less absenteeism from school and work, and acquisition of positive, health-related behaviors in the general population.

HISTORICAL CONSIDERATIONS

Nurses have been teaching patients for decades. In 1860, Florence Nightingale addressed patient education in her *Notes on Nursing*. In 1918, the National League of Nursing addressed the need to cover preventive and educational factors for visiting nurses in nursing schools' curricula.

The self-care movement that began in the 1960s greatly influenced the practice of educating patients. As the public sought to understand medical practices, the health care system was pressured to respond to the need for patient education. During the 1960s, a group of nurses developed a theory of nursing based on self-care. Through their concept, the patient was empowered through increased knowledge to become an integral part of the decision-making process.

As the benefit of patient education began to be documented in the literature during the early 1970s, the insurance industry, policy makers, and legislators became interested in the potential contribution of patient education to cost containment. Financial support was made available for research on patient education. Today, patient education is an important nursing responsibility in all health care settings. Changes in reimbursement by Medicare and other third-party payers, shortened inpatient hospital stays, and a shortage of nurses has decreased the amount of time nurses can spend educating patients and caregivers. However, in the inpatient setting, patient education is still necessary to provide the patient, family, and caregiver with an understanding of the patient's condition and therapeutic regimen. Nurses are also charged with preparing the patient for discharge from the hospital. The movement toward early discharge and the use of outpatient facilities for many procedures has changed the role of patients and their caregivers by increasing their responsibilities for self-care. Nurses in alternative health care settings, such as home care and ambulatory clinics, must ensure appropriate patient self-care through effective initial teaching and ongoing patient education.

All of these factors necessitate the effective use of valuable nursing time to facilitate patient education using all available resources. Guidelines for choosing and evaluating materials such as preprinted teaching guides and audiovisual media are presented later in this chapter.

PRINCIPLES OF PATIENT EDUCATION

The goals of patient education are to provide instruction to promote health, prevent illness, and cope with illness. The first step the IV nurse should take in understanding the principles

Box 25-1	Commonly Used Educational Terms
Learner	A person who acquires knowledge, skill, or behavior change as a result of instruction or study.
Learning	An interactive process that creates knowledge or skill and may bring about a change in behavior.
Learning style	The way an individual processes information. Preference for a particular style may change over time. There is no one preferred style of learning; all are of equal value if knowledge is gained by the learner.
Patient education	This is a planned learning experience using a combination of methods, such as teaching, counseling, and behavior modification techniques, that influence the patient's knowledge and behavior.[8]
Teacher	The person or program that facilitates learning.
Teaching	Communication specifically structured and sequenced to produce learning.[8]

and process of effective patient education is to become familiar with basic educational terms (Box 25-1).

To teach effectively, the IV nurse must understand the principles of patient education. These principles vary according to the age, condition, and cognitive abilities of the learner.

Pediatric patients

Patients require some education no matter what their age or developmental level. Children who receive adequate, age-appropriate instruction are often less anxious and more cooperative during procedures. The challenge of teaching children is gearing the instruction to the child's cognitive level. Table 25-1 provides general guidelines for age-appropriate approaches to pediatric patient education.[9]

By using these developmental guidelines, the IV nurse can design an educational plan that is age appropriate and patient specific. For example, consider the IV nurse charged with preparing a child for a procedure, such as peripheral IV placement. The nurse might address the key topics in different ways depending on the patient's age (Table 25-2).

Adult patients

Malcolm A. Knowles, often referred to as the father of adult education, noted that the adult's patterns of learning are distinct from those of the child. He suggested that, because of their extensive backgrounds and greater independence, adults bring more to a learning experience and that educators should serve more as facilitators, with an opportunity to benefit as much as the learner through their exchange. Knowles coined the term *androgogy* to describe the art and science of helping adults learn.[10] Table 25-3 presents practical recommendations for using these principles of adult learning to provide more effective patient education.

Table 25-1   **Pediatric Patient-Education Guidelines**

AGE	GENERAL CHARACTERISTICS OF PATIENT	PATIENT EDUCATION TIPS
Infant (0-12 mo)	Developing a sense of trust; attached to parent; stranger anxiety; rapid growth and development; sensorimotor phase	Instruct parents; keep parent in infant's line of vision; encourage parents to comfort child
Toddler (12-36 mo)	Limited understanding; striving for independence; egocentric; limited language skills; limited concept of time; unable to reason	Instruct parents; allow child to participate during instruction (e.g., hold dressing or open package); give simple explanations; explain procedures in relation to what child sees, hears, tastes, smells, and feels; emphasize aspects of procedures that require cooperation (e.g., lying still); communicate using behaviors; use play—demonstrate with dolls and small replicas of equipment; limit teaching sessions to 5-10 min; prepare child immediately before procedures
Preschool (3-5 yr)	Developing sense of initiative; increased language skills; limited concept of time; illness and hospitalization often viewed as punishment; fears bodily harm	Explain procedure in simple terms and in relation to how it affects the child; demonstrate use of and allow child to play with equipment; encourage "playing out" on a doll to clarify misconceptions; use neutral words such as "medicine under the skin" for "shot," "hurt" for "pain," and "tube" for "catheter"; avoid overestimating child's comprehension; encourage child to verbalize; limit each teaching session to 10-15 min; state directly that the procedure is not a form of punishment; point out on drawing, child, or doll where procedure is to be performed; explain unfamiliar situations such as noises and lights; involve child in instruction and care (e.g., allow the child to hold equipment, open packages, tear tape); instruct parents
School age (6-12 yr)	Developing a sense of industry; increased language skills; interested in learning; improved concept of time; increased self-control; developing relationships with peers	Explain procedures using correct terminology; explain reasons for procedures using anatomic drawings; explain function and operation of equipment in concrete terms; allow manipulation of and practice with equipment; allow questions and discussion; limit teaching sessions to 20 min; instruct in advance of procedures; suggest ways child can maintain control (e.g., deep breathing, counting, relaxation); include child in decision making (e.g., preferred site for venipuncture); may instruct in small groups or encourage teaching other peers; instruct parents
Adolescent (12-20 yr)	Developing a sense of identity; increasing capability for abstract thought and reasoning; conscious of appearance; developing peer relationships and group identity	Involve in all decision making and planning; provide reasons for and benefits of procedures; explain long-term consequences of procedures; encourage questioning regarding fears; discuss how procedures may affect physical appearance and what can be done to minimize it; suggest methods for maintaining control; be cognizant of adolescent's difficulty accepting authority; instruct in groups and encourage peer instruction; teaching session may be as long as 45 min

Adapted from Whaley LF, Wong DL: *Whaley and Wong's nursing care of infants and children,* St Louis, 1998, Mosby.

Table 25-2   **Examples of Age-Dependent Instruction**

AGE	TOPICS TO COVER	SAMPLE EXCERPTS FROM INTRAVENOUS TEACHING
Infant	Parents: ■ Procedure for IV placement ■ Why IV is needed ■ Possible locations for IV placement (especially scalp placement which tends to be upsetting to parents) ■ What to expect if they remain with the infant during the procedure ■ How to comfort the infant during and following the procedure Child ■ Offer comfort and reassurance in soothing tones	"Mr. And Mrs. B. as we discussed, Tiffany needs an IV so we can administer her antibiotics. For infants her age, we usually use a small, flexible IV catheter like this. If possible, we will place the IV in her hand or foot. However, sometimes we need to use a vein in the baby's scalp. If this is necessary for Tiffany, we will first have to cut a small portion of her hair from that area. I will be happy to save her hair for you if you wish. Often parents prefer not to stay and watch while the IV is placed. If you wish, you may wait here in the parent's room and I will bring her to you in about 20 minutes when we are done. You can have her blanket and bottle ready to comfort her."
Toddler	Parents ■ Why IV is needed ■ Procedure for IV placement and possible locations ■ Pros and cons of remaining with the child during the procedure ■ How to comfort the child Child ■ Demonstrate what to expect very simply using a piece of IV tubing and a doll or bear to demonstrate ■ Describe what the child can expect ■ Tell him why he is getting an IV	"Zachary, we need to give you an IV so you can get your medicine. The medicine will help make your leg better. See this little tube on this doll? We are going to put a tube just like this one in your arm. Then we can put your medicine in the tube. Zach, when we are ready to put this tube in your arm, we are going to take you to that room over there. You can lie down on the big table in there and your mom can sit next to you and hold your hand. After we put in the tube, we are going to put some tape on your arm, just like this. When we are all done you can come back to the playroom and we will watch a video. Do you have any questions?"
School age	Parents ■ Why IV is needed ■ Procedure for IV placement and possible locations ■ Pros and cons of remaining with the child during the procedure ■ How to comfort the child Child ■ Show the child the IV; describe its purpose using correct terminology ■ Explain the procedure for IV placement ■ Allow the child to handle and manipulate the equipment ■ Describe how the child can participate in procedure and expectations for behavior in specific concrete terms ("you can yell if you want but don't move") ■ Allow time for questions	"Jessica, can we sit down so I can show you something? This is called an IV catheter. We put them into veins like in this picture so that we can give people medication directly into their veins. Remember this morning when Doctor Rogers told you that you have pneumonia? Well, we need to put an IV in you so we can give you medication to make you better. The IV will go in your arm and will look just like the one Sarah has. Would you like to open this package to see what the tubing feels like? We will take you to the treatment room to put in your IV. While we are putting in the IV you will have to hold very still. Some kids find it easier to hold still if they squeeze a ball or count backwards from 100. Would you like to try one of these tricks? Also, you can let me know whether or not you want your mom to come in the treatment room with you.
Adolescent	Parent ■ Why IV is needed ■ Procedure for IV placement and possible locations ■ Pros and cons of remaining with the child during the procedure ■ How to comfort the child ■ Because one of the adolescent's developmental tasks is to establish his independence from his parents, he may wish to have teaching done apart from them Adolescent ■ Purpose of the therapy; pros and cons, risks and benefits of IVs ■ Procedure for IV placement, location of the IV, how it will look and what can be done to minimize the visibility ■ His feelings regarding the IV, his input as to where, when, and how to facilitate IV placement	"Jeff, as Dr. Gordon told you earlier you will require IV therapy to administer your antibiotics to treat your knee infection. I know you were hoping to be able to use oral antibiotics, but because of the location of the infection in the bone Dr. Gordon believes that the IV antibiotics will be more effective in clearing up the infection. In cases like this, we use peripheral IVs, like this one. Dr. Gordon would like us to get you started on your IV medication as soon as possible. So, as long as you are agreeable to this plan, lets talk about where and when we can put in this IV. Do you have any questions? Do you want to take a shower first? Do you want to talk to Dr. Gordon again before we go ahead with this?"

IV, Intravenous.

Table 25-3   Application of Knowles' Principles of Androgogy

ASSUMPTIONS	APPLICATIONS FOR ADULT PATIENT EDUCATION
1. Adults are independent learners.	Allow the adult to control the learning situation as much as possible (e.g., determine time frames, information addressed, and instructional techniques); show respect for the adult's independence.
2. Adults use their life experiences as a learning resource.	Assess the adult's past experiences before developing a teaching plan; draw on the adult's past experiences when possible throughout the educational process; show respect for the adult by giving credence to past experiences; provide opportunities for the adult to share knowledge and experience with others.
3. Adults' learning is oriented to developmental tasks of their role.	Assess the adult's current developmental stage and life tasks and problems (e.g., parenthood, career building, retirement); increase the adult's motivation to learn by applying the needed information to the adult's current life situation.
4. Adults' time perspective in learning is related to immediacy of application.	Be considerate of the many compelling and conflicting demands on the adult's time and thought processes; focus education on information that the learner views as being needed now.
5. Adults' orientation for learning is problem-centered.	Provide an opportunity for the adult to find answers to questions or problems; focus education on the adult's perceived needs.
6. Adults see themselves as doers.	Provide opportunities for the adult to apply learning through doing (e.g., return demonstration, restating information).
7. Adults resist learning under conditions that are incongruent with their self-concept.	Avoid learning situations that are potentially humiliating or detrimental to the adult's self-concept.

As with children, when designing a patient education plan for adults, the IV nurse should consider the patient's life stage or developmental stage. All adult age groups—young adults (ages 20 to 40), middle adults (ages 40 to 65), and adults in their later years (older than 65)—should be approached with an empathetic and nonjudgmental attitude while using the principles of adult learning. Additional considerations may also apply to older adults (Box 25-2).

The following case studies illustrate how to use different approaches when teaching the same material to adults in different life stages. In each of the following situations, the IV nurse in the outpatient clinic must teach the patient to self-administer IV antibiotics and flush the central venous catheter. Both patients have just arrived in the clinic for their 10-AM dose of IV antibiotics.

Case study one

Jack Gray is a 22-year-old college senior who had a central venous catheter placed for IV antibiotic administration. Jack arrives with his girlfriend and his fraternity brother. He states that they all have a class at 11:30, so he hopes "this will be quick." He states that he has already checked the Internet and found catheter flushing instructions from the University Medical Center. Jack says that his girlfriend used to draw up insulin syringes for her grandmother, so he thinks she might be a big help with this. He also wants his fraternity brother to see this procedure because they will be sharing a tent during the annual fraternity campout at the end of the month.

Case study two

Clara Barrett is a 78-year-old widowed grandmother who lives alone. She has had a central venous catheter placed for administration of IV antibiotics to treat a wound infection. She has insulin-dependent diabetes with associated visual problems and peripheral neuropathy. Clara has arrived in the clinic at 9:30 for her 10-AM appointment via the "senior shuttle," and appears very anxious. She says "I'll do anything you say but please don't make me go into the hospital or into a nursing home for this medication."

Box 25-2   Additional Educational Considerations for Older Adults

- Approach each patient as unique. Do not stereotype because of age. There is a wide range of functional levels within this population.
- Be aware that aging is a multidimensional process in which multiple factors affect functioning.
- Capitalize on the patient's strengths.
- Refrain from using first names unless invited to do so.
- Speak clearly and concisely.
- Avoid patronizing.
- Motivate the learner by showing how the acquisition of new skills and knowledge can improve their quality of life.
- Provide large-print reading materials.
- Limit teaching sessions to 20 to 30 minutes.
- Present one idea at a time and summarize often.
- Keep all training sessions well organized and slow paced.

The challenge for the IV nurse is to design teaching plans for these patients based on the principles of adult learning. The nurse must modify the approach for each learner to address individual learning needs. To accomplish this task, the nurse might ask questions similar to those in Table 25-4.

THE EDUCATIONAL PROCESS

Patient education is a process that includes thoroughly assessing the learner and teacher, developing a teaching plan based on the assessment, effectively implementing the teaching plan, and evaluating the results.

Assessment

Effective teaching depends on a complete and accurate assessment of both the learner and teacher. Philips describes the

Table 25-4   Addressing Individual Learning Needs

QUESTIONS	JACK GRAY	CLARA BARRETT
How do I allow Jack and Clara to control the learning session as much as possible?	Respect his need to limit the teaching session so he can get to class. Review the materials he obtained from the Internet to see if they can be used as part of the training. Enlist his help in designing his teaching session.	Approach her as early as possible. Call her Mrs. Barrett, not Clara. Assure her that the teaching will be provided at her own pace. Enlist her help in designing the teaching session. Ask her to describe her preferred method of learning.
How do I let Jack and Clara use their life experiences in the teaching plan?	Ask Jack's girlfriend to demonstrate her ability to draw medication into a syringe. Use the girlfriend's experience to help teach Jack. Explore with Jack whether audio-visual aids (e.g., videos, CD-ROM training) would be useful for him.	Ask Clara to describe her experience with drawing up and administering insulin. Explain the similarities to drawing up catheter flushes and administering IV medications. Ask her how she learned to draw up and give her insulin.
How do I orient the teaching plan to Jack's and Clara's current developmental stage, life tasks, and problems?	Jack is concerned with being able to do his therapy without it interfering with his college life. Support his use of friends as resources in the absence of his family. He may have a tendency to rush through the teaching. Set appropriate goals and time frames, providing opportunities to stop periodically and review the material (to improve retention).	Clara has some physical limitations related to her age and medical condition. Provide large-print teaching material. Speak loudly and slowly. Use video training prudently, because videos may be overwhelming and confusing to her. Allow extra time for return demonstrations because of her tremors and diminished dexterity.
How do I make the learning immediately applicable to Jack and Clara's lives?	Reinforce with Jack and his friends that successful return demonstration of the skills will allow him to be independent with the therapy. Let him set his own pace for the learning.	Reinforce with Clara that learning these skills will allow her to become independent with her therapy. Let her set a reasonable pace for the learning. Reassure her that she may have more than one training session.
How do I provide an opportunity for Jack and Clara to learn problem-solving skills?	Discuss with Jack how he can set up a schedule for administering his therapy that will not interfere with his classes. Help Jack figure out how to attend his fraternity weekend without missing doses of his medication.	Help Clara investigate resources such as neighbors or church members to assist or support her therapy. Offer Clara the option of administering the antibiotics using a syringe pump, because her poor vision limits her ability to count the IV drops.
How do I give Jack and Clara the opportunity to apply their knowledge?	Allow Jack the opportunity to demonstrate the entire procedure if he is ready. Offer constructive criticism and positive reinforcement. If he is ready, allow him to self-administer today's dose with his girlfriend, while being observed.	Have Clara demonstrate at least one of the skills in the teaching plan. Requiring her to demonstrate the entire procedure may be much too overwhelming for the first teaching session. Provide positive reinforcement.
How do I provide a learning experience for Jack and Clara in an atmosphere that is not damaging to their self-image?	Allow Jack to decide who will participate in the training and return demonstrations. Determine whether he wants his fraternity brother and girlfriend present during the entire training session. Be careful about correcting his behavior in front of his friends. Use encouragement, not criticism. Respect his confidentiality.	Don't ask Clara to participate in the same teaching session as Jack. These two will each learn at a different pace, which could be confusing and discouraging for Clara. Set small, reasonable, achievable goals. Provide encouragement and positive reinforcement when goals are met.

IV, Intravenous.

assessment process for the purpose of developing a teaching plan as "collecting a complete data base, identifying the client's strengths and weaknesses and determining personal characteristics, learning characteristics, and experimental characteristics of the client."[11] Phillips proceeds to describe the following four

dimensions to be assessed in a learner and the components of these dimensions: (1) the biophysical dimension (including age, visual acuity, manual dexterity, hearing, pain, fatigue, and medications), (2) the psychologic dimension (encompassing mild anxiety, defensiveness, signs and symptoms of stress response, adaptation to illness, and outlook on life), (3) the sociocultural dimension (pertaining to lifestyle, perception of hospital setting, perception of learning, occupation, education, income, housing, dietary pattern, sleep patterns, exercise, sexuality, coping mechanisms, and cultural issues), and (4) the environmental dimension (consisting of learning styles and the learning environment).[11]

Assessment of these areas becomes particularly important when developing an education plan for a home care patient or a patient who will be receiving outpatient therapy. For example, it is unrealistic to design a patient education plan that mimics the care the patient is receiving as an inpatient. Most patients cannot be expected to self-administer a 2-AM-dose of a medication just because the time was convenient for the hospital IV nurses to administer the dose.

To be effective, information imparted to the learner must be understood. There are various ways of assessing comprehension. Merely determining grades completed in school will not provide useful, complete information to assess comprehension levels. Many high school graduates do not possess a twelfth-grade level of comprehension. Direct methods for assessing comprehension include the Cloze test for reading comprehension, listening tests, and word recognition tests.[12] Indirect methods include asking the learner to read and restate information and, perhaps the least threatening method, allowing the patient a choice of instructional media.

If the learner is not ready or motivated to learn, no learning occurs. Many factors can affect learner readiness, including the patient's levels of stress, comfort, energy, and acceptance of diagnosis. Redman has stated that every patient is ready to learn something; it is up to the teacher to find out what it is.[8] Learner readiness may increase when even the smallest need is met. Explaining the importance of learning specific information may also improve readiness and motivation.

Although sometimes overlooked, it is also important to assess the teacher who is providing patient education. Being a nurse does not instantly qualify one as a capable teacher. According to Barnstable,[13] "Excellent teachers have one thing in common—a passion to keep improving their abilities. One does not 'arrive' at being an expert teacher. The drive toward excellence is an ongoing process."

Barnstable has described numerous techniques that creative teachers use to enhance their effectiveness (Box 25-3).[13]

The next important step in the educational process is developing the teaching plan. The time spent assessing learner needs is wasted unless these needs are included in an individualized patient teaching plan. Therefore the patient assessment, developed with active input of the patient whenever possible, should clearly present the patient's goals and objectives. This assessment is the basis for developing the teaching plan. Table 25-5 illustrates a patient assessment that can be used to develop a teaching plan.

Box 25-3   Techniques Used by Creative Teachers

- Present information enthusiastically.
- Use humor.
- Take risks.
- Deliver material dramatically.
- Use methods that match the topic rather than the teacher's personality.
- Engage the patient in problem-solving activities.
- Serve as a role model.
- Use anecdotes and examples.
- Use technology.
- Give positive reinforcement.
- Project an attitude of acceptance and sensitivity.
- Be organized and give direction.
- Elicit and give feedback.
- Use questions.
- Use repetition and pace the information appropriately.
- Summarize important points.

Table 25-5   Sample Assessment for a Teaching Plan for Home Infusion of Total Parenteral Nutrition (TPN)

Patient name	Mr. RY
Patient assessment	Mr. RY is 53 years old and a high school graduate. He is hospitalized and is to be discharged to the home on cyclic TPN infusion through a Hickman catheter. This is the first time Mr. RY has had a Hickman catheter and, before he was hospitalized, had never heard of it or TPN. He appears anxious to learn so he can go home, return to work on his farm, and spend time with his grandchildren. He has no medical education, but has worked closely with the veterinarians who care for his farm animals and has been trained to give injections to the farm animals. His wife is available to assist him, but he prefers to carry out as much of his care as possible. Mr. RY is a Methodist and is active in the small farm community where he has lived all his life. He is emotionally close to his family, all of whom live in neighboring communities. Mrs. RY has debilitating arthritis in her hands and appears nervous about having any responsibility for her husband's therapy.
Learner input	Mr. RY states that he was never a star student in school and does not read books because it takes too long. He reads the newspaper and farm magazines, and enjoys watching TV. He doesn't enjoy studying and related a bad experience he had when studying to become certified in CPR. Mr. RY states that he learns best when he can see things done and can then do them himself. He wants to learn everything he can about his therapy and hopes that he can remember everything and do the procedures correctly.

Planning

Once this assessment is complete, the IV nurse can use the information from assessment to develop a formal teaching plan. The components of the teaching plan are as follows:

1. The objectives, written in measurable terms
2. The content outline, developed from the objectives
3. The teaching method to be used to meet the objectives
4. The anticipated time frame for the teaching

Table 25-6 demonstrates a Patient Education Teaching Plan for Mr. RY based on the assessment presented in Table 25-5.

When possible, the teaching environment should be controlled and planned. A well-organized teaching plan can be ineffective if the environment is not conducive to learning. Environmental considerations include comfortable seating with good visibility, comfortable temperature, limited number of persons in attendance, adequate space for teaching supplies, equipment available for audiovisual materials, and limited distractions or interruptions from television, radio, other patients, and personnel.

There are many appropriate formats and resources for educating patients. The most effective teaching plan includes varied teaching approaches to match the learning style of the patient so that more of the patient's senses are involved in the learning process. According to Patterson,[14] people remember 10% of what they read, 20% of what they hear, 30% of what they see, 50% of what they hear and see, 80% of what they say, and 90% of what they say and do. Therefore, if patients' only source of education is a printed booklet, they will remember only 10% of the information read. The patient remembers only 20% of oral instruction, such as a lecture or audio tape. If the teaching session includes oral instruction and a demonstration, 50% of the information is likely to be retained. If the patient is given an opportunity to repeat the instruction, retention increases to 80%. The most effective instructional technique is return demonstration and instruction, where 90% of the information is retained.

Written education materials are often used to carry out and enhance patient education. Patient use of written educational materials must be considered carefully based on the patient's level of comprehension. Studies have shown that many printed patient instruction materials developed today require a comprehension level many grades higher than that of 60% of the U.S. population. To ensure that as many patients as possible comprehend the written instructions given to them, it is recommended that all printed materials be written at a fifth-grade level of comprehension. The readability of written materials can be assessed with readability formulas such as the Fry formula. At least 40 readability formulas exist, and most are based on just two factors: word difficulty and sentence length. "These formulas say that: 'The greater the number of multisyllable words, the greater the reading difficulty. Also, the longer the sentences, the greater the reading difficulty.' "[12]

Printed patient education materials may be written by the nurse on an individual basis for each patient, developed generically by the organization, or acquired from an outside source. With the necessary information, members of the nursing staff or education department can use readability formulas to evaluate educational materials. Some other tips for writing and evaluating patient education materials are listed in Box 25-4.

Product and service companies are good sources of free patient education materials. Requests can be sent directly to companies; addresses are usually included on the package labeling or can be obtained from the local sales representative. The Internet is also an excellent source of educational materials; however, the nurse must be sure to reference the source of any material obtained from the Internet because erroneous material is often found there.

Any patient education materials printed by an outside source should be evaluated carefully for teaching applicability (Box 25-5).

Oral instructions and demonstrations are the most commonly used approaches to patient education. The advantage of this one-on-one approach is the ability to immediately answer questions, reassess learning needs, and make changes in the teaching plan. However, one-on-one oral instruction is very time-consuming, which translates to being labor intensive. Also, as previously mentioned, oral instructions alone are ineffective; a patient will forget most of what was heard within minutes of leaving the educational session.

Audiovisual materials, such as videotapes, audio tapes, and television programs, are becoming more popular as teaching aids. Audiovisual materials ensure that a consistent message is delivered to patients, allow critical review of the message before it is presented, allow learners to stop the tape and proceed at their own pace, and demand less of the teacher's time. Drawbacks may include the cost of the tapes and equipment, inaccessibility of equipment, the inability to customize the material for the learner, and the lack of teacher-learner interaction.

Computer instruction (CD-ROM and Internet training) is also available for patient education. Benefits of this approach include interactive program capabilities and increased opportunities for off-site education. Drawbacks may include patient apprehension about computer equipment and cost.

In most instances, a combination of these methods provides the most effective learning opportunities for the patient.

Implementation

Good communication skills, teaching abilities, and organizational skills are key to the effective implementation of a teaching plan (Box 25-6).

Evaluation

"The actual intent of evaluation is not to place a value or worth on patients or nurses. Its purposes are to measure the degree to which goals have been met, to define specific outcomes, and to redirect patent care."[4] Evaluating the education plan requires the nurse to determine whether behavioral objectives were met and whether interventions (teaching methods) were effective. "Evaluation is closely related to assessment . . . Assessment refers to building a data base that includes nursing diagnoses and outlines the patient's needs or problems. Evaluation refers to the follow-up assessment that is continuously conducted as nursing

Table 25-6   Patient Education: Teaching Plan

OBJECTIVE	CONTENT	TEACHING METHOD	TIME FRAME
SESSION 1: INTRODUCTION TO HOME TPN			
On completion of teaching session, patient will be able to: Discuss goal and purpose of TPN therapy	I. TPN therapy 　A. Goals 　B. Purpose	Discussion: relate to usual eating habits	5 min
Discuss basic components of TPN solution	II. Components of TPN 　A. Protein 　B. Carbohydrates 　C. Vitamins 　D. Trace elements	Discussion: relate to oral nutrition	10 min
Explain roles and responsibilities of home TPN support team	III. The home care team 　A. Hospital 　B. Home care agency 　C. Nurse 　D. Physician 　E. Dietician 　F. Delivery person 　G. Home patient representative 　H. Pharmacist	Videotape from agency Discussion: relate to people that patient has already met	15 min
List emergency phone numbers	IV. Emergency phone numbers	Develop a list together with Mr. and Mrs. Y	10 min
Session 1 evaluation		Ask questions regarding content of session	10 min
SESSION 2: SAFETY AND INFECTION CONTROL	Review session 1		
On completion of teaching session, patient will be able to: Differentiate between "clean" and "sterile"	I. Definitions 　A. Clean 　B. Sterile	Discussion: apply to veterinary medicine Demonstration	5 min
Wash hands using proper technique	II. Hand washing 　A. Application to home TPN infusion 　B. Importance of hand washing 　C. Proper procedure 　D. How to accomplish this at home	Discussion Demonstration Videotape Printed materials with many pictures Return demonstration	15 min
Identify suitable work and storage areas in the home	III. Home work area 　A. Storage area 　B. Work space	Discussion regarding available work and storage space in home	10 min
Identify an appropriate way to dispose of medical waste at home	IV. Equipment disposal 　A. Needles 　B. Syringes 　C. Other	Discussion Demonstration Return demonstration	10 min
Session 2 evaluation		Return demonstration of hand washing and equipment disposal Ask questions regarding clean versus sterile	10 min
SESSION 3: SOLUTIONS AND MEDICATIONS	Review sessions 1 and 2		
On completion of teaching session, patient will be able to: Apply previously learned information and skills regarding solutions and medication	I. Review of solution and medication information	Patient demonstration of previously learned skills Patient discussion of solution and medication knowledge	15 min
Handle solutions and medications correctly	II. Solutions and medications 　A. Storage and preparation 　B. Warming 　C. Prescription verification 　D. Expiration verification 　E. Visual inspection 　F. Additives 　G. Use of syringes, vials, and ampules 　H. Injecting additives into the solution container	Discussion Demonstration Return demonstration	25 min
Session 3 evaluation		Discussion and demonstration of all procedures	10 min

Continued

| Table 25-6 | Patient Education: Teaching Plan—cont'd | | |

OBJECTIVE	CONTENT	TEACHING METHOD	TIME FRAME
SESSION 4: ADMINISTRATION TECHNIQUE			
	Review sessions 1, 2, and 3		

On completion of teaching session, patient will be able to: Prime tubing and filter	I. Priming
	  A. Tubing
	  B. Filter
		Demonstration
		Discussion
		Return demonstration
			15 min

Operate infusion pump	II. Infusion pump
	  A. Operation
	  B. Alarms
	  C. Troubleshooting
		Discussion
		Videotape from pump company
		Demonstration
		Return demonstration
			35 min

Session 4 evaluation		Set up and operate pump	10 min
SESSION 5: ADMINISTRATION TECHNIQUES			
	Review sessions 1 through 4		

On completion of teaching session, patient will be able to: Describe tapering	I. Tapering
	  A. Rate
	  B. Schedule
		Discussion
		Demonstration
		Return demonstration
			10 min

Administer fat emulsions	II. Fat administration
	  A. Purpose
	  B. Procedure
		Discussion
		Demonstration
		Return demonstration
			10 min

Connect TPN infusion	III. Connection procedure	Discussion Demonstration Return demonstration	10 min
Disconnect TPN infusion	IV. Disconnection procedure	Discussion Demonstration Return demonstration	10 min
Session 5 evaluation		Perform procedures without prompting	10 min
SESSION 6: CATHETER CARE			
	Review sessions 1 through 5		

On completion of teaching session, patient will be able to: Perform catheter dressing change	I. Dressing change
	  A. Purpose
	  B. Supplies
	  C. Procedure
		Discussion
		Demonstration
		Return demonstration
			20 min

Heparinize central catheter	II. Heparinization
	  A. Purpose
	  B. Supplies
	  C. Procedure
		Discussion
		Demonstration
		Return demonstration
			20 min

Session 6 evaluation		Perform procedures without prompting	10 min
SESSION 7: HOME MONITORING, COMPLICATIONS, AND EMERGENCY INTERVENTIONS			
	Review sessions 1 through 6		

On completion of teaching session, patient will be able to: Monitor TPN therapy at home	I. Home monitoring
	  A. Weights
	  B. Urine
	  C. Input and output
	  D. Documentation
		Discussion
		Demonstration
		Return demonstration of procedures and documentation
			20 min

Identify possible complications and interventions	II. Complications
	  A. Description
	  B. Interventions
		Discussion
		Review of written instructions
			20 min

Session 7 evaluation		Give correct answers to case study scenarios	10 min
SESSIONS 1 THROUGH 7			
Total teaching evaluation		Written evaluation form Patient explains each aspect of care while demonstrating Question patient regarding emergency procedures—use case studies related to farm environment	25 min

Box 25-4   Tips for Writing Patient Education Materials

Limit information to that which is absolutely necessary to know.
Use graphic images as often as possible (e.g., simple line drawings, when appropriate).
Break complex information into smaller parts.
Use a logical sequence to present information.
Put the most important points first.
Use a conversational, informal writing style such as "you will feel" rather than "the patient should feel."
Use short words (two syllables or less, when possible, and define longer words) and short sentences (fewer than 15 words).
Remove unnecessary words that obscure the main point.
Use headings to let the reader know what is coming.
Be consistent with wording (e.g., don't switch from "tube" to "catheter").
Consider the cultural and language needs of the patient population.
Test readability using accepted published formulas, such as the SMOG formula or the Fry Index of Readability.[11]
Summarize and review at the end of each section.
Have patients or other laypersons review and comment on the written material before printing.

Box 25-5   Useful Criteria When Selecting Preprinted Patient Education Materials

1. Are the facts, pictures, and subject matter accurate and up to date?
2. Is the material at the appropriate comprehension level for the patient population?
3. Are the learning objectives consistent with those of the teaching plan?
4. Is too little or too much information given?
5. Are the language and material as simple as necessary for the intended audience?
6. Do all procedures and directions follow hospital, clinic, or agency policy?
7. Is the information well organized?
8. Is the print clear and large enough to be easily read?
9. Are the illustrations appropriate and adequately labeled?
10. Do the pictures and drawings reflect a patient population with which the patient can identify?

Box 25-6   Recommendations for Providing Effective Instruction

- Establish rapport; reduce anxiety and fear.
- Incorporate a variety of teaching strategies (e.g., discussion, demonstration, written materials, audiovisual materials, return demonstration, peer instruction, restating) to respond to different learning styles and to take advantage of the synergy of complementary techniques.
- Speak the learner's language, avoid jargon, and clarify all terms.
- Divide the information into small steps.
- Be specific.
- Keep the information short, simple, and concrete.
- Address the most important information first.
- Stress the importance of instructions and expected benefits; explain the detrimental effects of inadequate treatment, but avoid fear tactics.
- Ask questions and encourage feedback to ensure comprehension of the information.
- Repeat the information as often as needed.
- Reward learning with oral praise.
- Take advantage of "teachable" moments when the learner is most likely to accept new information (e.g., when symptoms are present).
- Allow practice of a new skill or use of new information without delay.
- Express enthusiasm and concern through voice and body language.
- Allow the patient to share knowledge about the subject.
- Be flexible; adjust learning goals as necessary.
- Summarize often.

interventions are carried out."[4] The effectiveness of the teaching plan and the accomplishment of patient (learner) objectives should be evaluated throughout implementation and at the completion of the teaching sessions. The original teaching plan may be revised several times as a result of ongoing evaluation results.

DOCUMENTATION

As with all other nursing care provided to a patient, the action and results of patient education must be documented. Documentation is important for many reasons; it provides a complete picture of the patient's condition and progress, communicates educational progress to other members of the health care team, and provides information necessary for reimbursement.

Complete documentation should include the assessment of patient knowledge deficit and readiness to learn, learning objectives, implementation of the teaching plan, skills demonstrated, patient response to teaching, and an evaluation of the overall process. Documentation can be accomplished in narrative form or on a checklist.

THE TEAM APPROACH

Patient education is a collaborative effort of the health care team, patient, family, and caregivers. Patient education begins with admission or diagnosis and continues throughout the patient's hospital stay and, following discharge, in the home or alternative care setting. Each member of the team has expertise and knowledge that can strengthen and enhance the total education plan. The IV nurse must be constantly aware of the patient's immediate and long-term learning needs and should meet them through education or by planning patient instruction with other health care team members.

OTHER NURSING CONSIDERATIONS
Nursing diagnoses

Nursing diagnoses are used to communicate patient assessments. Those related to patient education include the following:

- Alteration in health maintenance
- Impaired home maintenance management
- Knowledge deficit (specify)
- Learning need (specify)
- Noncompliance (specify)
- Compliance (specify)

Patient outcomes

A compelling benefit of patient education is improved patient outcomes. Patient outcomes are the goals for which the teaching plan is designed and the indicators of its success. Measurable patient outcomes related to patient education are as follows:

- Improved adherence to a therapeutic regimen
- Increased patient satisfaction
- Enhanced patient self-determination with increased ability to handle symptoms

- Enhanced patient recovery after surgery
- Patient verbalization of understanding instructions and information given
- Correct patient demonstration of learned procedures

SUMMARY

Patient education is an important part of care provided by the IV nurse. Patient education must take precedence over nonnursing activities and should be part of the patient plan of care. Effective patient education requires the integration of education theory into nursing practice. Hansen and Fischer have summarized patient education strategies into five categories, represented by the acronym TEACH:

Tune into the patient by assessing his needs and the way he wishes to learn

Edit content by focusing on "must-know" information, being specific and unambiguous

Act on teachable moments by teaching at every opportunity

Clarify often by verifying your assumptions and seeking feedback often

Honor the patient as a partner by respecting him and building on his experience[15]

REFERENCES

1. Joint Commission on Accreditation of Healthcare Organizations: *Accreditation manual for home care,* Oakbrook Terrace, Ill, 1998, Joint Commission on Accreditation of Healthcare Organizations.
2. Joint Commission on Accreditation of Healthcare Organizations: *1996 Comprehensive accreditation manual for hospitals,* Oakbrook Terrace, Ill, 1995, Joint Commission on Accreditation of Healthcare Organizations.
3. Intravenous Nurses Society: Infusion nursing standards of practice, *JIN* (suppl) 23(6S), 2000.
4. Rankin SH, Stallings KD: *Patient education: issues, principles, practices,* ed 3, Philadelphia, 1996, Lippincott.
5. Knapp TA, Huff RL: Emerging trends in the physician's duty to disclose: an update of Cantebury v Spence, *J Leg Med* 3:41, 1975.
6. American Hospital Association: *A patient's bill of rights,* Chicago, 1980, American Hospital Association.
7. US House of Representatives: HR 3605: Patients' Bill of Rights Act of 1998.
8. Redman BK: *The process of patient education,* ed 7, St Louis, 1993, Mosby.
9. Whaley LF, Wong DL: *Whaley & Wong's nursing care of infants and children,* ed 4, St Louis, 1998, Mosby.
10. Knowles MS: *Modern practice of adult education: from pedagogy to andragogy,* ed 2, New York, 1980, Cambridge Books.
11. Phillips LD: Patient education: understanding the process to maximize time and outcomes, *JIN* 22:1, 1999.
12. Doak CC, Doak LG, Root JH: *Teaching patients with low literacy skills,* ed 2, Philadelphia, 1996, JB Lippincott.
13. Barnstable SB: *Nurse as educator: principles of teaching and learning,* Sudbury, Mass, 1997, Jones and Bartlett.
14. Patterson O, editor: *Special tools for communication,* Chicago, 1962, Industrial Audio-Visual Association.
15. Hansen M, Fisher J: Patient-centered teaching from theory to practice, *AJN* 98:1 1998.

BIBLIOGRAPHY

Baldwin EM, Stephenson LC: Notes: a system for defending patient education through effective documentation, *Home Healthcare Nurse* 16:253, 1998.

Brownson K: Improving patient education for poor readers, *Nursing Spectrum* 8:12, 1999.

Feuer L: The educated consumer is our prized possession, *Continuing Care* July/August:14, 1998.

Hansen M: Patient-centered teaching from theory to practice, *Am J Nurs* 98:56, 1998.

Phillips LD: *Manual of I.V. therapeutics,* ed 2, Philadelphia, 1997, FA Davis.

Redman BK: *The practice of patient education,* ed 8, St Louis, 1997, Mosby.

Trimble T: Discharge instructions—don't just show them the door! Emergency Nursing World Website (ENW.org) 1999.

Documentation

Brenda Dugger, RN, MS, CRNI, CNA*

nursing became organized and continuous. No one person contributed more to nursing than Florence Nightingale (1820 to 1910).[1] In her time, documentation was used primarily to communicate the implementation of physician's orders. Nursing notes were not viewed as an important part of the patient's medical record and were often discarded when the patient was discharged from the hospital. In her early writings, Nightingale advocated recording the patient's diet and environment as essential to the patient's chart, in an effort to collect and store data that could be used in patient care.

In the 1930s, a written plan of care was developed. In 1951, nursing standards became formalized, and the Joint Commission on Accreditation of Hospitals (now the Joint Commission on Accreditation of Healthcare Organizations [JCAHO]) was formed. In the mid-1960s, documentation in nurses' notes evolved as an essential method of evaluating nursing care that met the requirements of regulatory agencies, provided evidence in litigation, and delineated professional responsibility. When diagnosis-related groups (DRGs) were implemented in the early 1980s, documentation in the medical record served as a mechanism for determining reimbursement guidelines. In the 1990s, the emphasis was on quality improvement, with a focus on evaluating organizational and clinical performance outcomes. In the 2000s, documentation will emphasize outcomes. It will be important to emphasize activities that will improve clinical performance and facilitate the continuous collection and evaluation of statistical data to look for opportunities to improve care. Outcomes will be tied to costs, and health care providers and consumers will expect cost-effective positive outcomes. Documentation will continue to play a key role in providing the information necessary to track and evaluate patient care outcomes.

HISTORICAL OVERVIEW

Documentation of the nursing process has always been viewed as a necessary but time-consuming chore. Over the past 20 years, nursing documentation has become more important and has changed to respond to the requirements of state and federal regulatory agencies, changes in nursing practice, determination of reimbursement fees, and legal ramifications.

Until around 3000 BC, when a system of writing was developed in Egypt, no formal records were kept by attendants to the sick. With the advent of Christianity, patient care records of

PURPOSE AND SCOPE

Infusion Nursing Standards of Practice published by the Intravenous Nurses Society states that medical record documentation must provide a sufficient mechanism to record and retrieve significant information and to give evidence of the nursing process.[2] Documentation is required by many state statues and regulatory agencies. Several states have regulated the documentation of invasive procedures such as intravenous (IV) therapy. The underlying reason for these regulations is to protect the

*The author and editors wish to acknowledge the contributions made by Diane L. Baker, as author of this chapter in the first edition of *Intravenous Nursing: Clinical Principles and Practice*.

health care consumer by delineating professional responsibility and accountability. In 1985, the American Nurses Association (ANA) made the following statement in regard to the nursing process and the need for documentation:

> The nurse is responsible for data collection and assessment of the health status of the client; determination of the nursing care plan directed toward designated goals; evaluation of the effectiveness of nursing care in achieving the goals of care; and subsequent reassessment and revision of the nursing care plan.[3]

This statement forms the basis for nursing practice. It focuses on the nursing process, which all nurses are held accountable to for licensure. Responsible for data collection refers to the documentation process. A coherent record of the patient care event or encounter should be evident through the medical record. Documentation provides the pathway to continuity of care. Each professional specialty or point of service reveals a part of the patient's clinical picture or story. Documentation should clearly include the following:

- Diagnosis
- Assessment of the patient's condition
- Care given to the patient
- Any unusual circumstances or complications
- Interventions performed to correct the situation
- Interactions with the physician, supervisor, or other health care professionals
- Evaluation of all interventions
- Outcomes

The necessity of good documentation is an integral part of prudent patient care. The medical record is proof of the nursing process and the steps used to reach the resulting outcomes. Studies have shown that nurses often spend up to 30% of their time in the documentation process.[4] As nursing responsibilities expand, professional roles and accountability increase. With this expanded role, critical thinking becomes essential.[5] Hospital nurses often work by protocol to treat certain symptoms. For example, a protocol may direct the nurse to titrate a medication to obtain a certain effect. Home health nurses make independent decisions while working alone in the community. Infusion nurses are called on to lead other health care professionals in recommending catheter selection or improving catheter function. These activities are orchestrated by good communication and should be evidenced throughout the documentation.

No longer are episodes of illness viewed as separate. A focus on wellness chooses to look at the life of the individual in its entirety and all of the influences that affect the health of the individual. Good documentation of care in all settings provides invaluable information to guide future treatment.

DOCUMENTATION GUIDELINES AND TRENDS

Documentation should contain only factual information pertaining to the patient's condition, diagnosis, and treatment. Speculation, conjecture, or demeaning comments are inappropriate and may be damaging to the patient, nurse, and the institution. The medical record is confidential. Access to this documentation should be monitored and controlled according to organizational policy.

Written documentation

Written documentation in the medical record should be legible and concise. Illegible writing may become the focal point for a plaintiff's attorney, even if a mistake or error was not made. Scribbling, writing over another word or statement, and erasing an incorrect entry are unacceptable practices that can lead to dismissal in some organizations. In addition, writing over another word or statement or erasing an incorrect entry admits fault and can lead to serious consequences if the medical record ends up in court. Errors should be corrected by drawing a line through the incorrect word or words and writing "error" or "mistaken entry."[6] The entry should be accompanied by the initials of the individual making the entry.

Common terminology, approved by the organization and written into policy, defines the accepted terms and clarifies misconceptions about meanings or interpretations. For example, *SOB* may mean *shortness of breath* or *side of bed*. Abbreviations should be used only if accepted as the standard for the institution.

All observations should be recorded accurately. The date and institutionally accepted method of keeping time (military or regular) should be used for every entry. Liability cases have used the documented time of treatment to determine the appropriateness of nurse response time and judgment relative to patient care.

The propensity for accurate documentation often arises from fear of litigation. This mindset is positive because defensive charting (charting with the potential for legal review in mind) reminds the nurse that the medical record is often the deciding factor in malpractice suits.[7] Investigation, deposition, and testimony often occur months or several years after the questionable event. Failure to appropriately document nursing assessment, intervention, or outcomes may cast doubt on the nurse's actions. Careful, concise documentation may conversely show that the nurse is thorough in her actions and thought processes.[6]

A signature is mandatory after every entry. Chart reviews are difficult when entry ownership is not established or difficult to read. Initials are acceptable if the complete signature is on the bottom of the page or at the end of the documentation segment.

Flow sheets are often used for IV therapy records. They offer a concise list of IV fluids and medications given, the dates and time of IV insertion, and site checks. The flow sheet should include the type, length, gauge, removal, replacement, or rotation of the vascular access device. Degrees of phlebitis should be documented within the medical record each time a device is removed because of phlebitis. Considering the potency and venous irritability of newer medications, charting observations about a discontinued IV site may help identify a postinfusion phlebitis.

Computerized documentation

Many organizations have moved to an electronic form of documentation. Retrieval capabilities are greatly improved by use of an electronic record. Information is available from episode to episode, whether inpatient or outpatient. When the patient's entire clinical history is available, treatment can be more effective. Past illnesses may show potential trends and help reveal

FRACTURED HIP
DAY OF SURGERY
OUTCOMES

Pain control achieved with PCA/Epidural/IM medications	No evidence of DVT/PE
No evidence of skin breakdown	Patient/family verbalize knowledge of plan of care
No evidence of hip/pin dislocation	No falls or injury

Assessments	Medications	Treatments/IVs

Systems assessment q8h
Circulatory, motor, sensation, heel checks
   q2h to involved extremity
Assess pain per pain protocol
VS q1h × 2, then q4h × 24hr
Assess skin integrity every shift and initiate
   skin care protocol prn
Assess for risk of falls every shift
Intake and output every shift
Assess dressing with VS
	<u>Preop:</u> Antibiotics: as ordered
	<u>Postop:</u> Antibiotics: as ordered
	<u>Pain management:</u>
	IV PCA morphine (1 mg/ml)
	Loading dose: 2 ml
	Dose volume: 1 ml
	Lockout interval: 12 min
	4-hour limit: 20 ml
	<u>or</u> Demerol (10 mg/ml)
	Loading dose: 1 ml
	Dose volume: 0.5 ml
	Lockout interval: 15 min
	4-hour limit 10 ml
	<u>or</u> Epidural per anesthesia orders
	<u>or</u> Demerol 50-75 mg IM q3h prn
	<u>or</u> Vicodin 1 or 2 tablets PO q3-4h prn
	<u>Routine:</u>
	Coumadin 10 mg PO at 10 PM
	<u>or</u> Bufferin 2 tablets qAM
	MOM 30 ml PO qod
	Colace 100 mg bid
	Pepcid 40 mg PO qd
	<u>PRN:</u>
	Phenergan 25 mg IM q4-6h prn nausea
	Tylenol 650 mg q4h prn
	Ambien 5-10 mg qHS prn
	Maalox 30 ml q4h prn
	Laxative of choice prn
	Diphenhydramine (Benadryl) 25 mg PO/IM
	   q6h prn itching
		<u>Postop:</u> Record amount of hemovac
		   drainage q8h
		Foley catheter to straight drain; if Foley
		   catheter pulled out within first 48 hr
		   postop, reinsert
		Incentive spirometry or cough/deep
		   breathe q2h while awake
		Fleets enema prn
		D5.2NS at 50 ml/hr; if diabetic 0.45
		NS; reduce rate to KVO postnausea
		D/C IV when epidural/PCA or IV meds
		   are complete
		Knee immobilizer as ordered
		Plexi pulse as ordered

Nutrition	Diagnostics	Consults
<u>Preop:</u> NPO <u>Postop:</u> Full liquids		Notify patient's medical MD of admission PCC

Activity	Education	Discharge Planning

Overhead trapeze
Ankle pump exercises q2h while awake
Turn q2h on inoperative side with 1
   to 2 pillows between legs
Elevate FOB 30°, HOB lowered except
   when eating; do not elevate FOB for
   Dr. McDonald's patients
May lie on unaffected side with 1-2
   pillows between legs
Do not flex excessively at hip
	Reinforce teaching regarding:
	   Surgical procedure
	   Incentive spirometry
	   Pain management
	   Positioning
	   Safety
	   Hip precautions
	   Postop expectations
	
	Give Teaching Sheets:
	   Coumadin Therapy (if applicable)
	Pamphlet: After a Hip Fracture (If pt. did not
	   receive preop)	

FIG. 26-1   *Critical pathway based on surgical procedure.* (From Multidisciplinary Plan Resource Manual, High Point Regional Health System, High Point, North Carolina, 1999.)

5-DAY, 5 FU REGIMEN BASED CHEMOTHERAPY

Day 1

OUTCOMES

Pt/family will verbalize understanding of:

Plan of Care: Chemotherapy regimen, side effects of chemo (mucositis, diarrhea, nausea/vomiting), signs/symptoms of extravasation, signs/symptoms of mucositis, diarrhea control, strict I&O, diet, nausea control, no smoking policy, unit routine and D/C plan

Pt will demonstrate decreased level of anxiety

Pt will maintain adequate nutrition

Pt will have pain control

Pt will have stable vital signs

Pt will incur no injury during hospitalization

Assessments	Medications	Treatments/IVs
Admission assessment VS per unit routine Strict I&O q4h, ATC Assess for extravasation q1h while vesicant infusing, otherwise q2h ATC Assess pain using 0-10 pain scale, prn Assess oral hygiene every shift Assess nutrition and nausea Assess bowel function Informed consent for chemo, if first treatment	Tylenal 650-mg tabs/liquid PO q4h prn MOM/Mylanta 30 ml PO prn Temazepam (Restoril) 15-30 mg PO qHS prn Ambien (5 mg) PO qHS prn (Dr. Provatas pts) Compazine (3 mg) IV or 10 mg PO q4h prn Laxative of choice, prn Peri-Colace or Senokot 1-2 tab PO qd prn Magic Mouthwash 5-10 ml swish and swallow qid prn mouth discomfort	5 FU ___ mg/m^2 in 1 L D$_5$W IV over 24 hr × 5 L (calculate per ht. and wt.) Decadron 20 mg IV before Mitomycin day 1 Kytril 1 ml IV before Mitomycin/streptozocin Mitomycin ___ mg/m^2 in 100 ml NS IV over 30-60 min day 1 (or q8wk with streptozocin) Streptozocin 500 mg/m^2 in 250 ml NS IV over 1 hr qd × 5 days

Nutrition	Diagnostics	Consults
Diet as tolerated unless restricted	CBC, Chem 7 (unless obtained from office)	PCC—Oncology Nutritional Services prn Social Services prn Pastoral Care prn Financial Consult prn

Activity	Education	Discharge Planning
Up ad lib Offer reading materials, VCR for leisure (Obtain from Volunteer Services)	Review Plan of Care and expected LOS Verbal explanation of: • Medications and side effects • Diet and nausea control • Oral hygiene • Accurate monitoring of I&O • No smoking policy • Unit routine • Activity level • Bowel protocol • Chemo precautions • Pain management • S/S of extravasation Assess pt/family knowledge level of chemotherapy and disease process Give Chemotherapy Education Packet Allow pt/family to view video: "Chemotherapy: An Introduction to Treatment"	Identify caregiver Identify home support/resources needed by pt Identify support programs Identify discharge destination Assess D/C needs Make referrals as needed

FIG. 26-2   *Critical pathway based on a treatment regimen for intravenous therapy.* (From Multidisciplinary Plan Resource Manual, High Point Regional Health System, High Point, North Carolina, 1999.)

patterns of positive or negative outcomes from different courses of treatment.

The nurse's signature is attached to the record by an individual password that the nurse uses to gain access to the system. The password should never be shared or used by anyone other than the person to whom it is assigned. Passwords should be changed often to prevent misuse and protect the system. Confidentiality must be emphasized so that the information is not used in an illegal or inappropriate manner. Entrance to the

medical record can usually be tracked and an unauthorized chart entry may result in disciplinary action.

Using a computer, it is usually a simple process to document the selection of the insertion site and catheter gauge, purpose of therapy, degree of phlebitis or infiltration, and device removal; it can be accomplished simply by selecting the appropriate key words or phrases already programmed on the screen. The system should always allow narrative notes to further explain or describe abnormal or unusual events or situations. Home care

---

Charting by Exception

The following symbols are used when **Charting by Exception** assessments:
√ c = Comprehensive normal (Chart with the knowledge that these normals are already charted. Charting should reflect the abnormal/exceptions to these.)
√ = Abbreviated normal
* = Abnormal-refers to progress notes
→ = Continued abnormal, ↓ = continued abnormal for critical care
D = Deferred
N/A = Not applicable

Comprehensive Assessments: **1. On Admission, 2. After invasive tests and procedures, 3. On primary and secondary diagnosis related systems, q shift and prn, 4. Any system with an abnormality, q shift and prn, until it becomes normal.**

Neurological = Alert and oriented to person, place and time. Behavior appropriate to situation. Active ROM of all extremities with symmetry of strength. Facial symmetry. No paresthesia. Verbalization clear and understandable. Swallowing without coughing or choking on liquids and solids. Walks with steady gait. No visual field cut.

Neuro Checks = Glasgow Coma Scale 15 [eyes open; spontaneous (4), best verbal: oriented (5), best motor: obeys command (6)]. Pupils equal in size and reactive to light. Normal motor strength. Normal sensation. If any abnormalities in this category, use the *Neurological Assessment Flowsheet*.

Cardiac = Regular apical pulse within 60-100 beats/minute. S1 and S2 audible. Monitored patients: normal sinus rhythm.

Vascular = Peripheral pulses (radial, dorsalis pedis, posterior tibia) palpable and normal (scale: absent, doppler, weak, normal, bounding). No calf tenderness. CRT less than 3 seconds. NO edema. Extremities warm.

Respiratory = Respirations 12-20/min at rest. Respirations even and unlabored. Breath sounds clear bilaterally. No sputum or sputum is clear. Nailbeds and mucous membrane pink. Patent airway.

Gastrointestinal = Abdomen soft. Bowel sounds active. No pain with palpation. Tolerates prescribed diet. No nausea and vomiting. Having BMs within normal pattern.

Genitourinary = Able to empty bladder without dysuria. Urine clear and yellow to amber.

Integumentary = Skin color within patient's norm. Skin warm, dry, and intact. Mucous membranes moist and pink.

Musculoskeletal = Absence of joint swelling and tenderness. Functional ROM. No muscle weakness.

Psych/Social = Characteristics of appearance, behavior, and verbalizations appropriate to situation. Short and long term memory intact. Affect appropriate. No mood swings noted.

Pain = Without pain or experiencing pain that is managed effectively.

Surgical Dressing = Dressing dry and intact.

Incision/Wound = No evidence of redness, increased temperature, or tenderness in surrounding tissues. Sutures/staples/steri-strips intact. Wound edges well approximated. No drainage present.

Peripheral IV/INT/Central IV/Epidural = Insertion site is free of inflammation, induration, drainage, and tenderness. The IV line is functioning as expected. Dressing is dry and intact.

Where applicable: Reproductive = Female: Absence of vaginal discharge. Male: Absence of scrotal edema.

Abbreviated Assessment: **To be performed every shift unless a comprehensive assessment is required.**

Neurological = Alert and oriented to person, place, and time. Behavior appropriate to situation. *(Patient must be awakened to validate this assessment.)*

Cardiac = Regular pulse within 60-100 beats/minute. Monitored patients: normal sinus rhythm.

Vascular = Pulse normal. Extremities warm, no edema.

Respiratory = Respirations even, regular, and unlabored. Breath sounds clear bilaterally.

Gastrointestinal = Tolerates prescribed diet. BMs within normal pattern.

Genitourinary = Able to empty bladder without dysuria. Urine clear and yellow to amber.

Integumentary = Skin color within patient's norm. Skin warm and dry.

Pain = Without pain or experiencing pain that is managed effectively.

Surgical Dressing = Dressing dry and intact.

Incision/Wound = No evidence of redness, increased temperature, or tenderness in surrounding tissues. Sutures/staples/steri-strips intact. Wound edges well approximated. No drainage present.

Peripheral IV/INT/Central IV/Epidural = Insertion site is free of inflammation, induration, drainage, and tenderness. The IV line is functioning as expected. Dressing is dry and intact.

FIG. 26-3 *Charting by exception: comprehensive and modified assessments.* (Adapted from handout provided by Saint Joseph's Health System, Atlanta, Georgia.)

nurses often use handheld computers because they are convenient and easily accessible. Although computerized records are generally more readable than handwriting, the format is not always clearly delineated, especially when the record is not printed in color. At first, computer novices may be reluctant to enter a computerized system to retrieve data or enter personal orders.

Documentation of critical pathways

Critical pathways are multidisciplinary tools designed to encompass a plan of high-quality care at the lowest cost possible. Care is outlined, or "mapped," for a predictable length of stay and progression of recovery. Using critical pathways requires an increased interdisciplinary collaboration and efficiency facilitated by streamlined documentation procedures. The care plan

Box 26-1   Original Key Elements for Documentation by Exception

- Flow sheets
- Established institutional protocols reflecting standards of practice
- Nursing database
- Nursing care plans based on the nursing diagnosis
- SOAP progress notes

is designed for a specific episode of illness or surgical procedure. It provides data to track variances based on expected outcomes or failure to meet certain criteria.[8] Monitoring along the pathway may reveal areas of weaknesses in the care plan; this information can be used to improve recovery time or identify opportunities to improve patient care. Commonly used critical paths provide an outline of care for procedures with predictable outcomes and treatments, such as total knee replacement, hip replacement, or percutaneous transluminal coronary angioplasty.

Critical pathways often reflect the top 10 DRGs seen within an organization. However, some organizations have critical pathways for almost every diagnosis and procedure. Fig. 26-1 reflects 1 day of a pathway based on a surgical procedure, whereas Fig. 26-2 reflects 1 day of a pathway based on a treatment regime for IV therapy. Most pathways, which are diagnosis or procedure driven, include infusion therapy under "Medications: and/or "Treatments/IVs," as depicted in Fig. 26-1. Both pathways provide a plan of care for the patient on the stated day, and plans are provided for subsequent days until the patient is discharged (example of subsequent days are not provided because of space limitations).

Critical paths are usually documented with the *charting by exception* method, which records only abnormal findings and condenses normal findings. Normal findings are assumed unless otherwise indicated. Detailed descriptions of acceptable normal findings should be clearly defined in institutional standards of care.[8]

Documentation by exception, better known as *charting by exception,* was created in an effort to reduce documentation time and to make trends in the patient's status more obvious. Documentation by exception records only those events that do not reflect the normal. This form of documentation requires an understanding of what is normal so that the abnormal (exception) is recognized. Fig. 26-3 is a good example of a handout that can guide staff when charting by exception. It clearly delineates normal findings for comprehensive and abbreviated assessments.

The use of documentation by exception requires established guidelines based on the standards of practice to promote consistency in documentation. Originally, there were several elements that were necessary for this form of documentation (Box 26-1).

Currently, institutions using documentation by exception have modified the original set of elements to reflect the needs of their institution. Although most continue to use the first four elements, many use only some modified form of SOAP progress notes. Many have dropped the use of the *S, O, A, and P* with comments beside each.

Documentation by exception fits very well with computerized record keeping because normal findings can be identified in checklists; it is only the exception that has to be entered into the computer. Programs are now being developed to recognize abnormal findings.

Education about concise, accurate documentation is paramount. Statements should be specific and descriptive. Some indication in the record should refer to observations within normal limits, even if only a check mark or a symbol is used.

Charting by exception or abbreviated charting are new concepts for regulators and lawyers. The practice of assuming normal findings and routine care replaces the old rule of "if it wasn't charted, it wasn't done." Charting by exception does not negate the need for good documentation of assessments performed and unusual symptoms noted. Negative outcomes of infusion therapy, such as gross infiltration or severe phlebitis, often suggest that observations were *not normal.* In the absence of adequate documentation, such negative outcomes can imply insufficient observation by the nurse.

ACUTE CARE DOCUMENTATION

JCAHO requires certain documentation to establish or maintain accreditation. One requirement is that the hospital define patient assessment activities in writing so that scope, responsibility, and accountability are clearly delineated by the discipline. The initial assessment must be accomplished and documented within the first 24 hours of admission. Because most hospitalized patients have some form of infusion therapy, the assessment should also include an access device assessment, evaluation of current infusion treatment regimens, and discharge planning for future or continuing infusion needs. JCAHO also requires reassessment at regular intervals or in response to significant changes in the patient's condition or diagnosis. The patient's response to care may require reassessment, for example, when a malignancy is discovered and long-term venous access for chemotherapy is needed, or if the patient's condition worsens to cardiac arrest and an emergency central line is established during the code. The infusion needs changed in both situations, necessitating not only a change in the type of IV access but also a change in the plan of care for different IV therapy modalities. The standards indicate that care decisions should be based on identified patient needs and care priorities.[9]

The initial assessment documentation should include the patient's psychologic and social concerns as well as physiologic status. The level of family and caregiver support available for the patient in the home may determine the type of infusion therapy used and the type of catheter inserted. An implantable access device may be indicated if the patient needs intermittent therapy or daily flushing of an infusion device or if routine care is unavailable. Cultural influences, financial concerns, gender, age, and the availability of health care resources should be assessed. Documentation records should reflect external and internal restraints and provide justification for payment or future treatment decisions. A young male may be embarrassed about an exposed peripherally inserted central catheter (PICC), the use of heparin to flush a line may be too expensive, or a woman of ethnic origin may have cultural restrictions for catheter placement. Documentation of these concerns facilitates the decision-making process in developing the plan of care. Documentation may be accomplished on a separate form or on an interdisciplinary patient assessment form, such as a critical pathway.[8]

Successful continuity of care requires careful assessment and discharge planning. Infusion access must be appropriate to the level of care required and accessible to the patient. Managed care, insurance companies, governmental agencies, and other payers require precise, appropriate documentation, and the transfer needs must be justified to smoothly transition the patient from acute care to the home or other facility.

HOME CARE DOCUMENTATION

Requirements for clinical documentation are generally the same as those for acute care and home care settings except for environmental issues. In addition, documentation of home care services must include information that justifies the need for home care visits. Home care documentation should be multidisciplinary and require communication and documentation between disciplines. Although the principle diagnosis is critical for medical reimbursement, the record must reflect total patient care, including the assessment, care plan, evaluations, implementation of care, and outcomes. The principal diagnosis is key in determining payment under Medicare guidelines (e.g., Plan of Care HCFA 485).[10] It should reflect the most current acute condition or the diagnosis most closely linked with the plan of care. The diagnosis should justify the disciplines and services used, validate the need for prescribed medications and treatments, clearly indicate functional limitations, and include special precautions such as fluid restrictions or safety precautions.

Patient assessment

JCAHO standards for home care require an agency or organization to document the use of clinical practice guidelines, critical pathways, and standards of practice in the decision-making process. The documentation should include observations about safety of the environment, medications, storage and handling of supplies, use of medical gases, and instructions concerning handling and disposal of hazardous or infectious materials.[10]

Written assessments should also include the following:
- Medical history
- Pertinent physical findings
- Age- and gender-specific findings
- Laboratory results
- History of chemical dependency
- Psychologic and nutritional status
- Use of herbal and over-the-counter medications
- Condition of the home and surroundings
- Patient and family educational needs, abilities, and readiness to learn

There should be documentation about the environment indicating that it is safe and has water, electricity, and refrigeration.

The patient's learning needs, such as knowledge of their disease, prognosis, medication administration and schedules, procedure and treatments, personal access, emergency plans, infection control, and safety should be documented. Assessments should also include reporting victims of abuse or neglect. Discharge needs (termination of therapy) should be assessed

and a follow-up plan should be established to provide the patient with ongoing health care.

Infusion therapy

Additional documentation is required for infusion therapy patients. Documentation must demonstrate that the risks and benefits of the prescribed therapy or access device have been explained. Appropriate consents must be signed. The physician's orders must include the medication, dose, route, rate and volume, frequency of administration, and duration of the infusion therapy. Flush medication and frequency of flushing should be documented. Anaphylactic orders, if indicated, should also be included with the physician orders or outlined in organizational policy and procedure guidelines. Institutional policy should be specific as to the acceptability of administering medications that have not been approved by the U.S. Food and Drug Administration.

The patient or caregiver should receive written instructions about the infusion therapy. Interventions or treatments should be described. Documentation should include a description of written or verbal instructions with results of return demonstration for technical procedures.[10]

Subsequent documentation should include the following[10]:
- Changes in the initial assessment
- Procedure performed
- Local anesthetics, if used
- Description of device (gauge and length)
- Location of insertion site and number of attempts, if IV
- External length of catheter left outside the skin
- Location of catheter tip, if necessary (e.g., central venous catheter)
- Equipment used
- Infusate or medication and volume infused
- Patient's response and compliance
- Supply disposal procedures
- Unusual or unexpected sequelae

Documentation of catheter removal should include the integrity and length of the catheter, any complications incurred, and the dressing applied to the insertion site. Symptoms, interventions for complications encountered, and physician communications should be described and recorded, including the time. If extravasation has occurred, documentation should include insertion site appearance, amount of medication infused, amount and method of administering the antidote, and the patient's response to the interventions.

Documentation of periodic evaluations of therapy should include the patient's clinical status, complications and sequelae encountered, potential problems, the patient or caregiver's response and compliance to the therapy and care administered, telephone conversations that may support or reinforce education to the patient, and verbal communications between other members of the health care team.

Insurance requirements

Insurance companies look closely at the necessity for home care visits. Care is justified by specific descriptions of the patient's condition and the patient's degree of illness. Because the insurance case manager or reviewer may not have the complete chart, concise and pertinent documentation on the assessment form is imperative. Factual descriptions should be used, including details such as "redness extends 3 cm around insertion site in the left antecubital area." Documentation of patient teaching should be specific, such as, "taught patient how to use aseptic technique when attaching IV tubing to the catheter injection port," or "the patient will demonstrate how to clean and maintain PICC line dressing." The documentation of patient education should reflect, for example, that the patient knows the name, correct dose, and times the medication is administered. If reteaching is necessary, the reason for repeating instructions must be documented. Descriptions of patient progress should be specific, such as "the patient experiences nausea within 30 minutes from the start of the infusion."

Documentation must describe a chronic or acute problem. Payment may be denied based on the assumption that the care is custodial or maintenance in nature.

Evidence, including clinical diagnosis and significant clinical findings, must be given to justify the need for skilled care. A description of services should include the assessment, procedures needed, teaching activities, and the services needed to meet these requirements. Documentation should also include the patient's response, measurable outcomes, and progress as a result of the therapy or services delivered. The nurse should note appropriate and timely interventions related to identified nursing diagnoses, changes in condition, notification and communication with the physician, interventions made, patient response and progress, and evidence of coordination of other services.

NURSING HOME/SKILLED NURSING FACILITY

Infusion therapy is often delivered in extended care facilities. Documentation requirements are like those for home care if rehabilitation is needed, and similar to acute care documentation if IV therapy is temporary and short term.

INTRAVENOUS DOCUMENTATION
Assessment

The rationale for infusion therapy should be recorded to ensure the appropriateness of device selection and the purpose of the intended treatment. An accurate initial infusion therapy assessment documents the patient's general condition, skin, and reason for therapy. A PICC line may be inserted for long-term antibiotics, or a 16-gauge catheter may be placed for open-heart surgery. General information about the patient is helpful in determining the type of therapy that is most beneficial. The patient's cognitive mental condition, whether confused, combative, or restless, may affect placement preference.

Monitoring

It is imperative that infusion sites be monitored and that monitoring assessments be documented at frequent intervals, according to institutional policy. A site assessment that reads "site looks good" does not adequately describe a site that has "0+ phlebitis," which indicates no clinical symptoms of phlebitis or swelling. Any unusual symptoms noted, such as pain, tender-

ness, swelling, or poor function, should be addressed and followed throughout the documentation process. Skin condition should be assessed to document potential difficulties in placing, positioning, or securing the infusion device. Documentation for patients who are diabetic or have been taking steroids, anticoagulants, or chemotherapy should be specific because these patients may experience changes in skin fragility and thickness.

Many cases of legal liability hinge on the adequacy and timeliness of corrective action. Clearly, inadequate monitoring of an infusion site or incomplete documentation of monitoring activities can put the nurse and institution at a disadvantage in court. When vesicants such as dopamine or more irritating medications such as chlorpromazine are administered, site monitoring and documentation should be more frequent.

Treatment

Documentation of infusion therapy should include the type of access device, cannula gauge and length, location and condition of the insertion site, and date and time of insertion. There are many designs and materials used for catheters. Allergies to the cannula material may develop. If an agency or organization uses only one brand of catheter, documentation of brand is not as crucial as in facilities where many types are available. However, catheter care and use may be specific for a certain catheter type, or the patient may be transferred to another facility. In these instances, documentation of catheter type would help the nurse provide appropriate care. The cannula size and length provide important functional information; for example, blood products, surgery, chemotherapy, vesicants, or other special therapies require different catheter gauges.

Patient response to an infusion procedure should be documented. Excessive anxiety, patient movement, or an untoward response should be reported to others on the health care team. This information may forewarn subsequent infusion care providers that device dwell time may be adversely affected or that the next venipuncture may be difficult.

Documentation of the exact insertion site is essential in tracking appropriateness of site selection, phlebitis, and dates for cannula rotation. If therapy was established in the upper arm, fingers, or feet, additional documentation is needed to support limited or unavailable IV access in the hands, forearms, or antecubital fossa.

Infection control data and performance improvement activities require that all bloodstream infections and local peripheral infections be researched to determine, if possible, the cause of the infection. An accurate description of the insertion date and the condition of the insertion site will not only determine when the site should be rotated, but will also help track possible causes of any complications.

Observations and interventions

Observation of the patient and the delivery of infusion therapy provides the necessary information for documentation. Infusion sites should be observed and palpated, if possible. Documentation of infusion site observations should include the following:

- Tenderness
- Temperature at and around the site

- Discoloration
- Swelling
- Drainage

Institutional policy should quantify the frequency of required nursing observation and documentation. Home care policies should provide thorough education of the patient or designated caregiver in the importance of observing and caring for the infusion site and of documenting said observations and care.

Documentation of infusion device removal is crucial. Documentation of a peripheral IV device removal should include the site condition, date, time, and initials of the person removing the device. Documentation of a central venous catheter removal should include a description of how the device was removed, the length of time pressure was held on the insertion site after removal, the character and type of dressing applied, any ointment applied, the patient's response to the procedure, any patient restrictions after removal, and the initials of the nurse or name of the physician removing the device.

Complications

Complications associated with infusion therapy, such as pain, phlebitis, infiltration, extravasation, infection, and drainage, and any unusual symptom or event, should be recorded. For central lines, the lack of blood return or poor blood return, positional problems, catheter dysfunction (e.g., malposition), shortness of breath, or air embolism should be reported and documented. When interventions are necessary, the following should be documented:

- Date and time symptoms occurred requiring an intervention
- Assessment of the patient's condition
- Notification of physician
- Communication with patient and family, if necessary
- Treatment interventions taken
- Ongoing monitoring and further interventions
- Patient response until the problem is resolved

Outcomes

Positive and negative outcomes of infusion therapy should be addressed in the patient's record. Outcomes, or results of therapy, complete the procedure and indicate whether therapy was successful. Positive outcomes may be simple, such as "termination of therapy," or a bit more complex, such as "termination of therapy without complications." Negative outcomes should be described in detail, including interventions and sequelae. For example, extravasation documentation should include the following:

- Assessment of the site (e.g., degree of extravasation, discoloration)
- Estimation of the amount of drug infused into the tissue
- Notification of the physician
- Medications injected to reverse or minimize damage to surrounding tissue
- Device removal (how and by whom)
- Any other necessary interventions, such as application of heat or cold
- Patient response to the procedure

After an extravasation the nurse should observe the site often, and should document each observation until the site has healed or the patient is discharged.

COMMUNICATION

In addition to its other purposes, documentation is a way for health care professionals to communicate with one another. A medical record reveals the history, treatment, and outcomes for a given period. Documentation should include pertinent information about communication between patients, families, physicians, and other members of the health care team. Information about physician notification orders and directives should be noted. Communication to supervisors or others in authority should be noted if their response seems important to the patient's outcome.

PATIENT TEACHING AND UNDERSTANDING

Documentation should include the responses of the patient, family, and caregiver to teaching. All infusion therapy modalities should be explained to all those involved in patient care. The explanation should include the following:

- Purpose of the procedure
- Use of and care for the infusion
- Observation of the therapy and site
- Signs and symptoms of infection
- Recognition of other potential complications
- Interventions for problems and complications
- Any restrictions necessary while receiving therapy

Written information regarding infusion therapy is often given to the patient before the procedure. The information should be individualized and reflect the patient's specific needs. Receipt and understanding of the information by the patient, family, and caregiver should be recorded. Written instructions at discharge are necessary, especially for the patient receiving continuing therapy at home.

NURSING RESPONSIBILITIES
Accountability

Infusion nurses are accountable for their practices, including the elements of the nursing process: assessment, planning, implementation, and evaluation. Documentation needs to reflect these steps. Even if the infusion nurse's primary responsibility is working on an infusion team or in home infusion therapy, basic nursing skills and assessments are no less important.

Competency

Regulatory agencies require that staff competencies be evaluated and maintained. Written policies and standards are determined by the institution as to the frequency and depth of the validation process. Competency in infusion therapy should be assessed and documented. This may be accomplished by testing and return demonstration. Standards define acceptable practice guidelines for performance. Organizations should have written standards that establish the expectation for positive patient outcomes and should provide guidelines to accomplish those outcomes. Staff education and IV validation records should be kept in personnel files.

The Intravenous Nurses Certification Corporation established credentialing for IV therapy in 1983. Through testing designed to document the competency of practitioners of IV nursing therapies, an individual is awarded the credential, Certified Registered Nurse Intravenous (CRNI). The CRNI designation provides national recognition and documentation of competency for the infusion nurse. Courts of law recognize *Infusion Nursing Standards of Practice* as the basis for optimal infusion care. The signature of the registered nurse along with the CRNI designation indicates additional education and expertise in infusion therapy.

Performance improvement

Performance improvement activities are an integral part of the delivery of infusion therapy. Complications are not always avoidable; they should be investigated and issues should be evaluated to help prevent an unfavorable outcome. Efforts toward and results of performance improvement are part of the documentation of infusion therapy.

A study of the administration of dopamine through IV peripheral lines provides a good example of how documentation can lead to improved care. A study was initiated at St. Joseph's Hospital in Atlanta because of the high incidence of phlebitis noted when dopamine was administered through a peripheral vein. Further study of documentation revealed a 67% infiltration rate and an average dwell time of 14 hours before extravasation occurred. The problem and data provided an opportunity for improvement. The performance improvement process was used, and the results were reported to a multidisciplinary critical care committee. The physicians on the committee immediately confirmed that they had similar experiences with dopamine and validated the research findings. The committee designated dopamine for emergency use only.[11]

Documenting data and trends allows specific patient events to be retrieved and future developments to be predicted. JCAHO requires that all sentinel events, events that are life-threatening or have a life-limiting potential, be investigated for root and cause. When outcomes are unexpected or need to be improved, previous documentation provides important information and clues to help understand why the outcome occurred. An analysis of the root causes provides the basis for creating an action plan for improvement. Corrective efforts to improve infusion therapy outcomes may include education; changing policies and procedures, such as for dressing care or frequency of peripheral rotation; and product changes. *Infusion Nursing Standards of Practice* provides clearly stated standards and practice criteria information related to the practice of infusion therapy.

Any agency or organization delivering infusion therapy should maintain records concerning the infusion lines inserted (volume and type) and the rates of phlebitis, infiltration, and infection. These data are necessary to measure the effectiveness of infusion therapy.

REIMBURSEMENT

Organizations need financial support to stay operational. Therefore it is important to comply with payers' rules and guidelines. Appropriate diagnosis, treatment, intervention, and expected outcomes are reported to describe and justify payment. Poor documentation may result in denial of payment to the physician or the organization. Thorough knowledge and close monitoring is necessary to ensure proper coding to allow payment.

SUMMARY

Documentation offers a permanent record of events, behaviors, and responses to infusion therapy. It is the most important vehicle for validating the care performed by the infusion nurse. It provides the details necessary to understand the care given and the patient's response to that care. Documentation provides the information necessary for concurrent and retrospective reviews and information that allows the total performance of the infusion department to be evaluated and benchmarked against other organizations and national standards. Periodic concurrent and retrospective reviews of infusion practices provide medical information that can determine future treatment. The accuracy and completeness of infusion care documentation can help improve patient outcomes by adding pertinent information to the analysis of the patient's clinical picture. Documentation in the medical record is recognized in legal settings as proof of infusion care administered. Although it takes time, a commodity often in short supply, care must be taken to document all infusion care concisely, precisely, and accurately to create a valid, reliable medical record.

REFERENCES

1. Nightingale F: *Notes on nursing: what it is, and what it is not,* New York, 1986, Dover.
2. Intravenous Nurses Society: Infusion nursing standards of practice, *JIN* (suppl) 23(6S), 2000.
3. Iyer P, Camp N: *Nursing documentation: a nursing process approach,* St Louis, 1991, Mosby.
4. Stephens S, Mason S: Putting it together: a clinical documentation system the works, *Nurs Manage* 30(3):43, 1999.
5. Trott MC: Legal issues for nurse managers, *Nurse Manage* 29(6): 38, 1998.
6. Wilkinson AP: How to avoid your day in court: nursing malpractice, *Nursing 98* 28(6):34, 1998.
7. Schlmeister L: A complication of vascular access device insertion, *JIN* 21(4):197, 1998.
8. Aronson B, Maljanian R: Critical path education: nursing components and effective strategies, *J Contin Educ Nurs* 27(5):215, 1996.
9. Joint Commission on Accreditation of Healthcare Organizations: *Comprehensive accreditation manual for hospitals: the official handbook,* Oakbrook Terrace, Ill, 2000, Joint Commission on Accreditation of Healthcare Organizations.
10. Joint Commission on Accreditation of Healthcare Organizations: *1999-2000 Comprehensive accreditation manual for health care,* Oakbrook Terrace, Ill, 1998, Joint Commission on Accreditation of Healthcare Organizations.
11. Dugger B: Dopamine peripheral infusions: are they worth the risk? *JIN* 20(2):95, 1997.

Chapter
27

IV Therapy in the Acute Care Setting

Crystal Miller, RN, BSN, MA, CRNI*

ORGANIZATION STRUCTURE
   IV care delivery model
   Operational design
SCOPE OF SERVICES
MANAGEMENT CONSIDERATIONS
   Staff qualifications
   Workload standards
   Staffing
   Provision of services
   Human resources management
   Policies and procedures
   Quality management
   Financial management
SPECIAL CONSIDERATIONS
   Cost considerations
   Reimbursement
   Quality of care
   Risk management
   Justification

The challenge in the health care industry in the United States is to deliver the highest quality of care to the greatest number of people, using all available resources in the most cost-effective manner. With each advance in technology and each breakthrough in health care intervention, the challenge becomes greater and the solution more complex. In the past, budget management of a facility was often a matter of determining where and how to use the available funds. Payment was based on charges and fees for services, so attention to volume and operational costs was primary. Higher operational costs and decreased payment have changed the focus of management. As in the past, it is mandatory to the success of an institution for managers to be astute in all aspects of health industry standards. The emphasis for nurse managers has changed from managing only the delivery of care to managing the fiscal aspects as well.

A health care worker from 50 years ago might find our current health care system barely recognizable. We have seen a gradual decrease in the number of hospitals in this country. In 1989, there were 6720 hospitals, whereas in 1997 there were 6097 hospitals.[1] With projected closures, increased expenditures, and dwindling resources, reform was inevitable. Managed care and the Balanced Budget Act were implemented in an effort to decrease the gap between financial obligation and health care provider resources. These reimbursement measures offered hope for acute care facilities, but for a significant price. As the average patient days continues to fall and inpatient revenue sources dwindle, hospitals will continue to cut staff and find new ways to save money.[2]

The delivery of nursing care has been affected dramatically. One aspect that has felt the greatest impact is the delivery of intravenous therapy. Maintaining quality and cost-effectiveness in delivering this aspect of care alone is of great concern. Criteria for the justification of hospital admission often include the clinical necessity for an intravenous (IV) line or IV medications. Although it is not a criterion for remaining in the hospital after the acute phase of illness, as it once was, it is rare to find a patient who has not had IV therapy by the end of a hospitalization.

The impact of shortages of registered nurses (RNs), most of whom manage aspects of IV therapy administration and IV access, has led to changes in the way nursing care is delivered. Primary nursing and patient-focused care have placed more demands on the RN at the bedside. Many services that were formerly delivered by specialists, such as infusion therapy, are now the responsibility of generalist staff nurses and in some instances unlicensed support personnel. In addition to assessing patient needs in the hospital, the nurse has assumed the role of case manager, planning for safe and appropriate care beyond the hospital environment. High costs and decreasing reimbursements make earlier discharge to alternative settings a necessity. The demand for providing complicated intravenous therapies outside the zones of acute care has expanded the role of the infusion therapy nurse. Quality of care requires expertise in the specialty practice of IV therapy. Clearly, in the acute care environment, a benefit of the specialized skills of an IV team is enhancement of the process for managing patient care.

---

*The author and editors wish to acknowledge the contributions made by Leslie Baranowski and Edie Jonas, as coauthors of this chapter in the first edition of *Intravenous Nursing: Clinical Principles and Practice.*

Formerly, acute care facilities were reimbursed for the ancillary (versus routine) services provided by an IV team. This reimbursement provided an incentive for implementing hospital IV teams. Another impetus to establish such teams was the cost savings realized when IV care was managed by specialists; there were fewer clinical complications, fewer materials were used, and procedures were performed more quickly. With the institution of the prospective payment system, reimbursement could no longer be assumed. IV teams were at risk, and justification for their services came under the close scrutiny of cost-benefit analysis. Maintaining existing IV teams is sometimes a challenge for institutions, and establishing new teams even more so. This is true despite ample evidence of the potential benefits IV teams provide to patients and facilities. The commitment to quality in any setting requires careful analysis of how close adherence to standards of practice affects patient outcomes.

ORGANIZATION STRUCTURE

To maintain their viability, hospitals have become business savvy. In an arena of fierce competition, hospitals must anticipate the future and make cost-cutting modifications to survive the changes brought by reform initiatives.[2] Sweeping health care reforms such as the Balanced Budget Act of 1997 have forced hospitals to make drastic changes. Some facilities have become casualties, unable to maintain financial solvency with implementation of the reforms. Other institutions, recognizing the economic necessity and the potential benefit of changes, have merged to form multifacility health systems. Some hospital managers, in an effort to further control costs, have implemented reengineering plans that could undermine nursing's best efforts to maintain the quality and safety of patient care.[3]

IV care delivery model

Advances in health care delivery and related technologies, along with the adoption of more healthful lifestyles, have led to an increase in life expectancy, raising the average age of the hospitalized patient. This population has frequent and more acute illnesses, requiring complicated therapies, and these all affect the increasing need for complex care and nursing interventions. Models of care that offer relief for some routine, high-volume tasks a nurse must perform are being used. Such models often incorporate the use of unlicensed personnel to provide routine care under the direction of the RN. Computers are commonly used to help the RN document and communicate aspects of unit management and patient care coordination. The complex treatment modalities prescribed today almost always include IV therapies. Specialized nursing management of IV therapy has often been delegated to teams of IV nurse specialists. IV specialists offer the means for maintaining consistency and quality in IV nursing care throughout the acute care facility. Their early assessments and interventions have an impact on the discharge planning of IV therapy needs. Even the most complicated IV therapy needs can be met in the outpatient and home setting by these specialists.

With decreased lengths of stay, streamlined resources, and a reduced workforce, nursing is challenged to develop a care model that maintains both cost-effectiveness and quality of care. Reengineering and decentralization continue the transition of many services to the unit level. Skill-mix staffing has moved care delivery from the primary-care model to a patient-focused model. To enhance efficiency, the new care-delivery models are structured with increased numbers of unlicensed technical staff who are cross-trained to deliver services and care as directed by the professional nurse.

Today's professional-practice models focus on enhanced efficiency, improved quality, and desired patient outcomes.[4] It is important for the IV team to function within these models to have the most positive impact on patient care outcomes and prevent repetition of services. The mode of practice is setting and service dependent but contributes to the success of the IV team and the organization. Hospitals must strive for patient satisfaction, because quality care focusing on patient satisfaction costs less and is safer, more efficient, and less likely to result in legal complications.[5] Infusion therapy has moved beyond the realm of technical skills. Today's IV nurse provides clinical knowledge and serves as the primary resource for infusion therapy education. What better way to ensure positive outcomes than with a group of specialized nurses whose expertise benefits both the patients and the organization.

Operational design

Determining where to place an IV team within the organizational structure of an acute care institution is a strategic decision that can affect the functions and success of the team. Each organization is unique and requires individualized assessment of needs to make the best decision for placing the IV team so that it has the most positive effect on operations and outcomes. Because of the wide range of differences in institutional environments, the role of the IV team varies greatly from one organization to the next.

An IV team may logically report to any one of several overseers. For example, the team may report directly to administration, to a department (e.g., pharmacy, laboratory) or to a particular physician within the institution. It may be placed under the direction of the blood bank, the pharmacy, or the nursing service. Each organizational method is associated with distinct advantages and disadvantages that must be weighed carefully. The major consideration is to enhance the ability of the IV team to meet its own established objectives, goals, and standards of care while remaining cost-effective. The ability to positively affect the maximum number of patient outcomes must be preserved. The positive impact of an IV team directly relates to the scope of services offered. Autonomy, independence, and collaboration are vital for the existence of an IV department.

At first glance, because IV teams are made up of nurses, it would seem logical that the team should report to the nursing department or division. However, it has been found that an IV team's ability to achieve maximum function is enhanced when it can perform as an autonomous unit, distinct from general nursing services and responsibilities yet an integral part of the health care team. IV nurses are nurses, and they need to retain that professional identity, but it can be more effective to have the

IV team, with its specialized practice and levels of competency, report to a department other than nursing. A concern with having the IV team report to nursing is that a typical function and daily need of nursing services is to move or float nurses to other nursing departments within the hospital to resolve staffing problems or shortages. However, for the IV team to perform at an optimal level and to derive maximum benefit from the IV nurse's specialty skills to the patient and the organization, the IV nurse should be assigned exclusively to IV therapy–related functions, with no crossover into general nursing activities.

It is important to note that there are successfully operating, high-quality IV teams reporting to nursing departments. Advantages may be seen in retaining the IV nurse specialist's sense of participation with peers in activities and programs for nurses.

The concerns regarding the limitations encountered when IV teams are placed within the nursing division are significant. In many environments, it may be most advantageous for the IV therapy team to be established as an independent department that reports directly to administration or to a medical director. This allows the autonomy and independence critical for the team to achieve its objectives and goals, and to maintain its standards of practice. The structure of the IV therapy department is determined, to a great extent, by the services offered and the practice setting. When the IV therapy team is established as an independent department under administration, it is important that a close relationship be maintained with other departments, such as nursing, infection control, case management, and pharmacy.

This positioning has many advantages in terms of autonomy and maximum utilization of the IV team's expertise. One disadvantage that must be considered is how this positioning isolates the IV nurse from the nursing care team. It is essential that the IV nurse be an active participant in the nursing care team to meet the patient care objectives of providing timely and effective IV therapy in the most appropriate setting, without complications. The attention given to how and where the IV team should integrate with the health care team is ongoing.

It may also be appropriate for an IV team to report directly to a physician who has a specific interest in IV therapy. This physician should consult with the team and with patients receiving IV therapy. The physician should review and approve the IV therapy department policies and procedures, because most IV procedures are medical procedures requiring guidance only a physician can provide. Potential candidates for this role include the Chief of Staff, Chief of Medicine, Director of the Blood Bank, Director of Anesthesia, and Director of Infection Control. If a team does not report directly to a physician, it remains important that they have a physician designated as a medical advisor.

Other appropriate alternatives for placing an IV team are departments that provide a service, or multiple services, related to IV therapy practice. For example, the blood bank director may be a good alternative because of the way in which transfusion services relate to IV therapy. The complexity of transfusion therapy options and issues, along with advances in the technology available for its administration, make this an area with an increasing need for nursing expertise. Quality monitoring, utilization monitoring, and new approaches to transfusion therapy have greatly increased the necessity for the involvement of IV nurses in this aspect of care. If a team is not actively involved with the delivery and administration of blood components, reporting to the blood bank may not be a realistic or appropriate choice.

Many IV teams are placed under the pharmacy department because of the relationship between IV therapy and the administration aspects of IV admixtures, solutions, and medications. Delivering IV medications and solutions is an integral function of all IV teams. An association with the pharmacy affects the organizational structure and the workload responsibilities of the IV team in various ways. Some teams play an active role in preparing large-volume parenteral admixtures and piggyback medications. This can provide the pharmacy with more effective management of IV medications from the time they are ordered until they are administered. In contrast, many teams that report to the pharmacy are not involved with the actual preparation of medications, because this duty is often delegated to pharmacy technicians. There are other benefits afforded to the team reporting to pharmacy; for example, IV team nurses can gain expertise with regard to drugs.

There are many instances in IV drug and fluid administration in which drug compatibilities, characteristics, interactions, and filtration needs require specific administration supplies or intravascular access. The pharmacy staff benefits from the IV nurse's expertise with IV access devices and their use and maintenance requirements. Advanced knowledge of administering drugs intravenously prevents IV drug-related complications. An association with the pharmacy is valuable and necessary for the IV team that manages outpatient or home infusion therapies. Interaction with the IV nurse specialist gives the pharmacy staff the opportunity to participate more directly in IV-related patient care. The pharmacy director's membership on the Pharmacy and Therapeutics Committee is an asset to the IV therapy team, because the Committee is often the hospital's approval body for policies and procedures. The director of the pharmacy and the chairperson of the Pharmacy and Therapeutics Committee can be advocates for the IV team among the medical staff. Potential conflicts and problems that may be associated with reporting to the pharmacy include the fact that the pharmacy director, like the nursing department executive, cannot approve the medical policies and procedures that guide the IV team's practice. If there is not a strong commitment to the goals and objectives of the IV team, the department director's priorities, in time of conflict over resource allocation, might lean more heavily toward the needs of the pharmacists and pharmacy operational issues. There are successful IV teams that are part of the pharmacy department, and many home infusion agencies have a pharmacist as the general manager.

A close relationship with other hospital departments is essential for an IV team. In many hospital environments, establishing the communication necessary to ensure this close relationship may not be accomplished easily. In recent years, professional-practice models based on shared or collaborative governance have provided an alternative to the hierarchic management structures of most institutions. These practice models provide staff nurses with the opportunity to share the responsibility and accountability for the nursing organization. Committees are established in which nurses from the various areas of the hospital are responsible for activities such as setting standards for their practice, developing policies and procedures, and evaluating the quality of practice and its outcomes. Collaborative governance offers potential advantages for IV teams inside and outside the nursing division.

The IV team that actively participates in shared-governance models provides itself with associated opportunities and advantages. It also benefits from a strong communication system that would otherwise not be available to an ancillary department. Such involvement offers decision-making opportunities at the unit level and for hospitalwide concerns. Participation in shared governance activities strengthens the IV nurse's ties to the nursing structure, allows increased visibility, and enhances the team's value to the institution. It provides IV nurses with the opportunity to have a voice not just about IV issues, but about all facets of nursing. The viability of an IV team rests on the value the institution places on the department's contribution to hospital goals, and on meeting department-specific goals. Strong, unit-based groups for quality assurance, education, and policy and procedure formulation and review are developed.[6] When a shared-governance model is not practiced in an institution, it remains important that the IV team members interact with other members of the health care team to provide safe, high-quality IV therapy.

The Intravenous Nurses Society (INS) encourages IV nurses to collaborate with or participate in committees that regulate the practice of IV nursing.[7] The IV team must become actively involved on committees or task forces relevant to the specialty practice of IV nursing. For example, it is important that a representative from the IV therapy department participate in committees such as pharmacy and therapeutics, infection control, nutritional support, transfusion therapy, safety, quality assurance, and risk management.

SCOPE OF SERVICES

When establishing the scope of practice of the IV therapy department and the roles and responsibilities of the members of the IV team, it is important to evaluate the practice setting carefully, looking at current and potential demands for IV services. The present scope of services for IV therapies must be reviewed, the current demand for services and how that demand is being met must be ascertained, and the future demand for services must be carefully estimated. It is important to remember that as the IV therapy concept gains acceptance from medical and nursing staffs, the demand for services is likely to increase. This increase will affect the demand for existing services and will include requests for more sophisticated technologic procedures. Quality management data related to IV therapy are critical, providing valuable information for determining the essential functions needed to improve IV care. It is well known that IV teams deliver IV care with a higher level of expertise and have a positive impact on the quality of care, but it can be difficult to quantify the impact this has on the organization. Quality assurance data for evaluating the quality of IV care are not consistently kept in hospitals without IV teams and often

must be estimated from random checks of individual units or obtained from other facilities of comparable size. Consideration also needs to be given to the scope of pharmacy services currently in place and changes anticipated with the addition of the IV team. Once these have been determined, the desired team functions and service hours can be better defined.

The ideal IV therapy department should be staffed to provide the total spectrum of IV therapy services 24 hours a day every day. It has been documented that it takes the non-IV nurse up to three times longer than the IV nurse specialist to perform therapy. Adherence to standards is also ensured by using specialty nurses. The IV nurse should perform all functions connected with the administration of IV solutions, medications, chemotherapeutic agents, blood and blood components, and parenteral nutrition. The IV nursing team's responsibilities may include inserting IV cannulas; administering prescribed IV solutions, medications, and blood products; monitoring and maintaining IV peripheral and central access sites and systems; evaluating patient response to prescribed therapy; educating patients and families and evaluating their comprehension and competency; providing education about infusion therapy for non-IV staff nurses; documenting pertinent information on the patient's record; and participating in discharge planning. Compiling statistics to quantify and qualify IV therapy department services, productivity, and patient outcomes are an important function of the IV team staff. There are compelling data that specialized education lowers the risk of infection associated with vascular catheters.[8]

In addition to providing a full spectrum of IV therapy services, the ideal team should provide these services to all areas of the hospital. If this is not possible, a realistic alternative is usually for the critical care and emergency areas of the facility to provide their own IV-related care. However, it remains important for the IV team to be as involved as possible with these areas to provide whatever support is necessary and feasible. The responsibilities of the IV therapy services department are presented in the following outline:

I. *Hours:* The IV therapy department provides daily, 24-hour coverage, including holidays.

II. *Service areas:* The IV team routinely serves all patient care areas. Note that if the IV team is not staffed to provide service to all areas of the hospital, limited service to some areas may be necessary. In this case, departments such as the emergency department, labor and delivery, presurgery preparation areas, and critical care units may be responsible for their own IV care. With patient-focused care delivery models in place, some institutions have made IV therapy a unit-based responsibility for all departments and practice areas. This is highly variable from facility to facility. It is important that the IV team still provide limited service and support IV care needs on request, and to the extent resources permit, to departments responsible for their own IV care, and to ancillary departments such as radiology, nuclear medicine, and cardiology.

III. *Services* (note that possible services are listed, but any combination of services may be provided)
   A. Venipuncture (as needed)
   B. Routine peripheral catheter site changes

C. Initiation of blood components

D. Assistance to physicians in central venous catheter (CVC) insertion

E. Routine and as-needed CVC dressing care

F. CVC blood withdrawals

G. Daily peripheral site checks

H. Implanted port access

I. Declotting of CVCs and peripherally inserted central catheters (PICCs)

J. Insertion and maintenance of PICCs

K. Insertion and maintenance of specialty peripheral catheters

L. Consultation and teaching for long-term CVCs

M. Preparation of selected large-volume parenteral solutions and IV medications

N. Administration of intraspinal medications

O. Care of intraspinal catheters

P. Therapeutic phlebotomies

Q. Participation as member of code team

R. Chemotherapy administration

S. Care and maintenance of arterial catheters, obtaining blood gases

T. Administration of parenteral nutrition

U. Evaluation of IV therapy–related equipment

V. Data collection for IV-related statistics

W. In coordination with the pharmacist, consultation on pharmacokinetic scheduling and compatibility issues

X. Staff education through clinical validation and in-service training

Y. Patient teaching for catheter care and home or outpatient infusion therapies

Z. Provision of outpatient IV therapies, patient monitoring, and education

All functions of an IV nursing team should be established in policy and procedure and should be based on the team's objectives. The objectives should involve providing a systematic and consistent quality of IV therapy for the institution and its patients. Centralized responsibility and accountability should be built in for all IV services. Specific objectives for an IV team are presented in the following outline:

I. Philosophy

   A. The IV therapy department upholds the belief that each patient receiving IV therapy in a variety of settings should be provided with quality individualized care.

   B. It is believed that this care is best provided by RNs who have acquired specialized knowledge and developed skills specific to the practice of IV nursing.

   C. The IV therapy department supports a holistic approach to the delivery of patient care.

   D. The IV therapy department believes in exercising professional responsibility to provide patients with the preventive, curative, and restorative measures they need to achieve wellness.

   E. The IV therapy department strives for excellence through personalized, competent, and cost-effective care.

   F. The IV therapy department believes it has a responsibility to work with other hospital departments, health care professionals, and ancillary departments to coordinate patient services to ensure positive outcomes.

II. Objectives

   A. To provide standard, consistent, and progressive IV care to each patient receiving IV therapy by doing the following:

      1. Establishing performance measures for IV care and monitoring outcomes for all IV therapy department services

      2. Developing, implementing, and adhering to IV therapy policies and procedures according to the *Infusion Nursing Standards of Practice,*[7] with ongoing review

      3. Evaluating IV therapy equipment for utilization that best serves the needs of the patient and the facility

   B. To serve as role models, educational resources, and consultants concerning all aspects of IV nursing by doing the following:

      1. Providing IV therapy orientation and continuing education to appropriate health care personnel

      2. Investigating, validating, and developing the IV nursing specialty through research

      3. Using new technologies

      4. Continuously evaluating the performance and competency of all IV nursing personnel and others providing IV therapy

      5. Using the nursing process by collecting data, prioritizing problems and needs, developing a nursing care plan, and evaluating patient outcomes

An IV team's functions include some type of routine patient service rounds to designated areas of the institution. Rounds by the IV team or a specific IV nurse, such as the central line nurse, may be made routinely, at specific intervals, or a set number of times per shift or day, depending on such factors as the size of the facility, the workload type and volume, and staffing resources.

The IV team routinely reviews IV orders and maintains a patient profile, including IV solutions and medication orders and the IV access device in place. Current patient information should be maintained on IV profile cards (Figs. 27-1 and 27-2). The IV nurse uses the nursing process, which includes assessment, problem identification or nursing diagnosis, implementation, and evaluation, in the practice of IV therapy. A documented plan regarding routine and individual care needs is initiated and revised as needed. A communication system must be established between the IV team and other members of the health care team. If rounds are completed regularly, messages for the IV nurse can be left at designated areas. When rounds are intermittent or infrequent, some type of paging system is needed to communicate with the IV nurse.

Nursing staff responsibilities related to IV therapy vary with the institution and revolve around the functions of the IV team. The IV nurse should be responsible for the selection, initiation, and routine evaluation of the appropriate access device and site. This includes initiating the solutions, tubings, and devices required to administer IV therapies. With 80% to 90% of patients receiving IV therapy at any given time, the IV nurse is an integral part of the nursing process for each patient. The IV nurse's role is no longer viewed as a technical position but is one that consolidates knowledge regarding IV therapy and incorpo-

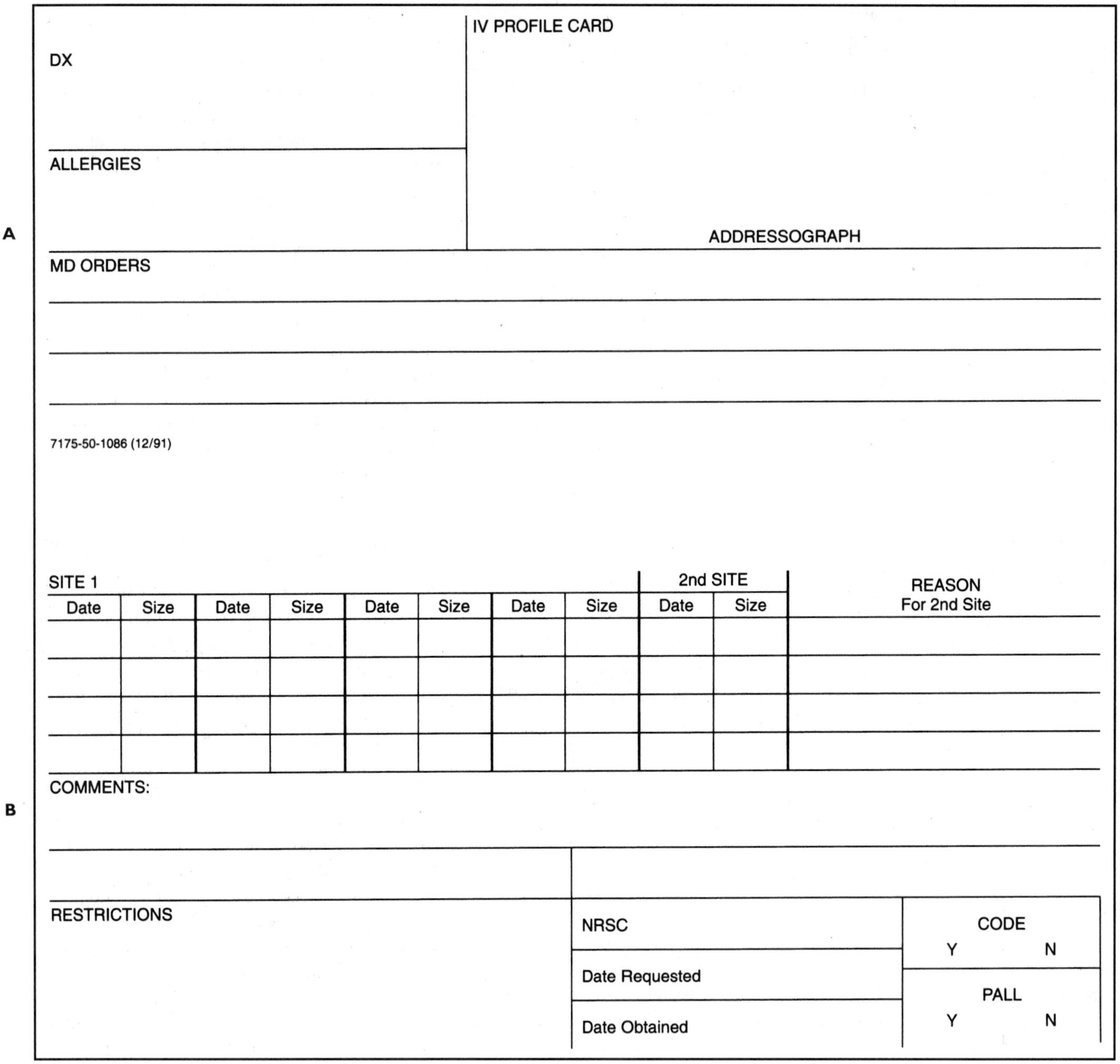

A

IV PROFILE CARD

DX

ALLERGIES

ADDRESSOGRAPH

MD ORDERS

_____

_____

_____

7175-50-1086 (12/91)

B

SITE 1								2nd SITE		REASON For 2nd Site
Date	Size	Date	Size	Date	Size	Date	Size	Date	Size	

COMMENTS:

RESTRICTIONS		
	NRSC	CODE Y N
	Date Requested	PALL
	Date Obtained	Y N

FIG. 27-1 *IV profile card for peripheral catheters.* **A,** *Front.* **B,** *Back.*

rates sound clinical assessment and intervention into the patient's care plan. It is essential that the IV nurse be given time for thorough patient assessment before preparing the patient's IV plan of care. If the IV team's staffing is limited, it may be necessary to designate some of the more routine technical portions of initiating and maintaining IV care to the staff nurse. The nursing staff must be educated regarding the functions of the IV therapy department and be clear as to their own responsibilities regarding their patient's IV therapy needs. Regardless of functions performed by the IV team, every nurse is responsible for routine, regular monitoring of a patient's IV site and infusions, and for ongoing patient assessment of the response to the therapies delivered. This monitoring, as described in *Infusion Nursing Standards of Practice,* should be related to the patient's condition, age, and practice setting and should follow established IV therapy policy and procedure. An IV team's functions may include routine site checks performed on each shift or selected shifts, but the staff nurse must perform site checks in the interim, with appropriate nursing interventions as necessary.

DX	CVC CARD	
ALLERGIES		
MD ORDERS	ADDRESSOGRAPH	**A**

TYPE	SIZE	INSERTION DATE
LOCATION	TIP PLACEMENT	CODE Y N

DRESSING	FREQ.	Huber Needle Date Size & Type
DISCONTINUED: Date & Reason		
DATE DSG. CHANGED		
COMMENTS:		**B**
		PALL Y N

FIG. 27-2 *IV profile card for central venous catheters.* **A,** *Front.* **B,** *Back.*

MANAGEMENT CONSIDERATIONS

The organizational structure and the roles of the various managers and staff members who constitute the IV team vary depending on the size of the department and hospital, functions and services provided by the team, hours of service, and budgetary constraints. It is critical to ensure that an IV team has precisely the right staff and is the right size to perform its services. Typically, IV teams consist of a management or supervisory position, nursing staff, and an educational coordinator.

However the team is organized, concise position descriptions for all members of the team are essential and should be reviewed annually and revised when necessary.

Staff qualifications

Entry-level requirements for the RN entering the IV nursing specialty include current licensure and minimum clinical experience of 2 years of recent medical-surgical nursing, including the opportunity to apply principles and practices of IV therapy.[7] The INS also recommends, but does not require, the Bachelor of Science degree in nursing. For entry at the specialist level, in addition to current licensure, it is suggested that the nurse have 1 year of experience in the specialty practice of IV nursing. One year of experience is defined as 1600 hours spent delivering IV therapies to patients within the last 2 consecutive years. It is also important for all IV team members to obtain national certification in the specialty of IV nursing through the Intravenous Nurses Certification Corporation. Although professional nursing certification is voluntary, certified team members validate the competency and advanced skill level of the staff; they are often used as a marketing tool by institutions. Certification enhances the professional credibility of the nurses and demonstrates their high level of commitment to their specialty practice. In a consumer-driven marketplace, credentialed professionals demonstrate an organization's dedication to professional development through continuing nursing education.

Because of the types of invasive procedures performed by IV nurses, IV teams are usually staffed with registered nurses. These procedures and activities require the level of theoretical and clinical knowledge and expert technical skill provided by RNs. The use of RNs on IV teams has been an especially important result of the patient-care delivery models implemented by many institutions in response to changes in the health care reimbursement structure. With much of direct patient bedside care often being delivered by unlicensed personnel, the extra support of an IV RN can be very valuable to the generalist RN who now has to manage many more patients than before. The educational background and skill levels of the IV nurse specialist who is an RN are needed more than ever to ensure quality of care in the delivery of IV therapies. Although the use of RNs may be optimal, to provide cost-effective services, many IV teams have also found it beneficial and necessary to use licensed vocational nurses (LVNs) or licensed practical nurses (LPNs). Consideration must be given to limitations in job functions of LVNs-LPNs when thinking of using them in the role of the IV nurse. IV therapy–related practice guidelines for the LVN-LPN vary by state and may be further restricted by institutional policy. When an LVN-LPN is a member of the IV team, all functions must, as defined in their licensure, be under the supervision of an RN. The supervising RN may be on the IV team or on the patient care unit where the LVN-LPN is performing IV care. LVNs-LPNs are limited in their role regarding IV therapy and may not perform advanced technical procedures such as PICC insertions. After completing education and training requirements, the LVN-LPN may be permitted to perform venipunctures, monitor IV lines and sites, and administer certain solutions and blood products.

Because of the specialized nature of IV therapy, the success of the department depends on the selection of nurses. IV nurses must be conscientious regarding all aspects of their duties and show evidence of good communication and teaching skills, integrity, reliability, accountability, initiative, and creativity. Mental and emotional stability are important characteristics because the IV nurse often needs to set priorities under pressure.[9] Presenting a professional image to patients and general staff is essential because IV nurses function throughout the institution. To operate an IV team successfully, it is important that the IV nurses function well independently, but they must also have a commitment to the team model concept both intradepartmentally and interdepartmentally. IV nurses' responsibilities are directed toward consistent positive patient outcomes, and a successful team must use a team approach when considering the tasks to be performed and the services offered. Because members of the team may find themselves tied up with various time-consuming or emergency procedures, it is imperative that there be constant and effective communication with other members of the team. The team must work together to assess the needs against available resources and determine how to effectively complete assigned tasks. The ability to meet care or access needs within a reasonable time is essential to avoid delays in therapy. The ability of the IV nurse to prioritize those needs and act on that judgment with clear communication with the IV team and other health care team members is essential. By selecting nurses who have demonstrated these qualities, the IV team's positive interaction with medical staff, other nurses, other departments, and patients is ensured. This level of professionalism will also enhance the value of team members and the IV team as a whole to the organization.

Typical position descriptions for the IV nurse include the clinical services provided, related responsibilities, and functional relationships within the institution. The following outline is an example of a position description for the clinical IV nurse:

I. Purpose of the department and role of the position within the department: fulfills the responsibilities and performs the duties of the IV therapy department, as allowed by the Nurse Practice Act; provides direct patient care using nursing process and is accountable for own practice; participates as patient care advisor; initiates and participates in patient and staff education; demonstrates leadership skills.

II. Licenses, certificates, degrees, or credentials required to perform the duties assigned to the position: RN with at least 2 years of recent medical-surgical or critical care experience— BSN preferred, CRNI (Certified Registered Nurse Intravenous) preferred, IV therapy experience preferred.

III. Functions
   A. Assessment
      1. Make rounds on nursing units to monitor IV devices in use.
      2. Assess patients with regard to diagnosis and special conditions that have any bearing on IV therapy services.
      3. Recognize abnormal conditions or potential problems, take appropriate action, and notify appropriate personnel.
   B. Planning
      1. Plan IV care for assigned patients.
      2. Build flexibility into daily routine to anticipate and handle unexpected situations.
      3. Integrate IV care with the nursing care plan.
      4. Develop individualized teaching plans for patients.
   C. Implementation
      1. Implement physician's orders according to needs and established nursing protocols.
      2. Implement standards of care identified at the unit level.
      3. Perform IV therapy procedures proficiently.

4. Respond to calls for IV therapy services.
5. Intervene in situations in which basic life support systems are threatened, untoward physiologic or psychologic reactions are probable, or changes in normal behavior patterns have occurred.
6. Document procedures, outcomes, and complications appropriately.
7. Demonstrate skills and knowledge as applied to advanced IV therapy (e.g., peripherally inserted central catheters, intraspinal catheters).

D. Evaluation
1. Evaluate patient response to care according to identified criteria.
2. Participate in unit-based quality management activities, as indicated.
3. Participate in product evaluation.

E. Communication
1. Interact with health care team to keep them informed of changes in patient condition.
2. Interact with others to promote and enhance positive relationships.
3. Document interventions and evaluations accurately and promptly.
4. Demonstrate understanding of policies and lines of communication within the institution.

F. Leadership
1. Identify problems in unit functions and either initiate solutions or inform appropriate persons.
2. Participate in ensuring that the nursing care provided is safe and of high quality, and act as a role model to other staff members.

G. Professional development
1. Participate in the evaluation of own performance by identifying strengths and weaknesses and developing a plan to improve weak areas.
2. Work toward patient care competence in specialties common to IV therapy.

H. Education
1. Identify and promote the level of clinical expertise required of staff to provide care to a specific patient population.
2. Serve as an educational resource for IV therapy education for staff nurses, physicians, and other members of the health care team.

I. Research
1. Participate in research projects in IV therapy.
2. Demonstrate awareness of documented research involving nursing practice.

IV. Skills, knowledge, and abilities. The IV therapy nurse must have the following:
A. Ability to establish and maintain effective interpersonal relationships.
B. Ability to set priorities and organize work.
C. Ability to read, write, speak, and understand the English language and use medical terminology appropriately.
D. Ability to assist in moving patients and stand on feet over extended periods.
E. Ability to track clinical skills through the use of outcome measurements.
F. Knowledge of medications, indications, dosage ranges, side effects, and potential toxicity.
G. Knowledge of legal implications for clinical practice.
H. Skills to perform cardiopulmonary resuscitation (CPR).
I. Ability to work accurately and quickly under pressure.
J. Judgment skills to be able to make independent clinical decisions in routine patient care matters.

V. Physical characteristics of critical job functions to be performed:
A. Possess physical strength to assist in lifting patients.
B. See well enough to read charts and gauges.
C. Speak well enough to communicate over the phone.
D. Hear well enough to take vital signs.
E. See well enough to start IVs.

VI. Special conditions of employment:
A. Current RN license for the state
B. Ability to work overtime and weekends
C. Degree from an accredited school of nursing
D. Two years of recent medical-surgical or critical care experience

Position descriptions must include educational requirements, licensing requirements, certification requirements, general nursing or IV therapy–related experience, accountability, and specific areas of responsibility. Position descriptions should be congruent with state statutes, measurable, and used in the evaluation process.[7]

IV nurses must provide an expert level of direct professional nursing care specific to IV therapy, establish standards for and monitor the quality of nursing care, and consult with and serve as an educational resource for patients and staff. They must have a clear understanding of the philosophy and standards of the institution, overall policies of the institution and department, functions of the department, and clinical and technical skills required for their role.

An IV therapy team should be managed by a licensed RN. Five years of recent experience in an acute care hospital setting is preferred, with a minimum of 2 years of experience in nursing management. Experience preparing and managing budgets is desirable. National certification in IV therapy (CRNI) should be required, or a candidate should at least meet the eligibility criteria for certification in the specialty of IV therapy. The individual must demonstrate good organizational and communication skills. To establish and maintain a successful IV team, the manager must have a high degree of interest and experience in the delivery of IV therapy. Maintaining skills and expertise in all aspects of the specialty is necessary for recognizing needs and implementing appropriate adjustments in services. The IV nurse manager should be well respected in the institution and be capable of dealing effectively with all hospital departments. The IV manager is held accountable for his or her own practice and work performed under his or her supervision. The title for this position (e.g., manager, director, supervisor, head nurse) may vary, depending on the department to which the team reports and the responsibilities of the position.

The IV therapy department manager's responsibilities are typically diverse and require good organizational and delegating skills. The manager's responsibilities include writing and reviewing policies and procedures based on current recommendations and standards, keeping abreast of the latest developments in technology, budgeting, and conducting performance evaluations. The IV therapy nurse manager provides IV therapy–related orientation and continuing education programs within and often outside the institution, keeps the staff motivated, and develops and maintains a quality management program. It is also crucial for the IV manager to serve on committees within the hospital related to IV therapy, such as pharmacy and therapeutics, infection control, product evaluation, nutritional support, safety, tumor board, and transfusion. Along with the clinical specialty rationales for membership on these committees, it is important that the IV therapy team participate in the evaluation, selection, standardization, and often servicing of IV-related equipment and supply items.

An IV therapy department manager must carefully design and implement an effective quality assurance and quality improvement program to ensure that acceptable care parameters are met. The program should address the delivery of necessary and appropriate care, achieving minimal complication rates and ensuring that all complications are investigated. It should evaluate negative outcomes to determine whether they are attributable to such factors as nurse practice, procedural or systems issues, equipment failure, or supply defects. The IV team staff can provide the data from IV therapy monitoring. The manager reports findings, assesses impact, and develops recommendations for corrective actions when necessary to improve outcomes. The following outline is an example of a position description for an IV therapy nurse manager. This formatting may be adapted to other positions.

I. *Position summary:* 24-hour administrative responsibility for the nursing and operational management of IV therapy services. The IV nurse manager reports directly to administration, physician, pharmacy, nursing, or blood bank. The IV nurse manager provides clinical supervision and administrative support for the members of the department. The IV nurse manager is responsible for coordinating services for patients, staff, and physicians according to approved hospital and departmental policies, procedures, and guidelines. The IV nurse manager maintains interdepartmental communication and relationships to ensure quality care, fiscal responsibility, optimal allocation of resources, and accurate, timely transmission of information. The IV nurse manager performs the duties of the IV nurse, as appropriate.

II. *Duties and responsibilities*
   A. Operational and administrative management
      1. Assume 24-hour responsibility for the clinical and administrative functions of IV therapy services.
      2. Develop and implement short- and long-term plans and goals for the department.
      3. Integrate IV therapy activities with other hospital departments to resolve identified problems, determine priorities, and provide direction related to patient care issues.
      4. Interpret and ensure compliance of the department with standards of the Joint Commission on Accreditation of Healthcare Organizations (JCAHO) and federal and state regulatory agencies.
      5. Direct and coordinate activities of IV therapy personnel; recruit and interview prospective employees; counsel, evaluate, and provide in-service training to IV personnel; and evaluate employees with the participation of the assistant manager or educational coordinator of IV therapy services.
      6. Plan and develop the budget; monitor revenue, reimbursement, and departmental performance reports; and prepare monthly variance reports.
      7. Develop and revise departmental philosophy, objectives, and policies and procedures based on the *Infusion Nursing Standards of Practice.*[7]
      8. Evaluate new products and procure supplies related to the IV therapy specialty.
      9. Ensure safe, effective patient care through collaboration with nurses, physicians, and other health care providers.
      10. Develop and plan new programs for the department.
      11. Conduct IV therapy classes and in-service training with the assistance of the assistant manager or educational coordinator.
      12. Promote a climate conducive to high-quality service and harmonious working conditions.
      13. Develop and interpret job descriptions and performance appraisals.
      14. Develop and maintain a quality management program, interpret quality management monitors, and report to the appropriate institution committees.
      15. Review and respond to patient and family complaints, including those that may result in litigation, take appropriate actions, and report outcomes to risk management; also, investigate unusual events and ensure proper documentation.
      16. Maintain clinical competency in IV therapy, provide clinical validation and perform all the duties and responsibilities of an IV nurse as required by the departmental workload.
   B. Financial management
      1. Develop departmental budget objectives consistent with the overall goals of the institution.
      2. Prepare departmental budget, allocating financial resources to meet departmental objectives, and prepare specifications for capital equipment requests.
      3. Review financial reports and use such control figures as variances and productive hours to provide timely evaluations of the department's conformance to budget; verify expenditures; monitor and evaluate staff productivity; and take action to meet budgeted productivity targeted.
   C. Personnel and resource management
      1. Develop workload standards to determine staffing requirements for the efficient use of personnel.
      2. Evaluate performance and clinical competency of the staff.
      3. Develop and revise job descriptions and performance standards, as necessary.
      4. Develop and submit monthly work schedules for all department employees.
      5. Monitor and direct corrective and disciplinary action

as appropriate to ensure standards of performance are met.

6. Respond to identified learning needs of staff and arrange for or provide educational programs.
7. Teach using lectures, discussion, and written materials on both general and specialized topics.
8. Plan, organize, coordinate, and direct in-service education and clinical training programs for nursing staff in coordination with the education department.
9. Validate nursing personnel in specialized procedures related to IV therapy.

D. Professional development

1. Assume responsibility for personal professional development; continuously update clinical skills, maintain required certifications, and keep abreast of current health care events.
2. Maintain association with professional and health-related associations and community groups.
3. Participate in professional seminars and workshops.
4. Maintain membership in professional organizations relevant to area of practice.

An important and challenging responsibility for the IV manager is ensuring technical and clinical expertise and maintaining staff morale in an arena in which most activities are carried out independently. It is crucial to hold regular staff meetings so that team members can openly share problems, questions, and educational needs. Staff meetings also provide an excellent opportunity for in-service training and reviewing procedures and equipment. Unit-based governing councils, which are part of a shared governance system, can also play an integral role in the success of the team and satisfaction of the staff. By empowering nurses and other staff, governing councils encourage greater commitment to the organization's goals and increased involvement and support to providing effective, high-quality health care.[10] The IV therapy manager must be aware of the aspects of shared governance that enhance the philosophy and meet the objectives of the IV team.

Larger and extremely active teams may require an assistant manager to assist with operational, clinical, and staff functions. The IV nursing specialist in this position could also serve as an educational coordinator, and share responsibility for staff development, competency reviews, and performance evaluation. The clinical qualifications for this role should be equal to those of the IV team manager, with some experience in nursing management functions desirable. Excellent communication skills are essential to this role, because this person is the primary liaison to nursing staff and other employees and departments within the facility.

An important supplemental role to be considered for inclusion in the IV therapy department is the educational coordinator. The educational coordinator's job description should include creating and maintaining an orientation program for new staff and providing continuing education and staff development programs and ongoing IV-related in-service training. The educational coordinator should also act as liaison to the medical and nursing staff and encourage staff to attend outside educational meetings and be active in their specialty organizations.

The educational coordinator should be responsible for teaching all clinical elements related to IV therapy practice. This individual either personally instructs or coordinates training classes or programs in management, supervision, consultation, technology, research, quality assurance, legal standards, communication, continuing education, patient and staff education, clinical judgment, and practice and procedures. The educational coordinator is responsible for orienting and assessing the clinical skills of new IV team members and providing clinical guidance to help all IV staff develop new skills. With organizational restructuring has come the additional responsibility of orienting the IV nurse to the role of educator. Providing in-service programs and assisting in skill validations have now become an integral component of the IV nurse's role. The educational coordinator shares learning principles that facilitate the IV nurse's transition to the role of educator. Encouraging IV nurses to participate in continuing education programs that are relevant to their specialty is an important aspect of the role. In addition, the coordinator is responsible for assisting the manager with personnel-related matters, including performance appraisals. The role could include responsibility for data collection, review and revision of policies and procedures, and planning and implementation of IV therapy–related competency reviews.

Teams in large facilities may find it appropriate to incorporate IV nurse specialists within the team who are dedicated to specific subspecialty areas of the discipline. The role could be defined as that of clinical resource person. For example, a staff member may be dedicated to all aspects of managing central venous catheters, nutritional support, or transfusion therapy or may be the validating agent for PICC insertion or chemotherapy administration. If there is a large and diverse pediatric population, there may be an IV team specialist for all aspects of pediatric infusion therapy. It is important to recognize the specialist as a valuable resource available throughout the institution for consultation.

Workload standards

To appropriately allocate resources and validate productivity of the IV team, some type of workload management system must be used.[11] This system must be specific for IV team activities and applicable to the institution. Workload standards provide a means for measuring productivity and help estimate staffing needs. Workload standards can be supported and customized by time and motion studies, or accepted, established standards can be used. Some IV teams have been able to develop systems or modify existing systems to include the specialty of IV therapy (Table 27-1 and Figs. 27-3 to 27-5).

A patient classification system (PCS) may also be used to justify and measure the IV workload. This type of system can be used to more accurately predict staffing requirements based on patient care needs, to validate the IV nursing team's productivity and cost-effectiveness, to prioritize the IV nursing workload, and to evaluate the quality of IV nursing care.[12] The following summarizes the steps for setting up a PCS for IV therapy.[13] Table 27-2 provides time values for IV therapy activities.

1. *Form a task force.* Participation of experienced IV nurses and nurse managers is essential to the development and acceptance of an accurate, workable system.

Table 27-1   **Inpatient IV Therapy Log Instructions**

ACTIVITY OR PROCEDURE	SAMPLE LOG ENTRY WITH COMMENTS	APPROXIMATE TIME SPENT (MIN)
New starts	# done. Simple start.	20
New starts (difficult)	# done. Difficult starts and/or 2 attempts.	45
Restart (RS)	# done. Simple restart.	20
RS (difficult)	# done. Difficult restart and/or 2 attempts.	45
Site check	# done. One for each patient. Includes site, bottle label and tubing labels, and "interventions."	10
IV push	# done. All meds pushed, including saline or heparin flushes.	5
Add-ons	# done. All solutions/piggybacks you hang. Does *not* include solution used for new start or blood product.	10
Blood products	Total # units. All blood products administered or delivered. Includes saline and tubing set-up.	
Blood	Blood	45
	Up to 10 units platelets (list platelets and cryo separately).	60
CVC dressing/discontinue CVC	Total # done.	20
Peripheral dsg	Total # done.	10
Change tubing	Total # done. Incl. CVC ext.	10
DC IV	Total # done. DC, no restart	10
Troubleshoot	Total # of times spent checking tubing problems, pump alarms, etc.	5
Port access	Total # done. Includes dsg.	30
Blood draws	Total # done. Periph and CVC	15
CVC insert assist	Total # done. Dsg. not incl.	45
Long-arm cath insert	Total # done. Dsg. not incl.	60
PICC insert	Total # done. Includes assessment. Dsg. not incl.	120
Admixtures	Total # prepared.	15
Code Blue	# codes responded to only.	30
IV cards	Total # prepared.	5
Janitorial/batching	Total time spent cleaning carts, stocking shelves, batching, etc.	
In-service, assist with patient care, pt. ed., nursing instruction	Total time spent in these activities.	
Extra time	Time spent over the allotted time for procedures. Anything not listed above, such as incident reports, searching for equipment, etc., policies and procedures.	

CVC, Central venous catheter; *DC*, discontinue; *PICC*, peripherally inserted cardiac catheter.

2. *Define IV therapy.* The goals and objectives of IV therapy must be reviewed and the scope of practice and service defined to provide a basis for workload measurement.

3. *Identify nursing activities.* Nursing activities include direct and indirect care. Direct care encompasses all nursing interventions provided directly to the patient, whereas indirect care consists primarily of supportive measures. Each activity is categorized and defined as to the necessary requirements.

4. *Develop time standards.* A time standard is defined as the amount of time required to perform an individual activity based on the definition. For direct care activities, time standards are determined by using the consensus method or by performing time studies (see Table 27-2). Indirect care activities are usually assigned a predetermined constant.

5. *Establish the frequency of activities.* Time and motion (frequency) studies provide a comprehensive database of activities performed, workload distribution, and staff utilization.

6. *Determine primary indicators.* Data from the frequency studies are instrumental in establishing major care activities, which represent approximately 90% of the total direct care workload. Workload measurement is limited to these primary indicators to offer an efficient, workable system. Time standards for these primary indicators are adjusted to compensate for excluded activities.

7. *Select system options.* IV therapy PCS can be based on prospective or retrospective data. Prospective data help predict activities to determine staffing need, whereas retrospective data offer a comprehensive workload measurement for productivity analysis. Other options include determining patient care hours per shift versus per day, using IV nursing care need codes versus actual time requirements, and implementing a manual versus a computerized system.

8. *Develop an IV care plan.* Based on the data determined by the previous steps, an IV care plan provides a format for recording data and calculating workload.

9. *Conduct a pilot study.* Testing the system on selected nursing units allows deficiencies to be identified and corrected before widespread implementation.

10. *Implement the system.* Educate the staff and implement the system on all nursing units.

	Date _____						Date _____						Date _____					
	Night	AM			PM		Night	AM			PM		Night	AM			PM	
		S	W		S	W		S	W		S	W		S	W		S	W
New starts (simple)																		
N.S. (difficult)																		
Restarts (simple)																		
R.S. (difficult)																		
Site checks																		
I.V. push																		
Add-ons																		
Blood products																		
CVC Dsg./DC CVC																		
Peripheral dressing																		
Change tubing																		
DC IV's																		
Troubleshoot																		
Port access																		
Blood draws																		
CVC insert-assist																		
Long arm cath insert																		
PICC insert																		
Admixtures																		
Code blue																		
IV cards																		
Janitorial/batch																		
Inserv/PT care/Ed.																		
Extra time																		
Initial																		
# Central caths																		
# PT on IV's																		
# Peripheral caths																		
Hospital census																		
QUALITY MANAGEMENT LOG																		
Phlebitis +1																		
+2																		
+3																		
Infiltrated																		
Clotted																		

FIG. 27-3 *Example of an inpatient IV therapy log.*

Staffing

To provide cost-effective patient care and reduce the incidence of complications related to IV therapy, an IV therapy team should provide full service with 24-hour-a-day coverage, 7 days a week.[7] The number of registered nurses on the team is determined by the number of hospital beds or patients served by the organization or agency, the type and volume of hands-on procedures performed, and IV therapies delivered. The ideal IV team is organized so that it consists of the management, educational, and IV nurse full-time equivalents (FTEs) needed to

STATISTICS: IV THERAPY (Inpatient)

The following statistical information is submitted for _____ .

	Actual Volume	Factor	Weighted Workload
Inpatient IV Therapy			
a. New starts (simple)	_____	× 1.33	_____
b. New starts (difficult)	_____	× 3.00	_____
c. Restarts (simple)	_____	× 1.33	_____
d. Restarts (difficult)	_____	× 3.00	_____
e. Site checks	_____	× 0.66	_____
f. IV push	_____	× 0.33	_____
g. Add-ons	_____	× 0.66	_____
h. Blood products	_____	× 3.00	_____
i. Platelets	_____	× 4.00	_____
j. CVC Dsg./DC CVC	_____	× 1.33	_____
k. Peripheral Dsg.	_____	× 0.66	_____
l. Change tubing	_____	× 0.66	_____
m. DC IV	_____	× 0.66	_____
n. Troubleshoot	_____	× 0.33	_____
o. Port access	_____	× 2.00	_____
p. Blood draws	_____	× 1.00	_____
q. CVC insert-assist	_____	× 3.00	_____
r. Long arm cath insert	_____	× 4.00	_____
s. PICC insertion	_____	× 8.00	_____
t. Admixtures	_____	× 1.00	_____
u. Code blue	_____	× 2.00	_____
v. IV cards	_____	× 0.33	_____
w. Miscellaneous	_____	× 0.33	_____
x. Administrative hours	_____	× 4.00	_____

(Unit of service: 1.00 factor = 15 minutes)

Total weighted units of service (UOS) = _____

FIG. 27-4 *Worksheet for determining weighted units of service for inpatient IV therapy.*

provide optimal service levels to all patients receiving IV therapy.

In reality, FTEs available for the IV therapy team are not always adequate to meet the ideal, and IV therapy department resources vary depending on the organization. Most IV teams probably do not have sufficient staffing resources to provide all specialty services and the related levels of care for their specialty. Having to work within such limitations, a choice must be made regarding how best to use the expertise of the team within the facility. A good approach is the phasing in of team functions over time. Initial services should address the most pressing needs and should be based on a realistic workload to establish the team on a firm footing. Once the team has been organized and is operating smoothly, successfully performing designated functions, additional services can be proposed as needs are recognized and resources allow. The managed care environment increasingly demands efficiency, improved productivity, and reduced costs.[14] As cost becomes an increasing concern, the use of IV nurse specialists allows increased quality and decreased cost to coexist.[15]

When a full-service team cannot be justified, a limited-service team, although not ideal, may be able to provide quality team services for some aspects of IV care. Budget considerations will define the limited-service hours. Limited-service teams can vary widely in the allocation of service hours. Typical options include covering day and evening hours, with no coverage during the night shift. Time studies related to workload volume help define the greatest hours of need. Some teams can flex their shift coverage into the late night and early morning hours, leaving only a 4- to 6-hour period without IV team coverage. This is obviously preferred when there are no resources for a full-service team because it offers the least interruption of service. Other teams may offer services only during expanded day-shift hours (i.e., early morning to early evening). This provides some consistent, quality care by IV nurses but leaves primary responsibility related to IV care to staff nurses during

STATISTICS: IV THERAPY (Outpatient)

The following statistical information is submitted for _____ .

(month)   (year)

Outpatient IV Therapy	Actual Volume	Factor	Weighted Workload
a. Starts	_____	× 2.00	_____
b. Site check	_____	× 0.66	_____
c. IV push chemo	_____	× 2.00	_____
d. CVC dressing	_____	× 2.00	_____
e. CVC blood draw	_____	× 2.00	_____
f. Port access	_____	× 2.00	_____
g. Med. Admin. IVP/IM/SQ (other)	_____	× 0.66	_____
h. Amb. pump (setup/DC/CassChn)	_____	× 4.00	_____
i. Chemo infusion	_____	× 3.00	_____
j. PRBC transfusion	_____	× 8.00	_____
k. Platelet transfusion	_____	× 6.00	_____
l. Gamma globulin infusion	_____	× 5.00	_____
m. Phlebotomy	_____	× 4.00	_____
n. Peripheral blood draws	_____	× 1.00	_____
o. PIC or PICC insertion	_____	× 3.00	_____
p. Hydration therapy	_____	× 2.00	_____
q. Janitorial/stocking	_____	× 1.00	_____
r. Teaching	_____	× 2.00	_____
s. Observation time	_____	× 1.00	_____
t. Insurance verification	_____	× 1.00	_____
u. CVC insertion assist	_____	× 3.00	_____
v. Infusaid refill	_____	× 3.00	_____
w. Miscellaneous	_____	× 0.33	_____
x. Pharmacy compounding (UOS)			_____

(Unit of service: 1.00 factor = 15 minutes)

Total weighted units of service (UOS) = _____

FIG. 27-5 *Worksheet for determining weighted units of service for outpatient IV therapy.*

the hours when there is no IV team coverage. This may lead to inaccurate data collection and inconsistent quality of care. When a limited-service IV team is in place, responsibility for IV functions during off-service hours must be clearly defined and understood to minimize the interruption of therapy. It is important to the ongoing collection of clinical data and to the workload management of the IV team that services to be performed by the general nursing staff are clearly communicated.

Initially, to secure the hours needed for core or basic staffing, many of the nurses and nursing hours can be transferred from the general nursing department and dedicated to IV therapy services. This eliminates the need for massive recruiting and hiring. There is a period of orientation and in-service training required during the initial phase. Ongoing monitoring of staff and systems at this time is crucial to address any problems that might arise. To determine staffing requirements, time studies must be completed for each IV function, keeping in mind that

Table 27-2	**Example of Time Values**		
Activity	**Adjusted Time (min)**	**Computer Time (min)**	**Kardex Points***
IV push	10.78	10.8	2
Site care	3.18	3.2	1
Piggyback	6.49	6.5	1
Venipuncture	16.08	16.1	3
Tubing change	7.08	7.1	1
TPN	5.24	5.2	1
CVC dressing	25.56	25.6	4
PCA	28.95	29.0	5
Chemotherapy	27.41	27.4	4
Blood	37.27	37.3	6
Indirect care	6.00	6.0	1

TPN, Total parenteral nutrition; *CVC*, central venous catheter; *PCA*, patient-controlled analgesia.
*1 point = 6 min.

productivity and efficiency improve after implementation. A time study should collect data on the average number of IV patients, the number of lines per patient, IV functions performed on each shift, and admixtures prepared for each nursing unit. With the average time for each activity determined from current literature or for each facility, staffing needs can be estimated. Subsequently, the number of hours spent to perform IV therapy can be determined, as can the number of FTEs. After selecting the team members, additional departmental costs can be predicted.[16] Using time study estimates and estimated volume data to define distribution of the workload, staffing levels for each shift can be determined. For greater accuracy, provisions for fatigue, delays, and travel time can be factored in. Orientation, vacation, holiday, and sick time relief can be estimated based on the benefits provided to team members and on historical data for even more accurate staffing estimates.

IV teams that are also responsible for outpatient therapy need to plan for additional staffing hours. Outpatient services may be provided in a dedicated room in the hospital setting or in an alternative setting. For smaller, hospital-based outpatient service operations, in-hospital IV nurses may be able to cover staffing needs, especially for scheduled services. Ideally, an IV nurse should be assigned exclusively to cover outpatient and home settings. To be cost-effective, all members of the IV team, whether in the hospital or an outpatient setting, should be able to function when needed in either environment. Twenty-four-hour service departments can also use their evening and night shifts in a cost-effective manner to cover off-hour calls from outpatients. They can be a valuable resource for the home health staff in problem solving when they are managing the patient in the home setting, and for the staff of skilled nursing facilities. Coordinating with the home health agency to make the necessary interventions in the home when the patient cannot come in to the IV nurse is an acceptable option. The initial contact and assessment for IV therapy–related issues should remain with the IV nurse specialist.

One problem encountered in staffing for the IV team is meeting emergency needs. How to cover that last-minute sick call or the extended illness of an employee is a dilemma that needs careful consideration by the IV team manager before it happens. It is more difficult for smaller teams that offer specialized services to maintain flexible staffing. For such teams, it is difficult to draw qualified staff from the general nursing population or even from outside agencies. Thought must be given to maintaining reliable on-call RN resources. One solution is to cross-train interested nurses from the critical care specialty or the emergency department, where venipuncture skills are most likely to be maintained. The workload distribution may need to be adjusted temporarily to integrate nonspecialist staff. For example, routine restarts should be assigned to the per diem staff and care of central line dressings to the IV nurse specialist. In areas where there are a number of IV teams or home infusion organizations that might provide IV nurse specialists, those resources could be used and shared. This practice will give IV nurse specialists a wide experience base and will meet the community's needs. The possibility for establishing community-wide adherence to standards in infusion care becomes more realistic with large numbers of specialists involved in the practice.

Of course, for organizations with 24-hour IV team coverage, staffing problems are magnified. Without careful attention to maintaining resources, the cost in overtime and the decline in levels of quality or service could be detrimental to the objectives of the IV team. Smaller teams should plan carefully for meeting staffing needs in many situations. Crisis staffing has a decidedly negative effect on the operations of the IV team.

Provision of services

Challenging aspects of managing the IV team include those associated with the selection, development, and retention of staff. The importance of those who staff the IV team cannot be overemphasized. They are often the most important ingredients for the success of an IV team. Each candidate must be viewed critically for the skills and qualities that are needed to enhance the department, organization, and profession.

Human resources management

Interview process. Determining the professional, social, and personal values that are shared by the manager and staff can provide the common bonds that make it easier to organize a team, design systems, budget appropriately, and move toward a common goal. The interview process provides an excellent opportunity to assess those values. It is important to have an interview tool or technique that yields the information necessary to make the right choices for meeting the team's needs. Thought should also go into how the individual can fit within the organization. Some interview models involve a panel composed of key staff members. These panels can be valuable, particularly when there are internal and external candidates; they can improve the likelihood of making the best selection.

The interview process becomes especially important when considering a candidate for work in a setting in which he or she has never functioned. For example, technical skills are important, but assessment and teaching skills are also essential and have a different focus in the outpatient or home infusion setting than in the acute care environment. It is important that the candidate's skills fit the setting and meet the requirements for the position. The following outline is an example of an interview tool to use for the IV nurse candidate.

Questions based on the following elements are suggested for interviews for IV nurse clinical staff. Because of the diverse and extensive level of knowledge required by the IV nursing professional, it is important to question the candidate thoroughly regarding IV-related experience and education. Examples of patient scenarios may be presented to help evaluate the candidate's IV abilities. Throughout the interview, it is also important to assess the candidate's personality and ability to work independently, yet still be a team player.

I. Previous experience
  A. Experience and areas worked related to IV therapy
  B. Number of years in acute care
  C. Last day worked in acute care

II. Education and training
  A. Nursing degree achieved/Public Health Nurse Certificate
  B. National certification
  C. Advanced cardiac life support/CPR
  D. IV-related education and training
  E. PICC certification
  F. Goals for certification or degree
III. IV therapy–related technical and clinical experience
  A. Peripheral catheter insertion: number of insertions/day
    1. Experience with pediatric and neonatal care
  B. Short-term central venous catheters
    1. Assistance with insertion
    2. Dressing changes
    3. Blood draws
    4. Patient education
  C. Long-term central venous catheters
    1. Assistance with insertion
    2. Dressing changes
    3. Patient education
    4. Blood draws
    5. Catheter repair and declotting
    6. Port access
  D. PICC catheters
    1. Experience with insertion
    2. Dressing changes
  E. Intraspinal catheters
    1. Dressing changes
    2. Medication administration
    3. Implanted pump refills
  F. Blood product administration
    1. Red cell products
    2. Platelets
    3. Fresh-frozen plasma
    4. Cryoprecipitate
    5. Use of microaggregate and leukocyte removal filters
  G. Admixtures
    1. Use of laminar flow hood
  H. Participation in Code Blues
    1. Familiarity with administering cardiac drugs
  I. Electronic monitoring device experience
    1. Pole-mounted infusion pumps
    2. Ambulatory infusion pumps
    3. PCA (patient-controlled analgesia)
  J. Experience working with chemotherapy agents
IV. Teaching
  A. Experience with patient teaching
    1. Was the experience positive?
  B. Staff education experience
    1. In-service training received in teaching strategies, among other programs
    2. Interest level in providing in-service training to staff and other IV nurses
V. Committee participation
  A. Previous committee participation
  B. Interest in committee participation
VI. Overall questions
  A. What qualifies a person for this position?
VII. Daily situation questions
  A. It is the end of the shift and your relief is not here; what action should be taken?
  B. A co-worker consistently does something that drives you crazy, such as leaving the IV cart a mess. How should this be handled?
VIII. Work schedule
  A. Shifts and hours preferred
  B. Number of days and pay period preferred
  C. Availability on short notice
  D. Feelings about reduction in work hours because of low patient census or overtime related to very high patient census
  E. Willingness to attend meetings

When that perfect candidate is elusive, the next best thing is to hire the potentially perfect IV nurse who may lack the required skills but has the required nursing experience and a great interest in the IV nursing specialty. The nurse's potential can be realized through a staff development program flexible enough to meet general needs, but that also addresses the individual needs identified for each new member of the team.

Performance standards. It must be the clear expectation that each member of the team is accountable for his or her own practice and performance. A system for measuring performance with clearly defined criteria must be established. It is valuable to have the participation of the IV team in defining the criteria.

The IV therapy team manager should be responsible for timely performance appraisals, required annually but also essential at intervals throughout the year; for coaching team members to higher levels of performance; and for submitting recommendations to strengthen performance. This can take place during informal coaching sessions to enhance performance and recognize success. The following outline is an example of criteria-based performance standards for evaluating IV nursing clinical personnel. It is the manager's responsibility to provide an equitable system for evaluating performance in relation to standards and expectations. In some instances, scenarios may be presented to further evaluate responses and interactions with others.

To facilitate objectivity and consistency in the evaluation process, each standard should be detailed with specific criteria for measurement.

I. Patient care management
  A. Actively communicates with physician.
  B. Reviews and interprets progress notes and appropriately implements physician orders.
  C. Exhausts all options to obtain appropriate and timely physician response.
  D. Maintains accurate diagnosis and current plan of care on IV therapy profile cards.
  E. Concisely communicates plan of care in shift report.
  F. Reviews patient tests, interprets results, and correlates this information with overall plan of care.
  G. Identifies potential problems related to patient diagnosis.

H. Complies with current medication administration policies and procedures.

II. Nursing process

A. Obtains an initial IV assessment; assesses patients with regard to diagnosis and/or special conditions that have any bearing on IV therapy.

B. Implements IV nursing measures to prevent potential problems related to patient's diagnosis and hospitalization.

C. Plans IV care for assigned patients; integrates IV care with the nursing care plan.

D. Communicates with medical and nursing colleagues, patients, patients' family, and allied health disciplines.

E. Assesses psychosocial needs and makes appropriate referrals.

F. Participates in quality assessment activities.

G. Fulfills the criteria for JCAHO and hospital nursing process requirements as evaluated by the process of five random chart audits.

III. Teamwork

A. Uses problem resolution skills to improve unit environment.

B. Observes and reports unsafe practices using notification system and appropriate channels of communication.

C. Manages time to complete assignments within time allotted on shift; when not possible to complete, informs manager of need for assistance.

D. Listens actively to patient and family complaints and endeavors to correct problem or refers to an appropriate authority.

E. Demonstrates flexibility as staffing needs change.

F. Assists as requested with orientation of staff members and teaching of general nursing staff and others.

IV. Discharge planning

A. Initiates referrals to IV therapy clinic, case management, or home health to plan for potential posthospital infusion care.

B. Implements patient education as related to outpatient IV therapy; develops teaching plans for individual patients.

V. Professionalism

A. Shares new knowledge with co-workers after attending programs such as director-approved continuing education classes and seminars.

B. Identifies own learning needs and pursues appropriate education.

C. Actively participates in evaluation of new products and equipment.

D. Reviews IV therapy policies and procedures during daily performance of duties.

E. Actively participates in new unit procedures and research projects.

F. Exhibits a positive attitude toward changes in the health care profession.

G. Participates in evaluation of own performance by identifying strengths and weaknesses and developing a plan to improve weak areas.

VI. Environmental safety

A. Demonstrates responsibility for patient safety by assessing need for safety precautions, instituting a safe plan of care, and providing a safe patient environment.

B. Demonstrates knowledge and application of infection control policies and procedures.

C. Demonstrates understanding of such emergency procedures as fire drills, evacuation measures, and disaster policies.

VII. Technical skills

A. Demonstrates competency in setting up, programming, and troubleshooting pumps, including the following:

1. PCA pumps
2. Ambulatory pumps
3. Syringe pumps
4. Pole-mounted pumps

VIII. Clinical skills

A. Follows proper policy and procedures with venipunctures.

B. Properly assesses IV sites and takes appropriate action to rectify any existing problems.

C. Follows proper policy and procedure when caring for short- and long-term central venous catheters.

D. Demonstrates proper policy and procedure and follows physician's orders when administering chemotherapeutic agents.

E. Follows proper policy and procedure when preparing admixtures.

F. Follows proper policy and procedure when administering blood products.

G. Demonstrates necessary knowledge and follows proper procedure in responding to codes.

H. Follows proper policy and procedure when caring for intraspinal catheters.

Performance recognition. There are several models for rewarding clinical experience and expertise. The preferred programs are those that recognize professional achievement and have a monetary incentive. The clinical ladder is a type of program that some facilities have customized to meet their criteria. It is a means for identifying competency, providing recognition and financial reward, promoting accountability and participation, and enhancing self-worth and positive morale.[17] It is an incentive and reward for the nurse who chooses to remain in a clinical role rather than advance into management. Successful clinical ladder programs for IV nurses can provide a system for recognizing and validating the expertise and higher clinical skill levels they have achieved. If the facility has a clinical ladder program, it can be customized for the IV team, no matter where the team is in the organization and whether the team is made up of RNs, LVNs, or both. It is essential to work with the human resources department to design and implement the program. The evaluation tools used can and must be adjusted to the clinical ladder.

Several types of clinical ladder programs have been used; the most common have three to five levels. These levels can include only education and experience, or, when considering criteria for the IV nurse specialty, can expand to include advanced skills, responsibilities, and certification. The following outline is an example of the basics of the clinical ladder levels:

I. Clinical Nurse I: entry level nurse or new graduate. RN with less than 1 year experience.

II. Clinical Nurse II

A. At least 1 year recent and relevant experience as a RN.

B. Clinical Nurse I may apply for the Clinical Nurse II level if employed as an RN for a minimum of 1 year and has received a "meets standards" rating on current evaluation.

III. Clinical Nurse III

A. Clinical Nurse II may apply for Clinical Nurse III level if a graduate of an accredited RN school of nursing, has worked a minimum of 1040 hours in each of the required years of experience specified in the following criteria, and meets one of the following criteria:

1. Baccalaureate degree in nursing with at least 3 years of RN experience in an acute care facility. Current evaluation must be above standards.

2. Baccalaureate degree in a field other than nursing with at least 4 years of RN experience in an acute care facility. Current full evaluation must be above standards.

3. Associate degree nurse or diploma program graduate with 5 to 10 years of experience in an acute care facility, 2 years of which must have been at the current facility. Also, the last evaluation must be above standards.

4. Associate degree nurse or diploma program graduate with 8 years of RN experience, based on anniversary date. Current evaluation must be above standards.

5. Master's degree in nursing (MSN) and at least 2 years of experience as a RN in an acute care facility. Current evaluation must be above standards.

6. Master's degree in a field other than nursing and at least 3 years of experience as an RN in an acute care facility. Current full evaluation must be above standards.

IV. Clinical Nurse IV: A Clinical Nurse II or III is eligible to apply for the Clinical Nurse IV level if a graduate of an accredited RN school of nursing, has worked a minimum of 1040 hours in each of the required years of experience specified in the following criteria, and meets one of the following criteria:

A. Baccalaureate degree in nursing with at least 6 years of RN experience in an acute care facility, 3 years while practicing with a degree, and 1 year of the 3 as a Clinical Nurse III. Current evaluation must be above standards.

B. Baccalaureate degree in a field other than nursing with at least 7 years of RN experience in an acute care facility, 3 years while practicing with this degree, and 1 year of the 3 as a Clinical Nurse III. Current evaluation must be above standards.

C. Master's degree in nursing (MSN) with 3 years of RN experience in an acute care facility, 1 while practicing with MSN. Current evaluation must be above standards.

D. Master's degree in a field other than nursing with 4 years of RN experience in an acute care facility, 1 year while practicing with the Masters degree. Current evaluation must be above standards.

In this model, there would be no level I nurses on the IV team. It is necessary to define the skill levels and the productivity criteria that make an IV nurse eligible for moving to another level on the ladder. The criteria are specific to each practice and each facility. Attainment of national IV nursing certification through the Intravenous Nurses Certification Corporation should be integral in the design or added to the evaluation tool. Credentialing is one of the most essential ways for IV team staff to validate their competencies and lend credence to their specialty.

Another essential role for the IV therapy team manager is competency review and assessment for adherence to policies, procedures, and standards. This review might be an expectation for anyone who is responsible for managing IV access or administration. It is a necessary part of the orientation to a new procedure or piece of equipment. The regular observation of routine skills helps ensure adherence to standards and enhances practice.

The clinical role the IV team manager assumes is service and resource dependent. It is critical that the manager maintain skills and expertise in all aspects of IV therapy. Changes in the delivery of IV therapy are occurring at an astounding rate. The effective manager needs to remain abreast of all these developments to maintain credibility as a resource and to adjust services appropriately.

Policies and procedures

The IV team manager is responsible for developing and continuously revising all IV therapy–related policies and procedures for the team and institution. Policies and procedures are the groundwork for departmental and clinical functions, serve as a guide to its operations, and give direction for safe, quality IV care throughout the facility.

It is important to carefully consider the format and content of these written documents, which are used as guidelines for practice. Policies describe the defined purpose and course of action and may be where the standard is described. There should be a detailed list of steps to be followed; the procedure, rationale for the action, expected result of the action, and steps to be followed when the expected result does not occur should also be presented. It is important to describe the products being used, including information on their effectiveness, safety, and risks. It is helpful to evaluate the format and content of the procedure by testing whether someone unfamiliar with the practice could complete the procedure appropriately by following the instructions. Standards covering principles of care should be used to achieve the end result or expected outcome. It is helpful, and in some facilities required, to list supporting references for the policy. This list can be a part of the document, or it might be included in a separate section. The dates of approval and implementation must be documented and a record kept of committee approval.

The manager must ensure that policies and procedures comply with state and federal laws and follow national standards and guidelines, such as those from the INS, Centers for Disease Control and Prevention, JCAHO, Occupational Safety and Health Administration (OSHA), and American Association of Blood Banks (AABB). The appropriate hospital committees must approve IV therapy policies and procedures. Because of the invasive aspects of IV therapy, many hospitals require physician approval. After procedures are written and approved, they must be made available to the nursing staff in addition to members of the IV team. Training and orientation programs used to implement procedures must be documented, including records of those in attendance. The education department is an excellent adjunct to the education and implementation process. In fact, everyone involved in administering IV therapy must be familiar with the approved policies and procedures, with appropriate updates as needed.

Quality management

Improving the quality of IV therapy administered to patients increases the rate of positive patient outcomes and supports the rationale for using an IV therapy team. Through monitoring, IV nurse specialists can provide the necessary information for determining that standards of care are being met. Criteria such as phlebitis, infection, clotted device, and infiltration rates are measurable indicators. The IV team manager assesses the impact, reports the findings, and makes recommendations for improving outcomes, as necessary.

The objective of therapy monitoring is to evaluate the quality of IV nursing as reflected in patient care records. Consequently, specific criteria or standards of care must be developed so that reviewers know precisely what constitutes quality IV nursing care. Evaluation standards and monitoring criteria for IV therapy can be developed and data retrieval methods implemented to help evaluate criteria. The following list suggests some criteria worth evaluating:

- Are needles disposed of in tamper-proof, leak-proof, puncture-proof, disposable containers?
- Are the principles of asepsis followed in setting up equipment?
- Is the patency of intermittent infusion devices verified before medications are administered?
- Are hands washed properly before patient contact?
- Are gloves worn during venipuncture and removal of IV catheters?
- Are approved skin-preparation practices performed?
- Is the IV access device properly inserted?
- Is the IV nurse attempting venipuncture more than twice?
- Is the nurse pushing IV medications using proper procedure?
- Does the nurse flush with saline before and after the IV push administration?
- Is documentation accurate, complete, and legible?

In addition to assessing whether these steps are actually being followed, the therapy audit must also judge how well they are being completed. Does the degree to which the step is accomplished fall far below, meet, slightly exceed, or far exceed the standard? On a less frequent schedule, the IV audit should be expanded to assess the team's performance in more detail, considering questions such as the following:

- Is the IV solution container labeled with the patient's name and room number, type of solution and additives, time and date mixed, and IV bag or bottle number?
- Is the IV administration set labeled with the appropriate date and time?
- Has the IV access site been labeled with the type, gauge, and length of device, date and time inserted, and initials of the person performing the insertion?
- Have all connections been secured?
- Is the documentation complete?

The data collection forms must allow objective ratings, identification of problem areas, random-data collection, and timely reporting. IV therapy must be monitored to ensure the quality of patient care, reinforce accountability, and enhance learning. Exceptional performance and exceptional patient outcomes are criteria for the success of IV team services. Monitoring not only discloses areas where patient care could be improved, but also identifies areas where the team is performing exceptionally well. In addition, properly conducted monitoring of IV therapy improves communication among professionals and encourages better documentation.

Perhaps the best measure of quality in health care is the customer's perception of the product or service provided. Quality can be achieved only when the provider knows and understands the patient's requirements, the variation among customers, and applicable standards of practice. The entire organization, from the top down, should be committed to quality improvement and the delivery of quality care. JCAHO has embraced this concept in its *Agenda for Change,* and by developing indicators that focus on quality improvement.

Continuing education and in-service programs related to IV therapy should be provided by IV nurse specialists. This is an important marketing tool for any IV team or infusion company and establishes the importance of the IV nurse and his or her specialized knowledge. When an IV nurse participates in the orientation of new staff nurses, a valuable opportunity is provided to discuss the benefits of the IV team to the institution and to their individual practices. Educational offerings provided by IV nurses also ensure that other nurses in the community are being provided with the same knowledge base and that the information provided is current and in accordance with established standards and guidelines.

The goal of any quality management program is to establish an organizational culture of excellent service that permeates administrative priorities, strategic planning, policies and procedures, physical design, and staff attitudes and behaviors.[16] It is possible that most IV teams already meet the objectives for this system. Actively soliciting patient/customer feedback is a component that the IV team can easily add to its services because personal contact is required for every service. It is essential that the results of that feedback, both negative and positive, be addressed. When the IV team manager responds to concerns, complaints, and compliments by immediately contacting the customer and staff, he or she can ensure that steps are taken to improve service, and can reinforce and reward behaviors that result in satisfaction and acceptable outcomes.

Financial management

The financial profile of the IV therapy department can be efficiently recorded and analyzed by establishing it as a separate cost center. This allows the IV team manager, accounting, and administration not only to measure the department's current status, but also to project its future impact on the institution's fiscal plan.

The budget, which is the fiscal or financial plan for a business, is necessary for examining the costs incurred for each department or service. It is one means for justifying the IV team. Costs, which include supplies and labor, are calculated as direct or indirect expenses. The IV team manager or director is responsible for developing the budget, which must include personnel, operations, and capital expenditures. Consideration should be given to indirect departmental costs, such as those for electricity, telephone, facsimile lines, computer and other equipment maintenance, food and office supplies, and personal protective equipment that might not be included in the operating budget. Items or programs included in the budget are determined by the organization. The more input the department manager has in the process, the easier it is to calculate the budget and determine the financial guidelines under which the department functions and by which it is judged.

For the operating budget, the calculations encompass all IV therapy department salaries, including those for managers, professional staff, and support staff, such as clerical workers. This is usually the highest cost item in the budget.

The cost items included for each employee are base salary plus any estimated raises, shift differentials, and other differentials, such as credentialing, where applicable. Benefits must be factored in, including each employee's accrued vacation, holiday and sick time, insurance, retirement, tuition assistance, education, and other paid benefits. This total is calculated using projected productive hours for each employee or each position. Overtime calculations for each position, holiday coverage, and any on-call hours anticipated for the department are estimated based on the projected hours needed. Departmental productive hours, hours needed for departmental functions, and nonproductive hours, such as education, sick time, and administrative time, are totaled and calculated at the rate determined by the mix of employees to make up the final budget dollar amount.

The operating budget also includes expenses for the supplies and equipment necessary for the department to function, which might not include patient chargeable items. This figure might include expenses for such items as pharmaceuticals, instruments, medical-surgical supplies, miscellaneous office supplies, forms, travel, and education programs.

The operating budget may be projected in several ways, as determined by the finance department. Examining historical costs for IV-related expenses and calculating a cost per procedure, per work unit, or per patient day may be used for these projections. It is important to include projections for new programs in the budgeting process.

The capital expenditure budget reflects purchases of major equipment such as office furniture and equipment, electronic infusion instruments, IV carts, beepers, and computers. There is usually a cap, such as $500, which must be exceeded for equipment to be placed in the capital expenditures budget. Construction project budgeting may also be the responsibility of the department manager.

Revenue projections are included in the operating budget. It is sometimes possible for the IV team to charge for services in addition to supplies; for an IV nurse placing an access device, for example, or other specialized services. Reimbursement is often determined by payer contracts and must always be investigated.

It is important that the staff be aware of and involved in the budget process, which is so important to the team's functions. With input in the decision-making process, there is more acceptance of responsibility for the outcomes.

The budget is the guideline used to examine the financial performance of the IV team. Each component of the budget should be reviewed and analyzed at least monthly. It is the manager's responsibility to explain any deviations between budget and actual costs and to implement corrective actions, when necessary. The monthly review is also a chance to report cost savings. If the department implements practices that result in savings, these should be recognized and reported, stating the dollars saved. For example, if the IV team selects needle safety devices for IV therapy and implements their use throughout the facility, the savings in needlestick costs can readily be identified. Unless the manager reports it, however, others may not attribute this improvement to the IV team.

Special Considerations

Fiscal restraints and organizational redesign necessitate that hospitals consider both internal and external environmental factors. An analysis of internal factors should begin by identifying the institution's priorities and then demonstrating how the IV team relates to those priorities. For example, if the facility has placed a high priority on improving the quality of IV care because of current deficiencies, the justification should focus on the advantages brought to the institution by the specialized knowledge and skill of the IV team. A complete internal analysis should also consider the institution's financial status and political structure, and the attitudes and perceptions of physicians, floor nurses, and patients. The external analysis should examine the effect of regulatory and demographic changes, changes in third-party payer reimbursement, competitor activities, limited human resources (e.g., shortage of nurses in the community), changes in availability or cost of supplies, and new technology.

Cost considerations

The significant rise in the cost of hospital care over recent years has prompted much discussion and action about cost containment efforts. Unfortunately, measures to contain cost impose limitations on revenues without addressing the issue of expenses. The new health care market requires nurses to partner with the institutions in which they work to provide high-quality, cost-efficient, care that promotes patient satisfaction.[18] It is essential that IV teams analyze the costs of delivering IV therapy to identify potential savings. Cost justification is an obvious and critical element in maintaining and justifying an IV team. Members of the team help achieve this goal by maintaining high productivity levels, reducing incidence of complications related to IV therapy, using products prudently, and producing revenue.

Clinical data have demonstrated that IV teams are cost-effective because of their efficient and effective use of equipment and because IV nurses practice at high productivity levels. Because it has already been demonstrated that an IV team can significantly improve patient care, the future of IV team services will be largely determined by the extent to which the team can support itself. The IV team can exist in the modern prospective reimbursement environment if it can become recognized as an important service, document the benefits it provides, and obtain patient and physician endorsement of its services. To justify, organize, and develop an IV team, it must be established that it is an important asset to a facility. It must also be shown that an IV team is well managed, has documented advantages, provides cost-effective services, and improves patient outcomes.

An IV therapy team controls costs by performing procedures and managing material resources efficiently. High productivity and thorough, accurate documentation have a positive impact on total costs. IV team managers must document the team's services so the associated costs and benefits can be quantified. If IV nurses, through specialization, develop expertise that reduces labor and material costs while decreasing the average length of stay and the incidence of IV-related complications, this information must be presented to administration, with figures that support these accomplishments.

The ability of specialized IV nursing teams to reduce labor costs can be an asset in any institution. Labor is the highest cost for most institutions and is obviously an area with tremendous potential for cost savings. In any given institution, a certain number of nurses must spend their time delivering IV therapy. Generalist nurses might be spending two, three, or four times longer than an infusion nurse specialist delivering the same therapy. It stands to reason that substantial hours could be made available and redirected to other areas if an IV team were developed and made responsible for all IV-related aspects of patient care. An IV team should be considered an integral part of whatever professional practice model the institution adopts. Because labor represents the highest cost associated with IV therapy, it is important to show that labor can become more efficient by using IV specialists. An IV therapy team saves time and decreases costs by assuming responsibilities and tasks formerly performed by staff RNs and performing them more efficiently. The time saved can be redirected to other patient care activities. Although the experience and statistics of IV teams in other hospitals may be used to justify a team, the relative amount of labor required for IV services in the specific institution should be determined and considered independently.

IV teams can also lower hospital costs by using supplies and equipment more efficiently. Supplies are often used ineffectively in hospitals. The IV nurse who uses IV therapy–related equipment is the best source for evaluating the institution's needs. An IV therapy team lowers expenses by standardizing and control-ling the use of IV-related materials and equipment and by controlling inventories of solutions and devices through a centralized system. The IV team should be responsible for purchasing products that are most suitable for the institution, considering the patient population and staff expertise, and for standardizing equipment as much as possible throughout the institution. Consideration must also be given to the amounts and types of products needed, product cost and quality comparisons, and the most cost-effective supply sources. When IV equipment is standardized throughout the institution, benefits result from cost savings available through manufacturer discounts for large-quantity purchases and the greater availability of equipment. The IV nurse should also actively participate in in-service training for new equipment with the company representative, not only to provide credibility to the new product but to assess reactions of the nursing staff and answer questions related to the institution and its policies and procedures. Should follow-up in-service sessions be necessary, the IV team may act as a readily available resource for the institution.

The demand for IV services should be assessed by using such figures as the number and type of IV services; number of patients receiving IV therapy; complexity of IV therapy procedures and materials used; and nurse time for each patient, department, and diagnosis-related group (DRG). The potential for IV therapy use should be quantified for each DRG by the percentage of patients receiving IV therapy, average IV costs and charges per patient, and total and average patient days. The severity of the illness of hospital patients should also be assessed because IV therapy needs increase with acuity as determined by secondary diagnoses, age, malnutrition, dehydration, and surgical versus medical stay.

Marketing is an essential component for the ongoing justification of IV services. The patient, our consumer, is a strong advocate for IV teams. The IV team has an important product to offer through its expertise, knowledge, and standardization of care. It is important to promote the benefits of the IV team and build a good reputation based on quality of service. An IV team should be marketed as a potential source for referrals or admissions. This includes inpatient and outpatient services, such as education and IV services for home care patients and clinics.

Reimbursement

Over the last decade, DRGs and the prospective payment system (PPS) have resulted in substantial changes in the overall plan for justifying IV teams. The PPS produces a list of prices that Medicare pays for services delivered for each DRG. With the advent of changes in Medicare payment, the institution is accordingly reimbursed at a prospectively determined rate for treating a specific case, irrespective of the charges accumulated during the patient's stay. Use of the PPS negated one of the reasons most IV teams were organized during the period of Medicare cost reimbursement: to maximize hospital reimbursement by establishing IV therapy as an ancillary service. Under government PPS, hospital administrators view all ancillary departments, including IV teams, as cost centers rather than as revenue centers. If an administrator determines that another cost center can deliver IV services more cost-effectively, the IV team concept may be discarded. In addition to documenting other potential and real cost savings, IV therapy teams have also tried to maximize revenue from other payers who are still willing to pay for services rendered by IV nurses. Services such as inserting access devices (e.g., PICCs and midarm catheters, which require special knowledge and expertise that the IV nurse specialist is most likely to possess) may be reimbursed. Contracting to provide those services to alternative settings may be another revenue source. Despite these revenue sources, it is clear that the primary justification for the IV therapy team is no longer as a source of revenue for the institution. Instead, the primary justification is that the IV therapy team is an exceptionally capable provider of cost-effective care.

With the advent of DRGs and managed care, length of stay has become a critical measure of a hospital's success. Consequently, departments or systems that can reduce the number of days a patient has to stay in the hospital may determine whether the institution operates profitably. Using an IV team ensures that therapy is consistently delivered as ordered. The team prevents delays in administering therapy because of its proficiency in starting IVs and its skill in preventing IV-related complications. A successful IV team also provides dedicated time for IV nurses to investigate physician orders, plan for therapy, and make recommendations for vascular access needs. This type of case management prevents the unnecessary continuation of IVs and ensures that the most appropriate type of infusion device is inserted for the reliable delivery of therapy. To determine how an IV team affects length of stay, the researcher should begin by identifying, for each DRG, patients with abnormally long stays and the reasons for those extended stays. Common reasons for extended stays include severity of disease, nosocomial infection, medical complication, lack of IV placement and resultant interruption of therapy, delayed laboratory results, and failure to discontinue IV therapy. The next step is to determine a percentage of cost savings that is attributable to the IV team (e.g., the number of patient days or supplies saved because of IV nurse intervention). It is also important to determine the number and percentage of patients discharged to home IV therapy services, the number of patients who could be discharged if outpatient or home IV services were available, the revenue potential based on current reimbursement policy and payer mix, and the cost of providing these services. By deducting costs from revenues, the profitability of an IV team can be estimated and promoted.[16]

Quality of care

Another reason for organizing an IV team is to enhance quality of care by using competent IV therapy specialists. However, this can be difficult to prove objectively. The philosophy of the INS is that IV nursing teams should be used to minimize patient risk and to ensure quality services.[7] Because 80% to 90% of all hospitalized patients require IV therapy, it makes sense that the clinical expertise of an IV nursing team be used to meet the increasingly complex needs of these patients. IV nursing teams provide high-quality patient care through more frequent monitoring of IV treatment modalities, thereby significantly decreasing the risk of complications related to IV therapy.[7] Because not all IV therapy complications are preventable, an administrator can question whether an IV team minimizes complications. Therefore, when presenting the case for cost savings attributable to quality, it is important to use an outcome-based audit tool to report decreased IV nosocomial infection and phlebitis rates. The data needed to quantify these savings, however, are not easy to accumulate. Information may have to be obtained from medical records, infection control program reports, and IV incident reports. In addition, a controlled study, either retrospective, concurrent, or prospective, may be necessary to provide more accurate documentation. The study can also determine additional costs that may occur because of nosocomial infections and phlebitis.

A 2-year study conducted at a 300-bed acute care facility supported previous data that personnel specially trained to maintain intravascular devices provide a service that effectively reduces catheter-related infections and overall costs.[19] After implementing an IV team on medical/surgical units, IV-related bacteremias decreased from 4.6% to 1.5% per 1000 patient discharges, with decreased morbidity and an estimated cost savings of $124,906.[20] Another study examined the incidence and cost associated with nosocomial bloodstream infections. A decrease in the occurrence of local complications from 21.7% in catheters inserted by medical housestaff to 7.9% in catheters inserted by the IV team was noted.[21] With a 35% overall infection decrease, including a 51% decrease in bacteremias associated with *Staphylococcus aureus,* this study clearly demonstrated how the presence of an IV team positively impacted the incidence of IV complications. The cost impact of complications associated with IV administration by nursing generalists may be convincing if the patient's length of stay is increased because of IV therapy complications such as phlebitis and infiltration.

Because it is difficult to quantify improvements in quality of care, IV teams may find it difficult to justify their existence in the face of increasing scrutiny during budget review. This presents a challenge to existing teams, and it will become more difficult for new teams to become established. It is therefore necessary to implement a comprehensive quality management program to continually justify the need for the specialty. Favorable statistics from a given institution provide ongoing justification when compared with national standards of treatment without teams. The administration of IV fluids, blood and blood products, and medications may be monitored for the following:

- Appropriate use of electronic infusion devices
- Infection rates
- Vascular access device complications
- Delays in therapy or extended lengths of stay attributable to lack of venous access or access complications

These criteria assess both the process and outcome variables of performance. If an institution determines that phlebitis rates and medication errors are high, filters and pumps are used incorrectly or inappropriately, IV sites are not rotated, tubing is not changed, and documentation and communication are poor, then that institution is a prime candidate for IV team implementation. In some cases, the medical staff is the driving force for assessing the possibilities of implementing an IV team. This usually occurs when the quality of patient care is threatened because of the lack of professional staff or a lack of expertise in the current staff.

Risk management

Risk management or liability issues for the institution are decreased by using an IV team. IV therapy specialists who are monitoring and delivering IV care are more expert in anticipating and preventing potential patient complications than generalist nurses. When IV therapy nurses manage or direct the use of advanced technologies and equipment for the delivery of care, safer product utilization results. Many lawsuits against hospitals are the results of complications that occur when equipment is improperly used, medications are administered incorrectly, or policies and procedures are not implemented. The potential for complications in IV therapy patients is greater when the hospital cannot provide specialized skill in and knowledge of the various aspects of IV therapy.

The presence of an IV team establishes that the institution adheres to professional and court-recognized standards such as the *Infusion Nursing Standards of Practice*.[7] IV therapy specialists operating in accordance with these and other national standards for IV therapy practice ensure that care is based on principles that have been established through expert development, review, and research. IV therapy–related complications lead to patient injury, increased hospital stays, and potential lawsuits. The ability to reduce these complications through the specialization provided by an IV team is a strong argument in favor of such teams. The first step in demonstrating that IV teams improve outcomes and decrease risks is to identify lawsuits that specifically involved IV complications. The total amount of legal fees, court costs, employee time, court awards, and settlements for these legal actions should be calculated. Plotting the frequency and costs of lawsuits may reveal trends that support the need for an IV team. Licensure allows and health care providers expect staff nurses to initiate IV therapy and perform specialized IV functions, but knowledge and experience levels in this nursing specialty vary greatly and may be limited. With the decentralization and transition of many services and the complex needs of acutely ill patients, it is increasingly difficult for the staff nurse to remain or become proficient in all required skills.

Justification

The justification for an IV team centers on the benefits associated with delivering IV therapy by a team of specially educated nurses. Benefits inherent in the use of IV teams include standardization of equipment, improved productivity with better utilization of nursing resources, fewer patient complications, and improved risk management because an expert is monitoring care. To justify the importance of maintaining IV teams or of creating IV teams based on enhanced patient care and cost savings, IV supervisors and managers should build their case on a foundation that addresses environment, demand, costs, and benefits. Each area must be thoroughly researched and carefully analyzed, and the findings of this study must be skillfully presented to the institution's decision makers. It is important to remember the reasons the team was established; those reasons should be assessed again when justifying the team's continued operation. Appendix I summarizes justification factors.

One way to justify continuation of the IV team is to evaluate and assess the performance of teams serving other institutions in the community. If the community standard is that IV teams are the rule rather than the exception, that standard provides tangible and immediate justification and support for maintaining the team. It is also helpful for IV team managers in a community to network to share clinical experiences, discuss practice issues, and evaluate technologies. When several IV teams practice in a community, it is natural for comparisons to be made regarding their services, staff qualifications, cost-effectiveness, and productivity. It is essential to keep the lines of communication open to share information and develop strategies for the continued success of the teams. When developing an IV team, it is important and helpful to use all available resources, including nearby teams and teams practicing outside the immediate area.

An IV team can have a positive impact on the morale of other hospital staff, such as the staff RNs or house officers who were previously responsible for IV-related duties. By relieving them of these duties, they experience fewer disruptions and a decrease in associated frustrations. The entire organization benefits from the knowledge that the patient has received the safest and most cost-effective IV care available.

Another strategy for maintaining an IV team is to take responsibility for highly specialized services that increase the team's value to the institution. In recent years, highly skilled procedures such as PICC insertions have become invaluable. Because the team is required to learn specialized procedures in addition to general procedures, it gains additional responsibility and authority. A hospital that eliminates a highly efficient, effective, and full-service IV team will have a difficult time providing the specialized services that had become standard for the IV team. Such a team would have established itself as an important part of the institution by continually doing more and producing more. Success, high productivity rates, and other measures of an IV team's importance to any institution must be tangible and quantifiable. The data must support the assumptions.

Marketing is an essential component for the ongoing justification of IV services. The patient, or consumer, is a strong advocate for IV teams. The IV team has an important product to offer through its expertise, knowledge, and standardization. It is important to present the benefits that an IV team offers and build a good reputation. An IV team should be marketed as a potential source for referrals or admissions. This includes inpatient and outpatient services, such as education and IV services for home care patients and clinics.

Consumer awareness has finally arrived in the health care arena, and patients have become *consumers* who expect quality care. It is not uncommon for patients to do some research on their own to satisfy their interest in having their health care needs delivered by institutions with a highly motivated and skilled professional staff. Patients are looking for caregivers who, through their interpersonal interactions and caring, demonstrate quality.[22] Whether an institution has a skilled IV team can be an important consideration for patients. It is vital for a hospital to demonstrate a genuine concern for improving an often distasteful aspect of hospitalization. When an experienced IV nurse delivers therapy, the incidence of complications are minimized. Consumer research shows that personal experience and word-of-mouth advertising create most of the image of a facility among consumers. Consequently, the competence and skill of nurses on the hospital staff is crucial to any hospital's marketing efforts. Hospitals can attract new patients by marketing the significance of IV specialization. The presence of IV nurse specialists results in positive outcomes and can help a facility meet patients' expectations.

The future of IV teams continues to depend on the issues of quality care and allocation of resources. For those committed to the philosophy of the IV therapy specialty, the challenge remains to provide rational and supportable justification for using their services. It is the challenge of the IV nursing specialists to provide this expertise efficiently and cost-effectively within a carefully managed health care system.

REFERENCES

1. American Hospital Association: *Hospital statistics*, Chicago, 1999, Health Forum and American Hospital Association.
2. Robertson KJ: The role of the IV specialist in health care reform, *JIN* 3:130, 1995.
3. Aiken LH, Sochalski J, Anderson GF: Downsizing the hospital nursing workforce, *Health Aff* 4:88, 1996.
4. Hoover KW: Nursing work redesign in response to managed care, *JONA* 11:9, 1998.
5. Curtain LL: Learning from the future, *Nurs Manage* 25(1):7, 1994.
6. Westrope RA, Vaughn L, Bott M, Taunton RL: Shared governance: from vision to reality, *JONA* 25(12) 45, 1995.
7. Intravenous Nurses Society: Infusion nursing standards of practice, *JIN* (suppl) 23(6S), 2000.
8. Sheretz R: Look before you leap: discontinuation of an infusion therapy team, *Infect Control Hosp Epidemiol* 20:99, 1999.
9. Weinstein SM: *Plumer's principles and practice of infusion therapy*, ed 6, Philadelphia, 1997, Lippincott-Raven.
10. McDermott K, Laschinger-Spence HK, Shamian J: Work empowerment and organizational commitment, *Nurs Mange* 27(5):44, 1996.
11. Baldwin DR: Workload management system for I.V. therapy, *JIN* 11(5): 308, 1988.
12. Baldwin DR: Patient classification system for I.V. therapy, *JIN* 12(5):313, 1988.
13. Kalafat J: A systematic healthcare quality service program, *Hosp Health Servs Manage* 571, 1991.
14. Brewer CS, Frazier P: The influence of structure, staff type, and managed-care indicators on registered nurse staffing, *JONA* 28(9): 28, 1998.
15. Intravenous Nurses Society: Position paper: the intravenous nurse specialist's role in the evolving healthcare environment, *JIN* 20(3): 19, 1997.
16. Burik D, Cramton CW, Holtz JM: A workbook approach to justifying I.V. therapy teams under prospective, *NITA* 7:411, 1984.
17. Pettno P: A four-level clinical ladder, *Nurs Mange* 29(7):52, 1998.
18. Elder KN, et al: Managed care: the value you bring, *AJN* 98(6)34, 1998.
19. Centers for Disease Control and Prevention: Guidelines for prevention of intravascular device-related infections, *AJIC* 24:262, 1996.
20. Miller JM, Goetz AM, Squier C, Muder RR: Reduction in nosocomial intravenous device-related bacteremias after institution of an intravenous therapy team, *JIN* 19(2)103, 1996.
21. Soifer NE, Borzak S, Edlin BR, Weinstein RA: Prevention of peripheral venous catheter complications with an intravenous therapy team: a randomized controlled trial, *Arch Intern Med* 158:473, 1998.
22. Williams SA: Quality and care: patients' perceptions, *J Nurs Care Qual* 12(6):18, 1998.

Justifying and Maintaining Intravenous Therapy Teams

Justification for IV teams centers largely on the benefits associated with delivering intravenous therapy by a team of IV nurse specialists. The following guidelines may be considered when establishing an IV team or justifying the continuation of an established team.

FUNDAMENTAL CONSIDERATIONS

Justification

To justify the need for an IV team, the external environment, internal institution environment, demands for services, cost factors, and associated benefits should be thoroughly researched and carefully analyzed.

Maintenance

An established team may have to research or analyze only specific areas as needed to justify its continuation. However, an established team should always be one step ahead and able to address all the factors used to justify a new team.

  I. Environmental analysis[16]

    To justify an IV team within an institution, first analyze internal and external environmental factors to assess any demands on the institution that can offset its ability to support new services, financially and professionally. The information may be obtained from administrators, financial managers, professional associations, and peer review organizations.

    A. External environment

      1. Impact of regulatory and demographic changes

      2. Payer and competition activities

      3. Worker supply changes

      4. Technologic changes

      5. Licensing changes

      6. Other area institutions (Do other local hospitals have IV teams? If so, how do the functions, responsibilities, and coverage of the teams differ? If not, what is different about a non-IV team hospital so that they do not require an IV team?)

    B. Internal environment

      1. Identify the priorities of hospital management and the IV team, and then show how the IV team's strengths and weaknesses relate to those priorities. For example, point out how an IV team can control costs while maintaining a high quality of patient care.

      2. Who makes decisions for the institution, and who influences the decision makers? Analyze the data from their perspective: what are their goals, what is important to them?

      3. Examine the hospital's financial status

      4. Consider the institution's internal power, political structure, and the overall climate for acceptance of services offered by the IV team, by floor nurses, and by physicians.

5. What is the hospital's mission?

6. How is the hospital performing financially? What changes are being implemented to control costs or improve reimbursement?

7. In what way is the existing or proposed IV team compatible with the goals of the hospital (i.e., improved, cost-effective quality care)?

8. What is the purpose of the IV team? Is this purpose recognized by administration?

9. What is the hospital's case mix? What are the implications for the IV team?

II. Demand for service analysis[16]

If the environmental analysis suggests that the IV team concept would receive support, the demand for services should be assessed to show the relative merits of an IV team to the institution. The following should be considered:

A. Evaluate the number and type of IV services that are being performed (e.g., starts, restarts, CVC maintenance procedures, tubing changes, infusion device manipulations, blood product administration).

B. Evaluate the number of patients receiving IV therapy and the intensity of IV therapy (e.g., days on therapy, procedures performed, materials and nurse time per patient, department, DRGs).

C. Quantify the potential for IV therapy for each DRG by the percentage of patients receiving IV treatment, average IV costs and charges per patient, and total and average patient days.

D. Assess the severity of illness of the hospital's patients. IV therapy increases with the severity of illness, as determined by secondary diagnosis, age, malnutrition, dehydration, and surgical versus medical stay.

III. Cost-benefit analysis reference[16]

Once an analysis of the institution and demand for services has been performed, the next strategy is to "sell" the concept of the IV team and its associated benefits. Major emphasis should be placed on the fact that IV teams can reduce hospital costs through savings in labor and materials.

A. Labor

1. Labor is the largest element of cost associated with IV therapy. It is important to show that labor can become more efficient by using IV nurse specialists.

2. Compare the workload unit requirements of IV specialists with those of non-IV specialists to demonstrate the efficiencies and salary differentials that provide savings. An IV team requires fewer workload unit requirements. Labor costs vary, depending on the salaries of the individuals providing IV therapy.

3. Emphasize that time saved can be redirected to other patient care activities and that improved efficiency can result in decreased FTE requirements on the units.

B. Supplies

1. Point out that IV teams can reduce material costs through more effi-

cient use of supplies and standardization of IV-related materials and equipment.

2. Evaluate the impact of an IV team in terms of total materials used and material usage efficiency. Compare this information with the materials that would be required without an IV team and then compare the total costs per procedure related to materials used with and without an IV team. It has been shown that an IV team may use as little as one third of the materials used by a non-IV team.[16]

C. Improved quality of care

1. Reports that IV teams improve quality of care may be regarded as subjective, rather than objective. It is important to define in quantitative ways the quality improvements offered by the IV team concept.

   a. Make a list of those items that define good or poor quality in IV care.

   b. Obtain information from medical records, infection control program reports, and IV incident reports. A controlled study, either retrospective, concurrent, or prospective, may be necessary for more accurate documentation.

   c. Select two similar nursing units for a quality study. Using your list of quality measurements, perform random checks of IV patients and establish quality indices on both units; then, on one unit, implement a pilot study using the IV team concept. After implementation, conduct a new study on both units and compare with previous results. Use statistical methods in the studies and use unbiased observers. Typically, phlebitis and infection rates are studied.

   d. Improved quality of care must provide clear cost savings.

2. For maintaining an existing team, it is important to establish a continuing quality management program, conduct studies to demonstrate the improvements the team has accomplished, and identify problem areas.

   a. All members of the team should log selected quality management data (e.g., number of patients with phlebitis, infiltrations, infections, clotted IVs). This should be done every shift and can be best accomplished while documenting daily workload data (see Table 27-1).

D. Length of stay

1. To determine how an IV team affects length of stay, identify patients with abnormally long stays and the reasons for those extended stays (e.g., severity of disease, nosocomial infection, medical complications, lack of IV placement and resultant interruption of therapy, delayed laboratory results, failure to discontinue IV therapy).

2. After considering reasons for extended stays, examine a population or DRG on which an IV team would have a major impact.

3. Call attention to the IV team's role in preventing extra patient days, and calculate the percentages of incremental preventable cost and incremental avoidable delays attributable to an IV team.

4. For existing teams, all staff members should log in, at the end of their shift, any interventions undertaken that would have an impact on length of stay or costs. This provides ongoing data for justification of the IV team. A simple way to collect data is to maintain a logbook in the department for each IV nurse to note these interventions quickly. For example, there could be columns for the date, room number, patient's name, intervention, results, time required by the IV nurse, and signature of the person carrying out the intervention.

E. Risk management
1. Plot the frequency and costs of lawsuits, which might disclose trends that support the need for an IV team.
2. Identify lawsuits that involved IV complications and then calculate the dollars spent for legal fees, court costs, employee time, court awards, and settlements for these suits against the hospital.

F. Marketing advantage
1. Market an IV team as a potential source of referrals or admissions. The IV team can be promoted as a time saver and more efficient source of IV therapy. The team can also provide outpatient services, such as education and IV services for home care patients and outpatients.
2. Emphasize the improved quality of care delivered by the institution with IV specialists providing care, based on national standards.
3. Work with the hospital's marketing department to investigate strategies for marketing to the hospital and community.

IV. Organization and functions of the IV team
Once the IV team concept has been proposed and accepted as a valuable service, several factors must be considered when establishing the organization and functions of the team.

A. Identify the organizational structure that best benefits and enhances the team within the institution. Each organizational structure is associated with advantages and disadvantages, depending on the institutional environment. It is important to look for a structure that allows the team to meet its objectives, goals, and philosophy of care while remaining cost-effective. Note that the INS recommends that the IV team be established as an independent department that reports directly to administration. Other departments or personnel to report to include the following:
1. Pharmacy
2. Blood bank
3. Nursing division
4. Medical director

V. Analyze current responsibilities
A. Compare current IV practice with the proposed practice of the IV team.
1. Admixture preparation
2. Venipuncture, maintenance, follow-up
3. CVC care

4. Blood product administration

5. IV-related activities performed by various classifications of employees

6. Current nursing policies regarding IV technique

VI. Volume of IV therapy activities

    A. Establish daily volumes of IV therapy activity for each nursing area. Sources of data include patient charts, pharmacy records, purchasing, and various documents maintained on the nursing units.

    B. Establish current volumes of IV therapy activities to provide information for comparison of the institution with other hospitals, and establish a baseline for comparison of growth and mix changes.

VII. Analyze hospital layout

    A. Look at the layout in the facility, including unit location and size, and types of IV therapy services that are required.

VIII. Resources and staffing

    A. What resources are available for designing an IV team? What role is played by a group such as the nursing division or education department?

    B. How many employees does the team need?

    C. Is there a significant shortage of nurses? Is it difficult to staff and provide 24-hour coverage?

    D. What role will an LVN-LPN play on your team?

    E. What resources do you have to train your staff?

IX. Functions of the IV team

    A. What services are most needed by the institution? If unable to justify all the services, it is desirable to provide an alternative and phase in functions over time.

    B. Is the team to provide a 24-hour, 7-day-a-week coverage? (Remember that this is preferred for optimal functioning of the team.) What are the implications if it does not? If the team is part-time, who is responsible for IV functions during the other hours?

    C. In what areas can the team provide services (e.g., general care areas, pediatrics-nursery, intensive care areas, emergency department, labor and delivery)?

    D. Possible team functions include the following (remember to identify those services that cannot be provided as readily without a team). These responsibilities should be emphasized, and provide the team with ongoing justification.

        1. IV equipment selection and evaluation

        2. Consultation

        3. Patient instruction

        4. Product defect reporting, reporting to the Food and Drug Administration (FDA)

        5. PICC and long-arm catheter insertion

        6. Cytotoxic medication administration

        7. Blood component administration

8. Plasmapheresis
9. Venipuncture
10. Medication administration
11. CVC care and maintenance
12. Therapeutic phlebotomy
13. Dialysis access
14. Arterial access
15. Blood draws
16. Code team member
17. Collection and documentation of infection control and quality assurance statistics
18. Extravasation management
19. Declotting catheters
20. Policy and procedure development and revision
21. Provide outpatient services
22. Provide home infusion services
23. Contracting external services (e.g., skilled nursing facilities, etc.)

  E. Be specific regarding functions. For example, when doing a new IV start, is the IV team going to hang only the first solution, or will they hang subsequent bottles?

X. Costs for the IV team (use the hospital accounting division as a resource)
  A. What are the projected costs of the necessary staffing (include salary, benefits, sick leave, vacation)?
  B. What are supply costs (projected or actual) for IV therapy activities?
  C. What are the methods for charging? Are they part of general nursing care charges or are they special charges? What is included in the charge structure?

XI. Analyze reimbursement and revenue
  A. Demonstrate how the IV team concept results in increased revenues—project potential increases. Check with other hospitals that have implemented teams for information.
  B. Look at current reimbursement issues, such as fee for service, discounted fee for user, per diem rate, per case rates, and capitation.

XII. Develop budgetary goals
  A. Organizational goals.
  B. Long-range objectives.
  C. For established teams, forecast levels of activity for the coming year.
  D. Continually analyze how the team's role can expand, and re-evaluate services provided. Remember that with the continual changes in health care and technology, the primary functions of the team may be altered.

XIII. Developing units of service
  A. Develop units of service standards for labor hours needed to provide particular services. These standards provide productivity data. Determine units of service through time estimates, historical data averages, service

logs, work sampling, predetermined accepted standards, and time and motion studies.

B. Units of service need to be logged by the IV staff daily on each shift. This can be accomplished efficiently by using computer and bar coding systems. Data can also be easily recorded manually on daily tally sheets. Each nurse can log procedures performed at the end of the shift and each procedure can then be converted to units of service.

XIV. Plan of care

A. It is important to establish the IV team's role in patient assessment and plans of care specific to IV therapy. Establish a system for integrating the IV nursing plan of care into the overall plan of care.

XV. Additional strategies for maintaining an IV team

A. Become indispensable.

1. Provide and be responsible for highly specialized services such as PICC insertions.

B. Provide educational and in-service programs.

1. Have members of the team be actively involved in nursing orientation, hospitalwide in-service training, and hospital and community educational programs.

C. Continually evaluate the function and success of other IV teams in the area.

D. Meet regularly with other IV team managers in the community.

Chapter 28

Intravenous Therapy in the Home

Rose Anne Waldman Lonsway, BSN, MA, CRNI*

This chapter gives a broad overview of home infusion therapy. It reviews basic concepts related to the field and describes its evolution and history, including the original model for providing home nutritional support and antibiotic therapy. It also describes the expansion of the original model by the nursing and pharmacy disciplines. This chapter describes the home care process and the roles and responsibilities of the service providers involved. Because health care providers must justify the services they provide, it also discusses the medical, professional, financial, and reimbursement benefits associated with home infusion therapy. The chapter reviews the most common infusion therapies provided in the home care environment and the resources—personnel and otherwise—needed to provide these therapies. This review includes the first home infusion therapies (total parenteral nutrition [TPN], antibiotic therapy, hydration, and pain management) and the newer therapies (complex chemotherapy, dobutamine therapy, transfusion therapy, alpha$_1$-proteinase inhibitor [Prolastin], tocolytic therapy, and the biologic response modifiers). Finally, special considerations are suggested, as are future directions for the field of home infusion therapy and its place in our health care system.

ORGANIZATIONAL STRUCTURE

Although home infusion therapy as we know it today is a relatively new field, home visitation by medical personnel, including physicians and public health nurses, dates back many years. The literature from the late 1970s cites cases in which the only reason for hospitalization was the extended need for intravenous (IV) nutritional support.[1] Now, however, modern technology, such as long-term indwelling catheters and ambulatory infusion pumps, makes it possible to provide highly technical infusion services in the home.

The federal government provided the biggest impetus for providing infusion services in the home when it implemented TEFRA, the Tax Equity and Fiscal Responsibility Act of 1982. TEFRA shifted Medicare reimbursement from a retrospective case-per-day payment system to a prospective payment system based on a fixed fee.[2] In 1983, the government established the

*The author and editors wish to acknowledge the contributions made by Linda Grace and Becky Tomaselli as coauthors of this chapter in the first edition of *Intravenous Nursing: Clinical Principles and Practice.*

fixed reimbursement amount for each of 467 diagnosis-related groups (DRGs). Under this system, the hospital knows in advance the exact amount the government will pay for a patient with a small bowel obstruction, for example. If the hospital provides the service for less than the diagnosis-related group (DRG) allowable, the hospital makes a profit. However, if care for a particular patient costs more than the amount allowed, the facility suffers a loss.

In 1984, health care costs rose 4.5%. This growth rate was considerably smaller than the 10% increase of 1983. This represented the first decline in U.S. health care costs in 20 years, leading many to conclude that the prospective payment system worked as intended.[2] For the first time, the health care system rewarded providers for efficiency and productivity and penalized them for inefficiency. The emphasis of the health care system changed from providing maximum quality regardless of cost to providing care in an atmosphere of efficiency, productivity, and cost-consciousness. In the earlier example of the patient with the small bowel obstruction, the hospital is now encouraged to discharge the patient as soon as feasible. Moreover, if the only reason for a patient to be retained in the hospital is to receive TPN, there is now a financial benefit for discharging the patient with a plan for home nutritional support. As the cost of health care has continued to rise over the years, the hospital-centered health care model of the 1980s has undergone great modification. Alternative sites, including the patient's home, are now considered the treatment settings of choice.

DEVELOPMENT OF THE INDUSTRY

The first two IV therapies to be self-administered in the home were TPN and antibiotics.[3,4] In the 1960s, the first description of the experimental use of parenteral alimentation in dogs using a fat emulsion of 10% was noted in the literature. In 1968, Dudrick experimented with parenteral nutrition using beagle puppies. In Dudrick's study, growth curves of two male puppies from the same litter were compared after one was fed orally and one parenterally.[5] Results showed similar growth curves in both animals. The same results were later found in pediatric and adult patients who, for whatever reason, could not use the gastrointestinal tract. Along with advances in medicine, technologic advances in equipment, such as long-term catheters, pumps (including ambulatory devices), and bags, have enabled patients to lead relatively normal lives by infusing essential nutrients parenterally. This advance, coupled with the need to control health care costs, led to the obvious alternative of providing infusion therapy in the home care setting.

The first report of the successful use of parenteral antibiotics was published in 1974 by Harrison, who treated a cystic fibrosis patient for acute pulmonary infection.[4] In 1979, the Cleveland Clinic developed a program to train patients in the self-administration of antibiotics. Poretz reported on 150 patients in the Cleveland Clinic Home Antibiotic Program. Results showed that adverse reactions were mild and infrequent, and demonstrated better than a 90% treatment success rate.[1,6] Based on these and other data from other similar programs, home parenteral antibiotic therapy was not only feasible, it was desirable. Patients were often well enough to be either at home or at work while receiving their therapy and were bored and frustrated by prolonged hospitalization. The impetus for the development of home programs came in response to DRGs and the encouragement of federal and state governments and private insurers, who were seeking to reduce the cost of health care.

Today, the home care industry is undergoing the same changes that the hospital industry experienced under TEFRA. The home care market as a whole expended $100 million in 1960. By 1997, that figure had grown to $32.3 *billion*. The escalation of costs in home care has brought increased scrutiny, regulatory oversight, slower growth, and decreased reimbursement. Home care expenditures increased by 30.7% between 1979 and 1980. Between 1996 and 1997, however, the increase had fallen to 3.7%.[7] The decrease has been and continues to be in response to initiatives such as managed care, fraud and abuse investigations by the federal government, and the Balanced Budget Act of 1997.

BENEFITS OF HOME INFUSION THERAPY

Home infusion therapy offers many benefits for patients, their families and caregivers, home care clinicians, and the health care system.

Patients

Patients experience psychosocial, emotional, financial, and health benefits. They are able to return to their own homes, which is a major benefit because the risk for acquiring nosocomial infections is decreased. Patients are also more comfortable in the privacy and familiarity of their own homes than the hospital. In addition, patients maintain a higher degree of control over their therapy and their lives with home care. Often, patients are able to return to work or other activities and still maintain their therapy regimen. Patients also experience financial benefits because home treatment is less expensive than hospital therapy. A study of the cost effectiveness of patients with class IV heart failure receiving care at home demonstrated a 27% savings over the cost of hospitalization.[8] This fact is extremely important in light of insurance costs and capitation initiatives, and the increasing life expectancy of patients with chronic or acute diseases.

Family members and caregivers

Home infusion therapy reduces the stress experienced by family members and caregivers when their loved ones are hospitalized. The primary caregiver is often a parent, spouse, or friend. Home care requires family participation. The home infusion program allows significant others to be active in the care of the patient to the degree they and the patient feel most comfortable. Assistance with care may be obtained based on the severity and acuteness of the illness and the financial resources of the patient. These options may include companions; skilled nursing care, either intermittent or continuous; and home health aides. Such assistance reduces time lost from work for family members and other caregivers.

In addition to the reduced cost of infusion therapy provided in the home, other financial benefits may be experienced by the family. Because the patient is treated in the home setting with clinicians going to the patient, the family members are no longer burdened with making special arrangements to transport their loved one for treatments and evaluations. Home infusion allows the family to spend time in their own home and eliminates the need for special arrangements for child care and other responsibilities often made difficult during periods of hospitalization. The home environment and activities return to as near normal as possible.

Home infusion clinicians

The IV nurse and pharmacist benefit from the home care environment because it allows more autonomous clinical practice and involvement in the design and provision of emerging home infusion therapies. Work schedules are often flexible and based on patient needs, visits, and therapies. Clinicians are allowed to expand their traditional roles and become more fulfilled. Nurses and pharmacists function as a team to provide highly technical, high-quality patient care in the home.

Health care system

The health care system benefits from home infusion therapy because it provides a cost-effective alternative for medical treatment. Payers are constantly searching for ways to reduce cost, and hospitals are attuned to DRGs and early discharge. Home infusion therapy has allowed an increasing number of patients to be treated without ever being admitted to the hospital, avoiding unnecessary costs and unnecessary psychologic stress related to hospitalization.

IV CARE DELIVERY MODELS
Pharmacy home infusion therapy model

The first established multidisciplinary approach for providing home care was Montefiore Hospital in New York in 1947. The concept of the visiting nurse was married with the physician's house call. Physical, occupational, and speech therapists were added to the team to provide total care to the patient in the home. Unfortunately, a physician shortage resulting from World War II made house calling a less efficient way of seeing patients, and this practice ended, along with the multidisciplinary home care concept.

The pharmacy home infusion therapy model, which was conceptualized in the late 1970s by entrepreneurial health care providers with a vision for providing high-technology infusion services, followed a similar multidisciplinary team approach using pharmacy, nursing, and ancillary services.[9] Early descriptions of the home infusion therapy model included two simply defined processes—admission and patient care (Fig. 28-1). *Admission* was the process by which the patient was admitted to the home infusion program. *Patient care* was the process of providing the prescribed therapy, after which the patient was discharged from the home infusion program. During the initial years of home infusion therapy, the number of patient diagnoses was limited. Most of the patients were treated with TPN for

short bowel syndrome, Crohn's disease, or ulcerative colitis; with antibiotics for subacute bacterial endocarditis; and with pain management for terminal cancer with intractable pain.[10,11]

Acceptance of home infusion therapy, largely as a result of community education and advances in pharmaceuticals, equipment technology, and medical treatment for chronic disease states, gave way to the development of the complex home infusion process known today. Although the basic home infusion therapy model of today has not changed significantly since its inception, many facets have become more complex with the addition of new therapies, the increasing severity of illness of the acute and chronic patients treated at home, the demands of third-party payers and regulators, and the increased number of communication channels, such as multiple case managers. However, the steps to achieve successful outcomes remain the same. Fig. 28-2 outlines the basic model.

The home infusion patient care model should provide a cohesive, multidisciplinary, team approach to patient care that respects the rights of patients, meets their needs, and effectively and efficiently manages the quality and cost of care.

The model endeavors to fulfill the following objectives:
- Facilitation of a smooth transition of care from the referring entity to the home
- Anticipation of potential problems, thereby allowing for early intervention by care providers and preventing or minimizing the need for rehospitalization
- Encouragement of patient comfort by allowing patients to receive care in a familiar environment and to live the lifestyle to which they are accustomed
- Maximization of independence and self-sufficiency by educating patients or caregivers in self-administration with minimal assistance from clinicians
- Facilitation of the patient's return to optimum health and independence

Realizing that return to optimal health and independence may not always be possible, the home infusion model acts as a conduit in the process of care management across the health care continuum. The model of care integrates clinical pharmacy and nursing services through four processes: admission/assessment, planning, patient care (including implementation, monitoring, and evaluation), and termination of care.

The pharmacy is responsible for the patient in this model. The pharmacy must be licensed as required by state and federal law. Nurses rendering patient care are employed by the pharmacy or obtained under a subcontract with a nursing agency appropriately licensed/certified to provide patient care.

Nursing agency home infusion therapy model

The nursing agency home infusion therapy model has evolved over time. In an effort to provide services in the most cost-efficient manner, the actual hands-on care of the infusion patient has shifted to the nursing agency. With the diminishing profit margins of nursing and pharmacy services and the high cost of professional salaries, agency administrators saw home infusion therapy as a way to survive. Home infusion therapy not only generates additional revenue for the agency from patient

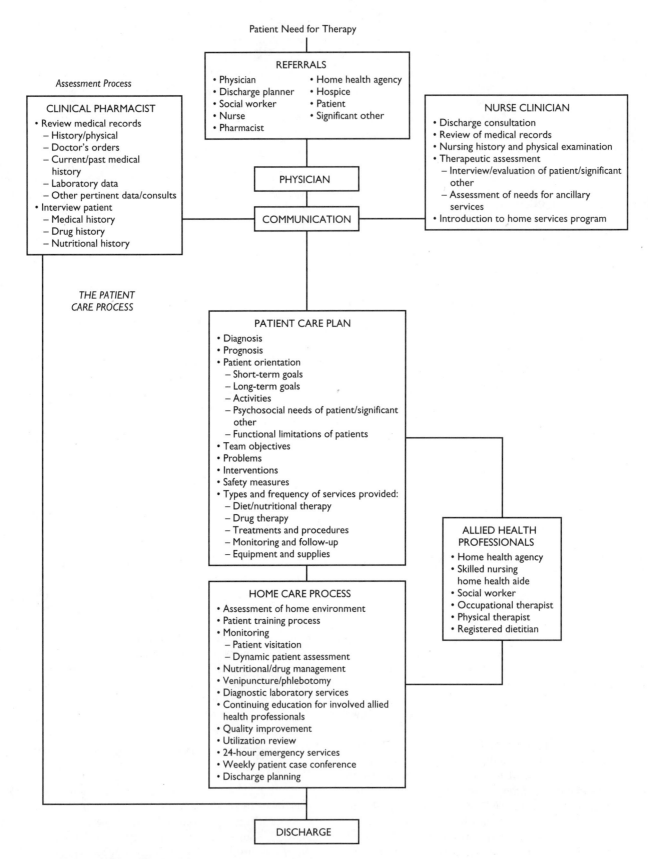

FIG. 28-1   *The admission process.* (Modified from Reid JS, Grace L, Venook S: *Patient care management system mode,* poster presentation, Nashville, Tenn, 1987, National Intravenous Therapy Association.)

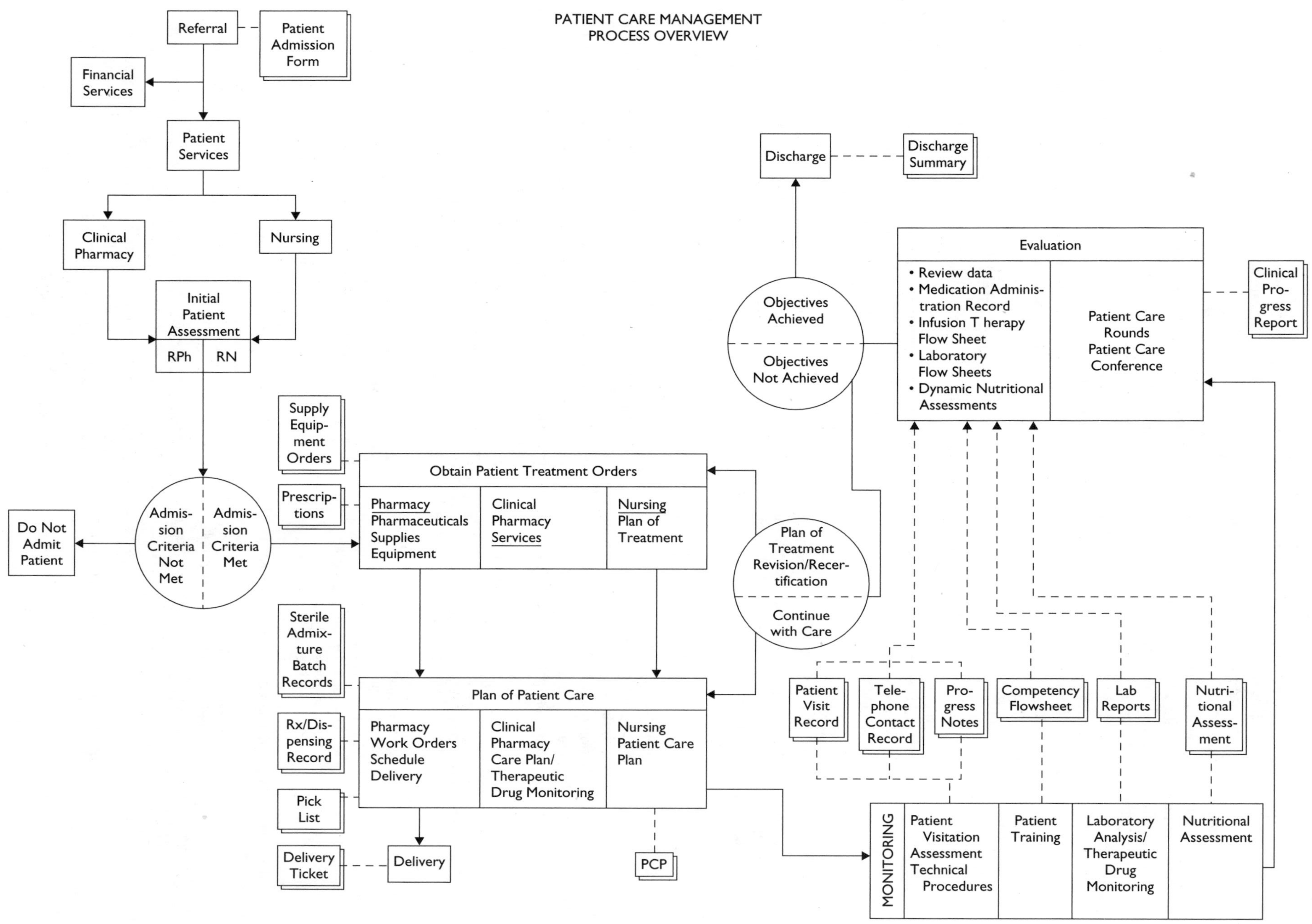

PATIENT CARE MANAGEMENT
PROCESS OVERVIEW

FIG. 28-2   Home infusion therapy patient care management system.

visits but ensures continuity of care by providing other professional services needed by the patient such as physical, occupational or speech therapy or the services of a medical social worker all from the same business entity. This model typically subcontracts for pharmacy services, either with a pharmacy that provides only the product or with a home infusion pharmacy that provides the full complement of pharmacy and nursing services. Some integrated health care systems have begun to use an on-site home infusion pharmacy in addition to a certified nursing agency. Often, pharmacies find the cost of seeking nursing agency licensure and certification beyond their financial reach. By working together with a nursing agency, however, the two entities can effectively deliver home infusion therapy.

The goal of both home infusion therapy models is to promote multidisciplinary collaboration, efficiency, and cost-effectiveness. It also allows a complete approach to patient assessment. Through an integrated assessment, a more accurate evaluation of the patient and improved recommendations for care are made. The collaborative process improves the level of care and services provided to the patient.

Involvement of ancillary services

Ancillary services are those services not provided directly by the home infusion therapy agency. These services usually include the provision of durable medical equipment (with the exception of infusion pumps), respiratory therapy, and in some cases, medical social work and physical therapy. These services are commonly provided, either by referral or subcontract, through the home care pharmacy or nursing agency that provides the infusion therapy. A list of direct and ancillary services can be found in Box 28-1. As the infusion pharmacy and nursing models merge, any combination of these services can be offered directly or indirectly. The multidisciplinary team concept for managing health care, in which the patient is central and all team members interact collaboratively, best accommodates the goal of quality patient care and services.

OPERATIONAL DESIGN
Home infusion patient care process

Although the medical community is equipped to provide home infusion therapy to almost any patient, not every patient is a home care candidate. The criteria that a patient must meet to be accepted into the home infusion program include clinical, financial, and technical issues. These issues are described in Guidelines for Patient Selection.

Therapies provided in the home setting

Historically, the most common therapies provided in the home care setting have been TPN, total enteral nutrition, antibiotics, chemotherapy, hydration, pain management, and aerosolized pentamidine. Catheter care is provided as well. Advances in medicine and technology have opened the door for the provision of several new home therapies, including biologic agents and blood modifiers, human growth hormone, immunoglobulin, blood products and blood factors, alpha$_1$-proteinase inhibitor, deferoxamine mesylate (Desferal), cardiologic agents, and continuous and complex chemotherapies. A list of common home infusion diagnoses and suggested therapies is provided in Table 28-1.

Patient admission process

The patient admission process begins with the referral. Many potential referral sources exist, including physicians, case managers, discharge planners, medical social workers, nurses, pharmacists, patients, and caregivers. In today's health care market, insurance companies must also be considered potential referral sources because of contractual relationships between insurers and medical providers, and via disease-state management programs. Although anyone can refer a patient, an order from the physician for pharmaceutical agents must always be obtained and verified by the pharmacy providing the therapy.

Guidelines for patient selection

Each patient undergoes an admission-criteria evaluation process to determine the appropriateness of the patient for the services offered by the provider. This process includes evaluation of clinical, technical, and financial criteria. When a pharmacy and a nursing agency share responsibility for a patient, the criteria for both agencies must be met before accepting a patient for service. A patient is admitted for services only when the criteria for services are met.

Clinical criteria. The patient must be considered medically stable for home infusion therapy as determined by his or her physician; however, because care at home has become so advanced, the criteria for medical stability have become very vague. *Medically stable* is usually defined as not requiring continuous intensive medical monitoring and intervention. Because services and care are now provided to more acutely ill patients in

---

Box 28-1   Direct and Ancillary Services

DIRECT SERVICES
Consultation for predischarge evaluation
Discharge planning and case management
Complete patient training (hospital and home)
Patient visitation in the home, clinic, or skilled nursing facility
Dynamic patient assessment and monitoring, including nutritional and physical assessment and therapeutic monitoring
Psychosocial support
Parenteral, intramuscular, epidural, and subcutaneous medication administration
Technical procedures by infusion specialists
Infusion control device implantation, monitoring, and removal
ANCILLARY SERVICES
Diagnostic and laboratory services
Social services
Diet counseling services
Physical therapy
Home health services, including skilled nursing care and home health aides
Durable medical equipment

Table 28-1   Potential Home Infusion Diagnoses and Suggested Therapies

Diagnosis/ICD 9 Description Code	ICD 9 Code	Suggested Therapy
Abscess, general	682.9	Antibiotic
Abscess, intracranial	324.0	Antibiotic
Abscess, pelvic	614.4	Antibiotic
Achalasia, digestive organs congenital	751.8	TPN
Achalasia, esophagus	530.0	TPN
Actinomycosis NOS	039.9	Antiinfective
Adhesions, intestinal or peritoneal with obstruction	560.81	TPN
Amyotrophia NOS	728.2	Antibiotic/TPN
Anemia	285.9	Blood
Aphagia	784.3	TEN
Arthritis, bacterial	040.89	Antibiotic
Arthritis, infective*	711.6-9	Antibiotic
Asthma*	493.00	Aminophylline
Atresia, alimentary organ or tract	751.8	TPN
Bacteremia	790.7	Antibiotic
Bacteremia caused by organism	038.8	Antibiotic
Blastomycosis	116.0	Antiinfective
Blood transfusion	V58.2	Blood
Bronchiectasis	494.0	Antibiotic
Bronchitis	491.0	Antibiotic
Cachexia caused by cancer	199.1	TEN/TPN
Cachexia caused by malnutrition	261.0	TEN/TPN
Candidiasis—unspecified site	112.9	Antiinfective
Carcinoma—intestinal	159.0	Chemotherapy
Celiac disease	579.0	TEN/TPN
Cellulitis	682.9	Antibiotic
Chemotherapy	V58.1	Chemotherapy
Coccidioidomycosis	114.9	Antiinfective
Colitis	558.9	TEN/TPN
Colitis, ulcerative	556.0	TEN/TPN
Congestive heart failure	428.9	Dobutamine
Cooley's anemia	282.4	Deferoxamine mesylate
Crohn's disease	555.9	TEN/TPN
Crush injury with infection	929.9	Antibiotic
Cryptococcoses	117.5	Antibiotic
Cytomegaloviral disease	078.5	Antibiotic
Deficiency, alpha$_1$-antitrypsin	277.6	Prolastin
Deficiency, antihemophilic factor	286.0	Blood product
Deficiency, growth hormone	253.3	Growth hormone
Deficiency, immunoglobulin	279.0	Gamma globulin
Decubitus ulcer	707.0	Antibiotic
Degenerative heart disease	429.1	Dobutamine

Diagnosis/ICD 9 Description Code	ICD 9 Code	Suggested Therapy
Dehydration	276.5	Hydration
Diabetes	250.0	Antibiotic
Diabetes with gangrene	250.7	Antibiotic
Diabetic ulcer	250.8	Antibiotic
Diarrhea, chronic	558.9	TEN/TPN
Diarrhea, infectious	009.2	TEN/TPN
Disease, pelvic inflammatory chronic	614.4	Antibiotic
Embolism, pulmonary*	415.1	Antithrombolytic
Encephalitis, viral	049.9	Antiinfective
Encephalitis, viral, arthropod borne	064.0	Antiinfective
Endocarditis, infectious	421.0	Antibiotic
Enteritis, viral	008.6	Antiinfective
Enteritis, bacterial	008.5	Antibiotic
Fibrosis, cystic	277.0	Antibiotic/TEN/TPN
Fistula, abdomen	569.8	TEN/TPN
Fracture, open	829.1	Antibiotic
Fungal disease	117.9	Antiinfective
Gangrene	785.4	Antibiotic
Gonococcal joint infection*	098.50	Antibiotic
Gonococcal pelvis infection chronic	098.39	Antibiotic
Hemophilia	286.0	Blood products
Herpes simplex, complicated	054.8	Antiinfective
Histoplasmosis—unspecified	115.9	Antiinfective
HIV type 2	079.53	Antiinfective/TEN/TPN
Hodgkin's disease—unspecified	201.9	Chemotherapy
Human immunodeficiency virus	042.9	Antiinfective/TEN/TPN
Hyperalimentation	783.6	TPN
Hyperemesis gravidarum*	643.0	TPN/Hydration
Hypogammaglobulinemia*	279.0	Gamma globulin
Ileus	560.1	TPN
Infarct, bowel	557.0	TPN
Infection	136.8	Antibiotic
Infection, atypical mycobacteria	031.9	Antibiotic
Infection bacterial—unspecified	041.9	Antibiotic
Infection, brain—unspecified cause of encephalitis	323.9	Antibiotic
Infection, cytomegalovirus congenital	771.1	Antiinfective
Infection, skin	686.9	Antibiotic
Ischemic, bowel—stricture of intestine	557.1	TPN
Ixodiasis	134.8	Antibiotic

Continued

ICD, International Classification of Diseases; *TEN,* total enteral nutrition; *TPN,* total parenteral nutrition.
*Requires further specification.

Table 28-1   Potential Home Infusion Diagnoses and Suggested Therapies—cont'd

Diagnosis/ICD 9 Description Code	ICD 9 Code	Suggested Therapy	Diagnosis/ICD 9 Description Code	ICD 9 Code	Suggested Therapy
Kaposi's sarcoma	176.9	Chemotherapy	Obstruction, intestine	560.9	TPN
Labor, premature	644.2	Tocolytics	Osteomyelitis	730.2	Antibiotic
Leukemia	208.9	Chemotherapy	Otitis, external malignant	380.14	Antibiotic
Leukemia, myelogenous*	205.9	Chemotherapy	Pain, bone	733.9	Pain
Lymph node removal*	40.2	Chemotherapy	Parkinson's disease	332.0	TEN/PEN
Lymphoma*	202.8	Chemotherapy	Pneumonia	486.0	Antibiotic
Malabsorption	579.9	TEN/TPN	Pneumonia, *Pneumocystis carinii*	136.3	Antiinfective
Malnutrition	263.9	TEN/TPN	Prematurity	765.1	PEN
Melanoma	172.9	Chemotherapy	Prostatitis	601.9	Antibiotic
Meningitis	322.9	Antibiotic	Pseudomonas	41.7	Antibiotic
Metaplasia, agnogenic myeloid	289.8	Antibiotic/TEN	Pseudo-obstruction, intestinal	564.8	TPN
Mycobacterium avium—intracellulare	031.0	Antibiotic	Pulmonary disease, chronic obstructive	416.9	Alpha$_1$-proteinase inhibitor
Mycosis	117.9	Antiinfective			Biologics
Myeloma	203.0	Chemotherapy	Purpura, idiopathic thrombocytopenic	287.3	Antibiotic
Myocarditis	429.0	Antibiotic	Pyelonephritis	590.8	Antibiotic
Neoplasm*	199.1	Chemotherapy	Septicemia	038.9	Antibiotic
Neoplasm, alimentary tract	159.9/197.8	Chemotherapy	Short-bowel syndrome	579.2	TPN
Neoplasm, bone	170.9/198.5	Chemotherapy	Sinusitis, chronic	473.9	Antibiotic
Neoplasm, breast	174.9/198.81	Chemotherapy	Stomatitis	528.0	PEN
Neoplasm, digestive organs	159.9/197.8	Chemotherapy	Thalassemia	282.4	Deferoxamine mesylate
Neoplasm, esophagus	150.9/197.8	Chemotherapy			
Neoplasm, intestine	159.0/197.8	Chemotherapy	Thrombophlebitis	451.9	Anticoagulants
Neoplasm, large intestine	153.9/197.5	Chemotherapy	Unspecified immunity deficiency*	279.3/D43	Antiinfective/TPN
Neoplasm, larynx	161.9	Chemotherapy	Wound, complicated	879.8	Antibiotic
Neoplasm, lung	162.9/197.0	Chemotherapy			
Neoplasm, metastatic	275.4	Chemotherapy			
Neoplasm, neck	195.0/198.82	Chemotherapy			
Neoplasm, prostate	185.0/198.82	Chemotherapy			

PEN, partial enteral nutrition.

the home, each patient's needs are evaluated individually along with the organization's ability to meet those needs in the home. The benefits of providing services in this setting are also evaluated.

Although geographic location is somewhat of a technical issue, it becomes a clinical issue when the accessibility of emergency medical services is evaluated. Moreover, proximity to the health care team is important, if not essential, to treatment. Proximity allows ongoing assessment to evaluate therapeutic progress, and timely intervention to prevent complications and emergencies. If clinical criteria are not met, alternative services may be arranged. The patient is then reevaluated according to the criteria of the alternative program. The patient acceptance/do-not-admit model describes this process (Fig. 28-3).

Technical criteria.

A vital component of successful home infusion therapy is the patient's desire and willingness to receive therapy at home. This element goes hand in hand with the patient's ability to learn to administer the therapy or to mobilize the support system if unable to administer the therapy. The home environment must have a telephone, electricity, hot and cold running water, refrigeration, and a clean, dry area for storing supplies and preparing medications and solutions.

Financial criteria and considerations.

When a patient is referred to the home infusion therapy provider, an assessment of financial resources is made. This includes evaluating the reimbursement potential for the therapy prescribed and verifying insurance coverage. Payment plans are arranged with the patient or guarantor of payment. If the therapy is not covered by insurance, the patient may pay for the therapy, receive the therapy in the hospital or physician's office, or obtain funding through charitable organizations. The organization's financial service representatives help the patient explore reimbursement possibilities and negotiate with insurance companies. Because insurance policies differ, this service assists the patient by interpreting and clarifying policy limits, negotiating rates and services covered under the policy, and determining which services are not covered.

It is important that clinicians be educated about the requirements of the various payers and understand that verification of insurance benefits does not equate to approval of visits. For most private insurers, visit approval is an ongoing process; it requires periodic updates to the insurer on the patient's condition and progress toward goals.

Initial patient assessment.

The initial patient assessment is the baseline evaluation of the patient against which all subsequent and future evaluations are compared. The assessment includes a medical, drug, and nutritional history; analysis of laboratory data and trends; a therapeutic assessment; a physical examination; a psychosocial and cognitive assessment; and evaluation of the admission criteria mentioned earlier. Ideally, this assessment is initiated before the start of care during a conference at which all members of the health care team, including the patient and members of their support system, discuss and develop the plan for care and services at home. The initial patient assessment is most commonly concluded at the first home visit, when the home environment and technical skills are observed.

Agencies that are Medicare certified must also complete an OASIS (Outcome and Assessment Information Set) assessment in addition to the routine home care assessment. The OASIS assessment gathers and quantifies information about the patient's functional status. This information is submitted to the state and the Health Care Financing Administration (HCFA) and will become a part of an outcome assessment database that will be used to measure and assess the quality of patient care and delivery of services.

The traditionally short interval from the referral to the initial infusion visit often prevents the luxury of a preadmission conference. More often than not, preadmission coordination of care and services occurs via telephone between the members of the health care team. The patient is not fully accepted into the program until all admission criteria have been evaluated and met, the initial patient assessment is complete, and the home environment is considered safe and appropriate for home infusion therapy. The nurse or pharmacist meet with the patient and family members or caregivers to develop the plan of care and complete the initial patient assessment. Ideally, orientation and patient education can begin at an introductory meeting in the hospital, before the assessment visit in the patient's home.

Patient care planning and initiation of therapy

Obtaining orders.

Although a referral can come from any discipline, most states require that physician's orders for prescriptions be verified by a pharmacist. An order can be taken from a physician's designated representative, and in most states, a verbal order taken by the pharmacist does not need a physician's signature. On the other hand, verbal orders taken by nurses must be signed in accordance with state nursing law and practice acts. If the organization is a state-licensed or Medicare-certified agency, state licensure and HCFA regulations must be followed and a physician's plan of treatment (Health Care Finance Administration form 485) must be completed as required.

Developing the plan of care.

Patient care planning begins when the referral is made and the physician's order is

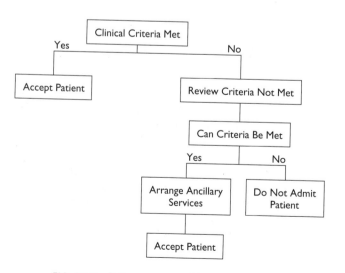

FIG. 28-3 *Patient acceptance/do-not-admit model.*

obtained. Planning continues throughout the course of therapy, sometimes even while the patient is not undergoing therapy. The multidisciplinary care plan is the most integral piece of the patient care process; it provides a road map for technical procedures and schedules, therapeutic monitoring, evaluation, treatment, and patient teaching. It establishes guidelines and goals for each patient, as well as scheduling requirements, and delivery system needs, and is updated as needed. The plan of care, including therapy scheduling, should be developed with the patient. It should be as convenient as possible for the patient and caregivers and meet the goals of therapy. If feasible, procedures should be provided during waking hours, interrupting the patient's rest period as little as possible. Long, cyclic infusions should be administered during sleeping hours, and short, intermittent infusions should be scheduled during waking hours. Delivery systems and equipment should be user friendly, safe, and trouble free. Lightweight ambulatory equipment should be used if the patient is mobile or needs around-the-clock infusion.

Initiating the plan: interdisciplinary communications and coordination of care.
Interdisciplinary communication and coordination are two important components of a successful home infusion program, second only to the patient component. Quality communication is the result of collaborative efforts, diligent management by the case coordinator, and interdisciplinary case conferences. Such communication enables a clear definition of the roles and responsibilities of each provider, ensuring the provision of quality patient care and services. Telephone conferencing, communication via facsimile machines, and computers with modems have enhanced communication and should be advocated for use in the home infusion therapy program. It is important, however, that while taking advantage of technology to improve and enhance communication, the patient's right to confidentiality is maintained at all times. For this reason, clinical information of patients with certain diagnoses should not be electronically transmitted. An example is a patient with a behavioral health diagnosis.

Performing the initial patient visit.
As mentioned earlier, the baseline patient assessment is usually completed during the initial home visit. The patient receives an intensive orientation to the service and instruction in the necessary procedures. The patient's psychologic status should be considered at this time because the patient likely has concerns other than the technical aspects of the home infusion visit. The patient may be under stress because of the illness and from issues related to family, work, or other responsibilities. How much information each patient can handle must be determined on an individual basis, realizing that only a portion of the information given will be retained on first hearing. For this reason, a teaching plan should be developed after the initial assessment and before the second visit (see Chapter 25). Important instructions should be given, repeated, and reviewed. Clearly written, step-by-step instructions reinforcing important information are left with the patient for reference. Telephone contacts should also be left with the patient in case questions arise or assistance is needed. Overwhelming a patient with too much information is counterproductive and can be harmful. Less important issues and details should be discussed on subsequent visits according to a predetermined education plan.

Orienting the patient to service.
General issues to be discussed during orientation include components of the service, roles of clinicians, ordering and delivery of equipment and supplies, and important telephone numbers and contacts. Addressed at this time are the more formal issues, such as service consents, assignment of benefits, receipt of goods, rights and responsibilities, and access to services in case of a medical emergency or a natural disaster. It is helpful to patients if emergency and contact numbers are placed by the telephone for easy accessibility. If that is not possible, a folder containing important information must be kept in one place known to all caregivers.

It is mandatory that advance directives be discussed with each patient. This mandate is a result of the Patient Self-Determination Act, passed by the U.S. Congress as a part of the Omnibus Reconciliation Act of 1990. It requires that home health care providers inform their patients of their rights to make decisions about their health care and to execute advance directives. Advance directives are documented instructions that relate patients' wishes for the provision of health care should they become incapacitated. It defines their choices and designates an individual who will make decisions on their behalf if they are no longer able to make their own decisions. These documents include a durable power of attorney for health care and a declaration pursuant to the Natural Death Act. Written material with this information should be left with patients for their reference.

If a patient has executed a do-not-resuscitate directive, it should be posted in the home in the event emergency personnel are called. The exact requirements for displaying this information vary from state to state. The clinician must ensure that there is a signed physician's order in the medical record confirming the do-not-resuscitate order. A verbal order is not sufficient in this circumstance.

Patient education.
Educating the patient about the home infusion therapy program involves providing information related to technical procedures and monitoring of therapy. The technical procedures that the patient is expected to learn and perform depend on several factors, including the patient's cognitive ability and willingness to learn, the complexity of technique, the organization's philosophy, the number of available visits, the patient's distance from the organization, and the standard of practice. Patients or their caregivers are commonly expected to administer solutions and medications, change dressings and infusion tubings, and give injections. They are not routinely expected to start IV lines or draw blood. The education process should progress according to the complexity of the prescribed therapy. Although no set standards exist for the number of visits required to teach a patient to administer therapy, some broad guidelines are provided in Table 28-2.

The length of teaching is customized and adjusted based on the patient's abilities and progress, and it should be documented in the care plan. Clinicians' communication skills vary, and not all are equally experienced in teaching the techniques of home infusion therapy. Some therapies are more complicated than others, such as those using programmable infusion devices, and take more time to teach and to learn. Therefore the teaching period should be as long or as short as the patient and clinician

Table 28-2	**Progressive Training for the Home Infusion Patient**

VISIT NO.	TEACHING ACTION
1	The clinician demonstrates preparation and administration of therapy.
2	The patient prepares and demonstrates use of the equipment, with the clinician's assistance and intervention.
3	The patient prepares the equipment independently. The clinician reviews the preparation and observes the demonstration with minimal intervention.
4	The patient prepares and demonstrates the equipment, using good technique without clinician intervention. The clinician observes.

Note: Each step in the process may be repeated as many times as necessary.

Table 28-3	**Potential Problems and Complications Encountered in Home Infusion Therapy**

PROBLEM	POTENTIAL COMPLICATIONS
MECHANICAL	
Blood back-up in tubing	Pump alarm signals
Inability to flush catheter	Noninfusing IV line
Fluid leakage	Pain or swelling at site
Catheter movement within the vessel	Redness or warmth at site (phlebitis)
SYSTEMIC	
Shortness of breath	Coughing
Respiratory distress	Chest pain
Rash	Itching
Fever	Chills
Muscle aches	Weakness
Exit-site drainage	Lethargy
METABOLIC	
Dizziness or fainting	Heart pounding
Increased thirst	Sugar in urine
Increased urination	Cold sweats
Abdominal or leg cramp	Flushing
Double vision	Headache
Confusion	Nervousness
Numbness	Twitching
Tingling in extremities	

feel is appropriate. When both feel comfortable, they sign a statement, usually a patient teaching checklist, documenting competency.

Monitoring and evaluating patient care. Monitoring is specific to the type of therapy, the patient's condition, and the goals of treatment. The patient or caregiver is generally expected to monitor and report any changes in condition or status. Therapy-specific issues discussed in the teaching sessions are also monitored, including vital signs, intake and output, weight, urine or blood glucose level, treatments, and medication or solution administration. A list of potential problems and complications is usually provided in the patient teaching material (Table 28-3).

The strategy for clinical therapeutic monitoring and evaluation of patients may vary depending on which model of home infusion therapy is being used, but the outcome should be the same. In the pharmacy home infusion therapy model, the nurse, pharmacist, or both communicate with the patient and caregivers to assess the patient's physical condition and therapeutic progress. They also evaluate the appropriateness of the prescribed therapy. The pharmacist analyzes laboratory data and reviews observations and physical findings. The pharmacy also assesses the appropriateness of the formulation or prescribed medication. These data can be analyzed to determine the patient's progress toward predetermined goals. At the same time, the nurse analyzes physical assessment findings, symptoms, laboratory data, and therapeutic response. The nurse and pharmacist then collaborate to make clinical recommendations for adjusting the plan. In the nursing agency home infusion therapy model, the process is the same, but collaboration usually occurs via telecommunications or during scheduled interdisciplinary meetings. In either case, the physician is contacted to communicate findings and to obtain new orders, if indicated.

Ongoing dynamic assessment

Physical systems. Clinical monitoring should be ongoing and dynamic. A commonly used tool for facilitating assessment is a physical systems review, during which the clinician reviews each system for subjective and objective signs and

symptoms and changes in condition. The patient's status is then measured against the baseline assessment.

Nutrition. Nutritional assessment is required for all home care patients but is more complex in the patient receiving nutritional therapies. Such patients require a combination of methodologies and is highly controversial among clinicians. Components of the evaluation include laboratory analysis of visceral proteins, such as total protein and albumin levels, and evaluation of somatic proteins, measured by anthropometric measurements and ideal body weight, usual body weight, and percentage of weight gain or loss over time. Other measures, such as transferrin levels and creatinine height index, are not usually performed in the home. Physical evaluation is also an important component of nutritional status. A course on general nutrition equips a clinician with the basic knowledge for determining signs and symptoms of nutritional deficiencies. For proficiency in the area of nutritional support, a residency or training period with a nutritional support team is recommended. Overall, the most reliable and commonly used measurement of nutritional status in the home patient is weight gain or loss (see Chapter 12).

Reporting and communications. Communication is the key to the success of the home infusion therapy program. Because members of the health care team do not share a common location (they may come from the physician's office, home infusion pharmacy, nursing agency, and equipment supplier), the desired frequency of interdisciplinary team meetings may not be possible. Alternative methods of communication should therefore be used. Advanced telecommunications have contributed to enhanced communications in the home infusion industry. Progress reports, physician's orders, and laboratory results are commonly faxed between physician's offices, infusion companies, nursing agencies, and laboratories. The telephone is used to discuss patient status, new or changed orders, scheduling and coordination of home visits, and various other activities.

Weekly patient-care conferences should be held to discuss new patients and changes in the care plan for patients already on service. Concise patient updates can be presented by each patient's primary clinician. The prescribed therapy, illness acuity, and patient status should be determinants of how often a patient's care and progress is discussed. For instance, a patient undergoing monthly IV gamma globulin therapy should be discussed the week before and after the monthly visit and when warranted by changes in status or condition. This method keeps weekly rounds manageable even if patient census is large.

All members of the health care team, regardless of their discipline or location, need to communicate outside of the patient-care conference. The better the communication, the better the continuity of care and service to the patient. The primary documents for communicating between the different disciplines are the clinical progress notes. Weekly patient-care conferences and communication among the physician, nursing agencies, patient, caregivers, and interoffice communication should be documented in these notes. The use of clinical progress notes and their content should be defined in organizational policy. Information such as laboratory analyses, clinical assessments, and documentation of progress toward outcomes may also be recorded in progress notes. Communication boards or computerized programs tracking schedules for deliveries, patient visits, and routing may be used; however, nothing replaces verbal communication among those involved in any aspect of care and service coordination.

Patient discharge and termination of care

Discharge planning takes time and should not be postponed until the last day of therapy. Discharge planning is initiated at the time of admission, when the duration of therapy is determined and discussed with the patient. It continues throughout the course of care as the nurse discusses discontinuation of therapy, postdischarge plans, and follow-up care or services. At a point close to discharge, usually the second or third visit from the discharge date, plans are finalized and the patient is provided with a written plan. Services are coordinated according to the physician's orders for postdischarge services as necessary. A written report describing the course of therapy, services delivered, achievement of goals, outcomes, and discharge instructions is then sent to the physician and other appropriate members of the health care team.

Postdischarge follow-up depends on the diagnosis and therapy. For instance, a patient with acquired immunodeficiency syndrome (AIDS) who has received a course of antibiotics may be closely monitored after therapy for recurrence of infection. After infusion, a chemotherapy patient may be monitored during the nadir of the white blood cell count for signs and symptoms of neutropenia-induced sepsis. Conversely, a patient who has had a successful course of antibiotics for subacute bacterial endocarditis may never be seen again by the home

infusion clinician once therapy is discontinued. The discharging agency must ensure the patient has the information necessary to move to the next step in the health care continuum. This may encompass ongoing care from another health care entity, such as an outpatient facility, or routine follow up by the physician.

SCOPE OF SERVICES
Therapies appropriate for home care

Antibiotics and antiinfective agents. The practice of administering antibiotics and antiinfective agents in the home originated in response to the demand for reduction of treatment costs to patients, third-party payers, and hospitals. Many patients have been trained to successfully administer their infusion antibiotics at home since the late 1970s.[6]

The most common diagnoses treated in the home care setting are disease states in which chronic or deep-seated infections are not effectively eradicated by oral antibiotics (Box 28-2).

Most commonly prescribed antibiotic and antiinfective agents. The selection of the antibiotic or antiinfective agent is of critical importance. Criteria reviewed by the physician and home infusion pharmacist when the medication is selected include efficacy of the medication against the offending pathogen or pathogens, tolerance of the patient to the medication, frequency of administration, stability of drugs and solutions, severity of toxicities, patient allergy history, presence of organ failure, duration of therapy, monitoring requirements, potential drug interactions, and availability of venous access.[6] Many antibiotic and antiinfective agents have been administered successfully in the home (Box 28-3).

Scheduling, dose frequency, and ease of administration are much more important considerations for home antibiotic therapy than for IV therapy administered in the hospital. Several antiinfectives (e.g., some cephalosporins) have extended half-lives that allow once- or twice-daily dosing, making it convenient for the patient and causing minimal interruption of daily activities. Antibiotics that have an increased ability to cause phlebitis should be considered carefully for peripheral adminis-

---

Box 28-2   Common Diagnoses for Which Home Intravenous Antibiotic and Antiinfective Agents Are Used

- Abscess
- Acute leukemia
- Bacterial endocarditis
- Candidiasis
- Cellulitis
- Chronic urinary tract infections
- Coccidioidomycosis
- Cryptococcal meningitis
- Cryptosporidiosis
- Cystic fibrosis
- Cytomegalovirus retinitis
- Hairy leukoplakia
- Histoplasmosis
- Lyme disease
- *Mycobacterium avium-intracellulare*
- Osteomyelitis
- Pelvic inflammatory disease
- *Pneumocystis carinii* pneumonia
- Sepsis
- Toxoplasmosis
- Wound infections

tration in the home because of the increased frequency of rotating peripheral IV access. Several options exist in this situation, including inserting a central venous access device, diluting the medication, slowing the infusion rate, or changing to another, less caustic, medication that is equally effective against the causative pathogen.

Common concerns and issues. A common concern of home infusion antibiotic patients and home infusion providers is reimbursement. Medicare payment has generally been denied for antibiotic therapy. In the past, vancomycin was the only antibiotic reimbursable under Medicare Part B because it was always administered via an electronic infusion device and coverage for home IV antibiotics is approved only in conjunction with a piece of durable medical equipment. In 1997, Medicare determined that it was not medically necessary for vancomycin to be delivered via a pump, and reimbursement for home administration of this antiinfective ceased.[12,13] Many third-party payers allow reimbursement of home infusion antibiotics after close review of the statement of medical necessity, the charges for the antibiotics and supplies, and the type of insurance coverage available. Because home administration of antibiotics is based on a culture and sensitivity test, and administration of antiinfective agents is based on diagnosis, a statement of medical necessity is completed to document the need, and the appropriateness of the medication for the causative organism. Because of the ever-changing health care environment and the

complexity of reimbursement issues, the home infusion provider must have an experienced billing and reimbursement specialist work with the patient, third-party payer, and home infusion team to obtain the best reimbursement possible.

A major concern for the patient and the health care team is achieving therapeutic goals. For this reason, time should be taken to teach the patient the importance of maintaining therapeutic blood levels of the prescribed medication. This can be accomplished only by diligent compliance with the dosing schedule. The home care team can help the patient schedule to minimize interruption of daily activities and rest periods. For multiple daily infusions, an infusion pump may be suggested, if appropriate for the drug. Hypersensitivity and allergic reactions are always of major concern, and these are discussed in detail under First-Dose Guidelines.

Some other concerns of home infusion antibiotic patients include their ability to self-administer medications and resolve problems, the frequency of rotating peripheral venous access sites, the frequency of administration, and the support available from the home infusion provider. Patients should receive thorough training from the home nursing and pharmacy clinicians regarding the diagnosis, medication prescribed, goals of therapy, aseptic technique, care and maintenance of the access device, set-up of supplies and equipment, and initiation and termination of an infusion. Information regarding possible side effects and complications, delivery of supplies and medications, and frequency of nursing visits should also be reviewed. This information is provided orally and in writing.

First-dose guidelines. Many patients are able to avoid hospitalization because of the advent of home infusion antibiotic therapy. This practice raises the controversial issue of first-dose administration in the home. In the past, the first dose of an antibiotic or antiinfective agent was given only in a controlled clinical environment, such as the hospital, physician's office, clinic, outpatient infusion suite, or emergency department. Although a controlled clinical environment remains the location of choice for first-dose administration, these drugs are often administered safely and effectively in the home. This change largely results from advances in technology and pharmaceuticals as well as specialization of home IV nurses and pharmacists. The availability of first-dose administration in the home does not negate the necessity for a controlled environment for highly sensitive or allergic patients. All patients who are to receive antibiotic or antiinfective agents need to have a thorough allergy history evaluation. The home infusion pharmacist reviews this information and performs a risk analysis. If the patient is determined to have low or minimal risk and no history of allergic response or cross allergies, the pharmacist may recommend that the first dose be administered in the home under the continuous supervision of the IV nurse. However, although the risk is low, a reaction can occur. Therefore an order for an anaphylactic kit and protocol should always be obtained and available. A few antibiotics, such as penicillin and cotrimoxazole (Bactrim), are known for having higher rates of allergic reaction. Clinicians should carefully evaluate the safety of these agents when considering giving a first dose in the home. Patients with allergies to penicillin may also have an allergic response to cephalosporins.

Box 28-3   Common Antibiotics and Antiinfective Agents Used in Home Care

- Acyclovir (Zovirax)
- Amikacin sulfate (Amikin)
- Amphotericin B (Fungizone)/amphotericin B lipid formulations
- Aztreonam (Azactam)
- Azithromycin (Zithromax)
- Cefazolin sodium (Ancef, Kefzol)
- Cefotaxime sodium (Claforan)
- Cefotetan disodium (Cefotan)
- Cefoxitin sodium (Mefoxin)
- Ceftazidime (Fortaz, Tazicef)
- Ceftizoxime sodium (Cefizox)
- Ceftriaxone sodium (Rocephin)
- Ciprofloxacin (Cipro I.V.)
- Clindamycin phosphate (Cleocin Phosphate)
- Fluconazole (Diflucan)
- Foscarnet sodium (Foscavir)
- Ganciclovir sodium (Cytovene I.V.)
- Gentamicin sulfate (Garamycin)
- Imipenem/cilastatin (Primaxin)
- Levofloxacin (Levaquin)
- Metronidazole hydrochloride (Flagyl I.V.)
- Nafcillin sodium (Unipen)
- Oxacillin sodium (Bactocill)
- Penicillin G aqueous (Penicillin G sodium) [or potassium]
- Piperacillin sodium (Pipracil)
- Piperacillin sodium/tazobactam sodium (Zosyn)
- Ticarcillin/clavulanate (Timentin)
- Tobramycin (Nebcin)
- Vancomycin (Vancocin)

Allergic and anaphylactic reactions can occur not only on the first dose, but also at any time during antibiotic therapy. The home IV nurse must be able to identify and differentiate allergic responses from anaphylactic reactions. IV nurses must train their patients to recognize and report signs and symptoms of allergic reactions and access emergency medical services in event of anaphylaxis. Although the practice of providing anaphylaxis kits for every home antibiotic patient is controversial, they should certainly be provided and readily accessible for all first-dose administrations. The kit should include epinephrine, diphenhydramine (Benadryl), hydrocortisone (Solu-Cortef), acetaminophen, 0.9% sodium chloride solution, an IV administration set, and the required needles, syringes, and swabs. Several commercially prepared kits are available. The home infusion pharmacist must review the anaphylactic kit and protocols with the physician and must obtain orders to dispense the kit and its contents. The home IV nurse must have knowledge of each medication in the anaphylactic kit and the protocols for intervention and must receive ongoing education on this issue. It is extremely important that the home infusion provider develops and implements policies and procedures for first-dose administration.

Delivery systems.

Home infusion antibiotics can be administered via a peripheral intermittent infusion device, central venous catheter, peripherally inserted central catheter (PICC), tunneled central venous catheter, or implantable port. The route of administration is determined by the patient, physician, and home infusion clinician based on diagnosis, duration of therapy, frequency of administration, venous access available, and medication prescribed. Antibiotics are usually administered via a gravity infusion device that uses minibags. Ambulatory infusion devices may be used for medications that need to be accurately controlled, such as amphotericin B, when patient compliance is a concern or if the frequency of the dose would lend itself to the use of such a device. In some situations, the infusion device is connected only intermittently. The access device is flushed after administration. In other situations, the infusion device may be connected continuously, with intermittent infusion of the medication at preprogrammed intervals. During the "off" cycle, the infusion device maintains positive pressure and administers a minute amount of solution to keep the infusion access device patent. Some pumps are also capable of delivering multiple antibiotics according to independently timed schedules.

Some home infusion programs are administering selected antibiotics IV push. Poole and Nowobilski-Vasilios have reported successful IV push administration of certain cephalosporins to selected patients. The study reported cost efficiency and no statistical difference in phlebitis rates between traditional administration methodologies and the IV push method. However, the authors caution against indiscriminate use of this delivery system and encourage carefully matching patient needs and safety to the methodology.[14,15] Another advance in therapy delivery in the home is the availability of lipid formulations of amphotericin B. The literature reports decreased rates of toxicity with this formulation, and infusion time is cut by as much as half. The result is the ability to administer higher doses of amphotericin, with less interruption of the patient's lifestyle and significantly lower incidence of untoward events.[16]

The cost versus benefit of each delivery system must be evaluated to identify the most appropriate and cost-effective method of administration.

Clinical monitoring.

Whether therapy is provided in the home, hospital, or outpatient setting, clinical monitoring standards are the same. Geographic logistics need to be considered. Routine visits by the home IV nurse are scheduled based on the access device and patient acuity. During these visits, the home IV nurse performs technical procedures related to the infusion access device and equipment, reinforces training, monitors compliance by counting inventory, draws blood, and performs a clinical assessment. Clinical assessment focuses on the development of adverse reactions and complications to the antibiotic, symptoms related to the patient's disease process, and progress toward the goals of therapy. Laboratory monitoring may include complete blood counts with differential, renal profile, electrolyte, liver enzyme, and antibiotic drug levels.

Some adverse reactions and complications include direct tissue toxicities, such as irritation to the veins (phlebitis) or intramuscular injection sites (pain, swelling, or hematomas). The gastrointestinal tract can also be irritated, causing nausea, vomiting, or diarrhea. Organs involved in metabolism or elimination can be directly affected (e.g., liver, kidney), which can result in reversible or permanent damage. Superinfections, such as yeast infections, can be caused when nonsensitive organisms are allowed to grow unchecked. Immediate or delayed hypersensitivity reactions may also occur and must be monitored closely. Patients should be cautioned against ingestion of alcohol or medications containing alcohol when taking some cephalosporins, such as cefamandole, cefoperazone, moxalactam, and cefotetan, because they may experience a disulfiram-like reaction. This reaction is an alcohol intolerance response and is exhibited by flushing, headache, nausea, vomiting, and tachycardia.

Total parenteral nutrition.

TPN, also known as *hyperalimentation* and when given in the home, *home parenteral nutrition,* was one of the first infusion therapies administered outside the acute care setting. Indications for TPN in the early stages of home administration were for nutritional deficiencies from the patient's inability to properly use the digestive system, which resulted in prolonged administration of TPN. The patients in the early stages recovered shortly after TPN was initiated or their only medical need was for TPN administration. Home parenteral nutrition was clearly a cost-effective alternative to extended hospitalization.

Indications.

Indications for TPN have expanded over the last 10 years. Initially, TPN, a total nutritional source providing all of the body's daily nutritional requirements, was prescribed when the patient could not eat because of a functional impairment, such as short-bowel syndrome or small bowel obstruction. It was also used when the patient was restricted from eating or when bowel rest was indicated, such as in the treatment of ulcerative colitis or Crohn's disease. As medical and technologic advances progressed and research found other indications for TPN, terms of reimbursement became more strictly defined by medical necessity. TPN was prescribed based on functional impairment and symptomatology rather than purely on diagnosis. For example, not all patients with a short bowel need TPN. However, a percentage of bowel resection patients have short-bowel syndrome and failure to thrive secondary to malabsorption, necessitating TPN administration.

Common diagnoses indicating TPN include short-bowel syndrome, massive bowel resection, mesenteric infarction, radiation enteritis, inflammatory bowel disease, intestinal obstruction, and motility disorders (e.g., intractable nausea and vomiting or diarrhea). In addition, the patient must be unable to absorb sufficient nutrients to maintain height and weight.

Although the potential indications for TPN have expanded, the use of TPN has decreased. Current scientific thought maintains that TPN should be used only if there is complete failure of the gut; "If the gut works, use it." In addition, studies demonstrate that there is a significant reduction in sepsis in critically ill patients fed enterally rather than parenterally.[17] The *Standards for Home Nutritional Support* by the American Society of Parenteral and Enteral Nutrition state that a patient who is a candidate for home parenteral nutrition should be unable to meet nutrient requirements via the gastrointestinal track adequately and safely.[18]

Routes of therapy.

Central venous access is generally the most common route used for administering home parenteral nutrition. TPN can be given centrally or peripherally. The peripheral route may be used provided that the final dextrose concentration is not greater than 10%.[18] Peripheral administration in the home setting is not generally recommended. With the advent of the PICCs and advances in permanent long-term access devices, use of peripheral access for TPN is rarely indicated in the home setting. There is no longer a need to subject the patient to increased risks of infiltration, phlebitis, and repeated infusion restarts.

Types of parenteral nutrition.

In addition to TPN, other parenteral nutrient admixtures prescribed for home infusion include partial parenteral nutrition and total nutrient admixture, also known as *three-in-one* or *all-in-one.* Partial parenteral nutrition provides a portion of the body's requirements and is prescribed as a supplement to oral or enteral nutrition. Although most commonly administered intermittently, three times a week or every other day, partial parenteral nutrition may be prescribed daily based on the patient's fluid needs. Total nutrient admixture is the same as TPN; however, the term indicates that patients are receiving part of their caloric source in the form of a fat emulsion and that a single-administration container system is being used. This system is recommended in the home care setting because it is easier to teach and to learn. The risks of contamination are reduced because there is only one line to manipulate.[5,17]

Intradialytic parenteral nutrition, which is parenteral nutrition administered to patients requiring hemodialysis, has been limited to date largely because of reimbursement issues. Intradialytic parenteral nutrition is administered over a 3- to 4-hour period, three to four times per week in conjunction with dialysis treatments. Other specialized formulas for hepatic or renal failure are not used as often in the home setting.

Common issues and concerns.

TPN in the home setting is one of the more complex therapies for several reasons, including TPN vascular access availability, duration and frequency of administration, mobility of the patient, complexity of the delivery system, and clinical and patient monitoring issues.

As with any home infusion therapy, psychosocial support and compliance are always important issues, especially in therapies of extended duration. Permanent vascular access devices, such as tunneled catheters and ports, are generally recommended for long-term TPN administration.[19] Intermediate vascular access devices, such as PICCs, can be used as well.[20]

Home parenteral nutrition is generally cycled or given over 12 to 16 hours, and most administrations occur during the sleeping hours. Ideally, the less time it takes to administer TPN safely, the easier it will be to integrate into the patient's life. Depending on the patient's diagnosis or disease process, the level of activity ranges from being completely bedridden to participating in normal daily activities, including work or school. Advances in ambulatory pump technology have minimized the concern about using such equipment while leading an active lifestyle. A small pump, able to be slipped into a backpack, can now be programmed to turn on, taper up, taper down, and turn off TPN.[21]

For some patients, clinical monitoring is one of the major concerns. The more acutely ill the patient, the closer the monitoring needs to be. The nurse and pharmacist need to pay particular attention to laboratory values, physical status findings, fluid requirements, and signs and symptoms of infection. The patient and the physician depend on the clinicians to communicate their observations between the patient's physician visits. Thorough training courses in advanced nutrition, physical and nutritional assessment, laboratory analysis, therapeutic monitoring, and nutritional support are recommended for home care clinicians caring for TPN patients.

Patient self-monitoring is as important as clinical monitoring. The patient must be taught to monitor vital signs, fluid status, glucose level (urine and fingerstick), and weight. The patient must be given guidelines for reporting outer limits.

Psychosocial support is another concern. As with any long-term therapy, family, friends, and caregivers provide important assistance and support during difficult times. Not all patients need assistance with the administration of their therapy, but most need some psychosocial support because nourishment by the IV route is not the norm. Patients who are more acutely ill or are diagnosed with a terminal illness may eventually need a full-time caregiver. It is generally recommended that along with the patient, a primary and an alternative caregiver learn and become involved in the home infusion program.

Because home infusion patients are not in a controlled setting, compliance with scheduling and daily administration is a concern. An excess number of bags in the refrigerator is usually the telltale sign of noncompliance. However, gross noncompliance may also be noted by fluctuations in laboratory values, both upward and downward, and loss of or failure to gain weight. Providing continual reinforcement and support and involving the patient and caregiver in the treatment plan reduces the chance of noncompliance.

Initiating TPN in the home setting.

Initiating TPN in the home setting requires the availability of skilled clinicians, especially a pharmacist with experience and education in the field of nutritional support, and a higher level of service. The patient is initially evaluated for nutritional and physical status as well as all other components of the initial patient assessment.

Baseline laboratory values are obtained and evaluated, and recommendations for TPN formulations are made. A modified formulation may be initiated, depending on the evaluation of the patient. The modified formulation is then adjusted upward to the final formulation as the patient's clinical condition permits. One or two bags are compounded at a time to limit waste. Obtaining laboratory values before the next bag is used allows one to make adjustments in the formulation until a stabilization point is reached. If uncomplicated, this process generally takes about 1 week. If complicated, stabilization can take several weeks. TPN is usually compounded for 7 days, at which time laboratory values are obtained and evaluated. Depending on the patient's stability, laboratory values may be obtained and TPN compounded twice a week, or in the case of the stable, long-term TPN patient, once a month.

Delivery systems. TPN is always administered by an infusion device in the home. The complexity of the therapy and the ambulatory status of the patient determine which pump is chosen. Usually, a programmable, variable-rate, volumetric pump that is safe, accurate, user friendly, and easy to troubleshoot is the device of choice.

Clinical monitoring. Clinical monitoring of home TPN patients should be no different from monitoring hospitalized TPN patients. However, although the areas monitored are the same, the logistics are quite different. Patients are taught to monitor vital signs, fluid intake and output, weight gain or loss, and blood or urine glucose levels. They are also taught to report outer limits to the home infusion clinicians. These outer limits commonly include temperature increases, weight gain of more than a half pound per day, spilling of glucose in the urine or abnormal fingerstick glucose level, and any changes in overall status. The home infusion clinician tracks and analyzes this information along with physical findings and laboratory analyses to evaluate progress, prevent potential complications, and make recommendations for achieving the goals of therapy. Areas that are generally monitored, tracked, and analyzed include vital signs, urine glucose level, weight, fluid status, complete blood count, and full chemistry panel (Table 28-4).

Chemotherapy. Chemotherapy has been prescribed for the treatment of cancer since the 1960s. As with other infusion therapies, the administration of antineoplastic agents has moved into the home care setting. The agents most commonly administered include fluorouracil and floxuridine. In the past few years, complex chemotherapy or multiple-agent chemotherapy regimens have been administered in the home under the care of trained oncology infusion specialists. With the support of these specialists, it is no longer necessary to admit these patients to the acute care setting for therapy.[22]

Indications. Although not all antineoplastic agents and protocols are amenable to home administration, single-agent therapy and continuous administration have been given safely and with good results. In the past, the diagnoses most commonly seen in the home were those for which continuous fluorouracil and floxuridine were prescribed. With advances in medical and clinical applications, as well as in technology, many patients with cancer are seen in home chemotherapy programs (Box 28-4).

The administration of chemotherapeutic agents in the home

Table 28-4　Laboratory Monitoring for the Home Total Parenteral Nutrition Patient

COMPLETE BLOOD COUNT	CHEMISTRY	
White blood cells	Sodium	Uric acid
Red blood cells	Potassium	Cholesterol
Hemoglobin	Chloride	Triglycerides
Hematocrit	Carbon dioxide	Bilirubin
Segmented neutrophils	Glucose	Alkaline phosphatase
Lymphocytes	Blood urea nitrogen	Lactic dehydrogenase
Band neutrophils	Serum creatinine	Aspartate aminotransferase
Eosinophils	Calcium	Alanine aminotransferase
Platelets	Phosphorus	Magnesium
	Retinol-binding protein	Ionized calcium
	Prealbumin	Albumin
	Transferrin	

Box 28-4　Common Indications for Chemotherapeutic Drugs Prescribed in the Home

- Bone cancer
- Breast cancer
- Chronic lymphocytic leukemia
- Hodgkin's disease
- Intestinal cancer
- Leukemias
- Lung cancer
- Metastatic cancer
- Multiple myeloma
- Head and neck cancer
- Non-Hodgkin's lymphoma
- Ovarian cancer
- Prostate cancer
- Stomach cancer

requires careful assessment of patients' ability and willingness to participate in their care and to learn and understand. Patients should be clinically stable and have family or significant others to assist with care as needed. Administration in the home requires appropriate levels of specialized clinical oncology support. A list of common chemotherapeutic drugs and combination regimens can be found in Table 28-5.

Routes of therapy. Safe, cost-effective chemotherapy can be given to the home infusion patient through many routes. This particular therapy, unlike some others, demands closer monitoring when the patient is *not* undergoing therapy. Chemotherapy infusions are most commonly given intravenously; however, they can be given by the intraarterial, intrathecal, intraperitoneal, or subcutaneous routes. These infusions may be given by bolus, continuous infusion, or periodic continuous infusion (5-day infusions).

Common issues and concerns. Patients are generally concerned with their quality of life during and after therapy. Issues related to side effects, such as nausea, vomiting, and hair loss, are the most common initial concerns. These concerns largely result from anticipation of the unknown and the media attention that these side effects receive. Other concerns that arise later include susceptibility to infection (as the patient reaches the nadir, the point at which the white blood cell count is at its

Table 28-5   **Commonly Used Chemotherapeutic Drugs and Combination Regimens**

COMMON THERAPEUTIC DRUGS USED IN THE HOME

Bleomycin	Carboplatin	Cisplatin	Cyclophosphamide	Cytarabine
Doxorubicin	Etoposide	Fluorouracil	Ifosfamide	Leuprolide depot
Levamisole	Methotrexate	Mitomycin C	Mitoxantrone	Tamoxifen
Vinblastine	Vincristine			

COMBINATION CHEMOTHERAPY REGIMENS PRESCRIBED IN THE HOME

ACRONYM	DRUGS	CANCER
PEF	Bleomycin, etoposide, cisplatin	Genitourinary
CAF (FAC)	Cyclophosphamide, doxorubicin, fluorouracil	Breast, metastatic disease
CAP	Cisplatin, doxorubicin, cyclophosphamide	Lung, non–small cell
CF	Cisplatin, fluorouracil	Head and neck
CFL	Cisplatin, fluorouracil, leucovorin	Head and neck
CHOP	Cyclophosphamide, doxorubicin, vincristine, prednisone	Non-Hodgkin's lymphoma
CV	Cisplatin, etoposide	Lung, non–small cell
CVI (VIC)	Carboplatin, etoposide, ifosfamide, mesna	Lung, non–small cell
EVA	Etoposide, vinblastine, doxorubicin	Hodgkin's lymphoma
FAC	Fluorouracil, doxorubicin, cyclophosphamide	Breast, metastatic disease
FAM	Fluorouracil, doxorubicin, mitomycin C	Colon, lung, non–small cell
FCE	Fluorouracil, cisplatin, etoposide	Gastric
F-CL	Fluorouracil, calcium leucovorin	Colon
FLE	Levamisole, fluorouracil	Colon
FMV	Fluorouracil, methyl-C	CNU, vincristine
IMF	Ifosfamide, mesna, methotrexate, fluorouracil	Colon
PFL	Methotrexate, cisplatin, fluorouracil, leucovorin	Breast
MVAC	Methotrexate, vinblastine, doxorubicin, cisplatin	Genitourinary
PFL	Cisplatin, fluorouracil, leucovorin	Genitourinary
VAC	Vincristine, doxorubicin, cyclophosphamide	Gastric, head and neck, lung, non–small cell
VIP	Vinblastine, etoposide, ifosfamide, cisplatin, mesna	Genitourinary
Wayne State	Cisplatin, 5-fluorouracil	Head and neck

lowest), nutritional status, and the ability to carry on routine activities of life without interruption.

While patients are not undergoing chemotherapy, a clinical concern is monitoring the nadir period. Approximately 14 to 21 days after therapy begins, depending on the drugs being administered, the patient reaches the nadir. During this time, the patient is most susceptible to infections. Neutropenic precautions, including scrupulous handwashing and hygiene, sterile accessing of infusion devices and infusion therapy technique, as well as crowd, injury, and dietary precautions, must be maintained.[23] Several biologic agents, such as the cytokines filgrastim (G-CSF) and sargramostim (GM-CSF), have been introduced to treat and prevent complications related to chemotherapy administration.[19] These agents, along with medical research that suggests new clinical applications and the reduction in risk of catheter-related infection resulting from advances in catheter technology, make home chemotherapy less intimidating and more acceptable. The newer-generation antiemetics, which control side effects without rendering patients unable to care for themselves, have also made home administration more desirable.[24]

The subject of permanent vascular access is usually encountered early by the home chemotherapy patient. The choice of access device is usually based on the frequency and duration of therapy, the medications prescribed, and the patient's prefer-

ence. Peripheral access for the administration of vesicant agents in the home is discouraged.

Psychosocial and physical support is important to the patient on chemotherapy. A new or reoccurring disease process places a major stress on the patient and family members. Toxicities and side effects also pose a potential for debilitation and a need for physical and psychologic support. For this reason, it is recommended that the patient have a strong support system and an alternative caregiver.

Delivery systems. Advances in technology that allow multiple-drug regimens to be delivered on multiple schedules via ambulatory devices have made chemotherapy administration in the home more easily achievable.[25] Whereas some patients receive chemotherapy by rapid infusion (bolus), a one-time rapid injection, others receive administration by continuous infusion that can last several days to several months. To date, the optimal schedule for most antineoplastic agents has not been established. Infusion devices are available that synchronize delivery of agents with circadian rhythms to allow maximum effectiveness and cell kill.

Clinical monitoring. Vital to the prevention of complications is ongoing monitoring of laboratory values, physical status, fluid status, and drug-related side effects and toxicities. Education and certification in chemotherapy administration and monitoring are strongly recommended. Knowledge about the drugs being administered helps clinicians monitor home chemotherapy patients. Although side effects are expected with this therapy, complications related to these side effects can be prevented. Therefore protocols and reporting guidelines should be established for physical and therapeutic assessment and for side effect and toxicity management. Protocols for use in home chemotherapy include hydration, therapeutic monitoring, antiemetic, laboratory, and patient monitoring. Extravasation, or escape of antineoplastic agents into the tissue, is not an expected event. Protocols should be readily available to treat extravasation promptly if it occurs. It is important to remember that a permanent catheter does not automatically preclude the occurrence of an extravasation. Camp-Sorrell describes a study in which 8 of 169 implantable ports used for the continuous infusion of vesicant agents extravasated. Possible causes noted were catheter tip migration, thrombosis, and catheter separation from the port body.[26] It is incumbent on the nurse to be diligent in monitoring and recognizing signs and symptoms of extravasation, paying particular attention to complaints of pain at and around the site of infusion. The treatment of extravasation remains controversial, and each organization providing this service must have agent-specific polices to direct the nurse in the event extravasation does occur. The most prudent course of action regarding extravasation is to employ skilled, experienced clinicians who will carefully monitor patients to prevent or minimize its occurrence.

Complex chemotherapy. A recent advance in home therapy is the provision of the complex chemotherapy regimens. This therapy includes hydration before and after treatment, antiemetic regimens, multiple chemotherapeutic agents, adjuvants, and if needed, biologic agents. Laboratory results and physical findings are monitored closely during and between treatments. Adjustments in therapy regimens and medications are made when complications and toxicities occur. Crisis can be avoided and preventive measures implemented only through diligent monitoring by clinicians specially trained in the field of oncologic infusion therapy. Providing complex chemotherapy in the home is not an undertaking for the novice home care clinician. An oncology residency or advanced oncology and chemotherapy certification is strongly recommended.

With the publication of new medical advances in continuous and complex chemotherapy regimens and the introduction of new drugs, chemotherapy is increasingly being administered in the home care setting. As patients become more acutely aware of the availability of home chemotherapy and with the success of new regimens, patients will seek not only quality of life but also an uninterrupted lifestyle. Predictably, referral sources will also realize the cost benefit of administering these complex therapies in the home versus the hospital, and the demand for cost containment will steer referrals into the home care program.

Pain management. Managing pain has always been an important focus in the hospital and has now become just as important in home care. Most of the pain management literature states that pain is untreated and underrelieved in most patients. Identified barriers to providing effective pain management include the cost of treatment, inaccurate perceptions of pain, poor pain assessment, inadequate knowledge of pharmacokinetics and equianalgesic dosing, and limited professional

accountability.[27] The one-to-one relationship of patient to clinician in the home and the interdisciplinary communication required of the team has proven effective in ameliorating these barriers. As Gorski and Grotham wrote:

> A collaborative interdisciplinary approach to pain management is necessary to create an effective treatment plan for a patient. A complete assessment of the patient's pain by the home care nurse, collaboration with the patient's physician in developing a pain management plan of care, and finally, comprehensive teaching to the patient and caregiver will help to ensure adequate pain management.[21]

It is now accepted that pain can cause physical harm to the patient and that patients need to have more involvement in the control of their pain.

Indications. Some of the most common diagnoses for home pain management include intractable pain of cancer or AIDS or following surgery, and chronic pain from causalgia, neuralgia, or reflex sympathetic dystrophy. The traditional response to debilitating pain associated with terminal disease is to administer oral medications, usually narcotic analgesics. When oral pain management results in poor pain control, other routes should be explored. Narcotic analgesics can be safely administered in the home by subcutaneous, IV, epidural, or intrathecal routes. These infusions may be intermittent, continuous, or continuous with patient-controlled bolus capabilities.[27,28] Better pain control and decreased central nervous system effects are experienced with a continuous infusion of a low-dose medication. Patients are able to manage their "breakthrough" pain by self-administering preset bolus doses.

Most commonly prescribed pain medications. The most common medications administered in the home for pain management are morphine sulfate, meperidine (Demerol), hydromorphone (Dilaudid), and fentanyl (Duragesic). It is important to note that meperidine (Demerol), because of its limited duration (2 to 3 hours) and the potential for central nervous system toxicity with repeated use, is not a drug of choice for chronic cancer pain.[29] The home infusion pharmacist collaborates with the physician to obtain the appropriate dose based on the route of administration. Thorough pain assessment by the home IV nurse should include location and distribution, timing and pattern, onset and duration, and quality and severity of the pain experienced (rated by the patient using an established scale). The home IV nurse uses these data to help the home infusion pharmacist and physician titrate the dosage to maintain adequate pain control. It is extremely important that the home infusion pharmacist, home IV nurse, physician, and patient work closely to obtain optimal pain management when medications or routes are changed. The home infusion pharmacist makes recommendations on equianalgesic doses to help stay within the same analgesic range. This analysis prevents inadvertent underdosing or overdosing, causing the recurrence of pain or excessive sedation.

Common issues and concerns. A successful home pain management program requires a motivated patient or caregiver, a conducive home environment, adequate support, and an appropriately prescribed medication, dose, and route of administration. Careful consideration should be given to the admission of patients with known IV drug abuse or those for whom the home environment poses a potential for drug abuse. Alternative arrangements need to be explored in these cases. Nursing management of the patient in pain is virtually the same regardless of the health care setting. Education plays an extremely important role in caring for the patient in pain. The patient and caregiver should be instructed in medication being administered, its side effects, and the route of administration. The basics of pain control, the pain rating system, and home self-monitoring should be explained. The teaching may include giving bolus dosing, determining precipitating events to pain, and handling side effects.

Many home pain management patients and caregivers have concerns regarding the administration of narcotics. One of the most common concerns is addiction. At this point in disease progression, many patients have been on narcotics orally for some time. Conversion to the parenteral route of administration does not lead to addiction, as some patients fear. Patients and caregivers should be reassured that addiction is of minimal concern and that bolus dosing should be administered as needed. Physical dependence and tolerance are expected and are easily managed by adjusting the dosage upward according to need, or conversely, slowly decreasing the dosage over time before discontinuing the narcotic.

Patients are also concerned about maintaining their mental capabilities. Through education, patients learn that by using the parenteral route, with the medication infusing continuously, a much lower dosage is required, therefore decreasing sedation. They are instructed to notify the home IV nurse if sedation does occur or if their pain is not being controlled. Such signs may indicate that the dosage should be adjusted or the route changed. Patients are instructed in the various parenteral administration routes. The patient and the physician decide on the route of administration that will be most effective for the degree of pain experienced and the condition and prognosis of the patient. The home IV nurse provides instructions for the care and maintenance of the selected route.

Patients are instructed on the clinical adverse effects of narcotics. Because constipation, nausea, and vomiting are relatively consistent side effects and are anticipated, they are treated concurrently with such drugs as stool softeners, laxatives, and antiemetics. Respiratory depression is of minor concern, because when dosages are titrated for pain relief, the respiratory depressant effects of narcotics lie above the sedation threshold, which lies above the pain relief threshold.[29] Patients also develop a tolerance to the sedative and respiratory depressant effects. Patients and caregivers are instructed that if the respiration rate decreases to half of what has been normal for that patient, the rate of infusion needs to be decreased and the home IV nurse notified. Sedative and respiratory depressant effects can be reversed with agents such as Narcan; however, it must be remembered that analgesia will be reversed as well.

Delivery systems.
The many technologic advances in infusion devices make administration of narcotics in the home relatively safe. These devices are designed for ease in ambulation. A built-in safety mechanism (lock-out function) prevents the rate of infusion and the programmed dose from being changed by unauthorized persons. Modern devices are able to infuse intermittently or continuously and allow the patient to administer bolus doses during continuous infusion. The remainder of the delivery system consists of the appropriate administration tubing for the infusion device, supplies, and a dressing change kit that is appropriate to the route of administration.

Clinical monitoring.
Clinical monitoring performed by the home infusion pharmacist and the IV nurse includes physical assessment, pain assessment, compliance check, equipment check, and psychosocial support.

Cardiac therapies.
Chronic congestive heart failure and its progressive degenerative course affects millions of people. Because of its prevalence, interest has increased in identifying alternative treatments that are relatively safe and cost-effective.

Indications and medications prescribed.
The use of parenteral inotropic agents in the home setting to manage terminal congestive heart failure was reported as early as 1984. The literature on this topic documents successful home IV infusions of dobutamine, dopamine, amrinone, and milrinone for the management of decompensated, terminal congestive heart failure in patients in whom conventional therapy was unsuccessful or for those who were awaiting heart tranplantation.[30-32]

Common issues and concerns.
The success of a home IV inotropic program depends on several factors. The first is patient stability before discharge. The patient must respond in the acute care setting to the IV inotrope and the dosage regimen to be administered at home. Another area of significant importance is the psychosocial evaluation, including assessment of patient acceptance, involvement, and compliance; identification of a patient caregiver to assist in the therapy; and knowledge of the limitations of the therapy. The patient, family, and caregiver must understand that this therapy is not a cure, but rather an attempt for improved quality of life compared with that which may be experienced in the cardiac care unit. Reimbursement for the home therapy should be verified before accepting the patient into the program. This is particularly true for the patient covered by Medicare. The patient must be end stage because of cardiac disease or be on a transplant list and must demonstrate response to the presence or absence of the drug with a failed trial of oral therapy.

Patient and caregiver training, as with any home infusion therapy, includes providing information regarding the disease state, prescribed medication, and goals of therapy. Education in the medication regimen includes expected therapeutic effects of the drug, side effects, and home self-monitoring. This information enables the patient to understand the rationale for increased urine output and the need for monitoring. Patient-specific information is provided regarding aseptic technique and the care and maintenance of the infusion access device. The patient and caregiver need to master set-up and initiation of therapy using an ambulatory infusion device. Troubleshooting pump malfunctions is also covered during training. Written patient training information is provided, and competency is documented on a patient-training checklist.

Some of the common concerns of the home infusion patient receiving inotropic therapy are adverse reactions, such as increased heart rate and blood pressure and ventricular ectopic activity; support from family members and the home health care team; and home self-monitoring. Identifying concerns early in the process and developing a plan of care will help allay these concerns. During routine nursing visits for physical assessment, the nurse should carefully monitor the results of vital sign assessment, draw blood, perform technical procedures, and reinforce teaching; these activities also decrease the patient's concerns.

Delivery route. Central venous access is preferred because of the need for continuous administration of the medication. Inotropes such as dobutamine have the potential to cause necrosis if allowed to infiltrate into the tissues. Central venous access is also more practical and cost effective for this long-term home infusion therapy. The pharmacist needs to dilute the drug to a concentration that is likely more concentrated than that used in the hospital. The strength of the dilution facilitates the use of ambulatory infusion devices and supports the goal of restricting fluid in patients with congestive heart failure.

Clinical monitoring. Infusing inotropes at home demands effective monitoring by the patient or caregiver and the home infusion clinician. Baseline vital signs are obtained and are used for comparison with all future vital signs, especially heart rate and systolic blood pressure. Once stable, vital signs are monitored three times a day or as per the physician's order. Patients record their fluid intake and urine output and their daily weight. The venous access site is monitored for signs of infection and for signs and symptoms suggestive of catheter occlusion or subclavian vein thrombosis. The clinician closely assesses for peripheral edema (location and severity) and determines respiratory status, heart sounds, daily weight, vital signs, and intake and output. Laboratory monitoring, which is established by the physician based on the severity of the disease, may include complete blood counts and electrolyte and chemistry profiles. Complications documented in the literature for home infusion inotropic therapy are primarily infections related to the infusion access device. Cases of drug intolerance have also been reported.

Biologic therapies. Biologic therapies are relatively new to home infusion. Advances in recombinant DNA technology have made therapies such as the hematopoietic growth factors (granulocyte colony-stimulating factor and granulocyte-macrophage colony-stimulating factor), erythropoietin, and interferon available for home use. This group of therapies, commonly called *biologics,* targets specific areas of the immune or hematopoietic systems that have been adversely affected by disease or a drug used in the treatment of a disease.[33] The biologics stimulate the proliferation or differentiation of specific cells in the hematopoietic system. Fig. 28-4 describes the biologics and diagnoses common to home infusion therapy.

Transfusion therapy. Home transfusion is a safe and effective treatment modality for providing blood and blood products to patients who require frequent transfusion but for whom hospitalization is not otherwise indicated. Blood transfusions can be performed at home provided that specific criteria are met.

As early as 1982 and 1983, home health care agencies were receiving inquiries regarding the availability of transfusions in the home care setting.[34] The American Association of Blood Banks (AABB) formally recognized the use of home transfusion

in 1988 when their Transfusion Practice Committee published a brochure entitled *Out-of-Hospital Transfusion.*

Blood components prescribed. The blood or blood products most commonly transfused in the home include packed red cells, washed packed red cells, frozen deglycerolized red cells, platelets, plasma, and cryoprecipitate or plasma derivatives. Other components need to be evaluated individually to determine their safety for administration in the home.

Indications. During the referral process and pretransfusion home visit, the home infusion clinician assesses the patient's candidacy for the home transfusion program. Admission criteria must be met before the patient is accepted into the program. The appropriateness of the diagnosis for transfusion must be assessed (Box 28-5). The patient's cardiopulmonary status and medical condition must be stable. The patient should be alert, cooperative, and able to respond appropriately to bodily changes that signal reactions and should be able to relate this information to the home transfusion nurse. The home environment should be conducive to the provision of home therapy. A capable adult is to be present during the transfusion, and telephone access must be available. Usually, the patient has physical limitations that make travel outside the home difficult. Last, there should be ready access to emergency medical services and the primary physician during transfusion.

Arrangements with blood bank. Each home infusion company and agency involved in providing transfusion therapy must identify a local blood bank from which to obtain blood products. In some areas, state regulations require that the home infusion company or agency *be* a licensed blood bank for limited transfusion services. The blood bank should be provided with a copy of the organization's transfusion program protocols, policies, and procedures for their review and recommendations. Clarification should be obtained regarding the blood bank's requirements for identifying patients, using identification bracelets, and transporting and storing blood products. The blood bank may also require specific equipment and supplies, such as microaggregate or leukocyte-depleting filters. The infusion company or agency must ensure that the home IV nurses are qualified in transfusion therapy.

Common issues and concerns. Home blood transfusion carries with it the same liability risk as hospital transfusion. During the pretransfusion visit, the informed consent and any other company-specific forms should be signed. The patient is educated on the purpose of the transfusion, their rights and responsibilities, and possible adverse reactions. A complete medical history is obtained, and a thorough physical examination, including evaluation of vascular access, is performed. An identification bracelet with the patient's full name and identification number is attached to the patient's wrist. The home IV nurse also obtains blood samples for baseline chemistry (if ordered), complete blood count, and type and crossmatch. All blood tubes must be labeled with the same full name and identification number found on the patient's identification bracelet. The sample is then returned to the blood bank for testing.

The blood product must be transported in a container that has an appropriate coolant for the component. The temperature should be recorded at the time of delivery or per blood bank or

FIG. 28-4 table — Biologics and diagnoses common to home infusion therapy.

	GM-CSF	G-CSF	EPOGEN	INTERFERON
DRUG	Sargramostim (Granulocyte Macrophage Colony Stimulating Factor-GM-CSF) Leukine (Immunex) Prokine (Hoechst-Roussel)	Filgrastim (Granulocyte Colony Stimulating Factor-G-CSF) Neupogen (Amgen)	Epoetin alfa (Erythropoietin; Epo) Epogen (Amgen) Procrit (Ortho Biotech)	Interferon Alfa 2a & 2b Intron-A (Schering) Roferon-A (Roche)
ACTIONS	A glycoprotein that stimulates the proliferation and differentiation of white blood cells in the granulocyte-macrophage pathways.	A glycoprotein that stimulates the production of neutrophils	A glycoprotein that stimulates red blood cell production	A sterile protein that has immunomodulatory and tumor antiproliferative activity.
INDICATIONS/USE	1. Acceleration of myeloid recovery in patients with non-Hodgkin's lymphoma (NHL), acute lymphoblastic leukemia (ALL) and Hodgkin's disease undergoing autologous bone marrow transplantation. 2. Bone marrow transplantation failure or engraftment delay. *Unlabeled uses:* a. Increase WBC counts in AIDS patients receiving AZT and patients with myelodysplastic syndrome. b. Correct neutropenia in aplastic anemia. c. Decrease nadir of leukopenia secondary to myelosuppressive chemotherapy.	Neutropenia in patients with non-myeloid malignancies receiving myelosuppressive anticancer agents.	1. Anemia secondary to chronic renal failure. 2. Anemia secondary to AZT therapy in HIV infected patients. 3. Unlabeled uses: a. Anemia in cancer patients receiving chemotherapy. b. Procurement of blood in presurgical patients.	Intron-A, Roferon A — Hairy cell leukemia in patients > 18 yrs old. Intron-A — AIDS-related Kaposi's sarcoma in patients > 18 yrs old. Intron-A — Chronic hepatitis, non A, non B/C. Non-approved use: Condylomata acuminata. Treatment of various tumors.
ADVERSE REACTIONS	Fever, headache, bone pain, chills, diarrhea, rack, malaise and asthenia	Bone pain—24%; Less frequently: Exacerbation of some pre-existing skin disorders (psoriasis, alopecia), hematuria, proteinuria, thrombocytopenia and osteoporosis; spontaneously reversible elevation in uric acid, lactic dehydrogenase and alkaline phosphatase have also occurred.	CRF patients: Hypertension 24%, headache 16%, arthralgias 11%, nausea 11%, edema, fatigue and diarrhea 95%, vomiting 8%, seizure 1.1%. AZT treated HIV patients: Pyrexia 38%, fatigue 25%, headache 19%, cough 18%, diarrhea 16%, rash 16%, respiratory congestion 15%, nausea 15%, SOB 14%	1. Flu-like syndrome. 2. Fatigue, dizziness, depression, sleep disturbances, paresthesia, nervousness, confusion, anxiety/agitation. 3. Nausea, vomiting, diarrhea, anorexia. 4. Rash, pruritus, alopecia, dermatitis, chest pain, arrhythmias. 5. Taste alteration, vision disorders. 6. Hypotension, edema, hypertension, chest pain, arrhythmia. 7. Anemia, leukopenia, thrombocytopenia.
MONITORING	• CBC with differential twice weekly • Physical assessment • Patient interview	• CBC with differential twice weekly during therapy • Physical assessment • Patient interview	• Baseline CBC and H/H twice weekly • Physical assessment • Patient interview • Monitoring BP closely on CRF patients	• Baseline CBC with differential and throughout therapy. • Baseline liver function tests and renal function test, and throughout therapy. • Physical assessment with close attention to: a. Cardiac status, b. Fever, sore throat, c. Signs of infection, d. Signs of bleeding, e. Neurologic status.
DOSAGE	250 mcg/m² over 2 hours for 21 days or until ANC reaches 20,000/mm³ or platelet count exceeds 500,000/mm³	5 mcg/kg/day SQ or IV × 2 weeks or until ANC reaches 10,000/mm³	Starting dose: 50 to 100 U/kg 3 times weekly, IV: dialysis patients, IV or SC: non-dialysis CRF patients. Reduce dose when: (1) Target range is reached or (2) Hematocrit increase > 4 points in any two week period. Increase dose if: Hematocrit does not increase by five to six points after eight weeks of therapy and hematocrit is below target range. Maintenance dose: Individualize. General dosage change: 25 U/kg/(3 times weekly). Target hematocrit range: 30% to 33% (maximum, 36%).	Roferon-A—Hairy cell leukemia—Induction dose: 3 M.I.U. for 16–24 wks SC or IM. Maintenance dose: 3 M.I.U. 3 times per week. AIDS related Kaposi's sarcoma—Induction dose: 36 M.I.U. daily for 10–12 wks, SC or IM. Maintenance dose: 36 M.I.U. 3 times a week. Intron-A—Hairy cell leukemia—2 M.I.U. per M² 3 times a week, SC or IM (maintain dose unless disease progresses rapidly or severe intolerance). Condylomata acuminata—1 M.I.U. per lesion 3 times a week intralesionally for 3 weeks. AIDS related Kaposi's sarcoma—30 M.I.U. per M² 3 times a week, SC or IM (maintain dose unless disease progresses or severe intolerance develops). Chronic hepatitis non A, non B/C—3 M.I.U. 3 times a week SC or IM for 6 months
COMMENTS	Caution in CHF or fluid retention, pre-existing cardiac, renal or hepatic disease. Therapy should begin two to four hours following autologous bone marrow infusion and not less than twenty-four hours following cytotoxic chemotherapy or twelve hours following radiation therapy.	Filgrastim should not be administered within 24 hours prior to or following the administration of cytotoxic chemotherapy.	1. Requires refrigeration at all times. 2. Patient may require iron supplementation.	1. Category C for pregnancy (potential risk to fetus). 2. Safety in children < 18 not established. 3. Interferon may have additive myelosuppressive activity with other antineoplastic drugs or radiation therapy. 4. Caution with aminophyllin. May decrease metabolism and increase aminophyllin levels.

FIG. 28-4 Biologics and diagnoses common to home infusion therapy.

Box 28-5   Diagnoses Appropriate for Admission to Home Transfusion Program

- Chronic gastrointestinal bleeding
- Anemia resulting from the following:
  - Bone marrow failure
  - Malignancy
  - Chronic renal failure
  - Sickle cell
  - Thalassemia
  - Acquired immunodeficiency syndrome
  - Chronic congestive heart failure
- Thrombocytopenia
- Bleeding related to congenital or acquired deficiencies in coagulation factors

---

agency policy. The blood products can be transported from the blood bank to the patient's home by the nurse performing the transfusion or by the blood bank. The blood product must be checked against the requisition by the blood center personnel and the home IV nurse. When the blood product is to be administered, the home IV nurse verifies with the caregiver the information on the blood product label and compares it with the patient's identification bracelet. All verifications should be documented on the transfusion visit form.

Safe transportation of blood components is critical. Insulated containers with wet or dry ice are used for transportation and storage in the home. A temperature-monitoring device is necessary to ensure maintenance of acceptable temperatures of the blood. The blood product should not come in direct contact with the coolant. Acceptable temperatures are 1° to 10° C for red blood cells and 1° to 6° C for fresh-frozen plasma. The patient's refrigerator is not to be used for storing blood components.[34]

Clinical monitoring. Once peripheral venous access has been verified or established and baseline vital signs obtained, the transfusion is initiated. Accurate records of vital signs and general patient condition should be maintained (Fig. 28-5). The home IV nurse remains with the patient during the entire transfusion and for at least 30 to 60 minutes after completion of the infusion. Organizational policy should delineate the frequency of vital signs during the procedure. Vital signs must be obtained before transfusion begins and every 15 to 30 minutes throughout the transfusion and for 30 to 60 minutes after the completion of the transfusion. Each unit of packed red cells is usually transfused over 1 to 2 hours, with a maximum time of 4 hours. If the transfusion must be performed more slowly, the units should be split to decrease the risk of bacterial proliferation, which occurs at room temperature. Usually, no more than 2 units of packed red cells or 10 units of platelets are transfused in a day. However, under certain circumstances and under a physician's direction, more than 2 units have been administered.

Between 30 and 60 minutes after completing the transfusion, the peripheral IV access device is removed or the central line is flushed. The blood container, administration set, and any other blood-contaminated supplies must be properly disposed of as per Occupational Safety and Health Administration (OSHA), city, and state waste management regulations. Some blood banks require that the empty blood bags and tubing be returned to them. Posttransfusion follow-up should be conducted via either telephone contact or a home visit. The physician may order follow-up laboratory studies. The patient and caregiver should receive further instructions on observing for transfusion reactions. Written information regarding reactions should be left with the patient.

Because each patient and each unit of blood is unique, every transfusion has the potential for adverse reactions. Patients are monitored frequently during the transfusion for symptoms of transfusion reaction (Box 28-6). The medications and supplies for the home transfusion reaction kit are the same as those for hospital transfusion. It usually includes diphenhydramine, hydrocortisone, acetaminophen (Tylenol), and epinephrine. The supplies include normal saline, an IV administration set, syringes with needles, blood-drawing supplies, urine specimen containers, and alcohol wipes. Orders for the transfusion reaction procedure should be obtained from the physician before the transfusion is performed.

A transfusion reaction kit and protocol should be available in the home during the transfusion (Box 28-7). In event of an urticarial reaction unaccompanied by other adverse effects, an antihistamine is usually ordered by the physician and administered. If the urticaria resolves, the physician may order the transfusion to be resumed slowly. Other nonhemolytic reactions may subside with prescribed therapy, without requiring hospitalization.

Reimbursement. Reimbursement for home transfusions varies between carriers. To verify coverage, each insurance carrier is contacted to describe the therapy, required nursing visits, and associated equipment and supplies. Many insurance carriers will reimburse for this therapy if it is "in lieu of hospitalization." A thorough investigation of resources is made, and all concerns (i.e., appropriate diagnosis, ability to transport) should be addressed. Only then can options be presented to the patient and the payers. Medicare does not currently reimburse for blood products.

Miscellaneous therapies

Deferoxamine mesylate therapy. Deferoxamine mesylate is an iron-binding agent that combines with iron in the body to produce a red chelate called *ferrioxamine,* which is then excreted in the urine and feces. Deferoxamine is prescribed to reverse iron overload. A common diagnosis for which the agent is prescribed in the home is *thalassemia,* which is also known as *erythroblastic anemia, Mediterranean anemia,* or *Cooley's anemia.* This disorder includes a group of hereditary hemolytic anemias in which the red blood cells are very thin and fragile. These anemias are thought to be caused by a deficit in hemoglobin synthesis, and they occur more often in people from the Mediterranean, South Asian, and North and Central African areas. The anemic symptoms of thalassemia usually appear early in life. Frequent periodic transfusions (every 3 to 4 weeks) of red blood cells, depending on hemoglobin levels, are required to correct the anemia. Iron overload occurs as a result of the blood transfusions, and unless reversed can cause damage to such vital organs as the heart and liver; iron overload can be fatal. Chelation therapy is begun when ferritin levels reach 1000 mg/L, signaling a complete saturation of circulating transferrin.[33,35]

TRANSFUSION PATIENT
VISIT/SHIFT RECORD

PATIENT NAME		PATIENT ID NO.		DATE		EMPLOYEE NUMBER	□ □ □ □ □

CLINICIAN NAME		CLINICIAN SIG.		VISIT TIME IN HOURS (Round to nearest ¼ hr.)	TIME ARRIVED	TIME LEFT	TO
CAREGIVER NAME		CAREGIVER SIGNATURE X		TRAVEL TIME IN HOURS (Round to nearest ¼ hr.)	TO	FROM	TO

SERVICE TIME: □ WD □ WED □ WE □ WEE □ WN □ WEN

SERVICE TYPE: □ INF NSG □ INF

LOCATION: □ HOME □ HOSP □ MD OFFICE/CLINIC
□ ECF/SNF □ OTHER _____

IPA DONE: □ YES □ NO

MILEAGE   TO   FROM   TO

CHARTING   MINUTES   SIG. PT.

□ BILLABLE □ NON BILLABLE   PAYOR SOURCE

DESCRIPTION

GENERAL: BASELINE H & H _____ V/S _____ PATIENT BLOOD TYPE _____

VENOUS ACCESS/CONDITION OF SITE _____

PHYSICAL ASSESSMENT _____

RX: NUMBER OF UNITS ON HAND _____

UNIT NO. ONE: TYPE _____ RH _____ BLOOD BANK NUMBER _____

UNIT NO. TWO: TYPE _____ RH _____ BLOOD BANK NUMBER _____

TRANSPORT: METHOD: _____ TIME _____ TEMPERATURE _____

TRANSFUSION

IV SOLUTION _____
BLOOD (No. of units, time started, time ended, rate, amount infused for each unit)

MEDICATIONS GIVEN _____

ANAPHYLAXIS KIT ORDERED? □ YES □ NO   PRESENT IN HOME? □ YES □ NO

V/S p̄ first 15 minutes, X2, then every 30 minutes, then 30 minutes after each unit.

	TIME	TEMPERATURE	PULSE	RESPIRATION	BLOOD PRESSURE		TIME	TEMPERATURE	PULSE	RESPIRATION	BLOOD PRESSURE
1						8					
2						9					
3						10					
4						11					
5						12					
6						13					
7						14					

TRANSFUSION REACTIONS

TRANSFUSION REACTION: □ YES □ NO   REACTION DESCRIPTION _____

ACTION TAKEN: _____

LABS DONE: _____

FOLLOW UP: _____

RESPONSE TO TRANSFUSION

FOLLOW UP LABS: _____

PATIENT EDUCATION

FIG. 28-5 *Record of vital signs and patient's general condition.*

Box 28-6 Symptoms of Transfusion Reaction

- Chills
- Chest tightness
- Headache
- Myalgia
- Pruritus
- Nausea
- Pain at infusion site, chest, or flank
- Fever

- Hemoglobinuria
- Restlessness
- Dyspnea
- Cough
- Vomiting
- Pink sputum
- Hypotension
- Tachycardia
- Bradycardia

PROCEDURE for Transfusion Reaction   Box 28-7

1. If reaction is suspected or observed, stop transfusion.
2. Change intravenous tubing and maintain patient's intravenous line with 0.9% sodium chloride solution.
3. Take vital signs and continue to monitor the patient until stable.
4. Administer medications as prescribed.
5. Verify match among the blood product identification label, requisition, and patient's identification bracelet.
6. Notify physician, as soon as patient's condition permits, for further instructions. Notify blood bank. Access local emergency services if a medical emergency arises.
7. Obtain necessary laboratory specimens:
   - Freshly collected urine
   - Blood samples, red top tube without separator gel and purple top tube
8. Monitor the patient until the reaction subsides or the patient is transferred to an emergency facility.
9. Document incident on transfusion flow sheet and transfusion reaction report.

Deferoxamine is prescribed based on the laboratory values of serum ferritin. It is most commonly administered via the subcutaneous routes and less commonly via the IV route by an ambulatory infusion pump over 8 to 12 hours. Because this is a lifelong therapy, patients are usually trained to mix and administer the drugs themselves. Side effects, although rare, may include disturbances of vision and hearing, vertigo, and respiratory difficulties.[35] Average life expectancy for the thalassemia patient is largely dependent on early detection of the disease, diligent monitoring, continuous treatment, and patient compliance. Home care has allowed these and other long-term therapy regimens to be administered with minimal disturbances of daily activities.

Alpha₁-proteinase inhibitor. Alpha₁-proteinase inhibitor is an enzyme indicated in the treatment of severe alpha₁-antitrypsin (AAT) deficiency with clinically demonstrable panacinar emphysema. AAT deficiency is an autosomal hereditary disorder characterized by low serum and lung levels of AAT. AAT is a protease inhibitor responsible for inhibiting neutrophil elastase. Emphysema is believed to result from an imbalance between the neutrophil elastase in the lung, which is capable of destroying elastin and other connective tissue components, and the antielastases that protect the lung from elastase. Therefore persons with AAT deficiency are at high risk for developing severe panacinar emphysema before 50 years of age. They are also at an increased risk for developing liver disease; however, this problem is usually seen in children. The first clinical symptom in adults is dyspnea on exertion and lower lung involvement.[33]

Treatment of this disorder is replacement therapy with alpha₁-proteinase inhibitor. Long-term replacement therapy should be considered only for patients who exhibit early evidence of the disease. It is not indicated for patients with emphysema associated with cigarette smoking who lack the positive phenotype. Alpha₁-proteinase inhibitor is prepared from large pools of fresh human plasma, usually from paid donors. It is heat treated to reduce the potential for transmission of infectious agents, such as the human immunodeficiency virus (HIV) and hepatitis virus. No cases of HIV transmission have been reported thus far. It is recommended by physicians, however, that before patients undergo alpha₁-proteinase inhibitor therapy, they be immunized for hepatitis using hepatitis B vaccination as per the manufacturer's recommendations.

Alpha₁-proteinase inhibitor is administered intravenously via peripheral intermittent vascular access device, tunneled catheter, PICC, or implanted port. The recommended dosage is 60 mg/kg once weekly to increase and maintain AAT levels. This dose can be administered at a rate of 0.08 ml/kg/min or greater.[35-37] The average infusion time is 30 minutes. An infusion device may be used if ordered. The drug concentrate must be refrigerated; the bottles should be brought to room temperature and then reconstituted with the sterile water that is provided. It may be diluted in 0.9% sodium chloride if necessary. The drug should not be refrigerated after reconstitution and should be used within 3 hours. Any unused solution should be discarded appropriately.

Alpha₁-proteinase inhibitor replacement is a lifelong therapy and may cause patient concerns. Lung function will not improve, but it is hoped that the progression of the disease can be halted with replacement therapy. Patients must learn to deal with the chronicity of their disease, and compliance often becomes an issue. Routinely skipped doses can lead to worsening of the disorder. The home IV nurse should educate patients regarding the IV access devices available for therapy. Some may decide to use a peripheral intermittent vascular access device or a long-term access device, such as a PICC or a tunneled catheter. Care and maintenance of the IV access device is a very important part of patient education. Because of the relatively short time the drug remains stable, patients are taught aseptic reconstitution procedures and IV administration. Some patients express concern over the possibility of acquiring hepatitis or HIV as a result of the method of preparing alpha₁-proteinase inhibitor. Educating the patient on the availability of the hepatitis B vaccine helps reduce their fear and the risk of acquiring hepatitis B.

Periodic pulmonary function tests may be needed to determine the progression of the disease and the patient's response to therapy. Effectiveness of therapy is demonstrated by slowing the destruction of lung tissue, as measured by increased serum alpha$_1$-proteinase inhibitor levels. Minimum serum concentration is 80 mg/100 ml.

Tocolytic therapy. Premature births are considered a major cause of morbidity and mortality. Several drugs have been prescribed to prevent preterm labor, including magnesium sulfate, terbutaline, and ritodrine. Recent studies using continuous subcutaneous infusion of terbutaline have proven efficient and cost effective, saving as much as $1000 a day. Study results of subcutaneously administered terbutaline have demonstrated fewer side effects than oral or IV administration.[38] They have also shown prolongation of pregnancy by an average of 8.5 weeks with 18% recurrence of preterm labor in a group receiving subcutaneous terbutaline, compared with an average prolongation of pregnancy of 2.4 weeks and 90% recurrence of preterm labor in patients receiving oral tocolytic therapy.[39] These effects are attributed to lower dosing levels, improved absorption into the subcutaneous tissue, and automatic and continuous delivery of the prescribed therapy.[40] The administration of terbutaline remains controversial. It cannot be expected to bring every pregnancy to term, but it may provide a longer gestational period and thereby improve the outcome of the pregnancy.

Home terbutaline therapy is given via a portable infusion pump, which is programmed to administer a continuous basal rate (0.05 mg/hr), scheduled bolus doses (0.25 mg) four to six times per day for peak periods of contractions, and unscheduled bolus doses (0.25 mg) should the patient experience two contractions in 10 minutes or four contractions in 60 minutes. The subcutaneous site is rotated every 3 to 4 days. The total daily terbutaline dose rarely exceeds 3 mg. The patient is instructed on caring for and maintaining the infusion site, reloading and reprogramming the pump, and self-monitoring, including counting fetal heart rate and uterine self-palpation for detecting contractions. The patient remains on bed rest for the duration of therapy. The home care nurse visits the patient weekly and as necessary to perform a physical assessment, including blood pressure, vital signs, weight gain, evaluation of clinical cervical dilation, and uterine contractions. The goals of tocolytic therapy are to stop labor, suppress contractions, and prolong gestation to at least 36 weeks. Terbutaline therapy is generally discontinued at the end of week 37.

Uterine monitoring equipment can send monitoring results via telephone to the home care agency or a contracted monitoring station. The patient initiates the monitoring and sends the results to the monitoring station at specified intervals.

Reimbursement for the therapy and associated monitoring varies between payers; it should be evaluated before beginning therapy.

Hydration. Hydration therapy has been successfully prescribed within the past decade for use in the home. Various conditions (Box 28-8) result in dehydration and fluid and electrolyte imbalance. Home hydration therapy has eliminated the need for hospitalizing patients with these conditions as long as they are medically stable and meet patient acceptance criteria. Hydration solutions are ordered by the physician based on the patient's diagnosis. Electrolytes may be added to correct electrolyte imbalance as indicated by laboratory data. The most effec-

---

Box 28-8   Common Diagnoses for Home Hydration Therapy

- Dehydration
- Fluid and electrolyte imbalance resulting from the following:
  - Cardiopulmonary disorders
  - Fistulas
  - Gastrointestinal dysfunction
  - Hyperemesis gravidarum
  - Intractable diarrhea
  - Chemotherapy (before and after therapy)
  - Radiation enteritis
  - Short-bowel syndrome

---

tive route of administration is determined by the physician, patient, and home infusion clinicians.

Short-term therapy, lasting from 1 to 7 days, is administered via a peripheral intermittent infusion device unless a long-term access device is available, such as in the chemotherapy patient. The delivery system is quite simple, consisting of the hydration solution and the IV administration set. The physician may order an electronic infusion device to regulate the rate of infusion. In most situations, an in-line flow regulator is all that is required. Hydration therapy patients are educated in the necessity for therapy, aseptic technique, set-up and administration of the solution, and possible complications.

Clinical monitoring of the patient includes physical assessment, closely monitoring weight and hydration status, and reviewing laboratory results. The frequency of laboratory tests depends on the diagnosis. Based on the degree of the patient's physical debility, other caregivers may be required to administer the therapy. Patients must be assessed for compliance because many discontinue their therapy before the prescribed duration because they feel better. Education and reinforcement help eliminate this tendency. To recover, the cause of hydration must be identified and corrected.

Epoprostenol sodium. Epoprostenol sodium, a naturally occurring prostaglandin, has been found effective in the treatment of primary pulmonary hypertension (PPH). The pathophysiology associated with PPH results in restricted blood flow in the small vessels in the lungs, which eventually leads to enlargement of the right ventricle of the heart and right-sided heart failure. Precipitating factors include infection with HIV, portal hypertension, pregnancy, and use of cocaine, certain appetite depressants, and methamphetamines. PPH may also be inherited.

There is an acute and chronic dosing phase for this drug. The home infusion patient should be in the chronic phase. There is no "right" dosage: the dosage is titrated to response. The drug has a short half-life and must be infused continuously via an ambulatory pump. Once initiated, this is a lifelong therapy, Therefore a central line is recommended.

Because of the complexity of epoprostenol sodium therapy, patient and caregiver education and involvement is crucial. Because of the short half-life, the patient must mix the drug and maintain the mixed solution at a controlled room temperature. The infusion should not be interrupted for longer than 2 to 3 minutes, and time to completion of a single dose should not exceed 8 hours at room temperature.

It is critical that the patient and caregiver know and be alert for side effects of this therapy because dosage adjustments and the patient's well being depend on this recognition.

Reimbursement is based on the payer. Because this is a lifelong therapy, coverage issues should be explored and confirmed before therapy is initiated. Because a pump is required to administer this therapy, it is covered under Medicare Part B under strict guidelines.[41,42]

Special pharmaceutical issues

Pharmaceutical issues can be broken to two types. The first, patient care management, was an added-value service until the past few years, when some state pharmacy laws and the Joint Commission on Accreditation of Healthcare Organizations (JCAHO) made it a requirement of retail and home infusion pharmacies. The clinical role of the pharmacist in patient care management has recently expanded and is discussed in more detail under Future Directions.

The second type of pharmaceutical issue relates to pharmacy operations management and has recently become increasingly important. As profit margins are squeezed, pharmacists need to become experts in business administration. Areas needing particular attention are procurement of pharmaceuticals and supplies, asset and inventory management, and cost of goods and services as compared with revenue generated. In other words, without sacrificing quality, the pharmacist must buy the best products at the lowest cost, produce and distribute them in the most cost-effective manner at the highest level of productivity, and get the highest return on dollars invested in the shortest possible time. Nurses also need to be astute in business and administrative issues and know how to contain costs through prudent product selection and judicious use of available supplies and equipment.

What does this mean to the home infusion industry? Not only will pharmacists have to be superior clinicians, but they will also have to master interactions and negotiations with insurers, case managers, and referral sources while also addressing the many issues of business management. Some state pharmacy laws already allow the use of pharmacy technicians and others are following suit. Soon, the impetus will be to use technicians in an effort to reduce the cost of service. This trend will require further education of pharmacists in personnel management. With the inevitability of cost containment, the home infusion industry will no longer be able to afford the luxury of an all-pharmacist staff.

MANAGEMENT CONSIDERATIONS
Staff qualifications

Because home infusion therapy is a highly specialized technical field, the qualifications for the nursing and pharmacy clinicians that make up the home infusion team are more specific.

Educational requirements. Educational requirements for IV nurses include graduation from an accredited school of nursing and professional licensure from the state in which they practice. Most IV nurses are registered nurses because there are still limitations on the role of licensed practical nurses (LPN) and licensed vocational nurses (LVN) in infusion therapy. Many state boards of nursing are closely reviewing the issues involved in expanding the role of LPNs and LVNs; some may allow more infusion therapy–related procedures in their scope of practice.[43] Although no established requirements exist regarding the degree or certification held by the home IV nurse, the Bachelor of Science degree in nursing is the preferred professional degree. At present, however, criteria are set by individual organizations or agencies based on job description and responsibilities.

Educational requirements for home infusion pharmacists include a Bachelor of Science degree in pharmacy from an accredited school of pharmacy and professional licensure from the state in which they will be practicing. Many clinical home infusion pharmacists have obtained advanced degrees such as a Doctor of Pharmacy or Master of Science in Pharmacy. Many pharmacy doctoral programs offer the pharmacist the opportunity to participate in specialized residencies that include nutritional support or home infusion therapy. Once again, the educational requirements are established by the individual organization or agency based on job description and responsibilities.

Experience. One of the key areas of qualification for nursing and pharmacy personnel is previous experience, not only in their respective profession, but in infusion therapy as well. The entry-level home IV nurse should have experience administering infusion therapies and inserting and managing venous access devices, as well as knowledge of the various infusion devices used to deliver the therapies. This experience may come from previous nursing positions on hospital infusion teams in critical care (intensive care, cardiac care, neonatal intensive care) or in specialty fields (oncology, pediatrics, hemodialysis, or outpatient infusion clinics). This background in general infusion therapy provides the IV nurse with a solid foundation on which to build home infusion experience. When practicing in home care, IV nurses must realize that although the standards of care are the same, they will practice in an environment that is more autonomous and less structured than the hospital or clinic. Independent decision making and effective communication skills are paramount. Some nurses find it difficult to make the transition to home practice and are not successful as home IV nurses.[44]

There are two levels of managers in home infusion therapy: the director and the supervisor. Whether the organization has need for one or both depends on the size of the facility and the number of staff needing supervision. In addition to the qualifications discussed earlier, the home IV nurse manager should have home care experience and should demonstrate management skills through previous experience as a charge nurse, head nurse, supervisor, or director of a nursing department. Organizational, time management, and communication skills are also important, as are personnel and financial management skills; these skills will ensure the cohesiveness and effectiveness of the nursing component of the team. Home infusion pharmacy managers should also possess management skills. They must be able to identify and prioritize operational and clinical issues to ensure successful operation in the home infusion pharmacy. Home care experience is also required.

Previous home infusion management experience is required for managers to hold a director position. Many organizations require at least 6 months to 1 year of home infusion management experience for the director of nursing or pharmacy. Experience in the delivery of complex therapies is desirable, as is advanced clinical experience in specialty areas such as chemotherapy, care for patients with AIDS, and nutritional support.

Personal attributes. Personal attributes and behavioral characteristics affect one's ability to become a successful home IV nurse or pharmacist. The home IV nurse should be independent, self-motivated, and flexible. Good decision-making abilities are important because clinical judgments must often be made independently. Impeccable communication skills are a must. The physician and other members of the home health care team rely on the home IV nurse and pharmacist for sound, thorough clinical assessment and communication of their findings. Prompt attention to detail is important. Home IV clinicians must be compassionate and empathetic. The ability to be a patient advocate is especially important in the home care setting, where the patient has more control over his or her therapy. The rules are no longer set by the clinician, but by the patient. The home IV clinician must always keep in mind that active patient participation and decision making is key to comprehensive home care. The clinician should have the skills to educate the patient in a manner that allows the patient to make sound judgments about his or her therapy.

The home IV clinician has a strong, well-rounded knowledge of general practice and his or her specialty area. Providing a specialist's expertise with a generalist's perspective allows a holistic approach to home infusion therapy. The home IV nurse must possess excellent physical assessment skills. Highly developed teaching skills are required, particularly the ability to present information clearly and confirm that it is understood. This educational process often extends to the medical community to provide information related to infusion therapies in the home.

Certification. Home infusion clinicians may receive advanced credentials as certified specialists. Certification requirements vary depending on the sponsoring professional organization and employer. Some employers require national certification by a professional organization, whereas others require their own internal certification. Many require both.

What are the advantages of national certification? There are many, and they work to the benefit of patients, nurses and their employers, and indirectly, the manufacturers of infusion products. The primary purpose of certification is to protect the public. Certification validates the advanced knowledge, skills, and competency that patients, as educated health care consumers, regard as a right rather than a privilege. There are also benefits to the nurse. National certification enhances personal development, promotes professional recognition and identification of clinicians as experts in the field, and can lead to better employment opportunities. Employers benefit because certification is a marketable quality and because certification requires a level of competency that translates into better service, fewer complications, and less liability exposure. Finally, certification benefits manufacturers of infusion products through proper use of products and equipment and expert input for product development and evaluation by certified nurses.[19,45]

Several professional organizations offer national certification related to home infusion therapy. The Intravenous Nurses Certification Corporation provides certification in infusion nursing. By documenting work experience and passing a comprehensive examination, the credentials CRNI (Certified Registered Nurse Intravenous) are awarded. The certification period is 3 years, after which the nurse may be recertified by testing or by earning recertification units through an approved Intravenous Nurses Society (INS) educational program or activity.

The American Society for Parenteral and Enteral Nutrition provides certification for nurses, dietitians, and physicians who desire to specialize in nutritional support. Certification for nutritional support pharmacists is available through the Board of Pharmaceutical Specialties. Certification is obtained by passing a comprehensive examination. The certification period for nurses and dietitians is 5 years.[46] Recertification for all disciplines is obtained by retesting. The Oncology Nursing Society also offers a credentialing examination for certifying oncology nurses, advanced oncology nurses, and pediatric oncology nurses. This certification is obtained by passing a comprehensive examination. The certification limitation period is 4 years, at which time recertification may be obtained by retesting or obtaining the specified number of recertification points.[47] Further information on these certification examinations is available through the sponsoring organizations.

Many home infusion companies and home health care agencies maintain their own internal programs to validate and document basic competency in the highly technical services they offer. One of the internal programs most often required is IV education. The INS recommends that such programs teach the theoretical aspects of the following areas: technology and clinical application, fluid and electrolyte balance, pharmacology, infection control, pediatrics, transfusion therapy, antineoplastic therapy, parenteral nutrition, and quality assurance.[19] The home IV nurse's knowledge of theory is assessed by a comprehensive examination. Along with the didactic portion of the program, a practicum should be completed to demonstrate technical proficiency. Other internal programs that may be offered to clinicians by home infusion organizations are transfusion therapy, chemotherapy, placement of PICCs, admixture, and pharmacokinetics. The aforementioned professional organizations recommend that theory and practical experience be a part of these internal programs.

Some home infusion companies and agencies provide additional internal programs that focus on advanced theory in certain specialty areas, such as complex home chemotherapy regimens, nutritional and metabolic support, and immunomodulating agents. By providing internal certification programs and ensuring that staff members achieve national certification, the home infusion company or agency decreases risk management concerns and assures patients that they will receive quality care from qualified, competent staff.

Responsibilities

IV nurse. The IV nurse's responsibilities include performing the initial patient assessment, reviewing systems, developing nursing diagnosis, reviewing medical history, conducting the psychosocial assessment, evaluating available support systems, and assessing functional limitations, environment, and cognitive and technical skills. Recommendations for care are based on the synthesis of knowledge gained through the previously listed activities. Ongoing responsibilities include patient training, therapeutic monitoring and evaluation, assessment of compliance with the medication regimen, performance of technical procedures of infusion therapy, psychosocial support, and 24-hour emergency availability.

Pharmacist. In some geographic locations, the pharmacist and the IV nurse visit the patient when necessary for evaluation and assessment. Whether the pharmacist provides home care depends on the philosophy of the organization and the demands of the marketplace. The pharmacist's responsibilities include reviewing medical records for current and past medical, nutritional, and medication history; reviewing laboratory data; obtaining physician orders; and conducting interviews with patients. The pharmacist also prepares, dispenses, and delivers medications, solutions, supplies and equipment; plans patient care; monitors therapeutic response; analyzes laboratory data; and is available 24 hours a day for emergencies. A therapeutic evaluation is made based on patient assessment (when possible), the physical examination and history, and information conveyed by nursing staff, patients, family members, caregivers, and other members of the health care team.

Nursing and pharmacy staff work together to formulate clinical impressions that are communicated to the physician. This process ensures that the best possible decisions are made and the highest quality of care and service is provided.

Other members of the health care team. A very important member of the health care team is the financial services representative (or reimbursement specialist), who is responsible for the financial aspects of services, such as verifying insurance coverage, negotiating with case managers, and discussing financial obligations with patients. Another member is the pharmacy technician, whose job responsibilities depend on state law. Some state pharmacy laws allow trained technicians to perform drug preparation duties, whereas others do not. State pharmacy laws, rules, and regulations can be obtained from the local state boards of pharmacy. A very visible and important member of the team is the delivery technician or driver. This member interacts with the patient often to deliver medications, supplies, and equipment.

Workload standards

Allocating staff resources begins by determining workload standards for each discipline. Home infusion workload standards need not only to encompass the different disciplines represented on the team, but should be modified to fit the services delivered. For example, the workload standard for initiating TPN in the home will be much different from the standard for a single course of antibiotic therapy. Other variables to consider include the delivery model used by the organization, the productivity level required to cover the cost of service delivery, the geographic area serviced and average travel time, and the patient case mix and acuity. Workload standards can be established by benchmarking with similar organizations, by performing time and motion studies, or by modifying an existing system.

Tasks to be considered for measurement when establishing workload standards include the following:

- Intake process, including obtaining orders and payer verification
- Preparation of medications and filling supply order, by therapy
- Interdisciplinary communication and information sharing
- Delivery of medication and supplies to the home (by discipline or provider responsible)
- Initial patient visit for assessment and education, by therapy
- Actual provision of care, by therapy, by discipline
- Documentation time
- Travel time

Each of the factors are broken into their component parts and assigned a time value. A flow chart helps ensure that all necessary factors and tasks are included in the calculations. It is often helpful to categorize tasks as direct and indirect care activities. Indirect activities should include time for documenting and coordinating care and for performance improvement activities. It is always prudent to involve the people actually doing the work in determining the tasks to be included; they perform the tasks daily and know them best.

Provision of services (staffing)

Once the workload allocations are established for each service line and discipline, staffing can be determined. For several reasons, consistently effective and efficient staffing levels are difficult to establish for home infusion services. Provision must be made to cover patient care needs 24 hours a day, 7 days a week, 365 days a year. Cases may need to be opened and visits made during off hours, when staff are paid at up to twice the usual rate of pay.

Decisions must be made regarding how the required full-time equivalents (FTEs) will be acquired. Will the staff be full-time permanent employees? Will they be paid a salary or on a per-visit basis? Will certain positions be filled with contract staff on an as-needed basis? If these alternative staffing methods are used, how will the desired level of quality patient care be ensured consistently?

Obtaining the correct mix of staff with the appropriate credentials and experience is critical. The practice of infusion nursing covers a wide range of nursing specialties, and care may be provided to patients with diagnoses covering all body systems and all age groups. This means that, in addition to nurses with a wide range of general nursing experience, the organization must hire employees with specialized competencies such as care of the pediatric, orthopedic, cardiac or oncology patient. Lack of specialized, documented competencies precludes accepting patients with corresponding care needs. The euphemism "a nurse is a nurse" has no application in the high-tech, high-risk world of home infusion therapy.

Policies and procedures

Organizational policies and procedures define and delineate the organization's scope of practice. Policies are developed based on applicable standards of care, certification and accreditation requirements, and state and federal law, and they are specific to the services and therapies provided by the organization. Procedures provide a road map for employees and establish acceptable care guidelines. The policies and procedures must be realistic and appropriate for the level of resources available to the organization. Policy and procedure manuals must be approved by the governing body of the organization, reviewed at least annually, and revised as necessary.

Quality management

The primary mission of the home infusion organization is providing care to patients requiring infusion therapy in their homes. Each home infusion provider needs to be able to demonstrate that it has a systematic approach to delivering services, identifying problems, resolving problems, and continually improving performance. Quality initiatives should focus on patient outcome criteria and concentrate on activities that occur often, affect large numbers of patients, and are at high risk for creating problems for either the patient or clinician. There may come a time when providers will be selected based on their history of achieving positive patient outcomes, as opposed to cost-effectiveness alone. Even payment for services may be based on outcomes some day. As patients move from one care setting to another more rapidly, it is important that the quality management program differentiate between adverse events resulting from care delivered in the home and adverse events with origins in another setting. Some examples of outcome criteria are unscheduled inpatient admissions, infection rates of central lines, monitoring appropriate elements of the patient's condition and response, and appropriate intervention in patients receiving parenteral nutrition.

Quality improvement is the process by which problems and opportunities for improvement are identified. Root causes are determined, and improvement and prevention systems and corrective actions are implemented continuously. All of these activities work together to ensure that quality care and services are provided to patients (see Chapter 4).

Standards of care. Standards of care have been in existence for many years. National standards have been developed to address infusion therapy in general and subcategories such as parenteral nutrition.[18,48] Although the setting for patient care may vary throughout the care delivery process, standards of care do not. Integrating nationally recognized standards into organizational policies and procedures helps facilitate the provision of appropriate, safe, high-quality care in the home.

Accreditation. JCAHO and the National League for Nursing have defined and issued home care standards. Both organizations offer a voluntary accreditation. One of the benefits of accreditation includes national recognition of compliance to standards. The HCFA has awarded deemed status to both organizations. With slight alteration in the accreditation process, the accrediting body may survey organizations for Medicare certification. Because payers tend to award preferred provider status to organizations that are accredited, home infusion organizations must give careful consideration to attaining and maintaining accreditation.

Accreditation helps define, measure, and validate an organization's form and function. It is an easy thing to say that services are high quality. However, accreditation makes that claim visible and is a value-added component of service delivery. As stated in the *JCAHO 1999-2000 Accreditation Manual for Home Care,* "Value in health care is the appropriate balance between good outcomes, excellent care and services, and costs. In order to add value to the care and services provided, organizations need to understand the relation among perception of care, outcomes and costs and how these three issues are affected by processes carried out by the organization."[49]

Many integrated health care systems are opting to seek accreditation for the integrated system. Home care providers affiliated with such an organization may affect the accreditation status of the entire health delivery system. Likewise, the home care provider's accreditation status can be impacted by the systems' performance. The integrated survey is thought to improve and promote continuity of patient care in every setting.

Translators. Many patients speak English as a second language or do not speak English at all. It is the home infusion provider's responsibility to ensure that patients understand their therapy. This goal can be accomplished by using bilingual clinicians or by using family members or friends as interpreters. A professional translator may also be used. A thorough assessment of the cultural populations in the provider's geographic service area will help identify translation needs and allow the provider to obtain appropriate translator consultants.

Documentation. Documentation is the primary communication tool among members of the home care team. Documentation has always been an accepted duty of the nurse in any health care setting. The home infusion pharmacist is responsible for documentation as well. This may be an expanded area of responsibility for many pharmacists entering the clinical realm of home infusion therapy. Continuous communication with all members of the team facilitates thorough documentation.

Nursing and pharmacy documentation includes initial and ongoing patient assessment and development of a patient care plan. Pharmacy documentation focuses on medication evaluation, therapeutic outcome monitoring, laboratory analyses, and recommendations to the physician. Nursing documentation focuses on physical and therapeutic assessment, especially as it relates to the disease process and the prescribed therapy, patient training, medication administration, skilled nursing services, technical procedures, and psychosocial evaluation and support. Nurses and pharmacists document communication with each other, members of the health care team, and the patient and caregiver. Routine patient care rounds and case conferences require documentation in the patient's medical records as well.

Documentation is important for securing reimbursement, and it has legal ramifications as well. The phrase "If it is not documented, it was not done" carries special emphasis for the home infusion team. The information in the patient's medical record should be structured in a way that allows someone unfamiliar with the patient (e.g., a Medicare or accreditation surveyor) to read the medical record and have a complete picture of the patient's medical and psychosocial needs and problems, goals for care, anticipated outcomes, services delivered, resources used, goals achieved, and outcomes of care. All elements of the documentation should be cohesive and suc-

---

Box 28-9   Potential Line Items in the Financial Management Plan

REVENUE
Gross revenue, by therapy
Contractual adjustments
Bad debt
Net revenue

EXPENSES
Payroll, payroll taxes, and related expenses
Gross salaries
Employer FICA and FUTA expense
Unemployment
Payroll-related employee benefits
    Sick pay
    Vacation pay
Employee benefits
    Health insurance
    Worker's compensation
    Educational assistance and conferences
    Professional affiliations
    Mileage reimbursement
Insurance
    Property
    Auto
    Liability
Utilities
    Telephone
    Gas
    Water
    Electricity
    Waste disposal
Advertising/promotional
Bank charges
Computer (software/hardware/communication)
Contract labor and associated costs
Due/subscriptions/books
Durable medical equipment
    Purchased
    Leased
Lease/rent
Licenses/taxes
Medical supplies
Minor equipment
Miscellaneous expenses
Nursing supplies
Office supplies
Postage
Printing
Recruiting/retention
Repair and maintenance
Depreciation

---

cinctly descriptive. Thorough documentation is a means to monitor care and services delivered and to find ways to continually improve services.

Financial management

Financial management in home care is no different from any other health care venue or business. Financial management begins with understanding the core function of the organization—what is it we are here to do? In most instances in this business, the answer will be provide the supplies, equipment and personnel that allows patients to receive needed infusion services in their home. Once the core function is identified, the associated financial requirements can be assessed and planned and a budget developed.

Current turmoil in health care financing makes planning and budgeting very difficult. This has become the era of rapid demands on resources, changes in reimbursement, and cost-cutting measures. Mozena, Emerick, and Black have observed that "We have evolved into a situation where we are obsessed with the manipulation of numbers, bottom lines and end results. Instead of focusing on the interaction of the core business systems within an organization, we are continually trying to produce short-term financial gains."[50]

Sound financial management involves having a thorough grasp of each system and process in the organization's core services and developing a working budget that supports those systems. Each system and process should be broken down into its component parts to determine the costs of the resources needed (e.g., supplies, equipment, services, personnel) to deliver the service.

Each department in the organization should have a separate line item budget that incorporates projected service income by therapy offered, contractual adjustments, and bad debt. Expenses include all costs associated with procuring supplies and equipment, including the cost of inventory turns and "just-in-time" stock levels, personnel costs, capital expenditures, and operating expenses.

Box 28-9 lists items that should be considered for inclusion in a financial management plan.

Each line item cost can be calculated as a cost per visit, cost per patient, or cost per therapy. Once this calculation is done, expenses can be projected and adjusted based on the volume of business and flexed with changes in volume. Each department must understand its contribution to the bottom line; this represents how departmental performance affects the entire operation. These budgeting activities are the crux of sound financial management and viability of the organization.

SPECIAL CONSIDERATIONS
Cost considerations

The home health care industry is and has been under intense scrutiny because of rapidly rising expenditures over the last 10 to 20 years. In the 1980s, diagnosis-related groups (DRGs) were implemented in the acute care setting. Hospitals had to change drastically to survive the changes in reimbursement. Patient lengths of stay and cost containment were the focus. As patients left the hospital "sicker and quicker," responsibility for their ongoing care fell to home care organizations. Home care providers adapted to meet the need and the number of patients cared for in the home grew exponentially. As patient numbers grew, the cost of care and dollars paid by governmental and private payers grew as well.

The home care industry is now in the position of the acute care setting in the 1980s. The reimbursement system is undergoing drastic change, moving from a cost-based system to an interim payment system, and anticipating implementation of the prospective payment system. The prospective payment system, like DRGs, sets a fixed amount of reimbursement for a particular diagnosis and a particular episode of care, currently defined as a 60-day period. There will be minimal compensation for patients requiring intense resource utilization. Although most of the changes are driven by Medicare, private insurers—by establishing health maintenance organizations, preferred provider organizations, and various forms of capitation—have had a significant impact on reimbursement. Many of these changes have occurred within a matter of 5 years. The major driving forces were the Balanced Budget Act of 1997 and fraud and abuse investigations initiated by the federal government.

The various changes mentioned have created new challenges and opportunities for home health care providers. It is now the home health provider that must dramatically recreate itself, finding new ways to meet patients' needs while managing its financial resources astutely. Home infusion therapy is by tradition a high-tech, resource-intensive business. Procuring pharmaceuticals and state-of-the-art infusion pumps and delivering them to the patient is expensive. Regulations and standards require that professional pharmacy and nursing staff be available to the patient 24 hours a day, 365 days a year. The cost of complying with regulatory and accreditation requirements is considerable and may be more than many providers are able to support. Each provider must prove the value and effectiveness of the care provided. Quality management principles help build and evaluate sound care delivery systems. Thorough analysis of the marketplace, in-depth knowledge regarding provision of infusion services, and ongoing statistical analysis of care and patient outcomes will serve well those home care providers who can provide state-of-the-art services cost effectively and efficiently.

Reimbursement

One criterion for accepting patients into home care is reimbursement for services. Many insurance policies cover home care; however, some policies limit services, such as nursing visits, equipment, or supplies. Patients with Medicare coverage need a thorough review of the diagnosis and prescribed therapy to determine reimbursement. The managed care environment continues to grow rapidly, exerting significant influence on reimbursement. Some payment systems are based on subjective review, which solidifies the need for meticulous and thorough documentation. Even with thorough documentation, this subjectivity leaves many uncertainties. During the insurance verification process, the carrier should be questioned regarding the required documentation, such as statement of medical necessity, physician orders or prescriptions, and clinical notes. This communication will help reduce the denial rate and expedite the reimbursement process.

Patients are provided with information regarding their portion of financial responsibility, which can often be a burden to the patient and family. The home infusion team works with the patient to develop financial arrangements and to research alternative sources for financial assistance.

Private insurance. Reimbursement for home infusion therapies has become more complex over the years because more and more therapies can be given safely and effectively in the home. Each patient should be evaluated individually for coverage, and the coverage should be verified with the payer, including specific information on the therapy and services covered by the insurer. The diagnosis, therapy, drug, duration of therapy, and covered services (e.g., nursing, pharmacy, laboratory, therapeutic monitoring, diagnostics) should be verified before providing a service.

Reimbursement for home care has traditionally been based on a fee-for-service or per-unit basis. In the past, payment was made after the services were provided. More often, now, reimbursement is negotiated by indemnity insurers before the start of therapy. Precertification is usually required before providing services. In addition, the provider must understand clearly which services, disciplines, and number of visits the payer approves. Services delivered without prior authorization will not be approved for payment. It is expected that treatment updates will be given to the payer's case manager at specified intervals. Once the approved services have been delivered, further approval must be sought from the payer for any additional services necessary. The advent of managed care has placed some care decisions in the hands of persons other than the physician. If the organization exceeds what is approved, that care will most likely not be reimbursed. Case managers working for the insurer will determine approval for the patient's plan of care. Insurers who are not using prospective methodology or for whom the infusion organization is not a preferred provider are reviewing cases for medical necessity and paying what is usually a negotiated price. Saladow states, "This growing influence of managed care may be the most important, broad based turning point in the delivery of health care in the United States."[51] Service providers should consider capitated payment agreements carefully before accepting a contract. It is imperative to understand the demographics of the covered group and extrapolate the potential resource consumption. Hastily agreeing to a capitated price just to secure business can put the organization in jeopardy if the cost to the home care organization is not thoroughly understood.

Medicare. Medicare pays for certain infusion therapies based on very specific medical-necessity guidelines. Short-term skilled nursing services are generally covered under Part A, if the home care company is a certified home health agency. Covered under Part B are infusion services, supplies, and some drugs. Payment for infusion medications, which is based on a predetermined rate or a prevailing charge, has not been consistent to date and generally has been denied for antibiotics. Under the prosthetic device benefit, Medicare pays the prevailing rate for medically necessary solutions and supplies. For infusion services to qualify for Medicare coverage, patients must meet not only the medical necessity requirement, but must be homebound. The homebound requirement means that considerable and taxing effort is required for the patient to leave the home, and any absences must be infrequent and of short duration. It is also important to remember that Medicare is considered an acute, short-term benefit and is not designed to cover chronic care. The exception to the intent of the acute care requirement is Part

B coverage for enteral or parenteral nutrition. Because these therapies are considered prostheses for the gut, they are considered a lifelong or permanent replacement and must meet a test of permanence. Details regarding medical necessity and Medicare benefit guidelines can be obtained through a Medicare intermediary.

Medicaid. Medicaid benefits vary from state to state. If Medicaid covers infusion therapies at all, its terms are restrictive; reimbursement rates are low, and eligibility criteria are strict. Medicaid reimbursement is generally an unreliable source for financing home infusion services. Medicaid follows the Medicare requirements for coverage with one major exception. The patient is not required to be homebound to receive Medicaid coverage for services. Information about Medicaid coverage can be obtained from the state programs.

Quality of care

Quality of care is a moving target. All organizations purport to provide their services with excellence; the highest level of quality. To do so, an organization's infrastructure must foster excellence in patient care and service delivery. The infrastructure consists of the following:

- Sound business practices and fiscal responsibility
- Expert, experienced, certified clinicians
- Integrated systems and processes
- Interdisciplinary communication
- Systematic, scientific collection and analysis of data

The present environment is one in which the only constant is change and the only variable is the speed with which it happens. Lowe-Phelps states that "The ultimate goal of any change activity should be to reduce variation in process, thereby improving its operation and outcome. When data analysis produces information that variation in a process exists, further analysis must be undertaken to reveal its nature related to either a common or special cause."[52] Organizations can be responsive to change by ensuring that all employees have a complete understanding of systems and processes, so that when change is necessary in response to the external or internal environment, where and how the change can occur is readily identifiable. Ongoing quality initiatives provide the basis for examining the infrastructure and ensuring each element of the organization is able to statistically document quality in patient care.

Risk management

The 20th century has been described as an era of professional autonomy. Along with autonomy have come regulations and legislation to help define the boundaries of practice. Despite these attempts to define practice boundaries, however, many gray areas remain. Organizations and staff must be cognizant of the potential liabilities in the home as responsibilities and therapies increase in number and complexity. Only clinicians trained and skilled in these new, complex therapies should undertake treatment of these patients. Home infusion providers are responsible for documenting the basic competency and advanced training of their clinicians.

Accurate assessment, ongoing communication, and meticulous documentation, coupled with strong problem-solving abil-

ities, are minimum requirements for the home infusion clinician. Although the home lacks the resources needed to manage medical emergencies, the home infusion clinician must use prudent clinical judgment in the management of such situations. Anticipating potential problems and taking proactive measures to prevent crises are qualities of a good home infusion clinician. Patient and family education also assist in the process of early problem detection and intervention.

All home infusion providers should have a system for risk management reporting, including incident, infection control, and adverse drug reaction reporting. These reporting mechanisms will indicate problem areas and allow early intervention, such as establishing a prevention system. This diligence, in turn, will reduce liability exposure.

Outcomes

Outcome monitoring is no longer a new concept; it is now expected by regulatory and accrediting bodies, payers, and the public. It is a requirement for accreditation through organizations such as JCAHO and the Community Health Accreditation Program (CHAP). JCAHO has initiated the ORYX program in which accredited organizations are required to select clinical indicators to monitor and report to the ORYX database for each service provided (nursing, pharmacy, and equipment).

There are two types of indicators measured: clinical and patient perception. The intent of clinical indicators is to measure care-related processes or outcomes. They encompass the appropriateness of clinical decision making and the processes that lead to clinical decisions. It is recommended that the indicators be "condition-specific, procedure-specific, or address important functions of patient care, such as medication use, infection control and patient assessment."[53] Patient satisfaction measures are classified as patient perception measures, gathering and analyzing data from the perception of the patient, their caregivers, and the family. Patient perception outcomes include aspects of care such as "patient education, pain management, communication regarding plans and outcomes of care, prevention and illness, and improvements in health status."[53] Outcomes for subcontracted services, such as rehabilitation therapist, social worker, and dietitian, must also be evaluated. These indicators can be interdisciplinary.

"The Joint Commission defines a performance measurement system as an interrelated set of process measures, outcomes measures, or both that facilitates internal comparisons over time and external comparisons of an organizations performance."[54] The organization must select and identify the chosen indicators and report them to JCAHO via ORYX-approved software vendors. Accredited organizations will be assessed with a type I recommendation for failure to meet the requirements of the initiative. There is concern on the part of providers that the cost of complying with the ORYX initiative will be too burdensome.[55]

Medicare-certified providers must use OASIS functional status assessment tools as a component of initial assessment, reassessment, resumption of care, or transfer to another venue of care or discharge. As with ORYX, data gathered from OASIS must be transmitted to HCFA along with other assessment data. Specified time intervals must be adhered to when submitting data. The HCFA is requiring that data for all patients served by the agency, even those who do not have Medicare as a payer, be submitted to HCFA. Health care providers must be vigilant to protect the confidentiality of patient information as data are transmitted to government agencies. Noncompliance with OASIS requirements results in deficiencies on Medicare survey.

The data recovered through ORYX and OASIS are used for benchmarking. The information is blinded, received, analyzed by the various vendors, and returned to the organization. The data allow the organization to compare its outcomes with similar organizations and thus determine which processes are effective and which require improvement.

Although accreditation by JCAHO or CHAP is a voluntary process, most third-party payers have made accreditation a requirement for reimbursement. The home infusion organization that has the ability to measure and analyze the outcomes of care it provides will be able to anticipate needed changes in operational and patient care processes. These data will provide the basis for a flexible and successful organization, capable of providing consistently excellent, cost-effective infusion therapy.

FUTURE DIRECTIONS

The home health industry is in a state of major flux. Changes in reimbursement have led many providers of home care to cease operations. This is coupled with the "graying of America" and the anticipated increase in demand for services because of the large aging population. As the condition of the home care patient becomes more acute, the clinical pharmacist and IV nurse will have to sharpen their skills. Therapeutic monitoring and patient care management by the nurse and the pharmacist is being demanded by payers and even required by law in some cases. One can only assume that as the care requirements become more complex and intensive, opportunities for the experienced, certified home infusion clinician will increase. Although it is difficult to predict what our health care model will look like in the future, one thing is certain: it will be radically different from today. The survival of the home care industry will depend on the flexibility and creativity of home care organizations. Increasing demand on rapidly shrinking resources will necessitate doing things differently, thinking "outside the box."

Advances in technology such as remote-access infusion devices and the maturing of telemedicine technology will allow clinicians to provide care in the home, preserving patients health care benefits by decreasing the amount of time spent in the home. "Tele-infusion devices are increasingly demonstrating cost-effectiveness and assist the client and caregiver to maintain the home-care industry's goal of client self management and independent handling of complex therapies in the supportive home environment"[56] Other advances, such as the ability to transfer data from the patient to the home care provider via telephone lines or wireless technology, will allow increased frequency of patient monitoring. If used as an adjunct to, not a substitute for, clinician interaction, it will preserve the patients sense of well being and independence.

Time and experience have proven that there are very few infusion therapies that, with care and some modification, cannot be delivered safely in the home. It is up to the industry to continue to be pioneers and calculated risk takers, while always acting in the best interests of patients. Advanced technology can never replace sound clinical practice and a desire to improve the services delivered to clients. The future of the industry is in the hands of those who embrace change and continuously use outcomes data to provide safe, effective care to their patients.

REFERENCES

1. Poretz DM: High tech comes home, *Am J Med* 91:453, 1991.
2. Darrow C: Hospitals seeking ways to cut costs, *La Crosse City Business* 3(19):1, 1985.
3. Paris E: Home remedies, *Forbes* January 9:143(1):58, 1989.
4. Rehm SJ: Home intravenous antibiotic therapy, *Cleve Clin J Med* 52:333, 1985.
5. Joyeux H: Background and development of the AIO concept, *Nutrition* 5(5):342, 1989.
6. Poretz DM: Home management of intravenous antibiotic therapy, *Bull NY Acad Med* 64(6):570, 1988.
7. National Health Statistics Group, Office of the Actuary: National health expenditures, 1997. Health Care Financing Review, vol 20 no 1, HCFA Pub no 03412. Health Care Financing Administration, Washington, DC, US Government Printing Office, March 1999.
8. Boger J, et al: Infusion therapy with milrinone in the home care setting for patients who have advanced heart failure, *JIN* 20(3):148, 1997.
9. Reid JS: *Clinical management resources guide,* Chattsworth, Calif, 1983, Community Alimentation Services, Department of Clinical Services.
10. Brown RB, Sands M: Outpatient intravenous antibiotic therapy, *Am Fam Physician* 40:157, 1989.
11. Herfindal ET, Bernstein LR, Kuzida K, Wong A: Survey of home nutritional support patients, *JPEN J Parenter Enteral Nutr* 13(3):255, 1989.
12. Schaffer C: Can we overcome the next set of hurdles? *Infusion* 4(12):27, 1998.
13. Kaplan LK: What's new in Medicare reimbursement for infusion services, *Infusion* 3(10):27, 1997.
14. Poole S M, Nowobilski-Vasilios A: Intravenous push medications in the home, *JIN* 22(4):209, 1999.
15. Poole S M, Nowobilski-Vasilios A: To push or not to push, *Infusion* 5(9):52, 1999.
16. Weissmann AC: Treatment of fungal infections with ABLC in the home care setting, *J Assoc Nurses AIDS Care* 10(3):43, 1999.
17. Breier SJ: Ethics and total parenteral nutrition, *JIN* 23(1):53, 2000.
18. ASPEN Board of Directors: *Standards for home nutritional support, nutrition in clinical practice,* 14:151, 1999, ASPEN.
19. Corrigan AM, Pelletier G, Alexander M: *Core curriculum for intravenous nursing,* ed 2, Philadelphia, 1999, Lippincott.
20. Carlson KR: Correct utilization and management of peripherally inserted central catheters and midline catheters in the alternate setting, *JIN* 22(6S):S46, 1999.
21. Gorski LA, Grothman L: Home infusion therapy, *Semin Oncol Nurs* 12(3):196, 1996.
22. Dougherty L, Viner C, Young J: Establishing ambulatory chemotherapy at home, *Prof Nurse* 13(6):356, 1998.
23. Bruchak KT: *Oncolink FAQ: bloodcounts,* University of Pennsylvania Cancer Center November 22, 1999 (Revised) Posted Feb 21, 1997, pp. 4-5.
24. Birmingham JJ: Decision matrix for selection of patients for a home infusion therapy program, *JIN* 20(5):260, 1998.
25. Saladow J: Infusion devices: where do we go from here? *Infusion* 4(9):27, 1998.
26. Camp-Sorrell D: Developing extravasation protocols and monitoring outcomes, *JIN* 21(4):235, 1998.
27. Falkenstrom MK: Pain management of the patient with cancer in the homecare setting, *JIN* 21(6):328, 1998.

28. Plaisance L: A stepwise guide to cancer pain management in the home, *Home Healthcare Nurse* 17(2):1, 1999.
29. Johnson DL: Pharmacologic pain management for cancer patients at home, *Home Healthcare Nurse* 16(3):10, 1998.
30. Boger JE, et al: Infusion therapy with milrinone in the home care setting for patients who have advanced heart failure, *JIN* 20(3): 150, 1997.
31. Gorski L: Cardiac infusion therapy. In *Best practices in home infusion therapy,* Gaithersburg, Md, 1999, Aspen.
32. Dugger B: Peripheral dopamine infusions: are they worth the risk of infiltration? *JIN* 20(2):96, 1997.
33. Ignatavicius DD, Workman ML, Mishler, MA: *Medical-surgical nursing across the health care continuum,* ed 3, Philadelphia, 1999, WB Saunders.
34. Friedman MM: Risk management strategies for home transfusion therapy, *JIN* 20(4):179, 1997.
35. Gorski, LA, Buxton HM, Czaplewski LM, Skurdal C: Additional home parenteral and infusion therapies. In *Best practices in home infusion therapy,* Gaithersburg, Md, 1999, Aspen.
36. Micromedix, Inc: Alpha 1-Proteinase inhibitor, human (systemic): www.nlm.nih.gov/medline plus/drug info/Alpha 1 proteinase inhibitor human.202022.html.
37. Scharnweber K: Alpha$_1$-antitrypsin deficiency and the impact of nursing interventions and treatment with intravenous therapy, *JIN* 22(5):259, 1999.
38. Lam F: The history and use of subcutaneous terbutaline pump therapy, *Triplet Connection* 15(2), 1998.
39. Newman RB: Subcutaneous terbutaline pump therapy, *Triplet Connection* 15(2), 1998.
40. Gorski LA, Buxton HM, Czaplewski LM, Skurdal C: Tocolytic therapy. In *Best practice in home health infusion,* Gaithersburg, Md, 1999, Aspen.
41. Skurdal C: Epoprostenol sodium infusion for the treatment of primary pulmonary hypertension, *Infusion* 4(12):35, 1998.
42. Gahart BL, Nazareno AR: *Intravenous medications: a handbook for nurses and allied health personnel,* ed 16, St Louis, 1999, Mosby.
43. Intravenous Nurses Society: Position paper, the role of licensed practical nurse and licensed vocational nurse in the clinical practice of intravenous nursing, *JIN* 20(2):75, 1997.
44. Coulter K: Nurses transition from hospital to home: bridging the gap, *JIN* 20(2):89, 1997.
45. Weinstein SM: Certification and credentialing to define competency-based practice, *JIN* 23(1):21, 2000.
46. National Board of Nutrition Support Certification at American Society of Enteral and Parenteral Nutrition web site: www.clinnutr.org.
47. Oncology Nurses Certification Corporation: 2000 Certification bulletin for OCN, AOCN and CPON certification, p. 18.
48. ASPEN Board of Directors: *Standards of practice for nutrition support nurses,* 1999, ASPEN. www.clinnutr.org.
49. Joint Commission on Accreditation of Healthcare Organizations: *CAMHC: 1999-2000 Comprehensive accreditation manual for home care,* Oakbrook, Ill, 1998, JCAHO.
50. Mozena JP, Emerick CE, Black SC: *Stop managing costs: designing healthcare organizations around core business systems,* Milwaukee, 1999, ASQ Quality Press.
51. Saladow J: History in the making, *Infusion* 5(9):16, 1999.
52. Lowe-Phelps K: Managing change while maintaining quality in home infusion therapy, *JIN* 19(1):42, 1996.
53. Barrell JM: ORYX: Outcomes measurement and accreditation, *Infusion* 4(8):37, 1998.
54. Popovich MA: Initiatives aim to integrate performance measures into the Joint Commission's accreditation process. In *Home health outcomes and resource utilization: integrating today's critical priorities,* New York, 1997, National League for Nursing.
55. Schmit C: ORYX, The unintended effects, *Infusion* 5(2):29, 1998.
56. McNeal G: Telecommunication Technologies in high-tech homecare, *Crit Care Clin North Am* 10(3):281, 1998.

Intravenous Therapy in the Alternative Care Setting

Nancy Mortlock, CRNI, OCN*

HISTORICAL PERSPECTIVE

Since the first reporting of outpatient intravenous (IV) infusion therapy in 1974, outpatient antimicrobial therapy has grown into an industry affecting millions of Americans and generating billions of dollars annually. It has demonstrated that IV therapies can be safely and effectively delivered in alternative settings while overall reducing health care expenditures. Reasons for this rapid growth include the many benefits outpatient therapy provides to patients, new technologies that make it possible, and well-documented cost savings.[1] Third-party payers, who were once satisfied with any savings afforded by outpatient care, allowed physicians a great deal of freedom in how care was provided. With the increase in the number of providers, however, payers have come to expect cost savings and attempt to control or manage the costs of outpatient care to maximize those savings. Cost-benefit assessments of outpatient therapy used to focus on decreasing hospital expense. Now, it is seen as a potential treatment option to prevent hospitalization altogether. Thus rather than being the central component of the health care system, the hospital seems destined to become a small specialty center for the sickest patients.

*The author and editors wish to acknowledge the contributions made by Debbie Benvenuto, Donna Baldwin, and David Scheutz, as coauthors of this chapter in the first edition of *Intravenous Nursing: Clinical Principles and Practice.*

In the early 1970s, Rucker and Harrison reported on outpatient IV medications used to manage children with cystic fibrosis. The first experience administering outpatient IV antibiotics to adults was in 1978, when Antoniskis described 13 patients who self-administered parenteral antibiotics, primarily for osteomyelitis. He demonstrated the safety of such therapy and showed significant savings compared with a control group that was treated in the hospital. Subsequently, the literature supports the efficacy, safety, and cost-effectiveness of treating patients with parenteral antimicrobics on an outpatient basis.[2]

Some alternative sites where IV therapy is now successfully delivered include outpatient infusion centers, physicians' offices, extended care facilities, home care programs, nursing homes, and psychiatric facilities. Therapy selection in the outpatient setting may be somewhat different from the hospital. Potent drugs with prolonged half-lives that allow ease of administration without sacrificing antimicrobial activity have now been developed. Cyclic total parenteral admixtures have been concentrated and given in combinations, making them easier and often quicker to self-administer. This convenience is very helpful to patients who wish to maintain their daily activities. In actuality, almost any antimicrobic that can be used in the hospital can also be used on an outpatient basis. In recent years, antifungal, antivirals, chemotherapeutics, narcotics, antiarrhythmics, and total parenteral nutrition (TPN) have been safely administered in alternative settings and appropriately monitored for side effects. As more procedures are being performed in the outpatient setting, physicians must now select patients for whom such care is appropriate and confirm that the quality of care being provided in specific alternative programs is high. The prescribing physician is the person held accountable and potentially liable for safety and efficacy, regardless of his or her level of direct involvement in the delivery of care.

The shift in the delivery of IV therapies to alternative settings has been accelerated by the following factors:

- Fixed or declining reimbursement for inpatient care
- Need to reduce financial loss by decreasing length of stay
- Emphasis on preventive care
- Patient desire to avoid hospitalization
- Potential revenue generation from outpatient clinic or home health care
- Availability of highly sophisticated vascular access and electronic ambulatory infusion devices
- Accumulation of scientific data supporting prolonged parenteral drug stability
- Newer antimicrobial agents
- Studies demonstrating the safe delivery of multiple IV regimens in alternative settings

Criteria that must be met before outpatient parenteral agents can be implemented include the following:

- The patient must have a disease that requires continued treatment beyond the anticipated period of hospitalization.
- There is no need for hospitalization.
- There must be no equally effective and safe oral agent or treatment regimen.[3]

Benefits

Patients treated outside the hospital, whether in an outpatient facility or at home, avoid problems inherent in the hospital system, including unfamiliar, sometimes frightening surroundings; isolation from friends and family, and lack of privacy. Avoiding or leaving the hospital setting also may facilitate the transition from the role of "sick patient" back to the familiar, functioning self, thus speeding adaptation and recovery.[1] Treatment can be adjusted to each patient's lifestyle or needs. After interviewing the patient, the most appropriate delivery system and unobtrusive dosing schedule can be determined. Children will benefit from early hospital discharge, returning to a more familiar environment and minimizing painful trauma or fear.

Delivery of outpatient infusion therapy requires that the team of professionals providing the care demonstrate proficiency and an advanced skill level in initiating, administering and terminating infusion therapy. Patient safety is the primary consideration of clinicians administering infusion therapy in all practice settings. Patients will experience numerous benefits from an outpatient treatment regimen that is based on accepted standards of practice.

Receiving infusion therapy at an alternative site helps avoid the ever-prevalent infections found in hospitals. Hospital-related infections are estimated to affect more than 5% of hospitalized patients, extending their hospital stays by an average of 4 days and directly causing 20,000 deaths a year in the United States.[4] Added health care costs in excess of $10 billion annually have been estimated as a result of nosocomial blood stream infections.[5] Although the risk of infection directly related to outpatient IV therapy has not been quantified, the incidence appears to be far less.[6] The phlebitis rate associated with IV antimicrobials is also greater in hospitalized patients than in those treated at home.[7] Another problem in the hospital is the increased prevalence of organisms that are highly resistant to the antimicrobials used against community-acquired infections. Multidrug-resistant enterococci and gram-negative bacteria typically lurk in hospitals. Infections related to outpatient therapy have not yet been given a descriptive name. However, the term *nosohusial* has been proposed.

DELIVERY MODELS

Outpatient parenteral therapy can be delivered in almost any setting. Each unique program is dictated by community needs and resources. Over time, the following basic models of outpatient infusion delivery have become increasingly standardized: the infusion center, the visiting nurse, self-administration, the emergency department, hospital-based programs, and the extended care facility. Each model has its own clinical and economic advantages and disadvantages.

The infusion center

An infusion center may be developed in a variety of medical settings, including a physician's office, hospital clinic, urgent care center, emergency department, or free-standing infusion clinic. Each of these settings has a medical staff on site and the ready availability of equipment and medications that may be needed to respond to vascular access problems or to change therapies. The clinic will probably employ a nurse, physician, pharmacist, social worker, dietician, and administrative staff, working together to provide an effective and efficient communication system for designing treatment programs and following the outcomes of therapy.

With staffing, equipment, and physician involvement similar to that of the hospital, the infusion center is a practical way to initiate extended outpatient care. Because of this similarity, the patient usually perceives the transition from the hospital to the infusion center as less traumatic and perhaps better supervised than going directly to home care and self-administration. One limiting factor of the infusion center model is the difficulty of treating patients who need parenteral therapy or nursing intervention more than once a day. For patients needing therapy more than once a day, a combination of self-administration in the home and visits to the infusion clinic may be helpful. It is important that patients and families who are going to be involved in self-administration are selected carefully.

Specialized infusion services provided in the infusion center may include catheter care, including implanted port access and removal; blood component administration; antimicrobial, antifungal, and antiviral infusion; continuous or intermittent chemotherapy; various intramuscular and subcutaneous injections; IV gamma globulin; hydration therapy; pain control; and TPN. The center should also educate patients and families about all of these services.

Significant savings can be realized when IV therapy is delivered in infusion centers rather than in other types of outpatient or home infusion programs or hospitals. Infusion centers allow excellent coordination of resources and efficient delivery of services. Several patients can be infused and monitored at the same time, saving money by using professional staff efficiently.

Hospital-based infusion center

In America and abroad, a large portion of outpatient infusion therapy is administered through a hospital-based infusion center. Often, the hospital infusion program is associated with a hospital-based home care agency. Under this model, the hospital's pharmacy either can provide the medicine and equipment and its nursing staff delivers the patient education and care or can use its own pharmacy, nursing, equipment, management, and delivery services separate from the hospital. A program of this nature can be organized as a division of the institution or as a separate affiliate company.

Hospital emergency department

Emergency departments can also serve as infusion centers. In other countries, this is the norm rather than the exception. A hospital emergency department can safely administer single daily doses of parenteral antibiotics; provide catheter care; insert, replace, or remove central venous catheters; taper TPN; monitor glucose levels; assess central venous catheter patency; initiate a new antimicrobial; or monitor for drug tolerance.

Although scheduled daily visits are planned and predictable, the traffic and flow in a busy emergency department is not. Some emergency departments find it difficult to staff adequately for infusion patients in addition to the unexpected trauma patients inherent to an emergency department. Other emergency departments have incorporated observation suites, allowing parenteral treatment to be initiated under skilled supervision while freeing up the department's beds for new emergency patients.

Visiting nurse

By definition, the visiting nurse model of outpatient infusion therapy is one in which the nurse administers medication in the home. These nurses must be specially trained and skilled to initiate a peripheral venous catheter and maintain a central venous catheter according to the standards of care. The agencies procedures and protocols, in conjunction with the physicians orders, dictate the care that the nurses administer in the home setting. Patients who have limited mobility—are bedridden, terminal, or difficult to transport—may require treatment at home. Individuals with advanced stage cancer or advanced acquired immunodeficiency disease may benefit from services provided by the visiting nurse.

One major advantage of home-based infusion is that it allows the nurse to evaluate the home situation. The nurse can assess physical limitations, environmental hazards, domestic issues, and any drug or alcohol abuse that would affect a patient's compliance with therapy or response to therapy. Problems in these areas are difficult to observe apart from a home visit. In addition, other skilled services can be instituted in the home, such as physical therapy, occupational therapy, and social or hospice services.

A limiting factor to this model of infusion delivery is the cost of a nurse's visit to the home. In some urban settings, one nurse can easily visit up to 10 patients per day, whereas in a rural area the time and travel involved may limit the nurse to two to three visits per day. In some cases, the cost may prohibit the nurse's visit. Also, if an antimicrobial needs to be given intravenously more than once per day, the cost advantage of nurse administration may be lost and other models of delivery become more beneficial.

Another problem associated with the visiting nurse model is nurse safety. As home health care expands, safety becomes an important issue—particularly in high-crime neighborhoods. Just how far a nurse or physician can or should go in visiting a home is unclear. Although there are very few recorded instances of injury or loss of life, the threat is certainly there. Security concerns must be considered in any home visit and should be reviewed carefully with staff so that risks are not overlooked. Key points to consider include those in Box 29-1.

Self-administration

Successful experiences with self-administration of IV infusions have propelled the industry and increased use of this model. Teaching patients and their families to provide long-term TPN, and in some circumstances to mix their own solutions, has

Box 29-1   Security Suggestions for Home Visits

1. Develop standards for what is reasonable for a home visit and what is not.
2. Use an infusion center rather than a visiting nurse if problems are anticipated.
3. Consider meeting the patient or family at a safe, convenient location other than the home.
4. Make visits in the morning rather than the afternoon or evening in troublesome areas.
5. Supply staff members with cellular phones.
6. Consider hiring a taxi and having them wait at the door.
7. Consider hiring escorts or guards.
8. Record any problems encountered so there will be no question if it is not reasonable to risk your personnel to provide the services.[8]

allowed the population of chronically ill patients to return to work or school and function as normally as their disease will allow. Patients with immune globulin deficiency and hemophilia have also been taught self-administration, as have patients with immunodeficiency virus who have cytomegalovirus retinitis, which often requires a long course of IV ganciclovir or foscarnet. The weeks of therapy required for severe infections, short gut syndrome, Crohn's disease, and analgesic pain control are now being safely administered by patients who receive IV administration education provided largely by the infusion nurse.

Children needing IV therapy may benefit from self-administration when a parent or responsible person is taught to administer the therapy. Parents can be remarkably adept when properly educated in the sterile procedures of IV administration but are often overlooked as caregivers.

Self-administration offers considerable financial savings, particularly for prolonged courses of treatment, afforded by significant reductions in personnel and overhead costs. An infusion center is still necessary to provide pharmacy services, initial doses of medications, vascular access, patient education, and physician oversight.

Consistent support is necessary for patients and caregivers who administer medication to ensure compliance with the prescribed treatment plan and to monitor patient response. Intermittent patient visits to the infusion center are necessary for ongoing assessment of the vascular access device, drug and supply distribution, and clinical assessment. A major liability concern and common criticism of the self-administration model is the perceived lack of medical supervision. Delayed or immediate anaphylactoid reactions may occur in any setting, but they are harder to manage when they are associated with self-administration. Medications may inadvertently be given too quickly, given too slowly, allowed to infiltrate, or not given at all. These errors can cause fluid overload, electrolyte imbalance, arrhythmias, harmful drug interactions, or continued infection. To prevent many of these self-administration problems, patients and caregivers need to be carefully selected, trained, and monitored for compliance with intermittent phone communications and spot home visits.

Home infusion company

The home infusion company has become the most common model of outpatient infusion therapy. Home infusion companies consist of nurses, pharmacists, dieticians, managers, equipment technicians, supply and delivery personnel, and sales representatives, who will promote their services to third-party payers and physician groups. Nurses are usually skilled IV nurses who have acquired nursing assessment, patient training, and organizational skills in previous employment. Commonly, nurses employed by home infusion companies have acquired substantial IV therapy skills working on a hospital-based IV team. In response to hospital staffing changes over the past decade and the termination of numerous hospital IV teams, many experienced IV nurses have joined the outpatient workforce, providing substantial advantage to home infusion companies in the areas of venous access, catheter placement, and infusion administration. Nurses who have prior critical care or medical surgical nursing experience have expert nursing assessment skills that, because of the rising acuity of home patients, are beneficial to home infusion.

Home infusion companies often have a contract with home health agencies to educate patients and perform the nursing functions necessary for the home patient. A home infusion pharmacist coordinates the patient's discharge, discusses the orders with the attending physician, and arranges nursing services for wound care, catheter and infusion management, and 24-hour call for emergencies with an outside agency. In the rare event that there are no patient care needs beyond the scope of pharmacy, the home infusion pharmacy will usually act as the primary provider. A pharmacy company may also turn to a home health agency if Medicare, Medicaid, or state law requires the nursing provider to be a licensed home health agency.

Although some patients welcome the visit from the nurse, some ambulatory patients prefer to get out of the house and visit the infusion center, rather than having to wait or schedule the nurse at home.

Most commonly, the greatest limitation of the home infusion model is the relative exclusion of the physician. Occasionally, infusion pharmacies and home infusion companies have managed the care of outpatient IV patients with minimal direction by the responsible physician. Physicians are approved to make home visits by most third-party payers, including Medicare, and home infusion companies should take advantage of this to keep physicians involved as fully as possible. Because fee schedules remain relatively low, regular home visits are cost prohibitive.

Long-term care facility

Long-term care facilities, nursing homes, or rehabilitation institutions provide another model for outpatient IV infusion therapy. With the cost of health care continuing to escalate, the need to find alternative sites at which to deliver antibiotic therapy has never been greater. The use of diagnosis-related groups as a reimbursement mechanism has forced hospitals and physicians to find other venues for treating stable patients. Because the Health Care Financing Administration (HCFA) has provided only limited support for outpatient antibiotic therapy, clinicians have been forced to provide these therapies in long-term care facilities.

The long-term care facility can provide many benefits to clinicians as they strive to maintain the quality of care outside of the acute care setting. In these institutions, physicians are able to control the patient's care through more aggressive personal supervision or by establishing an outpatient infusion therapy team. Personal supervision can occur in three different ways. The prescribing physician can admit the patient to a facility for infusion and serve as the patient's attending physician during his or her stay. All the duties and privileges of an attending physician, including the history and physical examination, daily progress documentation, and discharge summary are inherent in this model. Many long-term acute care hospitals require that a patient be seen daily by the attending physician, similar to an acute care hospital, regardless of the patient's needs. The obvious benefit of this model is that it provides the ultimate level of control and supervision. In the second model of physician supervision, the prescribing physician acts as a consultant to the attending. The follow-up and documentation requirements are fewer and there is less clinical control. In the final model, physicians may act as administrative consultants for the long-term care facility to provide medical and technical assistance to patients, physicians, and staff. This allows the physician to have input into policy development relating to the outpatient infusion aspects of the facility.[9]

Long-term care facilities are particularly appropriate venues for delivering IV therapy to patients with physical or mental limitations or patients insured by third-party payers who do not allow payment for home or office infusion therapy. They provide a safe environment for patients who require a substantial amount of monitoring, or those with substance abuse problems who are not sick enough to require hospitalization. Antimicrobials are among the most commonly prescribed pharmaceutical agents in long-term facilities, accounting for approximately 40% of all systemic drugs prescribed.[10] The point prevalence of systemic antibiotic use in long-term care facilities is approximately 8%, with a likelihood of 50% to 70% that a resident will receive at least one course of a systemic antimicrobial agent during a 1-year period. Because infections are common in these facilities, residents often are exposed to antimicrobial agents. These agents present some risk of adverse consequences even when they are prescribed and delivered appropriately.

The patient mix among long-term facilities is heterogeneous, ranging from healthy elderly in some nursing homes to debilitated, chronically ill patients in others. The population of nursing homes often includes more acute and subacute patients who may require multiple infusion therapies. Before the shift in staffing and patient acuity in the hospital, these patients were generally treated in hospitals. Occasionally, the nursing staff in a long-term care facility has not had adequate education or experience in IV nursing practices. The ratio of RNs is far lower in nursing homes than in most hospitals, creating difficulty for the RN who must administer, manage, and monitor residents receiving infusion therapies.

Commonly, an outpatient infusion pharmacy will provide the IV medications, supplies, and equipment to the long-term facility by contract. Experienced IV nurses often provide "back-up call" to the facilities because their staff nurses may not have sufficient IV experience and expertise.

Elderly nursing home residents are at increased risk of drug-related adverse effects by virtue of the physiologic effects of aging on kidney and liver functions, the presence of comorbid illnesses, and the concurrent use of other drugs to treat these diseases. Probably the most important adverse outcome of inappropriate IV antimicrobial use in long-term facilities is the promotion of antimicrobial resistance in this high-risk population and the increased opportunities for transmitting resistant organisms to other patients.

The limited availability of laboratory and radiology services in these facilities contributes to the difficulty in managing a course of treatment with IV therapies. It is often necessary to transport an infusion patient to a tertiary care center for laboratory monitoring, a chest radiograph to verify the location of a central venous catheter tip, or other diagnostic studies.

CHOOSING THE APPROPRIATE DELIVERY MODEL

Each IV infusion model is unique. A careful evaluation of the patient, disease state, venous access, and capabilities must be determined before choosing the appropriate delivery model.

The choice of delivery model depends on the individual patient, the provider's expertise, community resources, and geographic limitations. Third-party payers can also dictate the infusion model selected for their insured participants. Physicians experienced in managing outpatient therapies may prefer one delivery model. If a patient is unstable or is having difficulty with the infusions or venous access, the physician may prefer a model that provides acute monitoring and continuity of care between personnel caring for the patient.

Given the cost constraints of managed care, models that allow multiple patients to be infused simultaneously may be the most cost-effective. They require the least nursing time when the entire IV team is in the same building. Choice of an appropriate alternative setting depends on the specialized training and expertise of the programs' personnel and the resources available to them. Regardless of the model chosen, a continued and ongoing team effort among the medical professionals is crucial to the effectiveness and outcomes of treatment.

Clinical advantages and disadvantages

There are numerous considerations in determining which alternative setting is appropriate for the patient. The distinct advantages and disadvantages of the various models may have an effect on treatment outcome (Table 29-1).

SCOPE OF SERVICE
Patient selection

The patient is an essential member of the outpatient infusion team and should play many roles in his or her own care. Perhaps the most important role for the patient is reporting significant

Table 29-1   Advantages and Disadvantages of Alternative Care Settings for Infusion Therapy

ALTERNATIVE SETTING	ADVANTAGES	DISADVANTAGES
Infusion clinic	Team of professionals together in one place Physician oversight readily available Medications available in case a change is necessary Continuity of care	Patient must travel to infusion clinic Overhead costs Emergencies Storage of supplies and equipment Costs associated with space Nursing costs
Hospital emergency department	Available in rural communities Professionals available for emergencies First-dose monitoring	Patient must travel to facility Unpredictable census and staffing Lengthy wait for change in medication
Visiting nurse	Convenience to patient Environmental and home assessment Able to treat terminal or homebound patients	Costs of commuting time Intrusion on privacy Decreased physician oversight
Hospital-based infusion center	Safe environment for first doses Available medications and solutions May share experienced IV team nurses	Patient must travel to hospital May not be available rurally
Long-term care facility	Safe environment for patients with substance abuse Good for physically or mentally limited patients	Prevalence of nosocomial infections Lack of experienced IV nurses
Self-administration	Cost-effective Allows return to normal activities, school, and work	Possible noncompliance Follow-up and monitoring is more difficult Decreased physician oversight
Home infusion company	Convenience to patient Environmental and home assessment Able to treat terminal or homebound patients Appropriate for self-administered medications Home delivery of supplies and medications	Costs of commuting time Possible noncompliance Follow-up and monitoring is more difficult Decreased physician oversight

Table 29-2   Current Infusion Therapies/Diseases Acceptable for Outpatient Treatment

INFECTIOUS DISEASE	NUTRITIONAL DISORDER	CARDIAC DISEASE	HEMATOLOGIC ONCOLOGIC	OTHER
Endocarditis	Postsurgery nutritional deficit	Arrhythmia	Blood dyscrasias	Hydration
Osteomyelitis	Crohn's disease	Hypotension	Lymphomas	CVC care
Skin/soft tissue infection	Short-gut syndrome		Bone cancer	CVC insertion
HIV-related infections	Absorption therapy		Solid tumors	Blood/blood components
Wound infections				Factor VIII, IX
Respiratory infections				Pain control
Viral infections				

HIV, Human immunodeficiency virus; *CVC*, central venous catheter.

changes in vital signs and symptoms, including rash, nausea, vomiting, diarrhea, phlebitis, erythema, or purulence at the site of insertion. Educating patients to be reliable team members involves encouraging them to communicate often with the nurse, physician, and sometimes the pharmacist.

The criteria for patient selection and monitoring of patients who receive outpatient IV therapies have been gradually established by various professional groups. The Intravenous Nurses Society has developed standards of practice for the administration of IV medications and maintenance of vascular access devices. More recently, the Practice Guidelines Committee of the Infectious Disease Society of America has published practice guidelines for community-based parenteral antiinfective therapy. Other professional organizations, such as the Outpatient Intravenous Infusion Therapy Association and the Oncology Nursing Society, have produced publications stressing the importance of patient selection, monitoring, specific therapies, and outcome data for individuals being treated in alternative

settings.[2] All of these organizations have stressed the importance of a team approach consisting of patient, physician, nurse, and pharmacist.

Several essential interrelated criteria should be taken into account when patients are being selected as outpatient candidates. Clinical factors are the most important. The list of clinical conditions that can be effectively treated on an outpatient basis lengthens as sicker patients with more severe infections, cardiac arrhythmic problems, nutritional disorders, and cancers are assigned or discharged to outpatient care and newer, more potent medications become available.

Most infections can be treated, at least in part, in an alternative setting. Numerous hematologic or oncologic diseases are suitable for outpatient infusion. Table 29-2 details some of the current IV therapies and disease entities generally acceptable for outpatient treatment.

The selection of patients suitable for infusions in outpatient settings depends on a number of factors in addition to disease state and the patient's clinical status, including personal desires, attitudes, abilities, available support system for transportation, and support in the home. These issues must be evaluated because the success of therapy is fundamentally dependent on the patient's and caregiver's willingness to participate in the therapy, ability to understand its inherent complications and potential problems, and ability to learn the necessary skills.

The patient's mental and physical abilities, self-confidence, anxiety, and fears should all be assessed during discharge planning. Limitations on ambulation, prolonged sitting, and access to transportation may weigh heavily against outpatient treatment. The visiting nurse model may not be appropriate for patients who live alone and are not able to care for themselves even with the assistance of social services.

The risk of IV narcotic or other drug abuse must always be considered in patient selection. Although drug abusers may use a reliable IV line for other than prescribed IV medications, prolonged hospitalization may be difficult to justify and may not necessarily prevent the problem. Any suspicion of drug abuse should be tempered by the prescribing physician's judgment of the patient's ability to comply with the treatment plan.

Home circumstances must be evaluated carefully. Family support is particularly important if self-administration or family administration of IV infusion is planned. The presence of a family member who can be educated to recognize potential difficulties and evaluate the patient's condition is valuable for the patient and physician. The distance from a patient's residence to the nearest medical facility must also be considered. For example, a patient living several hours from a medical facility may find it harder to arrange for therapy administration. A supply of running water to ensure careful hand washing and a refrigerator to store the medication are essential if self-administration is planned.

Reimbursement requirements and limitations can play a large role in patient selection. Managed care and provider/payer contracts often direct the outpatient source of care that patients receive. The physician often is not allowed to choose the pharmacy or nursing agency that will administer the infusion or provide patient education and follow-up care. Third-party payers, through their medical directors and case managers, can determine which infusion providers can be used for certain patients.

Admission criteria

Admission criteria establish guidelines by which patients will be admitted to an alternative care setting and identify which alternative care setting can best meet the needs of the patient.

Acceptance of patients into an IV therapy program should be based on a reasonable expectation that the patient's medical, nursing and social needs can be met by the program. Acceptance should also be based on reasonable expectation that the program's staff, facility, and other patients will not risk physical harm nor be exposed to liability because of the patient's inability to comply with identified responsibilities. Determining whether the patient is a good candidate for self-administration at home should be based on an assessment of the patient's or caregiver's abilities, the suitability of the home environment, ease of

transportation to and from the home, and reimbursement requirements.

Patients should be admitted and cared for without discrimination on the basis of age, gender, mental or physical disability, race, color, religion, ancestry, or national origin. Documentation of the admission assessment and determination of place of service is the responsibility of the MD or RN admitting the patient to service. Criteria are written so that the final decision and accountability for admission to the program lies with the admitting physician.

The procedure for admission should include the following:

- Initial referral information is documented by the physician according to policy/procedure on an IV therapy intake form.
- Patient and physician will be informed of the patient's estimated financial responsibility for planned treatment prior to or within 24 hours of the start of care.
- Patient must be willing to accept responsibility for reimbursement.
- Every effort will be made to limit the patient's financial responsibility.
- Patients will be advised of other options of care, if appropriate.
- If a third-party payer is involved, limitations and requirements of the payer will be determined and considered in developing a plan of care.
- The patient or caregiver should understand the expectations and be willing to accept the responsibilities of participating in the outpatient infusion program.

The patient should have adequate venous access status to complete the planned course of therapy. All potential patients should be evaluated for history of IV drug misuse. If evidence of prior drug abuse exists, the patient can still be eligible provided there has no abuse for at least 1 year. Exceptions should be evaluated by the physician. Guidelines to assess the status of IV drug use may include the following:

- Patient statement denying use
- Patient's mental acuity
- Full venous assessment indicating no recent or current IV drug use
- Verbal or written verification by a rehabilitation program or primary physician that the patient has not misused IV drugs for at least 1 year or has completed or is currently enrolled in an approved rehabilitation program

A patient being evaluated for admission into a self-administration program should be evaluated against the following criteria before being admitted:

- Mental or psychosocial evaluation—the patient should be alert and oriented to person, place, time, and environment
- Demonstration of adequate memory, problem-solving skills, and abilities to manage
- Ability to demonstrate required tasks to comply with therapy
- Willingness and ability to accept responsibilities and risks involved in home infusion
- Demonstration of the manual dexterity and acuity of sight and hearing required to manage tasks and equipment and to seek help in the event of emergency

Box 29-2   Criteria for Assessing the Home Environment

- Reasonably safe for home infusion therapy
- Adequate area to prepare and administer IV infusion and perform dressing changes, if necessary
- Adequate refrigeration and storage space for medications and supplies
- Available intact electrical outlets if required for equipment
- Running water to wash hands
- Ability to store equipment, infectious waste, and medications out of reach of children
- Telephone access

Box 29-3   Educational Content of the Teaching Program

- Any activity that the medical team will expect the patient or caregiver to perform
- A demonstration of aseptic technique
- Typed information about each medication prescribed
- All infusion pumps, venipuncture devices, catheter irrigation supplies or dressing supplies
- Clearly stated instructions regarding when to notify the physician or nurse of any changes, signs, or symptoms
- Twenty-four hour phone numbers for support
- Adequate time to allow return demonstration of all procedures the patient will be expected to perform independently
- Detailed documentation in the patient record of all teaching that occurred.

Box 29-4   Essential Elements of Written Reference Materials

1. Use clearly stated, short sentences geared to a fifth grade reading level
2. Use illustrations whenever possible
3. Personalize the form when possible, and provide adequate space for written notes
4. Provide vital sign record keeping sheets for patient use
5. Use any appropriate videos and audio tapes
6. Practice arms and administration supplies for patients who will be participating in their own care

If the patient does not meet the admission criteria in terms of mental and physical capabilities, a primary caregiver must be identified who will be available to support home infusion. The home environment may be assessed via conversation with the patient in the clinic, hospital, or over the phone (Box 29-2).

Patient education

Patient enrollment in an alternative care setting, an initial step in discharge planning, usually takes place in the hospital and preferably before the day of discharge. Occasionally, patient education is delivered in the patient's home.

Thorough patient education can contribute to a favorable outcome. All patients entering an alternative setting infusion program should have education pertinent to their medications, vascular access device, infusion device, expected outcome, and any side effects. Patients who will be taught for self-administration will receive much more detail than the infusion clinic patient.

Education and patient training can be initiated before finalizing discharge plans (Box 29-3). It should be pertinent to the infusion device, the vascular access device, and the medication or solution the patient will receive following discharge. Written reference materials are essential (Box 29-4).

Documentation

A plan of treatment should be completed and documented with the physician's signature. Plans of care are often required by third-party payers and should be submitted to them as part of the preapproval process.

The patient's rights and responsibilities should be clearly communicated to the patient, caregiver, parent, and any significant care partner involved in the direct delivery of care. This document can prevent problems and is actually required by Medicare and by most state licensure regulations and accreditation standards. The patient should be informed of his or her financial responsibility for the infusion services and should sign any forms required to authorize payment of benefits to the physician.

Enrolling the patient into an outpatient infusion center involves several important steps to meet reimbursement and

risk management requirements and to ensure a successful course of therapy. These include the following:

1. The patient should review and sign a consent for treatment that states the risks associated with IV therapy and vascular access.
2. The patient should be advised of available providers of infusion service and any physician ownership in those providers should be disclosed.
3. The patient should sign an acknowledgement of training in self-administration, if applicable.
4. The patient should sign an acknowledgement of receipt of a list of patients rights and responsibilities.
5. The patient should sign a separate informed consent for each procedure anticipated for placing the IV line.
6. The patient should sign Medicare waivers, if applicable.
7. The patient should sign any forms required to authorize payment of benefits directly to the physician.

COMMON DISEASE STATES TREATED IN THE OUTPATIENT ALTERNATIVE SETTING
Malignancy

It has become quite common for chemotherapy to be given in an alternative infusion setting, either in an oncologist's office, at a free-standing infusion clinic, or, for continuous infusion with 5-flurouracil or other chemotherapy regimens, with an ambulatory infusion pump at home. The durability and dependability of long-term central venous catheters and ambulatory infusion pumps and a greater knowledge of the stability of chemotherapeutic agents has allowed tremendous freedom and flexibility for the patients with cancer. Infusion centers with private examination rooms provide an ideal alternative setting for immunocompromised patients. They are safe places to be examined by the physician, visit with the pharmacist, and have dressing changes, pump refills, or assessments performed by the nurse.

Malignancies commonly treated in alternative settings include leukemia and other blood dyscrasias, lymphomas, Hodgkin's disease, brain tumors, and breast, colon, pancreatic, ovarian, rectal, lung, throat, and neck cancer. The weighing of risks versus benefits of outpatient treatment is left to the discretion of the physician in consultation with the patient and family.

HIV

The immunocompromised person with human immunodeficiency virus (HIV) is susceptible to a variety of viral, bacterial, and fungal pathogens. Most bacterial pathogens need only short-term treatment, but many of the nutritional disorders and viral, fungal, and parasitic diseases require long-term therapy or suppression. Pharmacologic advances and better oral therapeutic regimens have lessened our dependence on infusion-based therapies. However, the treatments of choice and important backup therapies for some HIV-related complications still require infusion therapy. HIV-related conditions amenable to outpatient infusion therapy include *Pneumocystis carinii,* cytomegalovirus (CMV) retinitis, colitis, esophagitis, acute bacterial infections, dissemination of central nervous system cryptococcus, resistant esophageal candidiasis, resistant herpetic infections, wasting syndrome, and some hematologic abnormalities. Outpatient infusion therapy offers an important alternative to hospitalization for patients who need efficacious care for a variety of HIV-related infections, conditions, and complications.

The infusion nurse is an integral part of the team effort to provide an ongoing relationship with the HIV patient. One important task before therapy is started is to attempt to eliminate or minimize the fear associated with receiving infusion therapy in an alternative setting. The one-on-one relationship between the nurse and patient reinforces trust and provides the patient respect and privacy. Many patients with HIV appreciate this added privacy, which may not be possible with home health nurses visiting the home.

A sudden, acute, life-threatening opportunistic infection can isolate a person with acquired immunodeficiency syndrome (AIDS). If home care is selected, daily visits by concerned health care providers opens opportunities for social interaction. These visits provide the nurse with the time and relaxed atmosphere that allow extensive teaching and counseling. The infusion nurse must be knowledgeable about HIV in general, including psychosocial aspects, and about treatment modalities used not only for infusion but also for the overall treatment of HIV disease, including AIDS. The nurse should be aware of community resources and be able to coordinate assistance when appropriate. Because care is given at a single site, the patient witnesses open communication, immediate coordination of care, and direct interaction between health care providers.

Clinical criteria for receiving alternative setting infusion therapy requires that the patient be ambulatory and able to maintain many of the activities of daily living. The assessment process for the nurse includes evaluation of body systems, assessment of the IV access, and monitoring of laboratory results for adverse events related to treatment or disease progression.

Maintenance of venous access is performed by the nurse on a regular schedule, allowing the nurse to monitor for early signs of complications.

Infections

Like chemotherapy, the outpatient use of IV antimicrobials has proven to be an efficacious, safe, and preferred delivery modality for infectious diseases. The most commonly treated infectious diseases include skin and soft tissue infections, osteomyelitis, septic arthritis/bursitis, blood stream infections, endocarditis, respiratory infections, meningitis, Lyme disease, pelvic inflammatory disease, pyelonephritis, postoperative wound infections, CMV retinitis and other HIV-associated diseases, cellulitis, and abscesses. Physicians must make a final decision based on their assessment of the patient and their comfort level with available providers. At a minimum, the patient's vital signs should be stable and the infection should be stabilized and nonprogressive. Because deterioration is always a possibility, there should be a defined mechanism for timely reevaluation by the physician and contingency plans for access to emergency care. Patients who require other treatments, such as wound care, ventilatory support, physical therapy, or regular diagnostic studies, can often be managed outside the hospital with careful planning and adequate support systems.

THE INFUSION CENTER
Clinic design and space considerations

Acquiring the right kind of space for a free-standing infusion center allows flexibility in designing and building a work area that will provide adequate work space and facilitate good communication for all of the members of the outpatient infusion team. An infusion center should provide a reception area, private examination and counseling rooms, a pharmacy, administrative space, treatment areas for central venous catheter insertion and sterile procedures, and isolation rooms to separate patients who are immunosuppressed or who carry contagious disease and therefore should not be exposed to other patients. All rooms should be equipped with closable doors.

Experience has demonstrated that having a residential "group" infusion room can be therapeutic and provide an atmosphere for patients to visit and share their personal experiences. This area should be comfortable for patients who may spend 2 to 3 hours per day receiving infusions. It should be cheerful, soothing, and restful. Games, TV, a VCR, and magazines are helpful in providing the infusion patient enjoyable distractions. It is advisable to provide comfortable reclining chairs for elevating legs and feet when patients become light headed or nauseated during their infusion. State departments of health and Occupational Safety and Hazard Administration

(OSHA) provide information regarding acceptable upholstery fabrics, floor surfaces that can be easily cleaned and disinfected, and rules regarding eating and drinking in an infusion room. Natural light is important for accurate assessment of skin color. Ventilation and temperature control will add comfort and enhance a pleasing environment.

The pharmacy area should include an office for the pharmacists and pharmacy technicians, an anteroom where pharmacy personnel change into scrub clothing to prepare for mixing solutions, and a compounding or "hood room." The compounding room should be sealed off from traffic areas and vented, either to the outside or to the filtered duct system of the building. Each state's board of pharmacy provides certification specifications and regulatory requirements. The mixing hood manufacturers are helpful in providing installation information for these products. The Joint Commission for Accreditation of Healthcare Organizations (JCAHO) has guidelines to help develop policies and procedures for the pharmacy. State law dictates the legalities of physician involvement in dispensing medication through an office. In some states, the pharmacy cannot be owned and operated by a physician. A physician will often purchase compounding services from a free-standing pharmacy near the physician's office.

Communication and staff reporting is optimal if all members of the infusion team work in proximity. The nursing area, where nurses prepare IV bags, bottles, and tubings and stock IV start equipment and supplies, should be near the infusion area. Nurses should locate their work area within observation range of the patient; this will enhance productivity by allowing the nurse to document the treatment while it is happening. Supplies, phones, computers, nursing assessment equipment, and emergency equipment, such as oxygen tanks, masks, nasal cannulas, emergency medications, an Ambu bag, and resuscitation supplies, should be readily accessible.

If the infusion nurses are performing phlebotomies for laboratory studies, the state department of health provides guidelines for an acceptable blood drawing area and proper specimen handling. Often, the infusion nurse analyzes blood samples in the laboratory of the infusion clinic, thus eliminating the waiting period for the sample to be taken to an outside reference laboratory and analyzed.

Nurse productivity is enhanced when easy access to the pharmacist, physician, dietician, secretarial staff, and equipment and supplies is provided. Regular discussion about the patient's treatment, response to treatment, order changes, dietary needs, and laboratory findings can improve treatment outcomes.

Secretarial, billing and personnel offices should be positioned to enhance communication and reporting. Computer access, electronic billing and reimbursement capabilities, patient records, and a storage area for supplies and equipment should be located centrally to enable all staff access and availability (Fig. 29-1). The size of the infusion clinic should be based on the number of patient visits anticipated daily.

Physician oversight

The physician directed, alternative IV infusion clinic brings together a medical team comparable to that of a hospital

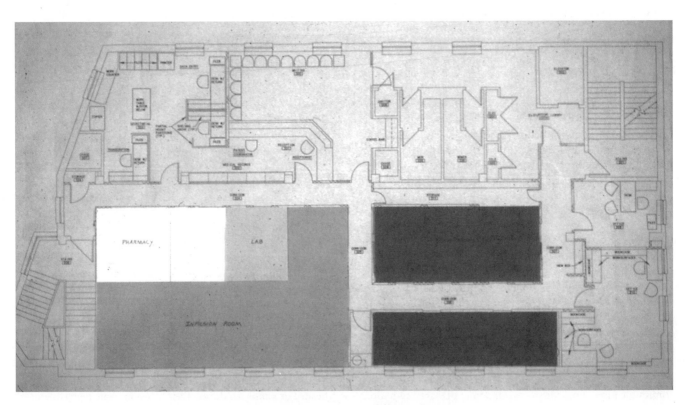

FIG. 29-1 *Design schematic of an infusion center.*

infusion center. Physician involvement is ensured in programs based in medical offices and multispecialty clinics.

The more involved and knowledgeable the physician is, the more appropriate the medical treatment plan. In the presence of clinical failure or intolerance, the physician can easily change the medication; if adverse reactions occur, closer follow-up can be provided. The duration of therapy can also be adjusted more easily with physician involvement. Laboratory results can be evaluated and the treatment plan altered while the patient is in the clinic. Finally, in the office or clinic model, the first dose of an antimicrobial can be administered under medical supervision, an option not always available for home infusion patients.

Unfortunately, there are numerous disincentives for physician involvement in the delivery of outpatient infusion therapy. Inadequate reimbursement for home visits, less frequent patient visits, and regulatory restraints regarding physician ownership of health care services, self-referral, and referral payments to other physicians all deter physician involvement.

Operational design

The professional team. Although the three primary team members, physician, nurse, and pharmacist, have distinct roles, they also have overlapping functions. As in constructing a workable design for the facility, it is imperative that the personnel be qualified, work as a cohesive unit, and have an advanced knowledge in infusion skills. Ongoing communication is an important element to improving treatment outcomes. In many outpatient situations, the care of the patient is fragmented because communication among professionals of the various organizations is too irregular.

Over time, the roles of physicians, nurses, and pharmacists in the delivery of outpatient parenteral therapies have evolved to include many activities and responsibilities. The physician continues to delegate responsibility, make the diagnosis, and act as the final authority for treatment, quality of care, and patient outcomes. The nurse, who provides direct patient care and evaluation, should be trained in vascular access and line maintenance and have knowledge about infusion devices. Pharmacists are experts in medication preparation, pharmacokinetic monitoring, and drug interactions and are knowledgeable about infusion devices.

Physician. Traditionally, the physician's role is one of initial patient evaluation. The physician takes a thorough patient history, performs a physical examination, and decides on the appropriate course of action. Concurrent disease states may be relevant to the treatment plan and response to the therapy. Ultimately, decisions regarding treatment, prescribing authority, and legal liability lie with the physician.

Physician involvement in alternative-site care is crucial in a number of areas. First, physicians must be instrumental in the development of practice guidelines. As treatment schemes for various disease processes are reengineered to become more efficient, physicians must have input into such factors as patient selection criteria, appropriate safety measures for alternative-site care delivery, and monitoring measurements for assessing the progress of treatment. Policy and procedure manuals should include the input of a physician.

In the event that a physician is not the provider of alternative-site infusion care, he or she should be familiar with the quality and capabilities of the provider. This assumes that there will be some objective benchmark of quality, such as accreditation by JCAHO, and meaningful data on outcomes and cost of services. Developing meaningful clinical outcomes data and integrating them into a continuous quality improvement program demands physician involvement. As care is transferred to a less expensive site, the physician is ethically obliged to ensure that medical outcomes are not compromised.

As managed care drives costs downward, the physician must help make decisions regarding resource utilization and ensure that low resource levels remain appropriate and adequate for safety and efficacy. Physicians make an important contribution to risk management in managed care organizations. In a system with some degree of vertical integration, physicians can provide leadership in identifying, developing, and coordinating multidisciplinary disease-management programs. All of these responsibilities, which physicians are in a unique position to assume, are crucial to managed care organizations in achieving their goal to provide the highest quality care at the lowest possible cost. As managed care continues to mature, it is imperative that physicians become actively involved, demonstrating their value to and demanding reasonable reimbursement from the system.

Nurse. Although some aspects of the nurse's role remain the same in any setting, responsibilities vary from one alternative setting to the next. Advanced knowledge and IV skills are essential for any nurse employed by an infusion service. The nurse must demonstrate an understanding and expertise with central venous catheters, insertion procedures, routine maintenance and standards of care associated with each device, peripheral IV starts, site selection, site management, and provision of medications and supplies. The nurse maintains the most regular contact with the patient and thus is pivotal in coordinating care and alerting the physician to problems. In all settings, the nurse provides a critical role in patient selection, education, vascular access, central venous catheter maintenance, helping patients deal with their illness and the prescribed plan of treatment, maximizing patient's self-care potential, evaluating patient progress, and monitoring and reporting of the patient's adaptation and response to therapy. The infusion nurse can be the catalyst between the patient and the other members of the health care team. The roles and responsibilites of the RN in an outpatient setting varies somewhat depending on the model. To a greater degree than the nurse in the infusion clinic, the visiting nurse makes observations and assessments that provide primary information on which the physician bases clinical decisions.

Assessment and planning include making initial decisions with the patient and the physician regarding appropriateness of the home setting, method of venous access, how and when the antimicrobial or solution will be administered, and determination of the patient's other needs. The nurse continually monitors the success of the treatment plan by evaluating the patient's compliance, clinical response, and reported satisfaction. The nurse may be responsible for selecting, initiating, and maintaining the vascular access device and for monitoring its status between doses, if necessary.

Box 29-5   Elements of the Expanded Nursing Role

- Assess performance improvement in the infusion practice setting.
- Educate patient, family members, caregiver, and staff.
- Review ethical matters.
- Collaborate with other health care providers, researchers, and case managers.
- Effectively use resources, including third-party payers and community resources.
- Investigate new devices to improve infusion therapy, medication delivery, venous access, and management skills.
- Build interdisciplinary, collaborative relationships.
- Support local, regional, and national efforts to influence the development and implementation of health care policy.
- Recognize the changing and expanded role of the registered nurse as a primary care provider, case manager, educator, triage coordinator, risk manager, benefit interpreter, and provider liaison.[12]

Administration of medications or solutions may be performed by the nurse, or the nurse may teach the patient or caregiver to infuse the drug and manage the infusion device between nurse visits. The nurse will often collect laboratory samples, evaluate clinical data reflecting the patient's response, and relay all information to the physician. Nurses share in the responsibility for distributing information to the other health care providers involved in the patient's care. With the expansion of managed care, quality improvement, and outcomes monitoring, the nurses role has expanded to include many of the duties in Box 29-5.

Infusion clinic nurses share much of the same responsibilities, but generally do not become involved in home visits and therefore are usually unaware of activities or concerns in the home. The nurses generally administer the medications; maintain venous access, change wound dressings; evaluate for healing and other clinical concerns; and draw blood samples for analysis. In other alternative settings, the nurse may choose to teach the patient or responsible friend or family member to administer the medication.

Nurses in all settings provide patients with information regarding possible side effects and adverse reactions associated with the medication and potential dangerous situations related to the vascular access device. Nurse availability should be provided 24 hours per day.

With the changes in reimbursement and managed care, it has become necessary for nurses to become knowledgeable in reimbursement, allowable charges, fee-for-service visits, capitated contracts, and the costs of providing nursing care in any model of infusion therapy. Seeking and receiving authorization for services and visits may fall within the scope of the infusion nurse.

Pharmacist. The pharmacist plays an important and often varied role in providing medications within the alternative care setting. He or she is probably the most knowledgeable about medication storage, preparation, dosing, and delivery.

Decisions and activities in which pharmacists should participate include the following:

- Developing research programs
- Researching and evaluating the direct or comparative efficacy, safety, and cost-effectiveness of specific drug delivery systems and administration devices
- Reviewing the patient's history of drug reactions and all medications the patient is taking
- Choosing and dispensing the particular drug and dosage delivery system or administration device and supplies for use in a patient's drug therapy
- Educating patients regarding side effects, drug interactions, kinetics, stability, and appropriate dosage and costs of medications
- Monitoring ongoing clinical information, laboratory data, and so on

Up-to-date policies and procedures for compounding sterile products should be written and available to all pharmacists. All pharmacy-prepared sterile products should bear an appropriate expiration date. The expiration date assigned should be based on currently available drug stability information and sterility considerations. Sterile products should be labeled with at least the following information: patient's name and other appropriate patient information; solution name; names, amounts, strengths, and concentrations of all ingredients; expiration date and time; prescribed administration regimen; appropriate auxiliary labeling; storage requirements; name of the person performing the admixture and/or the responsible pharmacist; device-specific instructions; and any additional information in accordance with state or federal requirements.

The pharmacist must inspect the container for leaks and integrity, and the solution for cloudiness, particulates, color, and volume; this inspection should be performed when the preparation is completed and again when the product is dispensed.

The pharmacist should be knowledgeable of pharmacokinetics and pharmacodynamics. To administer IV medications and solutions in any alternative setting, one must appreciate the important relationships between the pharmacokinetics and pharmacodynamics of these agents. *Pharmacodynamics* focuses on the actions of drugs on living organisms, whereas *pharmacokinetics* focuses on the therapeutic action and pharmacologic toxicity of the drug. Traditionally, in vitro susceptibility testing or the minimum inhibitory concentration (MIC) and minimum bactericidal concentration have been used to measure the activity of an antibiotic against bacteria. Although these observations are able to predict the potency of the drug-organism interaction, they do not describe the time course of this activity. The MIC does not establish whether there are enduring inhibitory effects following exposure to an antibiotic.

Knowledge of the pharmacokinetics of antimicrobials and the pharmacodynamics predictive of antimicrobial efficacy enables the pharmacist to design reasonable outpatient IV regimens for most agents. Understanding the characteristics of aminoglycosides, vancomycin, and the long half life beta-lactams, which allow once-daily dosing intervals, enables the pharmacist to help the physician develop a treatment plan for positive treatment outcomes.[11]

Documentation of the pharmacy's activities should be maintained on file and be sufficient to comply with state and federal laws and regulations and the institution's policies and procedures. State and federal law also establish how long records must be kept.

Selection and procurement of pharmaceutics, equipment, supplies, and services

Infusion equipment and supplies. Purchasing supplies and equipment can be a tremendous financial burden. Capital equipment, office furniture, and nursing, pharmacy, and secretarial supplies are expensive; purchase decisions must be prudent, especially in start-up infusion centers and centers that have not achieved a reliable revenue stream. A committee of end users, nurses, and pharmacists should be established to review the broad spectrum of infusion devices, vascular access devices, and supplies necessary to provide IV infusion services. This will greatly improve the outcomes of the program.

The appropriate vascular access device and medication delivery model for a patient depends on the purpose of the infusion, concentration and stability of the solution to be infused, condition and availability of venous access, patient safety features, and reliability of the patient.

Unlike the earliest venous access methods and infusion devices, which consisted of quills for needles and animal bladders for medication reservoirs, today's venous catheter systems and infusion devices are much more sophisticated, versatile, and sterile. Improvements in vascular access devices have resulted in soft, flexible, hypoallergenic materials of varied lengths, diameters, and gauges. Advancements in medication delivery systems allow complex or multiple therapies to be provided with little effort by the patient and make outpatient therapy available to a wider range of patients.

Central venous catheters. Peripherally inserted central catheters (PICCs) have provided flexibility in the choice of central access and a measure of comfort by limiting the number of painful, peripheral IV site rotations. The PICC is a well-recognized, safe, cost-effective, and less invasive avenue for dependable venous access in the outpatient setting, provided radiology resources are available to verify tip placement. PICCs provide the following benefits:

1. Eliminate the risks associated with traditional (surgical, anesthetized) central venous catheter placement
2. Reduce the potential for catheter sepsis
3. Facilitate self-administration because they are easy to use
4. Preserve the peripheral vascular system
5. Decrease the discomfort associated with peripheral, subclavian, or jugular catheter insertions
6. Allow insertion in the hospital and subsequent use in the alternative setting
7. Allow a wide range of medication administration, facilitating highly concentrated nutritional supplements and antimicrobials

Central venous catheters can be purchased from the manufacturer, local or district distributor, or local wholesaler. Qualified nurses or physicians should evaluate the style and quality of catheters before they are purchased. Because costs vary, comparison shopping is important, and catheters should be purchased by contract when possible.

Infusion pumps and devices. Infusion pumps, volumetric infusion devices, and syringe pumps should be procured through a purchasing contract, in batch purchasing if possible. The following criteria should be considered before purchase: (1) user friendliness, (2) patient safety, (3) air-eliminating or air-detection alarms, (5) durability, (6) accuracy and performance, and (7) pounds per square inch limitations.

Because each model is different, selecting a particular infusion device can be a complex process. If reimbursement is a significant issue, administering medications via IV push, syringe pump, or gravity system may be appropriate. Although administering medication via a syringe pump may be more expensive than via a gravity system, in the long run the cost of replacing syringe pumps that may be broken, lost, or not returned must be considered. A high number of unreturned pumps might be a factor significant enough to exclude their use.

Other capital expenses. The expense of computers, printers, furniture, and secretarial supplies must be anticipated. Great care should be taken to minimize expenses for the first 6 to 9 months in a new program; it will be approximately that long before sufficient revenues are generated to cover purchases, salaries, and operational expenses.

Laboratory services. In many alternative IV infusion centers, particularly in the physician-directed infusion clinic, an in-office laboratory is used to facilitate the routine and stat analysis of patient blood samples. In most states, chemistry, hematology, urinalysis, microbiology, and phlebotomy can be performed by nurses under the supervision of a physician. Like all laboratories, physician-directed laboratories must comply with the rules, regulations, biannual audits, proficiency testing, normal and abnormal control testing, and license and certification processes that have been established by local, state, and federal governments and agencies, including the Clinical Laboratory Improvements Amendments. Ownership of laboratories is regulated by the state. Physicians find the immediate availability of laboratory data an efficient way of monitoring patients while they are receiving an infusion. Most chemistry and hematology analyzers can compute results in 2 to 3 minutes, allowing the physician to make necessary changes immediately.

Quality assurance guidelines, state and federal regulatory bodies, and independent auditors hired by the Departments of Health in most states ensure that laboratory personnel are skilled and properly certified, and that they maintain the accepted standards of practice for phlebotomy, blood sample handling, preanalysis treatment, universal precautions, handling contaminated waste, storage, and reporting. A complete laboratory policy and procedure manual is mandatory and annual educational updates should be provided for staff members. Quarterly quality improvement monitors, billing and reimbursement tools, communication and reporting documentation, and patient record keeping are an essential part of an alternative infusion laboratory's operations.

LEGAL CONSIDERATIONS IN THE ALTERNATIVE SETTING

Historically, procedures, not limited to injections and infusions, performed in a physician's office by the office staff or the physician have been routine, customary, and legal. The Social Security Act defined the ability of physicians to provide services, including the administration and dispensing of prescription drugs.

The Stark legislation has complicated the physician's role in providing services to patients in the office, owning or sharing ownership in a laboratory, infusion center, radiology facilities (including magnetic resonance imaging [MRI] equipment), or any for-profit entity to which the physician may refer his patients for diagnostic services. Federal laws such as Stark apply only to Medicare and Medicaid.[13]

As managed care plans become dominant in many areas of the country, physicians are increasingly facing payers who are aggressively seeking to lower reimbursement rates and to exercise strict controls over how physicians practice medicine.

Federal laws and regulatory issues

The intent of Stark and similar laws is to prohibit any financial inducements that might lead physicians to inappropriately increase utilization of health care services, including home care, home infusion, MRI scans, and laboratory services.

Antikickback statute

The antikickback statute regulates certain activities of health care providers. Established in 1972, this criminal statute prohibits the intentional payment of *anything of value* to a physician in exchange for the referral of a Medicare or Medicaid patient. This statute affected joint ventures, wherein physicians would be part-owners of a separate diagnostic facility to which they would refer patients. Because some such arrangements may be technical violations of this law but not necessarily abusive, the Department of Justice compiled a list of "safe harbors" to protect entities that were not involved in abusive arrangements. The safe harbors were published in 1991, after Congress gave the Office of Inspector General civil-sanction authority regarding kickback violations.

Drug-dispensing limitations

Pharmacy. Any alternative setting providing infusion therapy should be aware that laws regarding compounding and dispensing to patients are state directed. Infusion centers usually have several choices in terms of how they acquire, compound, and dispense drugs. Rules vary state to state but generally include a nurse, or supervised technician, or a pharmacist who is an employee. A popular choice for pharmacy services is to contract for specific services, reimbursed by a fee per dose mixed or cost per hour.

There are distinct differences in the laws governing in-office infusion, physician's offices billing for dispensing drugs for self-administration in the home, infusion companies billing for dispensing drugs, and emergency departments or hospital-based infusion programs.

State laws address physician ownership of licensed retail pharmacies, physician's offices compounding or dispensing parenteral medications, physicians employing pharmacists, and physician office drug dispensing. State Boards of Pharmacy have current information regarding these matters.

Referral relationships. Under both the antikickback statute and Stark legislation, if a physician refers Medicare or Medicaid patients to an outside provider for outpatient infusion services, any financial arrangements with that provider must meet published safe-harbor or exemption regulations. Any compensation to the physician must be set at fair market value, in return for clearly defined and documented services provided by the physician to the provider. This also applies to the methods of compensation other than fee-for-service, such as stock, real estate, free rent, or services. Physicians are prohibited from referring patients to home health agencies for care if they receive more than a certain amount of compensation per year from the home health agency, hospital, or corporation that owns the home health agency, or if they have a significant portion of ownership in either organization. If services or products are furnished to the physician by that provider, they must be paid at fair market value.

Medicare fraud and abuse

Medicare fraud is defined as knowingly and willfully billing the Medicare program for services or products which were not actually provided, are not covered by the benefit, or are in excess of what would be considered usual and customary. This includes billing Medicare beneficiaries for services or products that are a covered benefit and should have been billed to Medicare. For an outpatient infusion clinic to bill for an hour of infusion, by definition the infusion must be provided by the physician or under the direct supervision of the physician. If the physician did not actually perform this service or was not present to supervise the services, it would be considered fraud to submit a bill under the physician's provider number.

Civil and criminal penalties are assessed when providers, audited by any federal or state auditing agencies, are found to have conducted fraudulent practices. In 1995, Operation Restore Trust was launched to uncover and punish fraud. The operation is a joint effort within the U.S. Department of Health and Human Services involving the HCFA, Office of Inspector General, and Administration on Aging. With help from the Department of Justice, Operation Restore Trust uses sophisticated statistical analysis methods to target providers for further investigation and audit. During an initial demonstration phase, these audits targeted home health agencies, hospice organizations, durable medical equipment providers, and long-term care facilities. The results were so impressive, however, that the investigation is being extended to include other health care providers.

Antitrust regulation

The basic premise of antitrust doctrine is that a vigorous competitive marketplace will produce the highest quality goods and services at the lowest possible price. Thus antitrust laws concern business practices from the consumer's perspective, generally with the single goal of ensuring that competition is not diminished. The courts have considered and rejected arguments that the practice of medicine is somehow different from other commercial endeavors and should be subject to a different antitrust standard. Little or no weight is given to arguments that anticompetitive practices are necessary to maintain quality of care or to preserve professional autonomy.

The federal antitrust statute most relevant to physicians is Section 1 of the Sherman Act, which generally prohibits "contracts, combinations . . . [and] conspiracies" that unreasonably restrain trade. Two elements must be present for the statute's proscription to be triggered. First, there must be an agreement—some concerted action—between two or more separate economic entities. Second, the conduct must unreasonably restrain trade (i.e., it must be anticompetitive). Certain types of conduct, such as "naked" price fixing agreements, group boycotts, and market allocation agreements, are considered so inherently anticompetitive that they are per se illegal. There is no acceptable defense to such conduct, and such activities risk criminal prosecution.

As in many areas involving application of complex legal principles, a small amount of advanced planning and analysis can help avoid very costly mistakes. Antitrust counsel should be retained to help health care providers determine whether such risks are serious and how they can be minimized.[12]

Medical liability coverage

Physician office–based alternative sites providing infusion therapy should advise their liability insurance carrier of this extension to their practice. There may be requirements or limitations involved to ensure coverage of all activities related to outpatient infusion.

Legal advisor or counsel

To interpret legislation, physicians and other health care providers should consult legal counsel with expertise in health care law. Physicians may also consult their own state medical association licensing board to determine the intended interpretation of bills in progress or passed into state law.

Nursing

State laws, usually enforced by a state Board of Health Care Licensure, and the Nurse Practice Act, will determine any limitations or restrictions in terms of the nurses role in an outpatient infusion clinic, physicians office, or alternative setting, just as it does in hospitals and other agencies. The specific duties and responsibilities of RNs, licensed practical nurses, and supervised technicians should be established in policies and procedures.

Regulatory bodies

It is important for any health care provider, agency, or physician's office to determine the state and federal guidelines affecting the organization. These laws, or the interpretation of these laws, may determine how the alternative outpatient infusion setting is structured, funded, and managed. Information regarding federal legislation and laws pertaining to fraud and abuse can be referenced in the Federal Register.

Table 29-3	**Most Common Infusion Therapies in Alternative Settings**		
Infusion Clinic	**Emergency Department**	**Visiting Nurse**	**Self-Administration (Home Infusion)**
Ceftriaxone	Ceftriaxone	Ceftriaxone	Ceftriaxone
Cefazolin	Cefazolin	Cefazolin	Cefazolin
Ceftazidime	Ceftazidime	Ceftazidime	Ceftazidime
Clindamycin	Clindamycin	Clindamycin	Clindamycin
Vancomycin	Vancomycin	Vancomycin	Vancomycin
Aminoglycosides	Aminoglycosides	Aminoglycosides	Aminoglycosides
Ganciclovir	Oxacillin	Oxacillin	Oxacillin
Acyclovir	Blood products	Factor therapy	Factor therapy
Oxacillin	Hydration fluids	Levaquin	Parenteral nutrition
PRBC	Chemotherapy	Pain management	Injections
Platelets	Antiarrhythmics	Parenteral nutrition	
IVIG	CVC placement	Chemotherapy	
Factor therapy	Injections	Injections	
Combinations		Ganciclovir	
Hydration fluids		Acyclovir	
Pain management		IVIG	
Parenteral nutrition		Hydration fluids	
Chemotherapy		Dobutamine	
CVC placement		Solu-Medrol	
Injections			
Solu-Medrol			
Antihypotensives			
Antiarrhythmics			
Anticoagulants			

PRBC, Packed red blood cells; *IVIG,* intravenous immune globulin; *CVC,* central venous catheter.

OUTPATIENT INFUSION THERAPIES

Alternative infusion therapy settings offer safe, efficacious, convenient, outpatient infusion with a wide range of treatments, IV medications, and solutions (Table 29-3).

Medications and solutions used in alternative settings must be selected by the prescribing physician after consideration of several factors, including dosing schedules, long-term toxicity, and medication stability. Such considerations may lead to the selection of alternative medications, differing forms of traditional agents, different treatment schedules, and different modes of delivery. Evidence of patient tolerance and a low incidence of toxic reactions are prerequisites for agents used outside the hospital, because patients are not monitored as closely. Prescribing physicians must be aware of the adverse effects associated with prolonged IV therapy.

An infrequent dose schedule is more convenient for the patient, facilitates compliance, and requires less staff time in terms of training and troubleshooting. Examples include cyclic TPN, and antimicrobials dosed once per day.

VENOUS ACCESS DEVICES

The advent of IV therapies administered in alternative settings has created a demand for soft, flexible, easily inserted, long-term IV catheters. A number of factors must be considered when selecting the appropriate vascular access device for outpatient infusion therapy. An experienced infusion team must have the clinical expertise and knowledge to assess all of the variables involved with a patient and choose the most appropriate option. Estimated length of therapy will usually be the first consideration in choosing venous access. Other variables include delivery model, infusate, potential for venous irritation, dosing frequency, infusion device options, concentration of infusate, flow rate, patient status and age, anticipated activity, convenience, patient choice, lifestyle, risk, and cost.

PICCs are suitable for long-term access and multiple therapies. A PICC insertion is an invasive, cost-effective procedure. This catheter has provided flexibility in central access and a measure of comfort by limiting multiple, painful, peripheral IV site rotations. A variety of PICC catheters are on the market today, offering choices of insertion techniques, sizes, lengths, composition, and single or double lumen capabilities. The PICC is less expensive to place compared with tunneled catheters, and can be placed without anesthesia. Millions of PICC catheters are placed annually in America today.

Midline catheters, which were introduced in the late 1980s, share many of the principles of the PICC, with exception of length. Midline catheters are manufactured using silicone and polyurethane. It is important for the nurse and physician to understand the differences in dwell time, concentration of infusate, and insertion and postinsertion maintenance.

Peripheral IVs, whether over-the-needle sets or winged steel needles, continue to provide quick, inexpensive, minimally invasive venous access. Many working patients receiving treatment in alternative settings prefer to have a peripheral IV started daily, usually using the winged steel needle. This device is removed after the infusion and the patient returns to work or school without a venous access device in place. Athletes, school children, and mothers responsible for carrying infants often prefer this method. Fortunately, with the convenience of small gauge sizes and topical anesthetic creams, the insertion of a winged steel needle causes very little discomfort.

In alternative settings where chemotherapy is the primary therapy infused, surgically placed tunneled catheters and implanted ports are more commonly used for outpatient infusion. Implanted ports designed for long-term outpatient use are reservoirs, with pierceable domes or septums, attached to a silicone or polyurethane catheter and surgically placed under the skin. Whenever necessary, the reservoir can be accessed by a nurse, physician or trained caregiver with a noncoring needle, which has an angled tip to prevent "gouging" or coring the port's septum. Implanted ports can provide continuous access when the needle is left in place and secured with a sterile dressing, but require intermittent needle changes. Tunneled central venous catheters are surgically placed under the skin to an exit site, creating a barrier to infection, facilitating patient access, and reducing the risk of dislodgment. Following initial healing at the site of insertion, these catheters can be maintained safely for long periods.

Other central venous catheters, such as a subclavian or jugular catheter, are less optimal and less commonly used. These catheters are difficult to secure, interfere with bathing, and are usually used only for short-term therapies. These catheters are generally placed by a physician via percutaneous or cut-down insertion into the jugular or subclavian veins. Made of polyurethane, they are manufactured with single, double, or triple lumens in various gauges. They are fairly easy to dislodge and make access difficult for patients who self-administer.

All central venous catheters require flushing to maintain patency. Central lines in the alternative setting can be used for infusion and blood sampling. These lines carry a certain amount of risk, but phlebitis and infiltration are uncommon.

INFUSION THERAPY DEVICES/MEDICATION DELIVERY SYSTEMS

Modern technology offers the alternative infusion setting a wide variety of medication delivery systems. Table 29-4 presents important features of many of these systems. Systems range from the simple minibag and straight IV tubing system to the high-tech, ambulatory, programmable, computerized pumps. Selecting the appropriate infusion device depends on the purpose of the infusion, concentration and stability of the solution, condition and availability of venous access, patient safety features, and reliability. Patient cooperation and teaching are important; explaining the procedure to the patient can eliminate problems during the course of treatment. Medication delivery systems vary in terms of cost, convenience, and reliability. Because of changes in reimbursement, there is a great deal of interest in infusion devices that are cost effective. For medications that require an electronic ambulatory infusion pump, the choice of a device should be made based on the types of therapies provided and the patient population served by the institution. If there is a risk of pump retrieval, disposable pumps may be attractive.

The minibag and gravity drip method of infusion has gained

Table 29-4   **Choosing an Appropriate Delivery System/Method**

DELIVERY METHOD	VENOUS ACCESS DEVICE	PROGRAMMABLE	AMBULATORY	MEDICARE REIMBURSED
Minibag and tubing	Peripheral catheter Midline PICC Central venous catheters	No	On IV pole	No
Electronic syringe pump	PICC Central venous catheters	Yes	Yes	No
Control Rate Devices	Peripheral catheter Midline PICC Central venous catheters	Yes	Yes	Limited
Electronic Ambulatory Pumps	PICC Central venous catheters	Yes	Yes	Limited

PICC, Peripherally inserted central catheter.

in popularity because of decreased reimbursement. Although IV push is suitable for a number of antibiotics, several therapies cannot safely be administered by this method. Safe delivery may require diluting the medication to avoid venous irritation, manipulating the osmolality, and adjusting the flow rate. It is important that practitioners be knowledgeable in selecting the appropriate IV infusion device to ensure compatibility with the therapy and the venous access device.

Electronic syringe pumps are equipped with alarms and setting mechanisms so that they can be programmed to deliver a concentrated medication in a prefilled syringe via a vascular access device. These pumps offer controlled delivery of medication and are less expensive than gravity systems, largely because of their durability, ability to be cleaned and reused thousands of times without maintenance, and the limited amount of supplies necessary for administration. Second to IV push, the syringe pump is the most economic delivery method available, excluding the cost of the pumps. Pump cost is quickly recaptured by the operational savings compared with other infusion delivery systems. These pumps are ideal for the alternative setting because several patients can be infused simultaneously under the supervision of the infusion nurse in attendance. The alarm system is designed to alert the patient, nurse, or caregiver in event of occlusion or completion of the dose.

Controlled-rate infusion devices are found in a variety of infusion systems. These devices typically have specialized tubing that controls the flow rate of medication from a reservoir. The reservoirs may be elastomeric balloons, pouches, or minibags. The flow rate is regulated by the internal tubing diameter or flow-restriction device. Spring-loaded devices are available and deliver medication using a compressed spring against a plate that applies pressure to the medication reservoir, creating enough force to deliver the infusate. These devices are not applicable for all medications, solutions, or volumes, nor are they appropriate for every venous access device (Table 29-4).

Pole-mounted volumetric pumps are still the standard delivery device for large volume infusions in alternative settings. Hydration therapy, amphotericin B, and TPN are often delivered by these pumps. Pumps offer a variety of features, including manual, battery-powered, electronic, digital, computerized,

auto-ramping, and keep-vein-open delivery. The pumps require an IV pole for ambulation, which are often considered a nuisance at the bedside or chair side because of the multiple-leg base. Pole-mounted pumps are cost-effective in that they generally can be used for several years with minimal preventive maintenance. The pumps are easy to clean, can be used for multiple patients, and are user friendly.

Electronic ambulatory infusion pumps are perhaps the most sophisticated delivery systems used in the alternative setting; they enable a large variety of therapies to be delivered via central venous catheters. Generally, the pumps are small and computerized. They can be programmed to deliver multiple doses over a 24 hour period, a range of intermittent catheter irrigation volumes, infusion intervals, and continuous infusion, and are able to record the total volume delivered, doses given, and reservoir volume remaining. These devices include single, double, multitherapy, or multiple channels. Batteries are necessary for operation. Disposable pumps are a new addition to the market. They can be programmed to deliver multiple therapies and multiple doses per day, and they can be set for a predetermined time- and volume-dependent period.

Most ambulatory pumps can be purchased or rented. Capital outlay for pumps may be a limiting factor for start-up infusion clinics, which may make rental attractive. Costs vary, but are usually negotiable depending on the volume purchased or contracted for rental.

MANAGEMENT CONSIDERATIONS
Staff qualifications

Physician. Physicians are required to have a current license in the state in which they practice. Continuing education at the category I, II, and III levels is mandatory for reissue of the physician's license. Information regarding continuing education requirements and qualified courses can be obtained from a local physician's organization or specialty association. A unique personal identification number and provider number are necessary to bill Medicare, Medicaid, the state Departments of Labor and Industries, and third-party payers. A Drug Enforcement Agency number is required for physicians who prescribe medication.

Pharmacist. Pharmacy personnel preparing or dispensing sterile products should receive suitable didactic and experiential training, and should undergo a competency evaluation through demonstration and testing, written, practical, or both. Training should include critical area contamination factors; environmental monitoring of facilities, equipment, and supplies; sterile product calculations; terminology; sterile product compounding documentation; quality assurance procedures; aseptic preparation procedures; gowning and gloving technique; and general conduct in the controlled area. The aseptic technique of each person preparing sterile products should be observed and evaluated as satisfactory during orientation and training and at least annually thereafter.

Beyond the personnel who prepare and dispense sterile products, even personnel involved in cleaning and maintenance of the controlled area should be knowledgeable about cleanroom design, the basic concepts of aseptic compounding, and critical area contamination factors.

Pharmacists bear a substantial responsibility for ensuring optimal clinical outcomes from drug therapy, and are qualified by education, training, clinical expertise, and practice experience to assume responsibility for the professional supervision of drug delivery systems and administration devices. As a natural extension of efforts to optimize drug use, pharmacists should participate in organizational and clinical decisions with regard to these systems and devices.

Nurses. All nurses are required to have a current state license issued by the state licensing agency. It is recommended that infusion nurses in alternative settings be certified in IV nursing.

The roles and responsibilities of the RN in an outpatient infusion setting varies somewhat depending on the model.

Policies and procedures

Practice guidelines. *Guidelines,* as defined by the Institute of Medicine, are systematically developed statements that can be used to assess the appropriateness of health care decisions, services, and outcomes. Practice guidelines relating to outpatient or home IV therapy have been published. These guidelines were developed as a result of the deliberations of a multidisciplinary panel of health care professionals and represent consensus recommendations. The participants included physicians, microbiologists, nurses, pharmacists, and administrators experienced in various aspects of outpatient IV therapy.

Likewise, the Intravenous Nurses Society has published *Infusion Nursing Standards of Care,* an authoritative document addressing standards of practice in all areas related in infusion therapy. All alternative settings performing IV infusion should base their policies, procedures, and documentation practices on these standards.

The accreditation process. Any U.S. health care organization may apply for a JCAHO accreditation survey as long as there are applicable standards for the organization. In addition to accrediting hospitals, JCAHO also has standards for non–hospital-based long-term facilities, home and ambulatory care organizations, and clinical laboratory services. An accreditation survey lasts for 3 to 5 days, and accreditation may be granted for up to 3 years. Categories of accreditation include: accreditation with commendation, accreditation, conditional accreditation, provisional accreditation, and not accredited. If an organization is found to have deficiencies that require a focused survey zeroing in on one or more areas of concern, the survey will generally occur within 6 months of the initial survey. In addition, a 5% random sample of accredited organizations now undergo an unannounced midcycle survey focusing on performance areas identified as being problematic nationwide within the past year.

In the past, a JCAHO survey was conducted in an office, where managers produced reams of policies and procedures. Surveyors now spend the majority of their time in patient care areas assessing the bottom line: Does the care provided make a difference for customers? Is the outpatient infusion clinic doing the right things and doing them well? Is the organization structured to improve the outcomes of patient care? Are patients satisfied with their care? Is the facility wasting precious resources because of unnecessary duplication of services? The outpatient infusion clinic, like others, is now assessed across the entire organization rather than as a separate department. Nursing and pharmacy quality performance is evaluated and surveyed on the basis of communication between the two departments and the expected outcome for the patients served.

JCAHO has identified nine dimensions of quality that can determine how a health care organization's functions may affect patients. They fall into two categories: doing the right thing and doing the right thing well (Box 29-6).

Policies and procedures for providing home infusion services must be consistent with published practice standards. Many third-party payers now require that eligible outpatient IV therapy providers participate in some formal accreditation. During the past decade, the JCAHO has expanded its certification process to include the outpatient and home care settings. The

---

Box 29-6   Nine Dimensions of Quality

DOING THE RIGHT THING
1. *Efficacy:* Did the care or intervention achieve the desired or anticipated outcome?
2. *Appropriateness:* Is the care or intervention provided relevant to and appropriate for the patient's clinical need?

DOING THE RIGHT THING WELL
1. *Availability:* Is the service or product available to meet the patient's need?
2. *Timeliness:* Is the care or intervention provided to the patient at the most beneficial time?
3. *Effectiveness:* Is the care or intervention provided in the correct manner, given the current state of knowledge?
4. *Continuity:* Is patient care or intervention coordinated over time with respect to other services and providers?
5. *Safety:* Are the risks presented by procedures and interventions, and by the infusion clinic itself, kept to a minimum for patients, visitors, and health care workers?
6. *Efficiency:* Is there a clear relationship between outcomes of care and resources allocated to deliver that care?
7. *Respect and caring:* Are patients and their families involved in decisions related to their care?

home care accreditation program is second in size only to the hospital program. Accreditation is also available for mental health care, long-term health care, and ambulatory health care. Thus programs based in physicians' offices and many alternative settings are now eligible for JCAHO accreditation. JCAHO's focus changed in 1995 to emphasize actual performance, and not simply the ability to perform as well as performance standards focusing on quality improvement. Indicators, defined as quantitative outcome or process measures related to performance, have now become an integral part of the accreditation process.[1]

Pharmacies providing infusion and other drug therapy to long-term care facilities are included in the accreditation process. Infusion centers and these pharmacies were previously excluded from home care accreditation because their services were not considered to be provided in the patient's home.

Most of the national infusion companies have acquired JCAHO accreditation. Other providers have been accredited through the National League of Nursing's Community Health Accreditation Program. A third agency, the Accreditation Association for Ambulatory Health Care, surveys intermediate-provider components of managed care organizations, such as surgical centers and multispecialty group services. The organization also accredits college and university health centers, employee health programs, and infusion centers.

Any accreditation process is costly, with fees based on a provider's gross annual revenue or a base fee plus a variable amount calculated on patient volume and number of sites. The incentives to pursue accreditation are strong. Most health insurance plans and managed care organizations require accreditation, and once accredited agencies can receive "deemed status," which allows them to be reimbursed by Medicare and Medicaid without undergoing a separate certification process.

Procedures. Written policies and procedures are necessary to provide consistency of care, a format for orienting new personnel, and a mechanism for demonstrating compliance for accreditation. These documents may be investigated by any accreditation body or Medicare. Qualified professional management staff must be responsible for directing, coordinating, and supervising all professional services.[14] Nursing, pharmacy, administrative, and safety and infection control policies should be included in the policy and procedure manual. Complete manuals are available for purchase, or they may be written by employees.

Documentation

In addition to a patient's medical record, numerous forms tracking all contributions to the plan of treatment are necessary. Each department in the alternative setting has forms documenting specific training, authorizations, consents, clinicians patient assessments, dates drugs are compounded, progress notes, interoffice communications, and so on. Ideally, the infusion record, specifically any clinical information, will be incorporated into the main medical record either during the course of treatment or at completion of therapy. Documentation requirements are listed in Table 29-5.

Additional forms may be required by specific accrediting organizations, payers, institutions, parent companies, referral sources, or other providers participating in the care of the patient. Interdisciplinary care plans, discharge summaries, quality improvement forms, adverse reaction event forms, and patient data forms for clinical studies and outcomes are optional.

Financial management

Clearly, a successful program for outpatient IV infusion is not feasible if it is not carefully planned in regard to capital expense outlay, personnel requirements, salary estimates, equipment purchases, and other miscellaneous startup costs. Instituting the business plan and maintaining tight control on inventory of medication and supplies, capital equipment, and personnel time are all critical to keeping a new business afloat in today's market. With delayed claim submission and claim denials by third-party payers, the accounts receivable for the first year can be financially devastating and very discouraging.

Analysis of health care costs is complicated by the fact that reimbursement is continually changing. In certain areas of the country, reimbursement to providers is still calculated on a fee-for-service basis, but most hospitals and thousands of

Table 29-5   Documentation Requirements

NURSING	PHARMACY	PHYSICIAN	ADMINISTRATION
Predischarge assessment	Oral medication profile	Consent for treatment	Financial information
Patient education	Prescriptions	Notification of ownership	Benefit authorization
Patient rights and responsibilities	Compounding record	Plan of treatment	Payment plan
Medicare disclaimer (waiver)	Dispensing records	Order sheet	Financial hardship
Checklist for admission criteria	Clinical monitoring	Lab flow sheet	Assignment of benefits
Self-monitoring forms	Interdepartmental communication	Progress notes	Release of information authorization
Guidelines for accessing help	Height and weight		Charge sheets/superbill
Visit schedule	Lab and clinical data		Certification of medical necessity
Infusion notes			
Graphic for vital signs			
Venous access flow sheet			
Progress notes			
Patient satisfaction survey			

physicians are now under managed care contracts, which translates to fixed reimbursement.

The single largest cost component is personnel. This change over the past decade has led to major restructuring or downsizing. Most hospitals are adjusting to lower reimbursement by developing strategies to shorten lengths of stay to improve the hospital's financial statement. Likewise, all health care providers are experiencing similar crises and are forced to evaluate the role of each employee.

As payers begin to search for more cost-effective ways of providing health care, organized delivery systems are being developed. An *organized delivery system* is a network of organizations that provides or arranges to provide a coordinated continuum of services to a defined population and is willing to be held clinically and fiscally accountable for the outcomes and health status of the population served. The central component of organized delivery is a complex medical care system integrated by a central database. Infusion therapy providers often participate in this capitation system. A structured health care delivery system will provide clinical integration, defined as the coordination of patient care services across the various personnel services and operating units of the system.

As health care reimbursement shifts to a capitated approach, hospitals and other health care providers, including infusion centers, are beginning to move into integrated systems in an effort to survive. Administrators are seeking ways of providing care that do not include actual hospitalization, which makes outpatient infusion therapy even more attractive than it was previously. In attempting to find new ways to handle patients, hospitals, physicians, and payers are looking for alternative treatment sites.

Health care delivery systems will continue to change because of the pressures of increased financial demands and changes in patient demographics. Organizations that will survive and continue to thrive in this environment will be those that develop models for patient care that take advantage of the efficiency and creativity of alternative care settings such as outpatient infusion.

Billing and collecting.
Dependable computers and applicable software for medical billing are the crux of a solid medical billing program. In a modern practice, the software must be able to analyze demographic information from personal patient data, store thousands of ICD 9 and CPT codes, electronically sort claims by payer, and electronically bill via modem. Several satisfactory medical billing software programs are on the market and should be tested and evaluated. Proving that a particular software package is right for a given facility is anything but easy. However, the time must be spent up front because once commitment is made and conversion of electronic files or entering historic data manually starts, it is too late to find out a mistake has been made.

Claim submission with a clear follow through in tracking misguided claims, denied claims and rejected claims is important to the survival of an active alternative-site infusion center. Each alternative setting should be aware that submitting claims is a complex procedure. It becomes even more complex with the rapidity of third-party payer changes, Medicare updates, insurance company mergers, and the continual movement of patients from one insurance plan to another. This responsibility should be shared by the manager of the clinic and the secretarial billing staff. It has proven very beneficial to have a clinical person involved in coding diagnoses for claim submission.

Before any claim submission, the administrative staff should become acquainted with the insurance providers who will handle large numbers of the facility's claims. Anticipating peculiarities of third-party payers and their routine claim submission guidelines and requirements will help facilitate a "cleaner" claim. This will naturally decrease the delay in being reimbursed for services.

Cost considerations.
With escalating costs for drugs, solutions, tubings, IV access devices, and delivery systems, evaluating the costs of supplies and equipment at regular intervals is essential. Without competitive purchasing contracts and regular evaluation of expenditures, financial liabilities soar. Purchasing power clearly relies on an aggressive search for discounted, bulk purchasing where possible. Buying groups have more influence than solo practitioners when negotiating the purchase of supplies, drugs, and equipment.

In deciding which infusion system or equipment to purchase, it is tempting to take the simplistic approach of merely looking at how much it costs to acquire the system. Providers and case managers involved in the selection process must take into account the overall cost of providing infusion care to the patient and not the up-front acquisition price. The infusion system that offers the lowest acquisition price does not necessarily provide the lowest overall cost of providing care; it may produce exactly the opposite result (Box 29-7).

Experienced, well-trained, and oriented staff can reduce unexpected revenue loss substantially. Hiring qualified clinical staff not only reduces orientation time but also the expense of providing supplies to train or refresh the clinical competencies of nurses. Hiring competent personnel will also reduce the IV supplies that are wasted when multiple attempts are required to obtain venous access.

Reimbursement.
Reimbursement for outpatient infusion therapy is in a state of flux. The initial cost savings afforded by outpatient infusion therapy were welcomed by most third-party payers in the early 1980s, allowing providers a great deal of

---

Box 29-7   Issues to Consider When Purchasing Infusion Equipment

- Overall product design
- Ease of staff and patient training
- Amount of nursing interaction required
- Ability to minimize complications
- Amount of pharmacy handling and filling time
- Ability to minimize waste
- Amount of storage space needed at the provider's facility
- Availability of the product and overall level of manufacturer and distributor support
- Ease of disposal and or retrieval of the product after discontinuation of therapy
- Ability to minimize down-time and repair costs
- Inventory costs
- Overall product reliability[15]

freedom in terms of methods and charges. As the infusion industry became more competitive, however, the payment mechanism has evolved into a bundling of goods and services and deep discounting. In addition, per diem rates have become the standard model of billing and collecting. Daily per diem rates were designed to eliminate line-item billing practices, condense billable services, procedures, drugs and supplies into one billing code, and sharply decrease the amount of claims and billing history on each patient. Some managed care organizations are now trying to transfer the risk of insuring subscribers to health care providers with a prepaid payment arrangement. Payer education, when possible, is an important practice that is often forgotten. Infusion and medication claims are often denied because a claim processor does not understand the claim. Whenever possible, the physician should invite case managers and utilization review personnel to make on-site visits to the infusion center. Nothing will educate a payer representative more quickly. Outcome data are helpful in educating case managers. Case managers should be reminded of the physician's responsibility and liability in directing the outpatient's care.

Some payers are attempting to include the professional services of the physician in the bundled infusion services. The decision to bundle or unbundle services is complex, having advantages and disadvantages. Before establishing a billing format, all of the options for billing services and supplies should be explored, keeping in mind the reimbursement practices of the biggest third-party payers.

Claim submission. A variety of products and supplies can be billed on a particular day of service. These may be billed as separate items, or bundled into one per diem charge. Either billing format should include the following items:

- Drug or solutions
- Compounding supplies and service
- Infusion supplies
- Nursing services, either infusions billed by the hour or a per diem rate for the entire infusion time
- Laboratory services
- Physicians services

Medicare. Outpatient IV antimicrobial therapy by the self-administered model is not a covered benefit by Medicare. In-office infusion, when administered through a physician-directed infusion center incident to the office visit, is a covered service through Medicare Part B, provided the physician is on site to directly supervise the administration of the medication.

The annual deductible for Medicare Part B is $100, payable by the patient. After the deductible is satisfied, Medicare will reimburse the provider 80% of what they consider to be allowable charges—medically necessary, reasonable, and customary. Following Medicare payment to the provider, the physician must make reasonable effort to collect the 20% patient balance. If the patient has supplemental insurance, the 20% can and should be billed to the supplemental plan.

A certificate of medical necessity must be completed and signed by the physician and submitted to the insurance company with the claims for infusion therapy. Diagnostic and procedure codes should accurately reflect the condition treated and the procedure.

Medicare coverage for outpatient infusion therapy is limited to the following under the Part B, Durable Medical Equipment (DME) benefit.

- A specific list of approved drugs that HCFA has determined require an infusion pump for administration to prevent rate-related toxicities
- Antibiotics or antivirals included on the approved list are amphotericin B, ganciclovir, acyclovir, and foscarnet
- A registered DME provider can furnish the pump to the patient, and be reimbursed for the pump, drug, and other supplies necessary for administration
- Charges are billed to the regional designated durable medical equipment carrier (Providers must have a provider number for DME and follow the DME guidelines for billing)

Medicaid. Claims submitted to Medicaid usually require itemization. However, this may vary from state to state. Each provider intending to bill Medicaid for outpatient infusion should investigate the proper, state-specific, billing format for Medicaid. Claims should itemize all supplies used or provided and should reflect correct codes to facilitate prompt payment.

Medicaid usually covers both home and office infusion. To qualify for reimbursement, home nursing services must be provided by a Medicare-certified home health agency. Preauthorization may be required by some state Medicaid programs for drugs, procedures, and supplies.

Private insurance. Billing requirements and reimbursement for outpatient infusion products and drugs vary greatly from one insurance carrier to another. Becoming familiar with large third-party payers, their personnel, and particular claim processing procedures may facilitate prompt payment.

Every billing office should be flexible and adapt quickly to continuous changes in procedure, billing codes, code descriptions, and ICD 9 codes and modifiers. The patient's financial record, including insurance benefits and copies of correspondence with payer and patient, should be kept in a separate file from the medical record, and should include the information in Box 29-8.

All negotiated per diems or billing rates should be documented in the patient's financial record and updated with each call or communication with the payer. A systematic collection effort and process should be clearly stated in the office policy and procedure manual. The information, although confidential, should be readily assessable to all administrative staff members in the billing office.

Box 29-8   Information to Include in Patient Financial Records

- Insurance company and billing address
- Benefits quoted upon preauthorization of therapy
- Usual benefits for physician services
- Case manager name and phone number
- Billing requirements
- Medical director
- Claims appeal process
- Patient financial responsibility

Infectious waste

All alternative-site providers of infusion must make provision for the proper handling and disposal of infectious waste. Advisories issued by the Environmental Protection Agency (EPA) have been developed as guidelines for correct disposal of infectious waste. In 1988, with the Medical Waste Tracking Act, the tracking of medical waste investigation was initiated by the EPA and mandated by Congress. Handling of medical waste must be addressed in institutional policies and procedures. Sharps disposal kits and prepackaged disposal systems are available from numerous manufacturers (see Chapter 34).[14]

Quality improvement

Quality improvement (QI) has been described as a process for evaluating patient care in a particular setting by developing standards of care and implementing mechanisms to ensure that the standards are met. QI has been defined by JCAHO as "the process for objectively and systematically monitoring and evaluating the quality and appropriateness of patient care, for pursuing opportunities to improve patient care, and for resolving identified problems." In addition, accrediting bodies, usually require the development and implementation of an active QI program. There are also standards of care that individuals within the community expect when seeking care.

QI is a highly flexible process that can improve the quality and cost-effectiveness of the complex and changing arena of health care, thereby providing customer satisfaction. QI is data driven. Quality improvement in health care can no longer survive as a soft science if it is to satisfy internal and external customers. Managing the future means continually looking for ways to improve quality. The alternative-site infusion provider must have an active quality improvement committee to administer and evaluate the QI program, evaluate outcomes, and institute appropriate corrective action.[16]

Outcomes measurement. Outcomes measurement, an essential process for providers of medical care, is intended to promote continuous improvement of care and demonstrate excellence to payers and patients. An *outcome* is an indicator of the results of a process, which is related to the content and delivery of health care and is used to determine the best approach to that care. Some outcome indicators follow a patient across several discrete encounters. Others do not look at patients at all, but rather at the system. Outcome data must be measurable. However, they are usually not useful indicators until they are transformed through analysis. Some outcomes are provider-driven, focused on physician or nurse goals, a particular diagnosis, medication delivery system, antimicrobial or treatment regimen, quality-of-life issues, or patient satisfaction. Data collection must be designed to answer specific questions and to be reliable, accurate, analyzable, and comparable between health care systems.

Quality improvement in medicine has been described as defining standards of care, reassessing those standards periodically, and continuously improving the medical systems that support those standards. Quality improvement is unlike the previously popular term *quality assurance,* which was punitive in nature and focused on finding the bad provider or the patient

service that was not functioning as it should. With quality improvement, if an aspect of care plays a central role in an organization, it should be studied and improved even if it is perceived to be good already.

Quality has been defined as the extent to which care provided is expected to achieve the most favorable balance of risks and benefits.[17] The concept of *value* has assumed increasing importance in the current health care environment. Although payers are using outcomes increasingly as a basis for making decisions about contracts and reimbursement, from a financial perspective good outcomes are not necessarily enough. Value weighs outcome in the context of the cost of care. If a large additional expense is necessary to improve an outcome, the value of the improvement must be considered.

Data collection and analysis. Data collection tools should be standardized, clear, concise, and completed accurately by all users. Definitions of data elements should be readily available to staff members inputting data or extrapolating data from patient records. The validity of the data should be continually monitored. Ideally, multiple data elements or sets can be compared and cause-and-effect comparisons can be made. Trending, or the viewing of data sequentially over time, is essential for seeing significant changes in a patient's condition or recovery.

Benchmarking is the term used to compare results with both internal and external standards. Internal benchmarking may involve setting standards and evaluating whether an organization meets those standards. Internal benchmarks may be used to differentiate providers within an organization and develop strategies for improvement. External benchmarking involves comparing an organization or elements within an organization with outside standards. For example, an organization's phlebitis rate may be compared with another institution's phlebitis rate or with the accepted standard published in *Infusion Nursing Standards of Practice.* External benchmarks are used to differentiate one program or one system from another.

Outcome evaluation in the alternative setting for infusion therapy is helpful in determining treatment effectiveness, efficiency, comparison of varied treatment regimens, outpatient versus inpatient care, comparison of different medication delivery systems, medication regimens, central venous catheters, or infusion care delivery models.[18]

Risk management

With the increasing shift of infusion therapy toward the alternative setting, the potential for associated risks is greater than in the past. The infusion therapy agency is responsible for the quality of care delivered by its agents. As the scope of outpatient services becomes more complex and specialized, nurses and pharmacists are sharing in administrative procedures formerly performed by physicians, many of which have legal consequences. An understanding of the legal principles and guidelines involved in modern health care practice may prevent unwanted malpractice suits. Understanding some important legal *terms* will help practitioners follow the legal guidelines.

Criminal law: The body of the law that deals with conduct considered so harmful to society as a whole that it is prohibited by statute and prosecuted and punished by the government.

Civil law: The body of the law that deals with conflict between private litigants (either individuals or legal entities) over personal wrongs, wherein the losing party generally compensates the prevailing party with money or property.

Tort: The body of the law that allows an injured person to obtain compensation from the person who caused the injury, whether by act or omission. Tort law serves as a deterrent by establishing community standards of unacceptable conduct.

Malpractice: The negligent conduct of professional persons.

Rule of personal liability: "Every person is liable for his own tortious conduct."

Incident report: Required documentation for any accident or error resulting in actual or potential injury or harm

Unusual-occurrence reports: Required documentation for reporting unexpected responses to therapy, such as an untoward outcome following administration of infusion therapy[14]

Minimizing the risks associated with infusion therapy involves careful initial and ongoing assessment. Many factors should be considered when evaluating a patient's home environment or family situation. Assessments must take into consideration lifestyles, likes and dislikes, and financial resources, all of which will vary from patient to patient. The home assessment is not an occasion to judge the personal aspects of a patient's life; the problems assessed should be limited to those affecting the patient's safety, competence, comfort, and recovery.

OSHA. Members of the health care team should be aware of hazards to health from chemicals that are used. The OSHA requires that medical office workers be trained to use these chemicals safely. All staff members have a right to a safe and healthful workplace. At the time of initial employment and at least annually thereafter, the staff must be made aware of the existence, location, and availability of medical and exposure records.

Hazards. A *hazard,* as defined by OSHA, is a source of potential danger or risk. Physical hazards and health hazards are the two largest groups of employee hazards. *Health hazards* refers to chemical or biologic agents that can damage a person's health through contact with the lungs, skin, eyes, mucous membranes, kidneys, marrow, or reproductive system. *Physical hazards* refers to causes of accidental injury. These hazards range from minor to major—from tripping over an electric cord to being burned as a result of misuse of flammable chemicals. The proper use of chemicals is essential for the medical office. Not all chemicals used in an infusion center or clinic are hazardous; however, some may be dangerous under certain conditions. Generally, the conditions under which chemicals cause harm are when they are not used according to the manufacturer's guidelines; mixed inappropriately, causing vapors; accidentally spilled or splashed; or used in confined, unventilated spaces.

OSHA requires that each health care worker be educated as to which chemicals are hazardous, the risks involved when working with a hazardous chemical, how to use the chemicals safely, and what to do in the event of an accident. OSHA also requires that each medical office or entity maintain a written hazard communication program. This program should include an inventory of hazardous chemicals, with product information and appropriate responses to accidental exposure, and attaching warning labels to all hazardous chemical and waste containers.

Exposure. Health care personnel can be exposed to a hazardous chemical if the chemical gets on the skin and is absorbed into the body. Although the skin is an effective protective organ that shields the body from most chemical agents, it is also permeable where cracks, wounds, and rashes allow passage of harmful chemicals. Even healthy skin can be damaged by exposure to highly corrosive or toxic agents. The skin can be exposed when a chemical is splashed or spilled or if it is accidentally touched without the protection of gloves.

To avoid skin contact with hazardous substances, techniques should be used that do not require direct handling of the chemical or drug. If direct handling is necessary, or if accidental contact is possible, protective gloves must be worn. Contact with hazardous chemicals through the mucous membranes of the eyes, nose, and mouth can be prevented by wearing a protective face mask or respirator and eye protection.

Inhalation exposure occurs when harmful chemicals release vapors that are breathed into the lungs. Some chemotherapy drugs and cleaning supplies may fall into this category. Chemical vapors can be kept to a minimum by replacing the caps on bottles and trays immediately after dispensing. This simple safety measure can help prevent chemical spills as well.

Exposure can also occur by ingesting harmful substances. This can occur if a chemical is touched by hand and then the same hand is put to the lips. It can also occur by accidentally eating or drinking a chemical or by eating food that has been contaminated with a chemical. To help prevent exposure through ingestion, food and drinks should not be allowed in areas where chemicals are prepared or infused.

Sharps containers. Handling sharps, working with lab materials, glass, scalpels, vials, and other objects that may penetrate the skin, must be performed per protocol and according to safety regulations. *Infusion Nursing Standards of Practice* provides criteria for the use and disposal of all sharps. The following guidelines should be established in policy and procedure.

- Needles should be discarded immediately after use into containers that are clearly marked, closable, puncture-resistant, and leak-proof on the sides and bottom.
- Sharps disposal containers should be replaced before they become overfilled.
- Needles are not recapped unless it is necessary, and then, only by using the one-handed "scoop" method.

Material safety data sheets. Material safety data sheets are provided by manufacturers for all chemicals, drugs, and potentially harmful substances. This printed sheet gives detailed information about each product containing hazardous chemicals. The sheets should be readily available to staff at all times.

Cleanup and disposal. After using a chemical or when a spill occurs, proper cleanup procedures must be followed. Caution should be exercised, and manufacturers instructions and guidelines such as those provided by OSHA should be followed when dealing with hazardous waste spills. Each infusion center should have a commercial hazardous waste disposal contract with a state-licensed provider. Requirements for commercial disposal may vary greatly from state to state. All patient care areas should be cleaned between patients in the event that something is spilled or contaminated. All surfaces should be cleaned, including furniture and work areas. Infusion devices should be cleaned with an industrial decontamination solution between each use and checked for any faults or damage.

Transfer and storage. All sharps containers, garbage cans, and materials contaminated with human or hazardous waste should be handled properly according to the standards, policies, and procedures of the organization and OSHA guidelines. When transferring containers or dispensers, careful consideration should be made to the proper handling, labeling, and disposal. It is important to maintain good housekeeping policies in the infusion room, pharmacy, patient care areas, and any area in which exposure may occur.

Emergency procedures. Each employee should know the location of emergency equipment, whether for patient care or general emergency. Employees should know how to use fire extinguishers. Eye wash appropriate for eye exposures should be kept in a convenient, accessible location for emergency use.

In addition to the general safety precautions described here, it is necessary to exercise care and responsibility with regard to hazardous chemicals. When working with hazardous chemicals, the worker should remain focused on the task at hand and follow safe procedures if interrupted. Finally, if a chemical is spilled or released into the environment, the proper authorities must be notified. Information regarding appropriate authorities should be provided in the organization's hazard communication plan.

Standard precautions. Standard precautions is a method for preventing the transmission of blood-borne infection. It is based on the concept that *control measures should be taken with all patients,* because there is no way to know for sure who is infected and who is not. Patients are often unaware that they are carriers of blood-borne pathogens. Consequently, standard precautions are based on the following:

- All human blood, any body fluids containing blood, and any other potentially infectious body fluids are handled as if they are known to be infectious for HIV or hepatitis B virus (HBV).
- All used needles or other sharps are handled as if they are contaminated.

Personal protective equipment. Although nurses, physicians, and pharmacists perform tasks where there is risk of exposure to blood-borne pathogens, they can work safely if they follow established precautions and use personal protective equipment such as gloves, face masks, and protective eyewear. Protective clothing placed between the health care provider and the source of infection can effectively diminish accidental exposure significantly.

Gloves should be worn whenever there is danger of touching or handling blood or other potentially infectious body fluids. Gloves prevent transmission of blood-borne pathogens through broken skin. To maximize protection, hands should be washed before and after using protective gloves. Selecting the correct size of glove will increase dexterity and reduce the clumsiness of oversized gloves. When donning gloves, they should be checked for holes and tears. Gloves should be changed as soon as is practical if they become contaminated, are torn, or are no longer effective because of sweat from your hands. It is important to remove used gloves properly to avoid skin contact with the outside of a contaminated glove.

Face masks and protective eyewear are used to protect the mucous membranes of the eyes, nose, and mouth. The infusion center's policy and procedures should reflect the mandatory use of these items. Masks should completely cover the nose and mouth, and be discarded after each patient or if they become soiled or moist. Eye shielding devices protect the eyes. Masks are available that are equipped with eye protective devices as well.

One-way valves on disposable Ambu bags provide safety for the health care worker while giving respiratory assistance to those in respiratory failure. These devices prevent fluids from entering the rescuer's mouth. These should be readily available in every infusion suite and any area where patient care is given.

Long-sleeved protective clothing must be worn when splashes of infectious materials are anticipated. Protective clothing should be removed as soon as is practical if it becomes soiled with blood or other body fluids. The soiled outside portion of the garment should not be touched; it should be held away from the body while rolling it up so that the contaminated area is in the center. Disposable gowns should be discarded after each use. Hands should be washed directly after removing the protective gown.

HIV and hepatitis B are blood-borne infections. This means that they are caused by the pathogens that are found in the blood of those infected. There are many blood-borne infections that pose risk to the health care workers. HIV and hepatitis B are found not only in the blood, but also in body fluids, including blood, body fluids containing blood, semen, vaginal secretions, peritoneal fluid, amniotic fluid, joint and spinal fluid, and body tissue. The three major modes of transmission in the workplace are as follows:

1. Puncture wounds from contaminated needles or other sharps
2. Skin contact that allows infectious fluids to enter the body through wounds, cuts, or broken or damaged skin
3. Infectious fluids that enter the body through the mucous membranes of the eyes, nose, or mouth (This can occur if the health care worker is splashed in the face with blood, or by touching the nose, lip, or mouth with a contaminated hand.)

Postexposure response. Policies and procedures should be readily available to anyone who may experience accidental exposure. OSHA recommends the following responses to exposure.

Hepatitis B. It is important for each employee to be aware of the potential symptoms associated with contraction of HBV. OSHA states that approximately one third of those infected do not experience any symptoms. Another third experience only a mild flulike illness that goes away. The last third experience abdominal pain, nausea, and fatigue. The skin and eyes become jaundiced, the urine darkens, and sometimes the recipient may experience rash, joint pain, and fever. Approximately, 6% to 10% of all those infected with HBV become chronic carriers of the disease. They may or may not have an active infection and they may have few or no symptoms, but they can transmit the virus to others. Carriers are at risk for chronic active hepatitis, a disease that affects the liver and can lead to serious illness and death.[19]

HIV. Puncture of the skin with a contaminated needle is the most likely cause of HIV exposure and contraction of the HIV virus in health care workers. The number of health care professionals reporting accidental needlesticks is increasing. A standard prophylactic medication regimen should be immediately available to the employee who has been accidentally exposed.

Hepatitis C. Hepatitis C (HCV) infection has been reported and carefully evaluated in virtually every country. This virus is commonly transmitted by percutaneous exposure to blood. Although blood transfusions were once important sources of HCV infection, most new infections are related to illicit injection drug use. Infection occurs in more than 90% of seronegative recipients who have been transfused with blood from donors who test positive to the HCV antibody. As a result, there is a high prevalence of HCV infection in thalassemic and hemophiliac patients who have had multiple transfusions. Transmission of HCV from patient to patient or patient to health care worker is uncommon in economically developed nations and most likely involves a lapse in infection control practices. Transmission to health care workers occurs after 2% to 8% of accidental needle-stick exposures involving infected patients. Studies of such accidents indicated that the risk of HCV transmission is intermediate. Despite these risks, the prevalence of HCV infection among dental and medical heath care workers is similar to that of the general population. HCV may also be transmitted from health care worker to patient.

Personal health and hygiene. Health care workers should take special care of their own personal hygiene and be aware of personal health issues that are impacted by the risk of blood borne exposures. Because it is possible for a pregnant woman to become infected and to transmit blood-borne infection to the unborn child, pregnant health care workers can protect themselves and their unborn children by adhering to safety precautions.[20]

Patient satisfaction

An important way to determine the success of any outpatient care program is to ask clients their feelings about the care they received. With the technologic advances in health care, it's tempting to assume that we know what our patients—our customers—need. Because we care and want the very best for them, it is easy to superimpose our values on those that we serve. Patient satisfaction is the degree of congruency between patients' expectations of ideal care and their perception of actual care received. Healthcare customers expect to receive quality care at the best monetary value available. They want professional competence, accurate diagnosis, state-of-the-art treatment, and no complications that might result in prolonged

therapy, delayed recovery, disability, or death. By and large, patient satisfaction with health care is related to the "ordinary" human virtues of communication, sensitivity, respect, dependability, trust, and personalized service.

Nurses play a key role in the health care system and make a critical impact in hospitals and alternative settings. Because nurses make up the largest and most visible group of health care professionals, the public tends to equate satisfaction with health care in general to the care nurses provide. Although patient satisfaction is a highly complex and individualized variable, patients always expect outstanding care from caring people.

In health care, the term *customer* is not limited to patients and families, but encompasses other staff and departments. It is important to accord people inside the workplace (coworkers, managers, insurance representatives, and physicians) the same degree of respect and consideration as those we care for daily.

Confidentiality

The principle of confidentiality requires that all providers in an outpatient infusion setting respect all privileged information about their patients. Nurses can inadvertently breach confidentiality when they really are trying to show concern. Friends and families that ask for information pose another problem. These issues should be handled tactfully and firmly. In part, being a patient advocate is protecting the patient's right to privacy. In any setting, it is important to maintain a private area where family and physician can meet for private discussions or where patients can simply be alone. A patient has a right to expect confidentiality within reasonable limits. Technical advances have made sensitive data more available to a host of people, and the right to confidentiality has become a real concern. All persons involved with patient-specific health information must be committed to an ethical code that protects patients' privacy.

Care should be taken to prevent release of sensitive information by telephone. Policies should address the issue of release of information. Staff should not discuss a patient within ear shot of those sitting in the infusion room. All patient records must be kept out of public areas and be maintained as confidential documents.

Staff rights and workplace ethics. At times a staff member may ask to be released from participation in an aspect of patient care. Such situations may involve cultural values or religious beliefs that are in conflict with treatment protocols. Organizational policies regarding staff rights should reflect fairness to all involved; they should foster a spirit of caring about each other and the profession and be helpful to everyone. Some accrediting bodies audit established policies regarding the rights of employees and the mechanisms for dealing with special requests.

Patient satisfaction surveys. Patients have a right to have their complaints to be taken seriously, investigated, and resolved. Patient satisfaction surveys can help identify common complaints and other opportunities for improvement. These surveys help determine patients' perceptions of an organization's care and services. Confidentiality of customer satisfaction surveys is also a patient right, and patients should always understand that the opinions they express will not affect the quality of future care.[21]

THE CHALLENGE OF CHANGE

There is no question that the American health care system is changing fast and furiously, and that money is a primary motivating factor of this change. The fact that former management models have not worked well is evidenced by skyrocketing costs, and by poor access to treatment for large groups of people. For IV nurses who gained most of their professional experience in the hospital, moving to an outpatient setting may be difficult. With hospital restructuring, cost containment measures, and mergers, new attention is given to alternative settings for providing quality IV therapy. All change is difficult. Even change perceived as positive may still be traumatic. Although health care is changing at a staggering rate, the basic sound concepts of caring, compassion, competence, and customer satisfaction will assume even greater significance, especially for nurses. The more prepared for change that nurses are, the more they will embrace the opportunities that such changes bring.[21]

REFERENCES

1. Tice A: Outpatient parenteral antimicrobial therapy: current status, *Sci Am Med* 84:2, 1997.
2. Poretz D: *Infectious disease clinics of North America,* Philadelphia, 1998, WB Saunders.
3. Gilbert D, Dworkin R, Raber S, Leggett J: Outpatient parenteral antimicrobial-drug therapy, *N Engl J Med* 337(12): 829, 1997.
4. Grachman P: Nosocomial infection control, *Rev Infect Dis* 3:640, 1981.
5. Wenzel E: *Infection control, principles and practices of infectious disease,* ed 4, New York, 1995, Churchill Livingston.
6. Graham D: Nosohusial infections: complications of home infusion therapy, *Infect Dis Clin Prac* 2:158, 1993.
7. Stiver H, et al: Self-administration of IV antibiotics: an efficient cost-effective home care program, *Can Med Assoc J* 127:107, 1996.
8. Nolet B: Outpatient parenteral antimicrobial therapy as an extension of the physician office based practice, *NW Mgmt* 1, 1997.
9. Petrak R: *Infectious disease clinics of North America,* Philadelphia, 1998, WB Saunders.
10. Nicolle LE, et al: SHEA long-term committee, Shea position paper, *Infect Control Hosp Epidemiol* 17:2, 1996.
11. Andes D: *Infectious disease clinics of North America,* Philadelphia, 1998, WB Saunders.
12. Itano J, Taoka K: *Core curriculum for oncology nursing,* ed 3, Philadelphia, 1998, WB Saunders.
13. Lawton S, Leibenluft R, Loeb L: Antitrust Implications of physicians' responses to managed care, *Clin Infect Dis* 20:1354, 1995.
14. Weinstein S: Plumers *Principles and practice of intravenous therapy,* ed 6, Philadelphia, 1997, JB Lippincott.
15. Slabadow J: Making sense of the options, ambulatory systems of IV antibiotic therapy, *Infusion* April:19, 1995.
16. Katz J, Green E: *Managing quality,* ed 2, St Louis, 1997, Mosby.
17. Kunkel M: *Infectious disease clinics of North America,* Philadelphia, 1998 WB Saunders.
18. Kunkel M: Outcomes measurement in OPAT: why and how, outpatient parenteral antimicrobial therapy: current status, *Sci Am Med* 50, 1997.
19. Universal Precautions, Medicom, Inc., 1992.
20. Federal Register, Rules and Regulations 64175.
21. Messner R: *Increasing patient satisfaction: a guide for nurses,* New York, 1996, Springer.

Chapter

30

Intravenous Therapy in Children

Anne Marie Frey, BSN, CRNI*

Starting and maintaining intravenous (IV) therapies in children poses unique challenges to the clinicians responsible for their care. Children are not only very different from adults, but they also display variations among their different age groups. These differences include physical, physiologic, developmental, cognitive, and emotional variables. When any type of infusion therapy is used in a child, a great responsibility is placed on the nurse. Accordingly, the nurse performing IV techniques in children should be highly skilled in the basic IV therapy applications and knowledgeable of the child's developmental stage. Most of the basic principles of safe administration of IV solutions and medications are the same, regardless of the patient's age. However, special considerations are necessary to safeguard the child undergoing these procedures; these measures include the need to calculate small doses and low infusion rates, to choose appropriate venipuncture sites and equipment, and to develop creative measures to distract curious little minds and hands.

This chapter focuses on the needs of children as they relate to infusion therapy and on the unique aspects of caring for children and their families.

ANATOMIC AND PHYSIOLOGIC DIFFERENCES IN CHILDREN

Children present a wide variety of physical characteristics different from those in adults. In addition, premature infants and newborns vary greatly from older children in their anatomy and physiology. These characteristics affect the ability of neonates and infants to cope with environmental stresses and to manage the metabolism, absorption, distribution, and excretion of medications and solutions. Although body systems in infants and children are different from those in adults, for the purpose of this text, only those related to infusion therapy are addressed in detail.

The newborn's adjustment to extrauterine life is a complex physiologic process. The first 24 hours of life are the most critical as the newborn makes the respiratory and circulatory transition to extrauterine life. During this period, there is a much higher incidence of death than in the remainder of the neonatal period. All of the body systems undergo change after

*The author and editors wish to acknowledge the contributions made by Corinne Wheeler, an author of this chapter in the first edition of *Intravenous Nursing: Clinical Principles and Practice*.

birth, and most of them remain immature for a while. During infancy (birth to 12 months of age), physical and developmental changes occur more rapidly than during any other period. The infant's head and body grow very rapidly during this period, and major body systems undergo a progressive maturation process. In healthy infants, the birth weight is usually doubled at 6 months and tripled at 1 year. During infancy, certain critical developmental tasks that affect nursing care are mastered. However, each child has his or her own pace of development; no two children of the same age are at the same exact stage of development and maturation.

Biologic development in the toddler period (12 to 36 months) is less dramatic than during infancy. Body systems continue to mature, resulting in many children reaching full maturation by the end of the toddler period. Growth slows during this time. Birth weight is quadrupled by 30 months, and the height at age 3 years is generally about half the adult height. Head circumference growth slows, and chest circumference exceeds the size of both the head and the abdomen. The toddler is able to participate in an increased number of activities as a result of gross and fine motor skill advancement. In toddlers, IV connections must be taped and secured and equipment kept outside of the child's reach.

Early childhood (36 months to 6 years), also referred to as the *preschool period,* is a time of growth stabilization. The average annual weight gain is about 5 pounds (2.3 kg); the increase in height ranges from 2.5 to 3 inches (6.4 to 7.6 cm). Most of the height growth occurs in the legs, leading to a more slender physical appearance. The preschooler's more mature body system enables him or her to tolerate moderate physiologic stress. Skills mastered during the toddler period are refined during this time and include a rapidly developing ability to understand and use language. Expected levels of growth and development must be attained for the child to refine these skills in preparation for the next stage of childhood, school age.

The school-age period (6 to 12 years of age) is a time of gradual growth and development until the end of the period, sometimes referred to as *prepubescence.* The school-age child will grow an average of 2 inches (5 cm) and gain 4.5 to 6.5 pounds (2 to 3 kg) annually. Until prepubescence, there is little difference in size between males and females; toward the end of this stage, however, a growth spurt occurs. Girls first surpass boys in both height and weight. Body proportions approach adult measurements by the end of the school-age period.

Adolescence is the period of transition from childhood to young adulthood. This period is divided into three substages: early adolescence (11 to 13 years), middle adolescence (13 to 15 years), and late adolescence (15 years and older). The changes occurring during adolescence are primarily puberty, growth, and personality. The central nervous system is inundated with hormonal activity, and dramatic and obvious growth changes are noted in both boys and girls. Both sexes develop secondary sexual characteristics and grow larger. Less obvious is the maturation of the reproductive system. This stage is often turbulent for adolescents because they are on a constant emotional roller coaster, attempting to master the developmental tasks for adulthood.

Physiologic system development in children

Thermoregulation. The large surface area in relation to volume, thin layer of subcutaneous fat, and unique method for producing heat predispose the neonate to excessive heat loss. Measures must be taken to protect the newborn from hypothermia during all aspects of care, including obtaining vascular access and site care. Unlike the adult, the chilled neonate does not shiver but uses the mechanism of nonshivering thermogenesis to increase heat production. In response to hypothermia, norepinephrine is secreted by the sympathetic nerve endings. This action stimulates the breakdown of brown fat to generate heat, allowing distribution of the heated blood through the body.

Increased metabolism as a response to hypothermia results in higher oxygen and caloric requirements. A healthy infant can usually tolerate increased oxygen consumption; however, a sick infant is predisposed to cold stress and hypoglycemia. Cold stress begins as the infant requires an increase in oxygen and caloric consumption. The activation of norepinephrine stimulates the metabolism, and anaerobic glycolysis results. The lactic acid produced by this process, combined with the acid end products of brown fat metabolism, can lead to acidosis.[1]

This process of thermoregulation continues throughout the infant's first several months of life. During infancy, the child's ability to shiver increases. The older infant usually has acquired the benefit of insulation by the gradual growth of adipose tissue. By early childhood, the skin is thicker, and the body has a higher percentage of fat and a decreased surface area/volume ratio; these factors enable the preschooler to better cope with environmental cold.

The nurse performing such procedures as venipuncture on an infant must maintain a neutral thermal environment for the infant to prevent the possibility of cold stress. A neutral thermal environment is one that permits the infant to maintain a normal core temperature with minimum oxygen consumption and calorie expenditure. The neutral thermal environment for smaller infants is 35.4° plus or minus 0.5° C (95.7° plus or minus 1° F) and for larger infants is 32.5° plus or minus 1.4° C (90.5° plus or minus 2.5° F).[2]

To help infants stay warm, nurses can use radiant warming panels, incubators, cotton blankets, and head coverings (e.g., a piece of stockinet knotted at one end) and ensure that only the extremity of the IV insertion site is exposed. Blankets can be warmed in warming units or in clean, unoccupied incubators. A warming lamp, placed at the recommended safe distance from the infant, can be used to prevent hypothermia if an infant must be removed from a neutral thermal environment.

Vessel size. The size of venous and arterial vessels in the infant and child are obviously smaller than those in the adult. Although the vessels are anatomically positioned in the same locations throughout life, their sometimes-threadlike characteristics and tendency to hide make them difficult to locate in the young patient. Applying heat to the extremity before performing venipuncture facilitates venous identification and catheter insertion.

Renal function. The newborn without congenital abnormalities has an anatomically complete renal system. However, all young kidneys have a functional deficiency in their ability to concentrate urine. In the infant younger than 6 weeks of age, glomerular filtration functions less precisely than in the mature child. Mature kidney function is complete by approximately 2½ to 3 years of age. The young infant's renal system has difficulty coping with changes in fluid and electrolyte status. Dehydration, conditions of hyperosmolality, and sometimes overhydration are problems for the infant. Not only are infants more prone to develop these conditions, but the effects progress more rapidly. Infants have a greater urine volume per kilogram of body weight and a smaller bladder volume capacity than older children. Expected urine output with adequate intake should be 0.5 to 1.0 ml/kg/hr for the newborn and 1.0 to 2.0 ml/kg/hr for the infant.[1]

Hepatic function. Decreased hepatic function because of liver immaturity in the newborn affects IV medication and solution administration. After the first few weeks of life, the liver is able to secrete bile and conjugate bilirubin. Throughout the first year of life, however, the liver remains immature in its ability to function. The infant's ability to metabolize drugs is dramatically less than that of the adult, as is the formation of the plasma proteins and ketones, the storage of glycogen and vitamins, and the capacity to break down amino acids. Digestive and metabolic processes are usually complete by the beginning of toddlerhood.[1]

Endocrine function. Like the renal system, the endocrine system in the newborn is fully intact anatomically; however, it functions at an immature level. The entire endocrine system interrelates and affects body homeostasis. Decreased functioning of this system affects the ability of the infant to cope with stress. For example, endocrine-secreted hormones that affect fluid and electrolyte equilibrium and metabolism include adrenocorticotropic hormone, antidiuretic hormone, and vasopressin. The immature endocrine system, in concert with other immature body systems, predisposes the infant to such conditions as dehydration and unstable blood glucose levels.

Body composition

Subcutaneous fat. The percentage of body fat gradually increases over the first 6 months of life. As shown in Table 30-1, the highest percentages of body fat are seen in the toddler and prepubescent years. Additional adipose tissue may add to the difficulty of locating veins for IV access. In addition, the percentage of body fat can affect therapeutic requirements of lipid-soluble IV medications such as diazepam (Valium), which is used as a sedative or anticonvulsant in children.

Circulating blood volume. In children, the circulating blood volume is much greater per unit of body weight than in the adult, but the absolute blood volume is small. Every child's total circulating blood volume should be calculated at admission to a pediatric intensive care unit (Table 30-2).

In a small infant, hypovolemia can occur from only a small amount of blood loss. The following equations compare the relative impact of an absolute-volume loss on a 7-kg infant and a 70-kg adult:

25 ml blood loss from 7 kg infant = 5% of total
circulating blood volume (500 ml)
25 ml blood loss from 70 kg adult = <0.6% of
total circulating blood volume (4150 ml)

When blood samples are obtained for laboratory examination, the smallest amount of blood required for accurate results should be removed. Blood replacement should be considered when blood loss is greater than 10% of the total circulating volume.[3] Blood sample amounts should be recorded in the output section of the intake and output record.

Fluid and electrolyte metabolism. The ratio of fluid to body mass is greater in the newborn than at any other time of life; this ratio decreases steadily with age (Table 30-3). The newborn has the largest proportion of free water in the extracellular spaces. This results in higher levels of total body sodium and chloride and lower levels of potassium, magnesium, and phosphate than in the adult. At a rate of exchange seven times greater than that of the adult, the infant exchanges approximately half of its total extracellular fluid daily. The basal metabolism rate is also twice as great in relation to body weight in the infant than it is in the adult. Insensible water losses are

---

Table 30-1   Percentage of Body Weight Made up by Fat

AGE	PERCENTAGE OF BODY FAT
Newborn	12
Toddler	23
Preschooler	12
Prepubescent	20
Adult	15

Table 30-2   Circulating Blood Volumes in Children

AGE	ML/KG OF BODY WEIGHT
Neonate	85-90
Infant	75-80
Child	70-75
Adolescent	65-70

From Hazinski MF: *Nursing care of the critically ill child,* St Louis, 1984, Mosby.

Table 30-3   Body Water in Proportion to Age

AGE	PERCENTAGE OF BODY WATER		
	TBW	ECF	ICF
Premature infant (1.2 kg)	81	59	22
Term infant (3.6 kg)	69	42	27
1 yr (10 kg)	60	32	28
Adult male (70 kg)	54	23	31
Adult female (60 kg)	49	23	26

Data from Mahan LK, Arlin MT: *Krause's food, nutrition, and diet therapy,* ed 8, Philadelphia, 1992, WB Saunders.
TBW, Total body water; *ECF,* extracellular fluid; *ICF,* intracellular fluid.

Table 30-4	Daily Caloric Requirements by Age
AGE	**DAILY CALORIC REQUIREMENT (CAL/KG)**
High-risk neonate	120-150
Term neonate	100-120
1-2 yr	90-100
3-6 yr	80-90
7-9 yr	70-90
10-12 yr	50-60

From Hazinski MF: *Nursing care of the critically Ill child,* St Louis, 1984, Mosby.

greater in infants because of their larger body surface/body weight ratio. These factors, in addition to the inability of the kidneys to concentrate urine in infants, can cause dehydration, acidosis, and overhydration.[4]

The daily fluid requirement (per kilogram of body weight) for an infant is three times greater than that of an adult and increases under stress. With each centigrade degree of temperature elevation, an additional 50 to 75 ml of fluid replacement is required. The normal daily caloric requirements are also greater than those of the adult because of the child's increased basal metabolism rate and rapid growth rate. Children who are ill, especially those with fever or who have had major surgery, require more calories than are required for regular maintenance (Table 30-4).

PEDIATRIC DEVELOPMENTAL AND ASSESSMENT CONSIDERATIONS

Successful pediatric IV therapy relies on more than technical skill and knowledge of the physiologic differences between children and adults. An understanding of the psychologic aspects of the child's growth and development and the application of appropriate interventions is essential when interacting with children. Table 30-5 outlines the various developmental stages of childhood and suggests nursing actions for each stage.

A complete health care assessment of a child has three main components: (1) health history, (2) physical assessment, and (3) review of diagnostic data. The urgency of the child's condition affects the order and the initial detail of these components. In emergencies, it may be necessary to obtain venous access and initiate IV therapy without a completed health care assessment. Routinely, however, the health care assessment is usually well under way before venipuncture, with the IV nurse contributing additional data.

History

Although in most cases the assigned nurse or nurse practitioner will obtain a nursing history, the IV nurse specialist can contribute to this ongoing database by assessing criteria related to IV therapy. This includes information such as IV history, current plan of treatment, expectations of the child and family, and special considerations that might affect IV access, such as hand dominance or thumb sucking if peripheral IV access in the upper extremities is considered.

Valuable information is collected not only during the initial assessment but also throughout the course of infusion therapy, whether in the hospital or in the home. In the younger child, the nurse should direct questions to the primary caregiver, including: (1) What are your concerns? (2) How is your child different from his or her normal or prior state? (3) What measures have been taken to alleviate the child's problem? and (4) How effective were the measures? When developmentally appropriate and possible, given the child's condition, questions should be asked directly to older children and adolescents. This practice provides them with an opportunity to actively participate in the process and to respond according to their own perceptions.

Knowledge of the child's age, preillness weight, fluid and dietary habits, and elimination patterns is useful for determining the child's current hydration status. Asking the parents if the child is thirsty or nauseated may also provide valuable information. Thirst in a child can be indicative of a fluid-volume deficit. However, nausea may blunt the desire to drink, even if the child is thirsty. The child's preferences for food and drink and any particular cultural and ethnic customs should also be considered.

Physical assessment

Before and during the course of infusion therapy, the clinical assessment of the child should include weight; height; vital signs; condition of skin, mucous membranes, and fontanels; urine volume; and neurologic status. Some elements of the clinical assessment may be performed simultaneously with the nursing history interview. When possible, the young child should be allowed to sit in the parent's lap or the parent should be allowed to be in proximity to the child. This helps the child feel more secure and enhances the child's ability to cooperate. The physician or nurse practitioner, along with the assigned staff nurse, obtain and document physical assessment data.

Height and weight. Height and weight measures are essential for accurate calculations to be made in fluid and medication administration. The comparison of prior weight with current weight is an accurate indicator of fluid-volume deficit or fluid-volume excess. Children younger than 2 years of age are more susceptible to weight changes resulting from fluid balance than from a change in body mass. In this age group, the proportion of body fluid to total body weight is greater (see Table 30-3), and most of this fluid is in the extracellular space.

Changes in weight must be monitored closely. Approximately 1 g of body weight is equal to 1 ml of body fluid. Thus weight loss or gain of 1 kg (2.2 pounds) within 24 hours represents 1 L of fluid loss or gain. Weight changes in a 24-hour period of plus or minus 50 g in an infant, 200 g in a child, or 500 g in an adolescent may be significant, and the physician should be notified. Infants should be weighed without clothing and consistently on the same scale. With small infants, the IV equipment should be weighed before venipuncture, and that amount should be subtracted from the total weight obtained. Calculations for fluid replacement are based on the percentage of weight lost; the amount of fluid restriction is based on the amount of weight gained.[3,5]

Table 30-5   Nursing Actions Appropriate for the Different Developmental Stages of Childhood

Age Group	Developmental Stage and Characteristics	Child's Response to Illness or Procedures	Preparation of Child	Family Involvement	Nursing Implications
Infant (birth to 1 yr)	Basic Trust vs. Mistrust Totally dependent on others for all needs. Trust develops as needs are consistently met. Mistrust develops as needs are not consistently met. Totally self-centered at birth. During infancy, begins to separate self from others. **Responses** Random communication skills (3 mo). Simple gesturing (12 mo). Exhibits early memory. **Fears** Separation Strangers **Rapid Motor Changes** Head control from poor to stable. Moves hand to mouth (birth-3 mo). Crawling (6-9 mo). Standing with support (12 mo).	Has the ability to resist with entire body. Recognizes primary caretaker and responds with fear of change. "Mirrors" emotional state of mother. Unpredictable response to repeated procedures. Uses cry to communicate all discomfort (not just pain)	Avoid feeding immediately before procedure (risk of vomiting and aspiration). Minimize separation from parents.	Encourage parental tactile contact and soothing verbal stimuli immediately after procedure and throughout duration of therapy. May be present during procedure but should not help restrain child. Demonstrate safe handling of infant. Encourage questions. Education directed to family.	Physical comfort is most effective. Keep infant warm. Use a pacifier. Talk in soft voice and call by name; cuddle infant. Avoid using infants preferred extremity for finger sucking. Distract with bright toys, and prepare equipment out of older infant's view. **Safety** Use assistants other than family to restrain infant. Monitor color and respirations during procedure. Protect site with half-cup or stockinet. Use elbow restraints over wrist restraints. Do not restrain all four extremities. Secure IV equipment out of infant's reach. Avoid using IV accessories with detachable parts. Restraining requires more than one person. Reassure during procedure with verbal and tactile stimulation. Provide toys to hit or throw. **Safety** Same as for infant. Note: Secure anchoring of IV site is essential for this age group. Use restraints minimally, because they may provoke increased fear and protest. Tape all IV connections and secure IV equipment out of reach to avoid choking hazard. Assess IV site a minimum of every 2 hr.
Toddler (1-3 yr)	Autonomy vs. Shame and Doubt *Preoperational thoughts:* Little understanding of past or present. Ritualistic. Explores self and world around him or her. Transitional objects provide comfort (blanket, toy). Differentiates self from objects. Can infer a cause while experiencing only the effect. Oppositional "No" stage. Early aggression and manipulative behavior. Has many fantasies. Enjoys new motor skills. Walking (12-15 mo) to running (24 mo). Indicates needs by pointing. Responds to sense of time.	Although often reminded "not to touch," is unable to comply. Gains comfort from parent's voice even if the parent is not in view. Misplaced objects of comfort lead to great emotional upset. Tolerates frustration poorly. Initial response to reason may be positive; however, without consistent effect. May regress to clinging, infantlike behavior. Attempts to "bargain" to avoid procedures.	Prepare immediately before procedure. Use concrete and immediate rewards. Use simple and honest explanations; tell child of impending "prick." Use calm, positive, firm approach. Do not give choices if a child does not have any.	Same as for infant. Encourage to decorate crib with pictures of family and pets. Use cassette tapes of family voices/ songs/stories.	

Continued

Table 30-5   Nursing Actions Appropriate for the Different Developmental Stages of Childhood—cont'd

AGE GROUP	DEVELOPMENTAL STAGE AND CHARACTERISTICS	CHILD'S RESPONSE TO ILLNESS OR PROCEDURES	PREPARATION OF CHILD	FAMILY INVOLVEMENT	NURSING IMPLICATIONS
Preschool (4-6 yr)	Initiative vs. Guilt Exhibits general interest and fears mutilation. Makes decisions, seeks companionship. Able to follow directions. *Preoperational thoughts:* "Magical thinking." Egocentric. Animalistic. Short attention span. *Fears* Bodily injury. Loss of control. The unknown, the dark, and being alone.	Illness or pain often perceived as punishment. Needs support to cope with intrusiveness of IV procedure. Curious about IV but able to keep from touching with frequent reminders. May appear compliant but may be withdrawn and resistant.	Give control when possible; child should be active in decisions. Explain procedure in simple terms. Explain relationship between cause, illness, and treatment (IV is not a punishment). Prepare just before procedure. Use equipment to teach (with dolls and stuffed animals). Encourage assistance by child (open Band-Aids, cleanse area). Explain that holding still is a big help and that it is OK to cry. Never bribe or threaten ("If you don't drink, you'll get an IV.") Praise cooperation.	Parents should provide comfort and support but should not help restrain. Child may be more cooperative if parent is not present.	*Safety* Same as for toddlers. Needs minimal restraints; needs maximum mobility to master surroundings. Address fears and misconceptions even if not expressed. Allow child to identify with you. Understand resistance as fear and reassure. Do not participate in discipline of child.
School age (6-12 yr)	Sense of Industry Enjoys learning. Struggles between mastery and failure. Wants to participate. Needs to know how things work. Concrete Operational Thinking Understands rules and directions. Ability to understand relationship between illness and treatment. Increased awareness of danger. Improved concept of time. Increased self control. Peer group increasingly important. *Fears* Body mutilation. Loss of control. Inability to live up to expectations of others. Death.	Important for child to feel a sense of control. May interpret illness as a punishment. Does not accept illness because of fear of death. Develops "magical" sense of denial (healthy for age).	Maintain privacy. Prepare several hours in advance. Use diagrams, models. Explain each step. Offer choices as much as possible. Allow child to help. Reassure that crying is OK. Reassure that you will help him or her to hold still. Games can be effective to gain cooperation. Give immediate tactile and verbal praise for cooperation. Provide distraction during procedure.	Parents present at child's choice. Prepare family and child together. Encourage family to arrange for peer visitation. Stress to parents the child's need for independence with self care. Parent can be "silent partner" in helping child understand.	Provide privacy. Allow child to assist with procedure. Offer encouragement and praise for cooperation. Allow child to assist with recording intake/output. *Safety* Impulsivity and playfulness may lead to accidents—remind child often of safe mobility with IV equipment connections. Provide distractions. Keep security objects close by. Allow as much mobility as possible.

| Adolescence (13-19 yr) | Sense of Identity Vacillates between dependence and independence. Questions authority figures. Strong need for privacy. Formal Operational Thought Able to understand abstract ideas. Able to consider alternatives. Little understanding of how body works. Peer acceptance important. **Fears** Loss of control. Altered body image. Separation from peers. | Hyperresponsive to pain; minor illness magnified. Regresses to lower developmental stage of behavior. Resistant to parent and authority figures. May be noncompliant with medication and treatment plan. Increased need for peer contact. Illness is threat to body integrity. Disease = ugliness. | Offer choices. Preparation several hours to days in advance is vital. Explain using adult terms. Show equipment, and explain function and allow time for questions. | Direct explanations to adolescent while parent is present. Reassure family of need for adolescent to participate and make decisions. Explain therapy as to an adult patient. Encourage family to bring friends. | Approach with sensitivity; adolescents react to "how" it is said rather than "what" is said. Provide privacy. Tolerate need to have "own stuff." Encourage to record own intake and output. Engage to help set up equipment. Set consistent behavioral limits, but allow some leeway in choices (e.g., if you want to take a shower now, I can start your IV later). Allow to wear own clothes. **Safety** May need supervision to ensure safety of IV site if "clowning around." Teach adolescent to report observations about IV. Monitor equipment; may tamper with pump rates. |

Vital signs

Temperature. Body temperature may initially be elevated during dehydration but becomes subnormal as dehydration progresses. With each degree of rise or fall in body temperature, the basal metabolic rate increases. This increase in basal metabolic rate results in additional fluid and caloric maintenance requirements of 10% to 12% above maintenance requirements (see Table 30-4). Upon admission to the hospital or home health care agency, a baseline body temperature should be assessed. In many health care settings, the traditional method of using the rectal route has been replaced by safer methods of body temperature recording. Rectal temperature assessment has the risk of perforating the wall of the rectum. This method is definitely contraindicated in conditions such as thrombocytopenia, neutropenia, and imperforate anus, or after rectal surgery.[6] Oral temperature measurement should be assessed on children older than 2 years of age who are cognitively able. More recently, devices that measure tympanic temperature in the ear have been used; these devices respond quickly and are comfortable but are accurate only if the probe fits well in the ear canal (usually in children older than 1 year of age). Axillary temperature measurements are often obtained in children up to 4 to 6 years of age or in any child who is uncooperative, is unconscious, is seizure prone, or has had recent oral surgery. The normal axillary temperature range is 36.5° to 37.0° C (97.9° to 98° F).

Pulse. The apical pulse is the best site for auscultation of the heart rate in an infant and child. Normal apical ranges for an infant are 120 to 140 beats/min. As the child grows older, the heart rate decreases to adult values of 60 to 80 beats/min. An apical rate in a resting infant of 80 to 100 beats/min is considered *bradycardia,* and an apical rate of greater than 160 to 180 beats/min is considered *tachycardia.* Changes in rate and rhythm may indicate changes in circulating blood volume or electrolyte imbalances. In the early stages of volume depletion, the pulse is usually tachycardic and becomes more rapid, weak, and thready as the condition worsens. The pulse bounds during fluid overload.

Evaluations of the presence and the quality of peripheral pulses and the adequacy of end-organ perfusion are key elements in the clinical assessment of shock in children. The carotid, axillary, brachial, radial, femoral, dorsalis pedis, and posterior tibial pulses are all easily palpable in the healthy child. A discrepancy between the central (apical) and peripheral pulses may result from vasoconstriction associated with hypovolemia or may be an early sign of diminished stroke volume. The pulse volume is directly related to blood pressure (BP). As shock progresses, the pulse pressure (systolic − diastolic = pulse pressure) narrows, resulting in a weak and thready pulse that may eventually become impossible to palpate. The rate of tachycardia also increases as the condition worsens. In septic shock or fluid overload, the pulse pressure widens and is represented by a bounding pulse.[7]

Respirations. The normal range of respiration in the infant is 30 to 60 breaths/min, and normal respiratory rate diminishes slowly during the toddler stage to near adult levels. An infant with a respiratory rate greater than 60 breaths/min is generally considered *tachypneic.* *Apnea* is defined as a 15- to 20-second or longer period without respiration. The infant's respiratory rate may be increased in either fluid depletion or fluid overload. Alterations in respiratory rate may represent inadequate oxygenation or an attempt to compensate for metabolic acid-base imbalances (i.e., respiratory rate is increased in acidosis and is decreased in alkalosis). The child who is hyperventilating either from anxiety or from a disease process is likely to develop respiratory alkalosis.

Breath sounds and rate should be noted when respirations are assessed. Moist breath sounds (rales) may be an indication of fluid overload.

Blood pressure. To accommodate the various sizes of children, BP cuff sizes range from newborn to adult. To obtain an accurate reading, the appropriate sized cuff should be used. The width of the BP cuff should be sufficient to cover 75% of the upper arm between the top of the shoulder and the olecranon. There should be enough room in the antecubital fossa to accommodate the bell of the stethoscope. The length of the cuff must completely surround the circumference of the limb with or without overlapping. Sites other than the brachial artery that can be used to obtain a BP measurement include the radial, popliteal, dorsalis pedis, and posterior tibial arteries.[5]

If an electronic BP monitor is used, the manufacturer's instructions and guidelines for correct cuff size should be followed. Even with an oscillometric device, movement interferes with the accuracy of measurement. The child should be quiet and the extremity stabilized during the procedure.

A listing of normal pediatric vital signs is provided in Table 30-6. BP readings in children normally run much lower than adult levels and vary upward with age.

Changes in BP may indicate a change in circulating blood volume. In fluid-volume deficit, the BP is usually decreased. When a fluid-volume overload exists, the BP is generally elevated. In infants and children, however, the BP should *not* initially be relied on as an accurate measurement of shock. Normal BP may be maintained as the circulatory system compensates with vasoconstriction, tachycardia, and increased cardiac contractility. The other assessment signs discussed, including skin color, temperature, fluid-volume, quality of peripheral pulses, mental status, heart rate, and urinary output, are the best status indicators. Hypotension, which occurs late and often suddenly, is a sign of cardiovascular decompensation. Once even a slight drop in BP occurs, it must be treated seriously because cardiopulmonary arrest often soon follows.[7]

Skin. Skin color, turgor (elasticity), temperature, moisture, and texture all relate to the child's state of hydration and nutrition. With fluid-volume deficit, the skin tends to be cool and dry and exhibits poor color return when pressure is gently applied to skin. Cyanosis and mottling usually occur in more advanced stages of fluid deficit. If fever is also present, the skin may be warm and moist. Skin turgor is generally a good indicator of fluid-volume status. Skin turgor is assessed by gently grasping the skin on the abdomen or inner thigh between the thumb and index finger and then quickly releasing. Good hydration is exhibited by an immediate return of the skin to its normal position. Fluid deficit may be present when the skin remains suspended (called *tenting*) for a brief period after being released.

Usually, the skin begins to demonstrate some sign of tenting

Table 30-6   Pediatric Vital Signs (Normal Values)

Age	Heart Rate/min	Respiratory Rate/min	Blood Pressure		Temperature	
			Systolic	Diastolic	Celsius	Fahrenheit
Infants	120-160	30-60	74-100	50-70		
Toddlers	90-140	24-40	80-112	50-80		
Preschoolers	80-110	22-34	82-110	50-78		
School-aged children	75-100	18-30	84-120	54-80		
Adolescents	60-90	12-16	94-140	62-88		
Any Age						
Oral					36.4-37.4	97.6-99.3
Rectal					36.2-37.8	97-100
Axillary					35.9-36.6	96.6-98

From Testerman EJ: Current trends in pediatric total parenteral nutrition, *JIN* 12(3):152, 1989.

with mild (less than 5%) fluid deficit. However, tenting is not consistently a reliable sign of hydration status. Variables such as hypertonic dehydration may be evidenced by doughy or rubbery skin, and conditions such as obesity, abdominal distension, and malnutrition may also affect the elasticity of the skin.[8]

Edema is a sign of fluid-volume overload or fluid shift from the intravascular space to the interstitial space. In infants, edema is most noticeable in the periorbital and scrotal areas, especially after the infant has been lying flat for a period. Occasionally, the eyes are so puffy that vision is impaired or eyelids are even swollen shut. As the child grows, the locations of visible edema shift to the abdomen and extremities. The presence and severity of edema can be assessed by indenting the skin with a finger and then releasing. The severity is indicated by the indentation (pitting) left by the finger.

End-organ perfusion is assessed via the skin, brain, and kidneys. Decreased perfusion in the skin is an early sign of shock. In healthy Caucasian children, the hands and feet are pink, warm, and dry. As cardiac output decreases, the most distal extremities become cool. In African-American children and children of other ethnic backgrounds, a grayish pallor may be indicative of poor perfusion and decreased temperature. As the condition progresses, the coolness advances toward the trunk. After the skin is blanched, a slow capillary refill (more than 2 seconds) indicates low cardiac output. Poor perfusion is also indicated by mottling, pallor, and peripheral cyanosis, except in newborns, who normally have acrocyanosis. Severe vasoconstriction is represented by pallor in older children and grayish color in newborns.[7]

Mucous membranes. Moistness of the mucous membranes provides information regarding the hydration status of a child. Dryness of the mucous membranes occurs early in dehydration. The area of the mouth where the gums and cheek meet is often the best place to assess moistness because it remains moist, even during mouth breathing. Longitudinal fissures on the tongue are an indication of dehydration, as is lack of tears in an infant older than 3 months of age. The lack of tears and the presence of dark circles around sunken eyes are signs of dehydration that occur later in the progression of the condition.[5,8]

Fontanels. The anterior fontanel remains open until the child is approximately 2 years of age. This characteristic pro-

vides an additional tool with which the hydration status of infants can be assessed. When an infant is in a normal sitting position, the anterior fontanel is either completely flat or slightly sunken. In states of fluid deficit, the fontanel is depressed. A bulging fontanel indicates increased pressure caused by either cerebral edema or fluid-volume excess.

Urine. An accurate record of urinary output is an important element in the management of fluid balance. Urine output that is greater than or less than the intake suggests a fluid excess or deficit. The time, amount, and color of urine and its specific gravity should be documented in the medical record. The frequency of monitoring of urine output (ranging from every hour to every 8 hours) is determined by the seriousness of the child's condition. In fluid homeostasis, 1 to 2 ml of urine output per kilogram of body weight per hour is expected.

A specific gravity value between 1.002 and 1.030 is usually an indication of fluid balance. Fluid restriction or deficit is reflected by a high specific gravity, whereas a low measurement reflects fluid retention or overload. In young infants, however, the immature renal system is less able to concentrate urine, causing the results of the measurement to be less accurate. This fact should be considered when specific gravity results are assessed; a normal measurement of specific gravity in an infant with fluid-volume deficit may be misleading.[5]

Children who are toilet trained present little difficulty in the monitoring of their urine output. Often, parents and older children can help record the time and amount. Children who are not toilet trained present a greater challenge. Pediatric urine collection containers are available; however, they are not easily applied and can be irritating to the skin. When hourly output records are necessary in critical care units, the child usually has a ureteral or urethral catheter in place. In pediatric units, the usual practice is to weigh the diapers. The weight of the dry diaper is subtracted from that of the wet diaper, allowing the nurse to determine urinary output. The weight in grams equals the volume voided in milliliters. A simple way to keep track of diaper weights is to write the weight on the clean diaper before placing it on the child. With this method, should another caregiver change the diaper, the comparison weight is readily available.

Urine can be obtained from a wet diaper by several methods. It can be aspirated directly from a wet diaper by using a syringe without a needle. However, ultraabsorbent disposable diapers, which contain a gel, can alter the results of some laboratory tests. If cloth diapers or ultraabsorbent disposable diapers are used, cotton balls or small gauze pads can be placed into the diaper. The urine can then be extracted by either aspirating the material with a needleless syringe or expressing urine with a gloved hand from the gauze or cotton ball into a container.

Neurologic status. In young children, neurologic status is more difficult to assess than in adults. Developmentally, young children are unable to respond verbally to questions regarding orientation to surroundings. Changes in behavior or mood, such as hyperirritability when touched or refusal to drink fluids, may indicate a change in the child's neurologic status. A child older than 2 months of age should be able to normally focus on his or her parent's face and be attracted by bright objects. Failure to recognize parents may be an early sign of hypoperfusion to the brain. The family is usually the first to detect this but may only be able to interpret this change as "something wrong." A usual sign of neurologic involvement in the infant is a high-pitched cry. Changes in the level of consciousness may be an indication of fluid-volume or electrolyte imbalance. Infants are more sensitive to excess sodium concentrations in the blood (hypernatremia) and abruptly demonstrate signs of lethargy, somnolence, and hypersensitivity to noise and touch. Twitching, tremors, or convulsions may be noted in more advanced cases. Cerebral edema caused by fluid retention can be displayed by vomiting, restlessness, irritability, and even convulsions, as well as complaints of headache in older children.[5,8]

FLUID THERAPY
Maintenance fluid requirements

Maintenance fluid requirements for a 24-hour period are based on the child's weight in kilograms. The regimen for normal maintenance fluids is based on water and electrolyte output via insensible fluid losses, gastrointestinal fluids, and urine. Because the metabolic rate in infants and children is higher than that in adults, fluid losses are also greater than in adults, and maintenance requirements are increased. The amount of fluid lost before treatment is determined by comparison of preillness and current weight and by clinical signs of deficit. Maintenance fluid requirements[4,5,8] for children are usually calculated by the guidelines in Table 30-7.

Example: Fluid maintenance for a 14-kg infant would be 1200 ml/24 hr:

```
1000 ml (for first 10 kg)
+200 ml (50 ml × 4 kg)
1200 ml/24 hr
```

Once the 24-hour maintenance fluid requirement has been calculated, the need for additional fluids must be evaluated. Conditions in which fluid requirements are increased include fluid loss before treatment (e.g., gastroenteritis), increased metabolism (e.g., fever, hyperthyroidism), concurrent losses (e.g., wound drainage, nasogastric suction), or the need to dilute urine (e.g., before chemotherapy).

Table 30-7   Maintenance Fluid Requirements for Children

Newborn (0 to 72 hr)	60 to 100 ml/kg/24 hr
0 to 10 kg	100 ml/kg/24 hr
11 to 20 kg	1000 ml for first 10 kg + 50 ml/kg/24 hr for each kilogram over 10 kg
21 to 30 kg	1500 ml for first 20 kg + 20 ml/kg/24 hr for each kilogram over 20 kg

Replacement (deficit) therapy

Replacement therapy is divided into phases. The first phase is initial management or rapid delivery of fluid therapy; the second phase, repletion or maintenance therapy; and the third, early recovery.

Phase I: initial management. In children with fluid-volume deficit, replacement of vascular volume is essential. These children require immediate infusion of fluids, especially with evidence of poor tissue perfusion or changes in vital signs and neurologic status. These symptoms or those associated with moderate to severe dehydration indicate the need for rapid fluid management.

A crystalloid solution (Ringer's lactate solution or 0.9% sodium chloride) 20 ml/kg is infused as rapidly as possible over 20 minutes. If the child has a documented normal blood glucose level or is known to have diabetes, dextrose solutions should be omitted to prevent hyperglycemia, which may induce an osmotic diuresis. Otherwise, Ringer's lactate solution is preferred because it prevents hyperchloremic acidosis, which may result from the infusion of large volumes of sodium chloride. The child's condition is then reassessed. If the response to the therapy is poor, an additional bolus of the initial solution is given. The child continues to be evaluated for the need of additional boluses, invasive monitoring, or the implementation of repletion (maintenance) therapy.[4,8]

The type of solution used for initial volume expansion for a child in hypovolemic shock is controversial. Crystalloid solutions are readily available, less expensive, and free from reactions and complications that can occur with blood and colloid products. Crystalloids expand the interstitial water space and replace sodium effectively; however, they are not efficient at expanding the circulating blood volume. Blood and colloids, such as 5% albumin, fresh-frozen plasma, and dextran, are much more effective at expanding the circulating blood volume than crystalloids. The major disadvantages to these products are the cost and the risk of potential transfusion reaction or complication. Therefore an initial bolus of 20 ml/kg is given, usually with a crystalloid solution. If further boluses are required, either a crystalloid or colloid solution may be given. Based on reassessment of the child's condition, repeated boluses are administered as needed. According to the *Textbook of Pediatric Advanced Life Support*,[7] a child with hypovolemic shock often requires at least 40 to 60 ml/kg in the first hour of resuscitation; occasionally up to 100 to 1000 ml/kg may be

Table 30-8   Replacement and Maintenance Requirements

Amount of Deficit	Formula for Calculating Amount of Replacement Fluid
Mild (5%)	Maintenance + (maintenance × 0.5)
Moderate (10%)	Maintenance + (maintenance × 1.0)
Severe (15%)	Maintenance + (maintenance × 1.5)

needed in the first few hours. In children with septic shock, at least 60 to 80 ml/kg is often required in the first hour. Regular reassessment of the child's condition and infusion of sufficient amounts of fluid are the keys to successful fluid therapy for hypovolemic shock.

Phase II: repletion and maintenance therapy. During this second phase (2 to 24 hours after onset of the deficit), replacement is combined with maintenance requirements. Acid-base and electrolyte disturbances are partially corrected. The simple formulas in Table 30-8 incorporate replacement and maintenance requirements for mild, moderate, and severe volume deficit.

Example: A 10-kg infant has a maintenance fluid requirement of 1000 ml/24 hr. The replacement amounts for 24 hours are shown in the following.

Mild (5%)	Maintenance + ½ maintenance
	1000 + (1000 × 0.5) = 1500 ml/24 hr
Moderate (10%)	Maintenance + full maintenance
	1000 + (1000 × 1.0) = 2000 ml/24 hr
Severe (15%)	Maintenance + 1½ maintenance
	1000 + (1000 × 1.5) = 2500 ml/24 hr

Note that the amount of fluid infused during the initial phase of replacement should be subtracted, and any ongoing losses sustained should be added to these amounts.

Phase III: early recovery. Early recovery, which can last from 24 to 96 hours, is aimed at correcting the remaining deficits occurring in hypertonic dehydration. These electrolyte deficits need to be corrected slowly so as not to impair neurologic status. By this time, the child usually is well enough to ingest some fluids orally.

Fluid-Volume Deficit

Any abnormal fluid loss or reduction in fluid intake can lead to depletion of fluid in the extracellular and intracellular compartments. The most common cause of fluid loss in children is gastroenteritis. Children with diarrhea accompanied by nausea or vomiting are at a greater risk for developing dehydration. In these children, oral fluid intake is reduced in response to the symptoms and therefore cannot balance the amount of fluid lost through the stools. A fluid-volume deficit results, and physiologic changes occur that progress as the condition worsens (Table 30-9).

Hypovolemic shock is a common problem in children who are in need of emergency care. Trauma and burns are obvious causes, but hypovolemic shock can also occur with gastroenteritis and diabetic ketoacidosis. Sepsis in a child can develop into septic shock, which is not classified as hypovolemic but equally requires fluid resuscitation. The initial therapies for hypovolemic and septic shock are similar, and both require immediate vascular access. In traumatic shock, large volumes of blood and fluid are required; therefore IV access sites should be adequate to meet these needs. In emergency situations in which large volumes of fluids are needed, two peripheral IVs, in 24, 22, or 20 gauge, or a short-term emergency central access device, such as a nontunneled femoral line, can provide adequate vascular access in a child.[7,9]

The clinical assessment and laboratory data determine the urgency and the type of therapy required. The degree of fluid loss is categorized according to the percentage of total body weight lost: mild (less than 5%), moderate (5% to 10%), and severe (more than 10%).

The infusion of IV fluids into infants and children with fluid-volume deficit requires an understanding of the various types of deficit and the specific therapies required. In addition to being characterized by degree of fluid loss, fluid-volume deficit (dehydration) is also categorized by type—isotonic, hypotonic, or hypertonic, depending on the changes in the child's serum sodium.

Isotonic

Isotonic fluid-volume deficit is the most common form of dehydration. In this form, the loss of solute and the loss of water are proportional. Dehydration is also considered isotonic when the losses are not proportional but the kidneys are able to compensate. Because the net fluid loss is isotonic, no redistribution between the intracellular fluid and the extracellular fluid occurs. The total loss is from the extracellular compartment, resulting in a reduction in plasma volume and circulating blood volume.

Correction of fluid and electrolyte imbalances is easily achieved in patients with this type of dehydration. Depending on the severity of the imbalance, an initial bolus of 0.9% sodium chloride or Ringer's lactate solution may be administered at 20 ml/kg of body weight. An infusion of maintenance fluids follows the bolus.

Hypotonic

Patients with hypotonic dehydration have a net loss that is hypertonic; that is, the loss of sodium is greater than the loss of water. This situation causes the extracellular fluid to shift into the intracellular space, where the fluid is less hypotonic. This phenomenon commonly occurs when a hypotonic solution (glucose in water, ginger ale) is given orally to the child in an attempt to replace fluid lost through vomiting or diarrhea. The sugar is taken up by cells and leaves the free water in the extracellular space. The child exhibits severer signs and symptoms of deficit in hypotonic dehydration than in the other forms of dehydration.

Treatment for this type of dehydration is similar to that for isotonic dehydration, except that extra sodium is added. With

Table 30-9   Clinical Assessment and Infusion Treatment for Types of Fluid-Volume Deficit (Dehydration)

DESCRIPTION	ISOTONIC	HYPOTONIC	HYPERTONIC
TYPE OF LOSS	Solute and water loss proportional	Greater solute loss than water	Greater water loss than solute
ICF and ECF fluid shift	None	From ECF to ICF	From ICF to ECF
Plasma volume	Decreased	Decreased	Maintained
Serum sodium level (mEq/L)	125-150	<125	>150
Cause	GI fluid loss Urine loss Decreased oral intake	GI fluid loss with hypotonic oral intake (glucose in water, ginger ale)	GI fluid loss with hypertonic oral intake (boiled skim milk) Diabetes insipidus Fever Hyperventilation
CLINICAL SIGNS			
Skin	Poor turgor, cold, dry, dusky	Very poor turgor, cold, clammy, dusky	Fair turgor; cold, thick, and "doughy" skin
Eyes	Sunken	Sunken	Sunken
Mucous membranes	Dry	Slightly dry	Parched
Fontanels	Depressed	Depressed	Depressed
Pulse	Rapid	Rapid	Moderately rapid
Blood pressure	Low	Very low	Moderately low
Neurologic status	Irritable or lethargic	Lethargic, coma, seizure	Hyperirritable, high-pitched cry, seizure
FLUID REPLACEMENT			
Resuscitation	Bolus of 0.9% sodium chloride or Ringer's lactate (20 ml/kg over 20 minutes)	Bolus of 0.9% sodium chloride or Ringer's lactate (20 ml/kg over 20 minutes)	None
Replacement	5% dextrose in water and 0.45% sodium chloride	5% dextrose in water and 0.9% sodium chloride If severely symptomatic, 3% sodium chloride (4 ml/kg over 10 minutes) with close monitoring	5% dextrose in water and 0.225%-0.45% sodium chloride If hypertensive, 0.9% sodium chloride or Ringer's lactate solution (20 ml/kg) over 1 hr
Infusion	Half of deficit replaced in first 8 hr, remaining over next 16 hr	Half of deficit replaced in first 8 hr, remaining over next 16 hr	Slow and gradual over 48 hr
Sodium (mEq)	2-3 mEq/kg/24 hr	2-3 mEq/kg/24 hr plus replacement. Sodium should only be increased ≤2 mEq/L/hr up to a serum level of 120 mEq/L	Sodium should not be reduced >2 mEq/L/hr
Potassium	2-3 mEq/kg/24 hr	2-3 mEq/kg/24 hr	2-3 mEq/kg/24 hr

ICF, Intracellular fluid; *ECF,* extracellular fluid; *GI,* gastrointestinal.

the addition of this sodium, the dehydration changes from hypotonic to isotonic. Maintenance fluids and replacement fluids for ongoing losses are administered in a similar fashion to therapy for isotonic dehydration. In severe cases of hypotonic dehydration, the child is treated with 3% sodium chloride solution, which is administered until the plasma level reaches 120 mEq/L. Hyponatremia should be corrected slowly, raising the serum sodium level no greater than 2 mEq/L/hr.[4]

Hypertonic

Hypertonic fluid-volume deficit has a proportionately greater loss of water than sodium; the net loss of fluid is hypotonic. Because of the hypertonicity of the extracellular fluid, the fluid in the intracellular space shifts into the extracellular space. Circulating blood volume remains relatively stable. Oral fluids

with high concentrations of sodium (e.g., boiled skim milk) fed to an infant with diarrhea, diabetes insipidus, fever, or hyperventilation can cause hypertonic dehydration.

Classic signs present in a child with hypertonic dehydration include doughy skin, irritability, high-pitched cry, and seizures. Subarachnoid and subdural hemorrhage may occur in more severe cases. Hyperglycemia and hypocalcemia are often associated with this type of dehydration.

Rehydration is performed slowly—rapid rehydration can lead to serious neurologic complications, including seizures. If the child is hypertensive, 0.9% sodium chloride or Ringer's lactate solution is infused over 1 hr (20 ml/kg of body weight). If the child is not hypertensive, a hypotonic solution (0.225% to 0.45% sodium chloride in 5% dextrose) with added potassium is infused. The calculated fluid deficit volume is infused over 48 hours.[4,8]

OTHER INTRAVENOUS THERAPIES

In addition to administration of fluids, IV devices in children are also used for such therapies as medication administration, parenteral nutrition, and transfusion of blood products. An overview of these therapies as they relate to children is provided in this section; see Chapters 9 and 10 for additional information on parenteral nutrition and blood component therapy.

Medication administration

The most commonly used calculations for pediatric medication administration are those based on body weight and body surface area (by use of a nomogram). Dosing of pediatric medications is usually recommended in terms of body weight, such as doses in milligrams per kilogram. This method is most often used to calculate drug dosages for infants and children. (See Chapter 19 for more details on IV dose calculations.) There are many intravenous medications that can be administered to children, some of which have not yet been approved for use in children. Because of documented need, medications that do not have U.S. Food and Drug Administration (FDA) approval for use in children are often used, based on research studies, prior experience, and efficacy in adults. The 1998 Pediatric Studies Rule requires that new drugs (prescription drugs, including biologics) that are important in the medical treatment of children include labeling information on safe pediatric use. The information would be required when a drug is approved. For drugs already on the market, the FDA can require children's studies in certain compelling circumstances—when pediatric labeling could avoid significant risks to children, for example.[10] IV medications commonly used in children include antibiotics, heparin, vasopressors, antineoplastics, and electrolytes.

Techniques. All methods of IV medication administration, such as IV bolus and intermittent and continuous infusion, are used in the pediatric patient. In children, however, the dose and volume can be different from those used in adults, depending on the age and the size of the child. In neonates and infants, medications are commonly calculated to the tenths of a milligram or milliliter. Continuous infusions are used primarily to replace fluid-volume and nutrition, administer drugs that require maintenance of a steady blood level, and administer potent drugs that must be highly titrated to individual needs. IV medications, especially antibiotics, should be infused in a timely fashion, but with an eye to preventing fluid overload, irritation to the vessel, and infiltration.[11]

Intermittent infusions can be administered by several different methods. The in-line calibrated chamber is commonly used in general pediatric settings. The medication is injected into the in-line calibrated chamber and infused at a prescribed rate. At the completion of the infusion, the usual practice is to flush the chamber with 10 to 20 ml (depending on tubing volume) of the IV solution or a solution of 5% dextrose in water or 0.9% sodium chloride. The advantage of this method is simplicity; however, there are several disadvantages to this technique. This method is not practical for small infants whose infusion rates are slow. Also, the drug must be compatible with the primary solution, or a second tubing set-up is required. Finally, flushing the chamber with solution often fails to clear the chamber of

medication or may provide more volume than the patient can tolerate.

The retrograde method of medication infusion is commonly practiced in the neonatal intensive care unit. A specific retrograde administration set is required for this purpose. The tubing volume varies but generally holds less than 1 ml. A three-way stopcock or access port is at each end of the tubing. The retrograde tubing is attached and primed along with the primary administration set. (Retrograde primary administration sets are also available.) To administer medications via the system, a medication-filled syringe is attached to the port most proximal to the patient, and an empty syringe is connected to the port most distal from the patient. The clamp between the port and the child is closed, and the medication is injected distally up the tubing (away from the child). The fluid in the retrograde tubing is displaced upward in the tubing into the empty syringe. Both syringes are removed, the lower clamp is opened, and the medication is then infused into the patient at the prescribed rate. The medication volume is then automatically incorporated into the regulated amount of fluid to be infused. This method is often used in infants who cannot tolerate a rapid infusion rate or additional fluid volume; in this method, the medication infuses at the same rate set for the IV infusion.

An increasingly popular and very accurate method of IV medication administration in infants and children is the syringe pump. The syringe pump can be connected via an extension set directly onto an intermittent vascular access device or in a piggyback fashion into the primary line. A syringe of diluted medication, prefilled by the pharmacy or by the nurse caring for the patient, is attached to microbore tubing, and the medication is then infused at a prescribed rate.

Several manufacturers of large-volume infusion pumps also provide a syringe-tubing set combination that is ideal for administering intermittent doses of medications. These set combinations reduce the flush volume required to clear the tubing and allow the large pump to act like a syringe pump.[11]

Parenteral nutrition

IV nutrition is administered when patients cannot or will not use their gastrointestinal tract or when they require supplemental calories for growth or healing. The goal of parenteral nutrition (PN) is to meet anabolic needs and allow normal growth and development. Because the metabolic rate of children is greater than that of adults, children require greater fluid and caloric intake per kilogram (see Table 30-4). Some indications for parenteral nutrition in children are congenital or acquired anomalies of the digestive tract (e.g., inflammatory bowel disease, Hirschsprung's disease, short-bowel syndrome, pancreatitis) and disease states that may increase the risk of starvation (e.g., cancer, cystic fibrosis, acquired immunodeficiency syndrome [AIDS]). Candidates for parenteral nutrition therapy are identified via the physical examination and nutritional evaluation, including such measurements as weight loss, falling behind normal percentile for height and weight on the growth chart, and abnormal laboratory values such as albumin.[9]

The parenteral nutrition solution is made up of several components, depending on the status of the child; these solutions can be individualized to fit specific pediatric calorie and nutrient needs (Table 30-10).[12] The basic components of PN are protein, carbohydrates, fat, electrolytes, vitamins, trace elements, and minerals. Protein, for growth, is administered in the form of crystalline amino acids; infants younger than 6 months require a special amino acid mixture that mimics breast milk to provide protein.[13] Dextrose is used as the carbohydrate source, providing energy so that the body does not break down protein or fat to meet metabolic needs.

When treating children, it is often difficult to balance fluid needs with calorie needs. A large volume would be necessary to infuse enough calories to meet a child's needs via the peripheral vein. Therefore PN is often concentrated in a smaller volume and administered via a central vein. A concentration of greater than 10% dextrose must be delivered via a central venous catheter (CVC) to prevent vein injury or extravasation, should infiltration occur. Dextrose 12.5% may be administered peripherally for short term to maximize calories; however, this solution tends to be irritating, and central access should be considered in the face of high carbohydrate needs.

The amounts of electrolytes, minerals, trace elements, and medications are individualized for the growth and nutritional needs of each child. For children receiving long-term PN, continued growth can change the nutritional requirements, so careful monitoring is essential. Fat emulsions or lipids provide a high calorie content per volume, making them ideal sources of calories for children.[13] Fat emulsions also buffer the irritating effects that glucose tends to exert on the vein. Lipids should be infused cautiously in patients with infections, compromised renal function, or hyperbilirubinemia. In premature infants younger than 30 weeks of age with hyperbilirubinemia, lipid hydrolysis releases free fatty acids that can displace bilirubin from albumin and increase the chance of kernicterus, or bilirubin encephalopathy. A smaller dosage (1 g/kg/day) and a long infusion time (15 hours or more) tend to reduce this risk in premature infants.[14]

PN can be administered in the hospital or the home; home PN is often administered via the central route and is cycled over 12 to 18 hours, usually at night, so that the child may function normally during the day. Home PN is usually initiated in the hospital. When the child is stable and the infusion process for home PN has been mastered by the caregiver or caregivers, with appropriate participation of the child (depending on his or her level of development), home PN may be instituted.

Continuous monitoring is required to ensure safe, efficacious infusion of PN that meets the changing needs of the child. This includes monitoring the infusion itself and assessing laboratory and nutritional measurements on a scheduled basis.

PN has its share of complications, which, as demonstrated in Table 30-11, can be divided into metabolic and catheter related. A multidisciplinary team approach can result in successful clinical application and monitoring of PN, with a minimal number of complications. Since the first documented success of infant PN in 1944[15] and the well-known efforts of Willmore and Dudrick in 1968,[16] the technique for infusing nutrition via the venous system has been continually refined over the past three decades, greatly improving the quality of life and chance for survival for children who undergo this therapy.

Transfusion therapy

The basic principles of blood component therapy for adults (see Chapter 10) also apply to children. Children are unique with regard to maturation of their hematopoietic system and special requirements related to their smaller vein size and volume of blood products to be infused. During the last few weeks of intrauterine life, maternal gamma immunoglobulin crosses the placenta into the fetus; therefore the mother's serum is used for compatibility testing during the first few days of life. The fetus does not produce its own antibodies until it is exposed to foreign substances after birth. After about 1 week of life, or sooner if the newborn underwent transfusion during the first week, serum from the baby may be used for compatibility testing.[17] Other differences between children and adults include blood volume (see Table 30-2), red cell life span, and hemoglobin. The red blood cell of the premature newborn has a life span of 35 to 50 days, and the red cell of a term baby survives 60 to 70 days, compared with 100 to 120 days in an adult.[17] At birth, infants have a high percentage of hemoglobin F, or fetal hemoglobin, which has such a high affinity for oxygen that release of oxygen into the system is hampered. The level of hemoglobin F declines rapidly after birth, and by 6 months of age, hemoglobin F is replaced almost entirely with hemoglobin A, or adult hemoglobin, which lets go of oxygen more rapidly. In premature infants, persistence of hemoglobin F can result in hypoxia and respiratory distress. Interestingly, because hemoglobin A is a beta-chain molecule, beta-chain defects such as sickle cell anemia and the beta-thalassemias were until recently not detected until 3 to 6 months of age. Now, with genetic testing, earlier diagnosis of these disorders is possible.[17]

Specific indications for transfusion therapy are similar to those of adults and are outlined in Chapter 10. General indications for pediatric transfusion therapy include acute hemorrhage, anemia, abnormal component function (either congenital or acquired), and the presence of toxic substances, such as caused by a decrease in bilirubin levels by exchange transfusion. The most commonly used products for transfusion in children are packed red blood cells and platelets. Hemorrhage can be defined as an acute reduction of blood volume (30% to 40%) or a 20% blood volume loss with chance for recurrence. A 30% blood loss may be linked with systolic BP readings as shown in Table 30-12.[17]

Young children, particularly neonates, may become anemic because of repeated blood withdrawals for laboratory testing. Blood withdrawal volumes, especially for neonates, should be recorded in the output section of the nursing flow sheet and monitored daily.

Hemoglobin and hematocrit values are considered less reliable indicators of blood loss. Activity level and cardiopulmonary status should be assessed before transfusion therapy is initiated in a child, because an unstressed child can tolerate hemoglobin levels of 3 to 6 g/dl without signs of heart failure or tissue hypoxia. Children usually undergo transfusion if hemoglobin levels fall below 6 g/dl.

Table 30-10   Components of Pediatric Total Parenteral Nutrition

COMPONENT	USE	DEFICIENCY	RECOMMENDED DAILY DOSE	COMPLICATIONS
Water	Vehicle for delivery of nutrients; helps meet daily requirements	Fluid deficit—decreased skin turgor, decreased weight, decreased tears, decreased CVP, lower temperature, increased heart rate, increased respirations	<10 kg, 100-150 ml/kg >10 kg, 1500-2000 ml/m²	Fluid excess, dilutional hyponatremia
Calories	Meet energy needs to promote growth and development (anabolism)	Catabolism—negative nitrogen balance, negative growth and development	<10 kg, 100-120 cal/kg >10 kg, 2000 cal/m²	
Glucose (1 g = 3.4 kcal)—most important macronutrient	Maintain positive nitrogen balance (anabolism); Preferred energy source for CNS and RBC	Protein catabolism, negative nitrogen balance	<10 kg, 20-30 g/kg >10 kg, 25-30 g/kg	Phlebitis, diuresis, hyperglycemia, hypoglycemia, hyperosmotic, hyperglycemic nonketotic acidosis
Protein (1 g = 4.0 kcal) Essential: lysine, leucine, isoleucine, methionine, phenylalanine, threonine, tryptophan, valine arginine, histidine Nonessential: proline, alanine, serine, tyrosine, glycine, cystine	Growth and tissue synthesis; provides energy if shortage of glucose and fat occurs; buffer in the extracellular and intracellular fluids	Kwashiorkor: edema, anemia, fatty degeneration of liver, scaling dermatitis, infection confirmed by serum transferrin; marasmus: adipose and skeletal muscle atrophy, weight loss, depressed skin test reactivity to antigens, lethargy, dehydration; mixed disorder: kwashiorkor and marasmus	<10 kg, 2-3 g/kg >10 kg, 1-2 g/kg	Azotemia, hyperammonemia, abnormal plasma amniograms, hepatotoxicity
Fats (1 g = 9 cal) Components: soybean or safflower oil Fatty acids: linoleic, palmitic, oleic, steric acid, egg yolk, phospholipids, glycerol	Energy—prevent fatty acid deficiency and provide concentrated caloric source	Mild diarrhea, dry and thickened desquamated skin, hair loss, brittle osteoporotic bones, thrombocytopenia	0.5-4.0g/kg	Altered pulmonary function, deposition of pigmented material in macrophages, kernicterus, coronary artery disease, spurious hyperbilirubinemia, spurious hyponatremia Adverse reactions: fever, chills, shivering, pain in chest or back, warmth, vomiting
Insulin	Regulates serum glucose level	Hyperglycemia		Hypoglycemia, hypokalemia
Potassium	Tissue synthesis; transports glucose and amino acids across cell membranes; regular heart rhythm; nerve impulses	Fatigue, drowsiness, decreased muscle tone, GI obstruction, flatulence, paresthesias	2-4 mEq/kg	Hyperkalemia, tissue sloughing and necrosis if infiltration present, hypokalemia, cardiac arrhythmias
Chloride	Acid-base balance	Excessive sweating, diarrhea, clouded sensorium, hypotonicity of muscles, tetany, decreased respirations	<10 kg, 3 mEq/kg >10 kg, 2-4 mEq/kg	Hyperchloremia, hypochloremia, metabolic acidosis or alkalosis

Continued

From Testerman EJ: Current trends in pediatric total parenteral nutrition, *JIN* 12(3):152, 1989; and Bilodeau JA, Poon C, Mascarenhas MR: Parenteral nutrition and care of central venous lines. In Altschuler SM, Liacouras CA, editors: *Clinical pediatric gastroenterology*, Philadelphia, 1998, Churchill Livingston.
CVP, Central venous pressure; *CNS*, central nervous system; *RBC*, red blood cell; *GI*, gastrointestinal.

Table 30-10   Components of Pediatric Total Parenteral Nutrition—cont'd

Component	Use	Deficiency	Recommended Daily Dose	Complications
Sodium	Fluid balance; acid-base balance; nerve impulses	Abdominal cramps, diarrhea, increased heart rate, apprehension, decreased blood pressure, cold and clammy skin	3-5 mEq/kg	Hypernatremia, febrile response, hyponatremia, phlebitis
Calcium	Clotting mechanism; muscle contractions; neuromuscular activity	Numbness, paresthesias, tetany	20-40 mg/kg	May cause tissue sloughing if infiltration occurs, hypercalcemic syndrome
Magnesium	Metabolism of carbohydrates and protein, enzyme activity, nerve conduction	Convulsions, tremors, increased blood pressure, increased heart rate, muscle cramps	0.25-0.5 mEq/kg	Magnesium intoxication, impaired kidney function, flushing, sweating, hypotension, respiratory paralysis, hypothermia, hypocalcemia
Folic acid	Cellular growth and development	Megaloblastic anemia	<10 kg, 0.2 mg >10 kg, 0.2 mg	Allergic reaction
Phosphates	Decrease paresthesias; regulate calcium metabolism	Muscle weakness, malaise, paresthesias, CNS irritability, confusion, seizures, obtundation, coma	2-3 mEq/kg	Reciprocal hypocalcemic tetany, hyperkalemia with potassium compound, phosphate intoxication
Acetate	Prevents acidosis	Acidosis	1-6 mEq	Alkalosis
Vitamin A	Prevents retardation of growth/visual adaptation	Night blindness, xerophthalmia, pyoderma, mucosal carotenization, drying of skin, lowered resistance to infection	1400 IU	Acute and chronic toxicity, anaphylaxis; overdose: nausea, vomiting, anorexia, drying skin and lips, malaise, irritability, headache, loss of hair
Vitamin B$_1$ (thiamine)	Absorption of protein and carbohydrates	Peripheral neuropathy, deep tendon reflex increase or absence, muscle tenderness, muscle atrophy, fatigue, decreased attention span, beriberi	0.3 mg	Warmth, pruritus, nausea, urticaria, weakness, sweating; hypersensitivity reaction
Vitamin B$_2$ (riboflavin)	Absorption of protein and carbohydrates	Cheilosis: lip inflammation, oral fissures, seborrheic dermatitis, corneal vascularization; ocular disturbances: itching, burning, corneal inflammation, dryness, dim vision, conjunctival redness, photophobia	<10 kg, 0.4 mg >10 kg, 1.1 mg	
Vitamin B$_3$ (niacin)	Absorption of protein and carbohydrates	Weakness, lassitude, anorexia, oral inflammation, indigestion, responsive dermatitis, irritability	<10 kg, 5 mg >10 kg, 12 mg	Toxic reactions: decreased glucose tolerance, skin rash, elevated uric acid levels, postural hypotension, flushing
Vitamin B$_5$ (pantothenic acid)	Absorption of protein and carbohydrates	Possible symptoms: malaise, headache, nausea, vomiting, fatigue	<10 kg, 5 mg >10 kg, 10 mg	
Vitamin B$_6$ (pyridoxine)	Absorption of protein and carbohydrates	CNS disorders, sideroblastic anemia, greater tendency to develop deficiency with vitamin B$_6$ antagonists isoniazid, penicillamine, semicarbazide, cyclosporine	>10 kg, 0.3 mg >10 kg, 0.3 mg	Paresthesia, somnolence, low serum folic acid levels

Nutrient	Function	Deficiency Signs/Symptoms	Dose	Adverse Effects/Toxicity
Vitamin B$_7$ (biotin)	Absorption of protein and carbohydrates	Fine-scale skin desquamation, anemia, anorexia, nausea, lassitude, muscle pain	<10 kg, 0.3 mg >10 kg, 0.3 mg	
Vitamin B$_{12}$ (cyanocobalamin)	Absorption of protein and carbohydrates	Pernicious anemia, glossitis, neurologic symptoms, constipation	<10 kg, 0.3 mg >10 kg, 1.5 mg	
Vitamin C	Wound healing	Scurvy, hemorrhagic petechiae, gingivitis, slow wound healing	<10 kg, 35 mg >10 kg, 40 mg	Large doses: diarrhea, renal stones
Vitamin D	Promotes absorption of calcium and phosphorus	Osteomalacia, low serum calcium level, low serum phosphate level, elevated alkaline phosphatase level, tetany resulting from hypocalcemia, rickets	<10 kg, 400 IU >400 kg, 35 IU	Weakness, headache, dry mouth, somnolence, nausea, vomiting, constipation, muscle pain, bone pain, metallic taste; hypercalcemia, hypercalciuria, hyperphosphatemia
Vitamin E	Protects red blood cells from hemolysis; enhances vitamin A; suppression of platelet aggregation	Anemia, excessive creatinuria, skeletal muscle lesions, increased platelet aggregation	<10 kg, 4 IU >10 kg, 9 IU	
Vitamin K	Promotes synthesis of active prothrombin	Prolonged prothrombin, bleeding, hematuria	<10 kg, 1.5 mg >10 kg, 2.5 mg	Anaphylaxis, pain and swelling at IV site, flushing, kernicterus
Chromium (trace mineral)	Glucose utilization and metabolism and peripheral nerve function	Insulin-resistant diabetes, neurologic changes (neuropathy)	0.14-0.2, mg/kg	Hypersensitivity, overdosage
Copper (trace mineral)	Formation of transferrin, and RBC and white blood formation	Anemia, leukopenia, neutropenia	<10 kg, 20 mg >10 kg, 300 mg	Hypersensitivity, overdosage
Manganese (trace mineral)	Activator for enzymes	Weight loss, transient dermatitis, occasional nausea and vomiting, changes in hair color	2-10 mg/kg	Hypersensitivity, overdosage
Molybdenum (controversial, trace mineral)	Unknown (part of enzymes)	In humans: impaired amino acid utilization; in animals: growth retardation, dental caries	0.2-0.25 µg/kg	Hypersensitivity, overdosage
Selenium (trace mineral)	Protects cells from oxidative damage	Muscle dysfunction (including cardiac muscle changes), muscle pain	2 µg/kg	Hypersensitivity, overdosage
Zinc (trace mineral)	Facilitates wound healing; skin hydration, senses of taste and smell	Scaling pustular rash, periorbital and nasolabial dermatitis, alopecia, change in taste or smell acuity, diarrhea, depression	<10 kg, 300 mg/kg >10 kg, 5 mg	Hypersensitivity, overdosage

IV, Intravenous.

Table 30-11   Complications of Pediatric Total Parenteral Nutrition

| METABOLIC | CATHETER RELATED | |
	CENTRAL	PERIPHERAL
Electrolyte imbalance	Bacterial or fungal sepsis	Sloughing of skin
Acid-base imbalance	Plugging or dislodgment	Phlebitis
Glycosuria	Local skin infections	Local infection
Hepatic disorders	Thrombosis of major vessel or embolism (vena cava	
Cholestasis	syndrome)	
Postinfusion hypoglycemia	Improper placement	
Essential fatty acid deficiency	Hemorrhage	
Hyperlipidemia	Extravasation of fluid	
Hyperammonemia	Pneumothorax	
Bone changes (demineralization)	Hemothorax	
Trace element deficiency	Perforation and/or infusion leaks (pericardial, pleural,	
Azotemia	mediastinal)	
Vitamin disorders	Hydrothorax	
Abnormal plasma amniograms	Arterial puncture	
Decreased pulmonary diffusion	Brachial plexus injury	
Eosinophilia	Catheter embolism	
Bleeding	Air embolism	
Adverse reactions to components	False aneurysm	
Anemia	Cardiac arrhythmia	

From Testerman EJ: Current trends in pediatric total parenteral nutrition, *JIN* 12(3):152, 1989.

Table 30-12   Effect of Blood Loss on Systolic Pressure

AGE	SYSTOLIC BLOOD PRESSURE WITH 30% BLOOD LOSS	NORMAL SYSTOLIC
<4 yr	<65 mmHg	75-110 mm Hg
5-8 yr	<75 mmHg	85-120 mm Hg
9-12 yr	<85 mmHg	95-135 mm Hg
Adolescent	<99 mmHg	100-150 mm Hg

Thrombocytopenia can result from maternally induced causes (e.g., aspirin ingestion during pregnancy), acquired disorders (e.g., idiopathic thrombocytopenia purpura), chemotherapy, or congenital dysfunction of platelets. Platelet transfusions are indicated when bleeding time is longer than 15 minutes or the platelet count is less than 20,000/mm^3 with active bleeding, less than 5000/mm^3 with or without active bleeding, or less than 50,000/mm^3 before surgery.[18,19]

Rarely is one whole unit used for a pediatric transfusion. Blood products are usually administered in increments of milliliters per kilogram based on body weight and estimated blood loss. Packed red blood cell dosage is 10 to 15 ml/kg; platelet dosage is 1 unit (50 to 70 ml) per 7 to 10 kg of body weight.[18,19] Transfusion equipment is similar to that for an adult; differences for children include use of smaller gauge needles for transfusion (27-, 25-, or 23-gauge winged-steel needles or 22- or 24-gauge catheters). Studies show that 27-gauge needles can be used to give packed red cells at a rate of up to 50 ml/hr without significant hemolysis.[20] Because of volume restrictions in many children, packed red blood cells are not usually diluted with saline; rather, a saline flush is given through the IV line to prevent mixing red cells with incompatible fluids that may cause hemolysis. In-line blood filters are used, which may be specially designed low-volume filters for children. In some cases, small aliquot bags or syringes of blood are transfused; these products are usually prefiltered by blood bank personnel during transfer to the smaller container. For accuracy, blood products are usually infused via an electronic infusion pump approved for use with blood and blood products. The rate of infusion for packed red cells is initially 5% to 10% of the total transfusion volume, given over 15 minutes.[18,19] If no adverse reaction is noted, the rate is then increased to 2 to 5 ml/kg/hr or as tolerated. Platelets are given by IV bolus or IV infusion over 30 minutes to 4 hours.[19] During transfusion, vital signs and monitoring guidelines are similar to those recommended for adults. In addition, small infants should be monitored for cold stress, hypoglycemia, and hypocalcemia. These reactions can occur because of the temperature of the blood product or the presence of a preservative in the blood, which can affect calcium and glucose levels. Another consideration in young infants and immunosuppressed patients is cytomegalovirus; it is important that the blood products be free of this virus. Although adults may also contract cytomegalovirus, infants who contract it suffer much greater consequences that can lead to death.[21]

Immunosuppressed pediatric patients, such as premature infants and children with malignancies, end-stage renal disease, or AIDS, are at risk of developing graft-versus-host disease (GVHD) if they receive transfusions of blood products that contain lymphocytes. GVHD can be prevented by giving these children transfusions with blood products that are rendered leukocyte poor, either by irradiating the product or by filtering or washing the cells before transfusion. Other transfusion reactions and complications are described in the chapter on transfusion therapy (see Chapter 10). Documenting transfusion in children is similar to requirements used with the adult patient.

Exchange transfusion

A type of therapeutic transfusion modality used almost exclusively in neonates and infants is exchange transfusion. The most common indication for exchange transfusion is hemolytic disease of the newborn, which is caused by ABO or Rh incompatibility. Hemolytic disease of the newborn caused by ABO incompatibility occurs when a mother with blood group O carries a fetus with blood group A or B, resulting in anti-A or anti-B maternal antibodies crossing the placenta and causing hemolysis of fetal red cells and mild-to-moderate anemia. This phenomenon can occur in the first child; it is not usually severe enough for exchange transfusion but instead can be treated with phototherapy or a single transfusion of red cells. In hemolytic disease of the newborn caused by Rh incompatibility, an Rh-negative mother carries an Rh-positive fetus (the father must be Rh positive for this to occur). At delivery, Rh-positive cells enter the mother's bloodstream, and Rh antibodies form in the mother. With subsequent Rh-positive pregnancies, these anti-Rh antibodies may cause hemolysis of fetal red cells that is severe enough to require exchange transfusion. This disorder rarely occurs anymore because it is preventable by the administration of anti-D immunoglobulin within 72 hours of delivery, abortion, or miscarriage. A baby born with hemolytic disease of the newborn caused by Rh incompatibility has moderate to severe anemia and can rapidly develop high serum bilirubin (unconjugated or indirect) levels, which may cause kernicterus or deposits of bilirubin in the brain tissue.

The goals of exchange transfusion are to correct anemia, lower bilirubin levels in the serum, and remove sensitized erythrocytes. Exchange transfusion is considered when bilirubin levels increase more than 1 mg/dl/hr or when they reach 15 to 16 mg/dl in the premature neonate or 20 mg/dl in the term infant. During exchange transfusion, part or all of the infant's blood volume is removed and replaced with plasma and red blood cells from one or several compatible donors. A two-volume exchange is usually performed, which replaces about 85% of the infant's blood volume and reduces the bilirubin level by approximately 50%. Albumin may be administered before the exchange to help bind bilirubin and increase the amount removed. One or two access sites, such as peripheral, central, or umbilical vessels, are used. Two sites are ideal because this allows simultaneous withdrawal and infusion of blood. Respiratory and cardiac status are monitored closely during the exchange, as is the potential for hypocalcemia and hypoglycemia. Complications of exchange transfusion include metabolic disorders, cardiopulmonary compromise, and catheter-related complications.

When transfusing a child, the child's and family's view of the transfusion, prior experience, and cultural and religious practices must be examined. Preparation should be age appropriate, as outlined earlier in this chapter. With proper preparation, close monitoring, and follow-up, IV nurses can ensure safe, efficacious transfusion therapy delivery.

PERIPHERAL ACCESS
Site selection

Whether the prescribed therapy is infused via the central or peripheral route, the main goal of therapy is to provide the treatment with the maximum amount of safety and efficiency while meeting the child's emotional needs and considering his or her developmental level. The characteristics of the prescribed therapy and the patient's physical and developmental aspects are important when the intravascular site is chosen in a child.

Characteristics of the therapy that must be considered include type and duration, rate of infusion, and expected site rotations. Physical considerations of the child include age, size, condition of the veins, reason for the therapy, general patient condition, and mobility of the child. Just as important are the child's developmental considerations: level of activity (e.g., turns, crawls, walks); gross and fine motor skills (e.g., sucks fingers, plays with own hands, holds bottle, draws, colors); sense of body image; fear of mutilation; and cognitive ability (i.e., understands and can follow directions).

The sites for peripheral IV site selection, as discussed pertaining to adults in Chapter 20, apply just as well to the pediatric patient. Although the anatomic location of the vessels are relatively the same in both children and adults, the child's smaller body and vessel size make it more difficult to successfully achieve access. However, the younger child has the advantage of additional optional site locations, including the scalp and the foot. Along with the individual preference of the clinician, each site has its own characteristics and its own advantages and disadvantages. Table 30-13 lists peripheral IV site locations and their advantages and disadvantages.

Peripheral sites

Scalp. The use of the scalp vein for IV access in infants is controversial. The veins are readily visible and easily accessed, but the cannula can be more difficult to secure. Scalp vein infusions tend to infiltrate more easily and, if not detected immediately, can cause the infant's head to appear distorted. This phenomenon results from the lack of surrounding tissue (which would help absorb some of the fluid) on the scalp. This appearance is temporary, of course, but can be alarming to the family. Using the scalp for an IV line is often most traumatic for the parents, in part because it is necessary to remove the infant's hair. This practice not only disrupts parents' perception of their beautiful baby, but can also interfere with their cultural beliefs and practices. It is important to fully explain the procedure to the parents before proceeding with scalp vein access and to give the removed hair to them as a keepsake. It is important to prepare the family for what the infant will look like once the scalp vein catheter is in place. To some parents, the visual impact of seeing a needle stuck into their baby's head is more traumatic than the reason for the treatment itself. Their lack of understanding can lead to additional anxiety and fear. Parents who do not fully understand the procedure commonly believe that the IV line is directly infusing into the child's brain.

Many pediatric facilities still use the scalp veins in neonates and young infants (Fig. 30-1), but often only after other sites have been accessed or if multiple IV sites are necessary to meet the short term plan of treatment. The scalp IV site can be stabilized while the extremities remain free from restraints. The infant can play with his or her hands or suck his or her fingers without interruption. On a very tiny infant, the clinician monitors not only the IV line but also numerous other elements,

Table 30-13   Intravenous Sites in Children

SITE	PATIENT AGE	VEINS USED	ADVANTAGES	DISADVANTAGES
Scalp	Infant, toddler	Superficial temporal, frontal, occipital, posterior auricular, supraorbital	Easily observed, readily dilates, no valves, hands kept free, head easily stabilized, allows accessibility to extremities	Hair must be shaved, arteries hidden, infiltrates easily, caudal disfigurement with infiltration, difficult to secure device, greater family anxiety
Foot	Infant, toddler	Saphenous, median marginal, dorsal arch	Readily dilates, hands kept free, less rolling, more visible in chubby infants, easy to splint	Decreases mobility with walking, limited to smaller-gauge sizes, more difficult to advance cannula, near arteries, increased risk of phlebitis in older patients
Fingers	Toddler through adolescent	Digital	Useful if unable to access other sites, easily stabilized on tongue blade in older child	Infiltrates easily, limited to smaller gauge sizes, dependent edema masks infiltration, difficult to stabilize in small infant
Hand	All ages	Metacarpal, dorsal venous arch, tributaries of cephalic and basilic	Easily accessible, readily visible, large enough for larger size catheter, distal location, bones act as natural splints	Increased nerve endings means increased pain, difficult to anchor catheter on infant, interferes with child's activity
Forearm	All ages	Cephalic, basilic, median antebrachial	Same as for hand, keeps hands free	Difficult to observe in chubby toddlers
Antecubital	All ages	Cephalic, basilic, median	Large veins visible and palpable, preferred site in infants	Elbow joint must be maintained in extended position, limits activity, limits sites for phlebotomy, limits sites for possible peripherally inserted central catheter placement

such as oxygen saturation, cardiorespiratory status, and body temperature. Extreme care and very frequent site assessments must be made if irritating solutions, with the potential for causing extravasation injury, are infused via a scalp IV line. An injury in this area may cause lifetime disfigurement. In severely ill infants, placing the IV line in the scalp allows maximum use of body space.

The superficial temporal, frontal, occipital, and posterior auricular veins of the scalp are most commonly used for IV access. Arteries are located near the veins and are sometimes hidden within the suture lines, which makes their pulsations difficult to feel. Scalp veins do not contain valves, a characteristic that reduces the risk of trauma to the vessel at insertion. Valves can obstruct the advancement of the IV catheter during insertion on a patient at any age.

The veins of an infant are fragile, especially the ones located in the scalp. Instead of a tourniquet, a rubber band with a piece of tape attached may be used as a tourniquet, or pressure should be applied with the finger proximal to the insertion site to distend the vein. During scalp IV insertion, the needle or catheter should be aimed downward, toward the heart, so that

the flow of the infusion can follow the same direction as the venous blood returning to the heart.

Scalp veins can be used in children as old as approximately 18 months, when hair follicles mature and the epidermis toughens.

Foot. The foot is commonly used in children as old as 2 years. However, it is generally avoided in the child who has mastered walking. Several veins are highly visible and easily accessible. The most commonly accessed veins are the large and small saphenous and median marginal veins and those of the dorsal arch. The curve of the foot, especially around the ankle, may make venous entry and catheter advancement difficult. Because the dorsum of the foot has little subcutaneous tissue, it is prone to extravasation injuries and should be avoided unless absolutely necessary.[22] Infants have great strength in their legs and kick their feet vigorously, so the site should be securely taped to an armboard, carefully maintaining normal joint configuration and site visibility. Foot vein sites are also used in children older than walking age for special circumstances, including children with spina bifida, who often have decreased or no leg and foot sensation, and in emergency or intensive care situations, where other access sites may be unavailable. After the

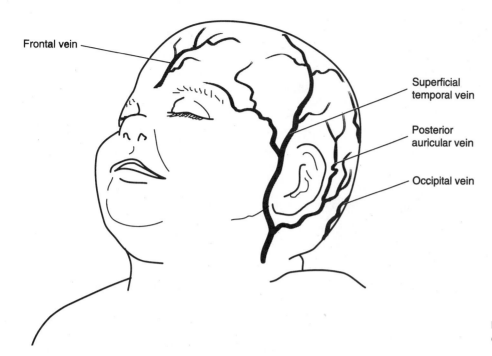

FIG. 30-1 *Scalp veins of an infant. These can be used as IV infusion sites.*

Frontal vein

Superficial temporal vein

Posterior auricular vein

Occipital vein

age of approximately 10 years, children start to experience phlebitis at rates approaching that of adults, and care should be taken to avoid using lower extremities for IV insertion unless the special circumstances identified above are documented; other access choices should be used as soon as possible.[23]

Upper extremity. As with adults, upper extremity sites are readily chosen for venous access in children. Similarly, the most distal part of the extremity is chosen first for access, choosing sites from hand to forearm, antecubital, and upper extremity veins. The dorsal metacarpal veins are smaller but sometimes may be the only vessels visible in the hand. Other veins of the hand, including the dorsal venous arch and tributaries of the cephalic and basilic veins, are generally easier to locate. The cephalic, median basilic, and median antebrachial veins in the forearm are sometimes difficult to locate in children, especially chubby babies and toddlers. Antecubital veins, although more easily located in children for emergent IV access, may need to be preserved for phlebotomy or peripherally inserted central catheter (PICC) placement.

Peripheral access devices

The guidelines for choosing the appropriate-gauge cannula are the same for children as for adults. Peripheral cannulas used in children range from 24 to 20 gauge. Peripheral access devices are available in various types and styles. Although personal preference for a certain type of device is a consideration, other factors, such as safety, patient comfort, type and length of therapy, and site of insertion, are all important.

Winged-steel needle set. The winged-steel needle set, also known as a *scalp vein needle* or *butterfly needle,* is available in odd-number sizes from 27 to 19 gauge, with the 23 gauge being the most common size used in children. Because these devices can easily become dislodged, causing injury to the child, they are best used for obtaining blood samples or for perform-

ing a one-time infusion of short duration. This set, once the only device available specifically for pediatric use, has been replaced by more contemporary types of peripheral venous access cannulas.

Over-the-needle catheter. These devices consist of a flexible catheter over an internal stylet. They are commonly used in children for peripheral short-term or intermediate-term therapy. The gauge used depends on the child's age and vein size; most sites described previously accommodate this type of catheter, including scalp veins. Gauge sizes range from 24 to 14; the size most commonly used for neonates is 24 gauge, and for children, 24 and 22 gauge, in lengths of 2 inches or shorter. Over-the-needle catheters are also available with built-in wings and extension sets. Newer devices also incorporate safety features that prevent needlestick injury, an important consideration when placing an IV in a moving target. However, when tested in actual clinical situations, early models of these devices proved awkward for placing IVs in children.[24]

Peripheral cannulas are available in many materials, including Teflon, polyurethane, and Vialon. The flexibility of over-the-needle catheters may add to the life span of the IV site. Peripheral IV sites should be rotated according to the *Infusion Nursing Standards of Practice*[25]; however, a recent research study in a large group of children demonstrated that IV catheters could be safely left in place up to 144 hours (6 days).[26] Guidelines issued by the Centers for Disease Control and Prevention regarding prevention of intravascular device–related infections make no recommendations regarding routine IV site changes in pediatric patients.[27] The condition of the site and the reason for not rotating the catheter must be documented in the child's medical record.

Midline catheter. The midline catheter is longer than a peripheral IV catheter and is intended for use in patients who require therapy of intermediate duration, from 2 to 6 weeks. It is inserted into a peripheral vein in the antecubital area and is advanced over a stylet into the upper arm veins, but not past the axilla. Because the tip is still located in a peripheral vein, manufacturers recommend infusing only isotonic and slightly hypertonic solutions and medications via midline catheters. In addition, because the midline catheter is still peripheral, site rotation recommendations related to peripheral cannulas may still apply. More published studies depicting outcome of midline catheters in children are indicated.

Venipuncture

The actual method of venipuncture is the same for children as for adults. However, certain techniques facilitate successful venipuncture in a small infant or child. Peripheral IV access in children can be made easier by following the measures described in Box 30-1.

Unlike adults, children fail to understand the need for venipuncture, may have a greater fear of pain, and generally do not hold still during the procedure. One should never attempt to start an IV line on an infant or a young child without extra help or a passive restraint device. Preferably, someone other than a family member should help hold and position the child. Child life therapists can assist with positioning-for-comfort techniques and help distract the child during the procedure. Some clinicians secure the extremity to a padded board before performing the venipuncture, whereas others apply the armboard after the IV has been placed, helping stabilize the extremity. One difficulty encountered when establishing venous access in the infant or child is unsuccessful access at the first selected site, resulting in the need for the board to be removed and reapplied at the next attempted site. Another difficulty is active resistance from the child during the insertion, resulting in dislodging of the newly inserted catheter.

Several options are available for inducing local anesthesia before venipuncture. Some institutions espouse the use of intradermal saline with preservative or lidocaine before venipuncture is performed on a child. A recent study conducted in the emergency department of a large urban pediatric hospital demonstrated that intradermal saline was as effective as lidocaine for site numbing in children 6 years of age and older.[28] The disadvantage of this practice is that an extra needlestick is involved. A eutectic mixture of anesthetic agents in cream form is now available for topical use 1 to 4 hours before the venipuncture is performed. Usually, the cream is applied to multiple sites in case the first attempt is unsuccessful. The length of time the cream must remain on the skin and reports of vein constriction may preclude its use in some situations.

The child's room needs to remain a "safe space." When possible, all attempts to start an IV line should occur in the treatment room or in an area separate from the child's room. The need to explain the procedure and completely prepare the child and family was discussed earlier in this chapter.

Because venous access in children, especially in young infants, is limited, every effort should be made to decrease the number of venipunctures necessary. A highly recommended measure to reduce the number of additional punctures is to collect the necessary blood sample for laboratory tests at the time of venipuncture for establishing an IV line. Once the blood

Box 30-1   Tips for Peripheral IV Access in Children

- Once the catheter is advanced into the vein and the stylet is removed, attach a small connector tube and a syringe prefilled with normal saline and flush a small amount into the vein. Correct position can be confirmed by nonresistant flushing and absence of swelling around the site at the tip of the cannula. The reason for this procedure is twofold: it confirms correct catheter placement, especially if a blood return was not present (in small infants, a blood return may not occur because of the size of the vessel and the gauge of the catheter), and it will keep the catheter from clotting before infusion is started.
- Collect laboratory specimens at the time of IV insertion, if possible, to prevent undue trauma and additional venipuncture.
- Surgical lubricating jelly works well as an adhesive, helping to secure tape around a scalp IV. Apply a small amount under the tape. When you are ready to remove the tape, apply warm water and the tape will lift off easily.
- A flashlight or transilluminator device placed beneath the extremity helps to illuminate tissue surrounding the vein; the veins are then outlined easier to see.
- Insert the cannula with bevel down in very small veins. This technique can help prevent puncturing the back wall of the vessel.
- Holding skin taut creates less pain and allows a smoother IV insertion.
- Spasms often occur in small veins; should "flashback" (blood return) cease, wait a second or two, then place a warm compress over the vein. Once the spasm stops, the cannula can be advanced.
- "Float" the IV cannula through the valves by flushing the catheter with normal saline solution as the cannula is advanced.
- Always have extra help and use positioning-for-comfort techniques. Infants can be held still for IV placement using a blanket as a "mummy" wrap (Fig. 30-2, A).
- Use a padded board to position areas of flexion (Fig. 30-2, B).
- Rubber bands or pieces of latex-free tubing can be used as tourniquets in small infants.
- If using the antecubital area, rotate the forearm while palpating. The tendon will roll, helping to distinguish the vein from the tendon.
- Wrap extremities in comfortably warm compresses before performing the venipuncture to assist in vein dilatation. (Commercially available warm packs applied for 10 minutes work well.)
- Use stickers or drawings on the IV site as a reward.
- A clear plastic IV house or stretch netting work well to protect the IV site or peripherally inserted central catheter site, especially for home IV patients (Fig. 30-4).

sample has been collected, the catheter is flushed with 0.9% sodium chloride and connected to the prescribed therapy, or flushed with heparinized saline or 0.9% sodium chloride to maintain patency.

The challenge of pediatric IV therapy is not over once successful venipuncture has been established. Keeping the IV catheter securely in place in an infant or child can be more

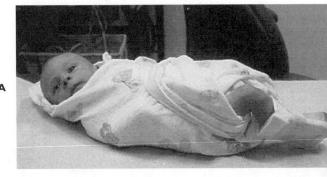

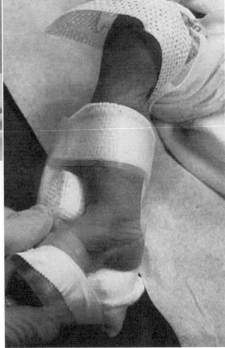

FIG. 30-2 A, *Baby wrapped in blanket "mummy" restraint before placing foot IV.* **B,** *Foot taped to padded board before IV placement, maintaining normal joint configuration and site visibility.*
(Courtesy Anne Marie Frey.)

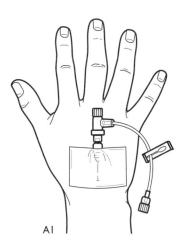

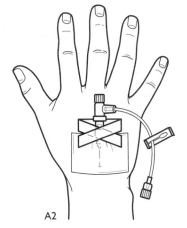

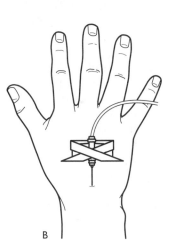

A1   A2   B

FIG. 30-3 *Securing an IV.*

difficult than the initial insertion. Sterile transparent dressings or gauze protection are required to effectively maintain an IV catheter in place (Fig. 30-3); occluding the area above the insertion site with tape should be avoided. The IV site needs to be visible for frequent assessments. Clear, plastic site protectors are available; these protectors are secured over the site and help prevent accidental dislodgment (Fig. 30-4, *A* and *B*). Roller bandages should not be used to cover or secure the cannula site; the cannula site should remain readily visible for inspection. Although some IV complications (e.g., dislodgment, infiltration) are expected to occur in infants and children, careful securing of the IV device and frequent observation of the site can minimize these complications.

Restraints should be avoided if possible, but they are some-

times required to keep the IV catheter secure. Elbow restraints are preferred to arm restraints. The restraints can be muslin squares, with pockets to contain tongue blades, or commercial restraints with Velcro closures. Restraints are rarely needed on all extremities. Should clove-hitch restraints be used, caution must be taken to attach the restraint correctly and not impair the circulation to the extremity. In all cases, especially when restraints are used, site assessment should be completed and documented at least once every 2 hours.[25]

Heparin locks versus saline locks

In many adults, 0.9% sodium chloride has replaced heparinized saline solution for the maintenance of intermittent vascular

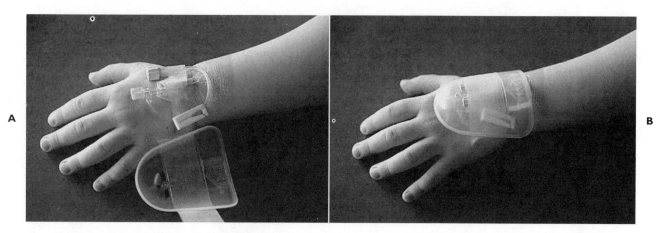

FIG. 30-4 A, *Peripheral IV site with microbore Luer-loking connector tubing and clear dressing fits under clear plastic IV HOUSE site protector in hand of patient.* **B,** *Peripheral IV site, protected by clear plastic IV HOUSE, in hand of pediatric patient.* (Courtesy I.V. HOUSE, Hazelwood, Mss, 800-350-0400.)

devices. In the early 1990s, published studies indicated that saline alone can be used to maintain patency of 22-gauge or larger catheters in children.[29-31] However, these results cannot be applied to all subgroups (e.g., neonates) or all gauges of catheter. More recent pediatric research revealed increased patency and less tenderness when IVs were flushed with 1 to 2 ml of 10 U/ml heparinized saline, whereas neonatal studies showed no difference between normal saline and heparinized saline as long as catheters were flushed every 4 hours.[32-35] Positive-pressure technique for flushing IVs, where the clamp is secured before removing the flush syringe, helped maintain patency. More research is needed in this area of practice, particularly with 24-gauge catheters and longer flush intervals.[32]

Effective heparin/saline ratios for maintaining the patency of peripheral IV lines range between 1 unit of heparin per 1 ml of normal saline to 10 units of heparin per 1 ml of normal saline. Heparin solution that does not contain benzyl alcohol should be used in neonates weighing less than 1200 g.

Complications

Complications related to IV therapy are discussed in detail in Chapter 24. Some complications occur more often or can be more serious in the pediatric population. Because of children's small vessels, the smaller-gauge IV cannulas, and the slow rates of infusion, clotting of the catheter can occur more often than in adults. Because of the smaller vessels and the higher levels of activity in young children, infiltration can be a problem.

When an irritating solution infiltrates, an extravasation injury, with swelling, blistering, and skin necrosis, may occur. These injuries can be devastating in children, causing loss of tissue and function of the affected area.[22] Generalized treatments, such as elevation and localized injection of hyaluronidase (Wydase), have been shown effective in diminishing an extravasation injury.[36] Specific antidotes are also recommended for some drug extravasations, such as phentolamine (Regitine) or nitroglycerin ointment applied to the site of vasopressor infiltration.[37] Phlebitis is seen less often in children than adults

until after the age of 10, when incidence of phlebitis begins to approach adult rates.[23] In addition, as discussed earlier, fluid-volume overload can be a serious complication in an infant and small child. Frequent site assessment, while an IV is infusing, is the recommended standard of care for preventing IV complications.[25]

CENTRAL ACCESS
Central venous catheters

A central venous catheter (CVC) is a device whose tip is located in a central vein, defined by the *Infusion Nursing Standards of Practice* as the superior vena cava, and in children with femorally inserted lines, the inferior vena cava.[25] Many catheter types and protocols for their care exist. Catheter type should be based on the age and size of the child, his or her cognitive ability, the length of the therapy, vein access, and body image considerations. Central catheters are usually considered when therapy is deemed necessary for longer than 2 to 3 weeks or when administration of hypertonic or irritating infusions is required.

Many controversies exist regarding flush protocols and dressing changes in central catheter care. Procedures described throughout this section are based on manufacturers' recommendations and the current literature. Protocols should be based on this information and on catheter type and volume, fluid balance, and patient condition; these criteria apply to both adults and children. More research is needed to substantiate uniform procedures that work for most patients.

Nontunneled percutaneous central venous catheters. Percutaneously placed CVCs are single or multiple lumen and are generally made of polyurethane. (*Note:* PICCs are discussed separately.) These catheters are placed directly into the superior vena cava by way of the right or left subclavian, the internal or external jugular veins, or the inferior vena cava via the femoral veins at the groin. Nontunneled catheters are usually placed by physicians and are used for short-term emergency access in critical care patients. Site preferences in children—in order of preference, safety, and accessibility—are the femoral

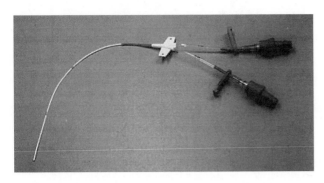

FIG. 30-5 *Pediatric-sized peripherally inserted central catheter.* (Courtesy Anne Marie Frey.)

Table 30-14	**Care of Nontunneled Percutaneous Central Venous Catheters**

Catheter volume: approximately 0.3 ml/lumen
Lumens: Single, double, triple
FLUSHING SCHEDULE

Intermittent (before and after medication administration):	3 ml of 0.9% sodium chloride followed by 1 ml of heparin solution (10-100 U/ml)
After blood infusion or withdrawal:	5-10 ml of 0.9% sodium chloride followed by 1-3 ml of heparin solution (10-100 U/ml)
Maintenance:	1-3 ml of heparin solution (10-100 U/ml) every 8-24 hours
Advantages:	Intended for short-term treatment, inpatient or outpatient insertion, usually secured with sutures, can be used for either intermittent or continuous infusion, access without needlestick to child
Disadvantages:	Limited placement time, requires aseptic dressing change, daily heparinization is required, disturbance in body image, cost of maintenance and supplies, easily occluded in femoral and jugular vein areas in infants, high risk of infection in proximity to diaper area

Table 30-15	**Care of Peripherally Inserted Central Catheters**

Catheter volume: 0.04-0.5 ml (depending on manufacturer)
Lumens: Single or double (see Fig. 30-5)
FLUSHING SCHEDULE

Intermittent (before and after medication administration):	2-3 ml of 0.9% sodium chloride, followed by 1-2 ml of heparin solution (10-100 U/ml)
After blood infusion or withdrawal:	5-10 ml of 0.9% sodium chloride, followed by 1-2 ml of heparin solution (10-100 U/ml)
Maintenance:	1-2 ml of heparin solution (10-100 U/ml) once or twice daily
Advantages:	Inserted at medical facility or in the home, longevity of catheters (weeks to months), accessed without needlestick to patient
Disadvantages:	Cost of maintenance supplies, disturbance in body image, child and family must learn catheter care, radiograph needed to confirm tip placement, higher infection rate in neonates than in children[39]

vein, internal jugular veins, and subclavian vein.[9] Table 30-14 describes the care of nontunneled percutaneous CVCs.

Peripherally inserted central catheters. Another type of percutaneously placed central catheter is the PICC. The PICC is a thin, single- or double-lumen catheter inserted via a breakaway or peel-away introducer or modified Seldinger technique. Sizes used in infants and children include 28 and 24 gauge, and 2, 3, and 4 Fr (Fig. 30-5). PICCs are inserted peripherally into one of several sites, including the basilic, cephalic, and median cubital veins of the antecubital fossa. In newborns and small infants, other choices include the large

saphenous, superficial temporal, external jugular, popliteal, and axillary veins.[38] Table 30-15 describes the care of PICCs. PICCs are inserted by highly skilled nurses as well as physicians. PICCs are used for intermediate duration of weeks to months, with the major indication being antibiotic therapy lasting several weeks.

Tunneled catheters. Surgically placed tunneled catheters are single-lumen or multilumen silicone catheters with one or two Dacron polyester cuffs. An example of this type of catheter is the Broviac catheter. These catheters are surgically tunneled under the skin of the chest into the superior vena cava.

Table 30-16   Care of Tunneled Catheters

Catheter volume: ≤1 ml (pediatric size)	
Lumens: Single and double	
FLUSHING SCHEDULE	
Intermittent (before and after medication administration):	3 ml of 0.9% sodium chloride, may be followed by 2-5 ml of heparin solution (10-100 U/ml)
After blood infusion or withdrawal:	5-10 ml of 0.9% sodium chloride, followed by 2-5 ml of heparin solution (10-100 U/ml)
Maintenance:	2-5 ml of heparin solution daily to weekly
Advantages:	Reduced risk of bacterial migration after tissue adheres to Dacron cuff or cuffs, inpatient/outpatient placement, longevity of placement (months to years), clean or sterile dressing technique used, repair of catheter possible, easily accessed by patient, accessed without needlestick to patient, child may swim in chlorinated pool after several weeks (depending on immune system status, site healing, and physician order)
Disadvantages:	Daily-to-weekly flushing required, disturbance in body image, child and family must learn catheter care, catheter is at risk for accidental removal or breakage if child is very active; infection also a risk[40,41]

Table 30-17   Care of Closed Tip, Pressure Valve, Tunneled Catheters

Catheter volume: Approximately 1 ml or less	
Lumens: Single or double for children	
FLUSHING SCHEDULE	
Intermittent (before and after medication administration):	5 ml of 0.9% sodium chloride
After blood infusion or withdrawal:	5 to 10 ml of 0.9% sodium chloride
Maintenance:	5 ml of 0.9% sodium chloride every 7 days
Advantages:	Same as for cuffed, tunneled catheter, daily heparinization not required, reduced risk of air embolism, reduced risk of clot formation, no clamping needed, easily repaired[40,41]
Disadvantages:	Disturbance in body image, surgical procedure required, child and family must learn catheter care, potential for accidental removal, infection, valve malfunction

Table 30-18   Care of Implantable Port

Reservoir volume: 0.33-1 ml	
Lumens: Single or double lumens for children	
FLUSHING SCHEDULE	
Intermittent (before and after medication administration):	5 ml of 0.9% sodium chloride, followed by heparin solution (10-100 U/ml)
After blood infusion or withdrawal:	5-10 ml of 0.9% sodium chloride followed by 5 ml of heparin solution (10-100 U/ml)
Maintenance:	5 ml of heparin solution (10-100 U/ml) every 30 days or after each use
Advantages:	Little site care and minimal flushing required, body image intact, longevity of placement, child may swim and bathe when needle is not in port, no catheter care required, low cost of maintenance supplies
Disadvantages:	Skin pierced with noncoring needle for access, pain associated with needle insertion unless topical anesthetic used, cost of surgical insertion and removal, possible displacement of port resulting from child's activity, vigorous contact sports (football, hockey) may not be allowed

An alternative site is the inferior vena cava, with the catheter tunneled to the abdomen, thigh, or back (Table 30-16). Tunneled catheters are used for longer-term indications such as long-term parenteral nutrition or cancer treatment.

Closed tip, pressure valve, tunneled catheters.
Another type of surgically placed tunneled catheter is a single-lumen or multilumen silicone catheter with a closed tip and a two-way, pressure-sensitive valve at the proximal end, inside the patient, or distal end, outside the patient. The backflow of blood into the catheter is prevented when the valve is closed. The valve opens for infusion into the venous system or for blood aspiration, which depends on the application of positive or negative pressure. An example of this type of catheter is the Groshong catheter (Table 30-17).

Implantable port. An implantable port is another surgically placed and tunneled device. It has a totally implanted metal or plastic dome that contains a self-sealing injection port. An implanted port may be sutured to the chest wall under the skin, and the catheter tip may be located in the superior or inferior vena cava. Another type of port can be implanted and positioned near the antecubital fossa in the arm. With the "arm" port, the catheter is threaded via the basilic vein to the superior vena cava (Table 30-18). Ports are also indicated for long-term intravascular access, particularly when intermittent IV therapy is needed, such as in children with cancer or cystic fibrosis.

OTHER INTRAVASCULAR ROUTES
Umbilical vein versus artery

The umbilical cord of the neonate provides an alternative route for vascular access. Because of the risk of complications associated with umbilical catheterization, it is reserved for emergency access in the delivery room and for hemodynamic monitoring in the neonatal intensive care unit. Three vessels are present in the umbilical cord: one vein (thin walled with a large-diameter lumen) and two arteries (thick walled with a small-diameter lumen). The goals of arterial catheterization versus venous catheterization differ, as do the techniques of insertion.

Because of its larger lumen, it is easier to catheterize the umbilical vein than other veins. Although the vessel may be accessed during the infant's first 4 days of life, an umbilical venous catheter is usually inserted in the delivery room in an infant whose condition is compromised. The purpose of venous catheterization is primarily emergency administration of medication and fluid, but central venous pressure measurement, venous blood sampling, and exchange transfusion are also accomplished through this line. The umbilical venous catheter (UVC) remains in place from several days to several weeks, but because the umbilicus is heavily colonized immediately after birth, long-term use of this site is not recommended.[42]

The most common reasons for establishing an arterial umbilical catheter are as follows: (1) monitoring arterial pressure, (2) obtaining blood samples for arterial pH and blood gases, (3) performing aortography, and (4) performing exchange transfusions. Although parenteral infusion of medications and fluid can be performed via the arterial catheter, it is not the primary reason for this catheter's placement. Placing an umbilical artery catheter (UAC) requires more time than venous cannulation and may not be the most appropriate choice for achieving access in an emergency.

With either umbilical access, aseptic technique is followed; the operator, usually a neonatologist, is scrubbed, gowned, masked, and gloved. Once the patient and equipment are prepared, the appropriate vessel is located, and a 3.5- or 5.0-Fr, flexible, rigid-walled, radiopaque, umbilical catheter is advanced into the vessel. For venous catheterization, the umbilical catheter is introduced upward toward the liver for 5 to 8 cm or until a blood return is noted. The line is flushed with 1 ml of a heparinized solution and is secured in place by suture or tape. Tip placement is confirmed by radiograph before the catheter is used. In some neonatal intensive care units and delivery rooms, specially trained nurse practitioners are instructed in the technique of venous umbilical catheterization.

Before a catheter is inserted into one of the umbilical arteries, the proper catheter length must be determined. This is accomplished by using a nomogram, or by calculating twice the distance from the umbilicus to the midpoint of the inguinal ligament. The umbilical catheter is advanced 1 to 2 cm at a time until the required length of the catheter has been inserted. After arterial blood aspiration, the line is slowly flushed with 0.5 ml of a heparinized solution. The catheter is temporarily secured, pending verification of tip placement by radiologic examination. Appropriate catheter tip placement should be between L3 and L4. Once correct placement has been verified by radiographic examination, the therapy may proceed.[42] The umbilical artery catheter may be sutured in place, secured with tape, or both.

Complications of umbilical catheterization include vascular compromise, hemorrhage, air embolism, infection, thrombosis, and vascular perforation. The risk of infection is similar for umbilical venous and arterial lines.[26] At higher risk for UAC bloodstream infection are low-birth-weight neonates receiving prolonged antimicrobial infusions; higher-birth-weight neonates receiving PN have a higher risk of UVC-related infection.[42] The nursing assessment for potential complications of the newborn with an umbilical catheter should include the following:

- Inspect lower extremities and buttocks often for blanching or sudden cyanosis caused by spasm or embolism. Circulatory compromise may be observed initially in the toes, and then advances upward toward the buttock. The catheter should be evaluated and possibly repositioned or removed if lower extremity circulation is compromised. Occasionally, warming of the opposite extremity may result in improvement in circulation of the compromised limb.
- Monitor the umbilical site often and ensure that the connections between attachments are secure.
- Monitor arterial waveforms. "Dampening," or alteration of waveforms from normal, requires reevaluation of tip placement and line set-up.
- Closely monitor respiratory status and peripheral pulse and check for edema, which may indicate emboli formation.
- Monitor the umbilicus daily for signs of infection during the treatment and for 12 hours after catheter removal; provide routine cord care daily.

Intraosseous route

The intraosseous (into the bone) route is an important adjunct to emergency measures used in infant and child resuscitation. This technique, which is used by trained professionals (physicians, nurses, and emergency personnel), does not replace conventional methods of venous access. Instead, the intraosseous route provides immediate vascular access in emergency situations when access by the IV route is unattainable (i.e., after 5 minutes of attempts) and fluid or medication administration is essential to sustain life. The needle is inserted into the bone marrow (medullary) cavity of a long bone (Fig. 30-6). The solution injected into the bone marrow cavity is rapidly drained into the central venous channel and exits the bone into the systemic circulation via the nutrient and emissary veins.

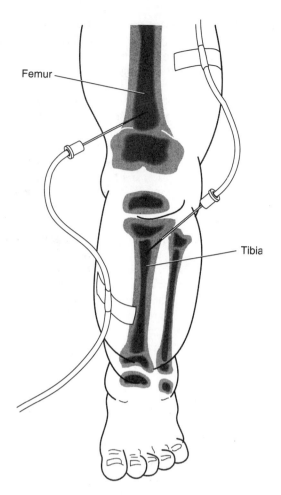

FIG. 30-6 *Intraosseous access sites for IV infusion.*

The optimal site for intraosseous needle placement in infants and children is the anterior medial aspect of the tibia; other sites include the distal medial tibia, midanterior distal femur, iliac crest, and humerus.[43]

As the child grows older, however, the cortex covering becomes tougher and can make penetration into the bone marrow more difficult. The distal femur is a larger bone to access, but it is usually padded more heavily with muscle and fat. Before 3 years of age, the sternum is *never* used; it is too thin to support an intraosseous needle.[44] Lower extremities that have had recent fractures or trauma are avoided. Other contraindications for needle placement include skin with infected burns or cellulitis and bone disorders, such as osteoporosis or osteogenesis imperfecta.

In emergency situations, an intraosseous needle is not required; intraosseous infusions have been successful with 16- or 19-gauge straight needles. Certain needle features, however, are preferable and contribute to the success of insertion. These features include (1) a short shaft, (2) a stylet, (3) a sturdy needle, (4) a handle, and (5) centimeter markings on the needle shaft.[45] All of these features are found on commercially available intraosseous devices and certain bone marrow aspiration needles.

Inserting the needle into the medullary cavity of a long bone and injecting a solution is rapid and simple. The leg is restrained and cleansed with an antiseptic, and in the awake child, 1% lidocaine is injected down to the periosteum. The needle is angled away from the joint space to avoid the growth plate and is introduced into the bone marrow with a downward screwing or boring motion, using firm pressure. Indications of proper placement include the feeling of a soft "pop" and a lack of resistance, the aspiration of bone marrow into a syringe, the needle standing upright without support, and a nonresistant flushing through the needle. Any standard syringe or IV administration set may be attached and medications or fluids infused by gravity or pressure. The rate of flow is regulated not necessarily by the gauge size of the needle but by the density and size of the bone marrow cavity. Medications, crystalloids, and colloids can be administered via this route.

The intraosseous route is intended for short-term use only. Once resuscitation efforts have stabilized the patient, an alternative route of venous access must be used. Because of the risk of infection, the intraosseous needle should not be left in place for longer than 24 hours. The most common difficulties encountered with the intraosseous technique are improper placement of the needle and needle obstruction with marrow.

Complications of intraosseous access are relatively rare but can include osteomyelitis, cellulitis, compartment syndrome, abscess, local necrosis, and tibial fracture. Embolization of fat or bony fragments is a potential complication, but to date has not been reported.[43,46,47]

The nursing responsibility regarding insertion of the needle varies from institution to institution. The primary responsibilities of the nurse are assessing the patient, administering medication and fluid, and monitoring equipment.

ADMINISTRATION EQUIPMENT
Containers

Infants and children can have boundless energy and curiosity, which can result in their pulling and tugging on IV lines and poles. A plastic rather than glass solution container should be used whenever possible to avoid breakage if the container falls off the pole. To prevent the risk of fluid-volume overload, the volume of the solution container should be based on the age and size of the child and the 24-hour volume needs.[25] In premature infants and neonates, smaller solution containers should be considered.

Administration sets

The IV set-up for infants and children is different from that of adults in that flow rate requirements are minimal, necessitating proper choice of tubing. Precise infusion rates are required to prevent the possibility of medication overdose or fluid-volume overload.

Microdrip (60 gtt/min) and microbore tubing are administration sets used for infants and children. IV tubing with an in-line, calibrated, volume-control chamber (50-, 100-, and 150-ml sizes are available) should be used on all children whose prescribed fluid rate is less than 100 ml/hr, unless another volume-control method, such as an electronic infusion pump, is used.[48] There is still debate over whether this chambered IV set

Table 30-19   Nursing Diagnoses and Desired Patient Outcomes in Children Receiving Intravenous Therapy

Nursing Diagnosis	Patient Outcome
Potential fluid-volume deficit because of vomiting, diarrhea, burns, hemorrhage, wound drainage, or diabetic ketoacidosis	The child's hydration status will demonstrate improvement by improved skin turgor, moist mucous membranes, stable weight, 1 ml/kg/hr of urine output, and serum electrolyte values within normal limits. Oral fluids will be tolerated. Urine specific gravity will be between 1.000 and 1.010.
Potential fluid-volume excess because of fluid overload, cardiac or renal disease, inappropriate secretion, or fluid shift	The child's weight will return to pre-illness status, edema will decrease, vital signs will return to normal, and no audible rales will be present.
Potential alteration in sensory perception because of electrolyte imbalance, cerebral edema, or fever	The child will respond appropriately for age (e.g, smile at parents, suck from bottle).
Potential impaired skin integrity because of diarrhea, edema, or dry skin	The child's skin will be free of signs of breakdown, excoriation in diaper area will decrease, and skin turgor will return to normal.
Potential diversional activity deficit because of environmental lack of activity; frequent, lengthy treatments; or long-term hospitalization	The child will participate in chosen activities and will express interest in surroundings and activity.
Potential fear because of separation from parent, unfamiliar environment, treatment, IV equipment, or normal developmental phobias	The child will demonstrate reduced fear behaviors (e.g., crying, wide-eyed gaze, tension, or hiding).
Potential knowledge deficit because of lack of exposure, information misinterpretation, cognitive limitation	The child and family will verbalize understanding of what was taught and demonstrate ability to perform new skills.
Potential impaired physical mobility because of restraints and IV support boards and decreased endurance and strength	The child will achieve maximum mobility within age and medical restrictions, no skin breakdown, no contractures, and maximum joint range of motion.
Potential altered nutrition resulting in less than body requirements because of nausea, vomiting, diarrhea, and inability to absorb nutrients	The child will tolerate feedings via oral route, feeding tube, or IV line without side effects, gain ___ g/day, experience an increased energy level, and participate in diet decisions, if age appropriate.
Potential self-concept disturbance or alteration in body image because of venous access device, illness, and effects of treatment (e.g., alopecia)	The child will participate in decision-making process about self-care, take initiative to do tasks, make eye contact, and interact freely with peers.
Potential altered patterns of urinary elimination because of fluid shift, diarrhea, inadequate intake, and chronic illness	The child will have adequate output that is in balance with intake and will have urine specific gravity between 1.000 and 1.010.

Data from References 1, 3, and 5.

is required when an electronic infusion device is used.[48] Use of an in-line chamber may provide an increased measure of volume control and also provides a mechanism for diluting and administering medication.

Because acutely ill patients often need multiple therapies, extension sets with three-way stopcocks are often used in the critical care unit; however, stopcocks can present infection and safety risks. In place of stopcocks, some institutions use multiple-arm connectors with two or more arms, each with its own clamp. These connectors provide a closed system for administration of multiple infusates via one IV site. In this case, it is advisable to consult with pharmacy experts regarding compatibility issues.

Electronic monitoring devices

As discussed throughout this chapter, the nurse caring for the child undergoing infusion therapy has a grave responsibility to ensure that the prescribed treatment is delivered safely and effectively. Most complications occurring in infants and children are attributed to dosing or fluid administration errors. The nurse must possess the knowledge necessary not only to verify, calculate, and administer the therapy, but also to accurately regulate the rate. The principles of safety and efficacy also apply

to the home setting, where many children now receive their infusion therapy. Today, infusion device technology is both sophisticated and simple. Ultratechnical devices found in critical care units can administer several infusions simultaneously or systematically, whereas small, portable, nonelectric infusion devices meet the needs of children at home.

Electronic infusion devices that help regulate fluid delivery are often used in infants and children. Infusion pumps used for infants and children must be very accurate ($\pm 5\%$ accuracy), guard against free flow, and have occlusion alarm ratings that fall within safety limits. Infusion pumps are necessary in infants and children who require arterial lines and highly accurate infusions, such as PN, chemotherapy, and vasoactive and other rate-dependent medications that must be delivered accurately to achieve desired effect. Pumps are available commercially in various styles and delivery options. Pumps exert varying degrees of pressure when they meet resistance during infusion. Careful evaluation of pressure and alarm features is important when a device is chosen. Considerations for evaluating a pump for pediatric use should include its ability to infuse tenths of a milliliter, variable pressure limits, low alarm limits, ability to be programmed by milliliters per hour, and tamper-proof features.

A popular volumetric pump often used for children is the syringe pump. This highly portable pump incorporates a syringe as the volume chamber to deliver the infusate. The syringe pump is indicated in children for infusion of intermittent doses of medications, such as antibiotics. A syringe pump that has rate and volume capabilities and can accommodate syringes from 1 to 30 ml or larger is most applicable for use in children.

Mechanical controllers, such as dial mechanisms on tubing, may help regulate flow rate; however, in the infant and child in whom flow rates are often only several milliliters per hour, their accuracy cannot be guaranteed. In addition, these mechanisms are often accurate only when used in conjunction with larger-gauge IV devices. Complete manufacturer's information should be examined before these devices are used.

In the home, children are more mobile and active. The best infusion device is one that is portable, requires little or no programming, and is easy for the child and family to operate. Such systems include syringe pumps and positive-pressure devices. One such device is an elastomeric infusion device that incorporates a fillable balloon inside a plastic housing. This system eliminates gravity flow concerns and delivers antibiotic and chemotherapy infusions at a constant rate. Each system has a different delivery rate, based on the volume infused. Advantages to the child and family are that these devices come prefilled by the pharmacy, the set-up time is minimal, and the devices are small and lightweight, a characteristic that promotes ambulation. For school-aged children or adolescents, such devices can be hidden in their clothes or be carried in a user-friendly pouch.

For other infusion needs, ambulatory pumps are commercially available. Individual patient needs and family and clinician's preferences determine which devices are best suited to the patient.

Examples of appropriate nursing diagnoses and desired patient outcome statements specific to the pediatric patient receiving IV therapy are detailed in Table 30-19. When documenting pediatric IV therapy, the caregiver needs to include clinical information, such as size of the catheter, patient response, and desired outcome of therapy.

ALTERNATIVE-SITE INFUSION THERAPY
Subacute care

In some cases, neonates and children may be transferred to a subacute care facility, usually for recovery from a long-term illness or injury. These facilities provide a step between hospital and home and in addition to nursing provide such services as physical, occupational, and respiratory therapy, and developmental and feeding teams. Children in subacute care may need short-term IV therapy intermittently, or continue on long-term therapies such as total parenteral nutrition via a tunneled catheter. In any case, nurses and other therapy providers need to be educated in care of the IV catheters and infusions when providing rehabilitative therapies.

Home infusion therapy

The fastest growing portion of the home care market is pediatric home care.[49] Home infusion therapy for the child is viewed as a positive alternative to hospitalization, but it certainly has its challenges for the child and family, as well as for the professional team responsible for the family's care. After discharge criteria have been met, the caregivers and the child (if appropriate) begin educational preparation for maintaining the prescribed IV treatment at home. Such therapies as antibiotics, antifungals, fluids, chemotherapy, blood and blood components, and medications can be delivered in the home. These therapies must be delivered using a team approach by a company "dedicated to pediatrics or with a strong pediatric division."[50,51]

More so at home than in the acute care setting, the psychosocial and developmental needs of the child and family are an issue. The child may be returning to school and will need assistance on how to deal with the curiosity and remarks from peers. Return to a sport or other activity may be important to the child, and he or she will need help to do so. If siblings are in the home, they may feel neglected because of their parents' attention to the child receiving therapy. Parents should be encouraged to spend private time with each of their children. At home, parents do not have the security of having nurses to rely on. Alternative caregivers should be identified early in the process so that the parents can have respite periods.

SUMMARY

Infusion Nursing Standards of Practice directs the practice of IV nursing in all settings in which IV therapy is delivered.[25] Therefore IV therapy services delivered in all environments are evaluated according to the same standards of practice. Individual policies and procedures in the hospital, outpatient department, subacute facilities, and the home should be developed according to these standards, keeping in mind the unique developmental needs of the child.

REFERENCES

1. Whaley L, Wong DL: *Nursing care of infants and children,* ed 6, St Louis, 1999, Mosby.
2. Merenstein GB, Gardner SL: *Handbook of neonatal intensive care,* ed 4, St Louis, 1997, Mosby.
3. Cahill-Alsip C, McDermott B: Hematologic critical care problems. In Curley MQ, Smith, JB, Moloney-Harmon P: *Critical care nursing of infants and children,* Philadelphia, 1996, WB Saunders.
4. Fann BD: Fluid and electrolyte balance in the pediatric patient, *JIN* 21(3):153, 1998.
5. Mott SR, James SR, Sperac AM: *Nursing care of children and families,* ed 2, Redwood City, Calif, 1990, Addison-Wesley.
6. Wilshaw R, Beckstrand R, Waid D, Schaalje GB: A comparison of the use of tympanic, axillary, and rectal thermometers in infants, *J Pediatr Nurs* 14(2):88, 1999.
7. Chameides L: *Textbook of pediatric advanced life support,* Dallas, 1988, American Heart Association.
8. Barkin RM: Treatment of the dehydrated child, *Pediatr Ann* 19(10):597, 1990.
9. Lavelle J, Costarino A: Central venous access and central venous pressure monitoring. In Henretig FM, King C, editors: *Textbook of pediatric emergency procedures,* Philadelphia, 1997, Williams & Wilkins.
10. Nordenberg T: Pediatric drug studies: protecting pint-sized patients, *FDA Consumer Magazine* (electronic article), 33(3), 1999.
11. Axton SE, Hall B: An innovative method of administering IV medications to children, *Pediatr Nurs* 20(4):341, 1994.
12. Testerman EJ: Current trends in pediatric total parenteral nutrition, *JIN* 12(3):152, 1989.

13. Bilodeau JA, Poon C, Mascarenhas MR: Parenteral nutrition and care of central venous lines. In Altschuler SM, Liacouras CA, editors: *Clinical pediatric gastroenterology,* Philadelphia, 1998, Churchill Livingstone.

14. Heird WC: Parenteral support of the hospitalized child In Suskind RM, Lewinter-Suskind L, editors: *Textbook of pediatric nutrition,* ed 2, New York, 1993, Raven.

15. Helfrick FW, Abelson NM: Intravenous feeding of a complete diet in a child, *J Pediatr* 25:400, 1944.

16. Willmore DW, Dudrick SJ: Growth and development of an infant receiving all nutrients exclusively by vein, *JAMA* 203:860, 1968.

17. Nathan DG, Orkin SH, editors: *Nathan & Oski's hematology of infancy and childhood,* ed 5, Philadelphia, 1998, WB Saunders.

18. Landier WC, Barrell ML, Styffe DJ: How to administer blood components to children, *MCN Am J Matern Child Nurs* 12:178, 1987.

19. Transfusion therapy guidelines for nurses. National Blood Resource Education Program, Public Health Service, National Institutes of Health, U.S. Department of Health and Human Services, 1990.

20. Keller S: Small gauge needles promote safe blood transfusions, *Oncol Nurs Forum* 22(4):718, 1995.

21. Yeager AS, et al: Prevention of transfusion acquired cytomegalovirus infections in newborn infants, *J Pediatr* 98:281, 1981.

22. Brown A S, Hoelzer D, Piercy SA: Skin necrosis from extravasation of intravenous fluids in children, *Plast Reconstr Surg* 64:145, 1979.

23. Nelson DB, Garland JS: The natural history of catheter associated phlebitis in children, *Am J Dis Child* 141:1090, 1987.

24. Friedland LR, Brown R: Introduction of a 'safety' intravenous catheter for use in an emergency department: a pediatric hospital's experience, *Infect Control Hosp Epidemiol* 13(2):114, 1992.

25. Intravenous Nurses Society: Infusion nursing standards of practice, *JIN* (suppl) 23(6S), 2000.

26. Garland S, et al: Peripheral intravenous catheter complications in critically ill children; a prospective study, *Pediatrics* 89:1145, 1992.

27. Pearson ML: Guideline for prevention of intravascular-device-related infections, *Infect Control Hosp Epidemiol* 17(7):438, 1996.

28. Fein JA, Boardman CR, Stevenson S, Selbst SM: Saline with benzyl alcohol as intradermal anesthesia for intravenous line placement in children, *Pediatr Emerg Care* 14(2):119, 1998.

29. Danek GD, Noris EM: Pediatric IV catheters: efficacy of saline flush, *Pediatr Nurs* 18:111, 1992.

30. Hanrahan KS, Kleiber C, Fagan CL: Evaluation of saline for IV locks in children, *Pediatr Nurs* 20:549, 1994.

31. McMullen A, et al: Heparinized saline or normal saline as a flush solution in intermittent intravenous lines in infants and children, *Matern Child Nurs J* 18:78, 1993.

32. Gyr P, et al: Double blind comparison of heparin and saline flush solutions in maintenance of peripheral infusion devices, *Pediatr Nurs* 21(4):383, 1995.

33. Kotter R: Heparin vs. saline for intermittent intravenous device maintenance in neonates, *Neonatal Network* 15(6):43, 1996.

34. Krueger-Paisely M, et al: The use of heparin and normal saline flushes in neonatal intravenous catheters, *Pediatr Nurs* 23(5):521, 1997.

35. Heilskov J, Kleiber C. Johnson K, Miller J: A randomized trial of heparin and saline for maintaining intravenous locks in neonates, *JSPN* 3(3):111, 1998.

36. Flemmer L, Chan SL: A pediatric protocol for management of extravasation injuries, *Pediatr Nurs* 19:355, 1993.

37. Denkler KA, Cohen BE: Reversal of dopamine extravasation injury with topical nitroglycerine ointment, *Plast Reconstr Surg* 84(5):811, 1989.

38. Oellrich RG, et al: The percutaneous central venous catheter for small and ill infants, *Am J Matern Child Nurs* 16(2):92, 1991.

39. Frey AM: Pediatric and neonatal PICC complications, *JVAD* 4(2 suppl), 1999.

40. Jones GR: A practical guide to evaluation and treatment of infections in patients with central venous catheters, *JIN* 21(5S):134, 1998.

41. Wiener ES, Albanese CT: Venous access in pediatric patients, *JIN* 21:S122, 1998.

42. Landers S, et al: Factors associated with umbilical catheter-related sepsis in neonates, *Am J Dis Child* 145:675, 1991.

43. Hodge D: Intraosseus infusion. In Henretig F, King C, editors, *Textbook of pediatric emergency procedures,* Baltimore, 1997, Williams & Wilkins.

44. Miccolo MA: Intraosseous infusion, *Crit Care Nurse* 10:35, 1990.

45. Dieckmann R, et al: *Pediatric emergency and critical care procedures,* St Louis, 1997, Mosby.

46. Manley L, Haley K, Dick M: Intraosseous infusion: rapid vascular access for critically ill or inured infants and children, *J Emerg Nurs* 14:63, 1988.

47. Simmons C, et al: Intraosseous extravasation complication reports, *Ann Emerg Med* 23(2):363, 1994.

48. Reiser DJ: *Intensive care nursery eliminates solusets, infusion management update,* Abbott Park, Ill, 1999, Abbott Laboratories.

49. Schuman A: Homeward bound: the explosion of pediatric home care, *Contemp Pediatr* 7:26, 1990.

50. Ringel M: For pediatric infusion, there's no place like home, *Infusion* 2(1):10, 1995.

51. Ringel M: Providing pediatric infusion therapies: putting the pieces together, *Infusion* 2(2):20, 1995.

Chapter 31

Intravenous Therapy in the Older Adult

Kathleen Walther, RN, BSN, CRNI*

THE AGING POPULATION

With medical advances, intravenous (IV) nursing faces the challenges of an ever-expanding aging population; the mean age of adults has increased to an unprecedented level. The older adult presents a unique set of concerns for which health care workers do not yet have a complete solution. Ironically, gerontology, the study of the aged, is one of the newest specialties in the medical world. Primary goals of IV therapy with the older adult include selecting the correct venous access device, type of therapy, and medication. To achieve these goals, the infusion nurse needs to have a broad-based understanding of geriatric assessment and the impact the aging and infusion processes will have on the older adult.

Gerontology has become a specialty in its own right with the development of gerontologic *Standards of Practice*.[1] A holistic approach must be incorporated throughout the continuum of care with the elderly patient to achieve the most positive outcome. The role of the infusion nurse is expanding to different health care delivery settings. Chronic diseases such as cardiovascular dysfunction, diabetes, and cancer continue to have a major impact on the world population. The elderly patient can present with all three diseases, thereby significantly increasing the challenges of infusion therapy. Accurate assessment of the older patient by health care professionals ensures timely and less costly interventions.

Statistics, projected growth

According to the World Health Organization, in the year 1900, the world's population was estimated to be 1650 million people.[2] By 1950, the population had increased by 53% to an estimated 2520 million people, showing a sharp reduction in mortality as a result of medical and pharmacologic advances.[2,3] It is projected that by 2050, the world population will exceed 9 billion people.[2-4] Currently, 580 million people in the world are older than 60.[2-4] This figure is expected to rise to almost 2 billion by 2050. The most dramatic increases will be in the less developed countries, where the older population is expected to grow from 171 million in 1998 to 1594 million in 2050.[3-5] This impact on the health care delivery system will tremendously affect the way that health care is delivered and the types of services that are offered. Infusion therapy will advance with various types of medical devices and will be a significant factor in maintaining the expanding (and aging) population.

Because of the sharp increases in life expectancy and the gradual decline in fertility rates, the proportion of older adults has now exceeded that of younger children for the first time in history. This phenomenon has been termed *population aging* and has required a shift in health care, focusing on the elderly.[2] Understanding the global implications of population aging will

*The author and editors wish to acknowledge the contributions made by Beth Fabian, as author of this chapter in the first edition of *Intravenous Nursing: Clinical Principles and Practice*.

empower the health care professional to provide the best possible care for older adults.

Aging theories

Many theories exist regarding the population and the process of aging. No one theory can fully describe the inevitable aging that the body endures. Eliopoulos describes the many theories of aging and categorizes them into two areas: biologic theories and psychosocial theories.[6] The common denominator in the theories is that currently, no single factor is responsible for the aging process.

Aging is unique for each individual, beginning at conception. Aging depends on nutritional, environmental, educational, genetic, societal, physiologic, and spiritual factors. Aging uses the life experiences and shapes the future needs of the older adult. Because of the complexities of the aging process, it is much more difficult to assess the older adult than the younger adult. When assessment is made even more difficult by acute or chronic cognitive deficits in the patient, the role of the infusion nurse becomes extremely difficult.

Older people are classified into three major groups:
1. Young old: 65 to 74 years
2. Middle old: 75 to 84 years
3. Old old: 85 years and older

The population experiencing the most change is the old-old age group. Advances in medicine and education provide the practitioner a wealth of knowledge about this group.[1,6]

LEGAL AND ETHICAL CONSIDERATIONS
Advance directives

To understand the requests of the older adult in the delivery of health care, there must be a clear understanding of advance directives. The desires of the elderly are often ignored, especially when a metabolic imbalance has rendered the older adult cognitively deficient. Chronic illnesses, medications, and fluid and electrolyte imbalances can impair the patient's ability to make clear-cut decisions about infusion therapy. The health care professional must advocate for the wishes of the patient. When an elderly person is treated, the entire family is affected. Many complex emotional and ethical issues arise regarding the treatment of the older adult. These issues need to be discussed in a controlled setting, before the onset of an acute illness that requires infusion therapy. The patient may have a variety of documents or persons designated responsible for the plan of care. These may include advance directives, which are legally binding documents set forth by the patient in anticipation of future health care needs. These documents are reviewed before providing any treatment. In the case of IV therapy, a review is particularly important if the practitioner is not familiar with the patient and has been called as the specialist to perform an invasive procedure.

The living will, a part of the advance directives, is a comprehensive document specifying the holistic aspects of the patient's care. Another document often used confers a durable power of attorney for health care to a friend, family member, advisor, or guardian. This person is appointed to make decisions when the patient is considered legally incompetent or incapable of making decisions regarding health care.[1,7]

Do-not-resuscitate orders

As with advance directives, do-not-resuscitate (DNR) orders are reviewed with the patient and family before the order is written. A DNR order must be written on the physician's order sheet and progress notes. A DNR order may be written in the absence of or in conjunction with a living will.[1,7] The patient or legal guardian must participate in the decision-making process. If the patient resides in a long-term care setting, cardiopulmonary resuscitation (CPR) must be available to the patient if the patient wishes. If the facility is unable to perform CPR, the patient must be informed. This is of particular importance to the health care professional consulting on an emergent basis to perform a venipuncture.

Informed consent

The initiation of IV therapy without consent is construed as assault and battery.[8] The older adult does not give up the right to refuse treatment. Health care professionals must recognize that the elderly person needs to feel a sense of independence and control over his or her environment. In the acute care setting, much of a patient's care and environment is out of his or her control. This circumstance must be met with reasoning and discussion, not force.

The patient who is confused does not necessarily relinquish his or her rights to refuse treatment. The determination of what is best for the care and safety of the patient must be weighed against a careful evaluation of the patient's mental and emotional ability to make rational decisions.[8] The patient's life and safety are always the first priority to the health care provider. If a patient cannot make these judgments, the patient, the family, or the hospital representative can ask the court to appoint a patient advocate to oversee the best interests of the patient. The determination of who will speak for the patient must be made early in the course of care so that proper therapy can be continued with the appropriate consent.

GERONTOLOGIC ASSESSMENT
Holistic approach to care

The older population is a very diverse group. Everyone ages differently, taking into consideration climate, geographic locations, family size, life skills, and experiences. Individual variations in biologic characteristics tend to be greater in the older population than in the younger population. This diversity makes it difficult to categorize most older people. The health care professional needs to do a complete, holistic assessment of the older adult before initiating therapy. All aspects of life need to be respected when an older person requires infusion therapy. It is important to take into account that this particular generation has survived many global changes and medical advances. This generation has seen the advances in antibiotic therapy and has witnessed the virtual eradication of diseases such as polio and whooping cough. Decisions regarding infusion therapy are very important to the process of completing therapy with the fewest complications and the most positive outcomes for the older adult.

Activities of daily living

Activities of daily living are a common criterion used by health care professionals to determine the care that an elderly person will require in event of an illness. Determining a patient's optimal level of functioning is a key component to this equation.

In the holistic plan for care, bathing, dressing, housekeeping, mobility, and cognitive function are factors in determining overall wellness. When infusion therapy is considered, other factors need to be identified before initiating therapy (Box 31-1).

If there is a question about the patient's cognitive level, many quick and easy assessments can be performed to determine whether the patient understands the impending therapy. It is important to have an understanding of the patient's entire 24-hour day. Issues such as insomnia, depression, or sundowning syndrome are some common examples that may complicate care.

THE AGING PROCESS
Cardiovascular function

One of the most important systemic changes that the health care professional needs to assess are the changes occurring in the cardiovascular system of the older adult. With advancing age, the left atrium enlarges to enhance ventricular filling. In most healthy older adults, a fourth audible heart sound can occur from the enlargement. The overall size of the heart increases in mass; the increase is estimated at 1 g per year in men and 1.5 g per year in women after the age of 30.[6,7,9] In both genders, the intraventricular septal thickness increases with age, creating a stiffness in the ventricular walls. This impedes the heart's ability to contract and relax. The heart valves may also become thicker and less flexible from lipid accumulation, collagen degeneration, and fibrosis. Decreased efficiency of the heart muscle reduces the cardiac output by approximately 1% per year in adulthood.[9] The vessels have greater peripheral resistance because of calcium deposits, cross-linking of collagen, and a reduction in elastin. The capillary walls are thicker, which may impede the effective exchange of nutrients. In older adults, the venous elasticity also slowly declines, making the veins more difficult for venipunc-

ture. The body's ability to store blood volume is reduced, and the peripheral valve efficiency is reduced. In areas of high venous pressure, the adult is at risk for varicosities. The older adult's lack of mobility may also impair venous return.

Respiratory function

Assessment of the respiratory system is paramount to providing the best possible care for the geriatric patient. The respiratory system changes begin with an overall decrease in vital capacity resulting from the loss of elastic recoil and decreased respiratory mass. There is an increase in dead space along with a decrease in the amount and effectiveness of the cilia along the tracheobronchial tree.[1,6,9] Because of the loss of elasticity and decreased effectiveness of the alveoli, the older adult is at increased risk for respiratory infections and dyspnea.

The older adult compensates for the flattening diaphragm and decrease in the capacity of respiratory muscles by using abdominal accessory muscles for respirations. These muscles make breathing increasingly difficult for the patient. Surgeries with anesthesia can make the older patient more prone to aspiration. The blood oxygen level decreases by 10% to 15%.[6] Oxygen perfusion decreases, and the elderly are more prone to hypoxemia. Care and consideration should be given to the amount of medication, number of infections, and comorbidity when determining respiratory function. Hypoxemia can result in cognitive impairment, which can be misconstrued in the older adult. Swallowing deficits can result in right lower lobe and right middle lobe pneumonia that is often undiagnosed and undertreated because of inadequate assessment skills.

Endocrine system

As people age, their normal immune system changes by becoming hyporesponsive to foreign antigens and hyperresponsive to self.[10] These changes can result in decreased resistance to infection, increased incidence of cancers, and increased autoimmunity. Infusion therapy nurses must consider that older adults may be more susceptible to infection and may not show the same signs and symptoms of infection they did when they were younger.[11,12] Because of this change, the use of aseptic technique and appropriate use of antimicrobial agents with all IV therapy–related procedures are essential.

The pituitary gland loses weight and vascularity with age, and there are changes in the thyroid gland. Hypothyroidism is a common diagnosis in the elderly that is often misdiagnosed because of its vague symptomatology, such as mild depression, weight gain, chest pain, atrial fibrillation, and cold intolerance.

Acquired immunodeficiency syndrome (AIDS) also affects older adults. Human immunodeficiency virus (HIV) may be misdiagnosed or missed entirely in the elderly because the early symptoms of fatigue, anorexia, and weight loss can be misinterpreted. Cognitive impairment, for example, is often diagnosed as Alzheimer's disease or dementia rather than a symptom of HIV.

The increased incidence of AIDS in this population has two significant causes. First, only one sixth of the older population surveyed used a protective barrier during intercourse.[13,14] Because the risk of pregnancy is eliminated, older adults need education on barrier protection. Second, the introduction of sildenafil citrate (Viagra) has led to a significant increase in sexual activity among older adults.[14] Care and consideration should be given to the older adult's sexual history when the early symptoms of HIV occur. The health care professional cannot be lax in using standard precautions such as wearing gloves during a venipuncture on the older adult.

Gastrointestinal function

The gastrointestinal function of the older adult can be complex and requires a comprehensive assessment. The life experiences and nutritional status of the older adult define and shape his or her future health and welfare. Comorbidity, such as a cardiovascular accident or hypertension, can lead to inadequate flow to the gastrointestinal tract or dysphagia.

The dentition of the elderly does not change with age.[1,6,9] However, studies have shown that by the age of 65, many elders are edentulous. Poor dental hygiene in younger years leads to loss of teeth, which impairs proper chewing of food. The salivary glands secrete less ptyalin and amylase as age advances and the saliva becomes more alkaline. The taste buds also atrophy with a decrease in discrimination between salt and sweet flavors.

By the age of 60, gastric secretions decrease by 20% to 30%.[6,9,15] A decrease in pepsin may hinder protein digestion and decrease hydrochloric acid, an intrinsic factor that can lead to malabsorption of iron, vitamin B_{12}, calcium, and folic acid. Pernicious anemia is also a concern for the older adult.

Constipation or diarrhea is not attributable to the aging process as was once commonly thought.[1] A slight decrease in intestinal motility comes with aging but does not lead to chronic changes in bowel patterns. The health care practitioner should pay attention to the medications that the patient is taking. Polypharmacy, the taking of multiple medications, in the elderly is a common problem; this practice can produce an array of side effects, including the loss of fluids and electrolytes.

Integumentary function

The integumentary system is the largest and most complex organ in the body. The skin can hold a wealth of information for the health care professional in terms of assessment. Accurate skin assessment can help determine hydration status, potential for infection, amount of sun exposure, and attention to personal appearance. The skin plays a key role in influencing self-esteem and appearance in the older adult.

The skin is the first body system affected by venipuncture. The changes in the texture, depth, and integrity of the skin result from the natural aging process and from the onset of certain disease states. Changes affect all layers of the skin, including the epidermis, the dermis, and the superficial fascia.[11,16]

The *epidermis,* the outermost layer of the integumentary system, has four cellular layers. The *stratum corneum* consists of dead squamous cells that form a protective barrier for the body. The *stratum granulosum* helps organize the keratin layer. The *stratum spinosum* produces the fibrous portion of the keratin layer. The *basal cell* layer is responsible for pigmentation. These layers play a role in thermal regulation of the body. With aging, the epidermis becomes thinner, thereby resulting in decreased healing rates and barrier protection. The cell replacement rate of the stratum corneum declines by 50% in the older adult.[9]

The *dermis* is the middle layer of the skin consisting of protein structures, blood vessels, nerve endings, and appendages such as hair follicles and nails. As the body ages, the dermis decreases in thickness by 20%.[6,9] The number of sweat glands and nerve endings also decreases. In regard to nerve endings, this is of particular importance in relation to pain perception and tactile sensation. The infusion nurse should consider the lack of sensation when performing a venipuncture and minimize catheter manipulation. This will help decrease the risk of a serious infiltration caused by the patient being unable to feel the pain or pressure caused by fluid leaking into the tissue. Because of the decreased thickness, the skin is at great risk for tears, which can lead to ulceration. Caution should be taken during insertion and removal of a venipuncture device and removal of the tape securing the device.

The subcutaneous layer of fat in the skin helps provide insulation from cold and serves as a shock absorber from blunt trauma. As the body ages, this layer becomes thinner and redistributes to the abdomen and thighs. With the thinning of this layer, the older patient is more at risk for hypothermia and skin tears.

Sensory function

Sensory functional changes occurring in the elderly can have a dramatic impact on quality of life. These changes, both normal and those associated with a disease process, can be misdiagnosed as a cognitive functional loss. Care and consideration should be given to accurate assessment of all functions when initiating infusion therapy.[17,18]

If the patient's visual acuity is impaired, the patient may appear withdrawn and unable to participate in the plan of care. Cataracts and glaucoma are easily treated with medications and surgery if detected in a timely manner.

Hearing deficits are also thought to be a part of the normal aging process. The deficits are usually part of the high-frequency range.[17,18] One of the most common reasons for hearing loss is increased cerumen in the ear canal. This can lead to gait disturbances and more commonly a withdrawal from daily activities. The ear canal curves as the person ages, and proper visualization is important in cleaning the ear canal.

Olfactory deficits can be another area for assessment in the elderly population. Some studies have shown an olfactory deficit in response to smells such as smoke. This is of importance to the patient at home, where the risk of fire is greater for the elderly population.

Tactile sensation is decreased and the skin is more susceptible to injury with aging. Infiltration may go unnoticed because of the skin's decreased integrity and loose skin folds. A large amount of fluid may infuse subcutaneously before the patient experiences pain. Phlebitis may develop without pain but with significant vein inflammation resulting from the decreased sensitivity of the skin's nerve endings.[11] Close monitoring of IV infusions, especially with potentially irritating medications, must be performed often because severe tissue necrosis, infection, or compartment syndrome can be the catastrophic result.[8]

The elderly person with a peripheral catheter may not be able to alert the nursing staff of pain at the insertion site resulting from chemical or mechanical phlebitis. Caution should be exercised in the selection of the appropriate venous access device.

The elderly may experience multiple sensory losses. The practitioner needs to be aware of any deficits when caring for the patient. Sensory deficits or disorders can also affect how the patient reacts and responds to the IV nurse and the delivery of infusion therapies. Sensory deficits can dramatically affect older patients' understanding of procedures, their independence, and their ability to cooperate with prescribed therapies. Therefore these changes must be kept in mind so that a personal connection is established with the patient and successful infusion therapies are administered.

Musculoskeletal function

Changes in the musculoskeletal function occur with age. Muscle mass gradually decreases with the muscle being replaced by fibrous connective tissue. The decreased elasticity in the ligaments, tendons, and cartilage can lead to a general overall stiffness in the older adult.[9,18]

Decreased density in bone structure may lead to osteoporosis and place the patient at risk for falls. Falls are a significant concern in the elderly population. Assessment of the patient's environment, medications, and history of disease is crucial in preventing potentially life-threatening falls.

Changes related to arthritis can have a particular impact on placement of an IV catheter. Areas of flexion should not be cannulated because of the impact of restricted movement on arthritic joints. Armboards should be avoided when possible for the same reason.

Fluid and electrolyte balance

Fluid changes in the elderly can lead to a significant imbalance because of the decrease in fluid ratios overall. As the body ages, changes occur in fluid to body mass ratios. Over the age of 65, overall body fluid gradually decreases to 33% in females and approximately 45% in males.[9,15] As a result, the elderly can exhibit significant signs of fluid and electrolyte loss within a 4-hour period. An accurate assessment is essential to promote well-being and prevent fluid and electrolyte imbalances.

A fluid and electrolyte deficit can result in behavioral changes. The elderly become inflexible to change, especially in the presence of cognitive impairment. If the patient with Alzheimer's disease paces the floor continuously and then appears lethargic and sits in a chair, this can easily be interpreted as tiredness or lack of interest. A quick fluid assessment should be performed to rehydrate the elderly patient without having to wait for significant electrolyte changes (Fig. 31-1).

Cognitive function

Psychologic factors in the older adult can affect how the patient responds to IV therapy. The cognitively impaired patient may have problems determining recent versus remote memory. For instance, the patient may understand the procedure while the IV catheter is inserted but an hour later may pull it out. Difficulties with short-term memory may also dramatically affect the older adult who is receiving instruction for home infusion therapies.[11] Depression may affect the older adult's attitude toward the IV line and decisions regarding the alternatives in the care and treatment of the illness. Causes for such behavior can be mental

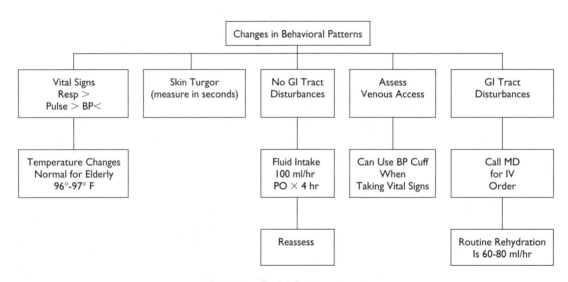

FIG. 31-1 *Fluid deficit assessment.*

deterioration, administration of medications, thyroid disorders, Alzheimer's disease, stroke, or electrolyte imbalances.

CONSIDERATIONS IN INFUSION THERAPY
Vein selection

Selecting the appropriate vein for IV access in the older adult can provide the IV nurse with a great clinical challenge. The IV nurse must possess clinical and anatomic knowledge specific to the older adult and must have the physical dexterity and high level of expertise needed to place an IV device into an appropriate vein.

Primary principles of IV site selection in the younger adult are applicable to the older adult. For instance, initial venipunctures should be in the most distal portion of the extremity, allowing for subsequent venipunctures to move progressively upward.[8] This method provides new IV access away from the previous site or area of complication. However, certain factors for site selection are specific to the older adult. For instance, the veins of the hands may not be the best choice for the initial distal site because of the loss of subcutaneous fat and the thinning of the skin. An IV device inserted into such a site could quickly lead to mechanical inflammation of the vein and infiltration.[8] In addition to this factor, one must take into account the number of venipunctures performed and the outcomes. Therapies that produce a high degree of phlebitis, such as medications with a high or low pH along with increased osmolarity, are factors to consider in determining vein selection.

Vein selection begins by evaluating the patient's peripheral access for potential sites that can accommodate the duration of the IV therapy. The entire surface of both arms should be inspected for potential sites. When possible, sites should be selected that will not hamper the performance of activities of daily living. Physiologic changes in the skin and veins should also be considered when an IV site is selected. For instance, stabilization of an IV catheter may be affected by decreased skin turgor; therefore areas where sufficient tissue and skeletal support exists should be selected if possible. The condition of the vein should be evaluated by careful palpation. The nurse should be aware of the more fragile nature of the vein and should begin at distal sites to preserve future access sites. The nurse should avoid previously used, bruised areas and articulating surfaces. In choosing a site, the nurse should also consider the need for future IV sites; vein conservation is a serious concern for the IV nurse.[8,19]

To help locate a vein, adequate lighting should be used. Bright examination lights located directly overhead may tend to obscure veins. The use of side lighting may highlight the skin's color and texture and allow visualization of the vein shadow below the skin.[10]

The use of a tourniquet may be helpful in distending and locating an appropriate vein. However, important considerations regarding the use of tourniquets for older adults should be kept in mind. The tourniquet should be applied in a flat fashion, snugly but not too tightly. Venous distension may take a few moments longer in the older adult because of the slower venous return in this population. Excessive distension of the vein must be avoided because it might cause vein damage when the vein is punctured, resulting in a hematoma. In addition, the tourniquet itself may create bruising. Because of these factors, it may be preferable to eliminate the use of a tourniquet in the older adult, especially if the vein to be used is visible and already somewhat distended without the use of a tourniquet.[12,19]

During venous distension, the veins should be palpated to determine their condition. Adequate time should be taken to carefully evaluate all potential IV sites. Palpation is the key to determining which veins have soft, bouncy vein walls. Resilient veins feel very different from those that are sclerosed and hard. Veins that feel ribbed or rippled may distend readily when a tourniquet is applied. However, these corded veins are enlarged as a result of thickening of the vein wall, which may be so thick that the lumen may be extremely narrow or occluded.[8] These sites are almost impossible to access, causing pain for the patient and frustration to the IV nurse.

The thickening that occurs in the vein wall also affects the function of the valves, which become stiff and less effective. In many elderly patients, these valves can be seen and palpated because of vessel sclerosis. The valves appear as small bumps along the vein path. The IV nurse must be aware of the potential problems associated with attempting vein access close to or through a valve area. For instance, venous circulation may be sluggish, resulting in slow venous return and distension, venous stasis, and dependent edema. These factors may inhibit the nurse's ability to thread a catheter into the vein. Inflexible valves can make catheter threading difficult or impossible. In these situations, it may be necessary to reduce catheter size by several gauges to thread a catheter through an inflexible valve. Sclerosed valves impede venous circulation and may result in slow or sluggish flashback, causing the IV nurse to advance the catheter too far, resulting in intima damage or vessel rupture.[8,10,19]

Small, surface peripheral veins appear as thin, tortuous veins with many bifurcations. Only a few short, straight branches may sustain an IV catheter. Appropriate catheter gauge and length selection are critical to achieve successful IV placement in these veins.

Vascular access device selection

When a patient's vascular access device needs are evaluated, a judicious analysis of many factors is necessary, particularly the type and duration of IV therapy. For instance, are hydration solutions, chemotherapy, antibiotics, total parenteral nutrition, or supplemental infusions such as potassium piggyback solutions to be administered? The nurse must recognize potentially irritating agents and consider decreasing the concentration or infusing into a larger vessel to promote hemodilution.[20] For example, continuous infusion of vesicant chemotherapy must be administered via a central access catheter to avoid the potential complication of peripheral extravasation. In addition, preparations containing greater than 10% concentrations of glucose, such as total parenteral nutrition solutions, must be administered through central venous access devices to prevent peripheral vein damage. The duration of therapy is also a factor in determining whether a patient's needs are best met by a central or peripheral IV line. If therapy is required for several weeks, central venous access may be the most cost-effective method for delivery, and it conserves the patient's peripheral access. Another indication for a central catheter is the patient who has no peripheral access available. The selection of the type of central catheter should be based on the evaluation of potential access sites and the anticipated duration of therapy.

In catheter selection, the skin and vein changes that occur with the older adult should be considered to enhance successful cannula placement and initiation of IV therapies. In particular, consideration should be given to catheter design and gauge size. The type of material the catheter is made of can make it more biocompatible as an indwelling IV device. This feature can determine where the catheter may be inserted and how long it may stay in place without developing secondary complications. Catheters can be made of silicone, various polyurethane formulations, or polytetrafluoroethylene (Teflon). Softer, more flexible materials may allow increased dwell time and reduce complications. In addition, the needle-bevel tip design of a peripheral catheter should be considered when selecting an infusion access device to provide the least traumatic insertion. The smallest possible gauge size appropriate for therapy and a vein that will provide adequate hemodilution around the catheter should be selected.[12,21] The use of 22- and 24-gauge catheters are appropriate for delivery of many IV therapies. These sizes are recommended when possible for the older adult to reduce insertion-related trauma and provide greater hemodilution, thereby reducing irritation of the intima of the vein resulting from catheter-insertion trauma or from medications.

When a midline or a peripherally inserted central catheter (PICC) is placed in an elderly patient, prehydration is often necessary beforehand. With the significant loss of fluid or the introduction of medications that have the potential for irritation or extravasation, this is important. On day 1 of therapy, assessment for intravascular depletion is performed with diagnostic tests such as blood urea nitrogen and accurate intake and output. If a 22- or 24-gauge catheter is inserted and slow rehydration occurs, the insertion of the larger venous access device, such as a midline or PICC, will be easier.

When a central venous access device is necessary, the need for a long-term versus a short-term device should be evaluated, as should the older adult's ability to care for the device. Percutaneously placed central venous catheters designed for short-term use may be appropriate for several weeks of therapy. A PICC may provide an excellent alternative for intermediate access and may reduce the complications associated with subclavian and jugular insertions. Tunneled catheters may be appropriate when long-term, frequent access is required; however, associated catheter care needs should be considered carefully. The patient and/or caregiver may have difficulty maintaining and coping with dressing and flushing procedures. In this instance, an implantable vascular access port may be a better alternative because of its limited catheter care requirements.

Administration equipment selection

Because of the dangers associated with overadministration or underadministration of IV therapies, the type of infusion equipment selected should provide safe, consistent delivery of required medications or fluids. To prevent fluid overload, the use of microdrip administration sets, if appropriate for the delivery rate required, should be considered. When rapid flow rates or more exact delivery are required, volume-controlled administration sets and electronic monitoring devices may be needed.[10]

Advanced technology in IV therapy uses stationary and ambulatory electronic monitoring devices, such as pumps, of all types and sizes to deliver IV therapies. Because of the fragile nature of the veins of the older adult, the nurse must recognize the potential complications associated with pressures generated by mechanical infusion devices. In addition, because of the dangers associated with overadministration or underadministration of prescribed therapies, monitoring devices must have safety features to protect the patient and still ensure delivery of the required medication or fluids.

An internal diagnostic system should evaluate the pump's basic programming to maintain a standard volume and rate of delivery. Variations from the settings should trigger alarms and stop the infusion until the problem can be corrected. Pump infusion pressures should be monitored carefully to ensure the appropriate delivery of fluids and medications. Pump line pressure can be calibrated in millimeters of mercury or pounds per square inch (psi).

Pump technical information may refer to pressure limits in terms of pounds per square inch. A pump with a fixed pressure alarm of 4 psi will sound an alarm when the peripheral venous pressure reaches 200 mm Hg (1 psi = 50 mm Hg).[8] This setting can result in a significant infiltration before any pump alarm sounds. Dramatic infiltrations can occur when pumps simply continue to pump or when gravity infusion is used because the loose peripheral skin of the older adult does not offer any peripheral tissue resistance to stop a subcutaneous infusion.[12,20]

An electronic flow control device is reliable only if it is used correctly. The device must not be so cumbersome that it inhibits the patient's movement. The older adult needs to maintain mobility to keep a sense of independence. If applicable to the type of pump and infusion, the pump should have a lock-out feature to prevent tampering with the programming once it has been set. This feature can be of significant importance with medications whose dosing can be critical. The older adult may feel overwhelmed by the prospect of home infusion therapy, and one of the most intimidating components may be the high-technology electronic monitoring device (see Chapter 15).

Special considerations for the older adult

Skin preparation. The first step in venipuncture is careful preparation of the proposed venipuncture site. The technique used to apply the cleansing agent can be as important as the antimicrobial effect of the agent. Application of cleansing agents should begin at the site and continue outward in a circular motion. Adequate friction is necessary to cleanse the skin. However, older skin is more delicate, and too vigorous an action may damage surface skin tissue.

Appropriate cleansing agents for skin preparation include alcohol, 2% tincture of iodine, 10% povidone-iodine, and chlorhexidine—as single agents or in combination.[21] Although practices vary, generally, preparatory cleansing with alcohol followed by an iodophor that is allowed to dry for 30 to 60 seconds is best for germicidal effect. For patients who are allergic to iodine, the site can be cleansed with alcohol pads until the pads no longer show soil after cleansing. Because older skin has lost some of its natural moisture as a result of aging, excessive use of alcohol may add to skin dryness and cracking.

Excessive amounts of hair over the IV site can be removed by clipping. Care must be taken to prevent nicking the skin. Shaving is not recommended to remove hair from potential IV sites because it causes microabrasions.[21] In the older adult, shaving could easily cause multiple cuts and nicks because of the fragile thinner skin layers; these cuts could provide an open pathway for bacteria to invade the tissue in and around the IV site.

Technique. A key factor for successful venipuncture for the older adult is absolute stabilization of the vein. In the older adult, the vessels may lack stability as a result of loss of tissue mass, and veins may tend to roll. Attempting to access such veins can result in the needle's tip nicking the vein or pushing the vein continually away. Skin tension is established by first determining the direction or axis of the vessel. Initial traction is accomplished by placing the thumb directly along the vein axis approximately 2 to 3 inches below the intended venipuncture site. The palm and fingers of the traction hand serve to hold and stabilize the extremity. The index finger of the traction hand can be used to further stretch the skin alongside the intended venipuncture site. Once traction has been initiated, it should be maintained throughout the venipuncture and catheter-threading procedure.[10]

The directional line of the vein should be observed. (Each vessel follows its own route.) By palpation, the IV nurse locates the vein and its route. When skin tension is established, palpating the vessel may be difficult or impossible. If the vein is a small, thin surface vessel, the venous distension may not be sufficient for extensive palpation. In these cases, the nurse should attempt to imagine the vein's track along the skin surface. This perceived path assists in aligning the catheter for insertion along the vein route after skin traction has been established.

As stated in *Infusion Nursing Standards of Practice,* 0.9% sodium chloride or lidocaine should not be routinely injected subcutaneously at the insertion site to anesthetize the area.[21] These preparations are most commonly used in anesthesiology before large-bore, 12- or 14-gauge catheters are inserted. In the elderly population, any additional needle puncture in the area for IV access may make successful venous access more difficult or impossible as a result of subcutaneous tissue swelling, vessel injury, or hemorrhage.

An IV catheter with a sharp, atraumatic bevel tip should be selected. The contour cuts on the bevel tip are designed for sharpness and ease of skin penetration. With the vessel held securely and the vein track visualized, the catheter should be aligned parallel to the vein track. The catheter should be brought close to the skin directly above the potential insertion site. The angle of insertion should be lowered to 20 to 30 degrees to reduce vein trauma on insertion.[8]

The insertion technique can be either direct or indirect.

When a direct technique is used, once skin traction is established, the vein is directly accessed at a 20- to 30-degree angle in a single motion, thereby penetrating the skin and the vein simultaneously. This method can be routinely used for patients with good vein access or those whose veins are easily stabilized. For patients with small, delicate veins or whose vessels are difficult to secure, an indirect or two-step insertion technique may be necessary.[10] With this technique, the skin is penetrated close to the vein by using the same firm motion as that used for a direct-access method. If a stabbing or thrusting motion is used with the catheter, there is a danger of going too deep or accidentally damaging the vein. Once the surface of the skin has been penetrated, the insertion angle of the catheter should be lowered to 10 to 15 degrees, the access vein should be restabilized, and the IV catheter bevel tip should be realigned to penetrate the vein wall. With a steady motion, the bevel tip should be advanced gently through the vein wall and into the lumen. The nurse should then check for backflow of blood into the flashback chamber of the catheter. As soon as the bevel and part of the catheter tip has advanced into the vein, the nurse should push the catheter forward off the stylet into the vein while stabilizing the stylet. During catheter-stylet separation, the nurse should observe the flashback chamber to ensure a continuing backflow of blood.[8] The stylet should not be pulled out of the catheter; rather, the catheter should always be pushed forward off the stylet into the vein. This method ensures that the bevel and part of the catheter are well into the vein before the stylet is removed.

If the veins are extremely fragile, it may be necessary to release the tourniquet as soon as a blood return occurs and catheter separation is achieved. This may prevent vein wall damage from high-pressure backflow of blood from the point where the catheter enters the vein.[8]

A "hooded" technique can be effectively used to advance the catheter into the vein. In this technique, the catheter is advanced forward over the bevel tip into the vein. This measure retracts the stylet tip inside the catheter. Then, the nurse threads the catheter into the vein by grasping the hub of the catheter and advancing the catheter-stylet as one unit up the vein, with the blunt catheter tip leading the way up the vessel. This process reduces the possibility of an accidental penetration of the vein wall during the threading. Vein stabilization and skin tension must be maintained from the time of insertion throughout the threading of the catheter. Only after the catheter has been advanced as far as possible can the tension from stabilization be eased slowly. The hooding technique can be essential to successfully threading the catheter without damaging or rupturing the fragile vessels of the older patient. If the skin tension is released before the catheter is threaded, the rebound of the skin and vein being released may cause the catheter to rupture the vein.[8,10]

IV access in the older adult may test all of the skill and knowledge of the IV nurse. However, the use of special techniques may enhance the success of venipuncture in these patients.

Device maintenance. Adequate stabilization of a vascular access device within a vein is essential to reduce the degree of mechanical irritation that results when the catheter shifts inside the vein. The key to maintaining an IV site in an older adult is to anticipate potential problems and to apply preventive measures before problems occur. Many IV protective devices can also be used to secure the catheter. The cost of these devices varies, and the degree of site protection must be carefully weighed on a cost-versus-benefit basis. Adaptations of products readily available can also be economically used to protect the IV site.

Site care begins with careful stabilization and application of a dressing. The decrease in subcutaneous fat and tissue in the elderly results in the catheter being unstable and in need of a secure dressing. To anchor the catheter, a ½-inch by 3-inch piece of tape with adhesive side up should be placed under the hub of the catheter. The edge of the tape should not be in contact with the IV site. The catheter rests on the adhesive strip, which helps anchor the catheter and protects the skin from the rigid plastic hub. The length of tape extending to each side of the catheter hub is then folded upward at a 90-degree angle to the catheter.[8] This modified chevron-taping technique can securely anchor the catheter with a minimum of tape. The use of soft-winged catheters also enhances the nurse's ability to stabilize and secure the catheter. These catheters offer another advantage; the extension tubing is a part of the catheter, thereby greatly reducing mechanical manipulation at the insertion site. IV devices that have stiff wings or flanges must be used with caution on the delicate skin of the elderly. Hard, stiff edges can cause skin irritation, soreness, or even ulceration. To prevent irritation when this type of device is used, any portion of the device that may cause irritation should be padded with a small gauze pad or sponge.

Securing the catheter to prevent accidental dislodgment is necessary; however, the amount of tape applied to the skin should be minimized in patients with delicate skin. Consideration should also be given to the kind of tape used on delicate skin. Some tapes may easily tear the fragile, thin skin of the older adult. Therefore the patient should be assessed carefully for any reaction to the tape product used. The patient should also be questioned about previous experiences with tape products before the tape is applied. Adaptations to the taping technique or product used should be implemented as necessary. To help reduce irritation or damage to the skin of the older adult, the additional protection provided by a skin polymer solution can be considered. This added skin barrier protects the skin from the effects of adhesives and from the drying nature of cleansing agents that occurs with repeated tape removal and dressing changes. While stabilizing the catheter, the nurse should apply the polymer solution in a circular motion around the site, starting ½ to ¾ inch out from the insertion point. The nurse should then allow the solution to air dry before applying the dressing. A gauze or transparent semipermeable membrane can be placed over the site to complete the dressing.

The IV nurse must anticipate potential hazards that could affect the continued successful delivery of the necessary infusion therapy. The older adult is not always as aware of his or her surroundings as other patients and is slower to adapt to environmental changes. These factors may result in accidents that might disturb or interrupt the patency of an infusion catheter. For example, the older adult may not remember that an infusion device is in place or may not have a good view of the set-up and may become tangled in the tubing, resulting in an accidental disconnection. Excessive lengths of tubing can become a physical hazard to the elderly patient who is trying to ambulate or to perform his or her own activities of daily living. The IV tubing should be long enough to give adequate range of motion but not to dangle on the floor or get caught under an IV pole or pump wheels. A segment of the IV tubing should be looped to the patient's arm so that inadvertent tugging pulls on the loop and not directly on the IV catheter site. Another important consideration is the type of administration sets connected to the catheter. A Luer-Lok connector provides a more secure connection and greater protection against accidental disconnection than do male-female interlocks, which can easily pull apart.

Occasionally, the catheter site may need to be covered to prevent the patient from inadvertently removing the catheter. An alternative method used to stabilize the catheter is to stretch properly sized site-protection material over the IV site. This measure provides coverage and stability for the site and protects the catheter from snagging on bed clothes, pumps, or other encumbrances. The site-protection material allows unimpeded peripheral circulation for the IV site while stabilizing the catheter and dressing. This material can also be used to help stabilize the device and minimize the need for tape. However, roller-type gauze, or any covering that is not easily removed should not be used because it decreases the ability to observe the site.

Another approach to covering an IV site is to place the patient in a long-sleeved gown or pajamas. If the IV is covered from the patient's view, the patient may not disturb it.

Armboards should be used with care to stabilize IV devices over areas of flexion. These boards must be padded and support the hand or arm in a functional position. The fingers should be allowed some motion to encourage circulation and to decrease the potential for dependent edema. The tape used to secure the board should be prebacked with gauze or tape so that the adhesive does not contact the patient's skin, thereby permitting good control of the extremity without circulatory impediment. The IV site and the vein path above the site should still be visible for frequent evaluation. When any extremity is immobilized, increased peripheral edema may occur as a result of slowed venous return in the restricted extremity. This problem can be critical in the older adult with peripheral vascular changes or limited mobility. Any decrease in activity to an extremity increases venous stasis and the resultant dependent edema; therefore these IV sites must be monitored often and the observations documented regularly.

Occasionally, some kind of immobilization device must be used to prevent the patient from dislodging the IV device. A physician's order is required for use of such a device. Immobilization policies vary between institutions, but regular monitoring and documentation are always required. Soft wrist immobilizers can be placed below an IV site but should never be placed directly over the IV site. If the IV site is in the wrist, hand, or fingers, the immobilizer should be placed around an armboard, and then the extremity should be secured on the armboard. The extremity with the IV is secured by the board while the board takes the pulling stress of the immobilizer. Mittens can also be applied, if necessary.[8] Dependent edema can develop below the immobilizer, where circulation can be impaired.

Site monitoring. The IV site should be observed regularly (as set by institutional policy) to ensure patency. In many hospitals, nursing practice policy recommends observing the area every 1 to 2 hours to verify site patency, condition, and flow rate and then documenting the observation in the patient records. Notation of IV site observations only once per shift is insufficient to validate 8 hours of patent IV flow, because complications such as phlebitis and infiltration, could go unnoticed for several hours. With the older adult, a small infiltrate could easily become a severe IV complication.

IV site rotation is recommended every 72 hours, according to *Infusion Nursing Standards of Practice.*[21] Variations from this standard may be acceptable if they are justified through documented and statistically substantiated clinical practice. The incidence of complications or phlebitis should be less than 5%, using a 72-hour site-change interval as the standard of care. If this standard is not met, the institution should return to a 48-hour site-change interval. If a routine site change is not performed because of limited access or patient condition, a full description of the site evaluation, dressing change, and reasons for the inability to rotate the IV site should be well documented in the patient's record.

Patient education

Family involvement. The patient education process begins with the physician's order for infusion therapy. It is important for the patient's self-esteem that all procedures be explained fully before they are performed. Such communication gives the patient a sense of participating in the process.

The nurse should speak slowly, clearly, and directly to the older adult. The patient should be addressed by name, and anyone who is involved in performing the procedure should be introduced by name and identification.[12] Steps in any procedure, such as infusion catheter insertion, should be described as they are performed. The patient will be more cooperative if he or she can anticipate the elements of his or her care and if trust is established.

Important ongoing infusion therapy–related considerations should be clearly and simply explained to the patient and family. For instance, while cleansing and dressing an IV site, the nurse should provide instructions on basic care to protect the IV site from infection or dislodgment. In this way, the patient and family can become partners in the maintenance of the IV site. If a pump or monitoring device is used, the nurse should explain potential alarms and how to prevent possible problems. The nurse should not use unfamiliar terminology, but instead should use clear, concise phrases that leave no doubt as to the meaning.[12]

Acute care considerations

Infusion therapy in the acute care setting can be a challenging experience for both the practitioner and patient. The rules of assessment for the younger adult are not appropriate for the elderly. The elderly are at an increased risk of misdiagnosis of a cognitive deficit resulting from acute illness, change in environment, or medications. Rapid decision making around the elderly can make them uncomfortable and withdrawn. The health care practitioner must not forget to include the elderly patient in his

or her own plan of care. The practice of placing large-gauge catheters also needs to be carefully evaluated. If the elderly patient is not to receive blood or large doses of fluid, a 22- or even 24-gauge catheter is a much better choice. Pathways and decision-making tools can address these issues with the least amount of conflict.

Home care considerations

The IV nurse must balance many elements when planning the delivery of infusion therapies in the home setting. The process begins with a physician's order for home infusion therapy. The IV nurse's role includes evaluating the type and duration of therapy and the infusion access and infusion delivery equipment required. These factors are all crucial to determining the appropriateness of home infusion therapy. Careful evaluation of the home physical environment, family members in the home, designated home health provider and other care providers, cost of the therapy, and insurance coverage must be performed. If these physical needs cannot be met, the environment for the patient and family may be too stressful for learning and retention.

Educating older adults in the administration of home infusion therapy presents certain challenges. As people age, they less readily adapt to environmental changes, especially those they cannot easily control or that affect their independence. Therefore the IV nurse must have a high degree of motivation and patience when instructing the older adult. Teaching the older adult complex drug admixtures, tubing connections, maintenance, pump programming, and accessing and deaccessing various IV devices is a step-by-step, individualized process. A progressively organized training program should include a written teaching manual or a program module using large print and, more importantly, direct demonstrations of specific procedures with return demonstration evaluated by the potential home care provider.

The medical knowledge and nursing care required of an older patient or family in a short time can be particularly overwhelming. The IV nurse must evaluate the older adult for the ability to perform and the willingness to comply with the required skills. With the older patient or designated primary care provider, time must be spent evaluating the emotional stability, intellectual capacity, and physical ability to perform the required skills. For instance, is the patient emotionally able to cope with care at home by a family member or a home health worker? The family members or significant others must be able to provide support for the patient and each other. In addition, can the learner understand the necessary health care concepts? A gap in comprehension may result from the aging process and language or cultural differences. The nurse should consider whether interpreters could be used to enhance learning. The use of pictorial step-by-step manuals can dramatically facilitate learning for those with a reading, language, or hearing deficit. Sign language interpreters and lip reading can help the hearing impaired. In addition, videotapes of procedures can permit the patient and family to refresh skills at home.

The number of IV nurses designated as patient educators should be limited to maintain continuity of the skills being taught. In patient education, the content must be taught in exactly the same way to each caregiver. Tasks can become easily confusing to the lay caregiver if different methods are used for procedures. Precise training examples should be used and repeated exactly the same way each time. This consistency and repetition will reduce the potential for errors or patient complications in the home.

The patient and family should have an understanding of what complications or problems could occur and the appropriate interventions for these problems. This information should be included in the patient teaching module and should be reviewed several times before discharge or independent administration. The information should include care of the infusion site and alternative access device (e.g., PICCs, implanted ports, and tunneled catheters), various pumps (intermittent, continuous, patient-controlled analgesia, ambulatory, stationary), medications and their side effects, total parenteral nutrition (cyclic or continuous), proper tubings and connections, medication incompatibilities, emergency procedures, emergency access to health care personnel, record keeping, storage of medical supplies, and proper disposal of medical wastes.

The impact of sensory changes that occur with aging, particularly changes in visual acuity, hearing, and manual dexterity, should also be considered. The importance of visual acuity is seen in the administration of small medication dosages for IV admixtures, the adjustment of pump rates, and the accessing of infusion devices and tubing connections. The primary care provider must be able to see and read the directions for medication administration and for the care and maintenance of infusion access devices. Changes in hearing may affect the patient's ability to hear and respond to pump alarms in a timely manner. Manual dexterity is another important requirement for many home infusion procedures. The older adult may have significant problems handling the necessary equipment because of illness-related changes resulting from arthritis, cardiovascular accidents, partial or full paralysis, amputation, or other physical impairments. For instance, the older adult may have difficulty attaching administration sets and handling the small caps attached to these sets. The older adult should be carefully observed working with the various devices, and alternatives should be used as are deemed appropriate. Needleless systems may be used with the older adult to eliminate the risk of needlesticks.

The IV nurse providing care in the home is a partner in the development of a safe, home-based, infusion delivery system. The concerns of the home care provider include the following:

- A clean, dry space for supplies
- A clean work preparation area
- Special refrigeration needs
- Pets
- Parasites and infestations in the home
- Necessary electrical outlets
- Batteries and sufficient supplies
- A telephone
- Names of people to call in an emergency

The hospital and home care provider must evaluate all of these factors to determine whether the home can provide a safe place for the administration of infusion therapy.

The desired outcome for any course of infusion therapy is to provide successful administration of a prescribed therapy for the duration required with no complications. The achievement of this goal is enhanced when care is provided by a highly skilled IV nurse. When the special needs of the older adult are addressed, the result will be atraumatic peripheral IV access; decreased complications through diligent infusion site monitoring, care, and maintenance; appropriate use of the newest techniques and care; quality patient education; coordinated transfers from the hospital or extended-care facility to the home; and successful delivery of home infusion therapies. Only through awareness of the special concerns can the IV nurse attempt to provide and care for vascular access for the older adult.

Long-term care considerations

The long-term care setting provides a unique set of conditions for the patient receiving infusion therapy. Prospective payment systems, managed care, and the drive for patients to be discharged from the acute care environment has placed patients with much higher acuity in settings that traditionally were not equipped to handle such patients. The lack of laboratory, x-ray, and on-call physician services once posed a barrier to acceptance of these patients in long-term care settings. However, long-term care is now seeing the influx of all types of therapies. Hydration and antibiotic therapy have been common in long-term care for many years. Recently, therapies such as inotropic medications and chemotherapy have made their way into the long-term care environment. These therapies require strict monitoring and staff members who have the validated competencies required to effectively manage infusion patients.

Educational requirements for the nursing staff and nursing assistants need to be defined. PICCs and midlines can be placed in this environment by qualified nursing staff. Currently, the model most commonly used is the pharmacy or outside agency contracting with nurses to place these lines. Because they are not considered emergency lines and the elderly often require prehydration before insertion, it may take 24 to 48 hours to place the line, depending on the patient's condition and geographic location.

OLDER ADULT COLLABORATIVE PATHWAYS

Pathway management of disease processes has been recognized as a cost-effective and vital part of the management of care. Disease state management of pneumonia, for example, has effectively reduced complications and length of stay for the older adult in the acute care setting. A collaborative pathway works on the same concept. However, it involves settings rather than disease processes. Patients, including the elderly, are no longer completing therapies in one setting and must rely on the health care professionals to ensure that their course is completed.

Clinical and critical pathways deal with disease-state management. The concept of a collaborative pathway takes this further by using the professional expertise found in different settings and building a strong bridge to the patient's recovery with the least amount of complications. Duplication of effort by a multitude of settings can greatly increase the cost of health care to the elderly consumer. This is of particular importance because the elderly are more likely to require health care and are often surviving on fixed incomes.

A number of variables must be considered when implementing a collaborative pathway. The education and expertise of the staff in handling simple or complex infusion therapy of the geriatric patient is of the utmost importance. All members of the health care team need to have education regarding the special needs of the elderly.

Regulatory differences also have a major impact on the collaborative pathway. Acute care settings and alternative care settings are governed by a variety of state and federal organizations. Health care workers should be familiar with regulations such as the Omnibus Budget Reconciliation Act of 1989 and the state Nurse Practice Act, and with organizations such as the Health Care Financing Administration and the Joint Commission on Accreditation of Healthcare Organizations.

Summary

Infusion therapy in the older adult is one of the most challenging responsibilities of the IV nurse. However, it can be one of the most rewarding. The ability to accurately assess and care for the older adult requires a very clear understanding of the aging process. Listening and learning from the older adult enables the infusion nurse to be the best possible patient advocate. The ability to communicate with other members of the health care team along the continuum of care regarding the patient's needs will ensure the successful completion of therapy and minimize complications. Society is aging—it is essential that health care personnel be prepared to deal with the specific issues of older adults.

References

1. Tyson SR: *Gerontological nursing care,* Philadelphia, 1999, WB Saunders.
2. World Health Organization: *The world health report 1999,* World Health Organization, Geneva, 1999, World Health Organization.
3. US Department of Commerce, Economics and Statistics Administration, Bureau of the Census: *World population profile: 1998,* Washington, DC, 1998, US Government Printing Office.
4. Campbell P: *Current population reports,* Washington, DC, 1997, US Department of Commerce, Economics and Statistics Administration, Bureau of the Census US Government Printing Office.
5. United Nations Population Division, *World population prospects: the 1998 revision,* New York, 1999, United Nations.
6. Eliopoulos C: *Manual of gerontologic nursing,* ed 2, St Louis, 1999, Mosby.
7. Stone J, Wyman J, Salisbury S: *Clinical gerontological nursing,* ed 2, Philadelphia, 1999, WB Saunders.
8. Weinstein SM: *Plumer's principles and practices of intravenous therapy,* ed 6, Philadelphia, 1997, Lippincott-Raven.
9. Lueckenotte AG: *Gerontologic nursing,* St Louis, 1996, Mosby.
10. Phillips LD: *Manual of I.V. therapeutics,* ed 2, Philadelphia, 1997, FA Davis.
11. Hazzard WR, et al: *Principles of geriatric medicine and gerontology,* ed 4, New York, 1999, McGraw-Hill.
12. Whitson M: Intravenous therapy in the older adult: special needs and considerations, *JIN* 19(5):251, 1996.
13. Centers for Disease Control and Prevention: AIDS among persons >/=50 years—United States, 1991-1996, *MMWR CDC Surveill Summ* 47:21, 1998.
14. High KP: AIDS: a disease of the young? *Infect Med* 15(12):832, 1998.
15. Chidester JC, Spangler A: Fluid intake in the institutionalized elderly, *J Am Diet Assoc* 97(1):23, 1997.
16. Gallo JJ, et al: *Reichel's care of the elderly: clinical aspects of aging,* ed 5, Philadelphia, 1999, Lippincott Williams & Wilkins.
17. Nusbaum NJ: Aging and sensory senescence, *South Med J* 92(3): 267, 1999.
18. Overcash J: Symptom management in the geriatric patient, *Cancer Control JMCC* 5(3S):46, 1998.
19. Roth D: Venipuncture tips for geriatric patients, *Nursing* 27(10): 69, 1997.
20. Powers FA: Your elderly patient needs I.V. therapy. . . can you keep her safe? *Nursing* 29(7):54, 1999.
21. Intravenous Nurses Society: Infusion nursing standards of practice, *JIN* (suppl) 23(6S), 2000.

Conscious Sedation

Lory Youmans, RN, MS

HISTORY

The use of nonanesthesiologists to manage patients receiving sedation has steadily increased over the past 20 years. As ambulatory surgery centers and outpatient procedure units have increased, so has the need for patients to achieve a speedy return to presedation levels of consciousness. More physicians and surgeons are choosing conscious sedation because it facilitates an early return to the basic routines of daily living.

Historically, patients had either general or local anesthesia. Procedures using local anesthesia were usually low risk and the patients were young and healthy. Local anesthesia usually involved injection of a localizing drug at the site of the procedure and sedative medications, such as diazepam (Valium), possibly in combination with a pain reliever, such as meperidine (Demerol) or morphine. The clinician assigned to the procedure usually monitored the patient and assisted the physician during the procedure as well. The patient would be transported to a postanesthesia care unit, monitored, dressed, and sent home or transferred to a nursing unit.

As newer, faster-acting medications came on the market, the need for regulating the practice of local sedation became evident because of the increased frequency and speed of patients' adverse reactions. Prompted by legal actions, liability became an issue in many states. The term *conscious sedation* was coined and became universally accepted.

As a result, many state boards of nursing issued position statements regarding the role of registered nurses (RNs) managing conscious sedation. Some statements consist of a mere paragraph, such as the North Dakota Board of Nursing's Declaratory ruling 89-1:

> Although RNs, under the direction of a physician, may administer narcotics, analgesics, sedative, and tranquilizing medications to patients, RNs may not administer any medication for the purpose of inducing general anesthesia. It is not within the authority of the board to determine how or for what purpose a specific drug with multiple uses is being administered at any given time. Institutional or agency protocol must address this.[1]

Other position statements are much more extensive and outline educational needs, medications that may be given, legal implications, and equipment required for safe administration and monitoring.

The Joint Commission on Accreditation of Healthcare Organizations (JCAHO) states that hospitals must have written policies and procedures and set guidelines regarding documentation requirements. The American Nurses Association, American Dental Association, Association of periOperative Registered Nurses (AORN), Society of Gastroenterology Nurses Association, Emergency Nurses Association, and American Society of Anesthesiology (ASA) are some of the professional organizations that have developed recommended practices for patients receiving conscious sedation/analgesia.

DEFINITION AND GOALS

Conscious sedation is produced by the administration of pharmacologic agents, by any route, that results in a depressed level of consciousness but allows the patient to independently maintain a patent airway and respond appropriately to verbal commands or physical stimulation. Conscious sedation enables the patient to tolerate unpleasant procedures by relieving anxiety, discomfort, and pain. Patients should be able to retain their protective reflexes.

An ASA task force on sedation and analgesia by nonanesthesiologists decided that the term *sedation/analgesia* more accurately defines this therapeutic goal than the term *conscious sedation*.[2] Patients whose only response is reflex withdrawal from a painful stimulus are sedated to a greater degree than desired from sedation/analgesia provided by nurses. This deeper level of sedation falls under the category of *monitored anesthesia care* (MAC) performed by licensed anesthesia personnel who have the knowledge to administer anesthetic agents in combination with sedation/analgesia medications.

Medicare, private insurers, and third-party payers have defined what procedures can be reimbursed under MAC versus nurse-monitored sedation/analgesia. The definition of MAC as established by the ASA is as follows: "Instances in which an anesthesiologist has been called upon to provide specific anesthesia services to a particular patient undergoing a planned procedure, in connection with which a patient receives local anesthesia, or in some cases, no anesthesia at all."[2] Although the procedure is performed under local anesthesia, licensed anesthesia personnel provide patient care. In these instances, the procedure is more extensive or the patient is more difficult to manage.

There are four levels of sedation. The first is *light sedation,* in which the patient is awake or arouses easily but is under the influence of the drug administered. The patient maintains normal respiration, normal eye movements, and intact protective reflexes. Amnesia may or may not be present. The second level is *sedation/analgesia.* This level is the goal of conscious sedation. At this level, the patient is in a pharmacologically controlled state of limited or minimally depressed consciousness. The patient independently and continuously maintains protective reflexes and a patent airway. The patient responds appropriately to physical stimulation and verbal commands. The third level is *deep sedation,* a controlled state of depressed consciousness or unconsciousness with partial or complete loss of protective reflexes, including the ability to maintain an airway independently and continuously. Although this level is not the intent of sedation/analgesia, the patient may occasionally achieve this level of sedation. The caregiver should be medically prepared to respond to this event. Level four is *general anesthesia,* or a controlled state of unconsciousness, loss of protective reflexes, and inability to respond to physical stimuli or verbal commands.

The primary goal of sedation/analgesia is to reduce the patient's anxiety and discomfort and to facilitate cooperation between the patient and the caregiver. The objectives for the patient receiving conscious sedation/analgesia include the alteration of mood, maintenance of consciousness, enhanced cooperation, elevation of the pain threshold, minimal variation of vital signs, some degree of amnesia, and a rapid, safe return to activities of daily living.[3] Patient selection criteria for receiving sedation/analgesia depend on meeting these objectives.

PATIENT SELECTION AND PREPROCEDURAL ASSESSMENT

A complete and thorough assessment is mandatory before the administration of sedation/analgesia. Pediatric and geriatric patients are suitable candidates for conscious sedation. The patient should be cooperative and have the ability to follow simple commands. In children and uncooperative adults, sedation/analgesia may expedite procedures that are not particularly uncomfortable but require that the patient remain still. A minimal loss of protective reflexes is recommended. Protective reflexes include the ability to breathe independently, the gag reflex, the ability to cough and swallow, and eye movements. Caution must also be exercised when a patient with a degenerative muscle disease is being considered as a candidate for sedation/analgesia.

The caregiver whose role is to monitor sedation/analgesia should be familiar with the relevant aspects of the patient's medical history. The initial assessment should include pertinent medical and anesthetic history, nothing-by-mouth (NPO) status

(Table 32-1), baseline vital signs, weight, current medications, allergies, mental status, and a history of tobacco, alcohol, and substance use or abuse. The patient's underlying medical condition should guide preprocedural lab studies.

Unsuitable candidates include patients requiring more extensive monitoring and sedation, as in high-risk patients with underlying medical problems, severe cardiovascular problems, severe respiratory problems, and extremely painful procedures. The ASA, which has established a classification system to help guide decisions (Table 32-2), recommends that sedation/analgesia be limited to ASA class I and II patients. An ASA class III patient may require consultation by the health care team, consisting of physician, anesthesia representative, and nurse, to determine whether anesthesia care is required.

The following list provides examples of the ASA classes:

ASA I: Healthy patient with no systemic medical problems undergoing a surgical procedure.

ASA II: Patient smokes and has well-controlled hypertension.

ASA III: Patient has diabetes and fairly stable angina. Takes medications, including insulin.

ASA IV: Patient has diabetes, angina, and congestive heart failure, dyspnea, and chest pain on mild exertion.

Table 32-1	**NPO Recommendations for Sedation/Analgesia***	
AGE	**MILK/SOLIDS**	**CLEAR LIQUIDS**
Adult	6-8 hr	2-3 hr
>36 mo	6-8 hr	2-3 hr
6-36 mo	6 hr	2-3 hr
<6 mo	4 hr	2 hr

Data from Reference 2.
NPO, Nothing by mouth.
*ASA-recommended practices.

Table 32-2	**American Society of Anesthesiology Patient Classification Status**	
ASA CLASSIFICATION	**MEDICAL DESCRIPTION OF PATIENT**	**COMMENTS**
ASA I	No known systemic disease	May have conscious sedation without other consultation
ASA II	Mild or well-controlled systemic disease	Same as above
ASA III	Multiple or moderate controlled systemic diseases	Consider medical consultation
ASA IV	Poorly controlled systemic disease(s)	Mandatory involvement of Anesthesiology Department
ASA V	Moribund patient	Same as above

Note: *E* connotes emergency and can be added to any of the classifications.
Data from Reference 4.
ASA, American Society of Anesthesiology.

ASA V: Patient is unstable. Not expected to survive without surgical intervention.

ASA I E: Unexpected surgical procedure in a healthy individual (e.g., healthy child bitten by a dog).

A thorough airway assessment is required, because positive-pressure ventilation may be necessary if respiration is compromised. Factors that may influence airway management include a history of stridor, snoring, or sleep apnea; significant obesity; previous problems with anesthesia or sedation; facial abnormalities; and advanced arthritis. Head, jaw, and neck deformities, including such findings as short neck, limited neck extension, neck mass, cervical spine disease, trauma, and tracheal deviation, may also create potential airway problems. An examination of the mouth may reveal a nonvisible uvula, tonsillar hypertrophy, small mouth opening, edentulous, protruding incisors, loose or capped teeth, or a high, arched palate. All of the aforementioned abnormalities may increase the likelihood of airway obstruction during sedation/analgesia.

MONITORING AND EQUIPMENT

Monitoring equipment required for sedation/analgesia must be in the room before the administration of any medication. This equipment should include oxygen and oxygen delivery devices, suction apparatus, noninvasive blood pressure device, electrocardiograph, and pulse oximeter.

It is important to remember that there are inherent limitations when using an oximeter. Oximetry readings are affected by vasoconstriction, hypothermia, vasoconstrictive drugs, and motion of the fingers. An oximeter measures the O_2 saturation at the capillary level. Hypoventilation and resultant hypocarbia follow a decrease in oxygen saturation by many minutes. The caregiver must monitor the rate and volume of respirations and not rely solely on oximeter readings.

Along with the respiratory rate and oxygen saturation, monitoring criteria should include blood pressure, cardiac rate and rhythm, level of consciousness, and skin condition. Undesirable changes in the patient's condition should be reported immediately to the physician.

The Ramsey sedation scale (Box 32-1) is commonly used to determine the patient's level of consciousness. Although it is most often used in intensive care units with intubated patients, it is appropriate for short-term therapeutic, diagnostic, or surgical procedures. In levels 1 though 3, the patient is considered conscious. Level 4 is approaching deep sedation, and level 5 is

deep sedation. Level 6 is considered beyond the intent and scope of practice for the RN administering sedation/analgesia.

Continuous intravenous (IV) access should be determined on a case-by-case basis. The facility's policy and procedures and the physician's preferences determine the type of IV access. If the patient is receiving sedation intravenously, IV access should be continuously maintained throughout the procedure. An individual with the skills to establish IV access should be immediately available in all instances.

Not all facilities require continuous electrocardiographic (ECG) monitoring throughout the procedure. Such monitoring remains controversial even in facilities that require it. The need to continuously monitor the ECG must be determined by the preprocedural assessment. Patients with a history of cardiac problems or other underlying diseases that may cause problems, such as hypertension or diabetes, should be monitored continuously.

Because diminished reflexes, depressed respiratory functions, and impaired cardiovascular function may occur within seconds or minutes after the administration of medications, an emergency cart must be immediately available whenever sedation/analgesia is administered. The cart should include resuscitative medications, including narcotic and sedative reversal medications, and equipment such as a defibrillator (Table 32-3). The caregiver must maintain a current certification in cardiopulmonary resuscitation (CPR) and maintain knowledge in the use of the emergency cart and the medication and equipment on that cart. There is debate as to whether the caregiver needs to maintain certification in advanced cardiac life support (ACLS).

The clinician monitoring the patient should have no other responsibilities. The patient should never be left unattended.

Table 32-3	**Emergency Resuscitative Equipment**
Oxygen	▪ A system of delivering 100% at 10 L/min for at least 30 min
Suction	▪ Apparatus capable of producing continuous negative pressure of 150 mm Hg
Airway management	▪ Face masks (all sizes) ▪ Oral and nasal airways ▪ Endotracheal tubes ▪ Laryngoscopes
Monitors	▪ Pulse oximeter with visible and audible displays ▪ Cardiac monitor ▪ Automated blood pressure device
Resuscitative equipment/medications	▪ Ambu bag ▪ Defibrillator with ECG recorder capabilities ▪ Emergency drugs, including naloxone (Narcan), flumazenil (Mazicon), ephedrine, and epinephrine ▪ Emergency drug card and ACLS protocols

Data from Reference 6.
ECG, Electrocardiogram; *ACLS,* advanced cardiac life support.

Box 32-1 Ramsey Sedation Scale[5]

▪ Level 1: Patient is anxious and agitated or restless, or both.
▪ Level 2: Patient is cooperative, oriented, and tranquil.
▪ Level 3: Patient responds only to commands.
▪ Level 4: Patient exhibits brisk response to a light glabellar tap or loud auditory stimulus.
▪ Level 5: Patient exhibits a sluggish response to a light glabellar tap or loud auditory stimulus.
▪ Level 6: Patient exhibits no response.

The nurse must be clinically competent to immediately identify complications and respond to adverse reactions during the procedure. The clinician should understand the pharmacology of the administered agents, and the role of pharmacologic antagonists for opioids and benzodiazepines. Anesthesia personnel would not be expected to hand the physician instruments or run out of the room for supplies, and neither should the individual monitoring the patient under sedation/analgesia.

Clinicians monitoring the patient during sedation/analgesia should demonstrate knowledge of anatomy and physiology, pharmacology of medications used for conscious sedation/analgesia, cardiac arrhythmia interpretation, complications related to the use of conscious sedation/analgesia, and respiratory functions. The practitioner must also have the skills necessary to assess, diagnose, and treat any complications that may arise during the course of care.

PHARMACOLOGY

Agents used for sedation/analgesia depend on the type, duration, and intensity of the procedure. The patient's health status should be considered when selecting and administering medications. Although the physician orders the type and amount of medication for administration, it is the caregiver's responsibility to validate the order, obtain the medication, and ensure proper administration. Proper administration includes the *five rights* of medication administration: right medication, right dose, right patient, right time, and right route. Any inconsistencies need to be resolved before medication is administered.

This section discusses the most commonly used medications: benzodiazepines, opioids, and their respective reversal agents (Table 32-4). Medications such as ketamine (a hypnotic), propofol, sodium pentothal, methohexital, and nitrous oxide are classified as anesthetic agents and should be administered only by physicians and nurses who have education and privileges in anesthesiology. They are not discussed in this chapter.

Benzodiazepines

Benzodiazepines can be administered as premedication, during the procedure for sedation/analgesia or general anesthesia, and during postprocedure care. They have anticonvulsant, antianxiety, sedative, muscle relaxant, and amnesic properties. Three benzodiazepines are used in sedation/analgesia. Midazolam (Versed) is the most commonly used benzodiazepine for sedation/analgesia because it has a fast onset of action, is short acting, and produces a high degree of retrograde amnesia. Diazepam and lorazepam are longer acting and are not as well suited for shorter procedures.

Midazolam. Midazolam (Versed), a short-acting benzodiazepine, is a central nervous system (CNS) depressant and a sedative-hypnotic. It may be administered intravenously, intramuscularly, orally, rectally, or nasally. The most common route is IV. The initial dose is 0.5 mg, and the dose should not exceed 2.5 mg in a healthy adult. The dose for a pediatric patient is 0.01 to 0.8 mg/kg for IV and intramuscular (IM) administration, and 0.3 to 0.7 mg/kg for oral (PO), rectal, or intranasal administration, with a maximum dose of 4 mg. Slurred speech is an excellent indicator of an adequate dose. Lower dosages should be given to patients who are older than 60 years of age, debilitated, chronically ill, or receiving narcotics. The onset of action is 3 to 5 minutes for IV doses and 10 minutes for IM or PO doses. The peak effect is 10 to 15 minutes, with a duration of 60 to 150 minutes. The half-life is 1.2 to 12.3 hours.

Midazolam is three to four times more potent than diazepam (Valium). It must be given slowly intravenously and never administered by rapid or single-dose bolus. Rapid or excessive IV doses may result in respiratory depression or arrest. The initial dose may be repeated every 2 minutes. The total dose should not exceed 5 mg in a 2-hour period. Premedicated patients usually need 30% less. If used with other CNS depressants, half the usual dosage should be given.

Doses of midazolam should be individualized, and the patients must be monitored carefully. It is difficult to foresee a patient's reaction to midazolam based on the history and physical examination. There can be serious and life-threatening respiratory depression and respiratory arrest. The best rule for administration of midazolam is to start with small doses and administer slowly. By following this simple rule, serious complications can be avoided.

Midazolam is contraindicated in patients with known benzodiazepine hypersensitivity or acute narrow-angle glaucoma. Adverse reactions from IV administration include hiccups, nausea, vomiting, over sedation, headache, coughing, and pain at the injection site.

Diazepam. Diazepam (Valium), a benzodiazepine used as an anticonvulsant, is a CNS depressant. It may be administered via the IV, IM, rectal, or PO routes, although IM administration is very painful and not recommended. The initial IV dose is 2.5 to 5.0 mg and may be repeated every 5 to 10 minutes. The maximum dose should not exceed 30 mg in 2 hours. When given intravenously, diazepam needs to be administered slowly over 1 minute for each 5 mg. Doses for the pediatric patient are 0.05 to 0.2 mg/kg intravenously and 0.5 mg/kg rectally, with a maximum dose of 10 mg. As with midazolam, slurred speech is an excellent indicator of an adequate dose. Lower dosages should be used in the elderly or debilitated patients. The onset of action is 1 to 5 minutes for IV, 15 to 30 minutes for IM, and 30 to 60 minutes for PO administration. The duration of action is 2 to 6 hours. Diazepam peaks in 10 to 30 minutes and has a half-life of 20 to 40 hours. This drug cannot be mixed with other medications or diluted because of the risk of precipitate formation. It must be injected as close to the IV injection site as possible because of the risk of thrombophlebitis.

Diazepam is contraindicated in patients with known hypersensitivity to benzodiazepines and must be used with caution in patients with impaired liver or kidney function. Adverse reactions include drowsiness, nausea, bradycardia, venous thrombosis, phlebitis, apnea, hypotension, headache, blurred vision, syncope, vertigo, skin rash, hiccups, and changes in salivation. There is a high risk of respiratory depression in the geriatric patient.

Lorazepam. Lorazepam (Ativan), a benzodiazepine used as an anxiolytic, is a CNS depressant and sedative-hypnotic. It is occasionally administered for its sedative effects during procedures that last more than 2 hours. The dosage is 1 to 2 mg

Table 32-4   Medications Commonly Used for Conscious Analgesia

NAME	DOSAGE	ONSET OF ACTION	PEAK ACTION	DURATION	CONTRAINDICATIONS	ADVERSE REACTIONS	SPECIAL CONSIDERATIONS
BENZODIAZEPINES							
Midazolam (Versed)	*Adult:* 0.5-2.5 mg IV initially to slurred speech *Pediatric:* 0.01-0.8 mg/kg IV/IM 0.3-0.7 mg/kg PO/rectal/IN Maximum 4 mg	3-5 min IV 10 min IM/PO/rectal/IN	10-15 min	60-150 min	Hypersensitivity to benzodiazepine, or with acute narrow-angle glaucoma	Hiccups, nausea, vomiting, oversedation, headache, coughing, and pain at injection site	Individualize dosages; serious life-threatening respiratory depression and arrest; start with low dosages and administer slowly
Diazepam (Valium)	*Adult:* Initial 2.5-5 mg IV for maximum 30 mg in 2 hr *Pediatric:* 0.05-0.2 mg/kg IV 0.5 mg/kg rectal Maximum 10 mg	1-5 min IV 15-30 min IM 30-60 min PO	10-30 min	2-6 hr	Hypersensitivity to benzodiazepine, acute narrow-angle glaucoma; use with caution in liver and kidney dysfunction	Drowsiness, nausea, bradycardia, venous thrombosis, phlebitis, apnea, hypotension, headache, bradycardia, blurred vision, syncope, vertigo, skin rash, hiccups, and changes in salivation	Use lower doses to combat a high risk of respiratory depression in the elderly and debilitated patients
Lorazepam (Ativan)	*Adult:* 1-2 mg IV 15-20 min before procedure 2-4 mg IM/PO 2 hr before procedure *Pediatric:* 0.02-0.05 mg/kg IV/IM for maximum of 2 mg	5-10 min	2 hr	6-8 hr	Hypersensitivity to benzodiazepine or acute narrow-angle glaucoma	Excessive sleepiness and drowsiness, hallucinations, dizziness, hypertension or hypotension, depressed hearing, diplopia, blurred vision, nausea and vomiting, partial airway obstruction, and skin rash	Maximum dose by all routes is 10 mg unless the airway is controlled; use with caution in older adults, in very ill, or when pulmonary reserve is limited; not suited for short-term procedures
OPIOIDS							
Meperidine hydrochloride (Demerol)	*Adult:* 30-150 mg IV in divided doses of 12.5-25 mg 50-100 mg PO/IM 30-90 min before procedure *Pediatric:* 1.0-2.0 mg/kg IV/IM Maximum 100 mg	1-5 min IV 15 min PO 10 min IM	10-20 min	1-4 hr	Known hypersensitivity to meperidine or on MAO inhibitors	Drowsiness, dizziness, confusion, headache, sedation, euphoria, convulsions, tachycardia, asystole, bradycardia, palpitations, hypotension, syncope, nausea and vomiting, anorexia, constipation, cramps, rash, flushing, blurred vision, respiratory depression	Watch for histamine release in IV doses that may cause tracking and red streaking of vein

Drug	Dose	Onset	Peak	Duration	Contraindications	Side Effects	Precautions
Morphine sulfate	*Adult:* 1-10 mg over 4-5 min *Pediatric:* 0.1-0.2 mg/kg for IV/IM/PO for maximum of 10 mg	Immediate to 7 min	10-20 min	2-4 hr	Known hypersensitivity to morphine or phenanthrene opioids (e.g., codeine, oxycodone)	Sedation, dizziness, delirium, seizures, euphoria, nausea, vomiting, constipation, urinary retention, blurred vision, bradycardia, tachycardia, palpitations, asystole, hypertension, hypotension, respiratory depression, rash, urticaria, flushing or diaphoresis	Use with caution in patients with supraventricular arrhythmia, head injury or increased intracranial pressure, during pregnancy, or with renal or hepatic dysfunction or pulmonary disease
Fentanyl citrate (Sublimaze)	*Adult:* 12.5-25 µg IV for maximum of 150 µg *Pediatric:* 0.5-1 µg/kg IV over 2 hr Maximum 4 µg/kg/hr	Immediate to 5 min	3-5 min	30-60 min	Known hypersensitivity to fentanyl	Sedation, dizziness, delirium, seizures, euphoria, nausea, vomiting, blurred vision, miosis, bradycardia, tachycardia, palpitations, arrest, hypertension, hypotension, respiratory depression, arrest, laryngospasm, apnea, or skeletal muscle rigidity	Administer with caution to any patient with supraventricular arrhythmia or bradycardia, head injury, renal or hepatic dysfunction, pulmonary disease, convulsive disorders, or physical addiction to this medication; reduce dosage 1/4 to 1/3 if used with other CNS depressants; rapid administration can lead to chest wall rigidity and difficulty breathing; watch for delayed onset of respiratory depression; not recommended if MAO inhibitors taken within 14 days

IV, Intravenous; *IM,* intramuscular; *PO,* orally; *IN,* intranasally; *MAO,* monoamine oxidase; *CNS,* central nervous system.

Continued

Table 32-4   Medications Commonly Used for Conscious Analgesia—cont'd

Name	Dosage	Onset of Action	Peak Action	Duration	Contraindications	Adverse Reactions	Special Considerations
REVERSALS							
Flumazenil (Romazicon) Benzodiazepine antagonist	0.2 IV every 45-60 seconds until desired effect Maximum 3 mg/hr	30-60 sec	6-10 min	Varies	Extreme caution in patients with seizure disorder	Nausea and vomiting, dizziness, injection site pain, agitation, headache, cutaneous vasodilation, paraesthesia, emotional lability, inflammation at injection site, abnormal vision, fatigue, and/or seizures	Chronic users of benzodiazepines are at risk of grand mal seizures; use caution with impaired hepatic or kidney function; does not reverse hypoventilation or cardiac depression
Naloxone hydrochloride (Narcan) Opioid antagonist	0.1-0.2 mg IV every 2-3 min until desired effect Maximum dose 10 mg	1-2 min	5-15 min	45 min	Known hypersensitivity to naloxone	Abrupt reversal may result in nausea, vomiting, sweating, tachycardia, increased blood pressure, tremulousness, seizures and cardiac depression	If this drug is administered to a patient with opioid drug dependence, severe withdrawal syndrome may result; administer with caution to patient with supraventricular arrhythmia, head injuries, or convulsive disorders

intravenously 15 to 20 minutes before the procedure, or 2 to 4 mg intramuscularly or orally 2 hours before the procedure. The dose for pediatric patients is 0.02 to 0.05 mg/kg intravenously or intramuscularly, with a maximum dose of 2 mg. The onset of action is 5 to 10 minutes, with peak action in 2 hours. The duration of action is 6 to 8 hours, and it has a mean half-life of 16 hours. Half the original dose may be repeated every 10 to 15 minutes. The maximum adult dosage by all routes is 10 mg unless the patient's airway is controlled.

Lorazepam is contraindicated in patients with known hypersensitivity to benzodiazepines or with acute narrow-angle glaucoma. It should be administered with caution in older adults, very ill patients, or patients with limited pulmonary reserve. Lorazepam is not suitable for short-term procedures. Adverse reactions include excessive sleepiness and drowsiness, hallucinations, dizziness, hypertension or hypotension, depressed hearing, diplopia, blurred vision, nausea and vomiting, partial airway obstruction, and skin rash.

Flumazenil. Flumazenil (Romazicon) is a benzodiazepine antagonist. The dosage is 0.2 mg intravenously every 45 to 60 seconds until the desired effect is achieved or until 1 mg is given. This dose can be repeated at 20-minute intervals. No more than 3 mg should be given in a 1-hour period. The onset of action is 30 to 60 seconds, and peak action is achieved in 6 to 10 minutes. The duration of this medication is influenced by the dose administered and the dose of the agonist. The half-life is about 60 minutes. This medication does not reverse hypoventilation or cardiac depression.

Flumazenil should be used with extreme caution in patients with a history of seizure disorders. Patients chronically receiving benzodiazepines are at risk of grand mal seizures with the use of flumazenil. It should not be used routinely and should be administered slowly with careful, continuous patient monitoring.

Flumazenil is contraindicated in patients with known hypersensitivity to benzodiazepines and patients undergoing long-term benzodiazepine therapy. It should be used with caution in patients with impaired hepatic or kidney function as it is metabolized in the liver and excreted in the urine. Adverse reactions include nausea and vomiting, dizziness, injection site pain, agitation, headache, cutaneous vasodilation, paresthesia, labile emotion, inflammation at injection site, abnormal vision, fatigue, and seizures.

Opioids

The terms *opioid, opiate,* and *narcotic* are used interchangeably to describe medications administered to help manage pain. Opioids provide analgesia and sedation and are effective in elevating the pain threshold. They are classified as agonists, mixed agonists-antagonists, or partial agonists, depending on their activity at the opioid receptors. They may be administered as a premedication or along with another medication during a procedure. Generally, an opioid and a benzodiazepine are administered along with local or regional anesthesia. Opioids are broken down by hepatic metabolism. Only the most common opioids are covered in this chapter. Other opioids, which might be used for sedation/analgesia but are not discussed in this chapter, include hydromorphone hydrochloride (Dilaudid), butorphanol tartrate (Stadol), and nalbuphine hydrochloride (Nubain).

Meperidine hydrochloride. Meperidine hydrochloride (Demerol) may be given orally, intramuscularly, or intravenously. The dosage is 50 to 100 mg orally or intramuscularly, given 30 to 90 minutes before the procedure, or 30 to 150 mg intravenously in divided doses of 12.5 to 25 mg for sedation/analgesia. The pediatric dose is 1.0 to 2.0 mg/kg intravenously or intramuscularly with a maximum of 100 mg. The onset of action is 1 to 5 minutes for IV, 15 minutes for PO, and 10 minutes for IM administration. The peak action is 10 to 20 minutes with IV administration and 1 hour for PO and IM administration. The duration of action is 1 to 4 hours, with a half-life of 2 to 6 hours.

Meperidine should be administered slowly intravenously because it causes histamine release at a greater frequency than other opioids; the patient may experience tachycardia and a red streak along the vein in which it was administered. It is contraindicated in patients with known hypersensitivity; it may interact with monoamine oxidase (MAO) inhibitors, resulting in hypertension, excitation, tachycardia, seizure, and hyperpyrexia. Adverse reactions include drowsiness, dizziness, confusion, headache, sedation, euphoria, convulsions, tachycardia, asystole, bradycardia, palpitations, hypotension, syncope, nausea and vomiting, anorexia, constipation, cramps, rash, flushing, blurred vision, and respiratory depression.

Morphine sulfate. Morphine sulfate (Astramorph PF, Duramorph PF, MS Contin, Roxanol) may be given intravenously, intramuscularly, or orally. The IV dosage is 1 to 10 mg, diluted in sterile water for injection, given over 4 to 5 minutes. The onset of action ranges from immediate to 7 minutes, with peak action in 10 to 20 minutes. The pediatric dose is 0.1 to 0.2 mg/kg for IV, IM, or PO administration, with a maximum of 10 mg. The half-life is 2 to 4 hours. If administered with another CNS depressant, the dosage is decreased by 30%.

Morphine sulfate is contraindicated in patients with known hypersensitivity to morphine or phenanthrene opioids (e.g., codeine, oxycodone). It must be administered with caution to any patient with supraventricular arrhythmia, head injury, or increased intracranial pressure; during pregnancy; or with renal or hepatic dysfunction or pulmonary disease. Adverse reactions include sedation, dizziness, delirium, seizures, euphoria, nausea, vomiting, constipation, urinary retention, blurred vision, bradycardia, tachycardia, palpitations, asystole, hypertension, hypotension, respiratory depression, rash, urticaria, flushing, and diaphoresis.

Fentanyl citrate. Fentanyl citrate (Sublimaze) is a synthetic opioid indicated for short-term analgesic action. It has a rapid onset of action and a short half-life. The dose is 12.5 to 25 µg intravenously, with a maximum dose of 150 µg. The pediatric dosage is 0.5 to 1.0 µg/kg over a 2-minute period for a maximum dose of 4 µg/kg/hr. The onset of action ranges from immediate to 5 minutes, with a peak action of 3 to 5 minutes. The duration is 30 to 60 minutes, with a half-life of 2 to 4 hours. The dosage must be decreased by one-fourth to one-third if used with another CNS depressant.

Rapid administration can lead to a rigid chest wall and

difficulty breathing, which can be reversed with naloxone (Narcan). However, a depolarizing muscle relaxant and intubation may be required. Fentanyl can be stored in fat and muscle tissue and consequently returned to the circulation, resulting in a delayed-onset respiratory depression.

Fentanyl is contraindicated in patients with known hypersensitivity. It should be administered with caution to any patient with supraventricular arrhythmia or bradycardia, head injury, renal or hepatic dysfunction, pulmonary disease, convulsive disorders, or physical addiction to the medication. It is not recommended in patients who have taken MAO inhibitors within 14 days of administration. Adverse reactions include sedation, dizziness, delirium, seizures, euphoria, nausea, vomiting, blurred vision, miosis, bradycardia, tachycardia, palpitations, respiratory and cardiac arrest, hypertension, hypotension, respiratory depression, laryngospasm, apnea, and skeletal muscle rigidity.

Naloxone hydrochloride. Naloxone hydrochloride (Narcan) is a narcotic antagonist; it works by competing for the receptor site, thereby reversing the effect of the narcotic. This means that naloxone reverses not only sedation and respiratory depression, but also analgesia. This sudden unmasking of pain may result in significant sympathetic and cardiovascular stimulation, resulting in hypertension, stroke, tachycardia, arrhythmia, pulmonary edema, congestive heart failure, or cardiac arrest.

The initial dose of 0.1 to 0.2 mg intravenously may be repeated every 2 to 3 minutes until the patient has a desired effect, to a maximum of 10 mg. The pediatric and adult doses are the same. The onset of action is 1 to 2 minutes, with a peak action of 5 to 15 minutes. The duration is 45 minutes, with a half-life of 60 to 90 minutes. Naloxone is contraindicated in patients with known hypersensitivity. If this drug is administered to a patient with opioid drug dependence, severe withdrawal syndrome may result. It should be administered with caution to patients with supraventricular arrhythmia, head injuries, or convulsive disorders. Abrupt reversal may result in nausea, vomiting, sweating, tachycardia, increased blood pressure, tremulousness, seizures, and cardiac depression. Because of the short half-life, patients can become narcotized after the effects of naloxone have abated, warranting close monitoring for renarcotization (see Table 32-4).

DOCUMENTATION OF CARE, REPORTABLE CONDITIONS, AND COMPLICATIONS

Documentation of nursing interventions ensures the continuity of patient care, improves communication among health care team members, and provides a mechanism for comparing actual versus expected patient outcomes. This documentation should include the following:
- Preprocedure assessment
- Dosage, route, time, and effects of all medications and fluids used
- Type and amount of fluids administered, including blood and blood products
- Monitoring devices and equipment used
- Physiologic data from continuous monitoring at 5 to 15 minute intervals and following significant events

- Level of consciousness
- Nursing interventions and the patient's responses
- Untoward significant patient reactions and their resolution[3]

The frequency of vital sign monitoring is determined by the medication, route of administration, and patient condition. At a minimum, baseline vital signs should be obtained immediately before initiating the procedure, after administering sedative/analgesic agents, upon completing the procedure, during initial recovery, and at the time of discharge. The frequency should increase if the patient's condition or level of sedation deteriorate. Equipment alarms should be set if recording is performed automatically.

The most common complications in the administration of sedation/analgesia are respiratory depression and respiratory arrest. The most common treatment for these complications is the administration of oxygen. The patient should be stimulated by verbal or painful stimulus and instructed to take a deep breath if the respiratory status becomes compromised. If spontaneous respiration does not occur, a head tilt–jaw lift maneuver should be initiated. Positive-pressure ventilation may be required if respiratory status does not improve. If the patient cannot maintain his or her own airway, an artificial airway is indicated. Although either a nasal or oral airway may be used, a nasal airway may be more tolerable for a conscious patient. Continuous observation of the patient's respiratory rate and monitoring of pulse oximetry may ward off the need for emergency measures.

Notify the physician immediately of the following:
- Rise or fall in systolic blood pressure (BP) of 30 mm Hg from baseline
- Tachycardia (>150 beat/min) or bradycardia (<50 beats/min)
- Rise or fall in respiratory rate (±6 per minute from initial respiratory rate)
- Oxygen saturation (Sao_2) less than 90% or significantly below presedation level
- Marked decrease in patient responsiveness to verbal or painful stimulation
- Signs or symptoms of medication intolerance or allergy
- Patient does not meet discharge parameters

POSTPROCEDURAL CARE

After the procedure, the patient is usually transferred to a room in an inpatient setting or to a recovery area until determined ready for discharge. This usually occurs once the patient's vital signs (e.g., blood pressure, pulse, respirations, Sao_2) have returned to and been maintained at presedation levels or at least 30 minutes since the last sedating medications were administered. Sedation/analgesia patients should be observed until they are no longer at increased risk for cardiorespiratory depression. The physician should remain immediately available to participate in the patient's postprocedural care until the risk of respiratory compromise is resolved.

When the monitoring caregiver is not the person providing postprocedural care, a report must be given to the receiving caregiver. This report should include the patient's preferred name and age, preexisting medical conditions, preprocedure vital signs, type of procedure performed, and the physician's name. It should also include type, dosage, route, and administration times of medications, plus allergies, intraprocedural monitoring values, dressings if applicable, intake and output, and complications.

Assessment of respiration, circulation, level of consciousness, skin color, and level of voluntary activity should continue and be recorded into the postprocedural phase of the patient's care. This care should be individualized and based on the level of sedation achieved, overall condition of the patient, and the nature of the intervention for which sedation/analgesia was administered. Several scoring systems are available to standardize documentation and the patient's readiness for discharge. Two of the most popular for sedation/analgesia and for ambulatory care patients are PADS (Post Anesthesia Discharge Scoring System) and PARSAP (Post Anesthesia Recovery Scoring for Ambulatory Patients System). Tables 32-5 and 32-6 present these systems.

A score in the PADS system of 9 or 10 is required for discharge, which means the patient must void or take fluids. For those institutions that have eliminated this requirement, the Modified PARSAP would be a better scale to use.

A postanesthesia scoring system is not mandatory as long as prudent guidelines for discharge are met. These include stable vital signs, mental status, and activity; relative freedom from pain, nausea, and vomiting; and the ability to void or take fluids. A physician must evaluate any patient who is unable to meet the discharge criteria. If any of these parameters are not met, instructions should be given to the patient and family or caregiver on what to do if the patient is unable to meet the parameters later.

DISCHARGE TEACHING AND INSTRUCTIONS

The patient who has received conscious sedation/analgesia should receive verbal and written discharge instructions and meet specified criteria for discharge. Because the medications administered may cause drowsiness and/or amnesia, discharge instructions should be given to the patient and significant other or escort. These instructions should be initiated in the preprocedural phase and repeated in the postprocedural phase before discharge. The instructions should cover home medication administration, dietary requirements, any limitations on activity, postprocedural care, signs and symptoms of complications, emergency numbers, physician numbers, and a follow-up appointment if applicable. The patient should not drive after the administration of sedation/analgesia medications, nor should the patient sign any important papers for 24 hours. The patient should be accompanied by a responsible adult.

Table 32-5   **Post Anesthesia Discharge Scoring System (PADS)***

VITAL SIGNS
2 = Within 20% of preoperative value
1 = 20%-40% of preoperative value
0 = >40% of preoperative value
ACTIVITY AND MENTAL STATUS
1 = Oriented × 3 or a steady gait
2 = Oriented × 3 and a steady gait
0 = Neither

PAIN, NAUSEA, AND/OR VOMITING
2 = Minimal
1 = Moderate, requiring treatment
0 = Severe, requiring treatment

SURGICAL BLEEDING
2 = Minimal
1 = Moderate
0 = Severe
INTAKE AND OUTPUT
2 = Postoperative fluids and void
1 = Postoperative fluids or void
0 = Neither

Data from Reference 7.
*Total score must be 9 to 10 for patient to be discharged home.

Table 32-6   **Post Anesthesia Recovery Score for Ambulatory Patients (PARSAP)***

ACTIVITY
2 = Ability to move four extremities voluntarily or on command
1 = Ability to move two extremities voluntarily or on command
0 = Unable to move extremities voluntarily or on command
RESPIRATION
2 = Able to breath deeply and cough freely
1 = Dyspnea, limited breathing or tachypnea
0 = Apneic or on mechanical ventilator
CIRCULATION
2 = BP ±20% of preanesthetic level
1 = BP ±20%-49% of preanesthetic level
0 = BP ±50% of preanesthetic level
CONSCIOUSNESS
2 = Fully awake
1 = Arousable on calling
0 = Not responding
O_2 SATURATION
2 = Able to maintain O_2 saturation >92% on room air
1 = Needs O_2 inhalation to maintain O_2 saturation >90%
0 = O_2 saturation <90% even with O_2 supplement

DRESSING
2 = Dry and clean
1 = Wet but marked and not increasing
0 = Growing area of wetness
PAIN
2 = Pain free
1 = Mild pain handled by oral medication
0 = Severe pain requiring parenteral medication
AMBULATION
2 = Able to stand up and walk straight
1 = Vertigo when erect
0 = Dizziness when supine
FASTING-FEEDING
2 = Able to drink fluids
1 = Nauseated
0 = Nausea and vomiting
URINE OUTPUT
2 = Has voided
1 = Unable to void but comfortable
0 = Unable to void and uncomfortable

Data from Reference 8.
*Total score must be 18 for patient to be discharged home.

The instruction sheet should be initiated preprocedurally and signed by the patient before the administration of conscious sedation/analgesia to verify the understanding of the basic postprocedural instructions. Before discharge, the instructions are reviewed with the escort or significant other. A copy of the instructions is kept as part of the patient's record.

Many facilities initiate postprocedural telephone follow-up within 24 hours of the procedure. This allows the caregiver to assess the patient's health status and recommend interventions if necessary. The patient should be informed that this will occur and be encouraged to write down questions as they arise, which can be answered during the subsequent phone call. This call should be documented either in the patient's record or in an ongoing unit logbook. This documentation allows the caregiver to assess patient care results and leads to increased patient satisfaction.

POLICIES AND PROCEDURES

Every practice setting should have policies and procedures in place. They should be written, reviewed periodically, and readily available within the practice setting. These policies and procedures provide guidelines for patient care, minimize risk factors, standardize practice, assist staff members, and establish guidelines for quality monitoring and quality improvement. The policies and procedures should include patient selection criteria, extent of and responsibility for monitoring, method of recording patient data, data to be documented, frequency of the patient's physiologic data documentation, mediations that may be administered by the caregiver, and discharge criteria.

COMPETENCIES

Webster defines *competent* as "properly qualified: capable" and "adequate for the stipulated purpose: sufficient."[9] When discussing the competency to administer and monitor conscious sedation/analgesia, the facility needs to define what those competencies entail. AORN states that "the RN monitoring the patient's care should be clinically competent in the function and in the use of resuscitation medications and monitoring equipment and be able to interpret the data obtained from the patient."[3]

The practitioner should be versed in anatomy and physiology, pharmacology of the medications used, cardiac arrhythmia interpretation (at a minimum, identification of lethal arrhythmias), possible complications, and respiratory functions, including oxygen delivery devices and oxygen transport and uptake. Along with these knowledge-based competencies, the practitioner should be able to demonstrate hands-on skills such as the proper use of an Ambu bag, head-tilt and jaw-lift maneuver, and insertion of nasal and oral airways. Because these high-risk skills are not used often, they should be reviewed and validated periodically, along with basic CPR or ACLS.

Each facility using sedation/analgesia needs to specify in their policy and procedures the competencies determined necessary for their staff members. An education/competency validation system should be designed to evaluate and document the demonstration of the knowledge, skills, and abilities related to managing the sedation/analgesia patient.

SUMMARY

As more and more procedures are performed on an outpatient basis, thereby returning patients to their daily activities at a faster pace, the need for trained and competent staff to administer and monitor sedation/analgesia will increase. This increases the demand for the skills needed to perform this task. A positive patient outcome is the primary goal. This can be accomplished only through education and safe practice by the entire health care team.

REFERENCES

1. Watson DS: *Conscious sedation/analgesia*, St Louis, 1998, Mosby.
2. American Society of Anesthesiology Task Force, et al: Practice Guideline for Sedation and Analgesia by Non-Anesthesiologists, *Anesthesiology* 82/2:459, 1996.
3. Reno D, editor: *Standards, recommended practices, and guidelines,* Denver, 1999, Association of Operating Room Nurses.
4. American Society of Anesthesiology: New classification of physical status, *Anesthesiology* 24:111, 1963.
5. Albany Medical Center: Guidelines for conscious sedation, *Crest* 108/5:543, 1995.
6. Wyman CI: Conscious sedation self study guide, Franklin Square Hospital Center, Internet article. http://gasnet.med.yale.edu/reference/protocols/sedation.
7. Chung F: New scoring system developed to assess readiness for phase II recovery discharge, *Anesthesia News* March:26, 1992.
8. Aldrete JA: Modifications to the post anesthesia score for use in ambulatory surgery, *Journal of PeriAnesthesia Nursing* 13(3):148, 1998.
9. Soukhanov AH, Ellis K, editors: *Webster's II New Riverside University dictionary,* Boston, 1994, Houghton Mifflin.

BIBLIOGRAPHY

Abranmo TJ: *Pediatric conscious sedation: module I, agents and procedures,* St Louis, 1966, Mosby.

American Society of Anesthesiologists: *Guidelines for sedation and analgesia by non-anesthesiologists,* Park Ridge, Ill, 1995, ASA.

Council on Scientific Affairs, American Medical Association, et al: The use of pulse oximetry during conscious sedation, *JAMA* 270(12): 1463, 1993.

Eubanks JR Jr: Midazolam: saint or sinner, *AORN J* 50(1):155, 1989.

Holzman RS, et al: Guidelines for sedation by nonanesthesiologists during diagnostic and therapeutic procedures, *J Clin Anesthesia* 6:265, 1994.

Messinger JA, et al: Getting conscious sedation right, *Am J Nurs* 99(2):44, 1999.

Murphy EK: Monitoring IV conscious sedation: the legal scope of practice, *AORN J* 57(2):512, 1993.

Sommerson SJ, et al: Insight into conscious sedation, *Am J Nurs* 95(6):26, 1995.

Watson DS: Clinical issues: issues surrounding intravenous conscious sedation, *AORN J* 54:105, 1991.

Watson DS: *Conscious sedation/analgesia,* St. Louis, 1998, Mosby.

Vascular Access in Interventional Radiology

Chapter 33

Gail Egan Sansivero, MS, ANP, AOCN

MINIMALLY INVASIVE TECHNOLOGY AND IMAGE GUIDANCE
VAD SITE SELECTION
USE OF FLUOROSCOPY
RADIOLOGIC APPROACHES TO VASCULAR ACCESS COMPLICATIONS
    Venous stenosis
    Withdrawal occlusion
    Catheter malposition
    Catheter embolism
INFUSION NURSING ROLE
WHAT'S IN THE FUTURE?

Since their introduction, vascular access devices (VADs) have played an important role in the management of health care problems in adults and children. These devices have made therapy safer to deliver and have positively affected the quality of life for millions of patients.

Today, more than ever, pressures exist to decrease cost and move procedures out of traditional surgical environments. Recent technical advances in interventional radiology practice and concern for reducing complications have resulted in the development of more percutaneous approaches to VAD placement and complication management. Interventional radiology can often achieve success when compared with traditional strategies based on landmark techniques.

Cost and morbidity comparisons of VAD placement in the angiography suite as compared with the operating room have been well documented.[1-3] McBride et al. evaluated 253 tunneled, cuffed catheters placed in the operating room or angiographic suite over a 2-year period. Procedure time was less than 1 hour in 85% of the procedures performed by radiologists, as compared with 60% for the surgical placements. General anesthesia was used in 67% of surgical cases, and 33% of radiology cases. There were no radiologic failures to adequately place a device; there were six (4.5%) surgical failures. A total of 17 (13%) of the surgical cases required two or more placements during the same procedure because of unexpected venous thrombosis/occlusion or inadequate vessel size at cutdown. The average catheter dwell time and infection rate were the same for both groups.[1-3] These data confirm earlier studies describing the improved accuracy of image-guided VAD placement and similar or superior performance of VADs placed by interventional radiology teams.

Currently, general anesthesia is rarely used by interventional radiology for vascular access. Interventional radiology placement is supplanting surgical placement of long-term, tunnelled, and implanted catheters because interventional radiology can place the lines more quickly, more accurately, with fewer complications, and with lower costs.

VADs have also become smaller, as engineers develop designs with a lower profile, which use materials that can maximize the inner diameter while minimizing the external diameter. In addition, some devices are placed using a more peripheral approach, in the arm, making the traditional placement by anatomic landmarks more challenging as placement is sight limited. Conventional sites for VAD placement can become exhausted in patients with chronic illness because of frequent VAD placement, VAD complications such as stenosis and thrombosis, and the effects of disease on the sites. These factors favor novel approaches, which are accomplished more successfully with microintroducer tools and image guidance.

The availability of image-guided technology such as ultrasound and fluoroscopy has supported the movement of VAD placement to interventional radiology, where personnel are skilled in the use of these modalities. Image guidance improves technical success and decreases complications.

MINIMALLY INVASIVE TECHNOLOGY AND IMAGE GUIDANCE

Microintroducer, thin wires, and sheaths are used daily in interventional radiology to obtain initial access to arteries and veins. This technology has been applied to the placement of VADs.

A standard microintroducer kit consists of a needle (usually 20 to 21 gauge), flexible tip wire (Cope Mandrill), and an introducer sheath. The needle, usually 2 to 5 inches long, may be scored near the tip, facilitating visualization with ultrasound. Access to the target vessel is obtained with this "skinny" needle, after which the guidewire is advanced. This guidewire can also be used to estimate the intended intravascular length of the VAD, with the VAD's catheter trimmed before insertion. Successive exchanges over the wire using different sheaths and introducers eventually allow the advancement of the VAD into position.

The microintroducer technique, particularly when paired with imaging techniques, can minimize tissue trauma and increase the likelihood of achieving target puncture with a single needle pass. In the case of nontarget puncture (e.g., inadvertent arterial puncture), the complication sequelae can be minimized because the puncture is relatively small.

Coupling microintroducer technology with image-guided equipment such as ultrasound provides the practitioner with additional tools to assess and target vessels. Ultrasound uses sound waves to distinguish structures in the selected area

Sample Vascular Access Consultation

Mrs. Jones is a 62-year-old woman who is referred for place-ment of an implanted port before beginning chemotherapy for recurrent, metastatic breast cancer. She is scheduled to begin chemotherapy with paclitaxel (Taxol) and carboplatin in 5 days.

Her medical history is remarkable for hypertension, arthri-tis, and type II diabetes mellitus. Mrs. Jones has never had a central vascular access device to her knowledge. She has been treated in the past with chemotherapy via peripheral veins.

Her surgical history is remarkable for a right modified radical mastectomy with lymph node dissection and a right breast reconstruction using a myocutaneous flap and appendectomy.

Mrs. Jones reports no known drug and skin preparation allergies. She has no known sensitivity to latex. Her current weight is 161 pounds. She has never smoked.

Current medications include metformin hydrochloride (Dimethylbiguanide Hydrochloride), lisinopril, and one aspirin (acetylsalicylic acid) a day.

Current laboratory data include a white blood cell count of 4500/mm³, hemoglobin (Hgb) of 14.0 g/dl, hematocrit of 39.6%, and a platelet count of 342,000/mm³. The blood urea nitrogen is 12 mg/dl, serum creatinine is 0.9 mg/dl, and the prothrombin time international normalized ratio is 1.1.

Physical examination reveals good skin turgor. There are cutaneous metastatic lesions overlying the reconstructed breast and right chest wall. There are no distended collateral veins over the chest wall.

The risks and benefits of implanted port placement and use are discussed with the patient. Potential target sites, particularly the left internal jugular or left arm veins, are reviewed. The patient is advised of preprocedure ultrasound examination to evaluate these sites. If these sites are all suitable, the patient prefers placement in the left arm.

The patient consents to proceed. The plan is to place a single-lumen low-profile implanted port via the left basilic or brachial veins or the left internal jugular vein. The patient will return to the office just before beginning chemotherapy for a site check and first-time access.

Glossary of Specialty Terms

Contrast: radiopaque solution injected into a vessel to opacify the intended target or anatomical structures in question

Sheath: a tapered plastic cannula, which is advanced over a wire and into the vessel; provides a channel for VAD advancement; measured in terms of the French size it will accommodate

French size: catheter size measured in outer diameter (3 Fr equals 1 mm)

Glidewire: a guidewire with a hydrophilic coating

Guidewire: a thin stainless steel or nitinol wire with a soft or "floppy" tip; used to provide structure for sheath and intro-ducer exchanges and guide an introducer or catheter into a vessel; most wires characterized by a central stiff core with a distal taper and are coated with Teflon, polyurethane, or poly-ethylene to reduce friction; designated by outer diameter in inches (e.g., 0.018 or 0.035) and overall length in centimeters; guidewire length *must* exceed the catheter length

Stent: a metal, tubular intravascular device placed in a vein or artery to help maintain patency

Transition: the quality of tapering between components of an introducer or sheath

Purchase: the length of wire or introducer placed within a vessel thought to be adequate to minimize the risk of acciden-tal withdrawal

Nitinol: a nickel and titanium alloy

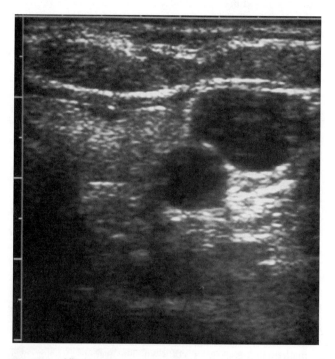

FIG. 33-1 *Ultrasound image of internal jugular vein (upper right) and carotid artery.*

(Fig. 33-1). Structures of different densities return inaudible sound waves to the ultrasound transducer, where they are translated into a visual image. Although arteries and veins will display similarly, they can be distinguished with a few simple steps. First, pressure can be applied against the site to compress the vessels. If patent, the vein should collapse, whereas the artery will pulse against compression. If thrombosed, the vein will not compress. In addition, Doppler can be added to the image, adding audible and visual assessment of vessel patency and flow. Arterial flow will be pulsatile, whereas venous flow should be continuous.

VAD SITE SELECTION

Historically, central VADs were placed via the subclavian veins using anatomic landmarks to guide puncture. However, the placement of a VAD in the subclavian vein is associated with an increased risk of stenosis and thrombosis when compared with placement via the internal jugular veins.

Cimochowski et al.[4] studied the access routes of 52 patients with subclavian and internal jugular permanent dialysis cath-eters. All patients were studied with venograms 1 to 27 months after VAD placement. There was a 50% stricture rate in patients with subclavian vein catheters, and no strictures were noted in patients with internal jugular catheters. In patients who had multiple catheters, the risk of stricture was higher. The presence of a stricture complicates subsequent VAD placement and impedes blood flow in patients with arteriovenous grafts and fistulas, whose flow rates are dependent on adequate return to the right atrium. In addition, the risk of pneumothorax is higher with the subclavian vein approach.[4]

Hirano and Yoshioka[5] evaluated internal jugular versus subclavian vein catheterization in 159 patients for procedure duration, incidence of catheter malposition, and complications. In the group of patients with internal jugular catheter placements, procedure time was shorter and the incidence of catheter malposition was significantly lower. Inadvertent arterial punctures occurred in 1% of the internal jugular punctures and 6% of the subclavian vein punctures. Of the subclavian vein puncture patients, 3% experienced pneumothoraces, compared with none of the internal jugular puncture patients. There was no difference in catheter-related infectious complications. All punctures were performed by anatomic landmarks only.[5]

Puncture of the internal jugular or subclavian vein via landmark technique is associated with the immediate complications of inadvertent carotid artery puncture, hematoma, subclavian vein puncture, and pneumothorax.[6] Although stenosis and thrombosis of the subclavian vein will make future VAD placement in the chest difficult or impossible, it also is a major cause of atrioventricular graft and fistula failure because flow depends on adequate return to central circulation.[7] In addition, puncture via anatomic landmarks makes placement in patients with unusual vascular anatomy difficult.

Ultrasound examination of potential target veins allows the practitioner to evaluate for exact location and patency, including presence of thrombus and location of neighboring structures (veins and arteries). Compression against the skin with the ultrasound transducer should demonstrate a decrease in vein diameter, whereas neighboring arteries will "bounce" back with arterial pressure. If the practitioner is still uncertain which vessel is arterial, Doppler can be added to assess flow. When a vein is thrombosed, it will be visible on the screen but will not compress with pressure applied against the skin. This preprocedure reduces the incidence of unsuccessful placement by eliminating unsuitable sites before the procedure is performed, and it allows selection of the most suitable site. Added as a real-time adjunct during device placement, ultrasound guidance is associated with a decrease in the risk of placement complications, number of attempts to achieve successful puncture, and procedure time.

Denys et al.[8] compared landmark puncture of the internal jugular with ultrasound-guided puncture and noted that the target vein was entered 78% of the time on the first attempt with ultrasound, compared with 38% on first attempt using anatomic landmarks. Inadvertent puncture of the carotid artery occurred in 1.7% of the ultrasound procedures and in 8.3% of landmark patients.[8]

Thompson et al.[9] compared the cannulation of the subclavian vein by inexperienced practitioners using ultrasound as compared with the landmark method. Although the success rate for cannulation with the landmark method was 44%, the authors were able to improve their success to 92% with ultrasound guidance. They were also able to salvage 80% of the landmark failures with subsequent use of ultrasound. Minor complications occurred in 40% of the landmark group, compared with

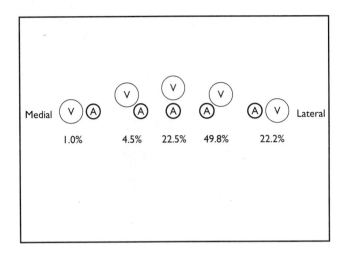

FIG. 33-2 *Five anatomic variants.*

4% in the ultrasound group. An average of 2.5 punctures were required in the landmark group, compared with 1.4 in the ultrasound group.[9]

Gordon et al.[10] prospectively evaluated the likelihood of successful internal jugular cannulation in a group of 869 adult patients requiring VAD placement, inferior vena cava (IVC) filter placement, or access for other angiographic procedures. Success was defined as ultrasound-guided cannulation of the internal jugular with needle placement sufficient for advancement of a guidewire. Successful punctures were obtained in 868 patients (99.9%). There were no pneumothoraces. Five anatomic variants were noted and are illustrated in Fig. 33-2. As might be expected, successful cannulation of the internal jugular by anatomic landmarks depends on the internal jugular residing in its expected position and its being patent and of normal caliber (Table 33-1).[10]

Some patients will have problems with stenoses and thromboses, which make conventional VAD placement difficult or impossible. Occlusions of the superior vena cava (SVC) and subclavian veins may result from previous VAD placement, tumor compression, hypercoagulable states, venous compression from other syndromes (e.g., Paget-Schroeter), radiation therapy, or previous surgeries. In these situations, novel approaches to VAD placement are necessary. A well-described approach for many patients is obtaining access directly into the IVC. Bennett et al.[11] described a series of 29 VAD placements in 22 patients in whom conventional VAD placement had failed. In each case, VADs were placed by direct puncture into the IVC and subsequently advanced successfully. Catheter tips were advanced to the junction of the IVC and right atrium. Catheter exit sites or port pockets were tunneled to the chest or abdominal wall.[11]

Access to the IVC can also be obtained via a transhepatic approach, as described by Patel.[12] Indeed, this approach can be used in patients with thrombosed IVCs. It is contraindicated in patients with uncorrectable coagulopathy and ascites. Using a subcostal approach to avoid traversing the pleura, the hepatic vein is accessed with a long, small-gauge needle. A thin (0.018-inch) wire is passed through the needle, into the hepatic vein, and advanced into the IVC, usually to the level of the right atrium. The standard steps for sequential dilation to VAD

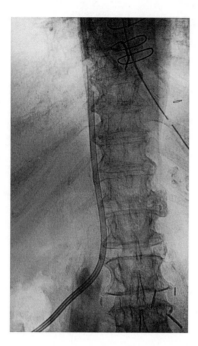

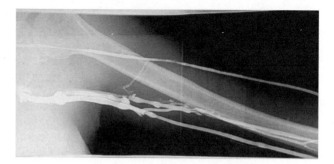

FIG. 33-4   *Normal left arm venogram.*

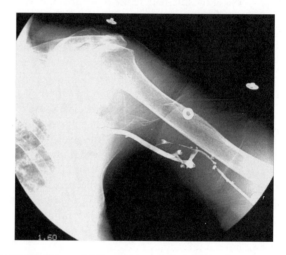

FIG. 33-3   *Translumbar hemodialysis catheter. Note the filling of the inferior vena cava with contrast.*

FIG. 33-5   *Abnormal left arm venogram. Initial puncture made into small collateral. Note partial filling of left basilic vein.*

Table 33-1	**Advantages and Disadvantages of Ultrasound**
ADVANTAGES	**DISADVANTAGES**
Provides excellent visualization of target vessel	Requires equipment investment
Visualizes neighboring structures	Requires special training
Assesses for patency	Some disposable materials additional
Is mobile	

Table 33-2	**Advantages and Disadvantages of Fluoroscopy**
ADVANTAGES	**DISADVANTAGES**
Provides excellent visualization of target vessel	Requires contrast agent for opacification
Assesses for stenosis, thrombus	Requires special equipment
Demonstrates collateral vessels	Is expensive
	Requires special training
	Exposes patient/staff to radiation
	Is not easily mobile
	Does not visualize arteries with veins

placement in other sites are then followed.[12] See Fig. 33-3 for positioning of translumbar and transhepatic VADs.

The common femoral veins can also be accessed directly, with catheters threaded into the IVC. This approach is used particularly for temporary catheters. Because of concerns about catheter flexion, iliofemoral venous thrombosis, and restricted patient mobility, a short-term, flexible device such as a Hohn catheter is a good choice for this site.

In patients with limited access, occluded veins can sometimes be recannulated by mechanical or pharmacologic techniques.[13] If a stenosed or thrombosed vein can be traversed with a guidewire, an angioplasty balloon may be advanced to the problematic area and inflated to reexpand the vessel and establish adequate flow. Infusion of thrombolytic agents or mechanical thrombectomy may also open a thrombosed vein. These interventions are used primarily in patients with limited access who require salvage of a preexisting VAD or who are expected to require new access for a prolonged time.[13]

USE OF FLUOROSCOPY

In addition to using fluoroscopy to guide wire advancement and confirm catheter tip positioning, fluoroscopy can also be used in conjunction with contrast or other opacifying agents to visualize vessels for device placement. Essentially a "live" radiograph, fluoroscopy will allow the practitioner to observe the needle, wire, and VAD. See Figs. 33-4 and 33-5 for fluoroscopic images of normal and abnormal vasculature.

Although some fluoroscopic equipment is mobile, the units are not practical for use outside the acute care environment. Most fluoroscopic units are dedicated to an individual x-ray or angiographic suite because they are used as an adjunct to many procedures. The operator must be shielded and monitored for radiation exposure. Young patients and pregnant patients should also be shielded (Table 33-2).

RADIOLOGIC APPROACHES TO VASCULAR ACCESS COMPLICATIONS

A number of VAD complications are amenable to management in the angiographic suite because of the need for excellent visualization of the device itself, the patient's vasculature, and the materials used to problem solve. Typical problems assessed and treated by interventional radiologists include venous stenosis, withdrawal occlusions, catheter malposition, and catheter embolism.

Venous stenosis

Over time, veins can become scarred and narrowed because of the constant irritation of a VAD. Many patients will be asymptomatic, particularly if collateral vessels have enlarged to assume venous blood return. Other stenoses may be discovered when VAD insertion becomes problematic. A stenosis is seen when contrast agents are injected into a vessel, demonstrating a narrowing (Fig. 33-6). The use of fluoroscopy and venography allows stenoses or occlusions to be evaluated and facilitates approach strategy planning.

Stenoses can be treated with angioplasty. A guidewire is advanced into position through the stenosis. An angioplasty balloon is then advanced over the wire to the area of narrowing. The balloon is inflated, reestablishing the intravascular lumen diameter (Fig. 33-7). Several inflations may be necessary to reestablish adequate flow. In some cases, the vein has a propensity to return to its stenosed state. If so, an intravascular stent may be deployed to maintain the vessel lumen (Fig. 33-8). The stent provides structural support for the vein, preventing future narrowing or collapse. VADs can be inserted through the stented vessel, if needed (Fig. 33-9). Stents are permanent devices.

Withdrawal occlusion

Withdrawal occlusion (the inability to obtain a blood return while being able to infuse) is a common VAD problem. Although this problem may be related to many factors, including partial intraluminal clot or narrowing or the formation of a drug precipitate, the presence of a fibrin sheath around the catheter's intravascular segment is a common culprit.

Both fibrin sheath and pericatheter thrombus can be assessed with the injection of a contrast agent through the VAD. With the patient under fluoroscopy, the VAD is injected with a small amount of contrast (usually no more than 20 to 40 ml). A "live" picture is captured, demonstrating flow out of the VAD's distal tip (Fig. 33-10). The presence of "fuzzy" looking flow near the tip, with or without retrograde flow, indicates the presence of a fibrin sheath or sleeve (Fig. 33-11). Sometimes, no definite catheter abnormalities are seen on injection. In these instances, if the vein appears normal and the catheter appropriately placed, the presumptive diagnosis of a partial fibrin sheath can be made. Filling defects at the distal tip are more characteristic of peri-catheter thrombus (Fig. 33-12).

If immediate restoration of catheter function is required, catheter stripping may be performed to remove a fibrin sheath. A snare, similar to a lasso, is inserted, usually from the common femoral vein and into the IVC. The open snare is used to encircle the VAD's distal tip and advanced up the catheter shaft. The

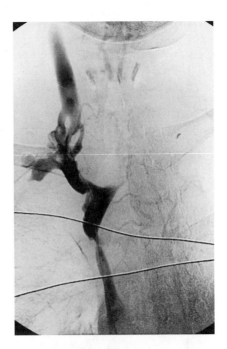

FIG. 33-6 *Stenosis of the superior vena cava.*

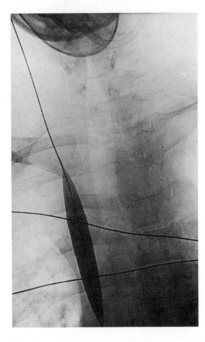

FIG. 33-7 *Angioplasty balloon inflated to treat superior vena cava stenosis.*

snare is cinched and then pulled down, grabbing and removing the fibrin sheath from the VAD (Fig. 33-13). This maneuver may be repeated several times.

Hemodialysis and apheresis catheters are particularly affected by fibrin sheath problems because the sheath may impede adequate flow rates needed for treatment. Because of the risk for catheter embolism, catheter stripping should be performed only on catheters with a large diameter, such as dialysis and apheresis catheters. It is not an option for smaller catheters such as

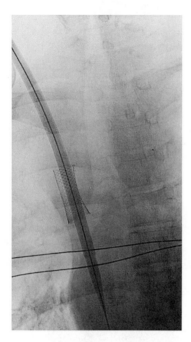

FIG. 33-8 *Superior vena cava stent (note sheath within stent).*

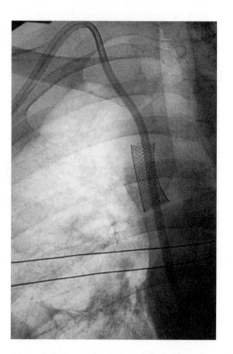

FIG. 33-9 *Hemodialysis catheter placed through superior vena cava stent.*

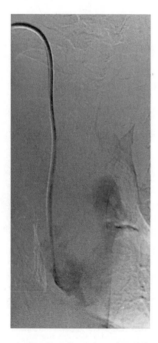

FIG. 33-10 *Contrast injection through catheter (note filling of pulmonary artery).*

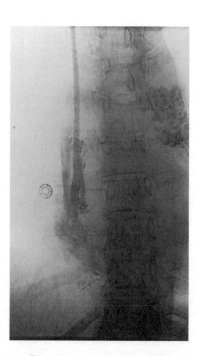

FIG. 33-11 *Fibrin sheath with retrograde flow of contrast.*

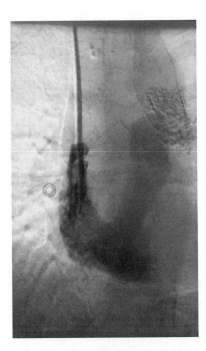

FIG. 33-12 *Contrast injection revealing pericatheter thrombus.*

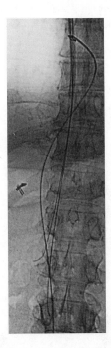

FIG. 33-13 *Snare in place around catheter. Note placement of two guidewires through catheter lumens.*

peripherally inserted central catheters (PICCs) and implanted ports. Function is restored immediately. However, this strategy may not produce long-term results, as a fibrin sheath may reaccumulate.

Brady et al.[14] evaluated the efficacy of percutaneous fibrin sheath stripping in 131 hemodialysis catheters. Their technical success, or ability to achieve dialysis flow rates of at least 250

ml/min immediately following intervention, was 95.6%. However, the overall median duration of poststripping patency was only 89 days. The site of catheter placement (e.g., internal jugular versus subclavian vein) was not significantly related to restoration of function.[14] Others have reported similar results. Haskel et al.[15] reported less success with 22 catheters in 20 patients, with 20 achieving no difference in dialysis flow rates by the fifth postintervention dialysis treatment. He included malpositioned and kinked catheters in his treatment group.[15] Rockall et al.[16] reported a median patency after stripping of 4.25 months in 17 of 22 catheters.[16]

Both fibrin sheath and pericatheter thrombus may be treated with the infusion of thrombolytic agents. Patients must be assessed carefully because the agents are infused systemically. Patients with hemorrhagic cardiovascular accidents, central nervous system lesions, recent surgical interventions, or bleeding disorders are generally excluded from this treatment option. The thrombolytic agent is infused directly through the VAD and into the clot or sheath using a slow infusion. The patient is monitored for signs and symptoms of bleeding for the entire infusion. The VAD is assessed for function at the conclusion of the scheduled infusion.

In patients with symptomatic thrombus formation in the central veins proximal to the VAD tip, a multiside hole infusion catheter may be targeted to the problem area for thrombolytic infusion, with or without heparin. The catheter is removed at the infusion's conclusion.

Angioplasty may be used to treat fibrin sheath. Guidewires are advanced through the tunneled VAD, and the VAD is removed over the wire. The angioplasty balloon is advanced over the wires to the area immediately within the sheath. The balloon is inflated, disrupting the sheath. The balloon is withdrawn, and a new VAD is advanced over the wires and into position.

An alternative to thrombolysis and stripping in poorly functioning hemodialysis catheters is catheter exchange. This option is desirable because it restores immediate function and preserves other sites for future access. In addition, placement-related complications such as nontarget puncture and pneumothorax can be avoided. In catheter exchange, two stiff glidewires are advanced through each catheter lumen and into the IVC. The old catheter is removed over the wires and the new catheter advanced over the wires into position.

Garafalo et al.[17] described the use of catheter exchange in 88 procedures performed for poor hemodialysis flow rates. Technical success was 100%, with a cumulative infection rate of 1.1 per 1000 catheter days. Patients with signs or symptoms of infection were not included. Secondary patency was 92% at 60 days and 82% at 120 days. These results compare favorably with success in de novo catheter placements.[17]

Catheter exchange can also be used in cases of unexpected device removal or dislodgement. Egglin et al.[18] described their experience with reinserting accidentally removed hemodialysis catheters in 13 patients. Of 13 catheters, 12 were replaced successfully through the preexisting catheter tunnel, the catheters having been removed for a median of 12 hours (range, 3 hours to 5 days). No infections were associated with use of the preexisting tunnels.[18] Patients with a history of central vein occlusions or tenuous access may be particularly good candidates for this procedure because it saves access sites.

Catheter malposition

Catheter tips may be inaccurately positioned on insertion, particularly when image guidance has not been used. Although all central VAD tips should be checked by radiograph, images may be of poor quality or misinterpreted. For example, a catheter tip in the azygos vein may appear to be in the SVC to an inexperienced practitioner. In other cases, catheter tips residing short of the SVC may be accepted as "good enough" when, in fact, the risk of poor catheter function and thrombosis increases when the catheter's tip is in the subclavian veins instead of the SVC. A catheter tip may also be malpositioned because of anomalous venous anatomy, preventing more optimal tip positioning. Occasionally, a VAD with good tip position on insertion becomes malpositioned over time. Forceful flushing, increased intrathoracic pressure (from coughing, vomiting, or tumor compression), extensive upper arm movement (e.g., in ballet dancers and construction workers), or simple chance may cause a catheter tip to coil back on itself or flip into the jugular veins (Fig. 33-14).

Catheter tip malposition may be corrected by internal manipulation. The catheter's tip is approached from the IVC via the common femoral vein. Using a tip deflecting wire, the clinician pulls the catheter tip back into position in the SVC (Fig. 33-15). This strategy provides no assurances that the catheter tip will not become misplaced again.

Catheter embolism

An embolized catheter fragment may result from forceful flushing, trauma, or pinch-off between the clavicle and first rib in VADs placed by a medial subclavian approach. The embolization may not be discovered for some time, particularly if a portion of the VAD remains intravascular. Although some patients may be asymptomatic, others will experience a change in their VAD function or complain of chest discomfort or palpitations. Any of these symptoms should be investigated immediately. Potential complications include infusate extravasation and tissue damage, arrhythmias, thrombus formation, and vessel perforation. A plain posteroanterior and lateral chest radiograph is suitable for initial evaluation. These studies will reveal the location of catheter fragments, most often lodged in the right ventricle or pulmonary artery (Fig. 33-16). Both the catheter fragment and remaining device require removal. The catheter fragment is approached with a snare directed from the common femoral vein through the IVC and into the right atrium. The snare is used to "lasso" the fragment. The fragment is then pulled out through a sheath that has been placed in the common femoral vein (Fig. 33-17).

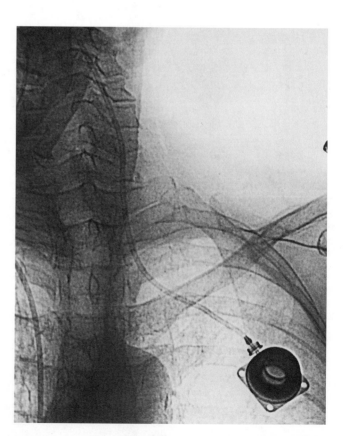

FIG. 33-14 *Implanted port with catheter in internal jugular vein.*

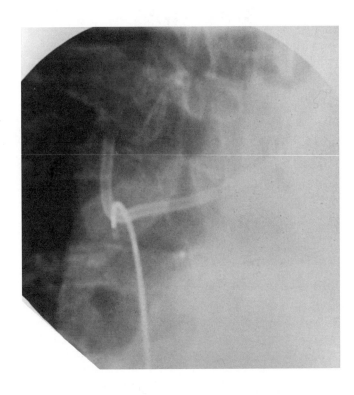

FIG. 33-15 *Catheter with tip deflecting wire in position.*

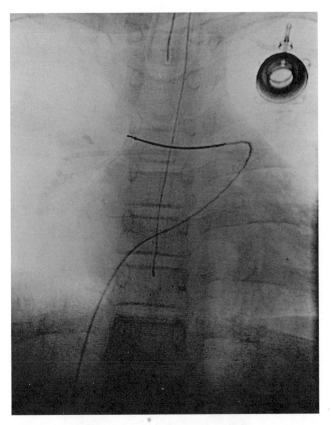

FIG. 33-16 *Embolized port catheter in pulmonary artery with snare capture.*

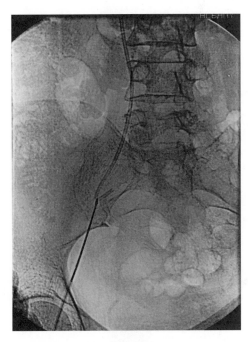

FIG. 33-17 *Catheter fragment with snare approaching sheath placed in the right common femoral vein.*

INFUSION NURSING ROLE

Nurses working in infusion therapy (e.g., intravenous [IV] team, PICC team, catheter care team) are often the first ones consulted when peripheral access is problematic. They are the ones who follow inpatients with central lines, including PICCs, whether placed by a nurse or interventional radiologist. These nurses are also often the first to recognize a problem or complication. Infusion nurses have the most contact with the inpatients and their families regarding catheter care, maintenance, and surveillance for complications. The input and suggestions of the infusion nurses regarding access options are important. It is imperative that the infusion nurses understand what interventional radiology can offer and, similarly, that the interventional radiologists understand the training and support that an infusion nursing team can offer. By supporting each other and keeping each other informed of advances, protocol changes, and other aspects of care, infusion nurses and interventional radiologists can work together collaboratively to provide quality service.

WHAT'S IN THE FUTURE?

As innovative and creative as VAD placement and management can be with current imaging modalities and specialized tools, the future promises even more dramatic changes that will promote optimal device placement in almost any situation. "Smart" wires and needles, loaded with Doppler ultrasound, are now being used for interventional radiology procedures. These devices simplify vessel targeting and tip placement by providing the practitioner with an audible signal of vessel flow. As flow tends to be continuous in a vein, the practitioner can differentiate between artery and vein. In addition, the wires can be used to distinguish the more turbulent flow of the right atrium from the flow in the SVC in landing VAD tips.

More portable and lightweight imaging tools, such as the SiteRite III (Fig. 33-18), will make ultrasound imaging available even for home VAD placement.

Novel VAD designs may not only promote optimal performance but also enhance quality of life. Two implantable dialysis ports are now in clinical trials (Fig. 33-19). These devices allow patients with renal disease the same opportunity to enjoy an active lifestyle as patients with other implanted devices.

Nurses are integral partners in the development of new devices, placement approaches, and use of accessory devices. In collaboration with manufacturers, nurses working in radiology and infusion nurses are in a prime position to advocate for both patients and professionals. Design innovation, modification of current devices for enhanced user safety, and investigation of novel management strategies are but a few of the focuses in vascular access where nurses' skills, knowledge, and experience are of critical importance.

In daily practice, nurses must not accept VAD complications as the "cost of doing business," but instead expect accurate VAD

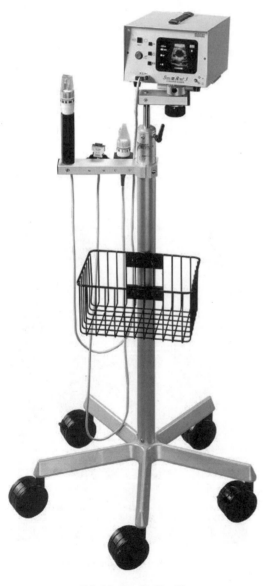

FIG. 33-18 *SiteRite III.*

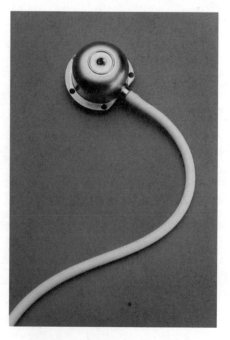

FIG. 33-19 *Implantable dialysis port.*

selection and placement coupled with optimal performance. Patients depend on it.

REFERENCES

1. Openshaw KL, et al: Interventional radiologic placement of Hohn central venous catheters: results and complications in 100 consecutive patients, *J Vasc Interv Radiol* 5:111, 1994.

2. Mauro MA, Jacques PF: Radiologic placement of long-term central venous catheters: a review, *J Vasc Interv Radiol* 4:127, 1993.

3. McBride KD, et al: A comparative analysis of radiological and surgical placement of central venous catheters, *Cardiovasc Interv Radiol* 20:17, 1997.

4. Cimochowski GE, et al: Superiority of the internal jugular over the subclavian access for temporary dialysis, *Nephron* 54:154, 1990.

5. Hirano T, Yoshioka H: Superiority of internal jugular venipuncture to subclavian venipuncture as a central venous catheterization, *Vasc Surg* 18(5):337, 1994.

6. Skolnick ML: The role of sonography in the placement and management of jugular and subclavian central venous catheters, *Am J Radiol* 163:291, 1994.

7. Uldall PR: Subclavian cannulation is no longer necessary or justified in patients with end-stage renal failure, *Semin Dial* 7(3):161, 1994.

8. Denys BG, Uretsky BF, Reddy PS: Ultrasound-assisted cannulation of the internal jugular vein: a prospective comparison to the external landmark-guided technique, *Circulation* 87(5):1557, 1993.

9. Gualtieri E, et al: Subclavian venous catheterization: greater success rate for less experienced operators using ultrasound guidance, *Crit Care Med* 23(4):692, 1995.

10. Gordon AC, et al: US-guided puncture of the internal jugular vein: complications and anatomic considerations, *J Vasc Interv Radiol* 9:333, 1998.

11. Bennett JD, et al: Percutaneous inferior vena caval approach for long-term central venous access, *J Cardiovasc Interv Radiol* 8:851, 1997.

12. Patel NH: Alternate approaches to central venous access, *Semin Interv Radiol* 15(3):325, 1998.

13. Kaufman JA, et al: Outcome of radiologically placed arm ports, *Radiology* 201:725, 1996.

14. Brady PS, et al: Efficacy of fibrin sheath stripping in restoring patency of tunneled hemodialysis catheters, *Am J Radiol* 173:1023, 1999.

15. Haskel ZJ, et al: Transvenous removal of fibrin sheaths from tunneled hemodialysis catheters, *J Vasc Interv Radiol* 7:513, 1996.

16. Rockall AG, et al: Stripping of failing haemodialysis catheters using the Amplatz goose-neck snare, *Clin Radiol* 52:616, 1996.

17. Garafalo RS, et al: Exchange of poorly functioning tunneled permanent hemodialysis catheters, *Am J Radiol* 173:155, 1999.

18. Egglin TKP, et al: Replacement of accidentally removed tunneled venous catheters through existing subcutaneous tracts, *J Cardiovasc Interv Radiol* 8:197, 1997.

Management of *Hazardous* Substances in *IV* Therapy

Mary R. Heisey, CRNI, and Maxine B. Perdue, CRNI, BSN, MHA, MBA, CNAA

REGULATIONS, STANDARDS, AND GUIDELINES
   Occupational Safety and Health Administration
   Environmental Protection Agency
   Centers for Disease Control and Prevention
   National Institutes of Health
   American Society of Health-System Pharmacists
   Intravenous Nurses Society
   American Association of Blood Banks
HAZARDOUS SUBSTANCES
   Biologic agents
   Chemical hazards
HAZARDOUS WASTES
INFUSION NURSING ISSUES
   Biohazards
   Chemical hazards and wastes
SUMMARY

The concern for management of hazardous substances is an issue that should not be taken lightly by infusion nurses and others involved in the delivery, preparation, administration, and disposal of hazardous substances, or in the performance of procedures that are associated with blood-borne pathogens. The potential risks are great, possibly resulting in lifelong problems or death. However, through research and the development of regulations and guidelines by the federal government, infusion nurses and others can protect themselves. Compliance with regulations for the delivery, preparation, administration, and disposal of hazardous substances and the use of standard precautions and engineering controls can help to eliminate exposure incidents. This chapter provides an overview of all regulatory bodies involved and then focuses on the issues relative to infusion nursing.

REGULATIONS, STANDARDS, AND GUIDELINES

Occupational Safety and Health Administration

In 1970, Congress established the Occupational Safety and Health Administration (OSHA) "to assure so far as possible every working man and woman in the nation safe and healthful working conditions."[1] Under the Department of Labor, OSHA

compiled a comprehensive set of rules and regulations that set standards for hazardous materials management and other areas of workplace safety through the establishment of the Occupational Safety and Health (OSH) Act. In terms of hazardous materials management, OSHA regulates numerous safety and health aspects, including material labeling and information communication, personal protective equipment, workplace monitoring, medical surveillance, and training requirements. In addition, numerous chemicals are regulated individually.

Hazardous Communication Standard. A key OSHA rule that has affected facilities managing hazardous materials and hazardous wastes is the Hazardous Communication Standard (HCS), which was passed by the U.S. Congress in May 1988. It requires every employer to develop, implement, and maintain a written, comprehensive communication program for the workplace. The standard identifies three areas that must be covered within each employer's comprehensive program[2] (Box 34-1).

General Duty Clause—Occupational Safety and Health Act. The OSH Act of 1970 and its amendments pertain mainly to workplace safety. Section 5, The General Duty Clause, establishes a set of regulations that set standards for both employers and employees. The clause stipulates that the employer must furnish each employee a place of employment that is free from recognized hazards that could cause death or serious physical harm and that the employer must comply with occupational safety and health standards given under this act. It further stipulates that each employee must comply with occupational safety and health standards and all rules, regulations, and orders issued by the act that apply to the individual's own action and conduct.

Noncompliance with the stipulations of the OSH Act can result in a fine being placed on the institution for the actions of both the employer and the employee. Therefore it is essential that institutions have well-developed policies and procedures for their employees to follow. In many institutions and agencies, compliance standards have been written into performance appraisals as safety standards. Employees are evaluated on their compliance to the standard.[3]

Work-practice guidelines for personnel dealing with cytotoxic (antineoplastic) drugs. In 1986, the Office of Occupational Medicine, a part of OSHA, developed a set of guidelines for health professionals to use during the course of handling hazardous substances to prevent exposure to cytotoxic drug therapy. They were not issued as mandatory standards, but rather as guidelines designed to assist all health

---

Box 34-1   Comprehensive Program for Management of Hazardous Wastes Areas Requiring Coverage

- *A means to identify and warn employees of hazardous chemicals:* Employers must post a notice (prepared by the Department of Labor) of employee rights under the act, and labels must be maintained on all chemical containers, including stationary containers.
- *MSDSs:* Material Safety Data Sheets are comprehensive data sheets that must be maintained on each hazardous chemical or medication. All medications must be classified to indicate a potential for significant health hazard. Each safety data sheet should provide information regarding proper handling and storage procedures, accident and fire prevention, special hazards, and emergency procedures for each chemical used in the work area. They must be available and accessible to employees at all times.
- *An employee information and training program:* The training program must be established in writing and kept at the facility. The program must provide education regarding the potential hazards, preparation, transportation, administration, management of accidental exposure, and disposal of all chemical agents used by the employee.

Box 34-2   Federal OSHA's Revised Compliance Directive, November 5, 1999

RECOMMENDATIONS FOR PREVENTION OF OCCUPATIONAL EXPOSURES TO BLOOD-BORNE PATHOGENS

1. Comprehensive Exposure Control Plan
   - Is a written plan to eliminate employee exposures to blood-borne pathogens
   - Is reviewed and updated annually
   - Reflects changes in technology
   - Emphasizes engineering controls
   - Includes procedures for identification and selection of safety devices and progress made in effort
2. Engineering Controls
   - Used to reduce (remove, eliminate, or isolate) employee exposure
   - Evaluated to reduce exposures before, during, and after use of products
3. Staff Education
   - Ongoing
   - Annual program to address what employees can do to eliminate potential exposures
4. Tracking and Follow-up of Injuries
   - Documentation of injuries (incident report log) with follow-up treatment
     - Includes employee job category, department, and body part affected
     - Includes type and brand of device, circumstances, and procedure
   - Documentation of procedure for evaluation of circumstances surrounding exposure incidents

---

care personnel, including physicians, nurses, pharmacists, aides, and the numerous and diverse health care support staff, who may be exposed to cytotoxic drugs through inhalation, skin absorption, or trauma. The guidelines were developed because of the concerns of health care personnel regarding the potential harm that may result from exposure to cytotoxic drugs.

Two elements were recommended as being essential to ensure proper workplace practices: (1) education and training of all staff involved in any aspect of cytotoxic drug handling and (2) the use of a biologic safety cabinet (BSC). The cost of implementing education and training and the installation of the BSC are relatively minor. The potential benefits are major.

Blood-borne pathogen standards. In the Federal Register of December 6, 1991, 29 CFR Part 1910.1030, OSHA published the Final Rule for rules and regulations for occupational exposure to blood-borne pathogens.[4] The detailed Register covers all aspects of the subject giving definitions of key words and phrases.

In 1992, OSHA issued a directive mandating that employers put into place certain rules and regulations when there is a potential for exposure to blood or other potentially infections materials. The mandate was comprehensive and included rules and regulations mandating everything from an exposure control plan to the use of a ducted exhaust-air ventilation system. This mandate required nurses to use personal protective equipment and engineering controls when performing venipunctures and when there was a potential for contact with blood-borne pathogens. The mandate defines *engineering controls* as sharps disposal containers and self-sheathing needles that remove the hazard from the workplace. The mandate further stipulated that these controls be evaluated and replaced on an ongoing basis.

On November 5, 1999, OSHA issued a new compliance directive to the Blood-Borne Pathogens Standard, CPL 2-2.44D, covering all U.S. employees at risk for occupational exposure to

blood or other potentially infectious materials.[5] The directive updates the regulations enacted in 1992 and contains a number of provisions that force health care facilities to take a more proactive approach to the prevention of sharps injuries. Although the directive does not place requirements on the employees, it does recognize and emphasize the advances made in medical technology and reminds employers that they must use readily available technology in their safety and health programs. Health care employers must begin replacing conventional needle devices with safer alternatives when possible—effective immediately. The directive does not mandate any specific devices but does require a comprehensive sharps safety program, including engineering controls, product evaluation and training, and documentation and reporting of all incidents of accidental needlesticks. The directive replaces the directive issued in February 1992 and is used by OSHA compliance officers to establish uniform procedures for enforcing the 1991 blood-borne pathogen standard.[6] Box 34-2 gives an overview of the major points addressed in this directive.

In September 1998, California passed state legislation mandating needle safety. In 1999, Tennessee, Maryland, and Texas followed with similar legislation. Since the new directive was issued November 1999, 12 other states have issued such legislation. At the time of this writing, a total of 18 states have mandated needle safety legislation; 6 other states have introduced legislation, 2 states are considering or drafting legislation, and 11 states have introduced or debated legislation that has failed or their fate is presently uncertain.[7]

Needlestick Safety and Prevention Act. Federal action to protect health care workers from the risks of sharps injuries passed the House of Representatives[8] and Congress in October 2000.[9] The act was signed by President Clinton on November 6, 2000.[10] The Needlestick Safety and Prevention Act (H.R. 5178) calls for revisions to the blood-borne pathogens standard (29 CFR 1910.1030) and directs OSHA to publish in the *Federal Register* changes to the standard. The changes affect four key areas imposing requirements on employers of individuals who have the potential for exposure to blood-borne pathogens.[11-13]

Redefine "engineering controls". The act redefined engineering controls to include safer medical devices such as sharps with engineered protections and needleless systems. The phrase *sharps with engineered sharps injury protections* is defined as "a non-needle sharp or a needle device used for withdrawing body fluids, accessing a vein or artery, or administering medications or other fluids, with a built-in safety feature or mechanism that effectively reduces the risk of an exposure incident." *Needleless systems* are defined as systems "that do not use needles for (a) the collection of bodily fluids or withdrawal of body fluids after initial venous or arterial access is established, (b) the administration of medication or fluids, or (c) any other procedure involving the potential for occupational exposure to blood-borne pathogens due to percutaneous injuries from contaminated sharps."[12,13]

Update blood-borne pathogens exposure control plans to reflect changes in technology. The act requires employers to update exposure control plans to reflect changes in technology that eliminate or reduce exposure to blood-borne pathogens. Employers will have to "document annually consideration and implementation of appropriate commercially available and effective safer medical devices designed to eliminate or minimize occupation exposure."[12,13]

Maintain a sharps injury log. The employer is required to establish and maintain a sharps injury log for the recording of percutaneous injuries from contaminated sharps. Information should be maintained in a manner to protect the confidentiality of the injured employee. The sharps injury log must minimally contain "(a) the type and brand of device involved in the incident, (b) the department or work area where the exposure incident occurred, and (c) an explanation of how the incident occurred."[12,13]

Solicit input from nonmanagerial employees. Employers required to establish an exposure control plan must "solicit input from non-managerial employees responsible for direct patient care who are potentially exposed to injuries from contaminated sharps in the identification, evaluation, and selection of effective engineering and work practice controls and shall document the solicitation in the Exposure Control Plan."[12,13]

Environmental Protection Agency

The Environmental Protection Agency (EPA) was established as an independent agency in 1970 to ensure that all Americans are protected from significant risks to human health and to the environment where they live, learn, and work.[14]

The following acts were developed through the efforts of the EPA. Although the EPA does not directly relate to infusion therapy, the infusion nurse is indirectly affected through the actions of EPA. Thus the acts and a brief description are listed here.

Toxic Substance Control Act. The intent of the Toxic Substance Control Act (TSCA) of 1976 is to ensure that chemicals manufactured or imported into the United States are registered and listed in the TSCA registry. To receive authorization to manufacture or import a new chemical for commercial purposes, a premanufacture notice (PMN) must be filed with the EPA.[15]

Resource Conservation and Recovery Act. In 1976, the EPA developed rules under the Resource Conservation and Recovery Act (RCRA) to regulate the management of hazardous solid waste from generation to final disposal, also termed *cradle to grave*. Under these regulations, the term *solid wastes* includes waste solids, sludges, liquids, and containerized gases. The regulations include criteria for defining hazardous wastes. In addition, the rules list several hundred toxic and acutely hazardous chemicals that if spilled or discarded, become hazardous waste. Included in the standards are requirements for facilities, transporter identification and tracking requirements, record keeping, and inspection requirements.

Medical Waste Tracking Act. The Medical Waste Tracking Act (MWTA), developed in 1988, requires the EPA to provide a demonstration program for characterizing and tracking medical waste and evaluating treatment techniques for this waste. The act made each facility responsible for properly disposing of all waste and legally responsible for the improper disposal of waste.

Comprehensive Environmental Response, Compensation and Liability Act. The Comprehensive Environmental Response, Compensation and Liability Act (CERCLA) of 1980, also known as the *Superfund Act*, and several other acts passed under the Superfund Umbrella, provide for liability, compensation, cleanup, and emergency response for hazardous substances released into the environment. The 1986 amendments to the act provided for $8.5 billion to be allotted for cleanup of Superfund sites over a 5-year period, as well as the requirement for potentially responsible parties to share in cleanup and associated costs.

Spill reporting, another part of this act, includes a list of hundreds of hazardous materials and reporting quantities requirements. This requirement for reporting allows the EPA to track hazardous waste incidents. Once reported, these incidents become part of the public record.

Superfund Amendments and Reauthorization Act. Under Title III for the Superfund Amendments and Reauthorization Act (SARA), the citizens of a community have a right to know what chemicals and wastes are stored at a facility and in what quantities.[15] Citizens also have access to reports detailing releases of certain chemicals into the environment. The Emergency Planning and Community Right-to-Know Act (EPCRA) of 1986 is often referred to as *SARA*, Title III, because the provisions of the act are incorporated in Title III of the Superfund Amendments and Reauthorization Act (SARA) of 1986. This act requires the establishment of local emergency planning and chemical release notification and to provide knowledge to the community about chemicals stored and released from facilities in the area.

Pollution Prevention Act. The Pollution Prevention Act of 1990 has changed the focus of "cradle-to-grave" management of hazardous waste to "cradle-to-cradle" management. The new cradle-to-cradle concept emphasizes prevention of waste through recycling, source reduction, elimination of toxic materials, and use of other methods to achieve environmentally conscious manufacturing. As a result, the act requires the EPA to develop programs to minimize pollution and to develop a list of priority chemicals to be targeted by minimization programs.

Centers for Disease Control and Prevention

The Centers for Disease Control and Prevention (CDC), headquartered in Atlanta, Georgia, is an agency of the Department of Health and Human Services. The CDC's mission is to promote health and quality of life by preventing and controlling disease, injury, and disability. The CDC performs many of the administrative functions for the Agency for Toxic Substances and Disease Registry (ATSDR), a sister agency of CDC. The Director of the CDC also serves as the administrator of ATSDR.

National Institute for Occupational Safety and Health. The National Institute for Occupational Safety and Health (NIOSH) was established by the OSH Act of 1970. NIOSH is part of the CDC and is the only federal institute responsible for conducting research and making recommendations for the prevention of work-related illnesses and injuries.

Although NIOSH and OSHA were created by the same act of Congress, they are two distinct agencies with separate responsibilities. OSHA is in the Department of Labor and is responsible for creating and enforcing workplace safety and health regulations. OSHA determines new and effective ways to protect workers from chemical exposure, dangerous machinery, and hazardous working conditions. NIOSH is in the Department of Health and Human Services and is a research agency that identifies the causes of work-related diseases and injuries and the potential hazards of new work technologies and practices.

In response to the 1999 OSHA directive, NIOSH published *NIOSH Alert: Preventing Needlestick Injuries in Health Care Settings.* This alert provides an overview of needlestick injuries in the United States, case reports, use of engineering controls in prevention strategy, recommendations for selecting and evaluating needle devices with safety features, and recommendations for employers and employees.[16]

National Institutes of Health

The National Institutes of Health (NIH) began as a one-room Laboratory of Hygiene in 1887. Today, the NIH is one of the world's foremost biomedical research centers and the federal focal point for biomedical research in the United States.

The goal of NIH research is to acquire new knowledge to help prevent, detect, diagnose, and treat diseases and disabilities that range from the rarest genetic disorder to the common cold.

American Society of Health-System Pharmacists

The American Society of Health-System Pharmacists (ASHP) is the national professional association that represents pharmacists in the organized health care setting. Based on published research, ASHP has offered guidelines that affect infusion nursing. An example is the guidelines concerning the handling of cytotoxic drugs published in 1990. The standards relative to intravenous (IV) nursing are reflected in *Infusion Nursing Standards of Practice.*

Intravenous Nurses Society

The Intravenous Nurses Society (INS) is very concerned with the safety of the infusion nurse as hazardous agents are prepared, transferred, and administered. *Infusion Nurses Standards of Practice* reflects this concern throughout all the standards. The standards have been written using federal regulations and input from experts within each field. Information about standard precautions appears in the infection control standard and the standards providing information directly related to the administration of antineoplastic agents appears in the standard on oncology/antineoplastic therapy.[17]

American Association of Blood Banks

The American Association of Blood Banks (AABB) publishes standards regarding the professional practice of blood donation, blood processing, and transfusion therapy. These standards address the safe and effective replacement of blood and blood components. The AABB standards that relate to infusion nursing are included in *Infusion Nursing Standards of Practice.*

HAZARDOUS SUBSTANCES

The definition of *hazardous* is dangerous, or full of risk.[15] Therefore *hazardous substances* are substances that have the potential for being dangerous or posing a risk from contact with the substance. This includes a wide range of substances, from drugs to blood-borne pathogens. OSHA more clearly defines *occupational exposure* as "reasonable anticipated skin, eye, mucous membrane, or parenteral contact with blood or other potential infectious materials that may result from the performance of an employee's duties."[5]

OSHA requires that infusion nurses and other individuals involved in any occupation in which contact or exposure to a hazardous substance is possible be given information on hazardous substances and any precautions necessary for working with them. Recognizing the potential risks for exposure, understanding how to minimize exposure, and knowing what to do if an exposure occurs are essential elements in preventing potential problems. The federal government has given OSHA the power to enforce the regulations and impose a fine on any institution or agency that is noncompliant.

The management of hazardous substances can be arduous and expensive. However, it is necessary to protect the patient, family, infusion nurse, other health care workers, and general public. This protection includes managing potential exposures to materials by their staff. These materials can be categorized as biologic agents and chemical agents.

Biologic agents

Biologic agents include human immunodeficiency virus (HIV), hepatitis B virus (HBV), hepatitis C virus (HCV), and the tubercle bacillus (TB). HIV, HBV, and HCV are transmitted by blood infected with the viruses, whereas TB is transmitted by contact with respiratory secretions infected with *Mycobacterium tuberculosis*. This chapter focuses on HBV, HIV, and HCV because they pose the greatest threat to the infusion nurse. Each is discussed as cases were documented.

HBV. The first documented case of occupational transmission of a blood-borne disease occurred several decades ago with hepatitis B.[18] In 1995, an estimated 800 health care workers became infected with HBV, representing a 95% decline from the estimations made in 1983.[16] The decline was the result of the widespread immunization of health care workers with the hepatitis B vaccine and the use of standard precautions and other measures required by OSHA.

The health care worker's chance of contracting HBV after an accidental needlestick on the job is 1 in 20.[19] Approximately two health care workers are infected each day with HBV.[20]

Such exposures are a risk only for heath care workers who are not immune to HBV. Immunity is obtained from antibodies to HBV developed from the administration of a preexposure vaccination or prior infection. Postexposure prophylaxis with hepatitis B immune globulin and initiation of hepatitis B vaccines is more than 90% effective in preventing HBV infection.[16]

About one third to one half of persons with acute HBV infection develop symptoms of hepatitis, such as jaundice, fever, nausea, and abdominal pain. Most acute infections resolve, but 5% to 10% of patients develop chronic infection with HBV that carries an estimated 20% lifetime risk of dying from cirrhosis and 6% risk of dying from liver cancer.[21]

HIV. The first documented HIV transmission occurred in 1984.[18] Between 1985 and June 1999, 55 cases of documented HIV after occupational exposure and 136 possible cases of occupational HIV transmission to health care workers within the United States were reported to the CDC. Most cases involved nurses and laboratory technicians. Needlestick injuries were associated with 49 (89%) of the documented transmissions. Of these, 44 involved hollow-bore needles, most of which were used for blood collection or IV catheter insertion.[16]

A health care worker's chance of contracting HIV after an HIV-infected needlestick is 1 in 250.[19] The risk of infection from a needlestick exposure to an infected patient depends on several mitigating circumstances. NIOSH lists the following factors that determine the risk for infection[16]:

- Pathogen involved
- Worker's immune status
- Severity of the needlestick injury
- Availability and use of appropriate postexposure prophylaxis

Studies by Cardo et al. show that the risk for HIV transmission is increased when the worker is exposed to a large quantity of blood from an infected patient, as indicated by a visibly bloody device, a procedure that involves placing a needle into an infected patient's vein or artery, or a deep needlestick injury to the health care worker.[22]

HIV is a complex disease that attacks part of the body's immune system and is thus associated with many symptoms. As the disease progresses, severe infection and other complications occur, which leads to acquired immunodeficiency syndrome (AIDS). Despite current therapies that only delay disease progression, most health care workers who become infected with HIV eventually develop AIDS and die.[16]

The CDC recommends postexposure prophylaxis for health care workers occupationally exposed to HIV under certain circumstances.[23] Limited data suggest that such prophylaxis may considerably reduce the chance of becoming infected with HIV.[16] However, the drugs used for prophylaxis have many adverse side effects. Currently, no vaccine exists to prevent HIV infection, and no treatment exists to cure it.[24]

HCV. Of the viruses, HCV is the most menacing because it has the ability to survive for long periods on various substances even when it is dry. Approximately 170 million people worldwide are infected with HCV.[18] HCV is currently the most common chronic blood-borne infection in the United States, with at least 4 million people affected by the disease.[25] At least 30,000 new cases of HCV and approximately 10,000 deaths occur annually from the disease.[18] The CDC predicts that the hepatitis C death toll will triple and surpass that of AIDS within the next 10 years.

The number of health care workers who have acquired HCV occupationally is not known. However, of the total acute HCV infections that have occurred annually, 2% to 4% have been in health care workers exposed to blood in the workplace.[16] Health care workers' chances for contracting HCV after an HCV-contaminated needlestick average 3.5 in 100.[19]

HCV infection occurs with no symptoms or only mild symptoms. However, unlike HBV, chronic infection develops in 75% to 85% of patients, with active liver disease developing in 70%. Of the patients with active liver disease, 10% to 20% develop cirrhosis, and 1% to 5% develop liver cancer.[25]

Prevention. OSHA provides guidelines, known as *standard precautions,* to minimize the risk associated with exposure to blood and body fluids by the infusion nurse and other health care workers while caring for patients. These recommendations emphasize that the blood and body fluids of all patients are potentially infectious and that health care workers should take necessary precautions when caring for all patients. Appropriate use of handwashing and protective barriers and care in the use and disposal of needles and other sharp instruments minimize the risk of HBV, HCV, and HIV transmission. The OSHA directive of November 1999 (as previously summarized in Box 34-2) is explicit and will prevent exposures if implemented within the workplace.

The CDC recommends that medical devices, such as endoscopes, contaminated by blood infected with HIV, HBV, or HCV be treated with a high-level disinfectant between uses.[26] Experiments have demonstrated the effectiveness of high-level disinfectants (e.g., glutaraldehyde, chlorine) to inactivate these pathogens.[27]

Spills of blood and blood-contaminated fluids should be

cleaned up promptly at the time of occurrence using an EPA-approved disinfectant. EPA-approved disinfectants include a tuberculocidal or a 1:100 solution of household bleach. Chemical germicide effectiveness is markedly decreased if gross amounts of body fluids are not first cleaned from surfaces or objects. Gloves should be worn when cleaning up spills, and the hands should be washed thoroughly after removal of gloves.

Linen soiled with blood or body fluids should be placed and transported in bags that prevent leakage. Personnel involved in bagging, transporting, and laundering contaminated linens should wear gloves.

Chemical hazards

Calculation of health risks. *Chemical hazards* relate to those hazards incurred by health care workers from chemicals with which they come in contact. Chemicals may have acute or chronic effects on infusion nurses and other health care workers. The effects vary depending on the following[28]:

- Chemical and physical properties of the substance
- Extent (duration and concentration) of exposure
- Route of exposure
- Presence of other chemical or physical agents
- Use of alcohol, drugs, or tobacco

A substance's exposure concentration is the mass per unit volume of air to which a worker is exposed. Airborne concentrations in the workplace usually are expressed in terms of milligrams of substance per cubic meter of air (mg/m^3) or parts of substance per million parts of air (ppm). The exposure dose is the amount of a substance that actually enters the body during the period of exposure. Until the substance is metabolized or eliminated, it remains in the body. Chemicals vary as to whether they are metabolized and excreted, excreted unchanged, or stored in the body.[28] Table 34-1 lists chemicals that are stored within the body.

Substances can enter the body through more than one route, but few can enter the body through all routes. An example is inorganic lead that can be swallowed or inhaled but that cannot penetrate the skin. Toxic substances can enter the body through several routes, including accidental needle puncture or through contact with skin, eyes, mouth (inhalation or ingestion), and respiratory system (inhalation).

The physical properties of both chemical and physical agents have numerous characteristics that affect the degree of exposure. Box 34-3 lists the properties of chemicals affecting the degree of exposure. These properties become relevant to exposure of the infusion nurse because they allow the substance to change from one form to another and give off harmful gases or vapors. Some chemicals have characteristics that can serve as a warning of the chemical's presence. The most common warning property is odor. The lowest concentration at which the odor of a chemical can be detected is called the *odor threshold*. Not everyone can detect odors equally well, and for this reason, infusion nurses should not rely on their sense of smell to warn them of the presence of a hazardous substance.

Dose time exposure. Infusion nurses and other health care workers are exposed to hazardous chemicals when preparing, administering, and disposing medications that are consid-

Table 34-1 Storage of Chemicals within the Body

Substance	Place of Storage
Solvents	Fatty tissues
Dust and fibers	Lungs
Lead and radium	Bone
Soluble gases	Blood

Box 34-3 Physical Properties of Chemical and Physical Agents

IMPACTING EXPOSURE
- Vapor pressure
- Solubility in water and organic solvents
- Boiling point
- Melting point
- Molecular weight
- Specific gravity
- Morphology

ered potentially hazardous, such as the antineoplastic agents. The degree of absorption that takes place during handling and the biologic effects that each individual encounters are difficult to assess and may vary depending on the hazardous substance. As a result, it is difficult to set safe levels of exposure on the basis of current scientific information. There is evidence that improper handling of hazardous substances create potentially toxic conditions. Therefore it is essential to minimize exposure to all hazardous substances because they either bind directly to genetic material in the cell nucleus or affect cellular protein synthesis, resulting in damaged growth and reproduction of normal cells as well.[28]

Antineoplastic agents. *Antineoplastic agents* are chemically unrelated classes of agents that are capable of inhibiting tumor growth by killing actively growing cells and interfering with cell division. The same mechanisms that are used for therapeutic treatment can also be carcinogenic, mutagenic, and/or teratogenic. There is evidence of biologic activity of some of these agents that has prompted research regarding potential reproductive hazards and the long-term health risks associated with persons handling these drugs. The risks to infusion nurses handling antineoplastic agents are a combined result of each drug's inherent toxicity and the actual exposure time to the drug.

Infusion nurses and other health care personnel handling antineoplastic agents can be exposed by three potential routes: accidental ingestion, percutaneous absorption, or inhalation of an aerosolized drug. The primary exposure route for all health care personnel is inhalation.[28] Although studies are limited, those available demonstrate the efficacy for using the vertical flow, BSC in decreasing the health risk from inhalation to medical personnel while mixing and preparing the antineoplastic agents. This knowledge provides the grounds for the mixing of antineoplastic agents within the pharmacy under a BSC instead of in a home care setting where such equipment is usually unavailable.

The dermal and ingestion routes also provide opportunities for exposure. These routes of exposure depend on contact with contaminated surfaces. Containers used to administer antineoplastic agents can be a source for surface contamination as a result of admixture accidents or the containers developing a leak onto a work surface or an individual.

Laundry contaminated with antineoplastic agents should be placed in a specially marked laundry bag and prewashed before regular washing. The purpose of the prewash is to remove as much of the drug as possible before mixing with the other laundry because laundering does not make cytotoxic medications harmless; it removes the drugs from the clothing. Institutions and agencies should establish guidelines for the treatment of uniforms worn by nurses when exposed to large amounts of antineoplastic agents. Some institutions require removal of the uniform, a shower, and application of clean clothing. In addition, they require that the uniform be placed in a laundry bag and labeled "Contaminated with Biohazard Substance." The uniform is then washed by the laundry within the institution and returned to the employee.

Other hazardous drugs. There are a number of drugs other than the antineoplastic agents that provide a potential for risks to infusion nurses and other health care workers, both acutely and/or through chronic low-dose exposure, even though they are beneficial in patient treatment. These medications are referred to as *hazardous drugs*. The 1995 OSHA Guidelines for Controlling Occupational Exposure to Hazardous Drugs provides a table of drugs considered hazardous.[29] Although the table does not reflect some of the newer drugs, it does provide a good list of those commonly used. Some of the drugs are extreme irritants and can cause significant skin damage on contact, whereas others are known carcinogens.

Other drugs considered hazardous include the antiviral agents ribavirin and ganciclovir, which have caused reproductive toxicity in animal studies. This raises a concern for exposed pregnant workers and female and male employees attempting to conceive. Pentamidine, used to treat *Pneumocystis carinii* pneumonia, has been linked to pulmonary effects. It is administered in aerosolized form as ribavirin. Its use has been known to cause environmental contamination in both occupational and bystander exposure.[29] Negative pressure rooms should be used when possible to treat patients with ribavirin.

Chemical disinfectants. Within the hospital, a number of different substances are used because of the variety of needs for disinfectants. The most important are isopropyl alcohol, sodium hypochlorite (chlorine), iodine, phenolics, quaternary ammonium compounds, glutaraldehydes, and formaldehyde. Although these substances may produce a substantial odor, workers should not rely on the odor as a warning of exposure for the reason previously stated. Workers should wear protective clothing such as gloves, splash-proof safety goggles, face shields, and clothing necessary to prevent skin contact. Areas of skin exposed to disinfectants should be washed thoroughly with soap and water to prevent contact dermatitis. When disinfectants are used, the area should be well ventilated to prevent mucous membrane and nasal irritation. Any clothing contaminated with disinfectants should be properly washed according to specific directions for contact with each type of disinfectant.

HAZARDOUS WASTES

Governmental regulators have spent nearly three decades defining what makes a material or waste hazardous. Generally, a *hazardous chemical* or *waste* is a material that is potentially dangerous to human health or the environment. The EPA defines a *waste* as hazardous if it is a solid waste that meets one of several definitions. The term *solid waste* might be somewhat misleading. *Solid wastes* are liquids, solids, and containerized gases.[15] Not all hazardous wastes are infectious. The CDC defines *infectious waste* as wastes that represent a significant potential risk of causing infection during handling and disposal. The CDC further qualifies this statement by stating that all wastes that have a potential for causing infection should be handled with caution using standard precautions.[30]

No epidemiologic evidence currently exists to suggest that most medical waste is any more infectious than residential waste. Moreover, there is no epidemiologic evidence that current disposal practices of medical waste have caused disease transmission. However, certain medical wastes do provide a potential for risks and should be handled and disposed of using standard precautions. These wastes include microbiology laboratory waste, pathology waste, bulk blood or blood products, and sharps, such as used needles or scalpel blades. In general, these items should either be decontaminated before disposal in a sanitary landfill or be incinerated. Secretions, bulk blood, excretions, and suctioned fluids may carefully be poured down a drain connected to a sanitary sewer.[30] Bloody secretions or fluids may also be solidified by using a biohazardous solidification system and then disposing as infected waste.

Regulated medical waste (RMW) is considered infectious waste because it can potentially transmit an infectious disease. This is also sometimes called *red-bag waste* or *biohazardous waste*. Only those items considered biohazardous should be red-bagged and specially processed. All other items should be placed in regular trash bags. The universal symbol for biologic hazards is fluorescent orange or orange-red[31] and is shown in Fig. 34-1.

Needles, syringes, and sharps should be disposed of in a puncture-resistant, leak-proof container that is easily accessible and appropriately labeled. Used or contaminated needles should not be bent or recapped unless using a one-handed technique. Needles and intravenous cannulas should be discarded into a puncture-resistant, leak-proof container labeled for disposal of needles and sharps. Industry currently manufactures various types of syringes and needles that have attached sheathing devices or attached covers that require minimal effort to engage; these devices prevent needlestick injuries when used according to the manufacturer's guidelines.

Hazardous waste from treatment with chemotherapy should be disposed of only in designated yellow or white (different color than red biohazard bags) plastic bags, and these bags should be placed in a rigid container designated for hazardous waste. All needles and syringes used in chemotherapy preparation and administration should be disposed of in a rigid container dedicated and labeled for the disposal of chemotherapy waste.

There are numerous administrative requirements for proper management of hazardous materials and hazardous waste speci-

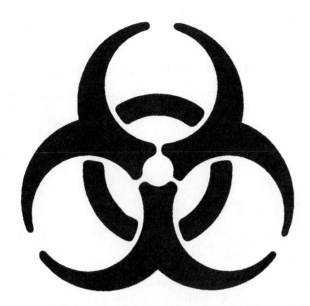

FIG. 34-1 *Universal symbol for biologic hazards. The symbol is fluorescent orange or orange-red. The background may be any color that provides sufficient contrast for the symbol to be clearly defined.*[25]

fied by governmental agencies. These requirements include proper container labeling, periodic training, container and containment inspections, and plans and controls for disposal.

Established policies and procedures for the management of hazardous waste are necessary to promote consistency and compliance. The Joint Commission on Accreditation of Healthcare Organizations (JCAHO) requires hospitals and home care agencies to have a documented management plan for hazardous materials and waste. Regardless of outside requirements, hospitals, home care agencies, and all those involved with hazardous wastes should have waste management plans in place to cover all wastes generated. The plan must include all departments within the institution or organization and must emphasize institution-wide/organizationwide goals and consistency among departments to be successful.

INFUSION NURSING ISSUES
Biohazards

Universal precautions, as defined by the CDC, are a set of precautions designed to prevent transmission of HIV, HBV, HCV, and other blood-borne pathogens when providing first aid or health care.[32] The use of universal precautions reduces employee exposure to blood-borne pathogens. Personal protective equipment provides a barrier to protect skin and mucous membranes from contact with blood and other potentially infectious material. However, personal protective equipment should not provide a false sense of security when using needles because needles can penetrate most barriers.

The primary route of exposure to blood-borne pathogens is through accidental percutaneous injury caused by needlesticks. Studies have shown that many of these injuries occur during disposal activities. Needlestick injuries occur in health care workers with the greatest involvement in direct patient care, especially the nursing staff and phlebotomists. Studies show that

these two groups sustain the highest percentage of reported injuries.[33]

Infusion nurses are particularly susceptible because their work involves procedures related to potential risks associated with being exposed to blood-borne pathogens. Infusion nurses tend to become relaxed in the performance of venipunctures because of their expertise. This is the time when mistakes can be made and injuries occur. Infusion nurses must always be on their guard, maintain caution, use devises that promote safety, and comply with policies and procedures that promote safety of the health care worker.

The correct and consistent use of puncture-resistant, rigid disposal containers in the health care environment reduces needlestick injuries. Disposal containers need to be functional, accessible, visible, and convenient to use. For optimal protective value, the container must be readily available and of sufficient size and capacity. Disposal containers should not be overfilled, and they should have a closure mechanism designed to minimize exposure to contents and injury to the hand during closure or transport.

Research shows that hypodermic needles and IV tubing assemblies inserted into a connecting Y site on a primary IV line (piggybacking) or directly into an IV access port (intermittent IV) have a greater risk of needlestick injury. The Needlestock Safety and Prevention Act of 2000 requires the use of needles with engineering controls to access IV lines. Industry provides numerous products that prevent needlestick injuries, including IV catheters, needleless IV tubing, Huber-Point needles, syringes, and disposable needle containers. These devices protect employees from occupational exposure to blood and other potentially infectious material.

Chemical hazards and wastes

The use of cytotoxic drugs to treat cancer began in the late 1940s with the use of nitrogen mustard. However, handling these drugs did not become an issue until individuals began to experience health-related problems. In the early 1980s, researchers began to look at the effects on health care workers handling these drugs. Research demonstrated that hazardous drugs can cause chromosome breakage in circulating lymphocytes, mutagenic activity in urine, and skin necrosis after surface contacts with abraded skin or damage to normal skin.[28]

OSHA established guidelines for the management of cytotoxic (antineoplastic) drugs in the workplace in 1986. At this time, engineering controls and personal protective equipment were not standardized. Although practices improved as a result of the guidelines, problems associated with the use of the drugs and other hazardous agents continued. In 1995, OSHA revised the guidelines to incorporate hazardous drugs. The guidelines stipulate that all health care workers in all settings must receive information and training to make them aware of the potential complications that hazardous drugs present in the work area.

Health risks from chemotherapy exposure are measured by time, dose, and exposure route (Box 34-4).

Although no information is available on the reproductive risks of handling chemotherapy drugs, employees who are pregnant, planning pregnancy, or breast-feeding may elect to

---

Box 34-4   **Three Main Routes of Exposure**

1. *Absorption through the skin or mucous membranes* after direct contact can happen during drug preparation or administration. Gloves should be worn when handling antineoplastic agents.
2. *Inhalation* of drug aerosols or droplets can occur during drug admixing or changing IV tubing. Only specially trained personnel should prepare drugs for administration. A class II or III biologic safety cabinet (BSC) or an OSHA-approved dust/mist respirator or face mask must be available to personnel for drug preparation.
3. *Ingestion* of food, beverages, or tobacco products accidentally contaminated by hazardous medications can cause exposure. Eating, drinking, smoking, applying cosmetics or lip balm, and handling contact lenses is prohibited in work areas where there is a reasonable likelihood of occupational exposure.[4]

CAUTION: CYTOTOXIC DRUGS

HANDLE WITH GLOVES, DISPOSE OF PROPERLY

FIG. 34-2   *Warning label for use on all containers containing cytotoxic drugs.*

Box 34-5   **Contents of Spill Kits as Recommended by OSHA[29]**

- One nonpermeable fabric gown with cuffs and back closure
- One pair of shoe covers
- Two pairs of latex gloves
- One pair utility gloves
- One pair chemical splash goggles
- One rebreather mask (NIOSH approved)
- One disposable dust pan (to collect broken glass)
- One plastic scraper (to scoop material into dust pan)
- Two plastic-backed absorbable towels
- Both a 250-ml and a 1-L spill control pillow
- Two disposable sponges (one to clean up spill and one to clean up floor after removal of spill)
- One sharps container
- Two large heavy-duty waste disposal bags

---

refrain from preparing, administering, or caring for patients receiving therapy with these agents.

To minimize the risk of exposure during preparation, administration, and disposal, infusion nurses and other health care personnel should use personal protective equipment. Latex powder-free gloves should be used for handling cytotoxic drugs. Glove thickness and time in contact with the drug are the major factors in permeability. Latex gloves are less permeable than nonlatex gloves. Individuals with a latex allergy should consider the use of vinyl or nitrile gloves or glove liners. Double gloving is recommended if it does not interfere with an individual's technique. Gloves should be changed regularly, at least hourly, or whenever punctured, torn, or contaminated with a drug. Gowns should be disposable and lint free and made from a nonpermeable fabric with a closed front and long, elastic or knit-cuffed sleeves. Cuffs on the sleeves of gowns should be tucked into the glove. Policies and procedures for the administration of chemotherapy are clearly defined by the INS in *Policies and Procedures for Infusion Nursing*.[34] Procedures for chemotherapy administration are reflected in Chapter 13.

Respiratory protection is best achieved with the use of a class II or III vertical airflow, BSC during preparation and mixing of drugs. An NIOSH-approved respirator should be worn when a BSC is not available. Eye and face barriers should be worn if splashes might occur or if sprays or aerosols are used. Regular eyeglasses with side shields are inadequate. Eye wash facilities should be available.

Infusion nurses should use only syringes and solution sets with Luer-Lok fittings for preparing and administering cytotoxic drugs because these fittings are less likely to accidentally separate. Syringes should be filled no more than half full with a cytotoxic agent to prevent spillage of a drug from a syringe or separation of the plunger from the syringe barrel. Syringes and needles used with cytotoxic drugs should not be crushed, clipped, or recapped in order to avoid drug aerosolization and/or needlestick injuries. They should be placed in a puncture-resistant, rigid container designated for "sharps" disposal. Drug administration sets should be attached to bags and primed in the BSC before the addition of the drug, or the IV tubing should be initially flushed with a solution not containing the drug so that the fluid in the tubing does not contain the drug. All containers with cytotoxic drugs need to be marked with a distinctive warning label. Fig. 34-2 provides an example of a label that can be used to designate cytotoxic drugs.

Materials transported from one area to another should be placed in resealable plastic bags marketed for transport of cytotoxic drugs and transported in a designated container to reduce the risk of breakage and contamination. Bags and solution administration sets should be discarded intact into resealable leak-proof and puncture-proof containers. Spill kits are necessary in all areas where cytotoxic drugs are mixed, transported, administered, and disposed. The same work practices are used in any setting where hazardous materials appear.

Spill kits can be assembled in the institution or purchased from a manufacturer, but they should include those items recommended by OSHA in 1995. Box 34-5 provides a list of those items recommend by OSHA for inclusion in spill kits.

Small spills are defined as spills of less than 5 ml or 5 g occurring outside a BSC. A volume greater than 5 ml or 5 g constitutes a *large spill*.[35] Infusion nurses should be knowledgeable in the use of spill kits. All spills should be cleaned up immediately by infusion nurses or other trained personnel wearing personal protective equipment, including two pairs of latex powder-free gloves; a disposable, impermeable gown; a face shield; and shoe covers. Liquids should be wiped and absorbed with absorbent gauze pads or towels and discarded into a large hazardous waste bag. Any broken glass fragments should be picked up and placed in a puncture-proof container using a small scoop. The spill area should be cleaned three times using a detergent solution, followed by clean water. Protective garb worn by employees cleaning spills should be placed in a cytotoxic waste disposal bag, sealed, and placed in a puncture-proof cytotoxic waste container.

SUMMARY

The management of hazardous substances is a critical component of infusion nursing. Nurses performing infusion procedures must be cognizant of what constitutes a hazardous substance and the risks associated with their use. Infusion nurses consistently perform procedures that either deliver hazardous drugs or provide exposure to blood-borne pathogens. Governmental regulations and guidelines have been developed to provide protection from these hazardous substances. Infusion nurses must be aware of these and be at the forefront for the development of policies and procedures that use and expand on developed guidelines. Infusion nurses must set the example for others in the use of personal protective equipment and engineering controls and in following infection control policies. Knowledge of hazardous fluids, medications, and chemicals being used and the use of personal protective equipment can minimize exposure of the infusion nurse and prevent the resulting complications.

REFERENCES

1. OSHA: *Strategic plan,* Occupational Safety & Health Administration, 1999.
2. Tools for Health-System Pharmacists. American Society of Health System Pharmacists, Bethesda, Md, 1998:HM-1.
3. High Point Regional Health System: High Point Regional Health System Employee Performance Development Program. Basic Job Expectations, Standard 5.
4. OSHA: Occupational exposure to bloodborne pathogens: final rule, *Fed Register* 56(235):29 CFR Part 1910.1030, 1991.
5. OSHA: Enforcement procedures for the occupational exposure to bloodborne pathogens. Directive CPL 2-2.44D; November 4, 1999.
6. Pugliese G, Bartley J: Federal OSHA's revised compliance directive: what will compliance officers look for? *Adv Exposure Prevention* 5(1):1, 2000.
7. Barlow RD: Needle-safety scoreboard by state: Massachusetts marches forward on needle safety, News and Analysis @ hospital-network.com, August 18, 2000.
8. House of Representatives passes needlestick prevention bill, Hosptial Network.com: Digital marketplace for health care induswysiwyg://664/http://www.hospitalne; October 5, 2000.
9. Senate follows House in passing federal needle-safety legislation, Hospital Network.com: Digital marketplace for health care industwysiwyg://662/http://www.hospitalne; October 26, 2000.
10. Clinton signs needle safety legislation, Hospital Network.com: Digital marketplace for the health care industwysiwyg://373/http://www.hospitalne; November 6, 2000.
11. OSHA guide for health care facilities (ISSN #1091-3432), Washington, DC, 2000, Thompson Publishing Group.
12. Needlestick Safety and Prevention Act (H.R. 5178). 106th Congress, 2nd session, Washington, DC, 2000.
13. Needlestick Safety and Prevention Act (introduced in the Senate), S. 3067 IS. 106th Congress, 2nd session, Washington, DC, 2000.
14. About EPA, US Environmental Protection Agency, 1999.
15. Woodside G: *Hazardous materials and hazardous waste management,* ed 2, New York, 1999, John Wiley & Sons.
16. CDC: NIOSH alert: preventing needlestick injuries in health care settings, Publication No. 2000-108, November 1999.
17. Intravenous Nurses Society: Infusion nursing standards of practice, *JIN* (suppl) 23(65), 2000.
18. Bockhold KM: Who's afraid of hepatitis C? *AJN* 100(5):26, 2000.
19. Duesman K, Ross J: Survey of accidental needlesticks in twenty-six facilities using VanishPoint® automated retraction syringe, *J Healthcare Safety Compliance Infect Control* March 1998, Available: http://vanishpoint.com/ARTICLE—Surveryof26Facilities.htm.
20. Hepatitis B Foundation: *Facts on Hepatitis B,* January 30, 1998. Available: www2.hepb.org/hepb/info.html#facts.
21. Shapiro CN: Occupational risk of infection with hepatitis B and hepatitis C virus, *Surg Clin North Am* 75(6):1047, 1995.
22. Cardo DM, et al: CDC surveillance group: a case-control study of HIV seroconversion in healthcare workers after percutaneous exposure, *N Engl J Med* 337(21):1485, 1997.
23. CDC: Public health service guidelines for the management of health care worker exposures to HIV and recommendations for postexposure prophylaxis, *MMWR* 47:RR-7, 1998.
24. CDC: Guidelines for the use of antiretroviral agents in HIV-infected adults and adolescents, *MMWR* 47:RR-5, 1998.
25. CDC: Recommendations for prevention and control of hepatitis C virus (HCV) infection and HCV-related chronic disease, *MMWR* 47:RR-19:1, 1998.
26. Abrutyn E, Goldmann D, Scheckler W: *Saunders infection control reference service,* Philadelphia, 1998, WB Saunders.
27. APIC: APIC guidelines for selection and use of disinfectants, Washington, DC, 1996, Association for Infection Control and Epidemiology.
28. Controlling occupational exposure to hazardous drugs, Chapter 21, OSHA Instruction CPL 2-2.20B CH-4, Directorate of Technical Support, 1995.
29. *Hazardous drugs/antineoplastic drugs,* Washington, DC, Office of Occupational Medicine, 1999:1.
30. Gruendemann B: *Healthcare waste management: a template for action,* Cary, NC, 1997, Association of the Nonwoven Fabrics Industry.
31. Guidelines for protecting the safety and health of health care workers, Chapter 6, National Institute for Occupational Safety and Health, 1998.
32. CDC: *Universal precautions for prevention of transmission of HIV and other bloodborne infections,* Atlanta, 1999, Hospital Infection Program, CDC.
33. DHHS: *Selecting, evaluating, and using sharps disposal containers,* Washington, DC, 1998, US Department of Health and Human Services.
34. Intravenous Nurses Society: *Policies and procedures for infusion nursing,* Cambridge, Mass, 2000, Intravenous Nurses Society.
35. Welch J, Silveira J: *Safe handling of cytotoxic drugs,* ed 2, Pittsburgh, 1997, Oncology Nursing Press.

BIBLIOGRAPHY

About CDC, Atlanta, 1999, Centers for Disease Control and Prevention.
About NIOSH, Atlanta, 1999, Centers for Disease Control and Prevention.
Elliott S, Walker D: *Safer needle devices: protecting health care workers,* Washington, DC, 1997, Occupational Safety and Health Administration.
Fahey JL, Flemmig DS: *AIDS/HIV reference guide for medical professionals,* ed 4, Baltimore, 1997, Williams & Wilkins.
Fishman M, Mrozek-Orlowski M: *Cancer chemotherapy guidelines and recommendations for practice,* ed 2, Pittsburgh, 1999, Oncology Nursing Press.

Groenwald S, et al: *Comprehensive cancer nursing review,* ed 4, Sudbury, Mass, 1998, Jones and Bartlett.

Guidelines for protecting the safety and health of health workers, Chapter 2, National Institute for Occupational Safety and Health, 1999.

Infectious waste, hospital infection program, Atlanta, 1999, Centers for Disease Control and Prevention.

NIH: *National Institutes of Health general background information,* Washington, DC, 1999, National Institute of Health.

OSHA seeks information on additional ways to eliminate or greatly reduce needlestick injuries, *OSHA National News Release,* 1998.

OSHA: *OSHA Revises Bloodborne Pathogens Compliance Directive,* OSHA U.S. Department of Labor, November 5, 1999.

Chapter

35

Ethics

Lorys Oddi, EdD, RN

The increasing complexity of biomedical decisions has created many ethical issues in health care. The unique role played by nurses in the health care system intimately involves them in these ethical issues. Long recognized as patient advocates, nurses sometimes feel uncomfortable with decisions made about patient care or with how the care is carried out. They may feel powerless, however, to articulate their concerns, or may be uncertain of how to—or if they have a right to—raise their concerns.

This chapter provides an overview of the unique role of nurses in recognizing and addressing questionable ethical practices, the multiple forces that affect nurses' ethical decision making, a sample framework that is useful for resolving ethical dilemmas, and some actions that can be taken by intravenous (IV) nurses to constructively address the ethical aspects of nursing practice.

UNIQUE ROLE OF NURSES IN THE ETHICAL ASPECTS OF PRACTICE

Ethics consists of moral judgments about the rightness or wrongness of actions in a specific situation. The nursing literature abounds with reports of situations encountered in nursing practice that raise questions about the *right* course of action that a nurse should take. In addition, ample evidence in the literature indicates that nurses may be unable to recognize ethical con-

flicts; even if conflicts are recognized, nurses may lack the knowledge and skill to approach such conflicts in a constructive way.

The involvement of nurses in ethical decisions has changed dramatically since Florence Nightingale introduced modern nursing in the latter part of the 19th century. The "Nightingale Pledge," which can be regarded as an embryonic form of the American Nurses' Association *Code of Ethics*, reflected society's view of nurses and the subordinate role they were expected to play in health care delivery.[1] Prominent ideas expressed in the pledge were the need for nurses to be obedient and to aide the physician in his work. Today's nursing ethics has moved beyond concerns about etiquette to emphasize nurses' responsibility to society and to patients, professional colleagues, employers, self, and family.

From its inception, nursing has continued to examine and articulate the importance of ethics to nursing practice. Furthermore, professional ethics have evolved to meet the changing needs of health care.

Some question whether such a thing as nursing ethics really exists; they suggest that the moral issues confronting nurses are identical to those of physicians and other health care workers. However, because of their intimate and ongoing contact with patients, their position in the health care hierarchy, and their opportunity to perceive the health care situation of patients and families, nurses are placed in unique ethical positions. Nurses must appreciate the ethical aspects of such practices as organ donation and transplantation, artificial prolongation of life, genetic engineering, and other biomedical advances. In addition, nurses are confronted by many critical issues for which they have professional autonomy to choose a course of action. For example, nurses must decide how, when, or if they should enhance the autonomy of a patient; whether to intervene if a professional colleague (nurse, physician, or other health care worker) is violating the rights of other individuals or is endangering patients; and how they can balance legitimate self-interest against the demands of the institution, patients, and physicians.

The nature of IV nursing and the different organizational structure under which IV nurses practice may further complicate their participation in ethical decision making. For this reason, IV therapy nurses must develop knowledge and skill to analyze the ethical aspects of care if they are to effectively fulfill their professional responsibilities.

INFLUENCES ON NURSES' PARTICIPATION IN ETHICAL DECISIONS

The activities and responsibilities of nurses in ethical dilemmas have their roots in the traditional patterns of nursing education and service. Although many changes have occurred since modern nursing began, the vestiges of outdated values and practices are still capable of affecting nursing behaviors. Some insight into these influencing factors may help nurses analyze their own behavior when they encounter ethical dilemmas and may provide a means of clarifying their ethical responsibilities in specific situations.

Patterns of education and service

Modern nursing was born in a military hospital, a fact that has traditionally exerted a strong influence on the practice of nursing. The military model of a hierarchy of command, with nursing at the bottom, has tended to dominate nursing. Nurses were, in effect, required to be "good soldiers" who obeyed orders without question and were prepared to make heroic personal sacrifices whenever needed or ordered to do so.

This early association with the military exerted a pervasive influence on patterns of education and service, traces of which are found in nursing education and practice today. The early training of nurses took place in hospital schools of nursing, which awarded a diploma on completion of an apprenticeship. Students, many of whom came from lower socioeconomic strata of society, were provided with training, room and board, and various necessities, such as uniforms and books, at little or no cost. Through their nurses' training, they were afforded an opportunity to earn a living and to advance their socioeconomic status after graduation. In exchange, the hospital had access to a source of relatively inexpensive labor that was totally subject to its control.

The reliance on student labor made it unnecessary for hospitals to hire graduate nurses to provide patient care. Instead, graduate nurses were independent practitioners of private duty nursing and obtained employment through registries and referral by individual physicians. Once employed by a patient, the nurse may have been put in a position of carrying out domestic tasks, such as baby-sitting and laundering the family's clothes, in addition to nursing duties. Thus, from the time they entered into training, nurses were subject to rigid control from the hospital school, on which they were dependent for education and sustenance, and from patients, who had considerable power to control the nurse through job opportunities. The need to submit to others' demands became a pervasive force in nursing.

Physicians also exerted a great deal of influence over nurses. Most physicians were men, who were viewed by society as having a dominant role over women. Physicians also were better educated and exercised strong authority in the hospital. Student nurses were expected to be deferential to physicians at all times, even to the point of standing whenever physicians came into a room. Such codes of behavior were rigidly enforced by the teachers and supervisors responsible for the training school. Moreover, after graduation, nurses were usually dependent on physicians for their very livelihood. Nurses perceived as being rebellious or disrespectful would not be recommended for private duty cases or could be removed arbitrarily from a case; future employment could thus be jeopardized. Nurses learned early to conform to the system and to placate physicians to survive.

The professional values stressed during the early development of nursing included self-sacrifice and loyalty to the physician and the hospital where one received training. The most important value, however, was unquestioning obedience to authority. The echoes of these early patterns of education and service still linger to a variable degree in nurses' education and employment environments today. Such influences exert an inhibiting effect on nurses' ability to participate meaningfully in ethical decisions in health care. Nurses who adopt the bureaucratic values of the workplace may view involvement in ethical aspects of care as antithetical to their role. They may have exaggerated views of physicians' authority in nonmedical decisions and may hesitate to question interventions about which they feel uncomfortable. They may fear that "making waves" will jeopardize their future.

MULTIPLE EXPECTATIONS IN CONTEMPORARY NURSING

Another potential influence on nurses' participation in ethical decisions lies in the fundamental expectations that nurses encounter in their personal and professional lives. These expectations create moral roles and duties that may exert opposing demands and may create ethical conflicts for the nurse. In addition to the expectations of the physician and the employing institution, the profession, the greater society, and the families of nurses have different claims on nurses' time and energy—to say nothing of nurses' duty to themselves.

Over the years, the nursing profession has been increasingly articulate in declaring the need for nurses to have autonomy in their professional practice. Improved education and the broadening of nursing responsibilities have certainly contributed to increasing this autonomy. Professional organizations also stress that nurses' primary responsibility is to their patients. Nurses are exhorted to be patient advocates. This professed autonomy model, which states that patients come first, may cause conflict if nurses practice in a situation in which they are expected to conform to institutional routines and practices regardless of their views of appropriate courses of action for patient care.

Whether the nurse is employed in a hospital, the community, a clinic, or a home, the employing institution exerts a significant effect on professional practice. Although they overtly promote the ideal of patients' needs as their primary concern, institutions may actually expect nurses to be primarily concerned with the agency's welfare. In today's climate of cost containment, nurses may feel pressure to "cut corners" in delivering care, to accept understaffing that they feel may jeopardize patient care, and to sacrifice their personal welfare and that of their families to work double shifts or forego earned days off when staffing problems arise. An employer does have certain legal and ethical rights that should be respected by the nurses they employ. However, when the demands of the institution appear to be excessive or in conflict with what the nurse feels are legitimate rights of patients or family, the nurse is placed in the uncomfortable position of having to choose whose rights are met. The institution expects nurses to be trustworthy and loyal and to work within its system. At times, these expectations conflict with the needs of patients, which puts nurses in the middle of two opposing demands.

Although their attitude toward nurses as collaborators in care has undergone remarkable improvement since the inception of modern nursing, physicians still may be more comfortable when nurses simply carry out their orders and refrain from questioning decisions they consider to be strictly their domain. Nurses who raise questions about ethical aspects of patient care with a physician may risk personal reprimand, verbal abuse, or disciplinary action within the institution or by the licensing board. Although physicians legitimately need nurses to carry out some medical aspects of patient care, they are not entitled to interfere with aspects of nursing practice that lie outside of their medical expertise, or to expect nurses to abandon their responsibility to patients and the institution because of a physician's demands.

Society's expectations of nurses can be somewhat ambiguous. Whereas general expressions of support for a more independent role for nurses and of trust and respect for nurses' expertise are documented in the literature, nurses are still often expected to function as "the lady with the lamp," to practice with limited financial reward, and to assume a subservient role to physicians in areas that society views as "medical." In the current economic environment, nurses may feel pressured to incorporate unlicensed personnel into the health care scene because of public concerns about the cost of health care. If the use of such personnel is viewed by the nurse as hazardous for patients, he or she faces another dilemma. To the extent that nurses feel they cannot fulfill the expectations of society, they may also experience confusion and conflict about such activities as providing artificial feeding, resuscitating terminal patients, and engaging in other life-prolonging efforts when such efforts appear futile.

The traditional view that nurses must sacrifice personal and family interests and concerns to meet the demands of patients and the employing institution may occasionally place nurses in ethical dilemmas. A nurse could feel obliged to work extra shifts and holidays to such an extent that primary commitments to family members (e.g., spouse, children, aged parents) would suffer. In these situations, the nurse's physical and psychologic health and well-being could be impaired. Nurses may also feel they are forced to give up other values and responsibilities to maintain the appearance of being a "good nurse." The era of nurses not being permitted to marry or not enjoying the benefits of a well-rounded life is gone. Although they are obliged to fulfill their professional responsibilities to their employer by reporting punctually and carrying out assigned tasks, nurses should realize that there are limits to how far they should go to compensate for their employers' deficiencies in planning and staffing. Rather than feeling guilty, angry, and devalued, nurses should refuse to engage in "codependent behavior" and should take constructive action to improve the working environment. Such action will ultimately benefit not only the nurse but also the institution, professional colleagues, and patients.

In summary, the traditional patterns of education and service and the conflicting expectations of multiple roles (professional, employee, family member, and individual) place nurses in ethical dilemmas. Nurses may feel they are obliged to be "all things to all people" and are adversely affected when they are unable to please everyone in a given situation. Feeling caught between opposing duties is stressful and demoralizing for the nurse, who may retreat into inaction in an effort to escape psychologic conflict.

CAN NURSES FUNCTION AUTONOMOUSLY?

The multiple professional demands on nurses lead to conflict. Because of legitimate rights of all parties involved in a situation, nurses cannot act with complete autonomy in every situation (this is true for any individual). Furthermore, if nurses fail to comply with demands or cannot meet the expectations of others, they may suffer consequences in their personal and professional lives.

Failure to act in accordance with one's beliefs violates one's conscience and places one in moral jeopardy. Unfortunately, the correct course of action is not always obvious. In addition, numerous other factors come into play, such as the seriousness of the violation of another's rights and well-being; the harshness of the consequences for all concerned; and the scope of the nurse's authority, control, and responsibility. For example, if a nurse risks negative repercussions from the institution or the physician by fulfilling perceived obligations to the patient, he or she may be tempted to avoid the risk and act in self-interest and for self-protection. Failure to act in accordance with one's conscience can cause acute discomfort and, as discussed later, can be very detrimental if it develops into an ongoing pattern of behavior.

Conflicting demands and potentially serious consequences mitigate nurses' moral responsibility for actions taken or avoided in a situation, however.

Nurses should not be required to be heroic in their disagreements with an institution, but rather need to develop a realistic view of others' duties in ethical dilemmas and to recognize the limits of their own responsibility. The consequences to all parties involved should be considered before any action is taken by the nurse, and the nurse must make every effort to make sound ethical decisions before choosing a course of action. Incurring a reprimand or the displeasure of a colleague is a small price to pay for taking appropriate action. However, harsh personal sacrifices, such as losing one's job or facing legal or professional disciplinary action, should not ordinarily be required to maintain one's moral integrity, unless the ethical violation involved is sufficiently grave to warrant such sacrifice. In other words, an important question to ask in nurses' ethical decision making may be, "How far must I go to resolve this situation?" In some cases the demands of other parties may be so unreasonable and the consequences of failure to comply with those demands so drastic that nurses may have to make a conscious choice about whether or not to continue to work in a given situation.

Fortunately, heroic sacrifice is not routinely required. Even if nurses cannot always successfully and openly confront issues, engaging in ethical analysis may clarify the issue and open the door for realistic efforts at resolution. In any situation, nurses can and must critically examine questionable health care decisions, analyze the constraints and contingencies involved, and ask for reasons or justification for actions taken. The nurse is not justified in standing by passively when ethical dilemmas arise.

Therefore, if nurses are responsible for recognizing and dealing appropriately with ethical conflicts, they must sensitize themselves to the ethical climate in which they work, recognize when ethical violations occur, and be prepared to take an active, constructive role in ethical decision making. Nurses who have knowledge and skills in ethical analysis can make a critical difference to health care. They are role models for colleagues, they enhance the sensitivity of professional colleagues to the rights of others, and they contribute significantly to changing the status quo in the ethical aspects of care.

EFFECTS OF VIOLATIONS OF ETHICS ON NURSES

Evidence exists in the literature that ongoing violation of nurses' values and beliefs has severe and far-reaching effects. Nurses who feel forced to act in opposition to conscience develop a sense of moral outrage. Internally, they are subject to feelings of rejection, disillusionment, hostility, and despair; their sense of frustration and powerlessness may be overwhelming. These negative feelings may pervade every aspect of life and interfere with a nurse's well-being.

Such intense emotions are capable of affecting the professional life of the nurse as well. To cope with the pain and guilt that accompany moral outrage, nurses may abdicate their professional ideals and ethical responsibilities and become totally compliant with the existing system, with detrimental consequences for the patient. The nurse's self-esteem and self-confidence suffer as a result. Some withdraw and regard patient care as "just a job"; they avoid any commitment and make no effort to go beyond the minimal requirements of the job. Others may make no conscious decision to withdraw. Instead, they drift into a series of small deferrals to decisions with which they disagree. Before they realize it, such nurses have developed a pervasive pattern of apathy and insensitivity to the ethical aspects of their practice. They can grow to tolerate almost any violation, regardless of its severity and consequences. Finally, some nurses either quit the job or leave the profession entirely. Although finding a new job may be necessary in some situations, a repeated inability to resolve conflicts is not a viable solution. Whatever the cause, repeated violations of one's integrity are harmful to oneself and, ultimately, to patient care. The whole reason for the existence of nursing is to contribute to the health of patients. Ultimately, all activities undertaken by the nurse must be measured against this standard.

PROCESS OF ETHICAL DECISION MAKING

Much of the process of ethical decision making is already familiar to nurses. The nurse need not be intimidated by this process, but rather should transfer already acquired skills to the ethical decision-making process and build on them.

Like the nursing process, ethical decision making requires a systematic approach; the nurse must collect facts from many sources, analyze those facts, and arrive at a conclusion. What may not be recognized by nurses is that values, which are inherent in ethical decision making, are also involved in the nursing process. Nurses ask themselves, "What *should* I assess?" "How *should* I do this procedure?" and "*Should* I consult the physician about this laboratory test?" "Should" questions are value questions. Within the nursing process, the nurse uses values that have been acquired through education and experience; these values are involved, perhaps unconsciously, in the day-to-day decisions the nurse makes about nursing practice.

The values involved in the ethical decision-making process may not be obvious to the nurse. Many of these values have their origins in the nurse's religious, cultural, and ethnic childhood experiences. They are an integral part of the nurse's personality and play a major role in the nurse's intuitive response to ethical dilemmas encountered in practice. Furthermore, each nurse has a different value system. Many of the beliefs, assumptions, and attitudes that contribute to the value system may need to be examined systematically before they are put into action in ethical decision making.

The process skills that nurses bring to ethical decision making are not sufficient to enable sound ethical decisions. Ethics is not intuition, personal preference, or what is popular in the culture at a particular time. Theories of the ethics of human actions have been studied for more than 2000 years in Western civilization. Individuals involved in the ethics of health care need to develop a basic understanding of this body of knowledge if they want to make sound, moral decisions. Following is a brief overview of fundamental concepts in ethics. Readers are encouraged to use this overview to orient themselves to the field of ethics so they can deepen their knowledge by further study.

Fundamental questions

Veatch and Fry[2] present a detailed discussion of the four fundamental questions that lie at the heart of any ethical decision. These questions address the nature of "right" actions, the kinds of actions that are right, the use of ethical principles, and decisions about actions to take.

What is right? The nature of right actions focuses on what determines the "rightness" of an action. Veatch and Fry conclude that the answer lies in the reasons for acting, according to universal values that consider others' welfare on an equal basis with one's own welfare.

Western culture is based on certain universal values, such as the value of human life and the harmful effects of lying or stealing. All humans are regarded as having worth and dignity, regardless of attributes such as race, religion, ethnicity, and wealth. Although humans may have the ability to commit a harmful act (e.g., murder), concern with universal values says that they should not put this capacity into action.

Kinds of right actions. Much is written in ethics literature about the kinds of actions that are right. The two broad philosophical approaches to this question are consequentialism and deontologism. *Consequentialism* maintains that the consequences of actions determine whether an act is right or wrong, whereas *deontologism* argues that the nature of the act itself determines whether it is right or wrong. Consequentialism tends to emphasize goals, wherein "the end justifies the means." Deontologism focuses more on doing one's duty and respecting the rights of individuals because by their very nature these are good things to do. In reality, aspects of both views may be needed in any ethical dilemma. Neither approach satisfactorily resolves all ethical conflicts, and each can be absurd if carried to extremes. Nurses who develop only a superficial understanding of these two approaches and try to apply them without sufficient analysis may become confused and frustrated. For this reason, the reader is encouraged to consult a basic ethics text, such as the ones listed at the end of this chapter,[3-5] to develop more insight into fundamental ethical theories.

Using ethical principles. Ethical principles should be used by nurses as a general guide to making decisions in a specific situation. As mentioned previously, no theory satisfactorily applies to all ethical conflicts. In other words, there is no "cookbook" to tell us step by step what to do and when to do it. This ambiguity is what makes the process of ethical decision making so frustrating for health care professionals. Each situation we encounter is unique because each patient and relevant circumstances are unique. A set of rules rigidly and automatically applied can lead to highly unethical decisions. The inability to apply rules rigidly leads some nurses to draw the erroneous conclusion that all ethical decisions are arbitrary and subject to personal whim. Nothing could be further from the truth: exercise of arbitrary and capricious decisions in the ethical aspects of care can create much harm and injustice. A consistent, thoughtful approach is mandatory for those responsible for the care of patients.

What action should be taken? The final question that underlies all ethical decision-making processes is, "How can we decide what action should be taken in a specific case?" To answer this question, one must systematically collect all the relevant facts and apply the ethical principles that one believes are appropriate to the situation. In short, one must systematically address the conflict.

Steps in the process

The numerous models and approaches to ethical decision making available in the nursing literature vary in complexity, practicality, and ease of application. For nurses engaged in active clinical practice, the steps suggested by Benjamin and Curtis,[4] outlined in this section, are the most practical; they form a common-sense approach that uses analytical skills already possessed by nurses.

Step 1: determine whether an ethical issue exists. Not every decision in health care involves ethics; those that do may not require in-depth analysis to determine a course of action. Most nursing actions can be implemented without fear of ethical violations. Nurses should sort out such actions and devote time only to serious ethical concerns.

An initial question for the nurse to ask is, "Is this strictly a matter of technical expertise?" Some matters do not fall within the realm of ethics because they relate solely to technical expertise. Diagnosis and prognosis are matters of technical expertise that require medical decisions, and physicians are educated to make such decisions. Such straightforward technical questions in themselves do not present ethical problems. Ethical problems may arise, however, when communication of technical informa-

tion is indicated. Nurses need to recognize that ethical issues arise, for example, if physicians use medical jargon that patients cannot understand, if they fail to provide enough information for patients to make appropriate decisions, or if they covertly or overtly discourage patients from asking questions about their diagnosis or treatment. Patients have the right to be informed so that they can make necessary decisions about their care. Any nurse has the expertise to recognize and address the ethical issues in this situation. However, based on their bias as to what is best for the patient, problems may arise.

In health care, many patients and health care workers label all or most matters as "medical." Patients and health care workers may regard physicians as the best or the only individuals who should make decisions because of their medical expertise. In reality, if the issue is nonmedical, there is a need to decide who has the right to make the decision. Without sound ethical analysis, personal values of health care personnel who make the decisions about patient care may be imposed wrongly on others, especially the patient.

A second question for the nurse to ask is, "Is a conflict of values operating in this situation?" As detailed in the preceding discussion of factors influencing nurses' participation in ethical decision making, physicians, patients, administrators, and colleagues bring different values to any situation. If a situation exists in which fundamental values are in conflict, ethical analysis must be undertaken to resolve conflicts so that important rights are not violated. One example concerns the withdrawal of fluids from a dying patient. Although a nurse may value the patient's right to "die with dignity," the physician may value a perceived duty to preserve life at all costs; discussing these different positions may facilitate a resolution of the issue in a way that respects the values of all concerned.

The key to identifying whether an ethical issue exists in a specific case, then, lies in the identification and elimination of questions that require only medical expertise to answer them. Next, nonmedical issues should be examined to identify conflicts in human values; when a conflict in values exists, ethical analysis must be performed to ensure that the most ethical approach to resolving the conflict is determined.

Step 2: engage in ethical analysis. To analyze an ethical conflict is to reflect critically on the facts and principles of the situation. Such reflection must be interactive rather than linear. That is, the nurse must evaluate the facts, consider different scenarios about the outcomes of different courses of action, and sort major issues from minor ones. This process requires the nurse to use imagination, see the situation as others may see it, analyze how different facts change the situation, avoid making hasty judgments until all aspects of the situation have been considered, and try to obtain a comprehensive perspective of the situation. Throughout the analysis, the nurse should be open to opposing views; in fact, opposition should be welcomed because it broadens one's view and forces one to examine other perspectives more thoroughly. A nurse may be angry that a physician provides what the nurse considers futile treatment for a terminal patient; however, talking to the physician may reveal that the patient requested such treatment in the hope of living to see a new grandchild. The nurse should be flexible enough to change position on an issue if convincing new evidence is presented that renders the position erroneous.

The author acknowledges the contributions of Lynda Trauner, practitioner of intravenous nursing, for examples in practice, and of her aunt, Mary E. Schell, a registered nurse for more than 60 years, for historical insights related to practice and education.

Collect and examine relevant facts. Sometimes, a conflict exists because individuals have different facts or do not have all the facts that bear on an issue. When the relevant facts are available, the conflict may disappear. Facts are not sufficient to resolve ethical problems, but they can significantly alter the ethical claims (rights and duties) of the individuals in the situation. Arriving at a decision without examining all available facts is foolish and may result in significant violation of patients' rights. For example, a nurse may fail to determine in advance whether a patient desires to be resuscitated should a cardiac arrest occur. Without knowing the patient's wishes, any course of action (to provide or withhold resuscitation) could violate the patient's wishes.

Clarify terms. The use of cliches and emotionally charged language, such as "right to die," "unfair," and "doctors cure, nurses care," can inhibit or prevent sound ethical analysis. Nurses may use terms imprecisely or assume that they understand what someone else means by a word or phrase, when, in reality, interpretations about what is meant may differ from individual to individual. So-called conflicts may evaporate when opposing parties discover that they both mean the same thing. Clarifying meaning helps resolve ethical conflict.

Determine pros and cons. Developing and justifying various positions regarding an ethical issue requires the ability to think logically and engage in philosophic analysis. Courses in logic or critical thinking may be required to improve one's ability in this respect. Nonetheless, logical thinking is necessary if nurses are not to rely solely on intuition to decide on a course of action, which would create the probability of treating others unethically. Such questions as, "Are there good grounds to support this action?" "Are my assumptions valid and true?" and "Is there a logical connection between these facts and my conclusions?" help sharpen thinking and clarify issues throughout the analysis.

Use a systematic framework. A framework is necessary to provide a common basis for discussion of everyone's rights and duties in any health care dilemma and of the goals to be achieved by any course of action. A framework is developed from the two major approaches to ethics described earlier: consequentialism and deontologism. Nurses should study the basic tenets of these approaches and clarify their own beliefs and guiding principles. Defending a position based on principle rather than on intuition and impulse gives credibility to that position. Others involved in the discussion can then learn how the nurse views the situation and can examine the logic of the nurse's position. In turn, they can then clarify their own positions to the nurse. Nurses, for example, may emphasize a patient's right to make autonomous decisions about receiving costly treatments, although the patient is receiving public aid. Management, however, may emphasize the "big picture" of allocation of scarce resources and the goal of having a financially viable institution.

Acting on principle is necessary if nurses are to exhibit integrity, which requires that one's actions be consistent with one's beliefs. People who lack integrity, who vacillate from one value system to another, quickly become known as unreliable, capricious, or untrustworthy among professional colleagues. They are dangerous because their actions, based on personal values, may violate the rights of those with whom they come in contact.

Reexamine your position as needed. Individuals must always remember that they may have inadequate or incorrect information about a situation. They may have engaged in faulty reasoning or may lack the insight or experience necessary to make the sound decision. Furthermore, health care situations are dynamic, and new developments may change the ethical aspects of any situation. These limitations mean that nurses must remain flexible and consider new information. Furthermore, nurses must respect others as moral agents who also have legitimate values and concerns. Respect for others is absolutely critical. If nurses enter ethical conflicts with a rigid and judgmental attitude, satisfactory resolution of conflicts will be delayed, inhibited, or prevented. In addition, interpersonal conflicts will develop if others feel devalued by the nurse's negative attitudes.

APPLICATIONS TO INTRAVENOUS NURSING PRACTICE

An examination of the nursing literature reveals that many rules, principles, and philosophies are available to help nurses in their ethical decision-making endeavors. Sometimes, this variety of information can be more a hindrance than help because the resulting detail and complexity can overwhelm the reader and lead to a sense of paralysis and despair. Each nurse should study and adopt a coherent approach that makes sense to him or her. It is useful, however, to have a starting point.

The principles involved with the framework presented in this chapter are not discussed comprehensively in the following paragraphs. Rather, discussion is limited to the essential elements of each principle, an overview of their importance, and examples of situations in which the IV nurse may encounter conflicts relating to the principles.

A framework for health care decisions

Two recognized experts in the ethics of health care, Beauchamp and Childress,[3] have evolved a "composite theory of ethical principles" that they believe is useful in most health care settings. The composite theory consists of the four ethical principles—autonomy, nonmaleficence, beneficence, and justice—that the authors encounter most often in their research.

The composite theory is a useful starting point for nurses in their study of ethical decision making because these four principles are easily understood and their underlying concepts are familiar and generally accepted in Western cultures. The principles are also broad in their application in that they apply to patients in addition to health care workers. A very practical feature of the composite theory is its flexibility; the relative priority given to each principle is determined by the context of the particular situation in which it is applied. Such flexibility is essential if the complex ethical dilemmas encountered in clinical practice are to be approached in a practical manner. Using a framework consisting of only four principles reduces the number of variables juggled by the nurse in what may be an already extremely complex dilemma, thus making the analysis more manageable. In addition, the principles are interrelated and often overlap.

Autonomy. The principle of *autonomy* is familiar to most nurses because it is the basis for the legal doctrine of informed consent. The American culture values independence and the right of individuals to be autonomous, that is, to be free from control by others and free from personal limitations that interfere with their ability to make meaningful choices in their lives.

Freedom from control by others means that one should not be coerced, forced, deceived, or manipulated into doing what another desires. Freedom from personal limitations means that one must have the mental capacity to consider the risks and benefits of any action, to anticipate the potential consequences of actions, and to choose in one's perceived best interests. Lack of adequate information, psychologic stress, and inadequate time to explore alternative courses of action are examples of personal limitations that interfere with autonomy.

The right of autonomy implies that others have a duty to respect and not interfere with the ability of an individual to exercise that right. Although health care professionals formerly deemphasized the autonomous rights of patients (because health care professionals believed that *they* should always act to promote patients' physical well-being), current trends in the legal and ethical aspects of health care give priority to patient autonomy. However, no one's autonomy is necessarily absolute. The rights of others and the inherent limitations of any situation make it necessary to balance individual autonomy against others' rights and duties.

As mentioned previously, nurses have the right of autonomy in their practice, and others should respect that right. Nurses exercise this autonomy in relation to ethical conflicts in health care by obtaining information necessary for them to make an informed decision, analyzing that information, and resisting others' attempts to force them to comply with unacceptable procedures. Remember, the nurse can always raise questions about any practice that causes discomfort or concern.

IV nurses may encounter potential violations of patients' rights of autonomy with every patient contact. Some obvious practices that may be questionable include the initiation, continuation, or discontinuance of total parenteral nutrition or experimental drugs; unusual dosages or combinations of drugs; and artificial hydration and similar procedures. To make autonomous decisions about undergoing any treatment, patients must be informed (using language and concepts that are appropriate to their educational level) about the associated risks, anticipated benefits, available alternative treatments, and the consequences of accepting or rejecting the treatment. Patients must be given adequate information with which to make their decisions; in addition, they must have adequate time to consider their choices without being pressured to comply, even if the staff believes that a certain treatment is the only choice a patient has. Remember, only the patient can choose what is best for him or her. The health care worker can only create the appropriate climate within which the decision can be made.

If patients lack decision-making capability (e.g., because of changes in level of consciousness, emotional distress, effects of age, inability to understand and judge alternatives), an attempt should be made to ascertain what the patient would choose if he or she were able. Advance directives, documentation of patient wishes before mental impairment, and information provided by significant others all make it easier for the system to respect patients' autonomy. These resources are available to IV nurses in any practice setting.

Health care workers must recognize that patients do not lose their rights of autonomy merely because their capacity to make decisions is impaired; therefore every effort must be made to discover the patient's preferences. In cases in which the patient's wishes cannot be determined, health care workers must rely on other ethical principles to guide care.

IV nurses have brief encounters with patients over varying lengths of time. In some respects, the nature of this contact is a disadvantage because the IV nurse may lack vital insight and opportunity to determine whether autonomy has been respected. Alternatively, these brief encounters over time enable the IV nurse to view the situation from a fresh perspective, free from activities on the unit that may have a desensitizing effect on the unit staff. In the community or home situation, the IV nurse may be the only health professional available to note changes in patients' conditions or attitudes. The IV nurse in any setting may be viewed by the physician as a collaborator whose expert opinion is valued because of his or her extensive knowledge and experience.

Thus IV nurses are often in a position to enhance the autonomy of patients they care for. The nature of their contact with patients and their unique perspective requires that they be sensitive to situations in which patients' rights of autonomy are in jeopardy. Sometimes, the conversation of a patient will suggest to the IV nurse that the patient does not fully understand the implications of a particular procedure. A patient's chance remark ("I don't want to go through all of this") may trigger a question about the patient's desire to begin or continue a course of therapy. A patient who lacks the mental capacity to understand what is being explained may appear to be suffering without hope of benefiting from a procedure. In all such instances, the IV nurse should explore the situation more fully— with the patient if possible. Collecting relevant data and raising questions based on personal observations can help clarify the existence of an ethical problem and provide additional facts with which the situation can be analyzed. Ethical analysis can then be used to resolve conflicts associated with the violation of a patient's autonomy.

Nonmaleficence. *Nonmaleficence* refers to the right of individuals to be free from the infliction of actual harm and the risk of harm by another person. *Harm* refers to physical and emotional damage. Often, health professionals may focus on avoiding harm, but forget that it is a violation of the right of nonmaleficence to act in a way that causes a *risk* of harm. The requirement of avoiding harm to patients has been a very strong mandate in health care for centuries. The mandate to avoid harm or the risk of harm is obviously not absolute in health care because numerous procedures can be "harmful," at least in the short term, but have an ultimately beneficial effect on the patient.

IV nurses can avoid causing physical harm to their patients by exercising care when performing procedures, administering proper dosages of IV medications and nutrients, keeping current with developments in the field, remaining alert to signs of untoward effects of treatments, and intervening early to prevent further damage when complications arise. Educating the patient, caregivers, and other staff about the specific care required for treatments provided by the IV nurse is another way of preventing harm. Physical harm may also be prevented when the IV nurse raises questions about poor care that he or she observes and takes action to promote safe care for patients. One group of IV nurses in a community setting was instrumental in changing policy regarding home administration of a chemotherapeutic agent that had a greater than 50% risk of systemic anaphylaxis. Their concerns about patient safety and their own ability to handle such a complication were expressed to their management and the physician. The expression of concern led to a resolution that was satisfactory for all.

Psychologic harm is a broad area of concern that may be less obvious than the threat of physical harm. Patients may be harmed psychologically by being cared for by nurses who convey a lack of concern and compassion. Indifference to patients as individuals can result in patients experiencing loneliness, despair, grief, anger, and other negative emotions, all of which are harmful or risk harm. The fidelity, veracity, and commitment of the nurse contribute to the avoidance of psychologic harm for patients. If nurses break faith with patients or deceive patients by lying to or misleading them, patients lose trust in their care givers—a disastrous situation when the patient is in most need of support.

Nurses should also appreciate the need for confidentiality in their relations with patients. Although nurses are strictly mandated to protect patients from unwarranted disclosure of intimate facts that are revealed in the patient-nurse relationship, sharing idle talk with patients about sensational aspects of patients' lives may lead nurses to share idle talk with others who have neither the need nor the right to know such details. The nurse should also not assume that the patient wants family members or significant others to know what has been told to the nurse. Much harm can result if a nurse inadvertently reveals sensitive information, such as a seropositive human immunodeficiency virus status, without the expressed consent of the patient. If disclosure is regarded as essential to the patient's care, the nurse should obtain the patient's permission to reveal the information to the appropriate individuals on the health team or should encourage the patient to make the disclosure. When disclosure of confidential information is mandated, such as the legal requirement to report suspected child abuse, the patient needs to know that the nurse will report information to the appropriate individuals.

Beneficence. The principle of *beneficence* goes beyond the mere avoidance of harm to taking positive action to help another person or to contribute to the well-being of that person. The principle of beneficence has long been the guiding force in health care. In fact, the past emphasis placed on beneficence over autonomy led to paternalism in health care; physicians and nurses felt justified in doing things to and for patients, even if patients objected, because it was "for the patient's own good." The fallacy of paternalistic thinking is that no one knows for sure what action is best for another individual; only that individual can weigh the positive and negative aspects of a recommended course of action to determine the best choice, which is one reason why autonomy has become an important consideration in health care.

Nonetheless, beneficence overlaps considerably with autonomy. Providing sufficient information about the risks, benefits, and consequences of a proposed course of treatment and its alternatives is an essential element of respecting a patient's autonomy. It also promotes the well-being of the patient by seeing that all available information is brought to bear on the decision.

IV nurses can contribute to the well-being of their patients by carrying out the patient's care in a safe, compassionate manner. Questioning management's decision to control expenses by using less expensive peripheral lines instead of central lines for patients on public aid is a beneficent action. Listening to patients' concerns and providing follow-up for problems also promotes beneficence. Intervening to ensure that the patient receiving nursing at home or in the hospital obtains the services of physicians, chaplains, or other resource personnel is also a means of actively promoting the welfare of patients.

Justice. *Justice* is the fourth and last principle of the composite theory of Beauchamp and Childress.[3] The principle of justice, as used here, involves fairness in dealing with others, or giving them that to which they are entitled or deserve. Treating all patients with respect is one manifestation of acting justly. IV nurses may encounter patients from diverse racial, ethnic, religious, and socioeconomic backgrounds, all of whom should be approached with a professional standard of care and concern. IV nurses may not personally approve of the lifestyles of some patients, and they may react with fear and repugnance when various situations (e.g., homosexual lifestyles, acquired immunodeficiency syndrome, criminal records) are encountered. Nonetheless, they must go beyond their personal preferences and deliver the same standard of care to all patients. Some employers may endeavor to have the IV nurse provide a lesser standard of care to patients who lack financial resources, in which case the nurse must take steps to ensure that the patient is treated fairly.

If IV nurses are aware of dishonesty in billing patients or governmental agencies for services, they may be required to take action to have such practices investigated. Ultimately, such practices may result in a loss of essential services to all because of the legal and professional sanctions that may result.

Actions to promote ethical practice

IV nurses can take many actions to improve their ability to practice ethically and ensure ethical care of their patients. First, IV nurses should actively improve their knowledge of and sensitivity to the ethical aspects of patient care. Attendance at workshops and conferences dealing with ethics is a good way to learn more about ethics. Continued independent learning (by reading texts such as those listed at the end of this chapter, for example) is essential to learning the theoretic basis for ethics. Professional nursing journals are increasing their publication of articles that deal with specific ethical conflicts through the presentation of case studies. Applying approaches for resolving ethical conflicts, such as the approach presented by Benjamin and Curtis[4] and summarized in this chapter, is useful. Using such approaches to review situations in which they have been involved will increase nurses' proficiency in analyzing ethical conflicts. Actions needed to promote ethical practice range from increasing one's ability to respond to ethical violations to informing relevant staff or organizations when ethical violations are identified.

Assessment. IV nurses need to develop insight and sensitivity to questionable practices that they encounter. Such insight requires a willingness to investigate further when one feels a sense of discomfort or questions some aspect of care. The nurse must embark on a systematic process of ethical analysis to determine whether an ethical conflict truly exists and to define the nature of the conflict.

However, reliance on a sense of discomfort is only one aspect of assessment. Serious violations of ethics may go unrecognized by the nurse whose value system is not attuned to the area of the violation. Thus the nurse is obliged to go beyond relying on an intuitive sense that ethical concerns exist and must make a conscious effort to learn more about the ethical implications of nursing practice. Such efforts include conducting a thorough review of the literature dealing with nursing ethics, attending meetings, discussing ethical issues with colleagues, investigating ambiguous areas, and consulting journal articles.

Role modeling ethical practice. IV nurses must show respect and faith in all members of the team as ethical practitioners who share concern for the ethical care of patients. In addition, the IV nurse must raise questions where doubt or insufficient information exists. Silence may result in the violation of another's rights. On the other hand, the nurse must appreciate the complexity of any health care situation and must not leap to conclusions without being certain that unethical practice is being used. The IV nurse's efforts to explore further any situation in which a patient's rights may be threatened or violated are an invaluable asset for ensuring ethical practice. Simple actions such as asking questions to see whether patients understand and accept their therapy, reminding physicians and other personnel to explain options fully to patients and families, and asking whether advance directives are available and encouraging their use are all means of anticipating and preventing ethical dilemmas throughout the course of an illness.

IV nurses should be especially alert to patients' comments that indicate their states of mind in relation to such issues as prolonging life with technology; these comments are invaluable should a patient lapse into coma and be unable to make necessary choices at a later time. Verbatim documentation of such comments in the chart is essential in case evidence of the patient's state of mind is required at a future date.

Problem solving. Ample evidence in the literature indicates that nurses are often reluctant to intervene when confronted with violations of ethics in health care. When IV nurses encounter practices that seem suspect, they should raise constructive questions about such practices. Further investigation may reveal that, indeed, an ethical problem needs to be resolved; conversely, the nurse may find that other colleagues have different ethical principles, that factors unrecognized by the nurse are influencing the situation, or that appropriate steps to resolve the issue have already been implemented. An open, problem-solving approach and avoidance of hasty judgments are necessary to promote the resolution of ethical dilemmas, as is persistence in confronting such dilemmas.

A useful approach that will increase sensitivity to ethical aspects of care is to copy information dealing with ethics for distribution and discussion among peers on the IV team. Group discussion can help sensitize everyone to the range of ethical issues involved in an area of practice. Open discussion may encourage a cohesive approach to resolving problems and helps develop consensus among the staff.

Resources available in the agency should be used to help define and address ethical concerns. Hospitals and nursing homes may have access to ethicists, legal counsel, or pastoral staff who can help clarify and facilitate resolution of ethical dilemmas. Nurses practicing in the community, who may not have ready access to such personnel, nonetheless can consult community religious leaders or the staff of the local hospital to obtain a referral for discussing such problems.

Volunteering to serve on the agency's ethics committee is an excellent way to gain knowledge and experience in the ethical aspects of care. Networking, which can widen the nurse's awareness of available resources, is an added bonus to such service. The creation of unit-based ethics committees, either for the IV team itself or for members of the unit staff with the IV nurse in attendance, may also be helpful. Such local ethics committees may improve problem solving, communication, and support for all individuals involved in patient care.

A critical mechanism for helping the individual nurse address ethical concerns in a systematic and constructive way is a personal diary. Any perceived problems or concerns should be fully and objectively described by the nurse. The situation, dates and times, and the people involved should be included. Diary entries can provide evidence of the prevalence and seriousness of problems. The continuing occurrence of some types of problems will become obvious through content analysis of the entries and can serve as an impetus for corrective action. When the IV nurse has prepared such an analysis, the next step is to ask a representative of the ethics committee or pastoral team or a risk manager to meet with the appropriate administrator to discuss the issue and to devise an approach for its resolution. Another important contribution of a diary is that it provides a reliable record of events that have transpired; thus it has a protective function for the nurse. The diary is a valuable legal record should litigation ensue from a breach of ethics in care.

Summary

The willingness and ability of IV nurses to participate in ethical decision making in clinical practice is influenced by numerous historical and organizational factors. The types of ethical dilemmas encountered and nurses' ability to intervene as autonomous practitioners are both affected by the values and the power of colleagues in the work situation. Nurses must be alert to the influence of these factors on their willingness to intervene. At all times, the nurse's primary obligation is to act to safeguard the patient's welfare, although other aspects of the situation must be investigated and balanced so that an ethically acceptable resolution is reached.

Although a concern for ethics is evident throughout the history of nursing, nurses may lack the knowledge and skills in ethical decision making that would give them the confidence and credibility to be full participants in this process. Nonetheless, nurses can and must always raise questions about the ethics of clinical practice. They should embark on a conscious effort to improve their knowledge of ethical theory and their ability to engage in ethical analysis. This chapter provides an overview of introductory material and suggestions for further study to improve the knowledge base of IV nurses in this area.

The pivotal position of IV nurses gives them an opportunity to recognize ethical problems in care that may not be evident to others on the health care team. Especially in the community, the IV nurse may be the only professional contact who has insights relating to ethical concerns. Hence IV nurses must assess possible ethical problems, act as a role model for ethical care, and adopt a problem-solving approach in situations that give rise to ethical concerns. IV nurses, like other nurses, have a critical role to play in ensuring ethical practice in today's health care environment.

REFERENCES

1. American Nurses Association: *The code for nurses with interpretive statements,* Kansas City, Mo, 1985, American Nurses Association.
2. Veatch RM, Fry ST: *Case studies in nursing ethics,* Philadelphia, 1987, JB Lippincott.
3. Beauchamp TL, Childress JF: *Principles of biomedical ethics,* ed 4, New York, 1994, Oxford University Press.
4. Benjamin M, Curtis J: *Ethics in nursing,* ed 3, New York, 1992, Oxford University Press.
5. Edge RS, Groves JR: *The ethics of health care,* ed 2, Albany, NY, 1999, Delmar.

Chapter 36

Research

Kimberly A. Christopher, PhD, RN, OCN*

A profession is identified by the unique body of knowledge possessed by its members. Continual development of this knowledge base is fundamental to the profession. When knowledge evolves from systematic inquiry based on the scientific approach, it is known as *research*. Research therefore enhances a profession by broadening the scientific body of knowledge essential to its practice.[1]

Research is vital to extend the base of nursing knowledge. Nursing intervention has traditionally been task-oriented, that is, nurses perform nursing activities. Nursing research is a pathway to improving patient care by identifying the unique properties of nursing. Research may substantiate traditional nursing interventions or may reveal the need to alter them.

The specialty practice of intravenous (IV) nursing requires research to validate and improve IV nursing care and treatment modalities and advance the professional practice.[2] Through research, nurses may validate current practices and develop new practices to facilitate optimal patient care outcomes. To promote IV nursing research, however, the nurse must understand basic research concepts and relate them to practice. The intent of this chapter is to broaden nurses' knowledge of research by applying research principles to IV nursing.

RESEARCH TERMINOLOGY

Scientific research has its own language and terminology. An understanding of this terminology is necessary to participate in the research process and comprehend the findings of others.

Concepts, constructs, and theories

Scientific research is usually concerned with abstract rather than tangible phenomena. *Concepts* are abstractions that help identify emotions or sensations characterized by a particular constellation of behaviors.[3] Examples of concepts are "pain" and "distress." In the research process, concepts are indirectly rather than directly measured.

The term *constructs* encompasses many related ideas. However, constructs differ from concepts in that the researcher deliberately constructs them for a specific scientific purpose.[3] Conceptual frameworks in nursing contain constructs that describe an abstract structure of the human response. For example, Dorothea Orem developed the construct of "self-care" to describe one's ability to care for oneself.

Polit and Hungler defined *theory* as "an abstract generalization that presents a systematic explanation about the interrelationship among phenomena."[1] A theory integrates findings to explain and predict phenomena. In this way, the findings become meaningful and can be generalized. For example, Selye's theory of stress presents a systematic explanation of adaptation to stress.

Variables

A *variable* is something that assumes different values.[1] *Quantitative variables* can be measured in specific units of measure and generally are analyzed through statistical procedures. In contrast, *qualitative variables* differ in quality or degree. They are measured in nonnumeric form and are described in terms of increased or decreased intensity.[1] An example of a qualitative variable is pain.

The purpose of most research is to establish a cause-and-effect relationship by examining the effect of the independent variable on the dependent variable. An *independent variable* is the variable that is manipulated; it is the presumed cause. A *dependent variable* is the unit of measure or the outcomes variable the investigator is studying to determine the presumed effect.[4] For example, the researcher investigates the effect of saline flushes (independent variable) on the maintenance of patency of an IV catheter (dependent variable). Additional examples of independent and dependent variables from published literature are listed in Table 36-1.

*The author and editors wish to acknowledge the contributions made by Carol Bolinger and Donna R. Baldwin, as coauthors of this chapter in the first edition of *Intravenous Nursing: Clinical Principles and Practice*.

Table 36-1	**Examples of Independent and Dependent Variables**	
RESEARCH QUESTION	**INDEPENDENT VARIABLE**	**DEPENDENT VARIABLE**
What is the effectiveness of various health care professionals inserting IV lines?[5]	IVs attempted by staff registered nurses, physicians, and IV nurse clinicians	Cost of procedures
What are the potential complications of midline catheters?[6]	Insertion of midline catheter	Complication rate
How does transparent polyurethane dressing compare with dry gauze dressing?[7]	Use of transparent polyurethane dressing	Condition of IV site
How effective is the Venoscope at detecting IV infiltrates?[8]	Intentional infiltration with normal saline	Venoscope ability to detect infiltration

IV, Intravenous.

The term *criterion variable* is sometimes substituted for dependent variable when criteria must be established to assess the success of an intervention.[1] For example, a phlebitis scale (criterion variable) measures the effects of a new IV catheter material (independent variable).

In research, all possible influences on the dependent variable should be controlled so that the true relationship between the independent and dependent variables is understood. Competing influences that interfere with identification of the underlying cause are known as *extraneous variables.* Failure to control these variables affects the validity of the research.[1] For example, an investigation of the dwell time (dependent variable) for five brands of peripheral IV catheters (independent variable) would be influenced by extraneous variables such as catheter gauge and length, insertion procedure, site maintenance, and patient characteristics. By standardizing catheter size and the type of patients included in the study, researchers are controlling these two extraneous variables.

Quantification of variables

Numbers may be used to represent measurements of the variable. The assignment of numbers to attributes of the objects follows a well-defined set of rules known as the *scale of measurement.* Four major scales used in research are nominal, ordinal, interval, and ratio. In a *nominal scale,* numbers are used strictly as labels to sort characteristics into categories. Demographic characteristics are often classified in this manner. For example, a male may be classified as a 1 and a female as a 2. When degrees of an attribute can be identified, an *ordinal scale* is used to order the objects on a continuum. This scale may be used to classify catheter dwell times in the following manner: (1) less than 12 hours, (2) 12 to 23 hours, (3) 24 to 47 hours, (4) 48 to 72 hours, and (5) greater than 72 hours. An *interval scale* is a scale of measurement where the distance between any two adjacent units of measurement (or "intervals") is the same but the zero point is arbitrary. An example of an interval scale is the Fahrenheit scale for measuring temperature. The last scale of measurement, the *ratio scale,* has the characteristics of an interval scale, but it also has a true zero.[4] A pain evaluation scale in which 0 represents the absence of pain and the numbers 1 to 10 depict increased pain intensity is an example of a ratio scale, as is the Kelvin temperature scale.

RESEARCH PROCESS

By means of the scientific approach, research moves in logical progression from posing a question to obtaining an answer. The question is reduced to its observable components so that possible answers may be tested and conclusions drawn. The research process consists of multiple steps that may be grouped into five sequential stages: conceptualization, planning, data collection, data analysis, and dissemination.[1] For clarification, the study presented in Box 36-1 illustrates each phase of the research process.[9]

Phase I: conceptualization

The research study begins when the researcher develops the question within a conceptual framework. Specific steps in this phase include identifying and describing the problem, reviewing the literature, selecting the conceptual framework, and formulating the hypothesis.

Identifying the problem. Selecting a problem for study requires identifying a question from an area of interest. Nursing situations that cause the staff to question their actions are a good basis for the formulation of research questions. When a nurse analyzes patient care quality or questions the standard, delivery, or outcome of care, the nurse is formulating a research question.

The most difficult step in research is developing a feasible research question. For years, IV nurses have been asked how much air is fatal if it is infused intravenously. Techniques are scrupulously followed to prevent any air from entering the IV line, but there are anecdotal accounts of air being infused without adverse patient outcomes. Investigation of this issue, however, would not be feasible because of the unethical demands it would place on study participants. Other considerations relevant to the feasibility of a research problem are timing, availability of subjects, cooperation of others, availability of facilities and equipment, finances, and experience of the researcher.[3] Box 36-2 lists some of the properties of a researchable problem.

Describing the problem. The research question is typically written as a problem statement, which summarizes the problem and identifies the key study variables. The problem may be written as either a declarative or an interrogatory

Box 36-1 The Reliability of Blood Sampling from Peripheral Intravenous Infusion Lines

The current study sought to establish parameters for choosing blood tests for which peripheral IVs may be effectively used, for testing a standard discard volume, and for evaluating the effects on testing outcomes of various IV infusates before developing a local practice standard.

Fifty-five adult inpatients, who consented to participate, were scheduled for morning blood tests, and had either an indwelling or saline locked IV line, were enrolled in the study. Four types of blood tests were evaluated, CBC, electrolyte panel, renal panel, and a general chemistry survey panel. Because subjects might have more than one of the target blood tests ordered, several test comparisons from a single source were possible.

Study subjects first underwent venipuncture by clinical laboratory personnel. Within 1 hour, a research nurse obtained a similar quantity of blood from each subjects' indwelling IV line. For patients with infusing intravenous solutions, the lines were turned off for 3 minutes before the blood draw. In all cases, the first 5 ml of blood was discarded. All cannulas were flushed with 5 ml of saline after the experimental blood draw. All blood samples were sent to laboratory via the hospital pneumatic system and each pair of samples underwent identical testing procedures. Additional data were collected from subjects' records on type and size of IV cannula, relative ease of the blood draw, and subjects' demographics.

Paired *t* tests were performed on all test results to measure statistical equivalence between each pair of blood samples. In addition, two hematologists independently evaluated the entire group of 110 paired sample results to evaluate whether any of the paired differences achieved clinical significance.

Modified from Mohler M, Sato Y, Wise L: The reliability of blood sampling from peripheral intravenous infusion lines, *JIN* 21(4):209, 1998.
IV, Intravenous; *CBC,* complete blood count.

Box 36-2 Properties of a Researchable Problem

- The outcome of the research will contribute to nursing practice and patient care in a meaningful way.
- The problem studied occurs often in a definable population.
- The methods currently used to address the problem are inadequate.
- The problem involves variables capable of being precisely defined and measured.
- The investigation of the problem is feasible.
- The research question is of interest to the researcher.

Box 36-3 Two Types of Problem Statements

Examples of researchable problems: Efficacy of using peripheral IVs for specific blood tests, establishing standard discard volume, and evaluating the effects of various IV infusates on testing outcomes.

Declarative statement: The purpose of this research is to determine the efficacy of using peripheral IVs for specific blood tests, to establish a standard discard volume, and to evaluate the effects of various IV infusates on testing outcomes.

Interrogative statement: What is the efficacy of using peripheral IVs for specific blood tests; what is the standard discard volume; and what are the effects of various IV infusates on testing outcomes?

IV, Intravenous.

statement. Box 36-3 contains an example research problem with each type of statement.

Reviewing the literature. Once the problem is formulated, the researcher needs to become familiar with previous investigations on the same or related topics. A review of the literature helps the researcher develop a more specific question. Often, the review reveals that the question has been adequately answered in the past, and further research may replicate and validate previous work on the subject. Replication studies are critically needed in nursing research because they add support to existing research findings.

Researchers may complete a literature review using sources listed in the *Index Medicus* and *Cumulative Index of Nursing and Allied Health Literature,* and social and psychologic indices. Computerized access to these two indices and other health-related indices is available. These sources drastically reduce the time invested in the literature search.

Once a cumulative list of articles of interest is developed, the laborious tasks of retrieving and reviewing these references ensue. The method of organizing reference articles is unique to each researcher. Many find it helpful to design a data management form or grid that lists key points, such as the statement of

the problem, the hypothesis, the methodology, the findings, and a full citation. It is also helpful to record any deficiencies noted by the reader or the author. The data grid is used when preparing the written literature review.

A written literature review is required for the research proposal and the future publication of the study results. It summarizes consistencies and inconsistencies in previous research (Box 36-4). Presenting inconsistencies emphasizes the need for further research and demonstrates that previous work has been considered in the formation of the current research study.

Developing the conceptual framework. The next step involves placing the problem within a theoretical or conceptual framework. Nursing scholars, such as Orem, Roy, and Neuman, have developed theoretical frameworks for nursing practice that describe the relationships between nursing, health, patients, and the environment. Theories allow nurses to make presumptions about the interaction of these elements so that the outcome of nursing interventions can be predicted.

Conceptual frameworks are less fully developed than are theories, but they also guide research. For example, Biggert and colleagues described the framework for pediatric home care in their article "Home Infusion Services Delivery Systems Model: A Conceptual Framework for Family-Centered Care in Pediatric Home Care Delivery."[10] This model can serve as a basis for research on the interrelationship of resources for families who care for their sick children at home.

Formulating the hypothesis. Initially, a researcher may have an intuitive feeling regarding the outcome, but the

Box 36-4   Literature Review Excerpt

Since the late 1970s, relatively few studies have tested the reliability of using indwelling peripheral IV lines for blood sampling. Seven studies that tested combinations of blood tests, IV infusions, wait times, and discard volumes were identified. Of the seven studies reviewed, none had more than 28 subjects and only three involved hospitalized patients. Only Ong et al. measured the reliability of indwelling IVs for common blood tests in hospitalized patients (1970). This study investigated whether accurate blood values could be obtained from an arm in which an IV was infusing. Blood was drawn above and below the IV infusion site. A control sample was obtained from the contralateral arm using standard phlebotomy. Findings demonstrated that samples taken from above the IV site varied greatly. For those samples taken below the IV site, statistically significant differences were found with hematocrit, carbon dioxide, and glucose. However, clinically significant differences were found only for glucose. These investigators concluded that blood sampling distal to an infusing IV was clinically reliable for all analytes except glucose. Watson et al. and Read et al., investigating similar combinations of blood tests and IV infusions, found similar results. They concluded that the greatest differences occurred among analytes related to the chemical composition of infusates.

Of the five studies sampling blood with an infusion in progress, no standard wait time between interruption of infusions and sampling was employed; hence there is no consistent evidence on which to base practice. Similarly, inconsistent procedures were associated with determining the relationship between discard volumes and test reliability. A 5-ml discard volume was determined sufficient in two studies, 3 ml in two other studies, and 1.5 ml in yet another study. Only Read et al. determined a minimum effective discard quantity by withdrawing and testing increments of 1 ml each.

Existing research failed to offer sufficient guidance for establishing safe guidelines for a clinical practice policy. Specifically, too few cases involving comparable patient populations had been evaluated. Data regarding discard volume and IV interruption lag times were inconclusive, and there was insufficient consistency among study findings of similar study designs.

Summarized from Mohler M, Sato Y, Bobick K, Wise LC: The reliability of blood sampling from peripheral intravenous infusion lines, *JIN* 21(4): 209, 1998.
IV, Intravenous.

hypothesis is not finalized. The hypothesis is derived after the problem is identified and the related literature is reviewed, and it predicts what the researcher expects to find.[1] Characteristics of a hypothesis, as defined in the Box 36-5, are illustrated in the following example.

HYPOTHESIS
Blood drawn from peripheral IVs provide as accurate a test result as blood drawn by venipuncture.

A *null hypothesis*, as its name implies, is not what the hypothesis states. Polit and Hungler describe a null hypothesis as "a statement that there is no actual relationship between variables and that any such observed relationship is only a

Box 36-5   Characteristics of a Hypothesis

- The hypothesis is in the form of a statement rather than a question.
- The hypothesis states the relationship between the independent and dependent variables.
- The hypothesis is testable.

function of chance, or sampling fluctuations."[1] A null hypothesis declares the lack of a relationship between the independent and dependent variables and is used as a tool to explain the statistical significance of study results. The null hypothesis for the preceding example is as follows:

NULL HYPOTHESIS
There is no difference in blood test results when blood is drawn from either a peripheral IV or from venipuncture.

Phase II: planning

The second phase in the research process involves planning the methodology to be used in the study. Methodology is simply the path the researcher plans to follow to get from the question to the answer. Formulation of the methodology depends on key factors related to the research problem. What type of study design best suits the question? What types of comparisons are being made? How often are the subjects available to the researcher? What type of conclusion is the researcher attempting to support? Answers to these questions determine the study design, the sampling methods, and the measures for research variables.

Study design. The term *study design* describes the framework the researcher plans to use to answer the research question. Many types of study designs exist, but some are more appropriate for certain types of questions and deal more effectively with certain types of data. The two main approaches in research are experimental and nonexperimental, and each has specific advantages and disadvantages.

An *experimental study design* is considered by many to be classic research because it meets stringent requirements (Box 36-6). The variables are under the control of the researcher and may be manipulated, one at a time, to enable evaluation of causal relationships.[1] Extraneous variables are present, but they are not studied. An example of experimental research published in the *Journal of Intravenous Nursing* is "A Randomized Study Comparing IV 3000 (Transparent Polyurethane Dressing) to a Dry Gauze Dressing for Peripheral Intravenous Catheter Sites."[7]

When the researcher is able to control the extraneous variables, the relationship between the independent and dependent variables is clearer. Identifying or controlling all of the extraneous variables is often impossible, and such control may not always be necessary. Only those variables that occur simultaneously with the independent and dependent variables require controls. The inability to regulate significant extraneous vari-

Box 36-6   Requirements for Experimental Studies

- The study must be prospective so that data are collected under experimental conditions as they occur.
- The researcher must be able to control extraneous variables and manipulate the independent variables. *Control* implies that extraneous variables are eliminated or controlled so that they do not affect the dependent variable.
- Study subjects are randomly assigned to groups.

Table 36-2   **Examples of Extraneous Variables and Controls**

EXTRANEOUS VARIABLES	CONTROLS
Personnel drawing the blood	All blood was drawn by study research nurse.
Blood-drawing technique	All blood was drawn within 1 hour of laboratory phlebotomy.
	First 5 ml of IV blood was discarded.
	Running IVs were stopped for 3 minutes before drawing blood.
	All IVs were flushed with 5 ml of normal saline after blood draw.
Testing procedures	All blood transported immediately using pneumatic tube system.
	All blood underwent identical testing procedures.

IV, Intravenous.

ables, however, introduces a contaminating effect on the data and produces misleading results. Examples of extraneous variables and controls in the study of blood sampling from IV infusion lines are listed in Table 36-2.

Investigation of relationships requires comparison. In an experimental study, a *control group* is compared with an *experimental group*. The control group of subjects participates in a study but never has the independent variable manipulated. In contrast, the independent variable is manipulated in the experimental group. Study subjects are assigned to the two groups randomly so that each person has an equal chance of being in either group. Once the study is completed, the results of the two groups are compared.

Blinding is a control method used to correct for investigator or participant bias. When both the investigator and the participants are unaware of the independent variable manipulation, the study is labeled double-blind. If only the subject or investigator is blinded, the study is considered single-blind.[11] In Yucha, Russ, and Baker's study, "Detecting IV Infiltrations Using a Venoscope," the research assistant was blinded to the infiltration process to avoid influencing the venoscope assessment results. This was a single blind study because only the research assistant was blinded.[8]

In nursing research, ensuring that the sample is randomized is often difficult. Because subjects may not be assigned to experimental or control groups on a random basis, each member of the sample may not have an equal chance of receiving the experimental treatment. When this occurs, the study is consid-

ered *quasiexperimental*. The research involves manipulation of the independent variables but lacks randomization. To compensate for the lack of random sampling, quasiexperimental designs introduce controls over the extraneous variables. An example is Loughran and colleagues' comparative study of guidewire use versus guidewire nonuse for inserting peripheral central venous catheters.[12] The researchers introduced controls by selecting study sites that had initiated their peripherally inserted central catheter programs at the same time. In this way, the site not using guidewires was comparable with the site in which guidewires were used.

Although experimental and quasiexperimental designs are highly effective for testing hypotheses concerning causal relationships between variables, some situations may prohibit the use of experimentation. In such situations, the *nonexperimental study design* is more appropriate. Because the researcher does not control the variables, causality cannot be established; however, associative relationships may be revealed.

The two broad classifications of nonexperimental research are descriptive and ex post facto. *Descriptive studies* do not focus on relationships between variables, but rather observe and describe phenomena. Goetz, Miller, Wagener, and Muder's[11] study of complications related to IV midline catheter use is an example of a descriptive study. The investigators observed the incidence of catheter-related bacteremia and hypersensitivity-like reactions.

Ex post facto studies examine relationships after the natural course of events, but they differ from experimentation because of the lack of researcher intervention. A type of ex post facto design often used in IV nursing research is the retrospective study. For example, Homer and Holmes[13] used a retrospective study design to evaluate the risks associated with 72- and 96-hour peripheral IV catheter dwell times.

Sampling plan. A *population* is the entire group of objects or people that are to be studied. Examples include all registered nurses working on hospital-based IV teams, all patients receiving total parenteral nutrition at home, or all patients receiving peripheral IV therapy. Because a population is generally too large to investigate each subject, the study is limited to a subset of the population, known as a *sample*. Sampling refers to the method by which this sample is drawn from the population, and it determines the extent to which the sample represents the entire population.[1]

Two classifications of sampling techniques are probability and nonprobability sampling. *Probability sampling* involves random selection of subjects from the population so that each member of the population has an equal chance of being selected. This is different from randomization, which is the random assignment of subjects to control and experimental groups. *Nonprobability sampling* relies on nonrandom selection procedures.[1] The probability approach is preferred, but most samples in nursing research are based on nonprobability techniques.

Three methods of nonprobability sampling exist. The first is *convenience sampling*, which relies on the subjects that are most available to study. The nurse who conducts an observational study of all peripherally inserted central catheters inserted in a metropolitan hospital during a 1-month period is relying on a convenience sample. With the second method, *quota sampling*, the researcher specifies characteristics of the sample to increase its representation of the population. The sample is subdivided into groups based on attributes such as age, sex, and diagnosis, and a specified number of subjects is selected from each group. For example, Moldowan divided the sample into men and women to study the outcomes of patients receiving intermittent bupivacaine by ambulatory infusion pump after undergoing thoracotomy.[14] The third method, *purposive sampling*, relies on the researcher's knowledge of the population to hand pick the sample. An example of purposive sampling is the Delphi technique, which is a tool for short-term forecasting. In this technique, a panel of experts is asked a series of questions in an effort to combine the expertise of the entire group.

To maintain homogeneity of the sample, the researcher may use inclusion and exclusion criteria, which limit the sample by including and excluding subjects who meet or do not meet the qualities defined by the researcher. A small sample is believed to be adequate if the population is relatively homogeneous. For most nursing studies, however, a fair degree of heterogeneity is preferred. In the study of blood sampling from peripheral IV infusion lines (see Box 36-1), the inclusion criteria were as follows:

- All inpatient adults
- Capable of giving consent
- Scheduled for early morning blood draw for complete blood count (CBC), electrolyte panel, or general survey
- Had an indwelling IV line either infusing or saline locked

Once the sampling method is determined, the next issue is the sample size. Most researchers recommend that the sample be as large as possible; if the sample size is not large enough, the results may not reflect the characteristics of the population. In Frisco and Bolinger's[15] study comparing saline with heparin in maintaining intermittent dwelling catheter devices, the sample size of 90 subjects was determined by means of a sophisticated, statistical determination known as *power analysis*.

Measurement of the research variables. Research requires the measurement of critical attributes of the object being studied. Because these characteristics need to be qualified, operational definitions of each attribute are developed. An *operational definition* is a description of the variable in terms of the procedures by which it will be measured (Box 36-7).[1]

Measurement of the variable based on the operational definition may be accomplished by several methods. The three methods most used by nurse researchers are self-report, observation,

and physiologic measures. *Self-reported data* are collected by directly questioning the subjects using an oral interview or a written questionnaire. Interviews and open-ended questions are unstructured means of data collection, whereas closed-ended and fixed-alternative questions limit the number of responses from which the respondents may choose. *Observational data* are obtained by direct examination and interpretation of the phenomena being studied. Frey[5] used observational data to demonstrate IV insertion success rates for various health professionals. In this study, data were collected on the time of day when most IVs were started, success rate of various health care professionals placing the IVs, and estimated time for the procedure. *Physiologic measurements* are often used in clinical studies because of their objectivity and validity.

Regardless of the measurement method used, the instrument used to collect data must possess certain attributes to obtain quality measures. *Reliability* is the ability of a tool to provide an accurate measurement each time it is used. The higher the reliability of a tool, the greater the accuracy of the data it obtains.[3] For example, a numeric phlebitis rating scale is often used to assess phlebitis. Because such scales are based on the assumption that the signs and symptoms observed at each stage always succeed those observed in preceding stages, researchers have questioned the reliability of a phlebitis scale as a measurement tool.[16] In fact, Maki and Ringer have suggested a more reliable alternative that defines phlebitis as the presence of two or more signs and symptoms from a standardized list.[17]

Validity refers to the ability of a tool to measure what it is intended to measure. Validity depends on reliability to the extent that an unreliable tool cannot produce valid results.[1] *Content validity*, the degree to which the tool adequately represents the content, is based a panel of experts' judgment. For example, Kaufman established content validity of an interview questionnaire regarding IV therapy education in associate degree nursing programs by having nursing faculty review the measurement tool.[18] In contrast, *construct validity* refers to the ability of the instrument to measure the abstract construct of interest. The more abstract the concept, the greater the difficulty in establishing construct validity.[1]

Validity is associated with the measurement tool, but it also reflects the adequacy of the research design. The research study must be evaluated in terms of the internal and external validity. *Internal validity* means that the study measures what it is intended to measure. If a study has internal validity, the findings are the result of the independent variable and do not reflect the effects of extraneous variables. For example, internal validity for a study of a new dressing material would require that extraneous variables, such as age, diagnosis, and dressing technique, be controlled so that the effects of the dressing may be determined. *External validity* is the extent to which the research findings may be generalized to the population. A study has external validity if the sample is representative of a broader population.[4] In Frisco and Bolinger's[15] saline-versus-heparin study, internal validity was ensured by controlling the extraneous variables. However, because the sample was limited to healthy male volunteers, the external validity of the study is limited.

Protection of human rights. An important consideration in the planning process is protection of the human rights

---

Box 36-7 Examples of Operational Definitions in Blood Sampling from Peripheral Intravenous Infusion Lines

Discard volume is defined as 5 ml of blood.
Wait time is defined as the 3-minute period that the IV is turned off before the blood is drawn.
Unit of evaluation is defined as one test of the four under scrutiny, including CBC, electrolyte panel, renal panel, and general chemistry.

IV, Intravenous; *CBC,* complete blood count.

of potential subjects. Because researchers may not be objective in their evaluation of the safety of the subjects they enroll in study protocols, institutional review boards (IRBs) may be used to objectively review the intended research. All research conducted by hospitals and universities that accept federal funding must satisfy guidelines set by their IRB to obtain funding. The IRB functions as an unbiased referee to assess the risk to participants and the benefit to scientific knowledge of research conducted in their domain. Legal and ethical implications of the proposed research are evaluated, and researchers may be required to modify portions of a project.

When an IRB is not available to the researcher, such as in a non–federally funded institution or an independent nurse researcher, the researcher may seek peer review from a professional organization or a research committee. The Intravenous Nurses Society has a research department geared to assist nurse researchers who are interested in projects related to IV nursing.

Nursing research that involves the cooperation of human subjects requires the consent of the subjects. Just as a hospitalized patient signs an informed consent before a procedure is performed, research subjects must also sign an informed consent to be observed, questioned, or exposed to experimental situations. Informed consent is obtained in the subject's native language and in language easily understood by nonmedical participants. All medical and legal terminology is described in simple terms, and subjects are fully informed about the nature of the research and its potential risks and benefits.[1] Basic components of an informed consent statement are listed in Table 36-3.

Because consent is voluntary, subjects have the right to withdraw from the study even after the investigation has begun. Subjects must be assured that withdrawing from the study will not affect the quality of their care.

Phase III: data collection

Collection of data is based on the planned methodology and procedures of the study. It may include obtaining the necessary consents, training those involved in data collection, scheduling subjects for interviews, and coding the results. In the study of blood sampling from peripheral IV infusion lines, data collection procedures were as detailed in Box 36-8.

Phase IV: data analysis

Data are collected to enable the investigator or investigators to draw conclusions about the population. To accomplish this, the data must be organized, summarized, and analyzed so that patterns and relationships may be detected. *Qualitative analysis* refers to the organization and interpretation of narrative data (nonnumeric) to determine themes or patterns. In contrast, *quantitative analysis* involves the manipulation of numeric data through statistical procedures.[1] These procedures range from the simple to the complex and may be classified as descriptive or inferential statistics.

Descriptive statistics. *Descriptive statistics* are used to organize, summarize, and describe collections of data in tabular, graphic, or numeric form.[4] One of the easiest such methods is

frequency distribution, which organizes data according to the number of occurrences of a phenomenon. Values are ordered from lowest to highest, and the frequency of each value is determined. Bar graphs and histograms are graphic representations of frequency distribution.

Table 36-3   Components of Informed Consent

COMPONENT	EXPLANATION
Subject status	Subjects are informed that information they provide is solely for the purpose of research.
Study purpose	The purpose of the research is stated in lay terms.
Potential risks	Any foreseeable risks associated with participation in the study are listed.
Potential benefits	Specific benefits from participation in the study are described.
Confidentiality	Subjects are assured that their privacy will be protected.
Voluntary consent	Subjects are informed that participation in the study is voluntary and that consent may be withdrawn without fear of retaliation.
Procedures	All procedures that will be used to collect research information are described.
Contact information	Information is provided regarding whom to contact for questions.

Box 36-8   Sample Data Collection Procedures

BEFORE STUDY
The study was explained to eligible patients the evening before testing. Those who agreed to participate gave written consent at that time.
STUDY DAY
Subjects first underwent venipuncture by clinical laboratory staff per institutional standard protocols. Within 1 hour of the first blood draw, a research nurse obtained a similar quantity of blood from each subject's indwelling IV line.
TREATMENT
Blood samples were obtained. Intravenous cannulas were flushed with 5 ml of saline after the experimental blood was drawn. All blood samples were immediately sent to the laboratory for processing using the hospital pneumatic system. Each pair of blood samples underwent identical testing procedures and the results were compared. Data were also collected on the type and size of IV cannula used, subject demographics, and relative ease of blood draw.
MEASUREMENT
Target blood tests included CBC, electrolyte panel, renal panel, and general survey panel. The unit of evaluation was one test of the four under scrutiny. Subjects' IVs were Teflon catheters in size 16, 18, 20, and 22. Ease with which blood was aspirated from IV catheters was rated on a three-point scale of difficulty.
METHODOLOGY
The study used a quasi-experimental design with each subject's blood serving as his/her control.

IV, Intravenous; *CBC,* complete blood count.

Measures of central tendency are also used to describe the data. The three measures commonly used are mode, median, and mean. The *mode* is the value that occurs most frequently in the distribution, the *median* is the middle score of a group that is arranged from lowest to highest scores, and the *mean* is the average distribution.[4] For example, Frey[5] used measures of central tendency to describe IV insertion success rates for various health care providers. In this study, the average reported time required to achieve successful IV access (mean) was 20 minutes per IV start.

Measures of central tendency report the average, but they do not describe the variability or dispersion of the values. Therefore the distribution also needs to be described in measures of variability, such as the range and the standard deviation. The *range* is the distance between the highest and the lowest values. In the study by Frey,[5] the range for catheter insertion time was 2 minutes to 90 minutes. The *standard deviation,* the most commonly used measure of variability, is an index of the spread of scores around the mean of a distribution (Fig. 36-1). It indicates how much the scores deviate from the mean. The further the value is from the mean, the more varied are the data. A small standard deviation implies tightly clustered data, whereas widely dispersed data are represented by a large standard deviation.[4]

Brown and colleagues[19] reported measures of variability in their study comparing patient-controlled analgesia (PCA) with traditional intramuscular analgesia. In the study, the duration of the PCA therapy ranged from 8 to 210 hours, the average length of therapy was 41.44 hours, and the standard deviation equaled 3.659. These results indicate that there was a wide range in the length of therapy and a significant variation in the scores in relation to the average length of therapy.

The significance of the standard deviation can be illustrated by the results from Frisco and Bolinger's saline-versus-heparin trial.[15] In phase I of the study, the mean (average) dwell time was 14 hours for catheters flushed with saline. When each dwell time for this group is plotted on a graph, the values form a "normal curve."

When a curve is normal, 68% of the population fall within one standard deviation (34% above the mean and 34% below the mean), 95% fall within two standard deviations, and 99.7% within three standard deviations. The standard deviation in the heparin-versus-saline study was 2.2, implying that 68% of catheters were patent for 11.8 to 16.2 hours, 95% were patent from 9.6 to 18.4 hours, and 99.7 were patent from 7.4 to 20.6 hours.[15]

Descriptive statistics are also used to describe the correlation between two variables. The statistic that describes the relationship and strength of association between the variables is the

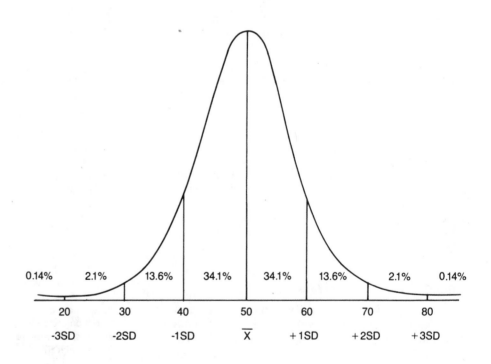

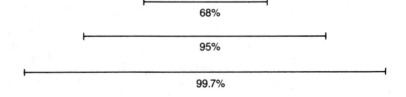

FIG. 36-1 *Standard deviations in a normal distribution.* (From Polit DS, Hungler BP: *Nursing research: principles and methods,* ed 6, Philadelphia, 1999, JB Lippincott.)

correlation coefficient. Many correlation coefficients exist, but the most widely used measure is the *Pearson r,* or the Pearson product-moment correlation coefficient. For example, a researcher studying the correlation of IV nursing experience and venipuncture proficiency would most likely use the Pearson r.

Inferential statistics.

Inferential statistics refer to procedures by which the researcher may draw inferences about the population based on data collected from the sample. Values are not simply described, but rather are used to make conclusions regarding the population. In this type of statistics, the validity of the inferences rests on the representation of the population in sample.

Hypothesis testing is a statistical approach by which the researcher objectively analyzes the results of the study. The null hypothesis, not the research hypothesis, is used to measure the significance of the findings. The findings are not significant if the researcher fails to reject the null hypothesis. However, errors may occur. Failure to reject the null hypothesis when it should be rejected is a *type II error.* In contrast, a *type I error* refers to rejection of the null hypothesis when it should not be rejected (Table 36-4).

Type I errors may be controlled by establishing levels of significance. The *level of significance* describes the risk of committing a type I error and is commonly referred to as the *p value.* The p value ranges from 0 to 1 and describes the probability that the findings are the result of chance.[4] The smaller the number for the level of significance (p value), the less likelihood of a type I error. The two most common levels of significance are .05 ($p < .05$) and .01 ($p < .01$). For a significance level of .05, the researcher is at risk of rejecting a null hypothesis that is true 5 of 100 times. When the .01 level of significance is used, the probability of a type I error decreases to 1 of 100. However, as the probability of a type I error decreases, the probability of a type II error increases.[4]

Research results are reported as either statistically significant or statistically insignificant. If the results are statistically significant, they are unlikely to be the result of chance. Insignificant findings imply that the results may be attributable to chance fluctuations.

Knowledge of the level of significance (p value) and the sample size *(n)* are important in the evaluation of the findings. A direct correlation exists between the magnitude of the p value and the size of the sample.[5] Madeo and associates[7] compared peripheral IV catheter sites using IV 3000 transparent polyurethane dressing (49 subjects) to sites using dry gauze dressing (31 subjects). The only statistically significant difference between the two groups was that the dressing condition of the IV 3000 group was better than the gauze group. The small sample size of both groups prohibits generalization of findings to the entire population.

Statistical tests.

The procedures used in inferential statistics may be classified as parametric and nonparametric. *Parametric statistics* test the significance of the differences between group means. They involve estimation of at least one variable, measurement of interval or ratio data, and assumptions about the variable under consideration.[1] Two common parametric tests are the *t* test and the analysis of variance (ANOVA).[4]

The *t* test is used in two-group situations, such as studies involving control groups, pretests or posttests, or paired samples. The means of each sample are compared to determine whether a statistically significant difference exists between the groups. If a significant difference exists, it is assumed to result from the influence of the independent variable. For example, Mohler and associates, in the blood sampling from peripheral lines, used the *t* test to measure the equivalence between each pair of blood samples. The *t* test failed to identify any differences among hemogram analytes. When electrolytes were measured, *t* tests determined significant differences between samples for chloride, carbon dioxide, potassium, and sodium.[9]

When the study involves three or more groups, *ANOVA* is used. ANOVA contrasts variation *between* treatment groups with variation *within* the treatment groups to determine the F ratio. If the differences between the groups are large relative to fluctuations within the group, it is possible to establish the probability that group differences are related to, or result from, the treatment.[1] For example, ANOVA would be the appropriate statistical technique to determine whether any of three different catheter materials contributed to phlebitis.

Nonparametric tests are used for nominal or ordinal data or when the normality of distribution cannot be assumed. The most common nonparametric technique is the *chi-square test,* which tests the presence of an association between two variables on the same subject. The chi-square statistic is computed to determine whether the observed frequencies in the categories differ significantly from the expected categories. If the chi-square value is substantially larger than what would be expected by chance, the value is determined to be statistically significant.[4] Chi-square analysis was used by Wood in her study comparing the use of two securement techniques for short peripheral IV catheters.[20] There was a 45% ($p = .002$) reduction in overall IV complications with transparent dressing and StatLock as compared with that of transparent dressing and tape.

Although the chi-square test is appropriate for samples of more than 30, *Fisher's exact test* may be used for smaller samples. Data are collapsed into cells to test the significance of differences in the size of the groups.[4] Bozzetti and colleagues[21] used the Fisher exact test to analyze groups of patients in their study of central catheter sepsis. The relationship between the results of hub cultures and clinical demonstrations of sepsis was statistically significant.

Because the phenomena of interest to nurses are generally complex, advanced statistical procedures, known as *multivariate tests,* may be used. The availability of computers to calculate the statistics has facilitated the use of these advanced statistical procedures. Two examples of multivariate statistical procedures are factor analysis and multiple regression.

When a large set of variables is being analyzed, *factor analysis* reduces them into a smaller, more manageable set of variables

Table 36-4	**Decisions Regarding the Null Hypothesis**	
Decision	**Null Hypothesis (H_0) True**	**Null Hypothesis (H_0) False**
Fail to reject H_0	Correct decision	Type II error
Reject H_0	Type I error	Correct decision

known as *factors*.[4] This multivariate procedure involves a higher degree of subjectivity but is nonetheless a widely used statistical technique. Yucha and associates[22] used factor analysis in their investigation of extravasation using common IV solutions. Differences in extravasation of the solutions were determined over time and were significant for factors such as pain, area of induration, and infiltrate volume.

Multiple regression analysis is used to study the relationship between two or more independent variables on a dependent variable. This method allows the researcher to make predictions about phenomena. From a set of independent variables, the researcher tests hypotheses about the relationship between the independent and dependent variables.[4] Lucas and colleagues[23] used multiple regression in their study of nosocomial infections in patients with central venous catheters. Among the study variables, the length of hospitalization and the number of intermittent infusions were the best predictors of central venous catheter infections.

Another procedure that may be used in research is *meta-analysis*. Meta-analysis applies statistical methods to findings from multiple research reports. The results of each study represent a single piece of data. Multiple studies are analyzed and the findings regarding the effectiveness of the interventions integrated.[1] Such an approach may help demonstrate the impact of IV teams on the quality of patient care outcomes (e.g., changes in incidence of phlebitis, infection, infiltration).

For statistical methods to render the quantitative data meaningful, the results must be understood. In this chapter, computation of the actual statistics was not discussed. Because explanation of the various techniques is far beyond the scope of this text, emphasis has been placed on the appropriateness of statistics in different research situations and their significance in regard to the findings. Table 36-5 is a summary of research problems and the appropriate statistical tests for each. Often,

one statistical method is insufficient based on the study design, and the answer to the research problem may require several statistical tests. For example, Goetz and associates used the *t* test, the chi-square test, and logistic regression model in their comparative study of IV midline catheter use.[6]

Interpretation. Analysis of the data provides the "results" of the study. However, this information must be interpreted to determine the implications of the findings within a broader context. Failure to reject the null hypothesis means that the findings support the research hypothesis. In Frisco and Bolinger's[15] saline-versus-heparin example, the null hypothesis (no differences in catheter patency relative to flush solutions) was not rejected; therefore the findings lend support to the research hypothesis (normal saline is as effective as heparin flush in preventing loss of catheter patency). If the null hypothesis is rejected, the research hypothesis is not supported. In this situation, methodologic weaknesses must be considered.

Statistical significance should not be confused with clinical significance. If the study is statistically significant, the results have occurred more often than if they had occurred by chance. In contrast, clinical significance would cause a change in nursing practice based on the findings. All too often, the statistical data reported have little effect on clinical practice and nursing interventions. Clinical significance means the study findings are relevent for patient care.

Phase V: dissemination

Publication in journals is the most effective route of dissemination for research findings. Journals reach a target group of professionals interested in the research topic and findings. For example, research studies relative to IV therapy would be expected to be published in the *Journal of Intravenous Nursing*. Often, it appears that a researcher has published the same article in several journals. Close inspection, however, reveals that minor alterations in the text have been made in a manner that does not infringe on the original copyright.

Professional meetings and conferences are another avenue for dissemination of information. Such meetings allow the researcher to target professionals who will be affected by the findings. The presentations may be formal lectures, abstracts, or poster presentations; the type of presentation selected depends on the material being presented and the preference of the researcher.

The Internet has had a powerful impact on the dissemination of research data. For example, subscription services will search for your key words of interest and then e-mail you every matching study published worldwide. Researchers are communicating instantly, sharing information on common interests, and working cooperatively to disseminate advance knowledge.

OVERCOMING BARRIERS TO RESEARCH

A comparatively small number of nurses perform research, often because of lack of experience, insufficient resources, inadequate funding, and time constraints. All of these reasons are obstacles that can be overcome.

Research has become a component of nursing curricula, and

Table 36-5	**Research Problems and Appropriate Statistical Tests**

RESEARCH PROBLEM	STATISTICAL METHOD
Cleansing the site with chlorhexidine will have an effect on decreasing the incidence of CVC site infections.	*t* test
Catheter dwell time differs in pediatric, adult, and elderly populations for two specific types of polymers.	ANOVA
Urban nurses are more satisfied with IV therapy responsibilities.	Factor analysis
Compliance regarding routine site rotations is higher in hospitals with IV teams than those without IV teams.	Chi-square test
A relationship exists between the use of an IV team and patient care outcomes such as the following:	Pearson r test
Phlebitis rate	
Catheter dwell time	
Infiltration rate	
Patient satisfaction	

CVC, Central venous catheter; *ANOVA*, analysis of variance; *IV*, intravenous.

nurses are learning how to apply research principles to their practice. Once the nurse identifies a problem for investigation, statisticians are available to help plan the research design and methodologies and analyze the results. Simply because the nurse is the principal investigator does not mean that all components of the research process must be performed by the nurse. Experts are available to help ensure the study's validity so results may be applied to practice.

In 1993, nursing gained a powerful ally when the National Institute of Nursing Research (NINR) was established at the National Institutes of Health in Bethesda, Maryland. The goal of the NINR is to promote excellence in nursing science by offering opportunities for continuing research training, career development, and research awards. The NINR meets these goals by offering assistance to nurses who conduct research. Fellowships offered by the NINR, as well as scholarships and grant funding, also encourage nurse researchers to expand their horizons.

Increasingly, nurses are participating in nursing research either as principle investigators or as members of a research team. Research offers nurses many exciting opportunities to advance the scientific basis of practice. It is through research that high-quality nursing care and positive outcomes will be achieved.

References

1. Polit DF, Hungler BP: *Nursing research: principles and methods,* ed 6, Philadelphia, 1999, JB Lippincott.
2. Intravenous Nurses Society: Infusion nursing standards of practice, *JIN* (suppl) 23(6S), 2000.
3. Burns N, Grove S: *The practice of nursing research: conduct, critique, & utilization,* ed 3, Philadelphia, 1997, WB Saunders.
4. Shavelson RJ: *Statistical reasoning for the behavioral sciences,* ed 3, Boston, 1996, Allen & Bacon.
5. Frey AM: Success rates for peripheral IV insertion in a children's hospital, *JIN* 21(3):160, 1998.
6. Goetz AM, Miller J, Wagner MM, Muder RR: Complications related to intravenous midline catheter usage, *JIN* 21(2):78, 1998.
7. Madeo M, Martin C, Nobbs A: A randomized study comparing IV 3000 (transparent polyurethane dressing) to a dry gauze dressing for peripheral intravenous catheter sites, *JIN* 20(5):253, 1997.
8. Yucha CB, Russ P, Baker S: Detecting IV infiltrates using a venoscope, *JIN* 20(1):50, 1997.
9. Mohler M, Sato Y, Bobick K, Wise LC: The reliability of blood sampling from peripheral intravenous infusion lines, *JIN* 21(4): 209, 1998.
10. Biggert R, Watkins J, Cook S: Home infusion service delivery systems model: a conceptual framework for family-centered care in pediatric home care delivery, *JIN* 15(4):210, 1992.
11. Jacobsen B, Meininger J: Seeing the importance of blindness, *Nurs Res* 2(1):54, 1990.
12. Loughran SC, Edwards S, McClure S: Peripherally inserted central catheters: guidewire versus nonguidewire use, *JIN* 15(3): 152, 1992.
13. Homer LD, Holmes KR: Risks associated with 72- and 96-hour peripheral intravenous catheter dwell times, *JIN* 21(5):301, 1998.
14. Moldowan C: Improved outcome for post-thoracotomy patients using intermittent bupivacaine with epinephrine by CADD-Plus ambulatory infusion pump, *JIN* 15(6):333, 1992.
15. Frisco R, Bolinger C: *Intravenous therapy: clinical principles and practice,* Philadelphia, 1995, WB Saunders.
16. Stoddard GJ, Ring WH: How to evaluate study methodology in published clinical research, *JIN* 16(2):110, 1993.
17. Maki DG, Ringer M: Evaluation of dressing regimens for prevention of infection with peripheral intravenous catheters, *JAMA* 258:2396, 1987.
18. Kaufman MV: Intravenous therapy education in associate degree programs, *JIN* 15(4):238, 1992.
19. Brown ST, Bowman JM, Eason FR: A comparison of patient-controlled analgesia versus traditional intramuscular analgesia in postoperative pain management, *JIN* 16(6):333, 1993.
20. Wood D: A comparative study of two securement techniques for short peripheral intravenous catheters, *JIN* 20(6):280, 1997.
21. Bozzetti F, et al: A new approach to the diagnosis of central venous catheter sepsis, *JPEN J Parenter Enteral Nutr* 15(4):412, 1991.
22. Yucha CB, Hastings-Tolsma M, Szeverenyi NM: Differences among intravenous extravasations using four common solutions, *JIN* 16(5):152, 1993.
23. Lucas JW, et al: Nosocomial infections in patients with central catheters, *JIN* 15(1):44, 1992.

Entrepreneurial Roles in *IV* Therapy

Lynn C. Hadaway, MEd, RNC, CRNI

the business world. Although clinical expertise will provide the foundation for a business, expertise in business development, marketing, and financial management is also needed. Nurses considering business opportunities should answer tough questions, such as the following:

- What do I want from a business—security, money, and/or power?
- Will the business affect my personal life, and if so, what effect will it have?

Nursing is a service industry and a service-oriented profession. There are three components to any service business: the customer or person receiving the service, the staff delivering the service, and the administrative group or manager. All three components are required, whether one takes on a business opportunity within an organization or creates an independent company. In this chapter, the required characteristics, skills, and processes for planning and starting a business are examined.

BUSINESS OPPORTUNITIES FOR IV NURSES

It may seem obvious, but the first question that potential business owners must answer is, "What business do I want to be in?" For IV nurses, the common answer is "The IV or infusion therapy business." However, there are other options; the infusion industry has a need for services other than the direct provision of IV therapy.

The first thing to determine is whether the business will sell a product, a service, or both. The following questions should be asked:

- How will the product or service be described?
- How does it look and feel?
- What are the features and benefits?

Features are what the product or service offers and are usually defined by the producer. On the other hand, the customer defines the *benefits* based on what those features actually provide for them. For example, a feature of a peripheral catheter is a needle protection device; the benefit is a dramatic reduction in accidental needlestick injuries and the subsequent performance improvements, such as reduced cost for chemoprophylaxis.

Through years of clinical practice, nurses are in a prime position to identify problems with existing products and to develop ideas for new products to solve those problems. A good example is the pediatric nurse who became tired of cutting and padding medicine cups to cover IV sites, and developed and now manufactures IV-site protectors. Another example is the nurse who created a device to safely remove port access needles because of concern over needlestick injuries while removing these devices. The device to house contaminated catheter stylets

Change, confusion, and often chaos mark our current health care system, leading many experienced nurses to doubt their ability to maintain employment. Mergers and acquisitions, re-engineering, and restructuring are the outcomes of the cost-containment strategies used today. The delivery and financing of health care is shifting from an inpatient, illness-based system to one where care is delivered in a wide variety of settings and health and wellness are emphasized. With intravenous (IV) teams being disbanded, hospital staffing levels reduced, and home care agencies going out of business or merging, many IV nurses are looking for other employment opportunities. Previously, the nursing role focused on patient care and advocacy, but the evolving system requires the roles of facilitator, coordinator, and integrator of services across the entire care continuum.[1]

Nurses' expertise lies in advanced skills of assessment and planning, making them suited for identifying opportunities in was also created by a nurse. Educational products from nurse entrepreneurs include videos, workbooks, computer-based learning tools, web-based continuing education, and anatomic models.

Service businesses started and managed by nurses include nursing, educational, and consulting services. IV nurses join a list of many other specialty practice nurses, including orthopedic, rehabilitation, oncology, and maternal-child nurses, who are taking an entrepreneurial approach. In infusion therapy, two approaches are found:

- Providing limited but highly technical skills, such as placing midline and peripherally inserted central catheters
- Providing complete infusion care to patients

Ambulatory clinics, infusion suites, and home care services are owned and managed by nurses, and other IV nurses are pursuing nurse-practitioner certification with the intent of starting independent practices.

Consulting services

Consulting services are provided by a number of nursing specialties. Block defines a consultant as "a person in a position of influence over an individual, a group, or an organization, but who has no direct power to make changes or implement programs."[2] Managers have direct control over actions and programs.

The result of consulting activities is known as an *intervention*. The first type of intervention produces a change in the organization's structure, policies, or procedures. For example, an IV nurse can apply his or her knowledge of *Infusion Nursing Standards of Practice* to revise policies and procedures for a variety of health care organizations. The second type of intervention teaches one or many people within the organization something new. For example, the consultant may conduct a thorough needs assessment of a hospital and present the data to the managers so that they can learn about their most prevalent infusion-related problems.

In clinical practice, consulting skills are needed daily. Explaining the types of vascular access devices to patients and allowing them to decide which will be used is a form of consulting. The skills necessary for this process include technical expertise in a particular area, interpersonal skills, and the skill to execute the consulting process. This process is very familiar to nurses because it is the same as the nursing process. First, the consultant meets the potential client, explores the problem, and contracts for services. The phase of data collection and diagnosis follows. The consultant then provides feedback to the client about the diagnoses and manages any resistance to the discussion. A collaborative decision is made about the actions to take. The implementation phase follows, and the project concludes with an evaluation and a successful termination of the relationship.[2]

Consulting services can be provided by an employee of the organization or someone external to it. Although the process remains the same, the internal consultant may encounter a different set of problems. Internal consultants enjoy employee status and therefore have knowledge of the workplace, employees, and internal systems. However, because they are part of the organization's hierarchy and have an established role in its political structure, they must meet management's expectations and face the possibility of being pushed into a role of direct responsibility for a plan of action (changing the role from consulting to management). In addition, they may possess the same biases as the rest of the organization and therefore have a difficult time identifying the true sources of a problem.[3]

Consultation opportunities abound in the practice of infusion therapy. Hospitals, home care companies, physicians' offices, institutional pharmacies, and ambulatory clinics may have an immediate need for infusion expertise on a short- or long-term basis. The IV nurse's knowledge base in infusion therapy has been evolving for many decades. Organizations without this knowledge will not be able to obtain it as quickly as they may need it. Simpson suggests that organizations are exhibiting arrogance when they think this additional knowledge is not necessary, and this attitude can destroy the organization.[4]

Nursing informatics and legal nurse consulting

Two other trends increase the consultation opportunities for IV nurses: nursing informatics and legal nurse consulting. As computer-based patient record systems become more prevalent in health care, nurse informaticians will be needed to effectively integrate this technology into the organization.[5]

Within the past 5 years, legal consulting has become recognized as a specialty in nursing.[6] Infusion therapy is an invasive, intense therapy with associated risks, including errors in medication administration, inappropriate use of devices, and failure to recognize and intervene appropriately for IV-related complications. These risks escalate with complex infusion therapy in patients with complicated disease and injury processes, especially under the current pressures for cost containment.[7] All of these factors lead to an increase in the number of IV-related legal cases and the subsequent need for IV experts.

Education and training services

The demand for infusion therapy educational services is growing. In prelicensure education, most nurses do not receive adequate education and training to practice infusion therapy. In addition, new products, medications, and practice expansion drive the need for training and continuing educational programs.

Training provides learning related to the current job and focuses on what the individual must know or be able to perform in the workplace. Continuing education programs relate to knowledge and nurses' needs to expand or enhance their professional performance. Educators may contract with manufacturers to provide product training or offer independent classes. An in-service presentation for a new brand of peripherally inserted central catheter (PICC) is an example of training, whereas a PICC course is an example of continuing education. Both processes require that the educator employ principles of adult learning.

Another business opportunity for IV nurse educators is distance learning. Distance education is characterized by separation of the place and/or time between the instructor and learner, among learners, or between learners and learning resources. It requires interaction between learners and instructors through one or more types of media (e.g., video conferencing, computer software, Internet-based instruction); this interaction can be accomplished in real time or through asynchronous methods.[8]

ENTREPRENEURS AND INTRAPRENEURS

An *entrepreneur* is a person who organizes, operates, and assumes the risk for a business venture. Nurses constantly identify patient needs and create and execute plans to meet those needs. The process is the same for nurse entrepreneurs; however, entrepreneurs use their unique knowledge and skills in the marketplace to meet those needs.

An *intrapreneur,* a concept less than 20 years old, takes direct responsibility for turning an idea into a new product or service within an organization. The intrapreneur reaps the benefit of bringing an innovation into practice without the challenges of starting a separate business or giving up the financial security of employment. Infusion nurses are often in this role, perhaps without realizing it. Examples of organizationwide innovations include starting an IV team, vascular access resource group, ambulatory infusion clinic, or vascular assessment program. Nurses constantly assume the role of introducing new products or services, or simply a new way of performing an infusion procedure. The nurse intrapreneur assumes responsibility for the business venture, takes ownership and manages the service as if he or she owned the company, yet maintains the security of employment.

Personal characteristics

Entrepreneurs and intrapreneurs share the same characteristics. Hard work over many long hours is common. A business requires a high degree of dedication and total commitment, demanding that the owner be in good health and have understanding family and friends. Many tasks will be needed—from executive decisions to mopping floors—and the entrepreneur must be willing to perform them all.

A high level of self-confidence is necessary. This confidence is demonstrated by a strong belief that the business plan is sound and that the nurse has the intelligence, dedication, and skills to make whatever adjustments are necessary along the way to create a successful business. The careful entrepreneur considers all options and chooses ventures with moderate risk. Nurse entrepreneurs have above-average intellect combined with common sense. Challenges and problems become opportunities instead of stumbling blocks.

The strong desire to create and a sense of urgency are critically important. The business is not just a "job," but an expression of a personal vision. This vision is based on high yet achievable goals, not starry-eyed dreams. Finally, the nurse entrepreneur must have a passion for excellence and feel the need to provide solutions to identified problems.

Necessary skills

To manage a business venture, certain skills are required. Technical competence in the profession is mandatory. Nurses must examine how long they have practiced in the specialty of infusion therapy and determine how well they are known by potential customers. Nurses who plan to apply their infusion knowledge and skills to another industry will also need technical expertise in that area. For example, if the nurse plans to provide educational products or services, an understanding of the training and development industry, principles of adult learning, and how to coordinate teaching strategies to learning styles will be necessary. If planning to manufacture a product, the nurse will need knowledge and skill about research and development, the process of making the product in sufficient quantities to meet but not exceed the demand, and the regulatory issues that affect the business.

Financial acumen is a strong requirement. Accountants and bookkeepers can be hired to keep track of the numbers, but the entrepreneur must know how to read and understand a profit and loss statement and a balance sheet.

Marketing is the management of the relationship between providers of products and services and potential customers. Marketing is similar to the nursing process; it involves assessing and diagnosing problems, planning the intervention, implementing the plan, and evaluating results. Marketing skills include knowing who the customers are, what their needs are, how to reach them through appropriate advertising, and how to properly price the product or services.[9]

The strengths and weaknesses of a company will depend upon the strengths and weaknesses of the people involved. A common method of analysis is the SWOT method—strengths, weaknesses, opportunities, and threats (Table 37-1). Strengths and weaknesses are the personal qualities of the people involved, particularly the owners and managers, that either enhance or limit their ability to perform the tasks necessary to create a successful business. Opportunities are personal and professional situations that may contribute to success. Threats are situations that pose increased risk. To obtain objective data, the assessment should include gathering data from people outside the business in addition to those who are starting the business.[9]

LEGAL, ETHICAL, AND REGULATORY CONSIDERATIONS

Although this aspect of starting a business may be the least interesting, the potential business owner must have a good understanding of local, state, and federal laws and regulations affecting the business. Ethical business practices provide numerous advantages in building a viable, healthy business.

Licensing, registrations, and permits

City, county, state, and federal governments may require certain licenses, registrations, or permits for the type of business being started. The Chamber of Commerce is a good place to learn about the applicable local government agencies for each situation. The business will probably need a permit or license, and a federal Employer Identification Number may be required for the permit application. If the business is not using the name of a

Table 37-1   Components of a SWOT Assessment for Infusion Nurses

STRENGTHS	WEAKNESSES
<ul><li>Years of experience in nursing</li><li>Years of experience in the infusion specialty</li><li>Years of experience in other industries that contribute to current goals (e.g., sales, customer service)</li><li>Job performance of the management team</li><li>Education of the company managers</li><li>Certifications of the company managers</li><li>Publications in the specialty</li><li>Presentations at national, regional, or local conferences</li><li>Experience selecting and training employees</li><li>Experience with cost-containment and quality improvement processes</li><li>Use of technology</li></ul>	<ul><li>Need for more education</li><li>Limited experience in infusion nursing practice</li><li>Lack of knowledge about the infusion industry</li><li>Lack of self-confidence</li><li>Comfort in present situation, reducing the need for change</li><li>Reluctance to take risks</li><li>Lack of perseverance</li><li>Lack of management experience</li><li>Laziness and/or complacency</li></ul>
OPPORTUNITIES	**THREATS**
<ul><li>Membership in local and national professional organizations in the infusion industry (e.g., INS, NAVAN, LITE)</li><li>Active participant in offices or committees in these organizations</li><li>Availability of a mentor</li><li>Networking with peers and leaders in the infusion industry</li><li>Participation in Internet-based listservers related to specific interests</li><li>Business courses at local colleges</li><li>Involvement in local programs related to the market being served (e.g., geriatrics, pediatrics, homeless)</li><li>Increased demands for infusion services in alternative sites</li><li>Changing regulations (e.g., prescriptive authority for advanced-practice nurses)</li></ul>	<ul><li>Changing trends in infusion therapy (e.g., decreased reimbursement for home care)</li><li>New or aggressive competition</li><li>Shortages of materials for the service (e.g., intravenous immune globulin, thrombolytic agents)</li></ul>

INS, Intravenous Nurses Society; *NAVAN,* National Association of Vascular Access Network; *LITE,* League for Intravenous Therapy Education.

real person, the owner must verify that no other business in the county is using the same name. A "doing business as" form may be needed to register the company name. If the business will sell products, a seller's permit for collecting state sales tax is needed. Some states collect sales taxes for services as well.

City and county governments establish rules concerning the types of activities that can be conducted in different geographical areas of their jurisdiction. Local zoning ordinances should be checked to be absolutely sure that the type of business being planned is not prohibited in the area chosen for the business. Some residential areas strictly prohibit all types of businesses, whereas others may allow small, nonpolluting businesses.

Local government agencies listed in the government pages of the telephone directory should be checked. Governmental agencies that regulate the activities of business include the taxation, planning, building and inspection, and health and safety departments. The state government has rules and regulations about licenses for certain types of businesses and professions. The obvious example is the state Nurse Practice Act requiring a nursing license. There may be other requirements for home health agencies or ambulatory clinics.

Taxes

City and county governments may levy taxes on business assets such as inventory, equipment, and furniture. The owner may be expected to complete an annual report of these assets and pay the taxes based on the value of that property. Sales tax on retail items may be paid to the state or local governments, or both. Most states require businesses to pay income tax also. Incorporated businesses and the owners of unincorporated businesses are required to file a federal income tax return. Quarterly state and federal income taxes are calculated on reasonable estimates of revenues, and are reconciled with the year-end tax filing.

A business with employees must have accounting processes to withhold state and federal personal income taxes and submit them to the appropriate agencies. An Employer Identification Number (EIN) from the local Internal Revenue Service (IRS) or Social Security office is necessary. Two other taxes must be withheld from employee paychecks. Social security tax, also known as *FICA,* is 6.2% of gross wages, and Medicare tax is 1.45%. The employer is required to pay an amount equal to the amount withheld from each employee.

Business owners may hire independent contractors rather than full- or part-time employees to simplify accounting processes. Independent contractors are considered self-employed; they are responsible for paying their own taxes and can deduct business expenses on their personal tax returns. However, the business owner is responsible for reporting the amount paid to the contractor. The IRS has written guidelines to distinguish between contractors and employees. In general, employees take direction from the employer about when and how the work must be performed, work on the employer's premises, and usually work for only one employer.[10] To qualify as independent contractors, workers must require minimal direction and supervision, have great latitude in determining where and when the work will be done, usually provide their own equipment to perform the job, and usually work for more than one employer. Information is available from the Internal Revenue Service to help distinguish between independent contractors and employees. It is strongly recommended that any employer considering using independent contractors seek advice from a certified public accountant first. The IRS looks at independent contractor relationships very carefully. If it determines that a worker has been wrongly classified as an independent contractor, the employer may be liable for back taxes. This can be a very costly error, especially if it involves multiple workers over a period of years. Unfortunately, the fact that honest error was to blame does not excuse the employer.

Contracts

Contracts, whether written or verbal, are legally binding agreements. If the business manufactures a product, contracts with raw material suppliers are necessary. Nurse entrepreneurs may contract with product manufacturers to provide education and training services. An ambulatory infusion center or home health agency need contracts with managed care organizations. Before signing a contract, the entrepreneur must understand the ramifications of what is written, which usually requires the assistance of a lawyer.

The format of a contract may be a simple letter of agreement, a memorandum of understanding, or a lengthy form full of legal language. The contract establishes the working relationship, the objectives of each party, and the scope of the project. Other components of the contract may include the responsibilities of each party, specifications for the product or service to be delivered, the time for production, any foreseeable delays, indemnification and liability limitations, insurance requirements, and a termination clause.[11]

Two issues commonly encountered by nurses in contract negotiation are confidentiality agreements and noncompete agreements. Confidentiality agreements may be required if the entrepreneur has access to information or property related to the client's business. This information may be in numerous forms, including studies, reports, pictures, charts, vendor or customer lists, blueprints, and financial records. The consultant will have access to proprietary information necessary for completion of a project. Good business practice dictates the need for appropriate control of information. The written contract may include specifics about how documents are stored and who has access to them.[11]

Noncompete clauses may present a dilemma in some circumstances. When an individual leaves an organization, they may be asked to sign a contract agreeing not to work for another competing company, or not to work as an independent contractor for clients they gained as an employee. Such agreements may severely limit an individual's earning potential. The courts tend to enforce these agreements conservatively. Such agreements must be reasonable in the following areas:

- Limited in time, usually 1 or 2 years

- Limited in geographic area, although industry-specific exclusions may cover a wider geographic area
- Limited to specific areas of competition, such as direct use of processes or procedures obtained entirely from the past employer

Because noncompete agreements can seriously limit one's ability to earn a living, they must provide something of value for the employee in return, such as additional compensation or a one-time fee paid by the employer.[11]

Intellectual property rights

Patents, trademarks, and copyrights are included in the area of law known as *intellectual property rights*. These laws are in constant evolution, but can be traced to the Constitution of the United States, which includes a provision for patent rights. Laws regarding intellectual property rights attempt to protect the interests of people and companies that develop new products or engage in creative arts. An interesting subspecialty of this area of law involves the balance between the rights of the organization, which invests heavily in the development of new ideas, and the rights of an employee to benefit from what he or she developed.[12]

Patents are issued by the U.S. Patent Office to protect an inventor's exclusive rights to manufacture, sell, and use the patented invention. *Trademarks* are issued to protect brand names, advertising slogans, and logos. *Copyrights* protect a wide range of creative works, including written materials (everything from product instructions and training materials to magazine articles and books), computer software, graphics, photographs, sound recordings, and audiovisual products.[10]

Nurse entrepreneurs who invent products should obtain a good patent attorney to protect against infringing on another's patent. They should file a patent to protect their own interests. Educators and trainers must apply the copyright notice to their original work to protect their interest. For example:

Copyright © (date and author's name). All rights reserved, including the right to reproduce these materials in any form, in whole or in part, with the express written permission of the copyright holder.

The author may register the work with the U.S. Copyright Office to establish the date of origin. Affixing the copyright notice to the original work before it is reproduced will protect the work from infringement; only the owner has the exclusive right to reproduce and distribute the materials. Educators, trainers, speakers, and instructors who fail to obtain permission to use copyrighted material are liable for copyright infringement.[11]

According to the copyright laws, the definition of "copy" applies to the entire document or a portion of it, such as a chapter in a book, or a journal article. It also applies to materials stored in printed or digital form. Reproducing copyrighted materials without the express permission of the copyright holder constitutes infringement (Box 37-1) and can lead to penalties under law. Copyright laws may also apply to reciting passages; faxing, copying, or electronically transferring copyrighted material; using material without authorization or violating a license agreement; and failing to keep documentation of license agreements and permission requests.[11]

Ethical issues

Nurses practice under a contract with society—a contract based in trust. Businesses operate under a similar social contract to meet society's needs for goods and services. When those needs are met, businesses flourish. However, when society restrains entrepreneurial activity, the supply of products and services decreases. The current market for IV nursing services and products is increasing to meet the demands of a growing number of clients.

Business practice, just like nursing practice, is guided by ethical standards. An examination of several codes of ethical conduct reveals similarities. The *Code for Nurses with Interpretive Statements,* written by the American Nurses Association, discusses the need for guarding clients' confidentiality, maintaining competence, adding to the current professional body of knowledge, and assuming responsibility and accountability for judgments and actions.[3] Although this was originally written with the patient as the "client," these points also apply to the individual or organization purchasing products or services in any business relationship. The Code of Ethics from the Institute for Management Consultants addresses confidentiality of client information, accepting engagements based on one's experience and competence, respecting the intellectual property rights of clients and other consultants, and reasonable and legitimate fee negotiation.[3]

Business ethics are based on common sense approaches to everyday issues such as delivering what one promises, neither withholding nor embellishing the truth, respecting confidences, honestly accounting for time and expenses, and engaging in professional conduct.[3]

Regulatory issues

The rise in the variety and number of advanced practice nurses (nurse practitioners, clinical nurse specialists, nurse midwives, and nurse anesthetists) is driving the need for increased knowledge of the health care reimbursement system. The Balanced Budget Amendment of 1997 made nurse practitioners and clinical nurse specialists eligible for direct reimbursement for nursing services from Medicare. Medicaid regulations for some nurse specialties vary from state to state; however, direct reimbursement is required to family and pediatric nurse practitioners and nurse midwives. The Federal Employee Health Benefit Program (FEHBP) and Civilian Health and Medical Program of Uniformed Services (CHAMPUS) are other public sources of health care reimbursement that provide direct payments to advanced-practice nurses.[13]

The U.S. Food and Drug Administration regulates the manufacturing and marketing of drugs, biologics, and devices in the United States. Nurses working in consultative roles with manufacturers must understand regulations governing how a product is brought to market and the methods used for postmarket surveillance. A thorough understanding of the product, labels and labeling, and appropriate product claims is required. For instance, the term *label* is used to indicate the written, printed, or graphic matter on the immediate container of an article. However, *labeling* includes the product labels and other written, printed, or graphic matter accompanying the product when it is delivered. The term *accompanying* is interpreted liberally to mean more than physical association with the product. It extends to posters, tags, pamphlets, circulars, booklets, brochures, instruction books, direction sheets, and fillers. Accompanying also covers labeling that is brought together with the device after shipment, including handouts and other instructional materials used in an educational course. When these materials are written, they are often reviewed by the manufacturer's regulatory affairs department.

PLANNING THE BUSINESS

Failure to produce a written plan for a business venture is one of the biggest mistakes made by entrepreneurs. Another mistake is considering the business plan as a tool exclusively for raising money. Although this may be an outcome of the process, written plans explain the logic behind ideas and the basic elements of business. Other purposes of a written plan include predicting profitability, projecting budgets, setting goals, and identifying potential problems and opportunities. The work involved in actually committing ideas to paper focuses thoughts and aids in making critical decisions.

The plan can be divided into three phases:
1. The feasibility plan, to evaluate the idea of launching the business
2. The business plan, for operating the business
3. The operational plan, for growing the business

This discussion focuses on the first two phases.

Feasibility plan

The first step, a feasibility plan, involves a thorough examination of all factors influencing the final decision to actually start the business or to forget the idea. Rather than basing the decision to move forward on the emotion and excitement of starting the business, this process will ensure that the decision will be based on careful thought, market research, and solid evaluation.

Components of the feasibility plan include sections on the product or service, the market, price and profitability, and a plan for additional action. The product or service section should explore the necessary stages of development and production, limitations and liabilities, and proprietary rights such as patents or copyrights. Customers—the people who will buy the product or service—create the market. This section examines the size of the market, the anticipated growth, trends within the industry,

Table 37-2	**Example of a Mission, Vision, and Values Statement**

MISSION

To advance, illuminate, and endow infusion therapy performance improvement

VISION

In the modern health care arena, infusion therapy is appreciated for its lifesaving potential and recognized for its capacity to produce life-threatening complications. Health care management in all settings regards infusion therapy as an invasive, complex intervention, demanding a high level of attention. Infusion services involve a collaborative effort between the health care disciplines of nursing, pharmacy, and medicine. Infusion therapy is no longer included within the scope of practice for all staff. Instead personnel deemed to be the most appropriate are charged with the responsibility for delivering the corresponding types of infusion services.

VALUES OR BELIEFS

To accomplish our mission and achieve our vision, we integrate the scope and practices of adult education with the principles and practices of infusion therapy.

INFUSION THERAPY	ADULT EDUCATION
We define infusion therapy as the art and science of parenteral administration of fluid and electrolytes, medications, nutrition, and blood and blood components. To safely accomplish positive patient outcomes, technology and its rapid advancement, quality and risk management, and infection control principles must be integrated with the delivery of therapy.	We define adult education as the art and science of facilitating learning in adults, including training and continuing professional education. Staff development processes are centered around performance improvement. Collaboration between instructors and learners and a spirit of critical reflection must be incorporated into a self-directed process.
We believe infusion therapy services:	We believe adult education services:
▪ Span all age ranges	▪ Place the decision to learn with the learner
▪ Should be carefully tailored to meet the individual needs of each patient	▪ Respect the uniqueness of each learner
▪ Should involve the patient and significant others in decision making	▪ Recognize the learner's volume and quality of knowledge and experience
▪ Should be delivered in a cost-effective process and setting	▪ Emphasize internal motivation to learn
We believe infusion therapy practice:	▪ Stimulate the development of critical thinking skills
▪ Requires a collaborative effort between the disciplines of nursing, pharmacy, and medicine	We believe adult education practice:
▪ Should be based on information obtained from a variety of resources, including the following:	▪ Requires the integration of staff development processes with the vision and mission of the organization
▪ Standards and guidelines published by professional organizations	▪ Integrates learners into the planning, implementation, and evaluation processes
▪ Documents from regulatory agencies	▪ Demands the use of innovative, interactive instructional strategies
▪ Published research using sound, scientific methods	▪ Requires the instructor's role to change from one of delivering content to one of facilitating learning
▪ Requires a continual assessment of patient populations, types of therapies, and staff competencies for each clinical setting	▪ Emphasizes the end result of performance improvement, not just training
▪ Requires continually expanding the individual's body of knowledge and skill	▪ Incorporates all levels of evaluation

From Lynn Hadaway Associates, Inc., Milner, Georgia.

benefits of the product or service, competition, and methods to reach potential customers. The price and profitability sections assess what customers will pay for the product or service and provide a forecast of sales, operating expenses, and start-up expenses. In the plan for action, the strengths and weaknesses, possible problems, needed licenses, capital requirements, and potential corporate partners are identified. The decision to proceed or stop is made after careful evaluation of the feasibility plan by the principals and any experienced business people who are willing to advise them.[14]

Business plan

After the decision to proceed with the business venture is made, the next step is to determine the mission, vision, and values of the business. Table 37-2 provides examples of these three elements of a business plan. The *mission statement* is a written reason for existence. It is a simple statement centered on the process of what needs to be done. It should be so short and simple that it can be understood by anyone and remembered

and recited quickly. The mission of any business is about the personal passion of the entrepreneur. It requires action verbs to state what one will do. It explains the principle, or cause for which one is willing to devote his or her life and implies that someone or some group is the beneficiary of the work.[15]

The *vision statement* is the result of what one intends to accomplish. It should capture how the world will change and what it will look and feel like when the mission is accomplished. This carefully crafted statement points the way to the future and increases one's motivation to accomplish the mission.[9,15]

Values are a set of beliefs or principles that guide the decisions, activities, and operation of the business. Everyone in the company must embrace these values and the incentive and reward systems must reinforce them.[9]

The legal structure of the business is important because it affects liability and taxation issues. The business may be set up as one of the following entities:

▪ Sole proprietorship
▪ Partnership
▪ Corporation

A *sole proprietorship* is owned and operated by a single person or a married couple. Most small businesses are sole proprietorships. This form of business is the easiest to start and pays the lowest taxes. However, growth is limited to the personal credit and assets of the individual. In addition, a proprietorship offers no protection against liability; personal property and assets are at risk to creditors.[10]

A *partnership* brings the skills, experiences, ideas, and money of at least one other person. Each partner shares equally in the risk and responsibilities. Although partnerships may provide a more solid foundation, they have also been known to cause rifts between friends. Sharing of ownership of a business can be a tricky prospect, especially if one partner is always working to make the business succeed, and the other has a "what will be, will be" approach. A successful partnership requires clear, consistent communication and good organization. The roles and responsibilities of each person can be divided according to their strengths. A partnership agreement is recommended to clearly address issues such as the duration of the partnership, the time and money each partner will invest, the methods for making decisions, the process and timing of sharing profits and losses, and the process for dissolving the partnership.[10]

A *corporation* becomes a separate legal entity, thus relieving the shareholders or stockholders of personal liability for the business's losses or risks. Although a corporation has greater fund-raising flexibility, it also requires a larger initial investment because of set-up costs. Shareholders may change at any time without affecting the legal status of the corporation or its operations. Also, having the image of a corporation may produce marketing advantages. If the owners do not incorporate when the business is founded, they will usually do so when it reaches the point where incorporation would provide a tax advantage.

There are two types of corporations: the C Corporation and the Subchapter S Corporation. The *C Corporation* offers greater liability protection and is chosen by most big businesses. This corporation pays taxes on the profits made, and the dividends paid to individual shareholders are taxed as ordinary income, resulting in double taxation. Costs for incorporation may be as high as $1000 in addition to attorney's fees and an annual tax required by some states. Smaller companies use a Subchapter S Corporation, named for the section in the Internal Revenue Code. The *S Corporation* provides liability protection but does not result in double taxation because income is taxed only as personal income.[10]

The business plan does not need to be lengthy or complicated, but it does need to be thorough and accurate (Box 37-2). It should be simple and easy to read. The use of technical jargon should be avoided so that someone outside the industry can understand the points being made. Financial estimates should be realistic and the plan should demonstrate that the owners have the necessary knowledge for operating the business.

Professional services needed

Although the first thought is usually to perform all work in-house, it may quickly become obvious that some tasks are better outsourced to other professionals. Assistance with financial management is one of the most important areas for profes-

sional advice. Bookkeepers collect the financial data of the company, accountants process the financial data to generate financial statements and prepare tax forms, and financial consultants use the financial data to project future growth and provide advice on major decisions.

Lawyers may be needed to form a corporation or partnership, to write or review contracts, or to manage human resource

---

Box 37-2   Components of a Written Business Plan

1. Executive summary (an abridged version of the entire plan)
   - Mission of the business
   - Product or service description
   - Overview of the marketing strategy
   - Revenue projections and future plans
   - Structure of the business
   - Biographical sketches of the management team
2. Business Description
   - Provide business name, address, names of all principals.
   - Explain the product or service in detail.
   - Describe how customers will obtain the product or service.
   - Explain how the product or service meets customers' needs.
3. Market Analysis
   - Define target customers using demographics.
   - Explain why customers will buy the product or service.
   - Discuss the potential size of the market.
   - Define economic, social, and regulatory factors that influence the market.
   - Identify important industry trends.
   - Discuss competitors and their relationship to the business.
4. Financial Plan
   - State how much equity financing will be provided by the owners.
   - State how much additional debt and equity financing will be needed.
   - Provide a projected income statement for 3 years.
     - First year by each month, second year by quarters, third year annually.
     - Explain the assumptions used to calculate the projections.
   - Provide a break-even analysis that shows when and at what sales volume the business will turn a profit.
   - Provide a statement about sources and uses of funds.
   - Provide a capital expenditure budget.
   - Provide an opening day balance sheet.
5. Management
   - Resumes of management personnel
   - Job descriptions
   - Organizational chart
   - Staffing projections, with explanation
   - List of professional team members
6. Supporting Documents
   - Resumes
   - Patents
   - Contracts
   - Letters of reference
   - Letters of intent
   - Market research studies
   - Logos
   - Designs

issues. Real estate specialists are needed if the business will need a specific location. Insurance agents are needed to advise about property damage or theft, workers' compensation and unemployment, errors and omission or malpractice, and health and disability policies. Bankers may be needed for assistance with cash flow problems. Experts in marketing, graphics design, advertising, and printing will be needed to get the message to potential customers in a manner that gets attention.

MARKETING THE BUSINESS

A large component of business planning is determining where potential customers are, what their needs are, and what motivates them to buy a product or service. Because customers create markets, marketing is the process used to create a customer.[3]

Customers hold the power to purchase the product or service. Marketing must target the person actually making the decision. Staff nurses may want the service of a skilled IV nurse to insert PICCs, but the decision to purchase the service rests with the person in charge of the nursing department, thus indicating this person as the customer.

Identifying customers

Analyzing the needs of customers will determine who is buying, what they are buying, and why they are buying. Wise decisions are based on good data. Demographic data help determine who is buying the product or service. Demographics include data on geographic, social, and economic factors of customers and potential customers, such as the following:

- Where do they live?
- What are their ages and education levels?
- How many are male? How many female?
- How large are their families?
- How much money do they earn?
- What are their occupations?

If the customers are other businesses rather than individuals, the size of the companies, the number of employees, their customers, and the number of years in business should be examined.

Next, it is important to know what the customers are buying. Features or characteristics, packaging, costs, and distribution affect customer decisions. What aspects of each will sway the customer's decision to buy the product or service?

The benefits of a product or service determine why the customer buys. Are they looking for ease of use or rapid access? It is critical to understand that the features yield benefits. Whereas features are defined by the business, the customer defines the benefits.[9]

Reaching the market

Marketing includes promotion, sales, distribution, and pricing of a product or service. *Sales* involves contacting customers and persuading them to purchase a product or service. *Distribution* is the channel through which the product or service reaches the customer. Services are usually distributed directly from the business to the customer, whereas products may use a direct

---

> **Box 37-3　Examples of Pricing Strategy Questions**
>
> 1. Is the product or service unique enough to command a high price? If so, how is this difference perceived?
> 2. Are there legal or regulatory limits on how much can be charged?
> 3. How will competitors respond to pricing?
> 4. Are there market conditions (pending legislation, new technology) that could affect the price?
> 5. Is it necessary to work through middlemen to get the product or service to the public? If so, what are their pricing policies?

---

channel or an indirect channel with some form of middleman, or agent, between the business and its customers.

Promotion is informing potential customers about the product or service. It includes advertising, networking, referrals, and publicity. *Advertising* is the placement of paid messages in a variety of media that will reach potential customers. To be effective, it must be repetitive and consistent. Business cards, letterhead, and product packaging are also forms of advertising. *Referrals* come from customers that have had a positive experience with the product or service. *Networks* are the contacts made through professional, business, or social organizations. Networking provides opportunities to promote the product or service and to learn from colleagues. *Publicity* includes announcements in the media about the product or services, usually obtained by sending news releases to the press. Articles published in appropriate journals or magazines and presentations given at organizational meetings are also forms of publicity.[10]

Pricing strategies

The final component of a marketing plan is the pricing strategy (Box 37-3).

Establishing fees can be a challenging and confusing task. Four major areas must be considered in calculating fees: base rate, variable costs, fixed costs, and profit. *Base rate* is the value of time in the marketplace. The hourly or daily salary of other professionals offering a similar service for another employer should be investigated. For nursing services, the pay for nursing staff from other infusion centers, home health agencies, and hospitals should be evaluated to arrive at a salary range. The number and types of competition in the proposed area should be identified. If the nurse's qualifications are scarce, it may be appropriate to use the higher end of the salary scale. For example, the market may allow charging a higher fee in one area if nurses are unavailable to perform specialized infusion therapy, such as placing a PICC.

For consultation services, not every workday is a billable day. Most services consider 10 billable days per month appropriate for calculating salary. For example, an annual salary of $50,000 would be divided by 120 billable days per year to yield $416.67 as the daily salary (Table 37-3).[3]

Variable costs are directly related to the sale of a product or service. They include raw materials and packaging, travel ex-

Table 37-3	**Calculating Fees for Consulting Services**	
ITEMS TO BE INCLUDED	**CALCULATION**	**EXAMPLE**
Desired annual salary of $60,000	Divide by 120 billable days per year	$60,000 ÷ 120 = $500 daily
Fixed costs = monthly overhead of $4250	Add the overhead of the business, including the following:	$4250 ÷ 10 = $425
	▪ Office rent	
	▪ Office equipment	
	▪ Utilities	
	▪ Telephone and pagers	
	▪ Insurance premiums	
	▪ Professional fees (e.g., accountant, lawyer)	
	▪ Marketing costs	
Profit for company	Add 10% to 20%	$92.50 to $185
Total daily fee		$1017.50 to $1100 (rounded down or up to an even number)

penses such as mileage and parking fees, and income and self-employment taxes. *Fixed costs* remain constant regardless of the amount of product or services being sold. They include communication services such as telephones and pagers, insurance, office space and equipment, utilities, professional fees, and marketing costs. Because the purpose of being in business is to make a profit, a reasonable profit margin should be built in to the fee schedule. For consultation services, this usually ranges from 10% to 20%.[3]

FINANCING THE BUSINESS

The primary reason for business failure is undercapitalization (not enough money!). According to Puetz, "most nurse consultants do not start their business on a sound financial footing."[3] A sound understanding of the financial aspects of running the business is therefore critical to its success. This includes the ability to read an income statement, interpret a balance sheet, and examine cash flow. Financing a business can be divided into two parts: initial financing and second-tier financing.

Initial financing

To open the doors of the business, money will be needed to cover personal expenses, seed money, and working capital. The business cannot be expected to produce an income for at least 18 months, maybe 2 years.

The amount of money needed each month to pay for household and family expenses should be closely examined. This includes the mortgage payment or rent, debt service, including principle and interest, tax payments, insurance, utilities, telephone, household maintenance, nonreimbursable medical costs, clothing, food, transportation or automobile costs, and entertainment. Any income from part-time employment should be subtracted from the monthly total, and the result multiplied by at least 18 months. This is the amount needed to ensure the family's security until the business can produce income.

Seed capital is the money needed to plan, prepare, open, and run the business until it reaches the break-even point. Small businesses are not considered "bankable" until a track record

has been established. That means the seed money, or a large portion of it, must come from the entrepreneur. Money can come from savings, home equity loans, or sale of stock, bonds, or other assets. There is always the danger that a home can be lost if the business is not successful. Seed money can also come from friends, family, and potential partners.[16] Seed capital should be thought of in two phases: initial cash outlay and working capital.

Initial cash outlay includes deposits on rent and utilities, insurance, machinery and equipment for manufacturing, office equipment, furniture, stationary, business cards, other office supplies, transportation equipment, professional fees for lawyers and accountants, and advertising and publicity costs.[16]

Working capital is the amount of money needed each month to operate the business. The monthly operating expenses and the amount of revenue generated each month should be considered. The difference between the two figures is the amount of working capital needed. When the amount of monthly revenue equals the monthly operating costs, the break-even point is reached.[16]

Second-tier financing

Once the business is operating, new needs become apparent. The possibility of a large contract could increase the demand for working capital. The business may have an opportunity to assume a commanding position in the market but not have enough cash flow to realize the opportunity. Financing at this level could require obtaining money from other sources.

Types of financing

Debt financing is borrowing money that must be repaid. *Equity financing* is money given to a business in exchange for some share of ownership.

Commercial banks provide debt financing if the business is "bankable," which is defined as one that shows a steady, sustainable, and predictable revenue stream. Banks may also need to see that the business has successfully managed one down cycle. Commercial lenders are companies that fill gaps left by the conservative attitude of banks. They take greater risks, offer longer terms for the loan, and have more flexible criteria. In exchange, they charge higher interest rates, have large prepayment penalties, and always require collateral. Although the Small Business Administration (SBA) offers guarantees for loans from a local bank, direct loans from the SBA are extremely limited.

Equity financing is derived from selling stock in an incorporated business, from venture capitalists, and from Small Business Investment Corporation investments. Venture capitalists are individuals who invest in small businesses with the potential for rapid growth and a good return on the investment. They almost always want to be part owner of the company. Small Business Investment Corporations are venture capital companies licensed by the SBA to invest in small businesses; they obtain part of the cash from the SBA.[16]

Summary

Challenges in the current health care environment present unique opportunities for nurses, including the chance to assume an entrepreneurial role. Just like the nursing process, business development requires careful assessment, planning, implementation, and evaluation. According to Tim Porter-O'Grady, health care is evolving into a continuum of care outside institutional parameters and is becoming more interdisciplinary. These changes will produce the need for "a more fluid and flexible set of supports and systems than is currently in place."[17] This should open the door for consultants to create changes in roles and organizational design. Nurses have the intimate knowledge of health care systems and the clinical experience to build the new health care continuum. For those with the desire to develop the necessary business and consulting skills, entrepreneurs with an IV nursing background can make a radical difference in health care as it is now known.

References

1. White R, Begun JW: Nursing entrepreneurship in an era of chaos and complexity, *Nurs Admin Q* 22(2):40, 1998.
2. Block P: *Flawless consulting: a guide to getting your expertise used,* San Francisco, 1981, Pfeiffer.
3. Puetz B, Shinn LJ: *The nurse consultant's handbook,* New York, 1997, Springer.
4. Simpson RL: Making the move from nurse to nursing informatics consultant, *Nurs Manage* 29(5):2, 1998.
5. Simpson RL: Technology and the potential for entrepreneurship, *Nurs Manage* 28(10):24, 1997.
6. Bowman P: Role of the legal nurse consultant in litigation, *J Nurs Law* 5(4):35, 1998.
7. Weinstein SM: Legal implications/risk management, *JIN* 19(3S): S16, 1996.
8. I.A.C.E.T: *Criteria and guidelines for quality continuing education and training programs,* Dubuque, Iowa, 1998, Kendall/Hunt.
9. Tiffany P, Peterson SD: *Business plans for dummies,* Foster City, Calif, 1997, IDG Books.
10. Tyson E, Schell J: *Small business for dummies,* Foster City, Calif, 1998, DG Books.
11. Eyres PS: *The legal handbook for trainers, speakers, and consultants,* New York, 1998, McGraw-Hill.
12. Lieberstein SH: *Who owns what is in your head?* Greens Farms, Conn, 1996, Wildcat.
13. Hadaway L: Navigating toward advanced nursing practice, *J Vasc Access Devices* 4(3):16, 1999.
14. Price C, Allen K: *Tips and traps for entrepreneurs,* New York, 1998, McGraw-Hill.
15. Jones LB: *The path: creating your mission statement for work and for life,* New York, 1996, Hyperion.
16. Pollan SM, Levine M: *The field guide to starting a business,* New York, 1990, Simon & Schuster.
17. Porter-O'Grady T: The private practice of nursing: the gift of entrepreneurialism, *Nurs Admin Q* 22(1):8, 1997.

Chapter 38

Future of Infusion Therapy

Sharon M. Weinstein, MS, RN, CRNI

Rapid advances in medicine and technology have contributed to the growth of the intravenous (IV) therapy specialty. The expanding number of clinical modalities and care settings will ensure the continued growth of the specialty practice. The structure and process of delivering patient care will continue to change in the future.[1] The health care environment will be affected by increased complexity in patient care and higher-risk patients and by the emphasis on health care reform and cost control. Despite the enormous turmoil the health care system has undergone—from the intensification of managed care to the development of integrated health systems—our model is still failing large numbers of uninsured and underinsured people. In addition, Friend has identified six major symptoms of a more general failure in our health care system (Table 38-1).[2,3]

The fiscal foundation on which hospitals were built has been turned upside-down, forcing hospitals to continually redesign themselves, closely scrutinizing operations and devising methods to more efficiently deliver patient care.[4] To remain viable, hospitals are faced with increased pressures to discharge patients as soon as their condition warrants and to decrease inpatient costs. As a result, we have witnessed significant downsizing, restructuring of internal operations, and the emergence of new patient care delivery models. Alternative sites and home infusion providers have not been immune to these changing forces and have had to significantly restructure as well. This trend will continue.

The health care environment at the end of the 20th century has presented the specialty of IV nursing with unprecedented challenges to not only survive, but to grow. The future of IV nursing revolves around the IV nursing specialty's response to change. In all practice environments, the IV therapy service program must be innovative and adaptable, and it must support and enhance collaborative practice.

EXAMINING THE PRESENT TO BUILD OUR FUTURE

To strategize for the future, we must examine the drivers of change in the profession. In the hospital setting, the major change affecting the IV therapy team concept has been work redesign models implemented by hospitals in response to increased pressures to contain costs. No universal redesign model is currently in place nationwide; the goal of *all* models is to improve continuity and reduce fragmentation by delivering patient-centered care.[1,4-6] This is being accomplished by cross-training staff and the increasing use of nonlicensed personnel. As a result, the use or need for ancillary services, such as IV teams, is challenged. Although the new care delivery models maximize the capabilities of every level of employee in an institution, ancillary services need not be made extinct. Many professional services, including IV teams, can be successfully integrated into these patient care models if they can demonstrate their support of the registered nurse and nonlicensed technical personnel care team members. To do so, the IV department must carefully evaluate how the team fits into the new structure and what benefits it can provide. This analysis requires a careful review of current services and a study of opportunities for new and more efficient ways to deliver IV care. Processes need to be carefully assessed, problems diagnosed, and action plans formulated to strategically direct an IV therapy service program.[6,7] An aging patient population and changing nationwide demographics present special challenges. For example, the number of immigrants and new Americans is growing, and we need to be more sensitive to cultural differences among patients. Diseases such as acquired immunodeficiency syndrome or infections related to bacteria-resistant medications will present many clinical, legal, and ethical problems.

*The author and editors wish to acknowledge the contributions made by Leslie Baranowski and Judy Hankins, as coauthors of this chapter in the first edition of *Intravenous Nursing: Clinical Principles and Practice*.

Table 38-1   Six Major Symptoms of an Ailing Health Care System

SYMPTOM	RATIONALE
Accelerating health costs	Managed care/profit pressure drive prices up
Uncertain level of quality	More data, yet consumer is confused
Decreasing consumer trust in providers	Proliferation of patient mismanagement and adverse events
Growth of liability issues	Changes in legislation may grant patients the right to sue health plans and employers who selected those plans on their behalf
Unknown impact of health care dollars on productivity	13% of gross domestic product is spent on health care, although it is difficult to justify the return on investment
Decreased consumer choice	Less competition leaves consumers vulnerable and frustrated

Adapted from Friend DB: *HealthCare.com: Rx for reform,* Boca Raton, Fla, 2000, CRC Press.

IV NURSING ACROSS THE CONTINUUM OF CARE

With the evolution of alternative and home infusion programs, IV therapy has developed into a multifaceted specialty practiced in many venues. The development of IV delivery in alternative settings has been characterized by extraordinary growth, not only in the number of patients treated but also in the diversity of therapies provided. The demand for alternative sites will continue to grow as hospitals are increasingly pressured to discharge patients as soon as clinically warranted. The proliferation of a capitated system, in which financial risk for patient care is shifted from payers to the providers, will grow. Health care systems that are capable of providing the full continuum of services will benefit under this system. Therefore the focus on establishing processes that allow patients to pass seamlessly from the inpatient setting to outpatient services will continue.[6] Hospital networks and integrated systems are already well positioned in the new health care environment. These networks will be able to provide continuous care delivery as patients are shifted between multiple care settings based on patient needs and cost differentials.[7] Many hospitals have recognized the alternative infusion business as a potentially profitable product line. The hospital-based IV nurse plays an integral role in planning patients' care to facilitate transition to other practice settings, including skilled nursing facilities, home care, ambulatory clinics, and infusion centers. The full-service IV team is a natural component of decentralized care, follows the patient-centered care model, and maximizes its benefit to the organization. Providers now have an incentive to control overall health care costs, in addition to controlling access to and use of alternative infusion services.

The key to survival in the future is flexibility. IV nurses need to remain flexible and carefully define *where* their expertise will have an impact on patient care no matter what setting is involved. The IV nurse is uniquely positioned and educated to manage subcutaneous, intraspinal, and intraosseous therapies. Expanding the scope of responsibilities to include these routes of administration in a profusion of practice settings is evidence of the IV nurse's commitment to meeting the needs of the health care institution in a changing environment.

Further emphasis on prevention is anticipated. Therefore the need for community outreach services provided by qualified health care practitioners will increase. The skills needed by these practitioners may include performing central line dressings on outpatient dialysis patients, or teaching venous access to occupational health nurses.

IV nurses need to market their services to clinics, dialysis units, and skilled care facilities where the volume of professional staff may be limited. Outsourcing programs for central line dressing procedures, IV outcome monitoring, and basic IV care to hospital-based IV nurses or entrepreneurs may be an effective and fiscally sound decision for alternative care sites.

With the expansion of IV therapy across the continuum of care, providers need to meet more sophisticated information requirements, including quality monitoring, outcomes studies, clinical benchmarking, and patient satisfaction surveys, in addition to better cost control and reporting. This necessitates an understanding of technology.

TECHNOLOGY

Infusion therapy has witnessed dramatic change in technology over the past 40 years. Evolving technologies can be anticipated to continue to affect IV nursing practice, safety, and patient outcomes.

New product development

Nowhere is change more evident than in the plethora of equipment and supplies used to deliver IV care. IV nurses should continue to collaborate with the health care industry to meet practice needs. Because of diminishing staffs, multiple care settings, and higher acuity levels, the industry will be challenged to develop more sophisticated equipment that is both user-friendly and incorporates safety features. Such changes may yield increased costs. Efficient use of products and supplies will enable manufacturers and health care facilities to contain costs.[7]

Impact of information technology

Advances in technology—particularly the Internet—have resulted in a new health care consumer who is armed with more information than ever before. Consumers today tend to know a great deal about their illnesses, their options, and the health care field in general.[8]

Nurses have always been in the information business, using tools that have varied over time.[9] Enhancements in information technology will continue. As practice areas become less bound by physical space or time, new opportunities and possibilities, never before imagined, will emerge. Technology will be used to teach via simulator, to monitor a patient's progress, and to support distance learning.

QUALITY IMPROVEMENT
Perceived value

Value has to do with the cost, quality, and service of the care provided; value is high on everyone's agenda.[2,4] Like price, quality is difficult to measure in health care. Analyzing only the charges associated with physician visits and hospital bills can be misleading because they omit utilization data, frequency of hospitalization, and provision of ancillary services. Charges in the 21st century are simply numbers that nobody pays. The true costs are more difficult to ascertain, even for providers themselves. To paraphrase Oscar Wilde in *The Picture of Dorian Gray*, nowadays people know the price of everything and the value of nothing.[8,9]

Quality is equally complex; the customer expects ease of access and good outcomes. Quality improvement tools such as total quality management and continuous quality improvement improve value in relation to cost, quality, and service.

IV team members need to reevaluate their current responsibilities to ensure a focus on outcomes rather than tasks. An annual assessment of all clinical departments will ensure an appropriate skill mix and optimum patient outcomes. The roles of the licensed practical/vocational nurse and nonlicensed assistive personnel should be assessed carefully to take greater advantage of the registered nurse's professional knowledge base, skill level, and guidance.[6]

Hospital redesign in the latter part of the 20th century evolved around whether specialization impedes the organization from delivering quality care. Labor represents the largest single component of the cost associated with IV services. The key to the success of an IV team is its ability to improve labor efficiency through the use of IV team specialists and resource personnel. Length of stay has become a critical measure of hospital success; each additional day in the hospital adds significantly to the costs. IV teams have contributed to decreased length of stay by ensuring timely delivery of therapies, better use of supplies, and decreased IV-related complications.[6,7] Now more than ever before, the IV team should be actively consulting with patient-centered care teams regarding recommendations for IV therapy–related plans of care. Consultation should include assessment for and coordination of outpatient services if appropriate.

Finally, the consumer expects acceptable service. IV nurses need to be responsible for the outcomes of IV therapy–related services. In assuming this responsibility, the nurse must remember that patient care succeeds in a collaborative practice model. Thus the nurse should integrate the expertise of individuals from other disciplines, including the pharmacy, nursing, laboratory, oncology, and outpatient units. Use of multidisciplinary practice committees can facilitate this goal. Such committees may take several forms. An IV therapy committee may be composed of members from many clinical departments. IV nurses can participate on institutional committees that might affect IV-related services, such as product evaluation, safety, and infection control. In addition to attending committee meetings, the nurse must review and update the IV therapy program to monitor and evaluate continuing quality improvement. This annual process encourages institutions to keep the system current because it includes reviewing the scope and important aspects of care.[10,11]

IV nurses must be cognizant of the institution's internal and external customers. Internal customers may be physicians, fellow health care workers, and ancillary support staff. External customers may be patients, other hospitals, alternative care facilities, and home care agencies. These customers need to be familiar with the quality of care that is delivered by IV nursing programs. The new health care consumer is educated, well-informed, and demands choices and competence.[9,12]

Ensuring clinical competencies

The IV nurse manager should be aware of the expertise of the IV therapy staff and their relationship to the mission of the health care facility. IV nursing leaders should continually assess and determine potential services that could be better provided by the IV staff. Nurses in today's health care environment must understand change to be able to function effectively. Hence the process of change should be an integral part of the IV nurse's continuing education program. Nurses involved in increasingly complex roles will also need to be educated and competent to assess patients, processes, and systems. The challenge will be to ensure that staff members feel competent in view of their increasing responsibilities for clinical management.[12]

Health care agencies will need to determine how to ensure that their staff are competent. New nurse orientation programs will need to be streamlined yet comprehensive, complying with age-specific clinical practice guidelines to meet the requirements of accrediting bodies such as the Joint Commission on Accreditation of Healthcare Organizations (JCAHO). Innovative ways to update staff in regard to procedural changes, including self-study packets, computer programs, or audiovisual techniques, will also be needed.

With rapid technologic advances, it is also going to be a challenge to provide IV equipment–related education in an efficient, effective manner. This task will need to be addressed by the health care industry and health care organizations.[12]

As patients migrate from the hospital setting, IV nurses will require a better understanding of adult and pediatric learning principles. They will need to ensure that patients, families, or significant others are competent to provide care and will need to educate them on the necessity of compliance if patients are to remain outside the hospital setting. Patients are reading more and are more proactive about their own care. Therefore tomorrow's consumers will more likely challenge their caregivers. Increased patient knowledge and expectations of quality increase the demand for specialists in IV therapy.

As rigid departmental boundaries become more fluid, the IV nurse's role will take on increased significance. It will be necessary for IV nurses to continue to focus on maintaining standards of quality IV care while yielding to a much-needed multidisciplinary approach to meeting the total needs of the patient.

The necessity of containing cost continues, and the possibility of restructuring responsibilities of health care personnel remains. IV nurses should be alert to the potential for acquiring new tasks. Therefore IV therapy managers must establish programs to ensure staff competencies to deliver services that will yield positive outcomes.

Competency-based orientation and training programs must be developed locally. However, given the diverse educational preparation, experience, and training of nurses, it is no longer realistic to assume that "a nurse is a nurse is a nurse."[6,13]

"There are a number of forces and influences, both external and internal, driving the development of formal nurse credentialing and privileging programs."[11,14] These include the JCAHO, the departments of health, state Nurse Practice Acts, the legal system, and the nursing profession.

The future of practice and education

The disparity in educational backgrounds among nurses is probably one of the best known and most problematic of the internal forces driving credentialing programs. Licensure to practice nursing may be acquired through associate degree programs, hospital-based programs, or baccalaureate programs. With the increasing complexity of health care, ensuring quality practice based solely on entry level licensure is becoming more difficult. Therefore national certification programs have been developed in an attempt to address the competency issue. Specialty organizations have been in the forefront of trying to protect the patient by ensuring competency via certification programs.[12]

This approach has certainly been true in the profession of IV nursing. IV nurses are following their patients into many alternative care sites. Often, the alternative care facility setting is less structured and less supportive when patient care problems arise. Therefore validating competency through national certification will continue to be valuable and possibly essential to help ensure that patient care will be provided by competent practitioners.

Nursing education must keep pace with the changes in health care. Significant changes will occur in curricula and continuing education programs. Nurses will need to be prepared to provide high-technology care in hospitals, and alternative care settings.

GLOBAL IV NURSING

Much of IV nursing's emphasis on the global health care environment comes as a result of collaboration with foreign nursing colleagues. As the professional society reaches out to schools, universities, and individual nurses, the globalization of IV nursing education expands. Nurses from Australia, Canada, Korea, Japan, the Russian Federation, and the People's Republic of China have expressed interest in the specialty practice, standards of practice, and certification. IV nurses have an opportunity and an obligation to work with their peers from abroad to improve and enhance the specialty practice. Global initiatives will continue throughout the worldwide IV nursing community.[12,14]

SUMMARY

The IV nursing specialty has established itself as an integral component of the multidisciplinary approach to quality care. From the critically ill neonate to the cancer patient receiving supportive therapy at home, the IV nurse's role in supporting multiple, extensive IV therapies has been well established. The IV nurse of the future needs to think strategically and to establish goals that closely reflect the institution's mission. Tomorrow's health care environment can be characterized by the following[3]:

- Rules change almost daily.
- Radical new care delivery models are developed.
- Multisite care is available across time and place.
- New payment models characterized by risk assumption across lifetimes are developed.
- Fewer resources are available.
- Far more accountability is required for clinical and financial outcomes.

The successful IV therapy program of the future will adapt to changing paradigms consistent with the pace of change, seeking and creating new opportunities for IV nursing. The challenge for the specialty of IV nursing in the coming years is to respond to the changes affecting health care and to design the new look of IV nursing.

REFERENCES

1. Henderson J, Williams J: The people side of patient care redesign, *Healthcare Forum* 42(4):44, 1999.
2. Friend DB: *HealthCare.com: Rx for reform*, Boca Raton, Fla, 2000, CRC Press.
3. Fralic MF: Planning for tomorrow's healthcare system. In Sullivan EJ, editor: *Creating nursing's future: issues, opportunities, and challenges*, St Louis, 1999, Mosby.
4. Griffith JR: *Designing 21st century healthcare*, Chicago, 1998, Health Administration Press.
5. Gannon K: Reach-out programs: hospitals expand into home care, *Hosp Pharm Rep* 8(6):1, 1994.
6. Baranowski L, Terry J: Future of intravenous therapy. In Terry J, editor: *Intravenous therapy: clinical principles and practice*, Philadelphia, 1995, WB Saunders.
7. Burik D, Cramton CW, Holtz J: A workbook approach to justifying I.V. therapy teams under prospective payment, *NITA* 7:411, 1984.
8. Chyna JT: The consumer revolution: an age of changing expectations, *Healthcare Executive* 15(1):7, 2000.
9. Weiner BE, Trangenstein PA: The third wave of information technology. In Sullivan EJ, editor: *Creating nursing's future: issues, opportunities, and challenges*, St Louis, 1999, Mosby.
10. Haugh R: The new consumer, *Hosp Health Netw* 73(12):31, 1999.
11. Sherer JL: The new medical team: clinicians, technicians, and . . . patients, *Healthcare Executive* 15(1):12, 1999.
12. Weinstein SM: *Principles and practice of intravenous therapy*, ed 7, Philadelphia, 2000, Lippincott Williams & Wilkins.
13. Archibald PJ, Bainbridge DD: Capacity and competence: nurse credentialing and privileging, *Nurs Manage* 25:49, 1994.
14. Vance C: Nursing in the global arena. In Sullivan EJ, editor: *Creating nursing's future: issues, opportunities and challenges*, St Louis, 1999, Mosby.

Index

Page numbers in italics indicate figures; t indicates tables; and b indicates boxes.